New Anticoagulants for the Cardiovascular Patient

Roque Pifarré, MD
Professor and Chairman Emeritus
Department of Thoracic
  and Cardiovascular Surgery
Loyola University of Chicago
  Stritch School of Medicine
Maywood, Illinois

Hanley & Belfus, Inc. / Philadelphia

Publisher: HANLEY & BELFUS, INC.
Medical Publishers
210 South 13th Street
Philadelphia, PA 19107
(215) 546-7293; 800-962-1892
FAX (215) 790-9330

Library of Congress Cataloging-in-Publication Data

New anticoagulants for the cardiovascular patient / [edited by] Roque
Pifarré.
    p.   cm.
        Includes bibliographical references and index.
        ISBN 1-56053-220-3 (alk. paper)
        1. Anticoagulants (Medicine)   I. Pifarré, Roque.
        [DNLM: 1. Anticoagulants—therapeutic use.   2. Anticoagulants—
pharmacology.   3. Antithrombins—pharmacology.   4. Antithrombins—
therapeutic use.   5. Cardiovascular Diseases—drug therapy.
QV 193 N532 1997]
RM340.N49   1997
615'.718—dc21
DNLM/DLC
for Library of Congress   96-51845
                                                                          CIP

New Anticoagulants for the Cardiovascular Patient   ISBN 1-56053-220-3

Last digit is the print number: 9   8   7   6   5   4   3

Contents

Contributors

V. Paul Addonizio, M.D.
Professor of Surgery, and Chief, Cardiac and Thoracic Surgery, Department of Surgery, Division of Cardiac and Thoracic Surgery, Temple University School of Medicine, Philadelphia, Pennsylvania

Eckhard Alt, M.D.
Professor, First Medical Department, Technical University of Munich, Munich, Germany

Joseph Arcidi, M.D.
Assistant Professor, Department of Thoracic and Cardiovascular Surgery, Loyola University Medical Center, Maywood, Illinois

R. J. R. Beijering, M.D.
Hemostasis, Thrombosis, Atherosclerosis, and Inflammation Research, Academic Medical Center, University of Amsterdam, Amsterdam, The Netherlands

Rodger L. Bick, M.D., Ph.D., FACP
Clinical Professor, Department of Medicine and Pathology, University of Texas Southwestern Medical Center, Dallas, Texas

Hans Klaus Breddin, M.D.
Professor of Internal Medicine, International Institute of Thrombosis and Vascular Diseases, Frankfurt, Germany

Diane V. Brezniak, M.A.
Chemist, Molecular Diagnostics, New York State Department of Health, Albany, New York

Andreas Calatzis
Medical student, Institute of Experimental Surgery, Technical University of Munich, Munich, Germany

Demetra D. Callas, Ph.D.
Fellow, Department of Pathology, Loyola University Medical Center, Maywood, Illinois

Alain F. Carpentier, M.D., Ph.D.
Professor and Chairman, Department of Cardiovascular Surgery, Broussais Hospital, Paris, France

Nickolay Chirgadze, Ph.D.
Senior Scientist, Macromolecular X-ray Crystallography, Lilly Research Laboratories, Eli Lilly & Company, Indianapolis, Indiana

Beng Hock Chong, MBBS, Ph.D., FRCP, FRCPA, FRACP
Associate Professor, Schools of Pathology and Medicine, University of New South Wales, Sydney, New South Wales, Australia

C. William Cole, M.D., FRCSC, FACS
Professor of Surgery, University of British Columbia, Vancouver, British Columbia, Canada

Trelia J. Craft, B.S.
Associate Senior Pharmacologist, Department of Cardiovascular Research, Lilly Research Laboratories, Eli Lilly & Company, Indianapolis, Indiana

Nicola D'Attellis, M.D.
Staff Anesthesiologist, Broussais Hospital, Paris, France

Volker Eschenfelder, M.D., Ph.D.
Professor of Biochemistry, Department of Biochemistry II, University of Heidelberg, Heidelberg, Germany

Jawed Fareed, Ph.D.
Professor, Department of Pathology and Pharmacology, Loyola University Medical Center, Maywood, Illinois

Sofia Farid, Ph.D.
Research Associate, Department of Psychiatry, Hines Veterans Affairs Hospital, Hines, Illinois

John W. Fenton, II, Ph.D.
Professor, New York State Department of Health, Albany, New York

Carol A. Fisher, A.B.
Research Instructor of Surgery, Director, Cardiothoracic Research, Department of Surgery, Division of Cardiac and Thoracic Surgery, Temple University School of Medicine, Philadelphia, Pennsylvania

Cornelius Förster
Medical student, Institute of Experimental Surgery, Technical University of Munich, Munich, Germany

Donetta S. Gifford-Moore, B.S.
Assistant Senior Pharmacologist, Department of Cardiovascular Research, Lilly Research Laboratories, Eli Lilly & Company, Indianapolis, Indiana

John E. Godwin, M.D., M.S.
Associate Professor, Department of Medicine and Pathology, Loyola University Medical Center, Maywood, Illinois

Eric D. Grassman, M.D., Ph.D., FACC
Associate Professor of Medicine, Department of Cardiology, Loyola University Medical Center, Maywood, Illinois

Sylvia Haas, M.D.
Professor of Medicine, Institute for Experimental Surgery, Technical University of Munich, Munich, Germany

Houria I. Hassouna, M.D., Ph.D.
Professor, Department of Medicine, Michigan State University, East Lansing, Michigan

Katherine P. Henrikson, Ph.D.
Assistant Professor, New York State Department of Health, Albany, New York

Debra A. Hoppensteadt, M.S., M.T. (ASCP)
Technical Specialist, Department of Pathology, Loyola University Medical Center, Maywood, Illinois

Omer Iqbal, M.D.
Research Associate, Department of Pathology, Loyola University Medical Center, Maywood, Illinois

Walter P. Jeske, Ph.D.
Postdoctoral Fellow, Cardiovascular Institute, Loyola University Medical Center, Maywood, Illinois

Lindsay C. H. John, B.Sc.(Hons.), M.S., FRCS
Department of Cardiothoracic Surgery, St. Bartholomews Hospital, London, United Kingdom

Sarah A. Johnson, M.D.
Professor, Department of Cardiology, Loyola University Medical Center, Maywood, Illinois

Brigitte Kaiser, M.D.
Departments of Pharmacology and Toxicology, Center for Vascular Biology and Medicine Erfurt, Friedrich Schiller University Jena, Medical Faculty, Erfurt, Germany

Evi Kalodiki, M.D., B.A.
Senior Vascular Research Fellow, Irvine Laboratory for Cardiovascular Investigation and Research, Academic Surgical Unit, Imperial College School of Medicine at St. Mary's Hospital, London, United Kingdom

Jeffrey R. Kappa, M.D.
Clinical Associate Professor, Department of Surgery, James H. Quillen College of Medicine, East Tennessee State University, Kingsport, Tennessee

Shukri F. Khuri, M.D.
Professor of Surgery, Harvard Medical School, Boston; Chief, Surgical Service, Brockton/West Roxbury VA Medical Center, West Roxbury; Associate Chief of Surgery, Brigham & Women's Hospital, Boston, Massachusetts

Jochen Kohn, Ph.D.
Professor, Rutgers University, The State University of New Jersey, Piscataway/New Brunswick, New Jersey

Michael J. Koza, B.S., M.T. (ASCP)
Department of Thoracic and Cardiovascular Surgery, Loyola University Medical Center, Maywood, Illinois

Bruce E. Lewis, M.D., FACC
Associate Professor of Medicine, Department of Cardiology, Loyola University Medical Center, Maywood, Illinois

Terry D. Lindstrom, Ph.D.
Research Advisor, Adjunct Assistant Professor, Department of Drug Disposition, Lilly Research Laboratories, Eli Lilly & Company, Indianapolis, Indiana

Vassyl Lonchyna, M.D.
Associate Professor, Department of Thoracic and Cardiovascular Surgery, Loyola University Medical Center, Maywood, Illinois

H. N. Magnani, M.D., M.Sc., Ph.D.
Medical Research and Development Department, NV Organon, Oss, The Netherlands

Fritz Markwardt, M.D., Ph.D.
Professor of Pharmacology, Erfurt, Germany

Simone Massonnet-Castel, M.D.
Staff Hematologist, Laboratory for the Study of Cardiac Prosthesis, Broussais Hospital, Paris, France

Harry L. Messmore, M.D.
Professor of Medicine, Loyola University Medical Center, Maywood, Illinois, and Hines Veterans Affairs Hospital, Hines, Illinois

Gert Mueller-Berghaus, M.D.
Professor and Head, Haemostasis Research Unit, Kerckhoff-Klinik, Max-Planck-Gesellschaft, Bad Nauheim, Germany

Andrew N. Nicolaides, M.S., FRCS, FRCSE
Professor of Vascular Surgery, Irvine Laboratory for Cardiovascular Investigation and Research, Imperial College School of Medicine at St. Mary's Hospital, London, United Kingdom

Götz Nowak, M.D.
Professor of Pharmacology and Toxicology, Pharmacological Hemostaseology Research Unit, Max-Planck-Gesellschaft, Friedrich Schiller University, Jena, Germany

Gregory A. Nuttall, M.D.
Assistant Professor, Department of Anesthesiology, Mayo Clinic, Rochester, Minnesota

Fredrick A. Ofosu, Ph.D.
Professor of Pathology, McMaster University, Hamilton, Ontario, Canada

William C. Oliver, Jr., M.D.
Assistant Professor of Anesthesiology, Mayo Clinic, Rochester, Minnesota

Ramadevi Parachuri, M.D.
Staff Physician, Hines Veterans Affairs Hospital, Hines, Illinois

Roque Pifarré, M.D.
Professor Emeritus of Thoracic and Cardiovascular Surgery, Department of Thoracic and Cardiovascular Surgery, Loyola University Stritch School of Medicine, Maywood, Illinois

Bernd Poetzsch, M.D.
Hemostasis Research Unit, Kerckhoff-Klinik, Bad Nauheim, Germany

Jerome Premmereur, M.D.
Director, Cardiovascular Development, Department of Research and Development, Rhône-Poulenc Rorer, Collegeville, Pennsylvania

Friedrich-Christian Riess, M.D.
Department of Cardiac Surgery, Albertinen-Krankenhaus, Hamburg, Germany

Kenneth J. Ruterbories, B.S., M.S.
Associate Senior Pharmacologist, Department of Drug Disposition, Lilly Research Laboratories, Eli Lilly & Company, Indianapolis, Indiana

Julie H. Satterwhite, Ph.D.
Research Scientist, Department of Pharmacokinetics and Bioavailability, Lilly Research Laboratories, Eli Lilly & Company, Indianapolis, Indiana

Gerhard Schmidmaier
Institute of Experimental Surgery, Technical University of Munich, Munich, Germany

Friedrich Schumann, Ph.D.
International Clinical Project Manager (retired), Bayer AG, Health Care, Pharmaceutical Division, Wuppertal, Germany

Richard P. Schwarz, Jr., Ph.D.
Vice President, Clinical Development and Regulatory Affairs, Texas Biotechnology Corporation, Houston, Texas

Gerald F. Smith, Ph.D., J.D.
Senior Research Scientist, Department of Cardiovascular Research, Lilly Research Laboratories, Eli Lilly & Company, Indianapolis, Indiana

Axel Stemberger, Ph.D.
Associate Professor, Institute for Experimental Surgery, Technical University of Munich, Munich, Germany

Mark R. Terrell, M.D.
Department of Anesthesiology, Loyola University Medical Center, Maywood, Illinois

Gaurav Upadhyay, M.D.
Research Assistant, Hines Veterans Affairs Hospital, Hines, Illinois

Jeanine M. Walenga, Ph.D.
Associate Professor, Departments of Thoracic and Cardiovascular Surgery and Pathology, Loyola University Medical Center, Maywood, Illinois

William H. Wehrmacher, M.D.
Clinical Professor of Medicine and Adjunct Professor of Physiology, Loyola University Stritch School of Medicine, Maywood, Illinois

Helmut Wolf, M.D., Ph.D.
Medical Department, Sandoz AG, Nuremberg, Germany

Jan Wouter ten Cate, M.D., Ph.D.
Professor of Medicine, Center for Haemostasis, Thrombosis, Atherosclerosis and Inflammation Research, Academic Medical Centre, Amsterdam, The Netherlands

Laura L. Wrona, R.N., CCRC
Research Coordinator, Department of Cardiology, Loyola University Medical Center, Maywood, Illinois

Foreword

Despite its lack of predictable dose response, need of monitoring, and high risk of bleeding complications, heparin has been the sole intravenous anticoagulant in surgical use for many years. These drawbacks, as well as the recognition of heparin-associated thrombocytopenia and heparin-induced thrombotic syndrome, warranted the development of alternative anticoagulants for patients undergoing surgery. Timely advances in recombinant technology led to the availability of recombinant hirudin for anticoagulant purposes. An understanding of the mechanism behind the anticoagulant actions of this antithrombin inhibitor subsequently led to the molecularly designed anticoagulants such as hirulog.

While synthetic antithrombin agents such as argatroban and efegatran were known for quite some time, the revived interest in antithrombin agents encouraged development of these products for clinical use. At the same time, improved synthetic methods continued to provide newer anticoagulants devoid of some of the side effects seen with heparins. The recognition of these agents as substitute anticoagulants is timely and will be extremely helpful in the management of large numbers of patients who otherwise would have suffered the consequences of either being treated with a drug with potential side effects or not being treated at all.

Parallel to the impressive progress in the understanding of the hemostatic and thrombotic processes, remarkable advances in the development of several classes of anticoagulant and antithrombotic drugs have occurred. The introduction of low-molecular-weight heparin has added a new dimension to the prophylaxis and treatment of thrombotic disorders. This and other drugs, such as the new agents used to maintain the patency of biomaterial used in cardiopulmonary bypass surgery, are discussed by several authors in this book. The importance of laboratory monitoring in the optimal use of these drugs also is discussed. Newer approaches to monitoring the antithrombin agents using ecarin clotting time and point-of-care testing are addressed as well. Thus, this volume provides timely and comprehensive coverage of new developments in anticoagulant and antithrombotic pharmacology, with particular reference to therapeutic approaches to cardiovascular surgery. Furthermore, the text contains information not only for surgeons and physicians but also for basic scientists conducting research in this field.

Dr. Roque Pifarré, a pioneering cardiovascular surgeon, and the contributing authors are to be commended for compiling an important book that readily fills a gap by providing much needed information—ultimately resulting in a direct benefit to patients. This book is undoubtedly a major and timely contribution toward the better understanding of the basic and applied aspects of anticoagulant and antithrombotic drugs.

Andrew N. Nicolaides, M.S., FRCS, FRCSE
Professor of Vascular Surgery
Irvine Laboratory for Cardiovascular
  Investigation and Research
Imperial College School of Medicine
  at St. Mary's Hospital
London, United Kingdom

Preface

Currently, unfractionated heparin continues to be the anticoagulant of choice in cardiovascular surgery. Although this drug has been very useful as an anticoagulant for cardiovascular patients, it may be associated with several serious complications. Potential problems include intraoperative and postoperative bleeding, heparin resistance, heparin rebound after heparin neutralization with protamine, and heparin-induced thrombocytopenia and thrombosis. Anyone who uses heparin in any form or by any route of administration should be aware of the syndromes of heparin-induced thrombocytopenia and heparin-induced thrombosis. Recognition of these complications casts shadows on the efficacy and safety of heparin as an anticoagulant. Thus, strategies to replace heparin have attracted great attention.

Alternative anticoagulants potentially can eliminate the use of heparin. Several newly developed anticoagulant agents are being evaluated experimentally, and some have been tested clinically. Low-molecular-weight heparin and heparinoids, hirudin, synthetic peptides, peptidomimetics, and snake venom such as ancrod are being carefully evaluated in clinical settings.

Despite impressive progress in the development of these new anticoagulants, a better anticoagulation approach for cardiovascular patients is not available at this time. Adjunct approaches to optimize the use of heparin by minimizing its toxicity and producing better means of anticoagulation are in progress at this time. Because of these developments, improved regimens for using heparin alone and/or in combination with the new anticoagulants may become available.

The contributors to this book represent both clinicians and basic scientists who have worked in specific areas related to the development of new drugs. Each chapter was prepared to provide an update on current developments, with specific references to cardiovascular relevance. Both the fundamental and clinical issues have been covered.

The purpose of this book is to provide a status report on recent efforts to avoid some of the complications that may result from the use of heparin. This book also provides a view of the future of anticoagulation by examining new agents pharmacologically and new techniques of genetic engineering in development. Furthermore, this book is intended to provide a current reference in this exciting field. It is hoped that the information provided here will be helpful to cardiologists and cardiovascular surgeons in choosing alternative approaches to anticoagulation in heparin-compromised patients.

Acknowledgments

I would like to thank my wife, Teresa, for her patience and consistent support. My gratitude goes to Mrs. Margaret Borgh for her invaluable assistance with the manuscript processing, correspondence, and communication. I thank the authors for their efforts, expertise, and cooperation. Ms. Linda Belfus is gratefully acknowledged for her editorial assistance.

Roque Pifarré, M.D.

CHAPTER 1

Clinical Disadvantages with the Use of Heparin as an Anticoagulant

ROQUE PIFARRÉ, M.D.
JEANINE M. WALENGA, Ph.D.
JAWED FAREED, Ph.D.

At present cardiac operations are performed routinely. The use of extracorporeal circulation with the heart-lung apparatus was made possible with the availability of heparin. Cardiopulmonary bypass (CPB) requires a high degree of anticoagulation and neutralization of the heparin with protamine at the conclusion of the procedure (Table 1). Unfractionated heparin continues to be the anticoagulant of choice in cardiovascular surgery. Heparin becomes effective in the presence of antithrombin III (AT III), a plasma protein with which it forms a complex. Heparin augments the activity of antithrombin III and neutralizes coagulation factors X, II, XII, XI, and IX.

The importance of using the proper dose of heparin cannot be overemphasized. The dose must be carefully balanced. Too high a dose leads to bleeding, and too low a dose may result in clotting. To obtain optimal anticoagulation during CPB, one must administer the proper dose of heparin and monitor the level of anticoagulation during the entire procedure. Protocols for anticoagulation vary significantly among different institutions. Likewise, great variation exists in techniques for monitoring anticoagulation during cardiopulmonary bypass (Table 2).

Although heparin has been highly effective as an anticoagulant in cardiovascular operations, its use may result in serious complications, including intraoperative and postoperative bleeding, heparin resistance, heparin rebound after neutralization, and heparin-induced thrombocytopenia and thrombosis (Table 3).

VARIATIONS IN ANTICOAGULATION EFFECTIVENESS

Different forms of heparin are derived from different raw materials and show differences in molecular structure, AT III affinity, and anticoagulation potencies.

The variations in AT III affinity among heparins from various sources result from the differences in molecular structure and specific binding sites. Bovine lung heparin has the lowest affinity for AT III, and porcine intestinal mucosa heparin has the highest.

The anticoagulation potency also varies. Porcine mucosal heparin has the highest potency, followed by bovine lung heparin. The anticoagulant effects on a given patient differ with the specific manufacturer and even the particular batch.

1

TABLE 1.   Heparin Neutralization with Protamine

Calculate protamine dose with Hepcon.
Give: 75% of dose at end of CPB
25% once all cell-saver blood has been reinfused
Repeat Hepcon once protamine is infused.
Repeat in 1–3 hours to rule out heparin rebound.
Usual dose: < 1:1

The dose of heparin for CPB must be carefully calculated. The size, age, previous exposure to heparin, and diagnosis of the patient must be taken into account. Because of the many variables involved, the level of anticoagulation during CPB must be carefully monitored.

ADVERSE REACTIONS TO PROTAMINE NEUTRALIZATION

Protamine, the only agent used to neutralize heparin, has a positively charged arginine. An ionic attraction binds protamine to heparin. Protamine forms large complexes with heparin that are digested by microphages of the reticuloendothelial system. This process takes place in the lungs when protamine is given intravenously.

The appropriate dose of protamine for heparin neutralization is a matter of great controversy. Most cardiovascular teams use a dose of 1–1.5 mg/100 U of heparin. In our institution the heparin dose is calculated with the Hepcon. The calculated amount is given as a split dose (Table 1). This method has helped to reduce the total amount of protamine given and to prevent heparin rebound.

Protamine is used extensively to neutralize heparin without complications. Nevertheless, an adverse response to protamine occasionally may be deleterious or life-threatening. The cardiovascular team members and anesthesiologist should be familiar with these adverse reactions in order to take prompt and adequate action.

Three major types of adverse response to the administration of protamine have been described. Type 1 is a hypotensive reaction that results from administering protamine too rapidly. This reaction, which is the most common of the three types, has been attributed to the release of histamine.[3] Hypotension is accompanied by a decrease in systemic vascular resistance and an increase in cardiac output.[4] In most patients such hemodynamic alterations are well tolerated and require no further treatment. Once the adverse reaction is recognized, the protamine should be stopped for a while and restarted slowly. In some cases, antihistamines may be indicated.

Patients with a history of fin-fish allergy may develop a type II reaction, which is a true anaphylactic response mediated by immunoglobins. Systemic and capillary leak due to the release of histamine and leukotrienes results in systemic hypotension, angioedema, anasarca, and noncardiac pulmonary edema.[4] Type II reaction requires vigorous treatment. Patients benefit from the administration of oxygen, fluids, and peak end-expiratory pressure (PEEP). In severe cases, antihistamines and steroids may be required.

Harrow[5] pointed out that type III reactions are related to heparin-protamine complexes. Pulmonary microphages activate complement and leukocyte aggregation, resulting in the release of free radicals and activation of the arachidonic acid pathway, which lead to

TABLE 2.   Loyola University Medical Center Anticoagulation Protocol

Without aprotinin	With aprotinin
Heparin loading dose: 200–250 U/kg	Heparin loading dose: 350 U/kg
Add 2,000–3,000 U as required to maintain	Maintain heparin concentration/Hepcon at 2.7 U/ml
ACT (celite) above 400 sec	ACT (celite) > 750 sec
	ACT (kaolin) > 500 sec

ACT = activated clotting time.

TABLE 3.   Disadvantages of the Use of Unfractionated Heparin

Individual sensitivities	Heparin rebound
Variations in anticoagulation effectiveness	Postoperative bleeding
Requires antithrombin III	Heparin-induced thrombocytopenia
Adverse reactions to protamine neutralization	Heparin-induced thrombosis
Inhibits platelet aggregation	Heparin-induced platelet dysfunction
Activation of neutrophils	Heparin-induced fibrinolysis
Heparin–protamine complex stimulates	Heparin resistance
complement activation	

the formation of thromboxane. The release of thromboxane into the pulmonary circulation causes an intense vasoconstriction, resulting in pulmonary hypertension and low left atrial pressure. Consequently, the right heart becomes dilated, and right-heart failure ensues. Once the diagnosis is made, the administration of protamine must be stopped, and a drip of isoproterenol is started. The administration of calcium may be useful. In some cases, the use of epinephrine may be necessary. The use of pulmonary vasodilators (prostacyclin) via the central venous line has also been recommended . Fortunately, type III reaction is rare.

The manufacturer recommends that protamine be given no faster then 5 mg/min. Morel et al.[35] demonstrated that the rate of protamine administration is an important factor leading to pulmonary vasoconstriction in sheep. They reversed the heparin dose with a 1:1 ratio of protamine. When protamine was given over 3 seconds, it resulted in thromboxane release, pulmonary vasoconstriction, pulmonary hypertension, increased systemic vascular resistance, and decreased cardiac output. When it was given over 30 minutes, no changes in the pulmonary hemodynamics were observed.

Although human studies to date have demonstrated no advantage to left-sided vs. right-sided administration,[36,37] most teams use right-sided administration. The rate of infusion—not the infusion site—is the important factor to prevent protamine reactions. More recently, Wakefield et al.[38] reported a significant drop in systemic oxygen consumption and declines in blood pressure, heart rate, and cardiac output with rapid administration of protamine to reverse heparin anticoagulation.

HEPARIN REBOUND

The term *heparin rebound* denotes the reappearance of clinical bleeding and prolonged coagulation times after heparin neutralization with protamine.[4] Satisfactory hemostasis is not accomplished if the reversal of heparin is only temporary. The rate at which heparin is metabolized, the amount of protamine necessary for its reversal, and the patient's response to heparin are subject to wide variations. Gallub[6] concluded that the hypocoagulability was due to reappearance of heparin in the circulating blood. More evidence now supports the accepted notion that heparin rebound is due to reappearance of circulating heparin.[7] The etiology of heparin rebound has not been clarified satisfactorily. Most likely heparin is deposited in extravascular tissues and reappears intravascularly after the neutralizing protamine has disappeared. It is recognized that heparin binds to endothelium. The current theory involves late release of bound heparin from endothelium.[8,9,10] Prolonged coagulation times occur as early as 1 hour after heparin neutralization and may persist as long as 6 hours.[2,11,12]

Regardless of the exact pathophysiology, heparin rebound seems to be due to the effect of heparin after it is neutralized with protamine. It has been suggested that enough protamine should be given to prevent heparin rebound and to ensure adequate neutralization.[11] We[2] and others[13] believe that it is not necessary to give a high dose of protamine to prevent heparin rebound. The amount of protamine can be calculated with the Hepcon and administered in two doses: 75% at the conclusion of CPB and the remaining 25% after all of the blood from the oxygenator and cell saver has been reinfused. Heparin rebound may take place up to 6 hours later, according to our experience; however, it most commonly takes place within the first 1–3 hours after administering the protamine.[14] We recommend that the Hepcon be repeated several times during the postoperative period, especially if the patient shows signs of bleeding after a period of dryness in the operative field.

HEPARIN RESISTANCE

Heparin resistance is decreased sensitivity to heparin. Higher-than-normal doses are needed to induce sufficient anticoagulation for the safe conduct of CPB. In some cases, excessive doses of heparin must be administered to prolong the activated clotting time (ACT) to a therapeutic level. The mechanisms for heparin resistance are not well understood; it may be due to decreased level of AT III or increased levels of platelet factor 4.[15]

AT III deficiency can be inherited or acquired. Congenital deficiency shows a reduced amount of normal AT III (< 50% of normal). It is seen in young people (15–30 years old) who suffer limb thrombosis or pulmonary embolism.[16,17] It may be precipitated by pregnancy, infection, and surgery. The primary clinical presentation may be either thrombosis after surgery or difficulty in achieving adequate anticoagulation for CPB.[18]

Acquired AT III deficiency is more common than the inherited form. Multiple conditions have been presumed to be associated with AT III deficiency. Prolonged preoperative heparin therapy, heparin-induced thrombocytopenia, thrombosis, disseminated intravascular coagulation, and oral contraceptive therapy are the most commonly mentioned.

Fresh frozen plasma has been used successfully to reverse heparin resistance in patients with AT III deficiency.[19] The introduction of a human AT III concentrate will make the use of fresh frozen plasma obsolete.[20,21]

HEPARIN-INDUCED THROMBOCYTOPENIA

The reported incidence of heparin-induced thrombocytopenia (HIT) varies between 5–28% of patients receiving heparin.[22,23] HIT, which occurs after 4–5 days of heparin administration, is thought to be immune-mediated. Thrombocytopenia is defined as a platelet count < 100,000/μl. The diagnosis of HIT is based on the finding of a platelet count < 50% of the pretreatment level or < 100,000/μl in patients receiving heparin therapy. HIT has persisted for 2 days or more.[24]

HIT may be due to the binding of IgG antibodies to platelet-bound heparin, which activates platelets and induces platelet clumping. There also may be an associated immune-mediated endothelial injury. Complement activation may set the stage for activated platelet clots. HIT may progress to intravascular thrombosis.[25,26] The incidence of thrombotic complications has been reported as high as 20%, with a mortality rate as high as 35%.[23]

The catastrophic complications of HIT mandate that heparin be used cautiously and only when clearly indicated. The development of new anticoagulants to replace heparin is an important priority. The management of patients with HIT and its complications is discussed in chapter 7.

HEPARIN-INDUCED PLATELET DYSFUNCTION AND FIBRINOLYSIS

It has been postulated that CPB results in loss of the platelet membrane receptors responsible for platelet adhesion and aggregation. Loss of platelet membrane receptors for both von Willebrand's factor (VWF) and fibrinogen has been reported during and after cardiopulmonary bypass.[27,28]

This assumption has been questioned by others,[29] and other factors, such as hypothermia and heparin, have been implicated. Khuri et al.[30] assessed platelet function by measuring the bleeding time and the level of thromboxane B_2. Both measurements showed a marked reduction in platelet function after administration of heparin. Others have also reported the inhibition of platelet function by heparin in postbypass bleeding.[31] Recently inhibition of VWF activity has been reported as another possible mechanism for the inhibition of platelet function by heparin.[32] The study demonstrated that the concentration and distribution of VWF were unaffected by the administration of heparin and concluded that heparin reduced platelet function by preventing VWF from binding to its receptor on the chlorophenoxyisobutyrate on the platelet.[32]

Heparin also can induce platelet dysfunction through its effect on plasmin, probably by facilitating the release of tissue plasminogen activator (tPA), which promotes fibrinolysis. Fareed et al.[33] reported an increase in tPA levels in human volunteers after administration of intravenous heparin.[33] Khuri et al.[32] demonstrated that the administration of heparin before institution of CPB resulted in an increase of fibrinolysis, as evidenced by an increase in plasmin and D-dimer levels. Fibrin degradation products and D-dimer levels increase during and after CPB.[30,34] The rise in plasmin and D-dimer levels after the administration of heparin indicates an increase in profibrinolytic activity. These two degradation products interfere with platelet aggregation and contribute to platelet dysfunction.

The study of Khuri et al.[32] confirms the need to continue to search for an alternative anticoagulant that does not interfere with platelet function or the fibrinolytic process.

POSTOPERATIVE BLEEDING

Patients undergoing cardiac operations are predisposed to increased postoperative bleeding by the combination of heparin anticoagulation and other factors. Excessive heparinization, heparin rebound, inadequate protamine neutralization, and protamine excess have been implicated in CPB-related bleeding. Other predisposing factors include (1) cyanotic heart disease, (2) prolonged perfusion time, (3) use of hypothermia, (4) preoperative use of warfarin-type drugs, (5) use of drugs that interfere with platelet function, and (6) reoperations.

The duration of perfusion time is highly important. The shorter the better! Prolonged perfusion requires higher doses of heparin, which in turn require higher doses of protamine for neutralization. Platelet dysfunction and fibrinolysis also increase. The need for expeditious operations and short perfusion times cannot be overemphasized.

The use of hypothermia to reduce oxygen and metabolic requirements is routine in current cardiac operations. When hypothermic CPB is used, it is difficult to rewarm the patient completely before leaving the operating room, and this contributes to blood loss and hemodilution. Hypothermia interferes greatly with platelet function and contributes to the postoperative blood loss in cardiac surgery.[41,42]

It has become customary to use warfarin for anticoagulation in patients who present with atrial fibrillation or dilated cardiomyopathy. Patients with mechanical valves are also anticoagulated with warfarin. Often, there is not enough time to reverse the anticoagulant effect of warfarin, which may be responsible for operative or postoperative bleeding.

Most patients diagnosed with coronary atherosclerosis are routinely given antiplatelet drugs. It is not well recognized that antiplatelet drugs affect all platelets; thus it takes 8–10 days for the antiplatelet effect to disappear. Every effort should be made to discontinue any drug that interferes with platelet function at least 1 week before surgery. If this policy is not followed, operative and postoperative bleeding will be increased. In such cases, the only solution is to administer platelets or to use aprotinin to restore platelet function.

The number of reoperations for congenital, valvular, or coronary procedures has increased steadily through the years. Reoperative patients have an increased tendency to bleed because of the dissection of adhesions from previous surgery, combined with antiplatelet medications and, in many cases, warfarin anticoagulation.

According to Bick,[39,40] all patients undergoing CPB have a platelet dysfunction. When bleeding occurs, Bick assumes that platelet dysfunction is the cause or a contributory factor. Platelets are ordered immediately for any patient with intraoperative or postoperative bleeding.

SUMMARY

Anticoagulation with heparin has made possible the use of the heart-lung machine to perform cardiac operations with CPB. Extracorporeal circulation requires a high degree of anticoagulation, which may cause severe complications. Postoperative bleeding and heparin-induced thrombocytopenia are not uncommon.

The complications associated with heparin anticoagulation can be prevented only if the amount of heparin is reduced or heparin is replaced by a new and better anticoagulant. The amount of heparin administered during CPB may be reduced significantly by adhering to a protocol that requires a lower dose. The initial dose of heparin is controversial. It may vary from 200–500 U/kg. Several institutions have demonstrated the safety of a loading dose of 200 U/kg, provided that more heparin is added during perfusion to maintain the ACT (celite) above 400 seconds. The authors are convinced that the more heparin administered to a patient, the greater the chances for postoperative bleeding. Frequent and careful monitoring of anticoagulation during CPB should prevent thrombotic complications.

Eliminination of heparin resistance, heparin rebound, and heparin-induced thrombocytopenia and thrombosis requires the elimination of heparin as an anticoagulant for CPB and its replacement by another agent that provides at least as effective anticoagulation without the disadvantages and complications described in this chapter.

REFERENCES

1. Babka R, Colby C, El-Etr A, Pifarré R: Monitoring of intraoperative heparinization and blood loss following cardiopulmonary bypass surgery. J Thorac Cardiovasc Surg 73:780–782, 1977.
2. Pifarré R, Babka R, Sullivan HJ, et al: Management of postoperative heparin rebound following cardiopulmonary bypass J Thorac Cardiovasc Surg 81:378–381, 1981.
3. Frater RWM, Oka HY, et al: Protamine induced circulatory changes. J Thorac Cardiovasc Surgery 97:687–692, 1984.
4. Horrow JC: Protamine allergy. J Cardiothoracic Anesth 2:225–242, 1988.
5. Horrow JC: Heparin reversal of protamine toxicity: Have we come full circle? J Cardiothorac Vasc Anesth 4:539–542, 1990.
6. Gallub S. Heparin rebound in open heart surgery. Surg Gynecol Obstet 124:337-346, 1967.
7. Kesteven PJ, Osborn A, Aps C, et al: Protamine sulphate and rebound following open heart surgery. J. Cardiovasc Surg 27:600–603, 1986.
8. Perkins HA, Acra DJ, Rolfs MR: Estimation of heparin levels in stored and traumatized blood. Blood 18:807–808, 1961.
9. Frick PG, Brogli H: The mechanism of heparin rebound after extracorporeal circulation for open cardiac surgery. Surgery 59:721–726, 1966.
10. Perkins HA, Osborn JJ, Gerbode F: The management of abnormal bleeding following extracorporeal circulation. Ann Intern Med 51:558–667, 1959.
11. Ellison N, Beatty P, Blake DR, et al: Heparin rebound. J Thorac Cardiovasc Surgery 67:723–729, 1974.
12. Kaul TK, Crow MJ, Rajah SM, et al: Heparin administration during extracorporeal circulation. J Thorac Cardiovasc Surgery 78:95–102, 1979.
13. Aren C, Feddersen K, Radegran K: Comparison of two protocols for heparin neutralization by protamine after cardiopulmonary bypass. J Thorac Cardiovasc Surgery 94:539–541, 1987.
14. Pifarré R, Sullivan HJ, Montoya A, et al: Management of blood loss and heparin rebound following cardiopulmonary bypass. Semin Thromb Hemost 15:2 173–177, 1989.
15. Esposito RA, Culliford HT, Colvin SB, et al: Heparin resistance during cardiopulmonary bypass. The role of heparin pretreatment. J Thorac Cardiovasc Surgery 95:346–353, 1983.
16. Nielsen LE, Bell WR, Barkon AM, Neill CA: Extensive thrombus formation with heparin resistance during extracorporeal circulation: A new presentation of familial anti-thrombin III deficiency. Arch Intern Med 147:149–152.
17. Thaler E, Ischner K: Antithrombin III deficiency and thromboembolism. Clin Haematol 10:369–390, 1981.
18. Towne JB, Bernhard VM, Hussey C, Garancis JC: Antithrombin deficiency—a cause of unexplained thrombosis in vascular surgery. Surgery 89:735–742, 1981.
19. Soloway H, Christiansen TW: Heparin anticoagulation during cardiopulmonary bypass is an antithrombin III deficiency patient. Am J Clin Pathol 73:723–725, 1980.
20. Hoffman DL: Purification and large-scale preparation of antithrombin III. Am J Med 87(Suppl 3B): 235–265, 1989.
21. Schwartz RS, Bauer KA, Rosenberg RD et al: Clinical experience with antithrombin III concentrate in treatment of congenital and acquired deficiency of thrombin. Am J Med 87 (Suppl 3B) 535-605, 1989.

22. King DJ, Delton JG: Heparin associated thrombocytopenia. Ann Intern Med 100:535–540, 1984.
23. Godal HC: Heparin-induced thrombocytopenia. In Lane DA, Lindahl U, (eds): Heparin: Chemical and Biological Properties, Clinical Applications. Boca Raton, FL, CRC Press, pp 533–548, 1989.
24. Bell WR: Heparin associated thrombocytopenia and thrombosis. J Lab Clin Med 111:600–605, 1988.
25. White PW, Sadd JR, Nensel RE: Thrombotic complications of heparin therapy. Including six cases of heparin-induced skin necrosis. Ann Surg 190:595–608, 1979.
26. Cines DB, Kaywin P, Bina M, et al: Heparin-associated thrombocytopenia. N Engl J Med 303:788–795, 1980.
27. Rinder CS, Mathew JP, Rinder HM, et al: Modulation of platelet surface adhesion receptors during cardiopulmonary bypass. Anesthesiology 75:563–570, 1991.
28. Wenger RK, Lukasiewicz H, Mikuta BS, et al: Loss of platelet fibrinogen receptors during clinical cardiopulmonary bypass. J Thorac Cardiovasc Surg 97:235–239, 1989.
29. Kestin AS, Valeri CR, Khuri SF, et al: The platelet function defect of cardiopulmonary bypass. Blood 82:107–117, 1993.
30. Khuri SF, Michelson AD, Valeri CR: The effect of cardiopulmonary bypass on hemostasis and coagulation. In Loralzo J, Schafer AI (eds): Thrombosis and Hemorrhage. Cambridge, Blackwell Scientific, 1051–1073, 1994.
31. John LCH, Rees GM, Kovacs IB: Inhibition of platelet function by heparin. J Thorac Cardiovasc Surgery 105:816–822, 1993.
32. Khuri SF, Valeri CR, Lorcalzao J, et al: Heparin causes platelet dysfunction and induces fibrinolysis before cardiopulmonary bypass. Ann Thorac Surg 60:1008–1014, 1995.
33. Fareed J, Walenga JM, Hoppenstead DA, Messmore HL: Studies on the profibrinolytic action of heparin and its fractions. Semin Thromb Hemost 11:199–207, 1985.
34. Giuliani R, Szwarcer E, Martinez Aquino E, Palumbo G: Fibrin-dependent fibrinolytic activity during extracorporeal circulation. Thromb Res 61:369–373, 1991.
35. Morel DR, Mo Costabella PM, Pitted JF: Adverse cardiopulmonary effects and increased thromboxane concentration following neutralization of heparin with protamine in awake sleep are infusion rate-dependent. Anesthesiology 73:415–424, 1990.
36. Milve B, Rogers K, Cervenko F, Salerno T: The hemodynamic effects of intra-aortic versus intravenous administration of protamine for reversal of heparin in man. Can Anesth Soc J 30:347–351, 1983.
37. Cherry DA, Chiu CJ, Wynands JE, et al: Intra-aortic versus intravenous administration of protamine: A prospective randomized clinical study. Surg Forum 36: 238–240, 1985.
38. Wakefield TW, Hantler CB, Wrobleski SK, et al: Effects of differing rates of protamine reversal of heparin anticoagulation. Surgery 119:123–128, 1996.
39. Bick RL: Hemostasis defects associated with cardiac surgery, general surgery, and prothesis devices. In Bick RL: Disorders of Thrombosis and Hemostasis: Clinical and laboratory Practice. Chicago, ASCP Press, p 95, 1992.
40. Bick RL: Physiology and pathophysiology of hemostasis during cardiac surgery. In Pifarré R (ed): Anticoagulation, Hemostasis, and Blood Conservation in Cardiovascular Surgery. Philadelphia, Hanley & Belfus, p 23, 1993.
41. Valeri CR, Faingold H, Cassidy G, et al: Hypothermia induced reversible platelet dysfunction. Ann Surg 205:175–181, 1987.
42. Khuri SF, Wolfe JA, Josa M, et al: Hematologic changes during and after cardiopulmonary bypass and their relationship to the bleeding time and nonsurgical blood loss. J Thorac Cardiovasc Surg. 104:94–107, 1992.

CHAPTER 2

An Overview of Blood Coagulation

WALTER JESKE, Ph.D.
ROQUE PIFARRÉ, M.D.
HELMUT WOLF, M.D., Ph.D.
JAWED FAREED, Ph.D.

Hemostasis, as defined by Virchow in the last century, is a fine balance between blood flow, humoral factors, and cellular elements of the vascular system. Current biotechnology has advanced our understanding of the thrombotic process and its regulation. Whereas in the past heparin and warfarin have been the only available antithrombotic agents, specific sites in the thrombotic network at both plasmatic and cellular sites can now be targeted. Antibodies against specific platelet receptors as well as specific antithrombin and anti-Xa agents are being developed. Mutations of endogenous inhibitors have been identified as causes of congenital thrombophilias. The use of heparin has also advanced. Heparin is no longer solely a surgical anticoagulant; it is used to treat a variety of conditions, including venous thrombosis, unstable angina, and myocardial infarction as well as in procedures such as angioplasty and stent implantation. The mechanism of heparin's action has become more complex with the discovery of tissue factor pathway inhibitor, selectins, and other cellular targets at which the drug is able to produce its effects.

Blood normally is maintained in the fluid state so that nutrients can be delivered to the various tissues of the body. When the integrity of the vascular system has been compromised, it becomes necessary for the blood to clot. The initial response to a break in the continuity of the vasculature is the formation of the platelet plug. Platelets in the flowing blood rapidly adhere to the exposed matrix of the subendothelial vessel wall and become activated. During this activation process, components of the platelet α and β granules (adenosine triphosphate [ATP], adenosine diphosphate [ADP], factor V, 5-hydroxytryptamine [5-HT]) are released, causing further platelet aggregation. Also during these morphologic changes, activated platelets express protein and cell receptors, and procoagulant phospholipids are expressed on their surface.

The negatively charged phospholipid phosphatidylserine is asymmetrically distributed in mammalian cell membranes, primarily on the inner leaflet. Upon exposure to collagen or thrombin, the distribution of phospholipids changes, with increasing phosphatidylserine in the external membrane leaf.[23] The increased expression of phosphatidylserine on the outer leaflet of the membrane creates a procoagulant surface on which several steps of the coagulation cascade take place.

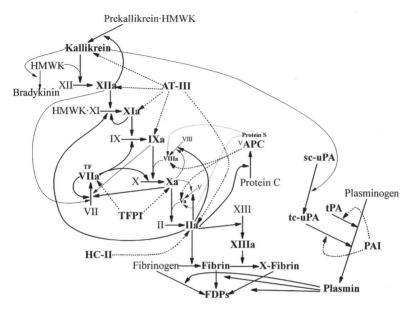

FIGURE 1.   The coagulation cascade. (Adapted from Callas D: Ph.D. dissertation. Loyola University Medical Center, May 1996.)

The platelet plug initially arrests the loss of blood. This, however, is not a permanent blockade. The formation of a fibrin-based clot acts to stabilize the initial platelet plug. The coagulation system is a complex network of zymogens, which must be activated to ultimately form the fibrin strands of the blood clot. On activation, most of these coagulation proteins are converted into active serine proteases that are similar to trypsin and chymotrypsin. Traditionally, coagulation has been viewed as having two distinct branches,[76,194] the intrinsic and the extrinsic pathways. Today it has been established that the two pathways are linked before the generation of factor Xa.[234] Figure 1 is a schematic drawing of the coagulation cascade.

INTRINSIC PATHWAY OF COAGULATION

In the intrinsic pathway, factor XII becomes activated in the contact phase of coagulation. This occurs when factor XII, factor XI, prekallikrein, and high-molecular-weight kininogen come together on a negatively charged surface. Although this reaction can take place in the laboratory on a negatively charged surface such as glass or kaolin, the physiologic surface is unknown. It has been proposed that the physiologic surface may be a tissue rich in collagen or sulphatides.[278] By binding to the negatively charged surface, factor XII is converted to its active form through an unknown mechanism. The formation of factor XIIa is amplified by a positive feedback loop. Factor XIIa is capable of converting prekallikrein to kallikrein. Likewise, kallikrein converts factor XII to its active form. Factor XIIa also converts factor XI to factor XIa, which in turn activates factor IX. Factor IX and its cofactor (factor VIII), along with calcium ions and phospholipid membranes, form the "tenase" complex, which converts factor X to factor Xa, thereby initiating the common pathway of coagulation. The phospholipid membrane in these complexes serves to lower the Km of the reaction. The phospholipid allows the enzyme to become saturated more easily and localizes the coagulation response to where it is most needed. The cofactor, factor V, increases the catalytic efficiency of the enzyme.[127] Factor Xa joins with its cofactor (factor V), calcium ions, and phospholipid membranes to form the prothrombinase complex. The prothrombinase complex then acts to convert prothrombin into the active enzyme thrombin. Factors V and VIII are activated through proteolytic cleavage by factor Xa or thrombin. They are not, however, active proteases. Factor V is believed to have two rate-enhancing effects on the prothrombinase complex. In the prothrombinase complex, factor Xa and factor V are present in stoichiometric amounts, resulting in an unknown alteration in the active site of factor Xa, which increases its catalytic efficiency.[197] Factor V also binds to prothrombin, thus sequestering it at the site of assembly of the prothrombinase complex. Overall, these two actions of factor V result in a 300,000-fold increase in the rate of prothrombin conversion.

Thrombin serves many functions in coagulation. First, thrombin cleaves the soluble protein fibrinogen to generate the insoluble fibrin monomer. Fibrinogen circulates as a disulfide-linked dimer containing two A-α chains, two B-β chains, and two gamma chains. Cleavage of fibrinogen by thrombin results in the release of fibrinopeptides A and B and the exposure of charged domains at opposite ends of the molecule. Exposure of these charged domains leads to polymerization of the monomers. The release of fibrinopeptides A and B occurs at different rates, with fibrinopeptide A preferentially removed in mammalian systems.[30,282] Removal of fibrinopeptide A leads to end-to-end fibrin polymerization, whereas loss of fibrinopeptide B allows side-to-side polymerization of the end-to-end linked monomers.[178] These monomers are cross-linked by the transaminase factor XIIIa to form the meshwork of the thrombus. Thrombin also acts to augment its own generation by being a part of several positive feedback loops in the coagulation cascade. In these loops, thrombin activates factors XII, XI, VIII, and V. By activating the precursors to its own generation, thrombin greatly amplifies its own generation. Thrombin also activates platelets[67] and the inhibitor protein C through binding with thrombomodulin[96] and stimulates activated endothelial cells to release tissue plasminogen activator.[231]

EXTRINSIC PATHWAY OF COAGULATION

The extrinsic pathway of coagulation is activated when circulating factor VII encounters tissue factor. Tissue factor is a transmembrane glycoprotein normally expressed by subendothelial fibroblast-like cells that surround the blood vessel. An intact endothelium normally shields the circulating blood from exposure to tissue factor. The tissue factor molecule consists of a 219-amino acid hydrophilic extracellular domain, a 23-amino acid hydrophobic region that spans the membrane, and a 21-amino acid cytoplasmic tail that anchors the molecule to the cell membrane.[9, 206] Other sites of tissue factor expression include activated monocytes, activated endothelial cells, and atherosclerotic plaques.

Factor VII exhibits a weak procoagulant activity on its own, typically accounting for about 1-2% of the total factor VII/VIIa activity.[208] On binding to tissue factor, a 10,000,000-fold increase in factor VIIa enzymatic activity is observed.[87] Both factor VII and factor VIIa bind to tissue factor with equal affinity.[216] How factor VII is initially activated is not known, although it is hypothesized that factor Xa can activate factor VII in a back activation reaction. The factor VIIa–tissue factor complex can then activate factor X, leading to the generation of thrombin and ultimately to the formation of fibrin strands.

It was shown in 1977 and more recently appreciated that the tissue factor–factor VIIa complex also activates factor IX to factor IXa, thus interacting with an intrinsic pathway enzyme.[234] This is believed to be important for maintaining the clotting process. Direct activation of factor X by factor VIIa–tissue factor can rapidly initiate coagulation, but both of these enzymes are quickly inhibited by the endogenous inhibitor tissue factor pathway inhibitor. By activating factor IX, the tissue factor–VIIa complex initiates two pathways for thrombin generation. The small amounts of factor Xa generated prior to TFPI inhibition are sufficient to cleave prothrombin and to generate a small amount of thrombin. This thrombin is capable of back-activating factors V, VIII, and possibly XI, thereby sustaining clot formation through generation of thrombin via the intrinsic pathway. It has been observed that the activation of factor X by the factor IXa–VIII complex in the presence of calcium and phospholipids is 50 times greater than by the tissue factor–VIIa complex.[198] Factor XI activation occurs in the presence of thrombin and a polyanion cofactor.[109,213] Activation with the cofactor has been observed to be poor. A physiologic cofactor has not been elucidated. It has been reasoned that if the direct activation of factor X by VIIa–tissue factor is the sole source of thrombin generation, there would be no manifestation of hemophilia, a genetic deficiency of either factor IX or factor VIII.

ROLE OF PLATELETS

Platelets are disc-shaped, anuclear cells that circulate in a nonadhesive state in the undamaged circulation.[238] These cells contain a contractile system and a number of storage granules. The α storage granules contain platelet factor 4 (PF4), β-thromboglobulin, platelet-derived growth factor (PDGF), fibrinogen, factor V, and von Willebrand factor.[164] The dense or β-granules contain ATP, ADP, and serotonin.[122,134]

The first step toward platelet aggregation is platelet adhesion. Normally, platelets do not adhere to the vessel walls because of the nonthrombogenic properties of the endothelium. Endothelial cells produce heparan sulfate (to activate antithrombin III), thrombomodulin (for activation of protein C), plasminogen activators (to induce fibrin degradation), and TFPI (to inhibit tissue factor activity). In addition, endothelial cells also produce prostacyclin (PGI$_2$), which inhibits platelet activation by raising platelet levels of cyclic adenosine monophosphate (cAMP) and endothelial-derived relaxing factor (EDRF, NO), which inhibits platelet activation through a mechanism dependent on cyclic guanosine monophosphate (cGMP). When this antithrombotic continuum of cells is interrupted by vascular injury, platelets adhere to the exposed subendothelial tissues.

Following adhesion, platelets become activated. In this activation process, there is a morphologic shape change in the platelet, and pseudopod formation is observed. This brings about a change in the conformation of the glycoprotein IIb/IIIa receptor on the platelet surface; this change allows fibrinogen binding.[238] Fibrinogen binding serves as a bridge that links individual platelets into larger aggregates. An increase in cytosolic calcium levels leads to activation of internal platelet enzymes with the subsequent release of platelet granule contents. The formation of these platelet aggregates is the process of primary hemostasis, the first step to arrest blood loss.

The release of platelet granule contents leads to further platelet activation and aggregation and activation of coagulation. Most of the known aggregating agents cause release of the platelet storage granule contents. These agonists include thrombin, ADP, collagen, thromboxane A$_2$ (TXA$_2$), platelet-activating factor, serotonin, epinephrine, immune complexes, and fibrinogen.[238] Thrombin is the most potent aggregating agent, capable of causing platelet aggregation with no contribution from TXA$_2$ or ADP.[238] Serotonin and epinephrine do not induce aggregation on their own but synergistically promote aggregation induced by other agents.[63, 142, 289]

Platelet membranes contain a variety of receptors for the various agonists, including the thrombin receptor, TXA$_2$ receptor, 5-HT$_2$ receptors, and α_2-adrenergic receptors. In addition, a number of glycoproteins (GPs) on the membrane serve as receptors for collagen (GP Ia/IIa), fibrinogen (GP IIb/IIIa), von Willebrand factor (GP Ib), and fibronectin (GP IIb/IIIa).[63,142,289] A high-molecular-weight chondroitin sulfate proteoglycan is released from the surface of the platelet during the aggregation process. This proteoglycan contains homopolymers of 4-O chondroitin sulfate that inhibit ADP-induced aggregation of platelets.

Activated platelets also provide a procoagulant surface on which several reactions of the coagulation cascade take place. Unstimulated platelets provide only a minimally effective surface on which the "tenase" and prothrombinase complexes can assemble,[102,339,349] primarily because of the bilayer partitioning of various phospholipids. In unstimulated platelets, the outer leaflet of the membrane consists of mostly phosphatidylcholine, whereas the inner leaf contains most of the phosphatidylserine. Two mechanisms have been proposed for maintaining this distribution.[271,305] When platelets are stimulated to release their granular contents, the procoagulant phospholipids are brought to the surface as the granules fuse to the membranes.[349] This expression of phosphatidylserine on the outer leaflet, along with factor V release from the α-granule, greatly accelerates the formation of thrombin.[154,207,313]

Platelet activation leads to the formation of microparticles derived from the platelet surface. These microvesicles typically account for 25–30 % of platelet procoagulant activity and factor V binding sites.[271,290]

ROLE OF PLATELET INTEGRINS

A number of the glycoproteins on the surface of the platelet belong to the superfamily of adhesive protein receptors known as integrins. Integrins are α/β heterodimer protein complexes that are present on the surface of adherent cells of most species.[33,82,199] These integrins mediate cell–cell and cell–matrix interactions involved in diverse biologic functions.[152,301] Integrins are divided into subfamilies based on the identity of the β-subunit. The first two subfamilies of integrins, the VLA complexes and the Leu-Cams, are found on white cells and mediate various leukocyte aggregation responses.[6,128] Platelets contain two members of the third subfamily of integrins, glycoprotein IIb/IIIa or P-selectin and the vitronectin receptor.[40,59,174,347]

Integrins function by interacting with a number of extracellular glycoprotein ligands such as fibronectin, laminin, collagen, vitronectin, fibrinogen, and von Willebrand's factor.[18] Integrins are capable of binding several ligands; the nature of the ligand specificity is not known.

Platelet membranes contain five integrin-like receptors that are involved in the formation of the primary hemostatic plug: VLA-2, VLA-5, VLA-6, glycoprotein IIb/IIIa, and the vitronectin receptor. Of these, GP IIb/IIIa is the most abundant.[246] VLA-2 (GPIa/IIa) is the binding site for collagen on the platelet surface.[297] VLA-5 and VLA-6 are responsible for the binding to vitronectin and laminin, respectively.[129,247] The extent to which these receptors contribute to platelet adhesion in vivo is not known. The physiologic function of the vitronectin receptor is not known.

Platelet aggregation requires activation of platelets by at least one platelet agonist, the presence of functional GPIIb/IIIa molecules, and the presence of at least one GPIIb/IIIa ligand.[283] Lack of GPIIb/IIIa complexes leads to the congenital bleeding disorder known as Glanzmann's thrombasthenia.[17] In nonactivated platelets, GPIIb/IIIa is capable of binding only immobilized fibrinogen. Platelet activation allows plasma-borne adhesive proteins to bind to GPIIb/IIIa complexes.[155] The activation of the IIb/IIIa complex occurs by an unknown mechanism; the number of receptors on the membrane is not altered by activation.[246] Fibrin polymers bind to the activated GPIIb/IIIa complexes and anchor the platelet plug in place.

Recent studies have shown that the binding of ligands to GPIIb/IIIa also activates a number of cellular processes important for platelet stimulation,[246] including the synthesis of 3-phosphorylated phosphatidylinositols, release of arachidonic acid, and increase in plasma calcium levels. Stimulation of these processes allows bidirectional signalling between the intracellular and extracellular compartments.

ROLE OF LEUKOCYTES

Leukocytes typically express minimal amounts of procoagulant activity in the unstimulated state.[84] Cytokines such as interleukin-1 (IL-1) and tumor necrosis factor (TNF) can elicit the expression of tissue factor on endothelial and mononuclear cells.[50] Monocyte procoagulant activity is also induced by endotoxin, the complement system, phorbol esters, prostaglandins, and a number of other agonists.[88] Procoagulant activity associated with leukocytes is not limited to the expression of tissue factor. Several monocyte/macrophage derived procoagulant activities have been characterized, including tissue factor,[114,203,273] factor VII,[57,202] and factor XIII.[337] In addition, some monocytes and macrophages have been shown to express functional factor V/Va[268] and to possess binding sites for factor X.[4] The factor Xa-binding site on leukocytes has been shown to be the integrin CD11b/CD18.[4] Not only does this integrin bind factor X, but it also proteolytically activates factor X to Xa, allowing initiation of coagulation on the surface of the monocytes and neutrophils.[5] Monocytes also contain a receptor for the factor IXa/VIII complex; this receptor allows the reactions of the intrinsic pathway of coagulation to take place on the surface of the monocyte.[204]

Prothrombin is efficiently activated on the cell surface of monocytes and lymphocytes.[311,312] As with platelets, the prothrombinase activity on monocytes is increased with activated monocytes compared with nonactivated cells.[264]

According to Altieri, when coagulation takes place on the surface of leukocytes, it "assumes the aspects of a broad inflammatory mechanism, directly influencing cellular motility and adhesion, phagocytosis, cell-cell communication, and normal or deregulated cellular growth."[5] Fibrin formation not only forms the basis for a blood clot but also serves to limit the inflammatory response. In addition, products of the coagulation process, such as thrombin, fibrinopeptides, and fibrin degradation products, have chemotactic and mitogenic properties.[240,281,284]

Studies have indicated that leukocytes play a critical role in the activation of coagulation in patients with septicemia and in animal models of acute lung injury.[49,229] One study has presented direct evidence of the role of tissue factor expression on activated endothelial cells during in vivo thrombogenesis.[214]

ROLE OF THE ENDOTHELIUM

The endothelium plays a relatively important role in the modulation of overall coagulation, fibrinolysis, and platelet-dependent processes. Endothelial cells react to various physiologic and pathologic states and release various mediators that modulate plasmatic processes. The role of endothelial function in mediating the overall coagulation process may be summarized by the following.

1. Regulation of thrombin function by binding to thrombomodulin
2. Release of fibrinolytic mediators in the regulation of the fibrinolytic system
3. Release of prostaglandin derivatives in the control of platelet function and vascular hemodynamics
4. Release of nitric oxide, TFPI, and other substances to mediate various functions

Under normal conditions, endothelial cells play a regulatory role in balancing the cellular and plasmatic reactions. However, in pathologic states, such as ischemia and occlusive states (thrombotic or restenotic), endothelial function changes markedly, and endothelial cells produce various substances that mediate the pathologic changes. These functions include the following.

1. Release of tissue factor to initiate the clotting process
2. Release of plasminogen activator inhibitor (PAI) to inhibit the fibrinolytic response
3. Generation of procoagulant proteins and von Willebrand's factor to activate thrombogenesis

Obviously the endothelium is a major player in the overall regulation of hemostasis.

ENDOGENOUS INHIBITORS OF COAGULATION

Antithrombin III

Antithrombin III (AT III) is a single-chain glycoprotein with a molecular weight of approximately 58,000 Da.[209] The primary structure of this serine protease inhibitor

(SERPIN) has been determined by protein and cDNA sequencing of clones from several species.[31,55,242,257,285,298] Normal plasma levels of AT III are approximately 2–3 μM.[65]

In the beginning of the twentieth century, it was suspected that a natural inhibitor of thrombin was present in the plasma.[143] The first hints of the existence of AT III were detected shortly after the discovery of heparin, when it was discovered that heparin required a cofactor to exhibit its anticoagulant activity.[45,144] At this point, the molecule was termed heparin cofactor.[45] It was not until the late 1960s that Abildgaard demonstrated that the proteins antithrombin and heparin cofactor were identical.[1]

AT III is a member of the SERPIN superfamily of proteins, which includes the inhibitors α_2-antiplasmin, α_1-antichymotrypsin, and α_1-proteinase inhibitor.[249] AT III is considered to be the primary inhibitor of coagulation[253] and targets most coagulation proteases as well as the enzymes trypsin, plasmin, and kallikrein.[26,316] Inhibition takes place when a stoichiometric complex between the active site serine of the protease and the ARG393-SER294 bond of AT III forms.[74,159,236,266]

The tertiary structure of AT III resembles α_1-antitrypsin in that it is folded into N-terminal domain helices and β-sheets. This tertiary structure is maintained by the formation of three disulfide bonds.[209] Four glycosylation sites exist on human AT III, two of which are suspected to contain carbohydrate chains. The glycosylation of these sites appears to effect heparin binding to the inhibitor.[41,42]

The efficient inhibition of proteases by AT III requires heparin as a cofactor. Without heparin, the inhibition rate constants for thrombin and factor Xa have been estimated at 1×10^3 and 3×10^3 L/mol sec^{-1}, respectively. In the presence of heparin, these rates of inhibition are accelerated to 3×10^7 and 4×10^6 L/mol sec^{-1}, respectively, for thrombin and factor Xa.[158] The binding site for heparin is located on the N-terminal domain of the molecule.

Two mechanisms have been proposed to account for heparin's ability to catalyze the antiprotease actions of AT III. The first model suggests that heparin binds to AT III and causes a conformational change at the active site.[266] The ternary complex or template model proposes that heparin acts catalytically by binding both AT III and the serine protease, thereby bringing them in close proximity.[26] Both models may be operative, depending on the serine protease that is inhibited. Conformational changes of AT III on heparin binding have been observed spectroscopically.[266,287,328] Furthermore, the ability of a pentasaccharide region of heparin to promote the AT III-mediated inhibition of factor Xa supports this model. The inhibition of thrombin appears to be better explained by the template model. Conformational changes induced by heparin binding do not alter the reactivity of AT III toward thrombin.[244] In addition, heparin pentasaccharides do not promote thrombin inhibition. Rather, chains of more than 18 saccharide units are needed for this inhibition. Kinetic studies indicate that heparin must bind both thrombin and AT III.[145,219] It is not clear if one binding must precede the other for optimal inhibition to occur.[115,251]

Deficiency of AT III predisposes the patient to thrombotic complications. AT III deficiencies can result from low protein levels or functionally abnormal molecules. Low protein levels can be brought about by reduced synthesis or increased turnover of the molecule. Functional deficiencies can be brought about by mutations in either the reactive site or heparin-binding sites. A number of such mutations have been documented.[32,35,56,94,169,177,235,300]

Heparin Cofactor II

Heparin cofactor II is a second plasma SERPIN that, like AT III, can be activated by glycosaminoglycan binding. This protein has also been called antithrombin BM,[342] dermatan sulfate cofactor,[2] and human leuserpin 2.[258] The existence of this second inhibitor and heparin cofactor was first shown by Briginshaw in 1974.[43,44] Whereas AT III has progressive antithrombin activity and also inhibits factor Xa, the second cofactor exhibits only weak progressive activity and does not inhibit factor Xa. Tollefsen observed two different thrombin inhibitor complexes, one of which could not be identified with antisera to known protease inhibitors.[306] Several clinical studies observed a discrepancy between levels of heparin cofactor activity and plasma AT III antigen.[107,116] The existence of the inhibitor was confirmed when the protein was isolated from human plasma[307] and from Cohn fraction IV.[342] The heparin cofactor II protein has a molecular weight of 62,000–72,000 Da, depending on the method used.[307,315]

Like AT III, heparin cofactor II inhibits proteases by forming a 1:1 stoichiometric complex with the enzyme. The protease attacks the reactive site of heparin cofactor II located on the C-terminus, resulting in the formation of a covalent bond. Heparin cofactor II has a higher protease specificity than AT III. Of the coagulation enzymes, heparin cofactor II is known to inhibit only thrombin.[316] In addition, heparin cofactor II has been shown to inhibit chymotrypsin[61] and leukocyte cathepsin G.[239] This protease specificity appears to be due to the active site bond in heparin cofactor II. Whereas AT III contains an Arg-Ser bond as its active site, heparin cofactor II is unique in containing a Leu-Ser bond. This suggests that another portion of the heparin cofactor II molecule may be required for protease binding.

As in the case of AT III, the inhibition of protease activity by heparin cofactor II is promoted by glycosaminoglycan binding. Whereas the activation of AT III depends on the presence of a specific sequence in the heparin chain, heparin cofactor II can be activated by a wide variety of agents. Heparins, heparans, and dermatan sulfate promote thrombin inhibition via heparin cofactor II. Agents with relatively little sulfation, such as chondroitin 4-O- or 6-O-sulfate, keratan sulfate, and hyaluronic acid, do not activate heparin cofactor II. Heparan sulfate containing 0.97 sulfates per disaccharide has been shown to be a better activator of heparin cofactor II than heparan sulfate containing 0.67 sulfates per disaccharide.[310] In addition, sulfated synthetic agents can activate heparin cofactor II. Both pentosan polysulfate[275,276] and dextran sulfate[343] have been shown to activate heparin cofactor II.

Both dermatan sulfate and heparin have been fractionated to study their heparin cofactor II-binding characteristics. In studies performed by Tollefsen et al., dermatan sulfate octasaccharides with higher negative charge were shown to bind to heparin cofactor II better than those with a lower charge.[309] Although these octasaccharides bind to heparin cofactor II, dermatan sulfate chains of 12–14 saccharides are required to promote thrombin inhibition. This finding is consistent with the template model of inhibition. Heparin has been fractionated by charge density and subsequently on an AT III-Sepharose column into high- and low-affinity fractions.[150] It has been observed that for a given charge density, AT III affinity is unrelated to the ability of the fraction to activate heparin cofactor II. High- and low-affinity fractions equally activated heparin cofactor II when charge density was constant. To date, definitive data supporting the existence of a minimally required sequence to activate heparin cofactor II have not been reported.

In the absence of glycosaminoglycan, thrombin variants recognize AT III and heparin cofactor II to a similar degree, indicating that neither the autolysis loop nor the β-loop of thrombin is required for SERPIN/protease interaction. Addition of heparin does not alter the interaction of AT III with the thrombin variants, suggesting the importance of the anion-binding exosite II for the heparin bridge between thrombin and AT III. The same studies indicate the importance of anion-binding exosite I for the inhibition of thrombin by heparin cofactor II; gamma thrombin, which lacks this site, is not inhibited. Based on these results, a complex double-bridge mechanism for heparin cofactor II-mediated thrombin inhibition has been postulated. Heparin or dermatan sulfate binds to the glycosaminoglycan-binding site on heparin cofactor II and anion-binding site I on thrombin. When heparin binds to heparin cofactor II, the acidic domain is displaced and is free to interact with the β-loop region of the anion-binding exosite of thrombin, facilitating its rapid inhibition.

The normal plasma level of heparin cofactor II is approximately 1.2 ± 0.2 μM.[308] Two patients to date have been described as having heparin cofactor II deficiency related to thrombosis.[288,314]

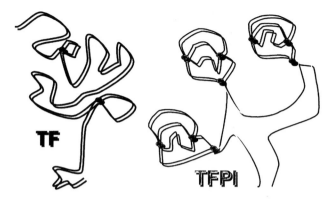

FIGURE 2.   Structure of tissue factor (TF) and tissue factor pathway inhibitor (TFPI).

Tissue Factor Pathway Inhibitor

Tissue factor pathway inhibitor (TFPI) is one of the coagulation protease inhibitors found endogenously within the vasculature. TFPI has also been known as lipoprotein-associated coagulation inhibitor (LACI) and extrinsic pathway inhibitor (EPI). This 42-kDa inhibitor has been shown to contain three Kunitz domains tandemly linked between a negatively charged amino terminus and a positively charged carboxy terminus.[110] The active site of the first Kunitz domain binds to the active site of the factor VIIa–tissue factor complex, whereas the active site of the second Kunitz domain binds to the active site of factor Xa. Mutation of the active site of the third Kunitz domain has no effect on the inhibition of either factor VIIa or factor Xa. Figure 2 presents a diagramatic version of tissue factor and TFPI. Both of these proteins are produced by recombinant methods and can be used for the study of thrombosis in simulated conditions. Modification of the second Kunitz domain has been shown to result in a loss of inhibition of tissue factor-VIIa activity. In experiments in which the third Kunitz domain is truncated, TFPI still inhibits factor VIIa–tissue factor complexes on cell surfaces in culture.[119] The carboxy terminus of TFPI is required for the optimal inhibition of factor Xa,[223,338] perhaps affecting the rate at which TFPI can bind to factor Xa. No difference is observed between the inhibition of factor VIIa–tissue factor complex by full-length TFPI or by a truncated form of TFPI.[338] Two studies have examined the kinetics of TFPI inhibition of factor Xa.[146,192] Both studies indicate that more than just the second Kunitz domain is required for factor Xa binding, because the association rate constants are higher for full-length TFPI than for carboxy-terminus or Kunitz 3-truncated TFPI. The third Kunitz domain has recently been shown to contain a second heparin-binding site.[93]

TFPI has been cloned from a number of species, including humans, rabbits, rats, and monkeys.[92,162,296,333,340] Monkey TFPI was observed to be similar in structure and function to human TFPI. Rabbit TFPI was shown to have a weaker antiprotease activity than human TFPI and not to associate with lipoproteins.[333]

In normal tissues of the vasculature, TFPI is produced by megakaryocytes and the endothelium. Once produced, TFPI is stored in three intravascular pools, which are located in the plasma, in platelets, and bound to the endothelium.[187] The smallest pool of TFPI is found in the platelets, accounting for less than 2.5% of the intravascular total. This small pool of TFPI is released on platelet activation.[225] The plasma contains 10–50% of intravascular TFPI. Most plasma-based TFPI is bound to plasma lipoproteins.[47,227] Approximately 5% of the plasma pool of TFPI circulates in the free form.[184,226] The lipoprotein-bound TFPI is reported to be of relatively low inhibitory activity.[183] The largest pool of TFPI is bound to the endothelial surface.[185,227,272] This pool accounts for 50–90% of total intravascular TFPI.

The TFPI pool bound to the endothelium has been shown to be heparin-releasable in a number of studies.[7,12,135,227,334] Venous occlusion[272] and agents such as 1-deamino-8-D-arginine vasopressin (DDAVP) that induce exocytosis of endothelial granular proteins[336] do not cause the release of TFPI. Repeated heparin administration is observed to release similar amounts of TFPI[7] with no tachyphylaxis. It is believed that the endothelial pool of TFPI is bound to glycosaminoglycans on the surface of the endothelium. Heparin injection is thought to displace TFPI from the endogenous glycosaminoglycans. The amount of TFPI in the plasma after heparin administration is determined by the heparin concentration. TFPI levels as high as 2–10 times baseline values have been reported after administration of heparin and low-molecular-weight heparin (LMWH). The chemical nature of the low-molecular-weight heparin also affects the degree of TFPI release. When different LMWHs are administered at the same anti-Xa unit dosage, plasma TFPI levels vary by as much as 30%.[329] Neutralization of heparin by protamine sulfate or protamine chloride results in a dramatic decrease in plasma TFPI levels.[121,141]

TFPI acts in vitro as an anticoagulant when measured by a number of assays. Both thromboplastin-induced clotting time and activated partial thromboplastin time (APTT) are prolonged by TFPI.[184,185] Factor Xa-based assays, such as the Heptest and the amidolytic anti-Xa assay, are also affected by recombinant TFPI.[170] Higher amounts of TFPI are required in the prothrombin time and APTT for prolongation of the clotting time than are needed in the Heptest. The prothrombin time (PT) is a more sensitive assay for the anticoagulant effects of TFPI than is the APTT, suggesting that the main in vitro inhibitory effect of TFPI is the inhibition of factor VIIa.[186] Cosupplementation of heparin and recombinant TFPI (rTFPI) to plasma in vitro has differing effects, depending on the assay used. Kristensen observed that heparin and rTFPI additively prolong the Heptest clotting time. Prolongation of the APTT and PT assays by heparin and TFPI is synergistic.[321,341] A study by Nordfang et al., however, suggests that the increased effect of TFPI in the presence of heparin is due to heparin–AT III complexes, because addition of heparin exhibited no effect in AT III-deficient plasma.[224] The rate of Xa inhibition by rTFPI was observed to increase 2.5-fold upon the addition of heparin,[48] although not with full-length TFPI.[338]

When administered to rabbits, TFPI had an antithrombotic effect when thromboplastin was used as a thrombogenic challenge.[78] TFPI was also shown to be an effective inhibitor when thrombosis was induced in rabbit jugular veins by endothelial destruction and restricted blood flow.[136] The antithrombotic and antiprotease actions of TFPI have been tested in several other animal models. Warn-Cramer et al. investigated the effect of immunodepletion of TFPI in factor VIIa- and factor Xa-induced coagulation in rabbits.[335] The rabbits were observed to be sensitized to the procoagulant effects of factor VIIa, but not factor Xa in the absence of factor VIIa. Two studies indicate that TFPI administration reduces the lethal effects of administration of *Escherichia coli* in a baboon model of septic shock.[51,68] These studies also indicate that TFPI may have an anti-inflammatory effect, because attenuation of the IL-6 response was also observed. Administration of TFPI has been observed to prevent reocclusion of arteries in dogs after clot lysis with tissue plasminogen activator.[122] Topical administration of TFPI has been shown to prevent thrombosis in a rabbit model of vascular trauma.[165]

Protein C

The protein C pathway is one of the natural anticoagulant systems that keeps blood in the fluid state. When thrombin is formed, it stimulates coagulation and its own formation by activating factors V and VIII through proteolytic cleavage.[156,163] Factors VIIIa and Va bind to negatively charged phospholipids on activated platelets and act as binding sites for factors IXa and Xa, respectively, allowing formation of the "tenase" and prothrombinase complexes.[198]

Thrombin can also act to limit its own procoagulant activity. When thrombin is in circulation, it binds a high-affinity receptor on the endothelium known as thrombomodulin.[97] The k_d for this binding is $0.2–0.5 \times 10^{-9}$ M.[237] Thrombomodulin is a membrane-spanning protein with multiple functional domains and a molecular weight of approximately 60,000 Da.[73] When thrombin binds to thrombomodulin, a change in substrate specificity is noted. Although this complex is a potent activator of protein C, the bound thrombin no longer cleaves fibrinogen, is not able to activate other coagulation proteases such as factors V and VIII, and does not activate platelets.[98,99] The thrombin–thrombomodulin complex is a 20,000-fold better activator of protein C than is free thrombin.[97,237] Thrombomodulin is present on the endothelium in most arteries, veins, and capillaries.[79,200]

Protein C is a vitamin K-dependent zymogen identified by Stenflo.[299] It is identical to autoprothrombin IIa.[280] On activation, protein C exhibits anticoagulant properties.[166,167] Alterations of the substrate specificity of thrombin on binding to thrombomodulin are thought to be due both to steric hindrance of thrombin's active site and to conformational changes in the active site.[138,211,344] Protein C is made up of disulfide-linked heavy and light chains and has a molecular weight of approximately 62,000 Da.[15,106] Protein C derives its anticoagulant properties from its ability to cleave and inactivate membrane-bound forms of factors Va and VIIIa.[100,101,332] Factors V and VIII and non–membrane-bound forms of factors Va and VIIIa are not cleaved by protein C.

Protein C requires two cofactors to express its anticoagulant activity—protein S and factor V. Protein S is another vitamin K-dependent plasma protein. Its free form expresses protein C cofactor activity for the degradation of factors Va and VIIIa.[71] Protein S is a single-chain, 70,000-Da glycoprotein[73] and has the highest affinity for negatively charged phospholipids among vitamin K-dependent proteins.[215] Protein S forms a 1:1 complex with protein C on the lipid membrane, which may account for its ability to increase the affinity of activated protein C for such membranes.[331,332] Although the mechanism of action of protein S is not completely understood, it may be related to its ability to make factors Va and VIIIa available for proteolytic cleavage by activated protein C.[261,295] Less is known about the role of factor V as an activated protein C cofactor, although it is hypothesized that factor V and protein S may act synergistically to localize protein C activity to the surface of membranes.[72,286]

Because low levels of protein C activation peptide are found in healthy individuals, it is suggested that protein C is constantly activated to a small degree.[14] Protein C administration has been shown to inhibit arterial or venous thrombosis in animal models.[8,117,330] Heterozygous protein C deficiency or activated protein C resistance due to factor V mutation are thought to explain 60–70 % of the cases of familial thrombophilia.[73]

Protease Nexins

Protease nexins 1 and 2 are endogenous serine protease inhibitors that have molecular weights of 43 kDa and approximately 100 kDa, respectively.[255,322] Both protease nexin 1 and protease nexin 2 have effects on the coagulation system. Based on cell culture studies, protease nexin 1 appears to be produced by fibroblasts, smooth muscle cells, and epithelial cells.[10,85,168] Protease nexin 1 has a 30% sequence homology with AT III and, like ATIII, has a high-affinity heparin-binding site. Heparin binding to protease nexin 1 accelerates protease inhibition.[11,171] Protease nexin 1 appears to be limited to the extravascular compartment, because human plasma contains only small amounts (20 pM).[255] Protease nexin 1 inhibits several serine proteases, including thrombin, urokinase, plasminogen activator, and activated protein C.[19,130,274] After formation of a stable complex with the target protease, the complex binds back to the cells, where it is internalized and degraded.[70] The physiologic role of protease nexin 1 appears to be related to protection of the extracellular matrix from degradation by urokinase and plasminogen activator.[260] This theory is supported by the fact that protease nexin 1 binds tightly to the extracellular matrix, thereby localizing its activity.[103]

Protease nexin 2 is identical to the secreted form of the amyloid precursor protein containing the Kunitz-type serine protease inhibitor domain.[233,322] Protease nexin 2 circulates in blood stored as a platelet α-granule protein that is secreted on platelet activation.[323] Protease nexin 2 inhibits trypsin- and chymotrypsin-like serine proteases and is also a potent inhibitor of factor XIa.[291,292,323,325,326] Its location in platelets and its ability to inhibit factor XIa suggest a role in regulating blood coagulation.

Other Inhibitors

A number of other serine protease inhibitors are known to play a role in modulating physiologic functions. Plasminogen activator inhibitors (PAIs) serve to limit the normal activation of the fibrinolytic process. High levels of PAI-1 are associated with an increased risk of thromboembolic disease.[262] PAI-1 also has been shown to regulate the degradation of extracellular matrix, which may be important in modulating cancer invasion. Alpha$_2$-antiplasmin rapidly inhibits the fibrinolytic activity of plasmin.[86] Alpha$_2$-macroglobulin has been described as a "panproteinase inhibitor" in light of evidence that it interacts with nearly any proteinase.[36] In addition, α_2-macroglobulin may play a role in inflammation and immune reactions through its ability to regulate the distribution and activity of numerous cytokines, including transforming growth factor ß, tumor necrosis factor α, platelet-derived growth factor, and several interleukins.[34,37,58,60,175] The complement and contact systems are regulated by c$_1$-esterase inhibitor through the inhibition of complement components C1r and C1s.[118,345] Deficiency of C1-esterase inhibitor is associated with angioedema.[52] Histidine-rich glycoprotein has been shown to bind to plasminogen and to interfere with its interaction with fibrin.[181,210] In addition, histidine-rich glycoprotein is known to bind to heparin and related glycosaminoglycans.[182] High levels of this protein have not been definitively linked to thrombosis.[91]

HEPARIN

Discovery

Heparin was discovered in 1916 by Jay McLean while he was studying the procoagulant actions of phospholipids.[205] Heparin was initially thought to be a phospholipid because it was isolated by using procedures designed to separate phospholipids. We now know that heparin is a glycosaminoglycan structurally related to the dermatans and chondroitins. More specifically, heparin has been defined as "a family of polysaccharide species, whose chains are made up of alternating, 1-4 linked and variously sulfated residues of uronic acid and D-glucosamine."[53] The uronic acid residues are either L-iduronic acid or D-glucuronic acid. The glucosamine residues are either N-sulfated or N-acetylated. Typically, the iduronic acid moieties are 2-O sulfated, whereas the glucosamine residues contain 6-O sulfate groups and a small proportion are 3-O sulfated. Molecular weight, oligosaccharide sequences, and charge density play crucial roles in the overall anticoagulant effect of heparin.

Chemistry

Heparin is synthesized by a number of tissues and mast cells as part of a high-molecular-weight proteoglycan (molecular weight = 750–1000 kDa). This proteoglycan consists of a peptide core composed of 20–25 residues each of glycine and serine.[263] Attached to the peptide are 15 polysaccharide chains with molecular weights ranging from 60–100 kDa. The polysaccharide chains are attached to the peptide core via a galactosyl-galactosyl-xylosyl trisaccharide sequence.[188]

The polysaccharide chains are formed by stepwise transfer of D-glucuronic acid and N-acetyl-D-glucosamine from UDP sugar nucleotide forms to the nonreducing end of the polysaccharide chain.[105,125,126] Presumably the sugar moieties are polymerized directly to the linkage region of the protein core. The alternating sequence of glucuronic acid and hexosamine is due to the substrate specificity of the glycosyl transferases.[191] After elongation of the polysaccharide chain, the polymer undergoes a series of modification reactions.

Heparin is structurally heterogeneous because of incomplete structural modifications. Four enzymatic modifications of the polysaccharide backbone occur after its synthesis. The majority of the N-acetyl groups on the glucosamine residues are removed.[139] The N-deacetylated glucosamines are subsequently sulfated. In the next step, D-glucuronic acid residues are epimerized to L-iduronic acid units by uronosyl C-5 epimerase.[189,196] During the epimerization process, most iduronic acids are 2-O sulfated. Finally, 3-O and 6-O sulfate groups are added onto the glucosamine units. Previous N-sulfation allows more efficient O-sulfation.[191] Several recent studies indicate that chain elongation and modification may occur simultaneously during heparin synthesis.

Nuclear resonance spectroscopy involves the measurement of radiofrequency radiation absorption by a given sample when it is placed in a strong magnetic field. The nuclei of many atoms act as magnetic dipoles in that they can be aligned either with or against the magnetic field. These nuclei include ^1H, ^{13}C, ^{19}F, and ^{31}P. ^1H and ^{13}C are the most commonly studied nuclei because of their abundance in organic materials. The ground state of a nuclei is the energy level when the dipole is aligned along the magnetic field. The excited state occurs when the nuclei are aligned against the magnetic field. Transfer of nuclei from the ground to the excited state occurs when nuclei absorb radiofrequency radiation. The amount of power that is absorbed depends not only on the molecular properties of the given sample but also on the surrounding magnetic field. The surrounding magnetic field includes the field produced by the instrument as well as any field produced by adjacent nuclei. Adjacent nuclei can either shield (decrease) or deshield (increase) the magnetic field produced by the instrument. Resonance frequencies of nuclei vary, depending on the chemical environment of the nuclei. This concept is expressed in terms of a chemical shift (δ). Chemical shift is usually given in ppm and is independent of the applied magnetic field. Because there is no way of measuring the strength of the magnetic field at a given nucleus without shielding, chemical shifts are determined relative to an internal standard. The chemical shifts of nuclei depend on the nearby chemical structures. Structural characteristics of a molecule can be elucidated with this technique because the various protons (^1H) and ^{13}C nuclei are present in different environments with respect to the local charge density and, therefore, are excited to different extents by the introduction of the radiofrequency pulse.

Monodimemsional spectroscopy of polysaccharides such as heparin is often of limited value because of the intrinsically broad signals and the large number of overlapping signals. Bidimensional spectroscopy is a more useful technique because it allows the correlation of two similar (^1H–^1H) or different (^1H–^{13}C) nuclei so that the signals relating to intramolecular interactions can be identified. These correlations are termed homonuclear and heteronuclear.

Biologic Effects—Nonanticoagulant

Heparin is a strongly anionic polyelectrolyte that at physiologic pHs contains three acidic functional groups that are fully dissociated: $-OSO_3^-$, $-NHSO_3^-$, and $-COO^{-221}$. As a result, heparin has a large number of pharmacologic properties, among which are its antilipemic and antihemolytic actions.[38,179] Heparin is also known to inhibit various enzymes, including myosin ATPase, RNA-dependent DNA polymerase, elastase, and renin.[69,220,279] Heparin also inhibits tumor growth.[104,193] In addition, heparin exhibits antibacterial and antiviral properties.[66,320]

Pharmacokinetics

Heparin is administered either by intravenous infusion or by subcutaneous injection. On entering the blood stream, heparin binds to various plasma proteins, thereby lowering its bioavailability and producing a variable anticoagulant response.[132] These proteins include histidine-rich glycoprotein, platelet factor IV, vitronectin, and von Willebrand factor.[77,137,176,182,243,255,293] Heparin exhibits complex pharmacokinetics and is cleared by two mechanisms. The rapid, saturable phase of elimination is thought to be due to receptor-mediated internalization of heparin by endothelial cells and macrophages.[108,111,195] A slower, nonsaturable renal mechanism also clears heparin from the plasma.[27,83,232] The anticoagulant effect of heparin is therefore not linearly related to dose in the therapeutic range.[133] The biologic half-life of heparin increases from 30 minutes after an intravenous bolus dose of 25 U/kg to 150 minutes after a dose of 400 U/kg.[27,83,232]

Clinical Use

Heparin is used in the therapy of several cardiovascular disorders, including prevention and treatment of venous thromboembolism, treatment of unstable angina and acute myocardial infarction, cardiac and vascular surgery, coronary angioplasty, stent implantation, and as an adjunctive agent during thrombolysis. Heparin is the anticoagulant of choice in pregnancy because it does not cross the placental barrier and is not known to cause unwanted effects on the fetus.[133,151]

Studies have demonstrated a reduction in mortality in patients receiving heparin for the treatment of pulmonary embolism.[13,29] In addition, recurrent thrombosis was not common during the heparinization period but increased significantly when heparin was stopped and no other anticoagulant therapy was used.[147,173] The effectiveness of heparin in treating venous thrombosis depends on the anticoagulant effect achieved.[148,318] Heparin is also effective prophylactically, reducing the risk of venous thrombosis and pulmonary embolism by 60–70%.[62,64] Heparin is effective for short-term prevention of acute myocardial infarction and recurrent refractory angina in patients with unstable angina.[218,302,303] This beneficial effect is lost after cessation of heparin therapy. In patients with previous myocardial infarction, heparin administration has been shown to reduce significantly both reinfarction and death compared with untreated controls.[217] Heparin has been tested as an adjunct in thrombolytic therapy and appears to increase patency during the initial stages of recanalization by preventing rethrombosis.[29,80]

Effect on Platelets

The effect of heparin on platelets is controversial. Studies by Ellison and Thomson have shown that heparin decreases the threshold for ADP- and epinephrine-induced aggregation and enhances platelet release reactions by both agonists.[90,304] Treatment with heparin was also observed to increase platelet retention on cellophane membranes. Other studies have indicated the opposite effects on platelets. Besterman showed that irreversible aggregation induced by collagen and epinephrine was reduced in patients treated with 2500–5000 U of unfractionated heparin.[22] In the same patients, no effect to a slight increase in aggregation was observed with ADP.[348] Heiden demonstrated a loss of [^{14}C]-5-HT release in platelet-rich plasma of patients treated with 100 U/kg heparin in response to collagen, epinephrine, and ADP.[123] An indirect mechanism was suggested to account for this observation because of the finding that in vitro addition of heparin caused no effect on aggregation.[89] Salzman et al. have shown that concentrations of heparin as low as 10 μg/ml induce aggregation in platelet-rich plasma but not in washed platelets.[270]

Heparin administration is also known to cause an adverse effect on platelets known as heparin-induced thrombocytopenia (HIT). Type I HIT occurs early in heparin treatment and causes a transient reduction in platelet count. Patients usually remain asymptomatic. Type II HIT is a more severe thrombocytopenia of delayed onset and often results in thrombosis; it is associated with a high rate of mortality. Although the exact mechanism is unknown, it appears that an IgG antibody is generated and that its F-ab portion binds to the heparin–platelet factor 4 complex. Optimal platelet activation occurs when heparin and platelet factor 4 are in near equimolar concentrations. The Fc portion of the antibody binds to the FcIIa receptor on the platelet surface and activates the platelets. The differences in response to these heparin–platelet factor 4 antibodies may be due to differences in the genotype of the FcIIa receptor. Studies have indicated that the IgG antibody–heparin–platelet factor 4 complex forms in solution and then binds to the FcIIa receptor on platelets.

Chemically Modified Heparins

Hypersulfated Heparins.   The anticoagulant and antithrombotic actions of heparins containing higher-than-normal degrees of sulfation have been examined in several studies. In a laser model of thrombosis, a supersulfated low-molecular-weight heparin (LMWH) was observed to require a 10-fold lower dose than native heparin or LMWH to achieve a comparable antithrombotic effect.[172] In another study, oversulfation of LMWH was observed to reduce the ex vivo anticoagulant activity relative to LMWH that has not been oversulfated. Addition of sulfate groups, however, did not affect the antithrombotic activity in a rat model of venous stasis-thrombosis and did not significantly increase the bleeding time.[212] The release of lipoprotein lipase by the supersulfated LMWH was twice that of heparin. In a pure biochemical system, the inhibition of thrombin via heparin cofactor II by supersulfated LMWH was approximately 100-fold stronger than for LMWH.[157]

Desulfated Heparins.   N- and O-desulfated heparins have been examined for a number of pharmacologic properties. In general, a reduction in the sulfation of heparin results in a decrease in the given biologic activity. N- and 6-O-desulfation significantly decreased the antiviral activity of heparin with respect to herpes simplex I binding.[131] Heparin potentiates the binding of vascular endothelial growth factor (VEGF 165) to its cellular receptors. O- and N-desulfated heparins potentiated this binding to a lesser extent.[294] Rajtar demonstrated that N- desulfated heparins were less effective at inhibiting platelet function than native heparin.[259] Both fully desulfated heparin and N-desulfated heparin lack the ability to bind heparin-binding growth factor.[16]

The anticoagulant and antithrombotic effects of desulfated heparins have also been examined. A partially N-desulfated heparin has been shown to have no measurable anticoagulant or antiprotease activity but to impair thrombogenesis in vivo in a dose-dependent manner.[269] A completely N-desulfated heparin derivative lacked both in vitro and in vivo activity.[153] Other investigators have shown that N-desulfated heparins have minimal anticoagulant activity.[28,75] N-desulfated heparin has been shown to be cleared approximately 6-fold faster than native heparin.[28] The weak anticoagulant activity is attributable to the lack of interaction with AT III.[75]

Low-Molecular-Weight Heparins.   The depolymerization of heparin either chemically by nitrous acid degradation, benzylation-alkaline hydrolysis, or peroxidative cleavage or enzymatically with heparinase results in the production of another clinically useful drug known as low-molecular-weight heparin. LMWHs exhibit several distinct properties that differentiate them from standard unfractionated heparin. Through the depolymerization process, the molecular weight is reduced to approximately one-third that of the parent material. This is important for two reasons. First, the largest heparin chains are not well absorbed after subcutaneous administration. The bioavailability of heparin is only 20–30%. The bioavailability of LMWH is nearly 100% when measured by an amidolytic anti-Xa assay. The smaller molecular size of the LMWHs also has an effect on the biologic activity of these agents. The LMWHs have a lower anticoagulant potency than unfractionated heparin. This is a reflection of their lower antithrombin activity. Heparin exhibits a 1:1 ratio of antithrombin to anti-Xa activity, whereas for LMWHs the ratio ranges from 1:2 to 1:4, depending on the molecular weight composition of the given LMWH.[133] Figure 3 demonstrates that heparin can be converted into various molecular forms, including the lower low molecular weight heparin fractions and defined oligosaccharides.

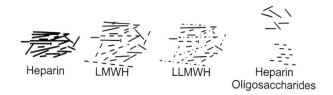

Heparin   LMWH   LLMWH   Heparin
Oligosaccharides

FIGURE 3. Comparison of heparin and its lower molecular weight derivatives.

LMWHs are the agents of choice in European countries for the prophylaxis of deep venous thrombosis because of their efficacy and safety. As a result of their high bioavailability, LMWHs exhibit a sustained pharmacologic effect; once-daily dosing is sufficient to keep the patient in an antithrombotic state. Heparin, in contrast, requires 2 or 3 daily injections to achieve a similar effect. Because of their nearly complete availability and limited plasma protein binding,[77,176,182,293] LMWHs have predictable clinical effects and do not require daily monitoring of plasma levels.[120] Heparin levels are monitored frequently with the APTT assay. It has also been suggested that LMWHs may cause lower rates of hemorrhagic side-effects, osteoporosis, and cytopenia than standard heparin.

LMWHs have been examined for efficacy in the treatment and prevention of venous thromboembolism. In general surgical patients, randomized trials indicate that LMWH is both effective and safe. Statistically significant reductions in thromboembolic mortality were observed without a significant increase in major hemorrhage. Most clinical trials indicate a bleeding effect that is equal to or less than that caused by heparin.[20,161,228,245] In orthopedic patients, LMWHs have exhibited equal or superior efficacy compared with low- dose heparin,[95,250] adjusted-dose heparin,[81,180] warfarin,[124] and dextran.[21] In medical patients, LMWHs have been shown to reduce the risk of thromboembolism relative to placebo[256,317] and heparin.[113,318] LMWHs have been shown to be effective in the management of established thrombosis by both preventing further extension of the thrombus and enhancing its regression.[149,252] Currently, LMWHs are undergoing several clinical trials for various cardiovascular and hematologic indications.

NONHEPARIN GLYCOSAMINOGLYCAN AGENTS

Heparan Sulfate

Heparan sulfate has a backbone that is structurally similar to heparin. Heparan sulfate generally contains more than 20% N-acetylated glucosamine and nearly equal amounts of N- and O-sulfation. In contrast, the ratio of O- to N-sulfation in heparin is almost 4:1.[191] Like heparin, heparan sulfate primarily inhibits proteases via activation of AT III and has been shown to catalyze the formation of thrombin–antithrombin complexes and also to exhibit anti-factor Xa activity. As it does not completely inhibit prothrombin activation, it is much less effective than heparin. The antithrombotic dosage of heparan sulfate is approximately 500–600 μg/kg compared with 60–70 μg/kg for heparin.

Dermatan Sulfate

Dermatan sulfate is a glycosaminoglycan polymer of iduronic acid and N-acetylated galactosamine. Because of a difference in the molecular backbone, dermatan sulfate is unable to interact with AT III; instead, it complexes with heparin cofactor II to mediate thrombin inhibition.[309] The anticoagulant potency of dermatan sulfate is less than that of heparan sulfate. Anticoagulant activity as measured by the APTT and thrombin time is nearly undetectable.[288] Dermatan sulfate inhibits thrombin as it is formed rather than prevents its generation. Thrombin generation inhibition by dermatan sulfate is much less than for an equigravimetric amount of heparin. At a dosage of 150 μg/kg, dermatan sulfate caused a 2% inhibition of thrombin generation compared with an 83% inhibition by heparin. Whereas dermatan octasaccharides bind heparin cofactor II, 12 –14 residues are required for thrombin inhibition. Dermatan sulfate chains with a higher charge density appear to bind to heparin cofactor II better than those with a lower charge.

Dermatan sulfate is active in vivo as an antithrombotic agent in the rabbit model of stasis-thrombosis but to a lesser extent than heparin. Although both agents inhibited thrombus formation to the same extent at an equigravimetric dosage of 150 µg/kg after 10 minutes of stasis, dermatan sulfate was ineffective at inhibiting thrombus formation after 20 minutes of stasis at a dose 8 times higher than that of heparin. The advantage of dermatan sulfate over heparin as an antithrombotic agent is a lower risk of bleeding complications. Dermatan sulfate has been shown not to increase bleeding significantly compared with a saline control at doses that are antithrombotically effective.

It is thought that the decreased bleeding seen with dermatan sulfate is a result of its minor effects on platelets. Sie et al. have shown that although thrombin-induced platelet aggregation is inhibited by dermatan sulfate in the presence of heparin cofactor II, aggregation induced by arachidonic acid, ADP, or collagen was not affected. In addition, dermatan sulfate has a smaller effect on heparin-induced thrombocytopenic serum-induced platelet aggregation than heparin.[140]

Chondroitin Sulfate

Chondroitin sulfate is a glycosaminoglycan that consists of alternating D-glucuronic acid and N-acetylated D-galactosamine residues. The galactosamine residues are typically 4-O or 6-O sulfated.[54] Chondroitin sulfate has a lower degree of sulfation than the heparin or heparan-type glycosaminoglycans, with a SO_3^-/COO^- ratio equal to 1. Because of the low degree of sulfation and the lack of iduronic acid moieties, chondroitin sulfate does not have strong interactions with the endogenous coagulation inhibitors, AT III and heparin cofactor II, or with lipoprotein lipase or low-density lipoproteins as heparin does.[54] Chondroitin sulfates are typically found in cartilage. Chondroitin sulfate has been used in the treatment of osteoarthritis because it inhibits elastase and hyaluronidase in the synovial fluid , both of which can damage joint cartilage. The anticoagulant activity of chondroitin sulfate is minimal; its potency is designated as less than 5 USP IU/mg and 5 anti-factor Xa U/mg by the Yin and Wessler test.[24]

The antithrombotic activity of chondroitin sulfate and its oversulfated derivatives was examined in a rat model of thrombosis and was observed to be minimal.[242] Oversulfation of the molecules did not enhance the negligible anticoagulant activity of the native chondroitin sulfate. The chondroitin sulfate present in ORG 10172 was not observed to enhance the antithrombotic effect of the high-affinity material in the preparation.[346]

Chondroitin sulfate has several biologic functions. Evidence indicates that chondroitin sulfate proteoglycans interact with the herpes simplex virus. Chondroitin sulfate offers neuroprotective effects against glutamate-induced neuronal cell death[230] and may play a role in neuronal patterning.[46] It has been shown in vitro to inhibit the activation of the complement system.[25] Potency was related to the sulfate content of the chondroitin. Chondroitin sulfate exhibits in vitro activity against human immunodeficiency virus-1.[160] When administered to cholesterol-fed rabbits, it suppressed cholesterol deposition in the aorta due to a decrease in plasma LDL cholesterol and to a change in arterial metabolism.[201] Chondroitin sulfate E is a weak activator of heparin cofactor II, accelerating the inhibition of thrombin approximately 200-fold. In addition, chondroitin sulfate may exhibit some anticoagulant activity through interference in the thrombin–fibrinogen interaction.[277]

CONCLUSION

The process of blood coagulation is no longer considered to be a simple transformation of fibrinogen to fibrin by the action of thrombin. Instead, this remarkably complex process is a result of several transformations that are mediated by enzymes, activators, inhibitors, and cellular contributors.The process of coagulation contributes significantly to thrombogenesis; however, it is no longer considered to be the sole event. The role of platelets, leukocytes, and endothelial cells has been gradually accepted as crucial in the overall regulation of thrombogenesis.

Surgical intervention—particularly cardiovascular procedures—inflicts a major stimulus for coagulation through the release of large amounts of tissue factor, enzyme, and platelet activation as a result of extracorporeal circulation and endothelial distress. This procoagulant environment necessitates the use of anticoagulant and antithrombotic agents to keep blood coagulation under control. Understanding of the activation processes has led to the development of newer approaches to inhibit the coagulation process. Furthermore, physiologic means, such as hypothermia and blood salvage techniques, have added to the restoration approaches during cardiovascular surgical procedures. Endogenous inhibitors such as AT III, protein C, and TFPI have also played a major role in the control of thrombigenesis. Heparin and its derivatives have been crucial in controlling the thrombotic process both during and after surgical procedures. Development of alternative anticoagulant drugs will continue to provide new ways to control the coagulation process.

REFERENCES

1. Abildgaard U: Highly purified antithrombin III with heparin cofactor activity prepared by disc electrophoresis. Scand J Clin Lab Invest 21:89–91, 1968.
2. Abildgaard U, Larsen ML: Assay of dermatan sulfate cofactor (heparin cofactor II) activity in human plasma. Thromb Res 35:257–266, 1984.
3. Agnelli G: Pharmacological activities of heparin chains: Should our past knowledge be revised? Haemostasis 26(Suppl 2):2–9, 1996.
4. Altieri DC, Edgington TS: The saturable high affinity association of factor X to ADP-stimulated monocytes defines a novel function of the Mac-1 receptor. J Biol Chem 263:7007–7015, 1988.
5. Altieri DA: Coagulation assembly on leukocytes in transmembrane signaling and cell adhesion. Blood 81:569–579, 1993.
6. Anderson DC, Springer TA: Leukocyte adhesion deficiency: An inherited defect in the Mac-1, LFA-1, and P150 glycoproteins. Annu Rev Med 38:175–194, 1987.
7. Ariens RAS, Faioni EM, Mannucci PM: Repeated release of the tissue factor pathway inhibitor. Thromb Haemost 72:327–378, 1984.
8. Arnljots B, Bergquist D, Dahlback B: Inhibition of microarterial thrombosis by activated protein C in a rabbit model. Thromb Haemost 72:415–20, 1994.
9. Bach R, Konigsberg W, Nemerson Y: Human tissue factor contains thioester linked palmitate and stearate on the cytoplasmic half cystine. Biochemistry 27:4227–4231, 1988.
10. Baker JB, Low DA, Simmer RL, Cunningham DD: Protease nexin: A cellular component that links thrombin and plasminogen activator and mediates their binding to cells. Cell 21:37–45, 1980.
11. Baker ME, French FS, Joseph DR: Vitamin K-dependent protein S is similar to rat androgen binding protein. Biochem J 243:293–296, 1987.
12. Bara L, Bloch MF, Zitoun D, et al: Comparative effects of enoxaparin and unfractionated heparin in healthy volunteers on prothrombin consumption in whole blood during coagulation, and release of tissue factor pathway inhibitor. Thromb Res 69:443–452, 1993.
13. Barritt DW, Jordan SC: Anticoagulant drugs in the treatment of pulmonary embolism: A controlled trial. Lancet 1:1309–1312, 1960.
14. Bauer KA, Kass BL, Beeler DL, Rosenberg RD: The detection of protein C activation in humans. J Clin Invest 74:2033–2041, 1984.
15. Beckman RJ, Schmidt RJ, Santerre PF, et al: The structure and evolution of a 461 amino acid human protein C precursor and its messenger Rna, based upon the DNA sequence of cloned human liver cDNAs. Acids Res. 13:5233–5247, 1985.
16. Belford DA, Hendry IA, Parish CR: Ability of different chemically modified heparins to potentiate the biological activity of heparin-binding growth factor 1: lack of correlation with growth factor binding. Biochemistry 31(28):6498–6503, 1992.
17. Bennet JS, Vilaire G: Exposure of platelet fibrinogen receptors by ADP and epinephrine. J Clin Invest 64:1393–1401, 1979.
18. Bennett J: Integrin structure and function in hemostasis and thrombosis. Ann N Y Acad Sci 614:214–228, 1991.
19. Bergman BL, Scott S, Watts S, Baker JB: Inhibition of tumor cell-mediated extracellular matrix destruction by a fibroblast proteinase inhibitor, protease nexin I. Proc Natl Acad Sci USA 83:996–1000, 1986.

20. Bergqvist D, Matzsch T, Burmark US, et al: Low molecular weight heparin given the evening before surgery compared with conventional low-dose heparin in prevention of thrombosis. Br J Surg 75:888–891, 1988.
21. Bergqvist D, Kettunen K, Fredin H, et al: Thromboprophylaxis in patients with hip fractures: A prospective, randomized, comparative study between Org 10172 and dextran 70. Surgery 109:617–622, 1991.
22. Besterman EMM, Gillett MPT: Heparin effects on plasma lysolecithin formation and platelet aggregation. Atherosclerosis 17:503–513, 1973.
23. Bevers EM, Rosing J, Zwaal RFA: Development of procoagulant binding sites on the platelet surface. In Westweek J, Scully MF, McIntyre DE, Kakkar VV (eds): Mechanisms of Stimulus Response Coupling in Platelets. New York, Plenum Press, 1985, pp 359–372.
24. Bianchini P, Osima B, Parma B, et al: Lack of correlation between "in vitro" and "in vivo" antithrombotic activity of heparin fractions and related compounds. Heparan sulfate as an antithrombotic agent "in vivo." Thromb Res 40:597–607, 1985.
25. Biffoni M, Paroli E: Complement in vitro inhibition by a low sulfate chondroitin sulfate (Matrix). Drugs Exp Clin Res 17:35–39, 1991.
26. Bjork I, Danielsson A: Antithrombin and related inhibitors of coagulation proteinases. in Barrett AJ, Salvesen GS (eds): Proteinase Inhibitors. Amsterdam, Elsevier, 1986,pp 489–513.
27. Bjornsson TD, Wolfram KM, Kitchell BB: Heparin kinetics determined by three assay methods. Clin Pharmacol Ther 31:104–113, 1982.
28. Bjornsson TD, Schneider DE, Hecht AR: Effects of N-deacetlyation and N-desulfation of heparin on its anticoagulant activity and in vivo disposition. J Pharm Exp Ther 245(3):80–88, 1988.
29. Bleich SD, Nichols TC, Schumacher RR, et al: Effect of heparin on coronary arterial patency after thrombolysis with tissue plasminogen activator in acute myocardial infarction. Am J Cardiol 66:1412–1417, 1990.
30. Blomback B, Vestermark A: Isolation of fibrinopeptides by chromatography. Arkiv Kemi 12:173–182, 1958.
31. Bock SC, Wion KL, Vehar GA, Lawn RM: Cloning and expression of the cDNA for human antithrombin III. Nucl Acids Res 10:8113–8125, 1982.
32. Bock SC, Harris JF, Schwartz CE, et al: Hereditary thrombosis in a Utah kindred is caused by a dysfunctional antithrombin III gene. Am J Hum Genet 37:32–41, 1985.
33. Bogaert TN, Brown N, Wilcox M: The Drosophila PS2 antigen is an invertebrate integrin that, like the fibronectin receptor, becomes localized to muscle attachments. Cell 51:929–940, 1987.
34. Bonner JC, Brody AR: Cytokine-binding proteins in the lung. Am J Physiol 268(6 Pt 1):L869–L878, 1995.
35. Borg JY, Owen MC, Soria C, et al: Proposed heparin binding site in antithrombin based on arginine 47. J Clin Invest 81:1292–296, 1988.
36. Borth W: Alpha 2-macroglobulin, a multifunctional binding protein with targeting characteristics. FASEB J 6:3345–3353, 1992.
37. Borth W: Alpha 2-macroglobulin. A multifunctional binding and targeting protein with possible roles in immunity and autoimmunity. Ann N Y Acad Sci 737:267–272, 1994.
38. Bradshaw RA, Wessler S: Heparin: Structure, function, and clinical implications. Adv Exper Med Biol 52, 1975.
39. Brandjes DP, Heijboer H, Butler HR, et al: Acenocoumarol and heparin compared with acenocoumarol alone in the initial treatment of proximal-vein thrombosis. N Engl J Med 327:1485–1489, 1992.
40. Bray PF, Rosa JP, Johnston JI, et al: Platelet glycoprotein IIb. Chromosomal localization and tissue expression. J Clin Invest 80:1812–1817, 1987.
41. Brennan SO, George PM, Jordan RE: Physiological variant of antithrombin III lacks carbohydrate side chain at ASN 135. FEBS Lett 219:431–436, 1987.
42. Brennan SO, Borg JY, George PM, et al: New carbohydrate site in mutant antithrombin (7ILE-ASN) with decreased heparin affinity. FEBS Lett 237:118–122, 1988.
43. Briginshaw GF, Shanberge JN: Identification of two distinct heparin cofactors in human plasma. Inhibition of thrombin and activated factor X. Thromb Res 4:463–477, 1974.
44. Briginshaw GF, Shanberge JN: Identification of two distinct heparin cofactors in human plasma. Separation and partial purification. Arch Biochem Biophys 161:683–690, 1974.
45. Brinkhous KM, Smith Hπ, Warmer ED, Seegers WH: The inhibition of blood clotting: An unidentified substance which acts in conjunction with heparin to prevent the conversion of prothrombin into thrombin. Am J Physiol 125:683–687, 1939.
46. Brittis PA, Canning DR, Silver J: Chondroitin sulfate as a regulator of neuronal patterning in the retina. Science 255:733–7336, 1992.
47. Broze GJ, Miletich JP: Isolation of tissue factor inhibitor produced by HEPG2 hepatoma cells. Proc Natl Acad Sci USA. 84:1886–1890, 1987.
48. Broze GJ, Warren LP, Novotny WF, et al: Lipoprotein–associated coagulation inhibitor that inhibits the factor VII-tissue factor complex also inhibits factor Xa: Insight into its possible mechanism of action. Blood 71:335–343, 1988.

49. Car BD, Suyemoto M, Neilsen NR, Slauson DO: The role of leukocytes in the pathogenesis of fibrin deposition in bovine acute lung injury. Am J Pathol 138:1191–1198, 1991.
50. Carlsen E, Flatmark A, Prydz H: Cytokine-induced procoagulant activity in monocytes and endothelial cells. Further enhancement by cyclosporine. Transplantation 46:575–580, 1988.
51. Carr C, Bild GS, Chang ACK, et al: Recombinant E. coli-derived tissue factor pathway inhibitor reduces coagulopathic and lethal effects in the baboon gram-negative model of septic shock. Circ Shock 44:126–137, 1995.
52. Carreer FM: The C1 inhibitor deficiency. Eur J Clin Chem Clin Biochem 30(12):793–807, 1992.
53. Casu B: Methods of structural analysis. In Lane DA, Lindahl U (eds): Heparin: Chemical and Biological Properties, Clinical Applications. London, Edward Arnold, 1989, pp 25–50, 1989.
54. Casu B: Structural features and binding properties of chondroitin sulfate, dermatan sulfate, and heparan sulfate. Semin Thromb Hemost 17(Suppl. 1):9–14, 1991.
55. Chandra T, Stackhouse R, Kidd VJ, Woo SLC: Isolation and sequence characterization of a cDNA clone of human antithrombin III. Proc Natl Acad Sci USA 80:1845–1848, 1983.
56. Chang JY, Tran TH: Antithrombin III Basel. Identification of a Pro-Leu substitution in a hereditary abnormal antithrombin with impaired heparin cofactor activity. J Biol Chem 261:1174–1176, 1986.
57. Chapman HA, Allen CL, Stone OL, Fair DS: Human alveolar macrophages synthesize factor VII in vitro. Possible role in interstitial lung disease. J Clin Invest. 75:2030–2037, 1985.
58. Chaudhuri L: Human alpha 2-macroglobulin and its biologic significance. Ind J Exp Biol 31:723–727, 1993.
59. Cheresh DA, Spiro RC: Biosynthetic and functional properties of an Arg-Gly-Asp directed receptor involved in human melanoma cell attachment to vitronectin, fibrinogen, and von Willebrand factor. J Biol Chem 262:17703–17711, 1987.
60. Chu CT, Pizzo SV: Alpha 2–macroglobulin, complement, and biologic defense: antigens, growth factors, microbial proteases, and receptor ligation. Lab Invest 71:792–812, 1994.
61. Church FC, Noyes CM, Griffith MJ: Inhibition of chymotrypsin by heparin cofactor II. Proc Natl Acad Sci USA 82:6431–6434, 1985.
62. Clagett GP, Reisch JS: Prevention of venous thromboembolism in general surgical patients: Results of meta-analysis. Ann Surg 208:227–240, 1988.
63. Coller B: Platelets in cardiovascular thrombosis and thrombolysis. In Fozzard UA, Haber E, Jennings RB, et al (eds): The Heart and Cardiovascular System, 2nd ed. New York, Raven Press, 1992, pp 219–273.
64. Collins R, Scrimgeour A, Yusof S, Peto R: Reduction in fatal pulmonary embolism and venous thrombosis by perioperative administration of subcutaneous heparin: Overview of results of randomized trials in general, orthopedic, and urologic surgery. N Engl J Med 318:1162–1173, 1988.
65. Conrad J, Brosstad F, Larsen ML, et al: Molar antithrombin concentration in normal human plasma. Haemostasis 13:363–368, 1983.
66. Corrigan JJ: Heparin therapy in bacterial septicemia. J Pediatr 91:695–700, 1977.
67. Coughlin SR, Vu TKH, Hung DT, Wheaton VI: Characterization of a functional thrombin receptor. Issues and opportunities. Clin Invest 89:351–353, 1992.
68. Creasey AA, Chang ACK, Feigen L, et al: Tissue factor pathway inhibitor reduces mortality from *Escherichia coli* septic shock. J Clin Invest 91:2850–2860, 1993.
69. Cruz WO, Dietrich CP: Antihemostatic effect of heparin counteracted by adenosine triphosphate. Proc Soc Exp Biol Med 126:420–426, 1967.
70. Cunningham DD: Regulation of neuronal cells and astrocytes by protease nexin-1 and thrombin. Ann N Y Acad Sci 674:228–236, 1992.
71. Dahlback B, Stenflo J: The protein C anticoagulant system. In Stamatoyannopoulos G., Nieuhuis AW, Majerus PW, Varmus H (eds): The Molecular Basis of Blood Diseases. Philadelphia, W.B. Saunders, 1994, pp 599–628.
72. Dahlback B, Hildebrand B: Inherited resistance to activated protein C is corrected by anticoagulant cofactor activity found to be a property of factor V. Proc Natl Acad Sci USA 81:1396–1400, 1994.
73. Dahlback B: The protein C anticoagulant system: Inherited defects as basis for venous thrombosis. Thromb Res 77:1–43, 1995.
74. Damus PS, Hicks M, Rosenberg RD: Anticoagulant action of heparin. Nature 246:355–357, 1973.
75. Danishefsky I, Ahrens M, Klein S: Effect of heparin modification on its activity in enhancing the inhibition of thrombin by antithrombin III. Biochim Biophys Acta 498:215–222, 1977.
76. Davie EW, Ratnoff OD: Waterfall sequence for intrinsic blood clotting. Science 145:1310–1312, 1964.
77. Dawes J, Pavuk N: Sequestration of therapeutic glycosaminoglycans by plasma fibronectin. Thromb Haemost 65:829, 1991.
78. Day KC, Hoffman LC, Palmier MO, et al: Recombinant lipoprotein-associated coagulation inhibitor inhibits tissue thromboplastin-induced intravascular coagulation in the rabbit. Blood 76:1538–1545, 1990.
79. DeBault LE, Esmon NL, Olson JR, Esmon CT: Distribution of the thrombomodulin antigen in the rabbit vasculature. Lab Invest 54:172–178, 1986.

80. DeBono DP, Simmons ML, Tijssen J, et al, for the European Cooperative Study Group: Effect of early intravenous heparin on coronary patency, infarct size, and bleeding complications after alteplase thrombolysis: Results of a randomized double blind European Cooperative Study Group trial. Br Heart J 67:122–128, 1992.
81. Dechavanne M, Ville D, Berruyer M, et al: Randomized trial of a low-molecular-weight heparin (Kabi 2165) versus adjusted-dose subcutaneous standard heparin in the prophylaxis of deep-vein thrombosis after elective hip surgery. Haemostasis 19:5–12, 1989.
82. DeSimone DW, Hynes RO: Xenopus laevie integrins. Structural conservation and evolutionary divergence of integrin beta. J Biol Chem 26:5333–5340, 1988.
83. DeSwart CA, Nijmeyer B, Roelofs JM, Sixma JJ: Kinetics of intravenously administered heparin in normal humans. Blood 60:1251–1258, 1982.
84. Drake TA, Morissey JH, Edgington TS: Selective expression of tissue factor in human tissues. Am J Pathol 134:1087–1097, 1989.
85. Eaton DL, Baker JB: Evidence that a variety of cultured cells secrete protease nexin and produce a distinct cytoplasmic serine protease-binding factor. J Cell Physiol 117:175–182, 1983.
86. Edelberg J, Pizzo SV: Lipoprotein (a) regulates plasmin generation and inhibition. Chem Phys Lipids 67–68:363–368, 1994.
87. Edgington TS, Mackman N, Brand K, Ruf W: The structural biology of the expression and function of tissue factor. Thromb Haemost 66:67–79, 1991.
88. Edwards RL, Rickles FR: The role of leukocytes in the activation of blood coagulation. Semin Hematol 29:202–212, 1992.
89. Eika C: On the mechanism of platelet aggregation induced by heparin, protamine and polybrene. Scand J Haemost 9:248–257, 1972.
90. Ellison N, Edmunds LH, Colman RW: Platelet aggregation following heparin and protamine administration. Anesthesiology 48:65–68, 1978.
91. Engesser L, Kluft C, Briet E, Brommer E: Familial elevation of plasma histidine-rich glycoprotein in a family with thrombophilia. Br J Haematol 67:355–358, 1987.
92. Enjyoji K, Em T, Kamikubo Y, Maki, S: cDNA cloning and expression of rat tissue factor pathway inhibitor (TFPI) J Biochem 111:681–687, 1992.
93. Enjyoji K, Miyaya T, Kamikubo Y, Kato H: Effect of heparin on the inhibition of factor Xa by tissue factor pathway inhibitor: A segment, Gly 212-Phe 243, of the third Kunitz domain is a heparin binding site. Biochemistry 34:5725–5735, 1995.
94. Erdjument H, Lane DA, Panico M, et al: Single amino acid substitutions in the reactive site of antithrombin leading to thrombosis. Congenital substitution of arginine 393 to cysteine in antithrombin Northwick Park and to histidine in antithrombin Glasgow. J Biol Chem 263:5589–5593, 1988.
95. Eriksson BI, Kalebo P, Anthmyr BA, et al: Prevention of deep-vein thrombosis and pulmonary embolism after total hip replacement: comparison of low molecular weight heparin and unfractionated heparin. J Bone Joint Surg 73A:484–493, 1991.
96. Esmon CT: The roles of protein C and thrombomodulin in the regulation of blood coagulation. J Biol Chem 264:4743–4761, 1989.
97. Esmon CT, Owen WG: Identification of an endothelial cell cofactor for thrombin catalyzed activation of protein C. Proc Natl Acad Sci USA 78:2249–2252, 1981.
98. Esmon CT, Esmon NL, Harris KW: Complex formation between thrombin and thrombomodulin inhibits both thrombin catalyzed fibrin formation and factor V activation. J Biol Chem 257:7944–7947, 1982.
99. Esmon NL, Carroll RC, Esmon CT: Thrombomodulin blocks the ability of thrombin to activate platelets. J Biol Chem 258:12238–12242, 1983.
100. Esmon CT: The protein C anticoagulant pathway. Arterioscler Thromb 12:135–145, 1992.
101. Esmon CT: Molecular events that control the protein C anticoagulant pathway. Thromb Haemost 70:29–35, 1993.
102. Esmon CT: Cell mediated events that control blood coagulation and vascular injury. Annu Rev Cell Biol 9:1–26, 1993.
103. Farrell DH, Wagner SL, Yuan RH, Cunningham DD: Localization of protease nexin 1 on the fibroblast extracellular matrix. J Cell Physiol 134:179–188, 1988.
104. Folkman J: Tumor angiogenesis. Adv Cancer Res 43:175–203, 1985.
105. Forsee WT, Roden L: Biosynthesis of heparin. Transfer of N-acetylglucosamine to heparan sulfate oligosaccharides. J Biol Chem 256:7240–7247, 1981.
106. Foster DC, Yoshitake S, Davie EW: Characterization of cDNA coding for human protein C. Proc Natl Acad Sci USA 81:4766–4770, 1984.
107. Friberger P, Egberg N, Holmer E, et al: Antithrombin assay—the use of human or bovine thrombin and the observation of a 'second' heparin cofactor. Thromb Res 25:433–440, 1982.
108. Friedman Y, Arsenis C: Studies on the heparin sulphamidase activity from rat spleen: intracellular distribution and characterization of the enzyme. Biochem J 139:699–708, 1979.
109. Gailani D, Broze GJ: Factor XI activation in a revised model of blood coagulation. Science 253:909–912, 1991.

110. Girard TJ, Warren LA, Novotny WF, et al: Functional significance of the Kunitz-type inhibitory domains of lipoprotein-associated coagulation inhibitor. Nature 338:518–520, 1989.
111. Glimelius B, Busch C, Hook M: Binding of heparin on the surface of cultured human endothelial cells. Thromb Res 12:773–782, 1978.
112. Gorog P, Raake W: Antithrombotic effect of a mucopolysaccharide polysulfate after systemic, topical and percutaneous application. Arznei Forsch 37:342–345, 1987.
113. Green D, Lee MY, Lim AC, et al: Prevention of thromboembolism after spinal cord injury using low-molecular-weight heparin. Ann Intern Med 113:571–574, 1990.
114. Gregory SA, Morissey JH, Edgington TS: Regulation of tissue factor gene expression in the monocyte procoagulant response to endotoxin. Mol Cell Biol 9:2752–2755, 1989.
115. Griffith MJ: The heparin-enhanced antithrombin III/thrombin reaction is saturable with respect to both thrombin and antithrombin III. J Biol Chem 257:13899–13902, 1982.
116. Griffith MJ, Carraway T, White GC, Dombrose FA: Heparin cofactor activities in a family with hereditary antithrombin III deficiency: Evidence for a second heparin cofactor in plasma. Blood 61:111–118, 1983.
117. Gruber A, Hanson SR, Kelly AB, et al: Inhibition of thrombus formation by activated recombinant protein C in a primate model of arterial thrombosis. Circulation 82:578–585, 1990.
118. Hack CE, Oglivie AC, Eisele B, et al: Initial studies on the administration of C1-esterase inhibitor to patients with septic shock or with a vascular leak syndrome induced by interleukin-2 therapy. Prog Clin Biol Res 388:335–357, 1994.
119. Hamamoto T, Yamamoto M, Nordfang O, et al: Inhibitory properties of full-length and truncated tissue factor pathway inhibitor (TFPI). J Biol Chem 268:8704–8710, 1993.
120. Handeland GF, Abildgaard U, Holm HA, Arnesen KE: Dose adjusted heparin treatment of deep venous thrombosis: a comparison to unfractionated and low molecular weight heparin. Eur J Clin Pharmacol 39:107–112, 1990.
121. Harenberg J, Siegele M, Dempfle CE, et al: Protamine neutralization of the release of tissue factor pathway inhibitor activity by heparins. Thromb Haemost 70:942–945, 1993.
122. Haskel EJ, Torr SR, Day KC, et al: Prevention of arterial reocclusion after thrombolysis with recombinant lipoprotein-associated coagulation inhibitor. Circulation 84:821–827, 1991.
123. Heiden D, Mielke CH, Rodvien R: Impairment by heparin of primary hemostasis and platelet [^{14}C]5-hydroxytryptamine release. Br J Haemost 36:427–436, 1977.
124. Heit J, Kessler C, Mammen E, Kwaan H, et al: Efficacy of RD heparin (a LMWH) and warfarin for prevention of deep-vein thrombosis after hip or knee replacement: the RD heparin study group. Blood 778:187A, 1991.
125. Helting T, Lindahl U: Occurrence and biosynthesis of ß-glucuronidic linkages in heparin. J Biol Chem 246:5442–5447, 1971.
126. Helting T, Lindahl U: Biosynthesis of heparin. Transfer of N-acetylglucosamine and glucuronic acid to low molecular weight heparin fragments. Acta Chem Scand 26:3515–3523, 1972.
127. Hemker HC, Kessels H: Feedback mechanisms in coagulation. Haemostasis 21:189–196, 1991.
128. Hemler ME, Ware CF, Strominger JL: Characterization of a novel differentiation antigen complex recognized by a monoclonal antibody (A-1A5): Unique activation specifies molecular forms in stimulated T cells. J Immunol 131:334–340, 1988.
129. Hemler ME, Crouse C, Takada H, Sonnenberg A: Multiple very late antigen (VLA) heterodimers on platelets. Evidence for distinct VLA-2, VLA-5 (fibrinogen receptor) and VLA-6 structures. J Biol Chem 263:7660–7665, 1988.
130. Hermans JM, Stone SR: Interaction of activated protein C with serpins. Biochem J 295:239–245, 1993.
131. Herold BC, Gerber SI, Polonsky T,et al: Identification of structural features of heparin required for inhibition of herpes simplex virus type 1 binding. Virology 206:1108–1116, 1995.
132. Hirsh J, van Aken WG, Gallus AS, et al: Heparin kinetics in venous thrombosis and pulmonary embolism. Circulation 53:691–695, 1976.
133. Hirsh J, Fuster V: Guide to anticoagulant therapy. Part 1: Heparin. Circulation 89:1449–1468, 1994.
134. Holmsen H: Platelet secretion. In Colman RW, Hirsh J, Marder VJ, Salzman EW (eds): Hemostasis and Thrombosis. Philadelphia, J.B. Lippincott, 1987, p 606.
135. Holst J, Lindblad B, Wedeberg E, et al: Tissue factor pathway inhibitor (TFPI) and its response to heparin in patients with spontaneous deep venous thrombosis. Thromb Res 72:467–470, 1993.
136. Holst J, Lindblad B, Bergquist D, et al: Antithrombotic effect of recombinant truncated tissue factor pathway inhibitor (TFPI$_{1-161}$) in experimental venous thrombosis. A comparison with low molecular weight heparin. Thromb Haemost 71:214–249, 1994.
137. Holt JC, Niewiarowski S: Biochemistry of a-granule proteins. Semin Hematol 22:151–163, 1985.
138. Holtin GL, Trimpe BL: Allosteric changes in thrombin's activity produced by peptides corresponding to segments of natural inhibitors and substrates. J Biol Chem 266:6866–6871, 1991.
139. Hook M, Lindahl U, Hallen A, Backstrom A: Biosynthesis of heparin. Studies on the microsomal sulfation process. J Biol Chem 250:6065–6071, 1975.
140. Hoppensteadt D, Walenga JM, Fareed J: Comparative antithrombotic and hemorrhagic effects of dermatan sulfate, heparan sulfate and heparin. Thromb Res 60:191–200, 1990.

141. Hoppensteadt DA, Fasanella A, Fareed J: Effect of protamine on heparin releasable TFPI antigen levels in normal volunteers. Thromb Res 79:325–330, 1995.
142. Hourani SMO, Cusack NJ: Pharmacological receptors on blood platelets. Pharmacol Rel 43:243–298, 1991.
143. Howell WH: The coagulation of blood. In The Harvey Lectures, vol 12. Philadelphia, J.B. Lippincott, 1918, pp 272–323.
144. Howell WH: The purification of heparin and its presence in blood. Am J Physiol 71:553–562, 1925.
145. Hoylaerts M, Owen WG, Collen D: Involvement of heparin chain length in the heparin catalyzed inhibition of thrombin by antithrombin III. J Biol Chem 259:5670–5677, 1984.
146. Huang ZF, Wun TC, Broze GJ: Kinetics of factor Xa inhibition by tissue factor pathway inhibitor. J Biol Chem 268:26950–26955, 1993.
147. Hull R, Delmore T, Genton E, et al: Warfarin sodium versus low-dose heparin in the long-term treatment of venous thrombosis. N Engl J Med 301:855–858, 1979.
148. Hull RD, Raskob GE, Hirsh J, et al: Continuous intravenous heparin compared with intermittent subcutaneous heparin in the initial treatment of proximal vein thrombosis. N Engl J Med 315:1109–1114, 1986.
149. Hull RD, Raskob GE, Pineo GF, et al: Subcutaneous low-molecular-weight heparin compared with continuous intravenous heparin in the treatment of proximal vein thrombosis. N Engl J Med 326:975–982, 1992.
150. Hurst RE, Poon MC, Griffith MJ: Structure-activity relationships of heparin. Independence of heparin charge density and antithrombin-binding domains in thrombin inhibition by antithrombin and heparin cofactor II. J Clin Invest 72:1042–1045, 1983.
151. Hyers TM: Heparin therapy: regimens and treatment considerations. Drugs 44:738–749, 1992.
152. Hynes RO: Integrins: A family of cell surface receptors. Cell 48:549–554, 1987.
153. Inoue Y, Nagasawa K: Selective N-desulfation of heparin with dimethyl sulfoxide containing water or methanol. Carbo Res 46:87–95, 1976.
154. Ittyerah TR, Rawala R, Colman RW: Immunochemical studies of factor V of bovine platelets. Eur J Biochem 120:235–241, 1981.
155. Jackson SP, Yuan Y, Schoenwaelder SM, Mitchell CA: Role of the platelet integrin glycoprotein IIb-IIIa in intracellular signalling. Thromb Res 71:159–168, 1993.
156. Jenny RJ, Tracy PB, Mann KG: The physiology and biochemistry of factor V. In Bloom AL, Forbes CD, Thomas DP, Tuddenheim EGD (eds)L: Haemostasis and Thrombosis. London, Churchill Livingstone, 1994, pp. 465–476.
157. Jeske W, Hoppensteadt D, Klauser R, et al: Effect of repeated aprosulate and enoxaparin administration on tissue factor pathway inhibitor antigen levels. Blood Coag Fibrinol 6:119–124, 1995.
158. Jordan RE, Oosta GM, Gardner WT, Rosenberg RD: The kinetics of hemostatic enzyme-antithrombin interactions in the presence of low molecular weight heparins. J Biol Chem 255:10081–10090, 1980.
159. Jornvall H, Fish WW, Bjork I: The thrombin cleavage site in bovine antithrombin. FEBS Lett 106:358–362, 1979.
160. Jurkiewicz E, Panse P, Jentsch K.D, et al: In vitro anti-HIV-1 activity of chondroitin polysulfate. AIDS 3:423–427, 1989.
161. Kakkar VV, Murray WJ: Efficacy and safety of low-molecular-weight heparin (CY216) in preventing postoperative venous thrombo-embolism: A co-operative study. Br J Surg 72:786–791, 1985.
162. Kamei S, Kamikubo Y, Hamuro T, et al: Amino acid sequence and inhibitory activity of Rhesus monkey tissue factor pathway inhibitor (TFPI): Comparison with human TFPI. J Biochem 115:708–714, 1994.
163. Kane WH, Davie EW: Blood coagulation factors V and VIII: Structural and functional similarities and their relationship to hemorrhagic and thrombotic disorders. Blood 71:539–555, 1988.
164. Kaplan KL: Platelet granule proteins: localization and secretion. In Gordon AS (ed): Platelet in Biology and Pathology, vol. 5. Amsterdam, Elsevier,1981 p 77.
165. Khouri RK, Koudsi D, Fu K, et al: Prevention of thrombosis by topical application of tissue factor pathway inhibitor in a rabbit model of vascular trauma. Ann Plast Surg 30:398–404, 1993.
166. Kisiel W, Canfield WM, Ericsson LN, Davie EW: Anticoagulant properties of bovine plasma protein C following activation by thrombin. J Biol Chem 16:5824–5831, 1977.
167. Kisiel W: Human plasma protein C. Isolation, characterization, and mechanism of action by a-thrombin. J Clin Invest 64:761–769, 1979.
168. Knauer DJ, Thompson JA, Cunningham DD: Protease nexins: Cell-secreted proteins that mediate the binding, internalization, and degradation, of regulatory serine proteases. J Cell Physiol 117:385–396, 1983.
169. Koide T, Odani S, Tokahashi K, et al: Antithrombin III Toyama: Replacement of arginine 47 by cysteine in hereditary abnormal antithrombin III that lacks heparin binding ability. Proc Natl Acad Sci USA 81:289–293, 1984.
170. Kristensen H, Ostergaard PB, Nordfang O, et al: Effect of tissue factor pathway inhibitor (TFPI) in the Heptest assay an in an amidolytic antifactor Xa assay for LMW heparin. Thromb Haemost 68:310–314, 1992.
171. Kruithof EKO: Plasminogen activator inhibitors—a review. Enzyme 40:113–121, 1988.
172. Krupinski K, Breddin HK, Casu B: Anticoagulant and antithrombotic effects of chemically modified heparins and pentosanpolysulfate. Haemostasis 20:81–92, 1990.

173. Lagerstedt CI, Olsson CG, Fagher BO, et al: Need for long-term anticoagulant treatment in symptomatic calf-vein thrombosis. Lancet 2:515–518, 1985.
174. Lam SC, Plow EW, D'Souza SE, et al: Isolation and characterization of a platelet membrane protein related to the vitronectin receptor. J Biol Chem 264:3742–3749, 1989.
175. LaMarre J, Wollenberg GK, Gonias SL, Hayes MA: Cytokine binding and clearance properties of proteinase-activated alpha 2-macroglobulins. Lab Invest 65:3–14, 1991.
176. Lane DA, Pejleer G, Flynn AM, et al: Neutralization of heparin-related saccharides by histidine-rich glycoprotein and platelet factor 4. J Biol Chem 261:3980–3986, 1986.
177. Lane DA, Lowe GDO, Flynn A, et al: Antithrombin III Glasgow: A variant with increased heparin affinity and reduced ability to inactivate thrombin associated with familial thrombosis. Br J Haematol 66:523–527, 1987.
178. Laurent TC, Blomback B: On the significance of the release of two different peptides from fibrinogen during clotting. Acta Chem Scand 12:1875–1877, 1958.
179. Levy SW: Heparin and blood lipids. Rev Can Biol 17:1–61, 1958.
180. Leyvraz PF, Bachmann F, Hoek J, et al: Prevention of deep vein thrombosis after hip replacement: randomized comparison between unfractionated heparin and low molecular weight heparin. BMJ 303:543–548, 1991.
181. Lijnen HR, Hoylaerts M, Collen D: Isolation and characterization of human plasma protein with high affinity for lysine binding sites in plasminogen. J Biol Chem 225:10214–1022, 1980.
182. Lijnen HR, Hoylaerts M, Collen D: Heparin binding properties of human histidine-rich glycoprotein: mechanism and role in the neutralization of heparin in plasma. J Biol Chem 258:3803–3808, 1983.
183. Lindahl AK, Jacobsen PBJ, Sandset PM, Abildgaard U: Separation of tissue factor pathway inhibitor by heparin affinity. Plasma from cancer patients and post-heparin plasma contain increased amounts of a fraction with high anticoagulant activity. Blood Coag Fibrinol 2:713–721, 1991.
184. Lindahl AK, Abildgaard U, Larsen ML, et al: Extrinsic pathway inhibitor (EPI) and the post-heparin anticoagulant effect in tissue thromboplastin induced coagulation. Thromb Res Suppl 14:39–48, 1991.
185. Lindahl AK, Abildgaard U, Larsen ML, et al: Extrinsic pathway inhibitor released to the blood by heparin is a more powerful inhibitor than is recombinant TFPI. Thromb Res 62:607–614, 1991.
186. Lindahl AK, Abildgaard U, Staalesen R: The anticoagulant effect in heparinized blood and plasma resulting from interactions with extrinsic pathway inhibitor. Thromb Res 64:155–168, 1991.
187. Lindahl AK, Sandset PM, Abildgaard U: The present status of tissue factor pathway inhibitor. Blood Coag Fibrinol 3:439–449, 1992.
188. Lindahl U, Roden L: Carbohydrate-peptide linkages in proteoglycans of animal, plant and bacterial origin. In Gottschalk A (ed): Glycoproteins: Their Composition, Structure, and Function. Amsterdam, Elsevier, 1972, p 491.
189. Lindahl U, Jacobsson I, Hook M, et al: Biosynthesis of heparin. Loss of C-5 hydrogen during conversion of D-glucuronic to L-iduronic acid residues. Biochem Biophys Res Comm 70:492–429, 1976.
190. Lindahl U, Backstrom G, Hook M, et al: Structure of the antithrombin-binding site of heparin. Proc Natl Acad Sci USA 76:3198–3202, 1979.
191. Lindahl U: Biosynthesis of heparin and related polysaccharides. In Lane DA, Lindah U (eds): Heparin: Chemical and Biological Properties, çlinical applications. London, Edward Arnold, 1989, pp 159–190.
192. Lindhout T, Willems G, Blezer R, Hemker HC: Kinetics of the inhibition of human factor Xa by full-length and truncated recombinant tissue factor pathway inhibitor. Biochem J 297(Pt 1):131–136, 1994.
193. Lippman M: A proposed role for mucopolysaccharides in the initiation and control of cell division. Trans N Y Acad Sci 27:343, 1965.
194. MacFarlane RG: An enzyme cascade in the blood clotting mechanism and its function as a biochemical amplifier. Nature 202:498–499, 1964.
195. Mahadoo J, Hiebert L, Jacques LB: Vascular sequestration of heparin. Thromb Res 12:79–90, 1978.
196. Malmstrom A, Roden L, Feingold DS, et al: Biosynthesis of heparin. Partial purification of the uronosyl C-5 epimerase. J Biol Chem 255:3878-3883, 1980.
197. Mann KG, Jerry RJ, Krishnaswamy S: Cofactor proteins in the assembly of blood clotting enzyme complexes. Annu Rev Biochem 57:915–956, 1988.
198. Mann KG, Nesheim ME, Church WR, et al: Surface–dependent reactions of the vitamin K-dependent enzyme complexes. Blood 76:1–16, 1990.
199. Marcantonio EE, Hynes RO: Antibodies to the conserved cytoplasmic domain of the integrin beta 1 subunit react with proteins in vertebrates, invertebrates and fungi. J Cell Biol 106:1765–1772, 1988.
200. Maruyama I, Bell CE, Majerus PW: Thrombomodulin is found on endothelium of arteries, veins, capillaries, lymphatics and syncytioblasts of human placenta. J Cell Biol 101:363–371, 1985.
201. Matsushima T, Nakashima Y, Suganp M, et al: Suppression of atherogenesis in hypercholesterolemic rabbits by chondroitin 6-sulfate. Artery 14:316–337, 1987.
202. McGee MP, Wallin R, Devlin R, Rothberger H: Identification of mRNA coding for factor VII protein in human alveolar macrophages. Coagulant expression may be limited due to postribosomal processing. Thromb Haemost 61:170–174, 1989.

203. McGee MP, Devlin R, Saluta G, Koren H: Tissue factor and factor VII messenger RNAs in human alveolar macrophages: Effects of breathing ozone. Blood 75:122–127, 1990.
204. McGee MP, Li LC: Functional difference between intrinsic and extrinsic coagulation pathways. Kinetics of factor X activation on human monocytes and alveolar macrophages. J Biol Chem 266:8079–8085, 1991.
205. McLean J: The thromboplastic action of cephalin. Am J Physiol 41:250–257, 1916.
206. McVey JH: Tissue factor pathway. Bailliere's Clin Haematol 7:469–484, 1994.
207. Miletich JP, Jackson CM, Majerus PW: Interaction of coagulation factor Xa with human platelets. Proc Natl Acad Sci USA 74:4033–4036, 1977.
208. Morrissey JH, Mack BG, Neuenschwander PF, Comp PC: Quantitation of activated factor VII levels in plasma using a tissue factor mutant selectively deficient in promoting factor VII activation. Blood 81:734–744, 1993.
209. Mourey L, Samama JP, Delarue M, et al: Antithrombin III: Structural and functional aspects. Biochemie 72:599–608, 1990.
210. Munkvad S: Fibrinolysis in patients with acute ischaemic heart disease. With particular reference to systemic effects of tissue-type plasminogen activator treatment on fibrinolysis, coagulation and complement pathways. Dan Med Bull 40:383–408, 1993.
211. Musci G, Berliner LJ, Esmon CT: Evidence for multiple conformational changes in the active center of thrombin induced by complex formation with thrombomodulin: An analysis employing nitroxide spin labelling. Biochemistry 27:769–773, 1988.
212. Naggi A, Torri G, Casu B, et al: "Supersulfated" heparin fragments, a new type of low-molecular weight heparin. Physico-chemical and pharmacological properties. Biochem Pharm 36:1895–1900, 1987.
213. Naito K, Fujikawa K: Activation of human blood coagulation factor XI independent of factor XII: Factor XI is activated by thrombin and factor XIa in the presence of negatively charged surfaces. J Biol Chem 266:7353–7358, 1991.
214. Nawroth P, Handley D, Esmon C, Stern DM: Interleukin 1 induces endothelial cell procoagulant while suppressing cell surface anticoagulant activity. Proc Natl Acad Sci USA 83:3460–3464, 1986.
215. Nelsestuen GL, Kisiel W, Discipio RG: Interaction of vitamin K dependent proteins with membranes. Biochemistry 17:2134–2138, 1978.
216. Nemerson Y: Tissue factor and haemostasis. Blood 71:1–8, 1988.
217. Neri Serneri GG, Rovelli F, Gensini GF, et al: Effectiveness of low-dose heparin in prevention of myocardial reinfarction. Lancet 1:937–942, 1987.
218. Neri Serneri GG, Gensini GF, Poggesi L: Effect of heparin, aspirin, or alteplase in reduction of myocardial ischaemia in refractory unstable angina. Lancet 335:615–618, 1990.
219. Nesheim M, Blackburn MN, Lawler CM, Mann KG: Dependence of antithrombin III and thrombin binding stoichiometries and catalytic activity on the molecular weight of affinity purified heparin. J Biol Chem 261:3214–3221, 1986.
220. Neuhoff V, Schill WB, Sternbach H: Microanalysis of pure deoxyribonucleic acid dependent polymerase from *Escherichia coli*. Action of heparin and rifanicin on structure and function. Biochem J 623–631, 1970.
221. Nieduszynski I: General physical properties of heparin. In Lane DA, Lindahl U (eds): Heparin: Chemical and Biological Properties, Clinical Applications. London, Edward Arnold, 1989, pp 51–64.
222. Niewiarowski S, Holt JC: Biochemistry and physiology of secreted platelet proteins. In Colman RW, Hirsh J, Marder VJ, Salzman EW (eds): Hemostasis and Thrombosis. Basic Principles and Clinical Practice, 2nd ed. Philadelphia, J.B. Lippincott, 1987, pp. 618–30.
223. Nordfang O, Bjorn SE, Valentin S, et al: The C-terminus of tissue factor pathway inhibitor is essential to its anticoagulant activity. Biochemistry 30:10371–10376, 1991.
224. Nordfang O, Kristensen HI, Valentin S, et al: The significance of TFPI in clotting assays—comparison and combination with other anticoagulants. Thromb Haemost 70:448–453, 1993.
225. Novotny WF, Girard TJ, Miletich JP, Broze GJ: Platelets secrete a coagulation inhibitor functionally and antigenically similar to the lipoprotein associated coagulation inhibitor. Blood 72:2020–2025, 1988.
226. Novotny WF, Girard TJ, Miletich JP, Broze GJ: Purification and characterization of the lipoprotein-associated coagulation inhibitor from human plasma. J Biol Chem 264:18832–18837, 1989.
227. Novotny WF, Palmier MO, Wun TC, et al: Purification and properties of heparin releasable lipoprotein-associated inhibitor. Blood 78:394–400, 1991.
228. Ockelford PA, Patterson J, Johns AS: A double-blind randomized placebo controlled trial of thromboprophylaxis in major elective general surgery using once daily injections of a low molecular weight heparin fragment (Fragmin). Thromb Haemost 62:1046–1049, 1989.
229. Okajima K, Yang WP, Okabe H, et al: Role of leukocytes in the activation of intravascular coagulation in Patients with septicemia. Am J Hematol 36:265–271, 1991.
230. Okamoto M, Mori S, Endo H: A protective action of chondroitin sulfate proteoglycans against neuronal cell death induced by glutamate. Brain Res 637(1–2):57–67, 1994.
231. Olsen ST, Bjork I: Regulation of thrombin by antithrombin and heparin cofactor II. In Berliner JJ (ed): Thrombin. New York, Plenum Press, 1992, pp 159–217.

232. Olsson P, Lagergren H, Ek S: The elimination from plasma of intravenous heparin: an experimental study on dogs and humans. Acta Med Scand 173:619–623, 1963.

233. Oltersdorf TL, Fritz LC, Schenk DB, et al: The secreted form of the Alzheimer's amyloid precursor protein with the Kunitz domain is protease nexin-II. Nature 341:144–147, 1989.

234. Osterud B, Rapaport SI: Activation of factor IX by the reaction product of tissue factor and factor VII: Additional pathway for initiating blood coagulation. Proc Natl Acad Sci USA 74:5260–5264, 1977.

235. Owen MC, Borg JY, Soria C, et al: Heparin binding effect in a new antithrombin III variant: Rouen 47 Arg to His. Blood 69:1275–1279, 1987.

236. Owen WG: Evidence for the formation of an ester between thrombin and heparin cofactor. Biochim Biophys Acta 405:380–3387, 1975.

237. Owen WG, Esmon CT: Functional properties of an endothelial cell cofactor for thrombin catalyzed activation of protein C J Biol Chem 256:5532–5535, 1981.

238. Packham MA: Role of platelets in thrombosis and hemostasis. Can J Physiol Pharmacol 72:278–284, 1994.

239. Parker KA, Tollefsen DM: The protease specificity of heparin cofactor II. Inhibition of thrombin generated during coagulation. J Biol Chem 260:3501–3503, 1987.

240. Perdue JF, Lubenskyi W, Kivity E, et al: Protease mitogenic response of chick embryo fibroblasts and receptor binding/processing of human a-thrombin. J Biol Chem 256:2767–2776, 1981.

241. Pescador R, Porta R, Mantovani M, et al: Pharmacologic profile of sulfamino-galactosaminoglycans. Semin Thromb Hemost 17(Suppl 2):74–79, 1991.

242. Petersen TE, Dudek-Wojciechowska G, Sottrup-Jensen L, Magnusson S: Primary structure of antithrombin III (heparin cofactor). Partial homology between α_1-antitrypsin and antithrombin III. In Collen D, Winar B, Verstraete M (eds): The Physiological Inhibitors of Coagulation and Fibrinolysis. Amsterdam, Elsevier, 1979, pp 43–54.

243. Peterson CB, Blackburn MN: Antithrombin conformation and the catalytic role of heparin II. Is the heparin-induced conformational change in antithrombin required for rapid inactivation of thrombin? J Biol Chem 262:7559–7566, 1987.

244. Peterson CB, Morgan WT, Blackburn MN: Histidine-rich glycoprotein modulation of the anticoagulant activity of heparin. J Biol Chem 262:7567–7574, 1987.

245. Pezzuoli G, Neri Serneri GG, Settembrini P, et al, for the STEP Study Group: Prophylaxis of fatal pulmonary embolism in general surgery using low-molecular weight heparin CY 216: A multicentre, double-blind, randomized, controlled, clinical trial versus placebo (STEP): STEP Study Group. Int Surg 74:205–210, 1989.

246. Phillips DR, Chaio IF, Scarborough RM: GPIIB/IIIa: The responsive integrin. Cell 65:359–362, 1991.

247. Pischel KD, Bluestein HH, Woods VL: Platelet glycoproteins Ia, Ic, and IIa are physicochemically indistinguishable from the very late activation antigens adhesion related proteins of lymphocytes and other cell types. J Clin Invest 81:505–513, 1988.

248. Pipitone VR: Chondroprotection with chondroitin sulfate. Drugs Exp Clin Res 17:3–7, 1991.

249. Pizzo SV: The physiologic role of antithrombin III as an anticoagulant. Semin Hematol 31(2):4–7, 1994.

250. Planes A, Vochelle N, Mazas F, et al: Prevention of postoperative venous thrombosis: A randomized trial comparing unfractionated heparin with low molecular weight heparin in patients undergoing total hip replacement. Thromb Haemost 60:407–410, 1988.

251. Pletcher CH, Nelsestuen GL: Two-substrate reaction model for the heparin–catalyzed bovine antithrombin protease reaction. J Biol Chem 258:1086–1091, 1983.

252. Prandoni P, Lensing AW, Butler HR, et al: Comparison of subcutaneous low-molecular-weight heparin with intravenous standard heparin in proximal deep-vein thrombosis. Lancet 339:441–445, 1992.

253. Pratt CW, Church FC: Antithrombin: Structure and function. Semin Hematol 28:3–9, 1991.

254. Preissner KT, Muller-Berghaus G: Neutralization and binding of heparin by S-protein/vitronectin in the inhibition of factor Xa by antithrombin III. J Biol Chem 262:12247–12253, 1987.

255. Preissner KT: Anticoagulant potential of endothelial cell membrane components. Haemostasis 18:271–276, 1988.

256. Prins MH, Den Ottolander GJ, Gelsema R, et al: Deep vein thrombosis prophylaxis with a low molecular weight heparin (Kabi 2165) in stroke patients. Thromb Haemost 58(Suppl):117, 1987.

257. Prowchownik EV, Markham AF, Orkin SH: Isolation of a cDNA clone for human antithrombin III. J Biol Chem 258:8389–8394, 1983.

258. Ragg H: A new member of the plasma protease inhibitor gene family. Nucl Acids Res 14:1073–1088, 1986.

259. Rajtar G, Marchim E, deGaetano G, Cerletti C: Effects of glycosaminoglycans on platelet and leukocyte function: role of N-sulfation. Biochem Pharm 46:958–960, 1983.

260. Rao JS, Kahler CB, Baker JB, Festoff BW: Protease nexin 1, a serpin, inhibits plasminogen-dependent degradation of muscle extracellular matrix. Muscle Nerve 12:640–646, 1989.

261. Regan LM, Lamphear BJ, Walker FJ, Fay PJ: Factor IXa protects factor VIIIa from activated protein C: Factor IXa inhibits activated protein C catalyzed cleavage of factor VIIIa at Arg 562. J Biol Chem 269:9445–9452, 1994.

262. Reilly TM, Mousa SA, Seetharam R, Racanelli AL: Recombinant plasminogen activator inhibitor type 1: A review of structural, functional, and biological aspects. Blood Coag Fibrinol 5:73–81, 1994.

263. Robinson HC, Horner AA, Hook M, Ogren S, Lindahl U: A proteoglycan form of heparin and its degradation to single chain molecules. J Biol Chem 253:6687–6693, 1978.

264. Robinson RA, Worfolk L, Tracy PB: Endotoxin enhances expression of monocyte prothrombinase activity. Blood 79:406–416, 1992.

265. Rosen SD, Bertozzi CR: The selectins and their ligands. Curr Opin Cell Biol 6:668–673, 1994.

266. Rosenberg RD, Damus PS: The purification and mechanism of action of human antithrombin-heparin cofactor. J Biol Chem 248:6490–6505, 1973.

267. Rosenberg RD, Lam L: Correlation between structure and function of heparin. Proc Natl Acad Sci USA 76:1218–1222, 1979.

268. Rothberger H, McGee MP: Generation of coagulation factor V activity by cultured rabbit alveolar macrophages. J Exp Med 160:1880–1890, 1984.

269. Sache E, Maillard M, Malazzi P, Bertrand H: Partially N-desulfated heparin: Some physico–chemical and biological properties. Thromb Res 55:247–258, 1989.

270. Salzman EW, Rosenberg RD, Smith MH, et al: Effect of heparin and heparin fractions on platelet aggregation. J Clin Invest 65:64–73, 1980.

271. Sandberg H, Bode AP, Dombrose FA, et al: Expression of coagulant activity in human platelets: release of membranous vesicles providing platelet factor 1 and platelet factor 3. Thromb Res 39:63–79, 1985.

272. Sandset PM, Abildgaard U, Larsen ML: Heparin induces release of extrinsic pathway inhibitor (EPI). Thromb Res 50:803–813, 1988.

273. Schwartz BS, Levy GA, Curtiss LK, et al: Plasma lipoprotein induction and suppression of the generation of cellular procoagulant activity in vitro. Two procoagulant activities are produced by peripheral blood mononuclear cells. J Clin Invest 67:1650–1658, 1981.

274. Scott RW, Eaton DL, Duran N, Baker JB: Regulation of extracellular plasminogen activator by human fibroblasts. The role of protease nexin. J Biol Chem 258:4397–4403, 1983.

275. Scully MF, Kakkar VV: Identification of heparin cofactor II as the principle plasma cofactor for pentosan polysulfate (SP54). Thromb Res 36:187–194, 1984.

276. Scully MF, Ellis V, Kakkar VV: Pentosan polysulfate: activation of heparin cofactor II or antithrombin III according to molecular weight fractionation. Thromb Res 41:489–499, 1986.

277. Scully MF, Ellis V, Seno N, Kakkar VV: The anticoagulant properties of mast cell product chondroitin sulfate Eur Biochem Biophys Res Comm 137:15–22, 1986.

278. Scully MF: The biochemistry of blood clotting: The digestion of a liquid to form a solid. Essays Biochem 27:17–36, 1992.

279. Sealey JE, Gerten JN, Ladingham HG: Inhibition of renin by heparin. J Clin Endocrinol 27:699–705, 1967.

280. Seegers WH, Novoa E, Henry RL, Hassouna HI: Relationship of 'new' vitamin K–dependent protein C and 'old' autoprothrombin II–A. Thromb Res 8:543–552, 1976.

281. Senior RM, Skogen WF, Griffin GL,Wilner GD: Effects of fibrinogen derivatives upon the inflammatory response. J Clin Invest 77:1014–1019, 1986.

282. Shainoff JR, Dardik BN: Fibrinopeptide B and aggregation of fibrinogen. Science 204:200–202, 1979.

283. Shattil SJ, Bennett JS: Platelets and their membranes in hemostasis: Physiology and pathophysiology. Ann Intern Med 94:108–118, 1981.

284. Shavit R, Kahn A, Wilner G, Fenton JW: Monocyte chemotaxis. Sheffield, WP, Brothers AB, Wells MJ, et al:Molecular cloning and expression of rabbit antithrombin III. Blood 79:2330–2339, 1992.

285. Sheehan JP, Tollefsen JP, Sadler JE: Heparin cofactor II is regulated allosterically and not primarily by template effects. Studies with mutant thrombins and glycosaminoglycans. J Biol Chem 269:32747–3251, 1994.

286. Shen L, Dahlback B: Factor V and protein C as synergistic cofactors to activated protein C in degradation of factor VIIIa. J Biol Chem 269:18735–18738, 1994.

287. Shore JD, Olson ST, Craig PA, et al: Kinetics of heparin action. Ann N Y Acad Sci 556:75–80, 1989.

288. Sie P, DuPouy D, Pichon J, Boneu B: Constitutional heparin cofactor II deficiency associated with recurrent thrombosis. Lancet 2:414–416, 1985.

289. Siess W: Molecular mechanisms of platelet activation. Physiol Rev 69:58–178, 1989.

290. Sims PJ, Wiedmer T, Esmon CT, et al: Assembly of the platelet prothrombinase complex is linked to vesiculation of the platelet plasma membrane. J Biol Chem 264:17049–17057, 1989.

291. Sinha S, Dovey HF, Seubert P, et al: The protease inhibitory properties of the Alzheimer's β-amyloid precursor protein. J Biol Chem 265:8983–8985, 1990.

292. Smith RP, Higuchi DA, Broze GJ: Platelet coagulation factor XIa-inhibitor, a form of Alzheimer amyloid precursor protein. Science 248:1126–1128, 1990.

293. Sobel M, McNeill PM, Carlson PL, et al: Heparin inhibition of von Willebrand factor-dependent platelet function in vitro and in vivo. J Clin Invest 87:1787–1793, 1991.

294. Soker S, Goldstaub D, Svahn CM, et al: Variations in the size and sulfation of heparin modulate the effect of heparin on the binding of VEGF165 to its receptors. Biochem Biophys Res Comm 203:1339–1347, 1994.

295. Solymoss S, Tucker MM, Tracy PB: Kinetics of inactivation of membrane-bound factor V by activated protein C. J Biol Chem 263:14884–14890, 1988.
296. Sprecher CA, Kisiel W, Mathewes S, Foster D: Molecular cloning, expression, and partial characterization of a second human tissue factor pathway inhibitor. Proc Natl Acad Sci USA 91:3353–3357, 1994.
297. Staatz WD, Rajpara SM, Wayner EA, et al: The membrane glycoprotein Ia-IIa (VLA–2) complex mediates the Mg^{++} dependent adhesion of platelets to collagen. J Cell Biol 108:1917–1924, 1983.
298. Stackhouse R, Chandra T, et al: Purification of antithrombin III mRNA and cloning of its cDNA. J Biol Chem 258:703–706, 1983.
299. Stenflo J: A new vitamin K-dependent protein. J Biol Chem 251:355–363, 1976.
300. Stephens AW, Thalley BS, Hirs CHW: Antithrombin III Denver: A reactive site variant. J Biol Chem 262:1044–1048, 1987.
301. Takada Y, Strominger JL, Hemler ME: The very late antigen family of heterodimers is part of a superfamily of molecules in adhesion and embryogenesis. Proc Natl Acad Sci USA 84:3239–3243, 1987.
302. Theroux P, Ouimet H, McCans J: Aspirin, heparin, or both to treat acute unstable angina. N Engl J Med 319:1105–1111, 1988.
303. Theroux P, Waters D, Lam J, et al: Reactivation of unstable angina after the discontinuation of heparin. N Engl J Med 327:141–145, 1992.
304. Thomson C, Forbes CD, Prentice CRM: The potentiation of platelet aggregation and adhesion by heparin in vitro and in vivo. Clin Sci Mol Med 45:485–494, 1973.
305. Tilly RHJ, Senden JMG, Comfurius P, et al: Increased aminophospholipid translocase activity in human platelets during secretion. Biochim Biophys Acta 1029:188–190, 1990.
306. Tollefsen DM, Blank MK: Detection of a new heparin dependent inhibitor of thrombin in human plasma. J Clin Invest. 68:589–596, 1981.
307. Tollefsen DM, Majerus DW, Blank MK: Heparin cofactor II. Purification and properties of a heparin dependent inhibitor of thrombin in human plasma. J Biol Chem 257:2162–2169, 1982.
308. Tollefsen DM, Pestka CA: Heparin cofactor II activity in patients with disseminated intravascular coagulation and heart failure. Blood 66:769–774, 1985.
309. Tollefsen DM, Peacock ME, Monafo WJ: Molecular size of dermatan sulfate oligosaccharides required to bind and activate heparin cofactor II. J Biol Chem 261:8854–8858, 1986.
310. Tollefsen DM: Heparin cofactor II. In Lane DA, Lindahl U (eds): Heparin: Chemical and Biological Properties, Clinical Applications. London, Edward Arnold, 1989, pp 257–274.
311. Tracy PB, Rorhbach MS, Mann KG: Functional prothrombinase complex assembly on isolated monocytes and lymphocytes. J Biol Chem 258:7264–7267, 1983.
312. Tracy PB, Eide LL, Mann KG: Human prothrombinase complex assembly and function on isolated peripheral blood cell populations. J Biol Chem 260:2119–2124, 1985.
313. Tracy PB, Nesheim ME, Mann KG: Platelet factor Xa receptor. Meth Enzymol 215:329–360, 1992.
314. Tran TH, Marbet GA, Duckert F: Association of hereditary heparin cofactor II deficiency with thrombosis. Lancet ii:413–414, 1985.
315. Tran TH, Lammle B, Zbinden B, Duckert F: Heparin cofactor II: purification and antibody production. Thromb Haemost 55:19–23, 1986.
316. Travis J, Salvesen GS: Human plasma proteinase inhibitors. Annu Rev Biochem 52:655–709, 1983.
317. Turpie AG, Levine MN, Hirsh J, et al: Double-blind randomized trial of Org 10172 low-molecular-weight heparinoid in the prevention of deep-vein thrombosis in thrombotic stroke. Lancet 1:523–526, 1987.
318. Turpie AGG, Robinson JG, Doyle DJ, et al: Comparison of high–dose with low–dose subcutaneous heparin to prevent left ventricular mural thrombosis in patients with acute transmural anterior myocardial infarction. N Engl J Med 320:352–394, 1989.
319. Tuszynski GP, Gasic TB, Gasic GJ: Isolation and characterization of antistasin. An inhibitor of metastasis and coagulation. J Biol Chem 262:9718–9723, 1987.
320. Vaheri A: Heparin and related polyanionic substances as virus inhibitors. Acta Pathol Micro Scand 171:7, 1964.
321. Valentin S, Ostergaard P, Kristensen H, Nordfang O: Simultaneous presence of tissue factor pathway inhibitor (TFPI) and low molecular weight heparin has a synergistic effect in different coagulation assays. Blood Coag Fibrinol 2:629:35, 1991.
322. Van Nostrand WE, Wagner SL, Suzuki M, et al: Protease nexin-II, a potent antichymotrypsin, shows identity to amyloid ß-protein precursor. Nature 341:546–549, 1989.
323. Van Nostrand WE, Schmaier AH, Farrow JS, Cunningham DD: Protease nexin-II (amyloid β-protein precursor): A platelet α granule protein. Science 248:745–748, 1990.
324. Van Nostrand WE, Wagner SL, Farrow JS, Cunningham DD: Immunopurification and protease inhibitory properties of protease nexin-2/amyloid ß-protein precursor. J Biol Chem 265:9591–9594, 1990.
325. Van Nostrand WE, Schmaier AH, Farrow JS, et al: Protease nexin-2 [amyloid β-protein precursor] is a platelet-specific protein in blood. Biochem Biophys Res Comm 175:15–21, 1991.
326. Van Nostrand WE, Schmaier AH, Farrow JS, Cunningham DD: Platelet protease nexin-2/amyloid β-protein precursor; possible pathologic and physiologic functions. Ann N Y Acad Sci 640:140–144, 1991.

327. Van Nostrand WE, Schmaier AH, Wagner SL: Potential role of protease nexin-2/amyloid ß-protein precursor as a cerebral anticoagulant. Ann NY Acad Sci USA 674:243–252, 1992.
328. Villanueva G, Danishefsky I: Conformational changes accompanying the binding of antithrombin III to thrombin. Biochemistry 18:810–817, 1979.
329. Vogel R, Welzel D, Bacher P, Wolf H: Die klinisch-pharmakologische Differenzierung von niedermolekularen Heparinen unter besonderer Berucksichtigung des Tissue Factor Pathway Inhibitor. Ph.D. Dissertation, Instituts fur Pharmazie der Universitat, Renensburg, 1995.
330. Wakefield TW, Greenfield LJ, Rolfe MW, et al: Inflammatory and procoagulant mediator interaction in an experimental baboon model of venous thrombosis. Thromb Haemost 69:164–172, 1993.
331. Walker FJ: Protein S and the regulation of activated protein C. Semin Thromb Hemost 10:131–138, 1984.
332. Walker FJ, Fay PJ: Regulation of blood coagulation by the protein C system. FASEB J 6(8):2561–2567, 1992.
333. Warn-Cramer BJ, Maki SL: Purification of tissue factor pathway inhibitor (TFPI) from rabbit plasma and characterization of its differences from TFPI isolated from human plasma. Thromb Res 67:367–383, 1992.
334. Warn-Cramer BJ, Maki SL, Rapaport SI: Heparin-releasable and platelet pools of tissue factor pathway inhibitor on rabbits. Thromb Haemost 69:221–226, 1993.
335. Warn-Cramer BJ, Rapaport SI: Studies of factor Xa/phospholipid induced intravascular coagulation on rabbits. Effects of immunodepletion of tissue factor pathway inhibitor. Arterioscler Thromb 13:1551–1557, 1993.
336. Warr TA, Warn-Cramer BJ, Rao L, Rapaport SI: Human plasma extrinsic pathway inhibitor activity. I: Standardization of assay and evaluation of physiological variables. Blood 74:201–206, 1989.
337. Weisberg LJ, Shin DT, Conkling PR: Identification of normal human peripheral blood monocytes and liver as sites of synthesis of coagulation factor XIII alpha chain. Blood 70:579–582, 1987.
338. Wesselschmidt R, Likert K, Girard T, et al: Tissue factor pathway inhibitor: the carboxy-terminus is required for optimal inhibition of factor Xa. Blood 79:2004–2010, 1992.
339. Wiedmer T, Esmon CT, Sims PJ: Complement proteins C5b-9 stimulate procoagulant activity through platelet prothrombinase. Blood 68:875–880, 1986.
340. Wun TC, Kretzmer KK, Girard TJ, et al: Cloning and characterization of a cDNA coding for the lipoprotein-associated coagulation inhibitor shows that it consists of three tandem Kunitz-type inhibitory domains. J Biol Chem 263:6001–6004, 1988.
341. Wun TC: Lipoprotein associated coagulation inhibitor (LACI) is a cofactor for heparin: Synergistic actor between LACI and sulfated polysaccharides. Blood 79:430–438, 1992.
342. Wunderwald P, Schrenk WJ, Port H: Antithrombin BM from human plasma: and antithrombin binding moderately to heparin. Thromb Res 25:177–191, 1982.
343. Yamagishi R, Niwa M, Knodo S, et al: Purification and biological property of heparin cofactor II: activation of heparin cofactor II and antithrombin III by dextran sulfate and various glycosaminoglycans. Thromb Res 36:633–642, 1984.
344. Ye J, Esmon NL, Esmon CT, Johnson AE: The active site of thrombin is altered upon binding to thrombocholine. Two distinct structural changes detected by fluorescence, but only one correlates with protein C activation. J Biol Chem 266:23016–23021, 1991.
345. Zahedi K, Prada AE, Davis AE: Structure and regulation of the C1 inhibitor gene. Behr Inst Mitteil 93:115–119, 1993.
346. Zammit A, Dawes J: Low-affinity material does not contribute to the antithrombotic activity of Orgaran (ORG 10172) in human plasma. ThrombHaemost 71:759–767, 1994.
347. Zimrin AB, Eisman R, Vilaire G, et al: Structure of platelet glycoprotein IIIa. A common subunit for two different membrane receptors. J Clin Invest 81:1470–1475, 1988.
348. Zucker MB: Biological aspects of heparin action: heparin and platelet function. Fed Proc 36:47–49, 1977.
349. Zwaal RFA, Bevers EM, Comfurius P, et al: Loss of membrane phospholipid asymmetry during activation of blood platelets and sickled red cells; mechanisms and physiological significance. Mol Cell Biochem 91:23–31, 1989.

CHAPTER 3

Inhibition of Platelet Function by Heparin

LINDSAY C. H. JOHN, B.Sc. (HONS), M.S., FRCS

Heparin has a multitude of clinical applications, but the universal underlying indication for its use is the prevention of thrombosis. It does so by its well-recognized anticoagulant activity, mediated principally through the action of antithrombin III. Although heparin is associated with a number of possible side effects, including hypersensitivity, skin necrosis, alopecia, hypoaldosteronism, and osteoporosis, the most common complication is hemorrhage. A common view is that the risk of hemorrhage is not associated with the anticoagulant action of heparin but instead with impairment of platelet function. Experimental evidence that heparin has an effect on platelet function is considerable.

METHODS FOR ASSESSING THE EFFECT OF HEPARIN ON PLATELET FUNCTION

Platelet Aggregometry

The two techniques of platelet aggregometry are optical and whole blood. Probably the most extensively used in vitro test of platelet function is optical aggregometry, which was first described over 30 years ago.[9] This technique assesses platelet clump formation in response to a stimulus by measuring changes in light transmission through platelet-rich plasma (PRP). The limitations of optical aggregometry include (1) the need for centrifugation to produce PRP, which reduces the number of larger, functionally more active platelets[68] and is associated with the synthesis and release of thromboxane;[19] (2) the requirement of at least 30 minutes for sample preparation time, which results in a variable response on aggregation by labile modulators such as thromboxane A_2 and prostacyclin;[74] and (3) the absence of white and red blood cells, both of which may be relevant for in vivo platelet function.[17,56,59] Whole blood aggregometry was developed to reduce some of the limitations of optical aggregometry[15] and measures changes in electrical impedance to assess platelet aggregation. It, too, has its limitations. Anticoagulation, which is necessary for both types of aggregometry, is known to influence platelet function. Citrate, the most commonly used anticoagulant in aggregometry studies, produces a nonphysiologic environment by lowering the calcium ion concentration.[53]

Both optical and whole blood platelet aggregometry have resulted in numerous reports of a significant effect of heparin on platelet function. Observations have varied widely. According to many reports, heparin promotes aggregation, both with the addition of agonists[58,67] and without (i.e., spontaneous aggregation).[11,18,20,61] However, a substantial number of reports indicate that heparin inhibits platelet aggregation.[23,41,65,66] A possible reason for this disparity may be related to the intrinsic disadvantages of platelet aggregometry as well as methodologic differences, including variations in platelet system, instrumentation, time of monitoring for aggregation, and type and dose of heparin preparation.[11] An alternative explanation may be individual variation in the effect of heparin on platelet function.

Measurement of Platelet Release Products

Platelet release reactions depend on the strength of the stimulus. Type I reactions are induced by weak, soluble agonists such as adenosine diphosphate (ADP) or adrenaline and involve the release of dense and α-granule products (e.g., platelet factor 4 [PF4] and α-thromboglobulin). Type II reactions are induced by strong agonists such as thrombin and result in lysosomal granule release products. Activation of platelets by heparin has been demonstrated by reports of release of PF4, α-thromboglobulin,[22] and serotonin[39] after heparin administration.

Platelet Morphology

The use of heparin has been reported to increase the number and length of platelet cytoplasmic processes,[43] indicating a direct effect by heparin on platelets.

Bleeding Time

Skin bleeding time (BT) is a test of platelet function that clinically correlates with "platelet-mediated bleeding"[44] and gives a measure of qualitative platelet dysfunction. Reports of an effect on BT measurements by heparin date from shortly after its first clinical use. In one review article,[33] 23 references were quoted on the subject between 1936 and 1958. Early reports noted either no prolongation, slight prolongation, or prolongation of the BT in some individuals. A number of more recent reports have also noted a prolongation of BT after heparin administration.[10,28,29,40,50,62] An interesting finding noted by some of these reports was the wide individual variation in the response of BT to heparin. In one study[28] a single dose of 100 U/kg of bovine lung-derived heparin was given intravenously to 34 normal volunteers. Ten minutes after injection the BT was prolonged beyond the normal range of 9 minutes in 43%; a change of 1 minute or less was reported in 43%; and bleeding continued at 20 minutes in 15%. In another study that measured BT 15 minutes after a bolus dose of 5,000 U of heparin,[40] some degree of prolongation was found in one-third of individuals, with marked prolongation in a few. It has been suggested that this variable sensitivity to the antiplatelet effects of heparin may indicate a major risk factor for hemorrhagic complications.[29]

Hemostatometry

The hemostatometer is a relatively recent innovation in assessing platelet function.[42,55] It aims at providing a more physiologic measure of platelet function than the alternatives by using flowing, nonanticoagulated blood with minimal damage to its cellular contents. In this technique, 2.5 ml of nonanticoagulated blood is perfused through polyethylene tubing by paraffin oil displacement, a method that has been shown to cause no measurable platelet damage. Holes are punched through the tubing, resulting in "bleeding" and a pressure drop. The pattern of the pressure recovery reflects the formation of hemostatic plugs in the holes. A typical "hemostasis curve" is shown in Figure 1. The initial recovery of the pressure represents platelet plug formation due to activation of platelets by shear stress and the release of ADP from the shear-damaged platelets and red blood cells. The later recovery is due to stabilization of the platelet plug secondary to thrombin generation, the subsequent increase in platelet aggregation, and the formation of fibrin so that it can resist the increasing pressure. The hemostasis curve is recorded and its area analyzed as H. The greater the value of H, the greater the inhibition of platelet function.

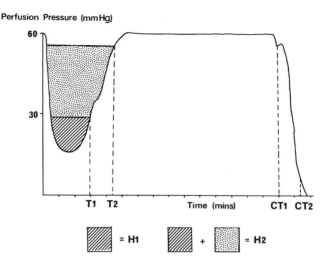

FIGURE 1. A typical hemostasis curve. The curve is a measure of the pressure against time from the initial bleed in the hemostatometer until the blood eventually clots. The area of the initial curve (shaded) gives a measure of the platelet function. (See text, where curve area is referred to as H).

Hemostatometry has been used to assess the effect of heparin on platelet function in cardiac surgical patients.[36] In a series of 290 patients, hemostasis curves were measured in vitro during the week before cardiac surgery, using a heparin concentration comparable to that required for cardiopulmonary bypass. A wide variation in the effect was noted (Fig. 2): 9% showed a proaggregatory effect (that is, the hemostasis curve was narrower with than without heparin; 59% showed a mild-to-moderate inhibition of platelet function in the presence of heparin (defined as a prolongation of the relevant hemostatometric parameter between 1–10 times that of a baseline sample without heparin); and 32% showed severe inhibition of platelet function (defined as a prolongation of the relevant hemostatometric parameter to > 10 times the baseline value). Representative examples of hemostatometric curves are shown in Figure 3.

ETIOLOGY FOR THE EFFECT OF HEPARIN ON PLATELET FUNCTION

Suggested etiologies for the effect of heparin on platelet function include the following:

1. Destabilization of platelet aggregates by impaired fibrin formation resulting from its anticoagulant action.[4]

2. Interaction between heparin and the platelet membrane leads to "perturbation" and internal calcium release.[12] Related to this suggestion is the evidence that heparin binds directly to platelets. A membrane-associated binding site for heparin was suggested by the isolation of a platelet membrane fraction that had "antiheparin activity."[51] In addition, platelets have been shown to bind with tritium-labelled heparin.[63] In one study using tritium-labeled heparin and different concentrations of unlabeled heparin to examine the binding of porcine heparin to platelets,[34] binding was shown to be readily reversible and included both saturable and unsaturable components. It has been suggested that electrostatic interaction is the dominant factor allowing binding between heparin and platelets.[64] Sulphate groups appear to be more important than carboxyl, if only because of a greater charge density. Molecular weight also may be important, because larger molecules present more negatively charged areas for binding. There are many potential candidates for a heparin-platelet binding site. Platelets contain a number of heparin-binding proteins, including thrombospondin,[1] platelet factor 4 (PF4),[14] von Willebrand factor (VWF), and fibronectin.[25]

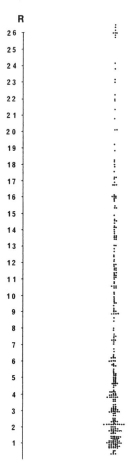

FIGURE 2. The variation in the effect of heparin on platelet function in 290 cardiac surgical patients as measured by hemostatometry. R refers to the ratio of the area of the hemostasis curves using blood with and without heparin. The greater the value of R, the greater the degree of platelet inhibition by heparin. A value less than 1 represents a proaggregatory effect. (From John LCH, Rees G, Kovacs I: Inhibition of platelet function by heparin. An aetiological factor in post bypass hemorrhage. J Thorac Cardiovasc Surg 105:816–822, 1993, with permission.)

All are secreted by platelets and then attach to the cell exterior. The platelet membrane surface receptor glycoprotein (GP) Ib has also been identified as a possible heparin-binding site by using affinity chromatography.[24,73] In addition, platelet α-adrenoreceptors have been suggested as a potential site.[72] However, many reports dispute the relevance of most of these potential binding sites. All of the heparin-binding proteins depend largely on divalent cations. The observation of the lack of importance of calcium ions for heparin-binding to platelets[35] makes them unlikely candidates. Specific monoclonal antibodies directed against GP Ia/IIa, IIb/IIIa ,and IV did not appear to affect the binding of radiolabeled heparin; thus they, too, are unlikely candidates. It has therefore been suggested[35] that heparin may bind directly to platelets without an intermediate receptor, possibly to a nonproteinaceous site or to a membrane protein protected from extracellular proteases by a carbohydrate or lipid.

The possibility that the direct binding of heparin to platelets may be related to its effect on platelet function is supported by the observation that aprotinin appears both to reduce inhibition of platelet function by heparin, as measured in vitro by hemostatometry, and to reduce significantly the binding of tritiumlabeled heparin to activated and nonactivated platelets.[38]

Impaired Function of von Willebrand Factor

Impairment of VWF function was first suggested from observations made during cardiopulmonary bypass.[54] VWF plays several crucial roles in platelet-mediated hemostasis.

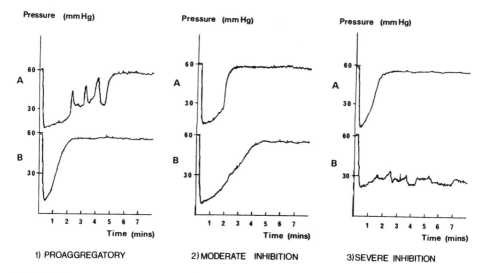

FIGURE 3. Examples of hemostasis curves showing the variation of the effect of heparin on platelet function. The curves labeled *A* are for blood without heparin; those labeled *B* are for corresponding samples with heparin added. The first pair demonstrates a proaggregatory effect, the second a moderate inhibition of platelet function, and the third a severe inhibition of platelet function by heparin. (From John LCH, Rees G, Kovacs I: Inhibition of platelet function by heparin. An aetiological factor in post bypass hemorrhage. J Thorac Cardiovasc Surg 105:816–822, 1993, with permission.)

Impairment of VWF after heparinization for cardiopulmonary bypass has been demonstrated;[65] the impairment related closely to plasma levels of heparin and not VWF. It has been suggested that this impairment may be related to heparin's interference with platelet adhesion to collagen.[49]

Lipase Release

A highly significant correlation between increased BT and lipase release has been demonstrated in a rabbit model in association with heparin.[6] One of the lipases, hepatic triglyceride lipase (HTLG), has a known anticoagulant effect.[5,26] It is also possible that lipases directly affect platelet function.

SIGNIFICANCE OF THE EFFECT OF HEPARIN ON PLATELET FUNCTION

The reported incidence of hemorrhage after clinical use of heparin varies between 1%[60] and 32%.[48] In a pooled analysis of randomized trials comparing different methods of heparin administration, the reported average incidence of major bleeding was 6.8% when heparin was given continuously and 14.2% with intermittent injection.[32] A number of factors may increase the risk of hemorrhage, including concurrent illness or recent surgery,[46] chronic heavy alcohol consumption,[70] concomitant use of aspirin,[75] and old age.[46] Serious bleeding may occur despite satisfactory monitoring and control of the anticoagulant effect.[60] In one prospective study,[7] activated partial thromboplastin time (APTT), which is widely used to monitor heparin treatment, failed to predict the excessive bleeding that occurred in 19 of 234 patients receiving heparin. The most common view is that the risk of bleeding is related to heparin-induced interference with platelet function[31,45,52] rather than to heparin's anticoagulant activity. As discussed above, considerable experimental evidence suggests a heparin-related effect on platelet function.

Although the absence of a relationship between measured parameters of the degree of anticoagulation and the risk of hemorrhage suggests that inhibition of platelet function

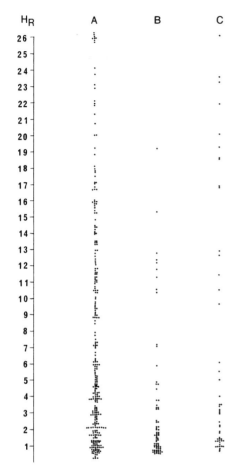

FIGURE 4.   The variation in the effect of different anticoagulants on platelet function as measured by hemostatometry (H_R corresponds to the parameter R of Figure 3; the greater its value, the greater the degree of platelet inhibition). Results labeled A are with unfractionated heparin (n = 290); those labeled B are with a low-molecular-weight heparin added (n = 74), and those labeled C are with hirudin added (n = 50). (From John LCH, Rees G, Kovacs I: Different anticoagulants and platelet reactivity in cardiac surgical patients. Ann Thorac Surg 56:899–902, 1993, with permission).

may be the relevant etiology, direct evidence has not been commonly reported. In a prospective study of the effect of a single intravenous dose of 100 U/kg of bovine lung-derived heparin on 34 normal volunteers, 15% were observed to have a BT > 20 minutes.[28] This study also reported the case of a patient who bled significantly on two occasions while receiving intravenous heparin. Two years later when the patient was readmitted, BT was markedly prolonged after intravenous heparin.[29] This case led the authors to suggest that variable sensitivity to the antiplatelet effects of heparin may indicate a major risk factor for hemorrhagic complications that is currently unappreciated and thus unmonitored.

A number of consequences of cardiopulmonary bypass (CPB) may potentially be involved in the cause of nonsurgical bleeding, including decreased platelet count, impairment of platelet function, hyperfibrinolysis, consumption of coagulation factors, changes in red cell deformability, inadequate heparin neutralization, and heparin rebound. The majority of reports, however, conclude that an acquired platelet dysfunction is the major cause of hemorrhage after CPB. Of particular relevance to the use of heparin in cardiovascular patients is a study attempting to relate the degree of inhibition of platelet function by heparin and the risk of bleeding after CPB.[36] The effect of heparin on platelet function was measured in vitro in 111 cardiac surgical patients by preoperative hemostatometry. As described above, this effect was measured by taking the ratio of the areas of the hemostasis curve of blood with and without heparin (R). This measure of the degree of platelet inhibition correlated significantly with total postoperative blood loss ($p < 0.0001$; $0.4 < r < 0.52$). A value of R

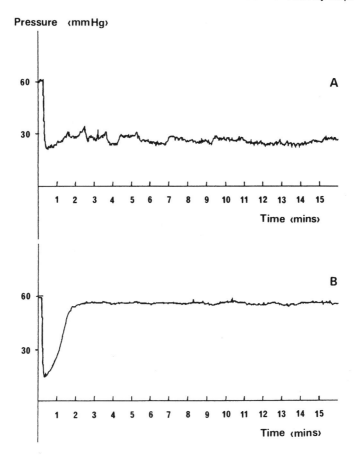

FIGURE 5.   Hemostasis curves demonstrating a reduction of heparin-induced platelet inhibition in the presence of aprotinin. Curve A shows the effect when heparin is added to blood in an individual who demonstrates severe platelet inhibition with heparin. Curve B shows the effect of adding aprotinin as well as heparin to blood from the same patient as for curve A. (From John LCH, Rees G, Kovacs I: Reduction of heparin binding to and inhibition of platelets by aprotinin. Ann Thorac Surg 55:1175–1179, 1993, with permission.)

between 1–10 was defined as demonstrating mild-to-moderate inhibition of platelet function, whereas a value > 10 was defined as demonstrating severe inhibition. Again, the difference in postoperative blood loss was highly significant: 713 ± 43 ml in the group with mild-to-moderate platelet inhibition vs. 1172 ± 76 ml ($p < 0.0001$) in the group with severe inhibition, as measured 18 hours postoperatively. It was concluded that platelet inhibition as a result of heparin is a previously unrecognized etiologic factor in bleeding after CPB.

POTENTIAL FUTURE DEVELOPMENTS

Alternative Anticoagulants

If the risk of hemorrhage as a complication of the use of heparin is related to an associated inhibition of platelet function, an obvious approach to reducing this risk is to use alternative anticoagulants that may have less effect on platelet function.

A number of platelet aggregation studies have suggested that certain low-molecular-weight heparin (LMWH) fractions may affect platelet function less than unfractionated heparin (UFH).[3,30,71] In rats LMWH may prolong BT to a lesser extent than UFH.[2] Animal studies have also suggested that certain LMWH fractions may cause less of a bleeding tendency than UFH.[13,16,21,47]

Another anticoagulant proposed as an alternative to UFH for cardiopulmonary bypass is hirudin.[69] The authors reported that in a canine bypass model hirudin caused a significantly smaller increase in BT than heparin, suggesting less platelet inhibition. Also of relevance to cardiovascular patients was a study comparing the degree of platelet inhibition by UFH, LMWH, and hirudin as tested in vitro by hemostatometry of blood from cardiac surgical patients.[37] The relative proportions of patients exhibiting enhanced platelet reactivity, mild-to-moderate platelet inhibition, and severe platelet inhibition, respectively, were 8.6%, 58.6%, and 32.8% for unfractionated heparin; 22%, 66%, and 12% for an LMWH (H-5640, Sigma, St. Louis, MO); and 6%, 66%, and 28% for hirudin (Fig. 4). At the concentrations examined, a significantly greater proportion ($p < 0.01$) of patients exhibited enhanced platelet reactivity, and a significantly smaller proportion ($p < 0.01$) showed severely inhibited platelet reactivity associated with LMWH vs. UFH. There was no significant difference between the patients treated with hirudin and UFH. Although the relevance of this study is limited because the clinically appropriate concentrations of the alternative anticoagulants and the comparative doses are unknown, it was inferred that LMWH may reduce the blood loss associated with CPB.

Prediction and Prevention of the Risks of Hemorrhage Secondary to Inhibition of Platelet Function by Heparin

A common finding among various methods for assessing platelet function is wide individual variation in the effect of heparin. Evidence suggests that individuals who demonstrate severe inhibition of platelet function with heparin are at greater risk of hemorrhagic complication.[29,36] Although the technique of hemostatometry is not widely available, it has demonstrated the possibility of predicting preoperatively which individuals are more likely to bleed after CPB as a result of severe inhibition of platelet function by heparin. It may be possible in the future to identify patients in whom alternative anticoagulants may be advantageous or in whom agents such as aprotinin may be indicated. Aprotinin, a protease inhibitor, has clearly been shown to reduce hemorrhage after CPB.[8,27,57] Aprotinin appears to reduce inhibition of platelet function by heparin, as measured by hemostatometry[38] (Fig. 5). In addition, aprotinin significantly reduces the binding of tritium-labeled heparin to both nonactivated and activated platelets. Interference with heparin-induced inhibition of platelet function by aprotinin may be one of its hemostatic actions in cardiac surgery, probably because aprotinin reduces the binding of heparin to platelets.

CONCLUSIONS

1. A number of different methods have demonstrated an effect of heparin on platelet function.

2. The effects appear to vary widely among individuals.

3. Individuals who demonstrate severe inhibition of platelet function with heparin appear more likely to have a greater blood loss after CPB. They also may be more likely to suffer from bleeding as a complication of heparin use in other clinical situations.

4. The etiology for heparin's effect on platelet function is unknown, but suggestions include (1) direct binding of heparin to platelets, (2) the anticoagulant effect of heparin, (3) inhibition of VWF function, and (4) lipase release.

5. Alternative anticoagulants may have different effects on platelet function, and it is possible that some may reduce the risk of bleeding.

6. Aprotinin may reduce inhibition of platelet function by heparin, and its prophylactic use may be indicated if at-risk individuals can be identified.

REFERENCES

1. Aiken ML Ginsberg MH, Plow EF: Divalent cation dependent and independent surface expression of thrombospondin on thrombin-stimulated human platelets. Blood 69:58, 1987.
2. Andrinoli G, Mastacchi R, Barbanti M, Sarret M: Comparison of the antithrombotic and haemorrhagic effects of heparin and a new low molecular weight heparin in rats. Haemostasis 15:324–230, 1985.
3. Barradas MA, Mikhailidis DP, Epemolu E, et al: Comparison of the platelet proaggregatory effect of conventional heparin and a low molecular weight fraction (CY222). Br J Haematol 67:451–457, 1987.
4. Barrett PA, Butler KD, Page CP, et al: Inhibition by heparin of platelet accumulation in vivo. Thromb Haemost 51:366–370, 1984.
5. Barrowcliffe TW, Gray E, Merton RE, et al: Anticoagulant activities of pentosan polysulphate (hemoclar) due to release of hepatic triglyceride lipase (HTGL). Thromb Haemost 56:202–206, 1986.
6. Barrowcliffe TW, Merton RE, Gray ME, Thomas DP: Heparin and bleeding : An association with lipase release. Thromb Haemost 60:434–436, 1988.
7. Basu D, Gallus A, Hirsh J, Cade J: A prospective study of the value of monitoring heparin treatment with the activated partial thromboplastin time. N Engl J Med 287:324–327, 1972.
8. Bidstrup BP, Royston D, Sapsford RN, Taylor KM: Reduction in blood loss and blood use after cardiopulmonary bypass with high dose aprotinin (Trasylol). J Thorac Cardiovasc Surg 97:364–372, 1989.
9. Born GVR: Aggregation of blood platelets by adenosine phosphate and its reversal. Nature 194:927–929, 1962.
10. Borowski A, Lauri D, Maggi A, et al: Impairment of primary haemostasis by low molecular weight heparins in rats. Br J Haematol 68:339–344, 1988.
11. Brace LD, Fareed J: An objective assessment of the interaction of heparin and its fractions with human platelets. Semin Thromb Hemost 11:190–198, 1985.
12. Brace LD, Issleib S, Fareed J: Heparin-induced platelet aggregation is inhibited by antagonists of the thromboxane pathway. Thromb Res 39:533–539, 1985.
13. Cade JF, Buchanan MR, Boneu B, et al: A comparison of the antithrombotic and haemorrhagic effects of low molecular weight heparin fractions: The influence of the method of preparation. Thromb Res 35:613–625, 1984.
14. Capitanio AM, Niewiarowski S, Rucinski B, et al: Interaction of platelet factor 4 with human platelets. Biochim Biophys Acta 839:161–173, 1985.
15. Cardinal DC, Flower RJ: The electronic aggregometer. A novel device for assessing platelet behaviour in blood. J Pharmacol Methods 3:135–158, 1980.
16. Carter CJ, Kelton JG, Hirsh J, et al: The relationship between the haemorrhagic and antithrombotic properties of low molecular weight heparin in rabbits. Blood 59:1239–1245, 1982.
17. Chignard M, Selak MA, Smith JB: Direct evidence for the existence of a neutrophil-derived platelet activator (Neutrophilin). Proc Natl Acad Sci USA 83:8609–8613, 1986.
18. Chong BH, Ismail F: The mechanism of heparin-induced platelet aggregation. Eur J Haematol 43:245–251, 1989.
19. Day HJ, Rao AK: Evaluation of platelet function. Semin Hematol 23:89–101, 1986.
20. Eika C: On the mechanism of platelet aggregation induced by heparin, protamine and polybrene. Scand J Haematol 9:248–257, 1972.
21. Esquivel CO, Bergqvist D, Bjork CG, Nilsson B: Comparison between commercial heparin, low molecular weight heparin and pentosan polysulfate on hemostasis and platelets in vivo. Thromb Res 28:389–399, 1982.
22. Flicker W, Milthorpe BK, Schindhelm K, et al: Platelet factor release following heparin administration and during extracorporeal circulation. Trans Am Soc Artif Intern Organs 28:431–435, 1982.
23. Giolami A, De Marcoh V, Virgolini L, et al: The effect of heparin on platelet aggregation by common inductors and ristocetin in congenital bleeding disorders due to factor VIII or fibrinogen defects. Blut 31:219–226, 1975.
24. Gogstad GO, Solum NO, Krutnes MB: Heparin-binding platelet proteins demonstrated by crossed affinity immunoelectrophoresis. Br J Haematol 53:563–573, 1983.
25. Gold LI, Frangione B, Pearlstein E: Biochemical and immunological characterisation of 3 binding sites on human plasma fibronectin with different affinities for heparin. Biochemistry 22:4113, 1983.
26. Gray E, Bengtsson-Olivecrona G, Olivecrona T, Barrowcliffe TW: Anti Xa activity of human hepatic triglyceride lipase. J Lab Clin Med 109:653–659, 1987.
27. Havel M, Teufelsbauer H, Knobl P, et al: Effect of intraoperative aprotinin administration on post operative bleeding in patients undergoing cardiopulmonary bypass operation. J Thorac Cardiovasc Surg 101:968–972, 1991.
28. Heiden D, Mielke CH, Rodvien R: Impairment by heparin of primary haemostasis and platelet (C14) 5-hydroxytryptamine release. Br J Haematol 36:427–436, 1977.
29. Heiden D, Rodvien R, Mielke CH: Heparin bleeding due to qualitative platelet dysfunction. Angiology 30:645–648, 1979.
30. Heinrich D, Gorg T, Schulz M: Effects of unfractionated and fractionated heparin on platelet function. Haemostasis 18(Suppl 3):48–54, 1988.
31. Hirsh J, Ofosu F, Buchanan M: Rationale behind the development of low molecular weight heparin derivatives. Semin Thromb Hemost 11:13–16, 1985.

32. Hirsh J: Heparin. N Engl J Med 324:1565–1574, 1991.
33. Hjort PF, Borchgrevink CF, Iverson OH, Stormorken H: The effect of heparin on the bleeding time. Thromb Diath Haemost 4:387–99, 1960.
34. Horne MK: Heparin binding to normal and abnormal platelets. Thrombos Res 51:135–144, 1988.
35. Horne MK, Chao ES: Heparin binding to resting and activated platelets. Blood 74:238–243, 1989.
36. John LCH, Rees G, Kovacs I: Inhibition of platelet function by heparin. An aetiological factor in post bypass hemorrhage. J Thorac Cardiovasc Surg 105:816–822, 1993.
37. John LCH, Rees G, Kovacs I: Different anticoagulants and platelet reactivity in cardiac surgical patients. Ann Thorac Surg 56:899–902, 1993.
38. John LCH, Rees G, Kovacs I: Reduction of heparin binding to and inhibition of platelets by aprotinin. Ann Thorac Surg 55:1175–1179, 1993.
39. Kappa JR, Fisher CA, Addonizio VP: Heparin-induced platelet activation; the role of thromboxane A_2 synthesis and the extent of platelet granule release in 2 patients. J Vasc Surg 9:574–579, 1989.
40. Kelton JG: Heparin induced thrombocytopenia. Haemostasis 16:173–186, 1986.
41. Kirby EP, Mills DC: The interaction of bovine factor VIII-associated platelet aggregation by heparin and dextran sulphate and its mechanism. Biochim Biophys Acta 585:416–426, 1979.
42. Kovacs IB, Hutton RA, Kernoff PBA: Hemostatic evaluation in bleeding disorders from native blood. Clinical experience with the hemostatometer. Am J Clin Pathol 91:271–279, 1989.
43. Kuzniewski M, Sulowicz W, Hanicki Z, et al: Effect of heparin and prostacyclin/heparin infusion on platelet aggregation in haemodialysis patients. Nephron 56:174–178, 1990.
44. Levine PH: Platelet function tests: predictive value. N Engl J Med 292:1346, 1975.
45. Levine MN, Hirsh J: Hemorrhagic complications of anticoagulant therapy. Semin Thromb Hemost 12:39–57, 1986.
46. Levine MN, Hirsh J, Kelton JG: Heparin induced bleeding. In Lane D, Lindahl U (eds): Heparin: Chemical and Biological Properties and Clinical Application. London, Edward Arnold, 1989, pp 517–532.
47. Ljungberg B, Johnsson H: In vivo effects of a low molecular weight heparin fragment on platelet aggregation and platelet dependent haemostasis in dogs. Thromb Haemost 60:232–235, 1988.
48. Mant MJ, O'Brien BD, Thong KL, et al: Haemorrhagic complications of heparin therapy. Lancet 1:1133–1135, 1977.
49. Messmore HL, Griffin B, Fareed J, et al: In vitro studies of the interaction of heparin, LMWH and heparinoids with platelets. Ann N Y Acad Sci 556:217–232, 1989.
50. Mikhailidis DP, Fonseca VA, Barradas MA, et al: Platelet activation following intravenous injection of a conventional heparin: Absence of effect with a low molecular weight heparinoid (ORG 10172). Br J Clin Pharmacol 24:415–424, 1987.
51. Moore S, Pepper DS, Cash JD: Platelet antiheparin activity. The isolation and characterisation of platelet factor 4 released from thrombin-aggregated washed human platelets and its dissociation into subunits and the isolation of membrane-bound anti-heparin activity. Biochim Biophys Acta 379:370–384, 1975.
52. Ockelford PA, Carter CJ, Cerskus A, et al: Comparison of the in vivo hemorrhagic and thrombotic effects of a low antithrombin III affinity heparin fraction. Thromb Res 27:679–690, 1982.
53. Packham MA, Bryant MN, Guccione MA, et al: Effect of the concentration of Ca2+ in the suspending medium on the responses of human and rabbit platelets to aggregating agents. Thromb Haemost 62:968–976, 1989.
54. Pekcelen Y, Inceman S: Heparin and ristocetin-induced platelet aggregation [letter]. BMJ 4:101–102, 1975.
55. Ratnatunga C, Rees G, Kovacs I: Preoperative assessment of hemostatic activity to predict excessive blood loss after cardiopulmonary bypass. Ann Thorac Surg 52:250–257, 1991.
56. Reimers RC, Sutera SP, Joist JH: Potentiation by red blood cells of shear-induced platelet aggregation: relative importance of chemical and physical mechanisms. Blood 64:1200–1206, 1984.
57. Royston D, Bidstrup BP, Taylor KM, Sapsford RN: Efficacy of aprotinin on need for blood transfusion after repeat open heart surgery. Lancet 1:289–291, 1987.
58. Ruggiero M, Fedi S, Bianchini P, et al: Molecular events involved in the proaggregating effect of heparin on human platelets. Biochim Biophys Acta 802:372–377, 1984.
59. Salvemini D, De Nucci G, Gryglewski RJ, Vane JR: Human neutrophils and mononuclear cells inhibit platelet aggregation by releasing a nitric oxide-like factor. Proc Natl Acad Sci USA 86:6328–6332, 1989.
60. Salzman EW, Deykin D, Shapiro RM, Rosenberg R: Management of heparin therapy: Controlled prospective trial. N Engl J Med 292:1047–1050, 1975.
61. Salzman EW, Rosenberg RB, Smith MH, et al: The effect of heparin and heparin fractions on platelet aggregation. J Clin Invest 65:64–73, 1980.
62. Schulman S, Johnsson H: Heparin, DDAVP and the bleeding time. Thromb Haemost 65:242–244, 1991.
63. Shanberge JN, Kabayashi J, Nakagawa M: The interaction of platelets with tritium-labelled heparin. Thromb Res 9:595–609, 1976.
64. Sobel M, Adelman B: Characterization of platelet binding of heparins and other glycosaminoglycans. Thromb Res 50:815–826, 1988.
65. Sobel M, McNeill PM, Carlson PL, et al: Heparin inhibition of von Willebrand Factor-dependent platelet function in vitro and in vivo. J Clin Invest 87:1787–1798, 1991.

66. Suzuki K, Nishioki J, Hashimoto S: Inhibition of factor VIII-associated platelet aggregation by heparin and dextran sulphate, and its mechanism. Biochim Biophys Acta 585:416–426, 1979.
67. Thompson C, Forbes CD, Prentice CRM: The potentiation of platelet aggregation and adhesion by heparin in vitro and in vivo. Clin Sci Mol Med 45:485, 1973.
68. Thompson C, Jakubowski J, Quinn P, et al: Platelet size as a determinant of platelet function. J Lab Clin Med 101:205–213, 1983.
69. Walenga JM, Bakhos M, Messmore HC, Fareed J, Pifarre R: Potential use of recombinant hirudin as an anticoagulant in a cardiopulmonary bypass model. Ann Thorac Surg 51:271–277, 1991.
70. Walker AM, Jick H: Predictors of bleeding during heparin therapy. JAMA 244:11, 1980.
71. Westwick J, Scully MF, Poll C, Kakkar VV: Comparison of the effects of low molecular weight heparin and unfractionated heparin on activation of human platelets in vitro. Thromb Res 42:435–447, 1986.
72. Willuweit B, Aktories K: Heparin uncouples alpha 2-adrenoreceptors from the Gi-protein in membranes of human platelets. Biochem J 249:857–863, 1988.
73. Wolf H, Glassl H, Nowack H, Wick G: Identification of binding site for heparin and other polysulfated glycosaminoglycans on human thrombocytes. Int Arch Allergy Appl Immunol 80:231–238, 1986.
74. Yardumian DA, Mackie IJ, Machin SJ: Laboratory investigation of platelet function: A review of methodology. J Clin Pathol 39:701–712, 1986.
75. Yett HS, Sallman JJ, Salzman EW: The hazards of aspirin and heparin. N Engl J Med 298:1092, 1978.

CHAPTER 4

Heparin as a Cause of Fibrinolysis and Platelet Dysfunction in Cardiac Surgery

SHUKRI F. KHURI, M.D.

The institution of cardiopulmonary bypass (CPB) elicits a hemostatic dysfunction that results in increased bleeding during and after cardiac surgery.[11] Heparin, a polyanionic glycosaminoglycan that binds to and catalyzes the action of antithrombin (AT III), continues to be the anticoagulant of choice in the prevention of thrombotic complications during and after CPB. Although its anticoagulant action is reversed with protamine at the termination of CPB, increasing evidence indicates that heparin independently contributes to the CPB-induced hemostatic dysfunction by inhibiting platelet function and promoting fibrinolysis. This chapter addresses the specific effects of heparin on platelet function and fibrinolysis and their contribution to the CPB-induced hemostatic dysfunction and postoperative blood loss.

CARDIOPULMONARY BYPASS-INDUCED HEMOSTATIC DEFECT

It has long been recognized that patients undergoing cardiac surgery have increased postoperative bleeding. This increase has been attributed to a CPB-induced hemostatic defect that was thought to be due mostly to platelet dysfunction and, to a lesser extent, increased fibrinolysis.[11,23] Because the magnitude of thrombocytopenia is not severe enough to account for the marked extension of the bleeding time observed during and after CPB,[12] investigations have focused on specific platelet abnormalities that may be induced by CPB. The platelet defect of CPB has been postulated to be due to a loss of the platelet membrane receptors responsible for platelet adhesion and aggregation. Loss of platelet membrane receptors for both von Willebrand factor (VWF) and fibrinogen were reported during and after CPB.[19,21,22] In these studies, however, the methods with which the platelets were prepared involved centrifugation and gel filtration of the platelets before assay and therefore introduced the possibility of an artifactual in vitro decrease in platelet surface glycoprotein Ib (GPIb)–factor IX complex (the VWF receptor) and GPIIb–factor IIIa complex (the fibrinogen receptor) as a result of proteolysis or activation. In a study of 20 patients undergoing cardiac surgery, we used a flow cytometric method that allowed us to study the platelet GPIb–IX and GPIIb–IIIa complexes in whole blood, thereby avoiding the potential artifactual reductions in platelet surface glycoprotein receptors. With this method, we demonstrated that CPB did not result in a decrease in the platelet surface expression of either the GPIb–IX complex or the GPIIb–IIIa complex.[10] This study underscored the possibility that factors extrinsic to the platelet may contribute to platelet dysfunction during cardiac operations.

Increased fibrinolysis is the second and more recently recognized component of the CPB-induced hemostatic defect. A number of pathways can lead to increased fibrinolysis during CPB, including activation of kallikrein and release of tissue-type plasminogen activator (tPA) from the endothelial cell.[11] Fibrin(ogen) degradation products (FDPs) and D-dimer increase during and after CPB.[7,11] Administration of aprotinin during CPB prevents the formation of FDPs and the reduction in α_2-antiplasmin activity.[3] It also reduces the bleeding time.[4] These observations, the mechanism of action of aprotinin,[15] and the clinical effectiveness of plasmin inhibitors such as aprotinin in decreasing blood loss[4] strongly suggest that fibrinolysis is important in the hemorrhagic diathesis associated with CPB.

EFFECTS OF HEPARIN ON FIBRINOLYSIS

Heparin and its fractions have been known to possess fibrinolytic activities for more than a decade. Fareed and associates reported an increase in tPA levels in human volunteers after the institution of intravenous and subcutaneous heparin over a period of 10 days (daily dose of 7500 U). They postulated a number of fibrinolytic actions of heparin and its fractions.[5] Several recent studies have shown that heparin and heparinlike compounds stimulated cell surface plasminogen activation by 10- to 17-fold.[18] Giuliani,[7] Kongsgaard,[14] and others underscored the profibrinolytic potential of heparin by demonstrating increases in D-dimer, tPA, and other fibrinolytic products during extracorporeal circulation. Their studies, however, did not separate the effect of heparin on the fibrinolytic system from the effect of the extracorporeal circuit. Based on a review of various in vitro studies,[1,6,16] Upchurch et al. postulated a number of mechanisms by which heparin is believed to facilitate fibrinolysis.[20] They include direct stimulation of the release of plasminogen activators from vascular and monocytic cells; facilitation of the activation of protein C; promoting the release of plasminogen activator; impairment of fibrin monomer polymerization; enhancement of the catalytic efficiency of plasminogen activation by urokinase-type plasminogen activators and tPA enhancement of plasmin-mediated activation of single-chain urokinase-type plasminogen activator; modulation of antiplasmin activities; catalysis of thrombin-induced neutralization of plasminogen activator inhibitor type 1; and potentiation of the effects of tissue factor pathway inhibitor, thereby reducing the modulatory prothrombotic effects that often accompany fibrinolysis.

Our group has conducted two studies aimed at elucidating the effects of heparin on fibrinolysis and platelet function. The first study included a total of 55 patients in whom hematologic measurements were made immediately before and 5 minutes after the administration of 4 mg/kg of heparin prior to the institution of CPB.[13] Baseline heparin concentration in plasma was 0.22 ± 0.11 IU/ml. Five minutes after heparin administration, it averaged 6.26 ± 1.53 IU/ml. Likewise, heparin administration elicited a rise in activated clotting time (ACT) from an average of 137.9 ± 19.2 seconds to 870 ± 168 seconds. Plasmin activity, which was measured in 19 patients using a chromogenic assay, increased in every patient after the administration of heparin. On the average, heparin elicited a 10-fold increase in plasmin activity (Fig. 1). In 51 patients in whom D-dimer measurements were made, the administration of heparin elicited an increase in D-dimer level in 43 (77%) and no change or a decrease in 12 (23%) (see Fig. 1). On the average, there was a modest but significant increase in the D-dimer level from a preheparin mean of 571.3 μg/ml to a postheparin mean of 698.5 mg/ml. The administration of heparin did not elicit significant changes in the plasma levels of fibrinogen, tPA, plasminogen, antiplasmin, or AT III. The failure to demonstrate a change in plasminogen with the administration of heparin was

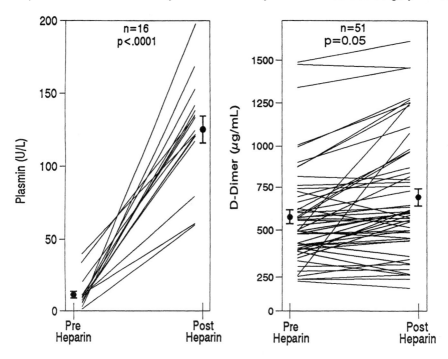

FIGURE 1. Plasma levels of plasmin and D-dimer in patients in whom paired measurements were obtained before and 5 minutes after administration of heparin. The mean ± standard error of the mean is shown for each time point. (From Khuri SF, et al: Heparin causes platelet dysfunction and induces fibrinolysis before cardiopulmonary bypass. Ann Thorac Surg 60:1008–1014, 1995, with permission.)

explained by the fact that the interaction between heparin and plasminogen has been shown to occur on the cell surface of plasminogen[13]; thus it is unlikely that the profibrinolytic effect of heparin would be reflected by the levels of plasminogen in the plasma. The lack of significant increase in tPA after the administration of heparin was also of concern. It was assumed that the plasma level of tPA antigen may not correlate with the functional activity of the molecule in patients undergoing CPB. Hence, although this clinical study provided convincing evidence of the profibrinolytic potential of heparin independent of the effect of the extracorporeal circuit, it was limited by clinical logistics, raising a number of questions and prompting a need for additional basic investigations.

To elucidate further the relationships between heparin and the fibrinolytic system, our group conducted study in 5 baboons to which increasing concentrations of heparin (ranging from 10–500 U/kg) were administered over a period of 60 minutes. A direct correlation (r = 0.65, p = 0.010) was demonstrated in vivo between plasmin activity, measured with the same assay used in the patient study, and plasmin light chains, as determined by densitometric quantification of Western blots of baboon plasma. When increasing heparin concentrations (1–10 U/ml) were added to baboon plasma in vitro (Fig. 2), a linear increase in plasmin light chains was observed as the concentration of heparin was increased (r = 0.71, p = 0.012). In vivo experiments in the baboons also demonstrated that increasing heparin doses resulted in a time-dependent increase in plasmin activity (Fig. 3). Other markers of fibrinolysis were examined over time. Fibrinogen decreased after heparin administration, but this decrease did not reach statistical significance. D-Dimer tended to increase from 123 ± 41 ng/ml at baseline to 140 ± 48 ng/ml (p = 0.09) after the

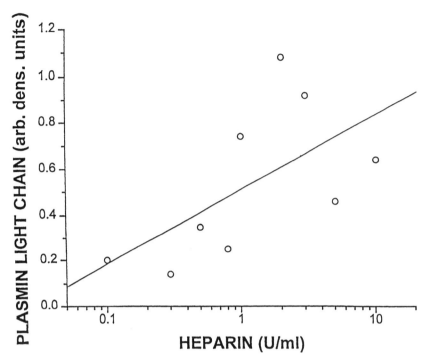

FIGURE 2. Effect of increasing doses of heparin on plasmin light-chain generation in vitro. This scatter plot, showing plasmin light-chain content after incubation of plasma with heparin (0.1–10 U/ml), demonstrates an increase in plasmin light chain as the concentration of heparin increases. (From Upchurch GR, et al: The effect of heparin on fibrinolytic activity and platelet function in vivo. Am J Physiol 271(40):H528–H534, 1996, with permission.)

administration of heparin. This finding reflected the modest increase noted in the patient study (see Fig. 1), in which better statistical significance was achieved because of a much larger sample size. D-Dimer, however, continued to be elevated at 24 hours after the reversal of heparin (441 ± 152 ng/ml). When a specific FDP, fragment E, was measured using quantitative Western blot techniques, the addition of heparin to baboon plasma in vitro resulted in a concentration-dependent increase. Linear regression analysis showed a correlation coefficient between fragment E and heparin concentration of r = 0.89 (p = 0.0067).

EFFECTS OF HEPARIN ON PLATELET FUNCTION

It has long been recognized that heparin prolongs bleeding time[8] and interferes with platelet aggregation.[2] However, recognition of heparin as an etiologic factor in postbypass hemorrhage is only recent.[9,11] After ascertaining that the factors responsible for CPB-induced platelet dysfunction were mostly extrinsic to the platelet (see above), our group conducted a number of studies aimed at understanding the mechanistic role of heparin as an extrinsic factor in the genesis of platelet dysfunction during cardiac surgery. In a study designed to elucidate the platelet function defect of CPB using whole blood flow cytometry, Kestin et al.[10] made observations before and 5 minutes after administration of heparin prior to institution of CPB. Heparin administration resulted in significant extension of bleeding time and a marked decrease in thromboxane B_2 levels in the blood emerging from a standardized bleeding-time wound. Heparin also abolished, almost completely, in vivo platelet reactivity, as assessed by the time-dependent upregulation of platelet-surface P-selectin,* which was measured in the blood emerging from the bleeding-time

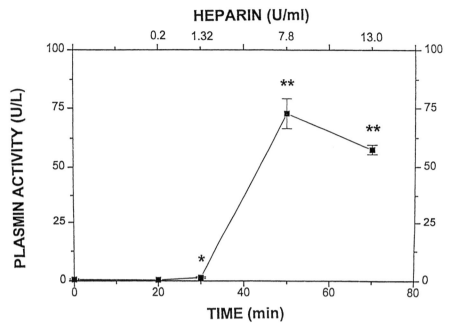

FIGURE 3.   Effect of progressive increase in heparin dosage on plasmin activity in vivo. Increasing heparin concentration over time causes an increase in plasmin light chain from 30 minutes to 70 minutes. Data are presented as mean ± standard error of the mean. (*p < 0.02 and **p < 0.0003). (From Upchurch GR, et al: The effect of heparin on fibrinolytic activity and platelet function in vivo. Am J Physiol 271(40):H528–H534, 1996, with permission.)

wound. Heparin administration, however, did not inhibit platelet reactivity in vitro, as determined by samples obtained from the same set of patients at the same time points using the same assays, performed in parallel with the same reagents. In fact, the administration of heparin in vitro appeared to augment the upregulation of P-selectin induced by the platelet agonist phorbol myrisate acetate (PMA). Heparin administration also appeared to augment in vitro the PMA-induced downregulation of the GPIb–factor IX complex. These findings were confirmed in the study by Upchurch,[20] which showed that heparin, administered to the baboon in vivo, augmented the ADP- and epinephrine-induced increase in platelet-surface P-selectin and concomitant decrease in platelet-surface GPIb (Fig. 4). In the absence of agonists such as PMA, ADP, and epinephrine, heparin administration to the baboon resulted in neither platelet degranulation, as determined by lack of expression of platelet-surface P-selectin, nor platelet activation, as determined by lack of decrease in platelet-surface GPIb (Fig. 4).

That the administration of heparin to patients before CPB causes significant platelet dysfunction was subsequently confirmed in our study of 55 patients undergoing various cardiac surgical procedures.[13] As in the Kestin study, administration of heparin caused marked extension of the bleeding time and significant reduction in the thromboxane B_2 level in the blood from the bleeding-time wound (Fig. 5). How can one reconcile this degree of heparin-induced clinical platelet dysfunction with the findings of Kestin and Upchurch that heparin in vitro causes *increased* agonist-induced platelet secretion and activation?

---

* P-selectin as contained in alpha granule inside the platelet. It is expressed on the surface membrane only when the platelet is activated and degranulation occurs.

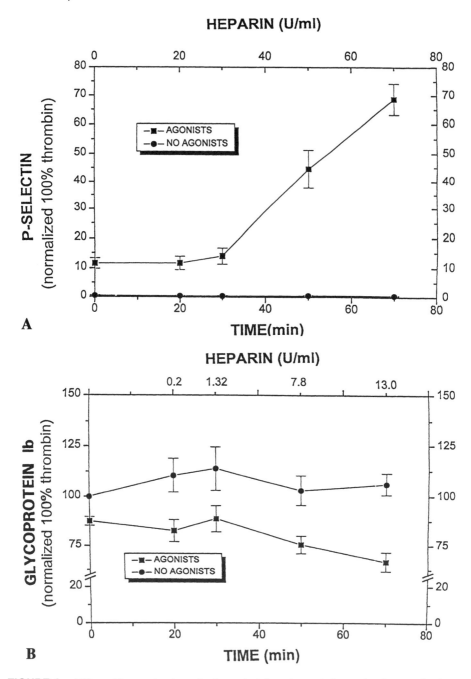

FIGURE 4. Effect of increasing heparin dose administration to baboons in vivo on platelet activation in vitro using whole blood flow cytometric analysis. Addition of subthreshold concentrations of ADP (1 μM) and epinephrine (5 μM) (squares) was accompanied by *(A)* an increase in S12 binding (P-selectin) and *(B)* a decrease in TM60 binding (GPIb) at concentrations of heparin greater than 1 U/ml compared with controls (circles). (From Upchurch GR, et al: The effect of heparin on fibrinolytic activity and platelet function in vivo. Am J Physiol 271(40):H528–H534, 1996, with permission.)

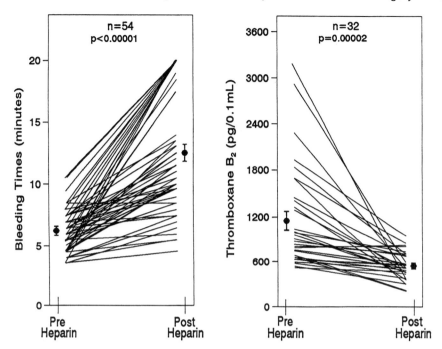

FIGURE 5.   Bleeding time and shed blood thromboxane B_2 in patients in whom paired measurements were obtained before and 5 minutes after the administration of heparin. The mean ± standard error of the mean is shown for each time point. (From Khuri SF, et al: Heparin causes platelet dysfunction and induces fibrinolysis before cardiopulmonary bypass. Ann Thorac Surg 60:1008–1014, 1995, with permission.)

Two mechanisms may explain this paradoxical decrease in platelet function after the administration of heparin to cardiac surgical patients. The first is related to the effect of heparin on thrombin and the second to the effect of heparin on fibrinolysis. Thrombin is the most potent endogenous agonist of heparin. Its inhibition by heparin suppresses platelet activation and function. The heparin-induced increase in fibrinolysis (see above) also affects platelet function. Plasmin, FDPs, and D-dimer have been shown to interfere with platelet aggregation, presumably through a proteolytic effect on the platelet GPIIIa in the case of plasmin[17] and by competing with fibrinogen for GPIIb/IIIa binding in the case of degradation products. Hence the generation of plasmin, stimulated by heparin, provides another possible mechanism by which heparin impairs platelet function. A confirmatory finding of this mechanism is the correlation between plasma plasmin levels and the bleeding time ($r = 0.75$, $p = 0.005$) that we observed after heparin administration to 12 patients before the institution of CPB.[20]

Hence, heparin has at least two distinct effects on platelet activation and function. Heparin augments in vitro platelet activation; yet, by inhibiting endogenous thrombin and stimulating fibrinolysis, heparin paradoxically suppresses in vivo platelet activation.

CLINICAL CORRELATIONS

The important clinical question is to what degree the effects of heparin on platelet function and fibrinolysis influence the intra- and postoperative blood loss in cardiac surgical patients, independent of the effect of the institution of CPB. The answer depends on yet another unanswered question: Are the heparin effects on platelets and the fibrinolytic system in patients undergoing cardiac surgery dose-dependent? The study in baboons by Upchurch et al.,[20] particularly its in vitro component, provides convincing evidence of dose dependence, which clearly needs to be verified in human studies. One method of addressing the dose-dependence issue in humans is to explore the efficacy of low-dose heparin in conjunction with heparin-coated circuits in reducing blood loss. Several ongoing studies are addressing this issue. Their results are preliminary, and it remains to be determined whether combining low-dose heparin with heparin-coated surfaces will suppress thrombin adequately and, at the same time, reduce the adverse effect of heparin on platelet function and fibrinolysis. It also remains to be determined whether an alternative anticoagulant that does not interfere with either platelet function or the fibrinolytic process can improve postoperative hemostasis in cardiac surgical patients.

Acknowledgment.   The author acknowledges the efforts of a large number of collaborators whose work was frequently quoted in this manuscript, particularly the efforts of Drs. C. Robert Valeri, Joseph Loscalzo, Alan Michelson, Anita Kestin, and Gilbert Upchurch. The author also acknowledges the superb help of Mrs. Nancy Healey, who coordinated the author's collaborative research and prepared the manuscript for publication.

REFERENCES

1. Anonick PK, Wolf B, Gonias SL: Regulation of plasmin, miniplasmin, and streptokinase-plasmin complex by α_2-antiplasmin, α_2-macroglobulin, and antithrombin III in the presence of heparin. Thromb Res 59:449–462, 1990.
2. Attar S: Discussion of Khuri et al: Heparin causes platelet dysfunction and induces fibrinolysis before cardiopulmonary bypass. Ann Thorac Surg 60:1008–10014, 1995.
3. Blauhut B, Gross C, Necek S, et al: Effects of high-dose aprotinin on blood loss, platelet function, fibrinolysis, complement, and renal function after cardiopulmonary bypass. J Thorac Cardiovasc Surg 101:958–967, 1991.
4. Bidstrup BP, Royston D, Sapsford RN, Taylor KM: Reduction in blood loss and blood use after cardiopulmonary bypass with high dose aprotinin. J Thorac Cardiovasc Surg 97:364–372, 1989.
5. Fareed J, Walenga JM, Hoppensteadt DA, Messmore HL: Studies on the fibrinolytic actions of heparin and its fractions. Semin Thromb Hemost 11:199–207, 1985.
6. Ghezzo F, Romano S, Mazzone R, et al: Heparin neutralizes serum antiplasmin inhibition of peripheral blood leukocyte fibrinolytic activity. Thromb Res 46:199–204, 1987.
7. Giuliani R, Szwarcer E, Martinez AE, Palumbo G: Fibrin-dependent fibrinolytic activity during extracorporeal circulation. Thromb Res 61:369–373, 1991.
8. Heiden D, Mielke CH, Rodvien R: Impairment by heparin of primary hemostasis and platelet (C14) 5-hydroxytryptamine release. Br J Haematol 36:427–436, 1977.
9. John LCH, Rees GM, Kovacs IB: Inhibition of platelet function by heparin. J Thorac Cardiovasc Surg 105:816–822, 1993.
10. Kestin AS, Valeri CR, Khuri SF, et al: The platelet function defect of cardiopulmonary bypass. Blood 82:107–117, 1993.
11. Khuri SF, Michelson AD, Valeri CR: The effect of cardiopulmonary bypass on hemostasis and coagulation. In Thrombosis and Hemorrhage. Cambridge, MA, Blackwell Scientific, 1994, pp 1051–1073.
12. Khuri SF, Wolfe JA, Josa M, et al: Hematologic changes during and after cardiopulmonary bypass and their relationship to the bleeding time and nonsurgical blood loss. J Thorac Cardiovasc Surg 104:94–107, 1992.
13. Khuri SF, Valeri CR, Loscalzo J, et al: Heparin causes platelet dysfunction and induces fibrinolysis before cardiopulmonary bypass. Ann Thorac Surg 60:1008–1014, 1995.
14. Kongsgaard UE, Smith-Erichsen N, Geiran O, Bjirnskau L: Changes in the coagulation and fibrinolytic systems during and after cardiopulmonary bypass. Thorac Cardiovasc Surg 37:158–162, 1989.
15. Mannucci PM: Nontransfusional modalities. In Thrombosis and Hemorrhage. Cambridge, MA, Blackwell Scientific, 1994, pp 1117–1135.
16. Markwardt FK, Klocking HP: Heparin-induced release of plasminogen activator. Haemostasis 6:370–374, 1977.
17. Ouimet H, Loscalzo J: Reciprocating autocatalytic interactions between platelets and the plasminogen activation system. Thromb Res 1996 [in press].
18. Rijken DC, de Munk GA, Jie AF: Interactions of plasminogen activators and plasminogen with heparin: Effect of ionic strength. Thromb Haemost 70:867–872, 1993.
19. Rinder CS, Mathew JP, Rinder HM, et al: Modulation of platelet surface adhesion receptors during cardiopulmonary bypass. Anesthesiology 75:563–570, 1991.
20. Upchurch GR, Valeri CR, Khuri SF, et al: The effect of heparin on fibrinolytic activity and platelet function in vivo. Heart Circ Physiol 271(40):H528–H534, 1996.
21. Van Oeveren W, Harder MP, Roozendaal KJ, et al: Aprotinin protects platelets against the initial effect of cardiopulmonary bypass. J Thorac Cardiovasc Surg 99:788–796, 1990.
22. Wenger RK, Lukasiewicz H, Mikuta B, et al: Loss of platelet fibrinogen receptors during clinical cardiopulmonary bypass. J Thorac Cardiovasc Surg 97:235–239, 1989.
23. Woodman RC, Harker LA: Bleeding complications associated with cardiopulmonary bypass. Blood 76:1680–1697, 1990.

CHAPTER 5

The Effect of Cardiopulmonary Bypass on Platelet Function

WILLIAM C. OLIVER, JR., M.D.
GREGORY A. NUTTALL, M.D.

Cardiopulmonary bypass (CPB) is commonly used in patients who require cardiac surgery, primarily for coronary artery bypass grafting (CABG). Advancements in surgical techniques and technology have reduced the mortality and morbidity associated with CABG to less than 4%.[30] However, excessive bleeding after CPB continues to occur in 5–25% of patients.[7] Approximately 5% of patients who undergo CPB require reoperation for bleeding.[24] A specific cause of excessive bleeding after CPB has been difficult to determine because of the complexity of the coagulation process and the many physiologic variables associated with CPB. Inadequate surgical hemostasis, acquired defects of coagulation, or both appear to be involved in most cases.[45] Half of all patients who require reoperation for bleeding are discovered to have inadequate surgical hemostasis.[67] For the remaining patients, acquired defects of coagulation include reduced clotting factors, inadequate heparin reversal, fibrinolysis, complement activation, and platelet dysfunction.[45] At the present time, fibrinolysis and platelet dysfunction are considered primarily responsible for bleeding after CPB.[51] Such patients are at risk for disease transmission,[31] increased costs,[49] and increased morbidity[39] due to transfusion of allogeneic blood products.

This chapter focuses on the effect of CPB on platelet function. A review of normal platelet function is also included to provide a foundation to understand platelet activity in abnormal physiologic situations such as extracorporeal circulation (EC).

NORMAL PLATELET FUNCTION

Successful hemostasis involves the vasculature (endothelium), coagulation cascades, and platelets. Platelets have a complex and important role in hemostasis, yet it is not clear exactly which functions of the platelet are essential for hemostasis. Platelets circulate in the blood but do not usually interact with the vascular endothelium.[25] When vascular injury has occurred, platelet response is rapid and localized to the injured area. Platelet activity can be separated into four components: adhesion, aggregation, granule secretion, and procoagulation. Platelets are activated initially by contact with the injured area, which exposes the platelets to certain stimuli.[4] Stimulation activates specific receptors on the platelet membrane and triggers intracellular effector enzymes. The activated platelets behave as catalysts in the hemostatic process; however, platelet activation is a graded response so that a minor stimulus will not result in complete intravascular coagulation.

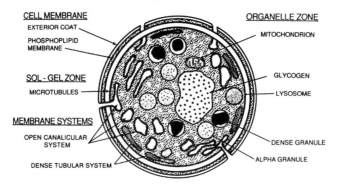

FIGURE 1.   Anatomy of the platelet cell in horizontal section. (From Gravlee GP, Davis RF, Utley JR: Cardiopulmonary Bypass: Principles and Practice. Baltimore, Williams & Wilkins, 1993, p 408, with permission.)

Once platelets arrive at the injured area, they adhere to the injured endothelium. This crucial event in hemostasis is referred to as platelet adhesion. More platelets are recruited to the injured site by compounds that attract platelets and cause vasoconstriction. Platelets begin to attach to each other—a process referred to as platelet aggregation. The result is the formation of a "plug." The plug becomes fortified with fibrin strands within minutes of injury. Fibrin can be generated at the surface of the platelet by the intrinsic pathway of coagulation. The localized nature of the reaction also makes it easier to control. Although a strong plug is necessary to prevent hemorrhage, it is important to prevent unopposed coagulation that would cause thrombosis. Therefore, continued platelet activity is inhibited by endothelial production of prostacyclin and a fibrinolytic system that dissolves the platelet plug.

Platelet Morphology

Platelets are membrane-encapsulated fragments of megakaryocyte cytoplasm that consist of a nonuniformly constructed trilaminar phospholipoprotein membrane[68] (Fig. 1). The external membrane is composed of primarily neutral phospholipids, whereas the inner membrane is more negatively charged. The external membrane becomes more negative when the platelet is activated because the distribution of the phospholipids is altered. The negatively charged external membrane enhances the activation of other coagulation processes that increase the platelet's procoagulant activity. The surface of the platelet is particularly suited for involvement in various aspects of coagulation (Table 1). The membrane provides sites for adhesion, aggregation, platelet factor 3 (PF3), and receptors for agonists (adenosine diphosphate [ADP], collagen). The platelet membrane is also a major source of arachidonic acid which is necessary for synthesis of prostaglandins and platelet activating factor (PAF). Both compounds are important for normal platelet function.

In the unstimulated state, the platelet is disc-shaped with a diameter of 2–3 μm (Fig. 2). Because there is no nucleus to synthesize protein, the platelet's life span is only 10–14 days. Platelets contain an array of specialized structures that include microtubules,

TABLE 1.   Platelet Functions Involved in Coagulation

Platelet receptors catalyze prothrombin to thrombin
GPIIb-IIIa thrombin-induced receptor for von Willebrand factor
Enhanced activation of factor X
Receptors for factors XII and XI
Inhibited activation of factors Va, Xa, thrombin, and VIIIa

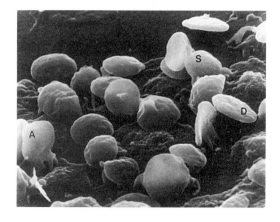

FIGURE 2. Human platelet morphology. Scanning electron micrograph depicts platelets in various stages of activity on a fibronectin-coated surface. Disc-shaped platelets *(D)* are basically unstimulated. Spherical platelets *(S)* are activated. Some platelets *(A)* have pseudopodia extended onto the fibronectin surface. (From Rossi EC, Simon TL, Moss GS: Principles of Transfusion Medicine. Baltimore, Williams & Wilkins, 1991, p 182, with permission.)

organelles, and an internal network of canaliculi (see Fig. 1). The organelles include mitochondria, Golgi bodies, ribosomes, and granules. There are four types of granules: lysosomes, α-granules, dense granules, and microperoxisomes.[5] Lysosomes contain a variety of acid hydrolases. Microperoxisomes contain peroxidases such as catalase. The α-granules contain fibronectin, von Willebrand factor (VWF)/factor VIII, fibrinogen, platelet factor 4 (PF4), ß-thromboglobulin (BTG), factor V, and thrombospondin (TSP) as well as other secretory proteins.[68] Dense granules contain serotonin, ADP, adenosine triphosphate (ATP), histamine, and calcium. Approximately 65% of the total ATP and ADP of the platelet is contained in the dense granules. The α-granules and dense granules are more important for platelet function. Congenital deficiencies of these granules cause mild bleeding tendencies.[8]

Besides secretory granules and organelles, the platelet has an extensive system of microtubules to communicate with the external environment and to maintain internal access to enzymes and ions. There are two well-defined membrane systems in the platelet (see Fig. 1). The canalicular system is an open and elaborate array of microtubules that communicate with the external environment. This open system increases the surface of the platelet in contact with the blood. The canalicular system also increases the number of receptor sites that are available and facilitates granule secretion.[40] The other system of membranes is the dense tubular system found randomly within the platelet. These tubules connect with the open canalicular tubular system. The dense tubular system is a calcium reservoir analogous to the sarcoplasmic reticulum of muscle cells as well as a site for enzymes involved with arachidonic acid metabolism and prostaglandin synthesis.

Actin is an important component of platelet structure. Actin polymerization and cytoskeleton reorganization are responsible for platelet shape changes in response to certain stimuli.[40] During platelet inactivity, these contractile proteins are in the nonpolymerized state; with platelet activation, they polymerize to form pseudopodia (see Fig. 2). These calcium-mediated, actin-catalyzed myosin components contract and thus change the platelet's shape. The change in shape of the platelet is necessary for effective platelet adhesion.

Platelet Activation

Normally, the vascular endothelium is a neutral environment for the blood and its formed elements. Platelets circulate primarily in a nonactivated condition. They usually react to damaged vascular endothelium but also may react to foreign or charged surfaces and certain compounds called platelet agonists. When the integrity of the vascular endothelium is disrupted, subendothelial connective tissue is exposed to the blood. The subendothelium contains collagen, VWF, fibronectin, and proteins that recruit platelets to

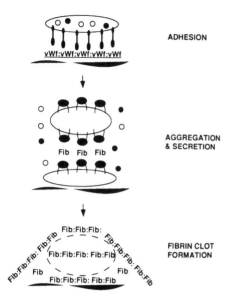

FIGURE 3. Illustration of platelet activity in clot formation. Rod with nodules at letter end = GPIb/IX; VWF = von Willebrand factor; wavy lines = extracellular matrix (subendothelium); O = α-granule; • = dense nodule; nodules with two arms = GPIIb/IIIa; Fib = fibrinogen; Fib:Fib:Fib: = fibrin; dashed oval = platelets undergoing autolysis. (From Bennett DA, Evans DA: Disorders of platelet function. Dis Month 38:590, 1992, with permission.)

the damaged site. The initial and crucial step in hemostasis and formation of a platelet plug is platelet adhesion to the subendothelial molecules at the damaged site (Fig. 3). Platelet adhesion is the affinity of platelets for nonplatelet surfaces.[4] Adhesion to the subendothelium is mediated by specific platelet membrane receptors[5] (Fig. 4). Certain glycoprotein platelet receptors recognize a specific part of a subendothelial compound. This

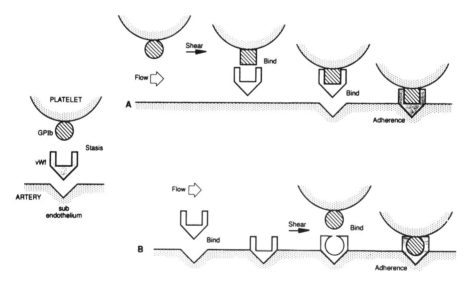

FIGURE 4. Mechanisms of adhesion. During low blood flow (venous), no interaction occurs between von Willebrand factor (VWF) and GPIb. During high blood flow and high shear force (arterial), a change occurs in GPIb or VWF or both. *A,* With shear, platelet GPIb undergoes a conformational change that allows attachment of VWF. *B,* VWF binds to the subendothelium, undergoes a conformational change secondary to shear that results in the binding of platelets through GPIb. (From Roth GJ: Developing relationships: Arterial platelet adhesion, glycoprotein IB, and leucine-rich glycoproteins. Blood 77:7, 1991, with permission.)

part of the subendothelial compound (fibrinogen, fibronectin, vitronectin, and VWF) is a specific amino acid sequence that is most commonly a tripeptide, arginine-glycine-aspartic acid.[25,37] After undergoing a conformational change,[43] the platelet receptors bind to the subendothelial compounds[37] (see Fig. 4).

Blood flow determines which subendothelial matrix molecule will bind to a specific platelet receptor.[5] Under conditions of low blood flow (venous), glycoprotein (GP) GPIa/IIa receptor[25] binds to collagen and GPIc/IIa[40] binds to fibronectin. The GPIa/IIa is the major collagen platelet receptor.[35] During high blood flow and increased shear (arterial), attachment of platelets with collagen or fibronectin is inadequate. Therefore, platelets bind to VWF (see Fig. 4) through the interaction with platelet receptor GPIb.[40] Although GPIIb/IIIa receptors can be substituted for GPIb, GPIb is the major VWF-binding protein.[25,55] This complex of VWF and GPIb is a critical component in the role of platelet adhesion. An abnormality in this receptor complex may result in bleeding tendencies.[8]

The origin and multimeric composition of VWF are unique to sustain platelet–vessel wall interactions in conditions of high shear.[23] VWF is found in plasma, platelets, and endothelial basement membrane. The VWF that binds to platelets is not the circulating VWF; it originates in the subendothelium. VWF has no interaction in unstimulated platelets.

Platelet adhesion is a prerequisite for platelet aggregation and formation of a platelet plug in vivo. Once activated, platelets begin to adhere to the injured site. They become "sticky" as their discoid shape becomes more spherical through centralization of cytoplasmic organelles and extension of pseudopods[68] (Fig. 5). At this point during platelet adhesion, platelets degranulate and induce vasoconstriction, which attracts more platelets. As

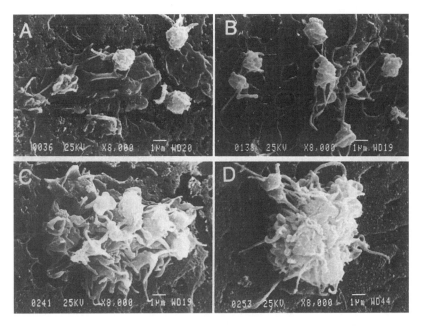

FIGURE 5.   Scanning electron micrographs of four aggregation grades of platelets on the extracellular matrix. *A,* Platelets are discoid. No pseudopodia. *B,* Initial signs of activation with slight signs of pseudopodia. *C,* Prominent signs of aggregation: platelet spread, multiple pseudopodia, and clustering. *D,* Aggregate. No individual platelets can be identified (magnification × 8000). (From Golan M, et al: Transfusion of fresh whole blood stored (4 degrees C) for short period fails to improve platelet aggregation on extracellular matrix and clinical hemostasis after cardiopulmonary bypass. J Thorac Cardiovasc Surg 99:355, 1990, with permission.)

platelets adhere to each other, the process is referred to as primary platelet aggregation. Primary aggregation is reversible and reflects the affinity of platelets for one another.[4]

If a platelet plug is to evolve, platelet activation and aggregation must continue. Platelets are activated at a rate that depends on the eliciting thrombogenic stimuli. The shape and membrane changes associated with platelet activation and aggregation make the platelet surface more attractive to other platelets (see Fig. 5). As the stimulus becomes stronger, platelets degranulate, and irreversible changes in the platelet occur. As more platelets are attracted to the site, the platelet plug is formed. Activated platelets provide a good thrombogenic surface for fibrin formation, which is necessary for a stable platelet plug. Once irreversible platelet aggregation has occurred, a solid and dense collection of platelets and fibrin will form. If the stimulus is insufficient to produce irreversible platelet aggregation, the platelet will revert to its original state and assume a discoid shape. The ability of the platelet to revert from primary aggregation to the unstimulated state is protection against a full hemostatic response to a minor stimulus.

The process of activation within the platelet is complex. It occurs by a process known as stimulus–response coupling. Activation requires G-proteins, which are found in the platelet membrane. G-proteins are involved in the enzymatic pathways that generate platelet shape change, granule secretion, and prostaglandin synthesis.

Granule Secretion

An important aspect of platelet response to injury is release of its granules. Granule contents attract platelets to the injured site to form platelet thrombi. In addition, degranulation causes acceleration of the coagulation cascade, local vasoconstriction, and increased vascular permeability.

Granules are secreted in response to various stimuli. Epinephrine, ADP, and thrombin stimulate degranulation. Arachidonic acid metabolites are also usually necessary to stimulate granule secretion except in the presence of a strong platelet agonist. Alpha granules and dense granules are released in response to low levels of stimulation and weaker agonists. Thrombin is a potent stimulus for dense granule secretion. The release of lysosome granules requires a major stimulus, such as high concentrations of thrombin and collagen.

Granules are secreted through exocytosis, which is a calcium-dependent, active process that requires ATP and platelet microfilament contraction. Platelet agonists raise the cytoplasmic calcium concentration. The rise in calcium level stimulates microfilament contraction, which forces granules to the surface of the platelet to be released.

Platelet Aggregation

In contrast to platelet adhesion, platelet aggregation requires platelet stimulation, active platelet metabolism, and fibrinogen. Aggregation is initiated in three related but independent pathways.[68] It may occur after platelet activation by one of several agonists that bind to a specific platelet membrane receptor during activation.[37] A second messenger system transfers information to the platelet membrane so that receptors can be prepared[50] and intracellular enzymes can be activated. Preparation involves a conformational change in the receptor that exposes a fibrinogen-binding site.[43] The receptor must be altered to bind with fibrinogen. This receptor-specific preparation that occurs after stimulation[40] not only alters platelet receptors to bind with fibrinogen but also increases intracellular calcium. The increased cytosolic calcium facilitates activation of phospholipase A_2 and mobilizes free arachidonic acid (Fig. 6). Arachidonic acid is mobilized and converted to labile endoperoxides by the enzyme cyclooxygenase. Thromboxane synthetase converts most of the endoperoxides into thromboxane A_2 (TxA_2)[50] (Fig. 7). The generation of TxA_2 is important for normal platelet function. TxA_2 is a vasoconstrictor that recruits other platelets to aggregate and lowers the activation threshold of other weaker agonists that will trigger granule secretion.[50]

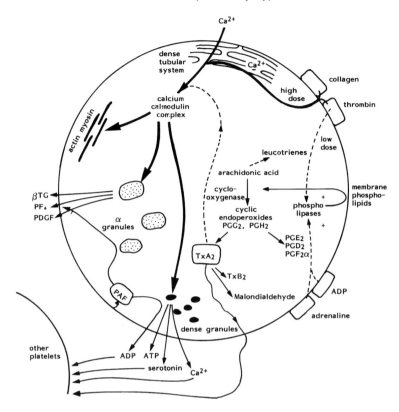

FIGURE 6.   Representation of the pathways for platelet activation. Ca^{++} = calcium ions; PGG_2, H_2, E_2, D_2, and F_{2a} = prostaglandins G_2, H_2, E_2, D_2, and F_{2a}; TXA_2 = thromboxane A_2; TXB_2 = thromboxane B_2; β-TG = β-thromboglobulin; PF4 = platelet factor 4; PDGF = platelet-derived growth factor; ADP = adenosine diphosphate; ATP = adenosine triphosphate. (From Yardumian DA, Mackie IJ, Machin SJ: Laboratory investigation of platelet function: A review of methodology. J Clin Pathol 39:702, 1986, with permission.)

Another pathway to platelet aggregation is independent of arachidonic acid metabolism. Certain agonists, such as thrombin, ADP, or collagen, can produce a significant enough rise in the concentration of intracellular calcium to cause granule release. Increased calcium leads to liberation of arachidonic acid and subsequently TxA_2.

The third pathway for platelet aggregation involves release of PAF, which aggregates platelets. PAF is released from the platelet membrane in response to activation of phospholipase A_2. This activates platelets independently of calcium and TxA_2.

The likelihood of platelet activation and aggregation depends on the potency and concentration of the platelet agonists.[41] Collagen and thrombin are potent platelet activators. They do not require platelet aggregation to induce platelet secretion.[5] Weaker platelet agonists are ADP, epinephrine, prostaglandin endoperoxides, TxA_2, PAF, and serotonin.[41] Some weaker agonists can potentiate the effect of stronger agonists such as thrombin and collagen.

Platelet aggregation involves a calcium-dependent fibrinogen binding between platelet receptor and adhesive proteins[25] (see Fig. 3). The major platelet receptor for aggregation is GPIIb/IIIa,[29] which is distributed throughout the platelet plasma membrane.[20] The GPIIb/IIIa receptor is considered the fibrinogen receptor. The binding of the fibrinogen to GPIIb/IIIa receptors permits crosslinking of adjacent platelets that facilitate

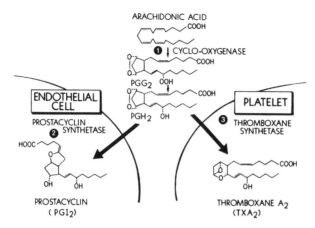

FIGURE 7.   Arachidonate metabolism. Arachidonic acid conversion to prostacyclin and thromboxane A2. (From Rossi EC, Simon TL, Moss GS: Principles of Transfusion Medicine. Baltimore, Williams & Wilkins, 1991, p 184, with permission.)

aggregation. Fibrinogen is not the only compound involved in aggregation. The GPIIb/IIIa receptor has an affinity for VWF, fibronectin, and vitronectin.[43] VWF can bind with GPIIb/IIIa receptors when platelets are activated by thrombin, ADP, or collagen.

Besides the ability of platelets to adhere, aggregate, and form a platelet plug, the platelet surface can activate the intrinsic coagulation pathway.[65] On the platelet surface, factor XI can be converted to factor XIa. This localizes the conversion of factors IX and X. Factor Xa can be bound to the platelet by factor V and PF3. Because factor Va is present on the platelet surface, large amounts of thrombin can be generated.[25] Thrombin has a pivotal role in the formation and strengthening of the platelet plug because it cleaves fibrinogen into fibrin monomers that can polymerize nonenzymatically to provide a solid gel network and stabilize the platelet plug.

Regulation of Platelet Activity

Platelet activation and aggregation are regulated primarily at the site of each platelet. Platelets do not normally adhere to the endothelium. One reason is that the endothelium manufactures prostacyclin, a potent platelet inhibitor. Prostacyclin does not circulate continuously but is released in response to local stimulation.[68] It acts by binding to adenylate cyclase in the cell membrane, which increases the concentration of cyclic adenosine monophosphate (cAMP), an inhibitor of platelet activation.[41] Increased cAMP lowers the concentration of intracellular calcium, which is critical to platelet activity. Endothelial production of prostacyclin provides a balance between thrombosis and platelet inhibition.

Calcium is involved in practically every facet of platelet function and regulation of platelet activation.[50] Calcium mobilization and changes in calcium flux affect the activation of enzymes, reactions in the cytoskeleton, shape changes, and expression of receptor binding sites. Furthermore, extracellular calcium is required for cell-to-cell interaction and fibrinogen binding to platelet membranes during aggregation. Most of the calcium in a platelet is found in the dense granules.

Platelet Membrane Glycoproteins

Platelet membrane surface receptors are important in platelet adhesion and aggregation. Six major platelet surface glycoproteins have been characterized: GPIb, GPIc, GPIIb, GPIa, GPIIa, and GPIIIa. Of the several different groups of receptors that are found on the platelet membrane, integrins are a family of immunologically and structurally related cell

FIGURE 8. Platelet-extracellular matrix receptors. $\alpha_{IIb}\beta_3$ is also known as GPIIb/IIIa. COLL = collagen; FB = fibrinogen; FN = fibronectin; LM = laminin; TSP = thrombospondin; VN = vitronectin; VWF = von Willebrand factor. (From Hyne RO: The complexity of platelet adhesion to extracellular matrices. Thromb Haemost 66:40, 1991, with permission.)

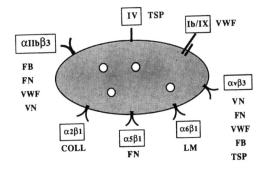

surface glycoproteins (Fig. 8). Integrins are a combination of two glycoproteins. There are five integrins that function as platelet surface receptors, but GPIIb/IIIa, GPIc/IIa, and GPIa/IIa are the most important (Table 2). These receptors have a strong affinity for adhesive proteins such as fibrinogen, VWF, fibronectin, and vibronectin.[43] Each receptor has an affinity for several extracellular matrix proteins.[29] As mentioned previously, GPIIb/IIIa receptor is important in the cohesion of platelets with fibrinogen.[23] In the absence of fibrinogen, compounds such as fibronectin, vitronectin, and VWF[37] may bind to GPIIb/IIIa. Another receptor, GPIa/IIa heterodimer complex, mediates adhesion to extracellular matrix (collagen).[35] Adhesive proteins such as collagen and fibrinogen do not interact with receptors of inactivated platelets.[29]

Other receptors on the platelet membrane are not integrins. For example, GPIb is bound to another smaller protein, GPIX, to form a noncovalent complex.[55] The binding of VWF to GPIb-IX leads to platelet activation, attraction, and attachment. GPIb-IX is the primary receptor that binds VWF during platelet adhesion.

An important receptor in the α-granules is P-selectin (platelet activation-dependent granule-external membrane, granule membrane protein 140). This glycoprotein is expressed on the platelet surface after platelet activation by thrombin.[20] It is a marker for platelet activation and also may function to mediate the reaction between platelets and polymorphonuclear leukocytes.[18]

TABLE 2. Platelet–Extracellular Matrix Adhesion Receptors

Integrins		
GPIIb-IIIa	$\alpha_{IIb}\beta_3$	FB, FN, VWF, VN (TSP, COLL)
	$\alpha_v\beta_3$	FB, FN, VWF, VN, TSP
GPIa-IIa	$\alpha_2\beta_1$	COLL
GPIc-IIa	$\alpha_5\beta_1$	FN
GPIc-IIa	$\alpha_6\beta_1$	LM
Others		
GPIb/IX	VWF	
GPIV	TSP	
Ligands		
COLL	Collagen	
FB	Fibrinogen	
FN	Fibronectin	
LM	Laminin	
TSP	Thrombospondin	
VN	Vitronectin	
VWF	von Willebrand factor	

From Hynes RO: The complexity of platelet adhesion to extracellular matrices. Thromb Haemost 66:41, 1991, with permission.

TABLE 3.   Laboratory Evaluation of Platelet Function

Peripheral smear evaluation	Platelet lumiaggregation
Platelet count	Platelet antibodies
Template bleeding time	Platelet membrane glycoproteins (flow cytometry)
Platelet aggregation to	Platelet factor 4
Adenosine diphosphate	Beta-thromboglobulin
Epinephrine	Thromboxanes
Collagen	Hemostatometer
Ristocetin	Clot reaction test
Arachidonate	Thromboelastogram
Thrombin	Sonoclot

Assessment of Platelet Function

Laboratory assessment of platelet function is summarized in Table 3. Platelet function must be assessed in the context of platelet count. The mean platelet volume and the morphology of the platelets may also be helpful to explain clotting problems. In general, the bleeding time (BT) is more useful as a screening test for platelet function than as a diagnostic tool; however, it may be useful to diagnose platelet dysfunction after CPB.[8] The BT is affected by skin temperature and minor inconsistencies in technique. Platelet aggregometry measures the amount of light that passes through a spectrophotometric chamber as platelets aggregate in response to a certain agonist. Platelet aggregation tests are excellent indicators of platelet function, but they are expensive and impractical in clinical situations. The thrombelastogram and sonoclot have been reported to represent platelet function, but they are not platelet-specific. More recently, the hemostatometer[34] and the clot retractor[22] have been noted to quantitate platelet function successfully. The platelet activated clotting time also has become available to measure platelet function. This test uses the Hepcon HMS machine to perform a titration of PAF in whole blood. The test is easy to perform, and the results are rapidly obtained. It is currently under investigation.

The development of an easy and reliable method to quantitate platelet function in the clinical setting will be a significant advance in the diagnosis and treatment of coagulopathy associated with CPB.

EFFECT OF CARDIOPULMONARY BYPASS ON PLATELET FUNCTION

Platelet dysfunction is considered one of the major hemostatic disruptions associated with CPB[24,39] and may account for a large percentage of all nonsurgical bleeding after cardiac surgery.[22,24] Bleeding is associated with increased postoperative morbidity.[22,39] When there is a generalized ooze in the surgical field, platelet dysfunction is frequently suspected. Extracorporal circulation exposes the formed elements of the blood to contact with a large synthetic surface area. The duration of this contact has recently been shown to be significant predictor of platelet dysfunction.[39] However, the critical defect in platelet physiology and the most important factors involved in the platelet dysfunction are unclear.

Platelet dysfunction associated with CPB can be classified as an extrinsic or intrinsic defect. Extrinsic defects include heparin,[33] medications, hemodilution, hypothermia,[44,67] and fibrinolysis.[39] Intrinsic platelet defects include abnormalities in platelet membrane receptors and degranulation. Platelet dysfunction associated with CPB adversely affects platelet function both qualitatively and quantitatively.[7,39] As a result, platelet transfusions are frequently administered in response to excessive postbypass bleeding.[7]

Extracorporeal Circulation

The EC circuit of CPB consists of an oxygenator, roller pumps, cardiotomy suction, plastic tubing, and filters. Most of the hemostatic effects of CPB are thought to result from exposure to the large synthetic surface area of the oxygenator.[11,17] During CPB, the blood is in prolonged contact with a nonbiologic surface that activates platelets, plasma proteins, and the fibrinolytic system.[16] The response of platelets to exposure to a nonbiologic surface is similar to their response to a weak agonist. Platelets undergo activation, adhesion, aggregation, and degranulation. These detrimental effects occur during the first minutes of CPB.[16,59] In laboratory studies in which human blood is recirculated in an EC system, platelet counts fall, plasma levels of PF4 rise, and platelet response to an agonist such as ADP is diminished.[1] In addition to the platelet response, plasma proteins are also affected by the nonbiologic surface. A layer of fibrinogen is deposited on the synthetic surface that provides an excellent area for platelet reactivity.[16] Activated platelets expose their GPIIb/IIIa receptors and adhere more easily to the fibrinogen. Subsequently, some of the platelets degranulate, thus attracting additional platelets and coagulation proteins. As platelets continue to accumulate at the sites, the number of circulating platelets is reduced and overall platelet function is compromised.[3] Platelet destruction has been verified at the surface of the cardiotomy suction and oxygenator through radioactive labeling of platelets.[46]

The synthetic surface of the EC has also been shown to damage the platelet membrane both functionally and morphologically.[17,67] George et al.[20] demonstrated circulating membrane fragments during CPB. The damage may result from shear stress, surface adherence, or turbulence within the oxygenator. Gas bubbles within the oxygenator may also damage platelets.[17] The complex interactions and mechanisms that characterize the interface between platelets and the EC are not completely understood; however, the overall effect is that the number of functioning circulating platelets is significantly reduced during CPB.

Thrombocytopenia

During the first 5 minutes of CPB, there is a predictable decrease in platelet count of 30–50%[1,45,64] (Fig. 9). However, the platelet count usually remains above 100,000/μl.[26] Hemodilution is primarily responsible for the decreased platelet count,[1] but other possibilities include liver sequestration of platelets, platelet adhesion to synthetic surfaces, formation of platelet aggregates,[64] and platelet trauma.[46] The degree of thrombocytopenia is not significantly influenced by the choice of oxygenator.[7] Initially the platelet count may decrease more with a membrane oxygenator than with a bubble oxygenator, but it continues to decrease with the bubble oxygenator throughout the duration of CPB.[17]

CPB-associated thrombocytopenia is not highly significant in regard to bleeding and overall platelet function; however, the combination of thrombocytopenia and platelet dysfunction may contribute to excessive bleeding and increased BT.[64] A platelet count of 100,000/μL in adults is usually adequate for hemostasis. Furthermore, the platelet count correlates poorly with postoperative bleeding.[7,51] The value of the platelet count compared with platelet function in relation to CPB-induced bleeding has been demonstrated in a study comparing the administration of preoperative single-donor apheresis platelets or aprotinin to patients undergoing CPB.[56] Preservation of platelet function improved hemostasis and transfusion requirements more than platelet transfusion and higher platelet counts. Similarly, in another study, patients undergoing CPB were randomized to receive donor platelets or placebo. There was no difference in blood loss, transfusion requirements, or clinical outcome between patients who received platelets and those who did not.[57]

In assessment of the platelet count, the mean platelet volume (MPV) is important (se Fig. 9). Platelets are continuously removed from and added to the circulation during CF so that a heterogenous population of new and old platelets exists.[16] Younger and lar

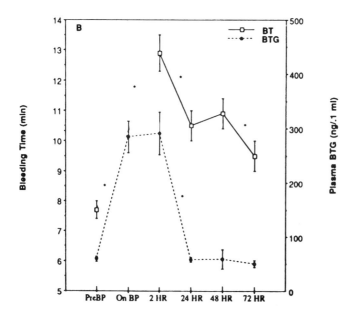

FIGURE 9. Platelet parameters measured preoperatively (PreBP), on bypass (BP), and 2, 24, 48, and 72 hours after CPB in patients having coronary artery bypass graft operations without receiving tranfusions. *A,* Platelet count (PC) and mean platelet volume (MPV). *B,* Bleeding time (BT) and plasma β-thromboglobulin (BTG). (From Khuri SF, et al: Hematologic changes during and after cardiopulmonary bypass and their relationship to the bleeding time and nonsurgical blood loss. J Thorac Cardiovasc Surg 104:97, 1992, with permission.)

platelets are more hemostatically active.[47] A lower MPV is associated with more bleeding after CPB[47] and reduced platelet aggregation.[11] The nadir for platelet size occurs five minutes after CPB;[11] size usually increases over 2–24 hours after CRB with the arrival of larger platelets.[39,45] BT and platelet aggregation to ADP also return to baseline during this 24-hour period in most patients. The improvement in MPV parallels an improvement in maximal platelet aggregation to ADP but not necessarily to decreases in blood loss and use of allogeneic blood.[11]

Platelet Dysfunction

In contrast to thrombocytopenia, platelet function can be correlated with postbypass bleeding.[22,39,51] Onset of CPB results in a prolongation of the BT that represents platelet dysfunction.[26] The progressive nature of this platelet dysfunction is demonstrated by an increase in the BT to more than 30 minutes as the duration of CPB is increased to two hours.[26,39] Immediately after termination of CPB, the BT decreases to 15 minutes and usually normalizes within 2–4 hours[26] (see Fig. 9). However, in patients who bleed excessively after CPB, platelet dysfunction may persist.[14] Harker et al.[26] found that a BT greater than 20 minutes after CPB was associated with excessive bleeding and improved with platelet transfusions. Blood loss and transfusion requirements have also been correlated with the BT two hours after CPB.[39]

Another indication of platelet dysfunction besides the BT is reduced platelet aggregation to weak and potent agonists[12,45] upon initiation of CPB.[47] These defects in aggregation persist for several hours after CPB and correlate with excessive bleeding in the immediate postbypass period.[51] More significantly, preoperative studies of platelet aggregation identified patients more likely to bleed excessively after CPB.[51] An abnormal preoperative or postoperative measurement of platelet aggregation was associated with a fourfold increase in the risk of bleeding. Such studies provide more evidence for the relationship between platelet dysfunction and bleeding after CPB.

The mechanism for platelet dysfunction is not completely understood. Reasons for the occurrence of CPB-induced platelet dysfunction include platelet activation and degranulation, platelet membrane alterations and abnormalities, and extrinsic defects of platelet function.

Platelet Activation and Cardiopulmonary Bypass

Platelet activation begins in the initial moments of CPB as contact with the synthetic surface occurs; however, the significance of platelet activation in regard to platelet dysfunction and postbypass bleeding is uncertain. Harker et al.[26] found a rise in plasma and urine levels of PF4 and BTG in association with a loss of α-granules and increased BT in humans and baboons during CPB. The progressive rise of these platelet secretory products in the plasma was cited as evidence for ongoing platelet activation during CPB.[59] However, PF4 and BTG are less specific markers for α-granule release than P-selectin.[53] Based on P-selectin levels, platelets undergo progressive activation during CPB with α-granule release[52] (Fig. 10A). However, Rinder et al.[52] could not correlate maximal platelet dysfunction based on platelet aggregation to ADP with peak platelet activation (Fig. 10B). Furthermore, neither peak activation nor peak aggregation of platelets predicted postoperative bleeding.[52] The use of drugs, such as prostacyclin, that inhibit platelet activation during CPB slightly improves the platelet count, decreases plasma levels of PF4 and BTG, and reduces chest-tube drainage compared with controls.[3] Nonetheless, the cause of platelet dysfunction associated with CPB appears to be more than α-granule depletion.[17]

Some investigators have questioned the degree of platelet activation during CPB.[69] Zilla et al.[70] believe that platelet activation is not sustained throughout CPB despite elevated plasma levels of PF4 and BTG. They found minimal concentrations of PF4 and BTG in plasma on initiation of CPB and only 3.4% of the available PF4 in the plasma at the end of CPB. They dispute previously reported increases in plasma levels of PF4 and BTG[26] as minor in comparison to the potential for granule release. The actual platelet content of α-granules does not support significant degranulation during CPB.[17] Elevated plasma levels of α-granules may be secondary to platelet trauma and lysis without necessarily representing activation. An association between bleeding, platelet dysfunction, and α-granule release is further strained with the knowledge that the BT normalizes several hours after discontinuation of CPB, but a deficiency in PF4 and BTG remains. This suggests that α-granule depletion and platelet dysfunction may be independent events.[52]

Another reason that Zilla et al.[70] maintain minimal activation of platelets during CPB is based on ultrastructural analysis of platelets during CPB. Platelets change shape with activation. Ultrastructure analysis of platelets detects the reversible phase of platelet activation. The release of α-granules and dense granules in the plasma usually represents irreversible aggregation—not simply platelet activation. Zilla et al.[70] found that at the beginning of CPB, almost half of the platelets were activated, as determined by shape changes, but granular secretory products did not rise (Fig. 11). Therefore, the initial exposure of platelets to CPB is sufficient to induce activation but not sufficient to cause irreversible secondary aggregation. Many believe that the loss of platelet aggregability—not activation—is the most important consequence of CPB. Zilla et al.[70] also found that platelet morphology gradually recovered, yet platelet reactivity to ADP and collagen did not improve. This finding suggests that factors other than platelet activation are responsible for platelet dysfunction after CPB.

Other causes for platelet activation during CPB besides platelet contact with the nonbiologic surface of EC include release of PAF[16] and plasmin. Plasmin activation of platelets impairs hemostasis after CPB.

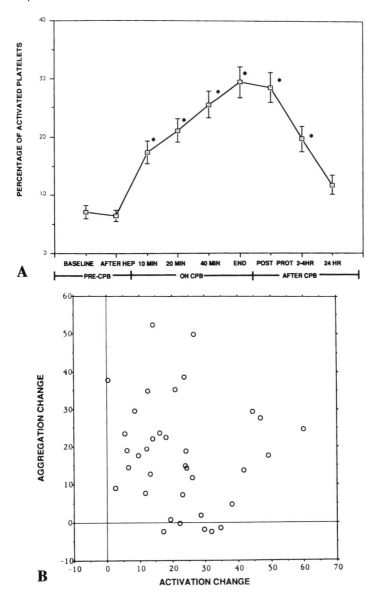

FIGURE 10. *A,* Percentage of circulating activated platelets in whole blood at each of the various time points before, during, and after CPB. Data are mean ± SEM. HEP = heparin, PROT = prota-mine. Samples are compared with baseline by ANOVA (*p < 0.05). *B,* Correlation between change in activation and change in aggregation (absolute value) between baseline and the end of CPB. No correlation was observed at r = 0.03. (From Rinder CS, et al: Platelet activation and aggregation during cardiopulmonary bypass. Anesthesiology 75:391, 1992, with permission.)

Platelet Membrane Receptors

The role of platelet glycoprotein receptors is established in normal hemostasis. The effect of EC on these receptors and their significance in postbypass bleeding are unclear.

An essential step in the formation of a platelet plug is the binding of platelets to one another with fibrinogen as the bridge. The platelet receptor that binds fibrinogen is

SEM - PLATELET MORPHOLOGY - DISCOID, SMOOTH SURFACE
(mean±sd; * p < 0.05)

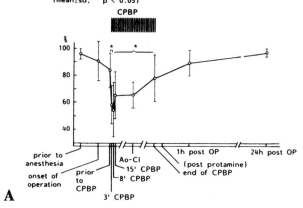

FIGURE 11. Schematic presentation of quantitatively measured parameters. Significant changes (p < 0.05) are indicated by the asterisk. *A*, Platelet morphology—discoid, smooth surface. *B*, Platelet morphology—shape changed. CPBP = cardiopulmonary bypass; Ao-Cl = aortic cross-clamp. (From Zilla P, et al: Blood platelets in cardiopulmonary bypass operations. Recovery occurs after initial stimulation, rather than continual activation. J Thorac Cardiovasc Surg 97:382, 1989, with permission.)

SEM - PLATELET MORPHOLOGY - SHAPE CHANGED
(mean±sd; * p < 0.05)

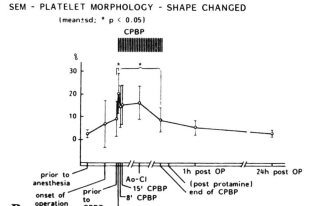

GPIIb/IIIa. A reduction in GPIIb/IIIa receptors during and after CPB has been reported in some studies[54,66] but not in others.[36] The reduction in GPIIb/IIIa receptors was not associated with platelet activation[54] (Fig. 12A). In contrast, a loss of GPIb receptors during CPB has been associated with platelet activation (Fig. 12B). The decrease in GPIIb/IIIa receptors may be a detachment of the membrane receptors from previously activated platelets that have separated from platelet aggregates.[66] However, reduction in GPIIb/IIIa receptor is not the result of shear forces alone during CPB because the GPIV receptor for thrombin-sensitive protein (TSP), which stabilizes the platelet aggregate, increases simultaneously with a decrease in the GPIIb/IIIa receptor.[54]

Loss of GPIIb/IIIa receptors may impair platelet-to-platelet interactions and has been postulated as a cause for platelet dysfunction after CPB. A 20–30% reduction of the GPIIb/IIIa receptor after CPB is unlikely to impair hemostasis significantly (see Fig. 12A). However, there is great interpatient variability in the number of platelet receptors destroyed. The actual reduction in membrane receptor loss may not be appreciated because new platelets enter the circulation and are not absorbed onto the protein-coated EC surface. At the end of CPB, there is a heterogeneous platelet population as the damaged platelets are replaced. This may offset any reduction in platelet function associated with CPB secondary to receptor loss. It may also explain a lack of correlation in some patients between bleeding and receptor loss.

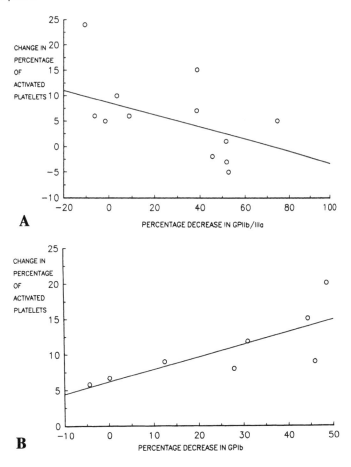

FIGURE 12. *A,* Correlation between the change in the percentage of activated platelets and the percentage decrease in GPIIb/IIIa in samples of whole blood taken after heparinization and at the end of CPB ($r = 0.6$; $p < 0.05$). *B,* Correlation between platelet activation and the percentage decrease in GPIb. The x-axis is the percentage decrease in GPIb in samples of whole blood taken after heparinization and 2–4 hours after the end of CPB. The y-axis is the increase in the numbers of circulating activated platelets between the same time points ($r = 0.76$; $p < 0.05$). (From Rinder CS, et al: Modulation of platelet surface adhesion receptors during cardiopulmonary bypass. Anesthesiology 75:566, 1991, with permission.)

A new nonpeptide that acts as an antagonist to GPIIb/IIIa receptors has been shown in dogs to prevent the significant drop in platelet count that usually accompanies the onset of CPB.[13] In a similar experiment, dogs were given a short-acting antagonist to GPIIb/IIIa receptors before CPB. It failed to prevent a decrease in platelet count after initiation of CPB; however, postbypass bleeding was significantly improved.[61] A platelet receptor antagonist prevents platelet attachment to synthetic surfaces as well as membrane fragmentation. A reduction in postbypass bleeding supports a role for these receptors in platelet dysfunction and CPB. Protection of platelets during CPB has been further advanced by combining therapies directed at different levels of platelet activity. By using a combination of prostaglandin and platelet receptor antagonist, platelet function and activation were preserved in vivo.[6] The clinical utility and potential of these therapeutic measures may soon be realized.

The adhesive receptor GPIb has been reported to decrease during CPB.[54,63] Rinder et al.[54] found a 28% decrease in GPIb only at the end of CPB (see Fig. 12B). Some patients had GPIb levels as low as 41%. The loss of GPIb was greatest in patients with the greatest platelet activation, but platelet activation was not the only explanation for decreased GPIb receptor, because inactivated platelets also experienced a decrease in GPIb receptor.[54] Plasmin reduces GPIb in association with a reduction in ADP-induced platelet aggregation in vitro and in vivo.[2,67] Van Oeveren et al.[63] found that patients who received aprotinin, an antifibrinolytic agent, did not experience a 50% fall in GPIb in the initial 5 minutes of CPB, unlike the control patients. Aprotinin administration and GPIb preservation also correlated with significant reductions in transfusion requirements and postoperative chest-tube drainage. In contrast, Kestin et al.[36] found no reduction in GPIb receptors during CPB. The difference between their findings and the findings of Rinder et al.[54] is attributed to a difference in technique. Kestin et al.[36] used whole blood flow cytometry. Whole blood cytometry may avoid a potential artifactual decrease in platelet receptors that may accompany centrifugation. Some in vitro experiments have reported degradation and relocation of the GPIb receptor by plasmin, but the receptor is replenished rapidly once plasmin attack has ceased. This finding may partially explain the recovery of platelet function several hours after CPB.[60] The results of aprotinin administration to patients undergoing CPB support the importance of plasmin and the adhesive receptor GPIb in regard to hemostasis and CPB; however, other factors associated with CPB may be as important.[36]

Two other receptor abnormalities are associated with CPB. In vitro preparations with simulated CPB have demonstrated reduced fibrinogen binding.[48] Moreover, within two minutes of initiation of CPB, there is a significant decrease in the number of α_2-adrenergic receptors.[64] This finding supports the initial loss of platelets through a process of adhesion to the surface of the CPB circuit. It may also explain any benefit from the infusion of an antiplatelet adhesive agent such as PGE_1.

The platelet membrane appears to be involved in postbypass platelet dysfunction, but the contribution of activation and platelet membrane loss is unclear. Kestin et al.[36] found no reductions in adhesive and aggregatory platelet receptors when using a different method for determining platelet receptors. When this observation is coupled with investigations of platelet degranulation, the cause of platelet dysfunction during CPB may be shifting toward an extrinsic rather than intrinsic platelet defect.

Heparin Inhibition of Platelet Function

Platelet dysfunction after CPB may be an extrinsic defect of the platelet.[36] Recently, Kestin et al.[36] reported no loss of GPIb/IX and GPIIb/IIIa receptor complexes and a lack of platelet degranulation in patients undergoing CPB. They attributed platelet dysfunction after CPB to heparin inhibition of thrombin. Ferraris et al.[19] reported a diminished response to thrombin in platelets after CPB, which normalized in 2–24 hours (Fig. 13). The platelet receptor for thrombin may be temporarily unavailable after CPB.[19] This unavailability may contribute to the platelet function defect as characterized by Kestin et al.[36]

The effect of heparin on platelet function has recently been evaluated with a new instrument called the hemostatometer. The hemostatometer uses non-anticoagulated blood in the measurement of platelet function. John et al.[34] found that 58.6% of cardiac patients showed a mild inhibition of platelet function after heparin administration. Another assessment with hemostatometry in cardiac surgical patients attempted to correlate clinical indices of bleeding with platelet dysfunction and heparin.[33] The study found that patients who exhibited severe platelet inhibition with heparin (Fig. 14) also experienced significantly greater chest-tube drainage at 4, 12, and 18 hours after bypass. The investigators were also able to correlate the in vitro effect of heparin on platelets and the in vivo effect after heparinization and before sternotomy, suggesting that hemostatometry is a valid measurement of platelet function. These findings support a significant effect of heparin on platelets.

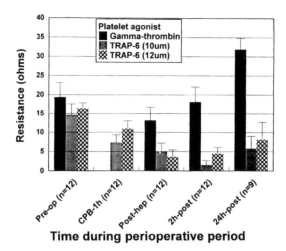

Time during perioperative period

FIGURE 13. Whole blood aggregometry response to γ-thrombin and to a six-peptide thrombin receptor agonist (TRAP-6). Whole blood samples were taken from heparin-free arterial lines in patients undergoing routine cardiac procedures. Aggregation is expressed as ohms as measured on whole blood aggregometry. Aggregation was independent of platelet count above 80,000/μl. The dose of agonist used was the dose that induced 50% of maximal aggregation in a series of normal individuals. Pre-op = preoperative response to agonists; CPB-1h, response to agonist after 1 hour of cardiopulmonary bypass; Post-hep, response to platelet agonists 15 minutes after complete reversal of heparin; 2 h-post, agonist response 2 hours after end of cardiopulmonary bypass; 24 h-post, agonist response 24 hours after end of cardiopulmonary bypass. (From Scott CS, et al: Blood 83:299, 1994, with permission.)

More recently, Greilich et al.[22] demonstrated platelet dysfunction with CPB using a new instrument called the clot retractor, which measures platelet force development within a clot and appears to be platelet-specific. Greilich et al.[22] found nearly complete abolition of platelet force during CPB with high-dose heparin (Fig. 15). In vitro studies also show the suppression of force development in a dose-dependent manner with the addition of heparin.[22] This technique also reveals a lack of return of full platelet force development after reversal with protamine, which is consistent with the prolongation of the BT after CPB.[39]

The discovery of platelet inhibition secondary to heparin is not a totally new concept. In 1977 Heiden et al.[27] demonstrated a reversible inhibition of platelet function with heparin based on prolongation of the BT, but they could not explain their finding. More recently, Khuri et al.[38] demonstrated that administration of heparin before CPB leads to platelet dysfunction, as determined by a temperature-controlled prolongation of the BT and a reduction in the TxA_2 level in the shed blood at the BT site. This finding provides more evidence that heparin contributes to postbypass hemorrhage through its effect on platelets.

A mechanism for platelet dysfunction with heparin has not been established. Mechanisms that may account for heparin's effect on platelets include direct binding of heparin to activated platelets, inhibition of adenylate cyclase or release of intracellular calcium through a platelet membrane interaction,[33] or inhibition of thrombin, one of the most potent platelet agonists. Heparin may also impair VWF activity.[58] None of these mechanisms for heparin-induced platelet dysfunction have been proved.

The role of heparin in CPB-induced bleeding is still being defined; however, the possibility that another anticoagulant may be used for CPB anticoagulation with less platelet dysfunction has been considered. Unfortunately, large clinical trials with alternate anticoagulants have been disappointing for various reasons.[32] However, alternate anticoagulants may be a way to reduce bleeding associated with CPB.

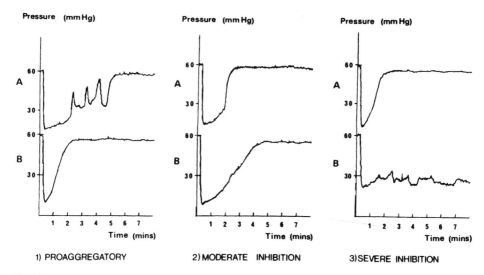

FIGURE 14. Hemostasis curves demonstrating different degrees of heparin effect on platelet function with the hemostatometer. A, Baseline sample. B, Heparinized sample. (From John LCH, et al: Effect of heparin on in vitro platelet reactivity in cardiac surgical patients: A comparative assessment by whole blood platelet aggregometry and haemostatometry. J Thorac Cardiovasc Surg 105:820, 1993, with permission.)

Other Platelet Inhibitors

There are additional causes for CPB-induced platelet dysfunction. Hypothermia can impair platelet function.[62] Hypothermia causes abnormal platelet morphology and platelet activation and reduces platelet aggregation,[21] perhaps secondary to inhibition of TxA_2 synthesis. Platelet aggregation is greatly affected by temperature less than 33°C in vitro and continues to worsen as the temperature is lowered. Certain medications are known for their platelet inhibitory actions, such as nitroglycerin, nitroprusside, calcium channel blockers, and aspirin. The effect of aspirin on platelet function can be significant. Platelet function may be abnormal for more than 24 hours. Postbypass blood loss and transfusion requirements have been reported to be higher in patients who have been taking aspirin.[10] It is also possible that an unidentified platelet inhibitor is circulating in the blood.[24]

The use of autologous blood salvage may affect platelet function through mechanically induced platelet damage or transfusion of platelet inhibitory products such as fibrin degradation products. Boldt et al.[12] recently reported that platelet aggregation was diminished most markedly in patients undergoing CPB who had autologous blood salvage compared with hemofiltration. The additional trauma related to washing and centrifuging the red blood cells was postulated as the cause.

The oxygenator is the largest nonbiologic surface area of the EC. It is considered a major contributor to coagulation abnormalities. The bubble oxygenator causes platelet dysfunction secondary to air–blood interface.[17] Studies have been divided concerning any advantage to platelet function based on choice of oxygenator.[9,17,39] Platelets may be less damaged with a membrane oxygenator compared with a bubble oxygenator, although this difference has not resulted in less postoperative blood loss when experimental conditions are equal.[9]

Cardiotomy suction, a part of the EC, adversely affects platelet function.[17] The damage is caused by air–blood interface and mechanical trauma. The amount of aspirated blood correlates directly with platelet loss. Cardiotomy suction may reduce any potential

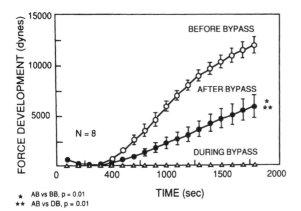

FORCE DEVELOPMENT (dynes)

BEFORE BYPASS

AFTER BYPASS

*
**

N = 8

DURING BYPASS

TIME (sec)

* AB vs BB, p = 0.01
** AB vs DB, p = 0.01

FIGURE 15. Response of platelet force development to cardiopulmonary bypass. Samples were taken before surgery (before bypass), during bypass, and after the administration of protamine sulfate (after bypass). Clotting was initiated at time 0 by the actions of calcium and batroxibin. (From Greilich PE, et al: Reductions in platelet force development by cardiopulmonary bypass are associated with hemorrhage. Anesth Analg 80:463, 1995, with permission.)

advantage to platelet preservation associated with a membrane oxygenator. Filters may also affect platelet function (Fig. 16).

Fibrinolysis-induced Platelet Dysfunction

The effect of fibrinolysis on platelet function is becoming increasingly accepted as a major factor in platelet dysfunction associated with CPB.[15,38] The major component in fibrinolysis is tissue plasminogen activator (tPA), which activates plasminogen and thus leads to formation of plasmin. Plasmin activity is known to cause platelet damage and dysfunction, expressed primarily by the downregulation of the GPIb receptor. The ristocetin-agglutination response, which depends on adequate GPIb receptors, is markedly reduced after in vitro exposure to tPA and fibrin monomers. This process is fibrinolytic-induced platelet damage.[15] Evidence for fibrinolytic-induced platelet dysfunction is found in many double-blinded, randomized trials involving CPB and prophylactic administration of antifibrinolytic agents such as aprotinin, tranexamic acid, and aminocaproic acid.[28,42]

CONCLUSION

Normal platelet function is a complex and essential process of successful hemostasis. CPB causes a multifactoral temporary platelet dysfunction. Despite knowledge of the causes and mechanisms involved in platelet dysfunction, many questions are still unanswered. Greater knowledge about the mechanism of platelet dysfunction may allow more

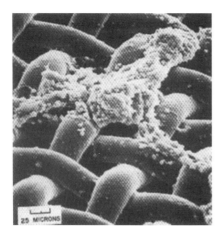

FIGURE 16. Platelet aggregate emboli trapped on a 40-micron arterial line filter during CPB. (From Edmonds LH: Blood–surface interactions during cardiopulmonary bypass. J Card Surg 8: 407, 1993, with permission.)

specific therapy to reduce the bleeding associated with CPB. Also needed is a rapid and accurate clinical test of platelet function to diagnose and guide therapy in patients with platelet dysfunction. As additional prophylactic measures are devised to reduce the incidence of postbypass hemorrhage, indicators of platelet function need to be developed to predict the risk of postbypass bleeding. Furthermore, efforts to develop more physiologically compatible extracorporeal circuits to reduce CPB-associated blood loss are ongoing. If some of these goals can be achieved, the risk of platelet transfusion and blood products can be reduced in cardiac surgery requiring CPB.

REFERENCES

1. Addonizio VP: Platelet function in cardiopulmonary bypass and artificial organs. Hematol Oncol Clin North Am 4:145–155, 1990.
2. Adelman B, Michelson AD, Loscalzo J, et al: Plasmin effect on platelet glycoprotein Ib-von Willebrand factor interactions. Blood 65:32–40, 1985.
3. Aren C, Feddersen K, Radegram K: Effects of prostacyclin infusion on platelet activation and postoperative blood loss during coronary bypass. Ann Thorac Surg 36:49–54, 1983.
4. Barrer MJ, Ellison N: Platelet function. Anesthesiology 46:202–211, 1977.
5. Bennett JS, Kolodziej MA: Disorders of platelet function. Dis Month 38:577–631, 1992.
6. Bernabei A, Gikakis N, Kowalska MA, et al: Iloprost and echistatin protect platelets during simulated extracorporeal circulation. Ann Thorac Surg 59:149–153, 1995.
7. Bick RL: Hemostatic defects associated with cardiac surgery, prosthetic devices, and other extracorporeal circuits. Semin Throm Hemost 11:249–280, 1985.
8. Bick RL: Platelet function defects associated with hemorrhage or thrombosis. Med Clin North Am 78:577–607, 1994.
9. Boers M, van den Dungen JJ, Karliczek GF, et al: Two membrane oxygenators and a bubbler: a clinical comparison. Ann Thorac Surg 35:455–462, 1983.
10. Boldt J, Knothe C, Zickmann B, et al: The effects of preoperative aspirin therapy on platelet function in cardiac surgery. Eur J Cardiothorac Surg 6:598–602, 1992.
11. Boldt J, Zickmann B, Benson M, et al: Does platelet size correlate with function in patients undergoing cardiac surgery? Intens Care Med 19:44–47, 1993.
12. Boldt J, Zickmann B, Czeke A, et al: Blood conservation techniques and platelet function in cardiac surgery. Anesthesiology 75:426–432, 1991.
13. Carteaux J-P, Roux S, Kuhn H, et al: Ro 44-9883, a new nonpeptide glycoprotein IIb/IIIa antagonist, prevents platelet loss during experimental cardiopulmonary bypass. J Thorac Cardiovasc Surg 106:834–841, 1993.
14. Czer LS, Bateman TM, Gray RJ, et al: Treatment of severe platelet dysfunction and hemorrhage after cardiopulmonary bypass: Reduction in blood product usage with desmopressin. J Am Coll Cardiol 9:1139–1147, 1987.
15. de Haan J, Schonberger J, Haan J, et al: Tissue-type plasminogen activator and fibrin monomers synergistically cause platelet dysfunction during retransfusion of shed blood after cardiopulmonary bypass. J Thorac Cardiovasc Surg 106:1017–1023, 1993.
16. Edmunds LH: Blood-surface interactions during cardiopulmonary bypass. J Card Surg 8:404–410, 1993.
17. Edmunds LHJ, Ellison N, Colman RW, et al: Platelet function during cardiac operation: comparison of membrane and bubble oxygenators. J Thorac Cardiovasc Surg 83:805–812, 1982.
18. Evangelista V, Piccardoni P, White JG, et al: Cathepsin G-dependent platelet stimulation by activated polymorphonuclear leukocytes and its inhibition by antiproteinases: Role of P-selectin-mediated cell-cell adhesion. Blood 81:2947–2957, 1993.
19. Ferraris VA, Rodriguez E, Ferraris SP, et al: Platelet aggregation abnormalities after cardiopulmonary bypass [letter]. Blood 83:299–300, 1994.
20. George JN, Pickett EB, Saucerman S, et al: Platelet surface glycoproteins: Studies on resting and activated platelets and platelet membrane microparticles in normal subjects, and observations in patients during adult respiratory distress syndrome and cardiac surgery. J Clin Invest 78:340–348, 1986.
21. Golan M, Modan M, Lavee J, et al: Transfusion of fresh whole blood stored (4 degrees C) for short period fails to improve platelet aggregation on extracellular matrix and clinical hemostasis after cardiopulmonary bypass. J Thorac Cardiovasc Surg 99:354–360, 1990.
22. Greilich PE, Carr ME, Carr SL, and Chang AS: Reductions in platelet force development by cardiopulmonary bypass are associated with hemorrhage. Anesth Analg 80:459–465, 1995.
23. Hantgan RR, Hindriks G, Taylor RG, et al: Glycoprotein Ib, von Willebrand factor, and glycoprotein IIb:IIIa are all involved in platelet adhesion to fibrin in flowing whole blood. Blood 76:345–353, 1990.
24. Harker LA: Bleeding after cardiopulmonary bypass. N Engl J Med 314:1446–1448, 1986.
25. Harker LA: Acquired disorders of platelet function. Ann N Y Acad Sci 509:188–204, 1987.

26. Harker LA, Malpass TW, Branson HE, et al: Mechanism of abnormal bleeding in patients undergoing cardiopulmonary bypass: Acquired transient platelet dysfunction associated with selective α-granule release. Blood 56:824–834, 1980.
27. Heiden D, Mielke CH, Rodvien R: Impairment by heparin of primary haemostasis and platelet [14C]5-hydroxytryptamine release. Br J Haematol 36:427–436, 1977.
28. Horrow JC, Hlavacek J, Strong MD, et al: Prophylactic tranexamic acid decreases bleeding after cardiac operations. J Thorac Cardiovasc Surg 99:70–74, 1990.
29. Hynes RO: The complexity of platelet adhesion to extracellular matrices. Thromb Haemost 66:40–43, 1991.
30. Warm Heart Investigators: Randomized trial of normothermic versus hypothermic coronary bypass surgery. Lancet 343:559–563, 1994.
31. Jet JR, Kuritsky JN, Katzmann JA, Homburger HA: Acquired immunodeficiency syndrome associated with blood-product transfusions. Ann Intern Med 99:621-624, 1983.
32. John LC, Rees GM, Kovacs IB: Different anticoagulants and platelet reactivity in cardiac surgical patients. Ann Thorac Surg 56:899–902, 1993.
33. John LC, Rees GM, Kovacs IB: Inhibition of platelet function by heparin: An etiologic factor in postbypass hemorrhage. J Thorac Cardiovasc Surg 105:816–822, 1993.
34. John LCH, Rees GM, Kovacs IB: Effect of heparin on in vitro platelet reactivity in cardiac surgical patients: A comparative assessment by whole blood platelet aggregometry and haemostatometry. Thromb Res 66:649–656, 1992.
35. Kainoh M, Ikeda Y, Nishio S, Nakadate T: Glycoprotein Ia/IIa-mediated activation-dependent platelet adhesion to collagen. Thromb Res 65:165–176, 1992.
36. Kestin AS, Valeri CR, Khuri SF, et al: The platelet function defect of cardiopulmonary bypass. Blood 82:107–117, 1993.
37. Khaspekova SG, Vlasik TN, Byzova TV, et al: Detection of an epitope specific for the dissociated form of glycoprotein IIIa of platelet membrane glycoprotein IIb-IIIa complex and its expression on the surface of adherent platelets. Br J Haematol 85:332–340, 1993.
38. Khuri SF, Valeri CR, Loscalzo J, et al: Heparin causes platelet dysfunction and induces fibrinolysis before cardiopulmonary bypass. Ann Thorac Surg 60:1008–1014, 1995.
39. Khuri SF, Wolfe JA, Josa M, et al: Hematologic changes during and after cardiopulmonary bypass and their relationship to the bleeding time and nonsurgical blood loss. J Thorac Cardiovasc Surg 104:94–107, 1992.
40. Kieffer N, Guichard J, Breton-Gorius J: Dynamic redistribution of major platelet surface receptors after contact-induced platelet activation and spreading: An immunoelectron microscopy study. Am J Pathol 140:57–73, 1992.
41. Krishnamurthi S, Westwick J, and Kakkar VV: Regulation of human platelet activation—analysis of cyclooxygenase and cyclic AMP-dependent pathways. Biochem Pharmacol 33:3025–3035, 1984.
42. Lemmer JH, Stanford W, Bonney SL, et al: Aprotinin for coronary bypass operations: Efficacy, safety, and influence on early saphenous vein graft patency. J Thorac Cardiovasc Surg 107:543–553, 1994.
43. Lewis JC, Hantgan RR, Stevenson SC, et al: Fibrinogen and glycoprotein IIb/IIIa localization during platelet adhesion. Localization to the granulomere and at sites of platelet interaction. Am J Pathol 136:239–252, 1990.
44. Lisi G, Sani G, Maccherini M, et al: Platelet function and hypothermic cardiopulmonary bypass [letter]. Ann Thorac Surg 56:1442–1443, 1993.
45. Mammen EF, Koets MH, Washington BC, et al: Hemostasis changes during cardiopulmonary bypass surgery. Semin Thromb Hemost 11:281–292, 1985.
46. Martin JF, Daniel TD, Trowbridge EA: Acute and chronic changes in platelet volume and count after cardiopulmonary bypass induced thrombocytopenia in man. Thromb Haemost 55–58, 1987.
47. Mohr R, Golan M, Martinowitz U, et al: Effect of cardiac operation on platelets. J Thorac Cardiovasc Surg 92:434–441, 1986.
48. Musial J, Niewiarowski S, Hershock D, et al: Loss of fibrinogen receptors from the platelet surface during simulated extracorporeal circulation. J Lab Clin Med 105:514–522, 1985.
49. Nightingale CH, Robotti J, Deckers PL, et al: Quality care and cost-effectiveness: An organized approach to problem solving. Arch Surg 122:451–456, 1987.
50. Rao GH: Signal transduction, second messengers, and platelet function [editorial; comment]. J Lab Clin Med 121:18–20, 1993.
51. Ray MJ, Hawson GA, Just SJ, et al: Relationship of platelet aggregation to bleeding after cardiopulmonary bypass. Ann Thorac Surg 57:981–986, 1994.
52. Rinder CS, Bohnert J, Rinder HM, et al: Platelet activation and aggregation during cardiopulmonary bypass. Anesthesiology 75:388–393, 1991.
53. Rinder CS, Bonan JL, Rinder HM, et al: Cardiopulmonary bypass induces leukocyte-platelet adhesion. Blood 79:1201–1205, 1992.
54. Rinder CS, Mathew JP, Rinder HM, et al: Modulation of platelet surface adhesion receptors during cardiopulmonary bypass. Anesthesiology 75:563–570, 1991.
55. Roth GJ: Developing relationships: Arterial platelet adhesion, glycoprotein Ib, and leucine-rich glycoproteins. Blood 77:5–19, 1991.

56. Shinfeld A, Zippel D, Lavee J, et al: Aprotinin improves hemostasis after cardiopulmonary bypass better than single-donor platelet concentrate. Ann Thorac Surg 59:872–876, 1995.
57. Simon TL, Akl RF, Murphy W: Controlled trial of routine administration of platelet concentrates in cardiopulmonary bypass surgery. Ann Thorac Surg 37:359–364, 1984.
58. Sobel M, McNeill PM, Carlson PL, et al: Heparin inhibition of von Willebrand factor-dependent platelet function in vitro and in vivo. J Clin Invest 87:1787–1793, 1991.
59. Stratta P, Canavese C, Costa P, et al: Biological stress induced by extracorporeal circulation: Comparison between cardiopulmonary bypass, hemodialysis and plasma exchange. Trans Am Soc Artif Intern Organs 30:502–507, 1984.
60. Tabuchi N, de Haan J, van Oeveren W: Rapid recovery of platelet function after cardiopulmonary bypass [letter]. Blood 82:2930–2931, 1993.
61. Uthoff K, Zehr KJ, Geerling R, et al: Inhibition of platelet adhesion during cardiopulmonary bypass reduces postoperative bleeding. Circulation 90:II269–II274, 1994.
62. Valeri C, Feingold H, Cassidy G, et al: Hypothermia-induced reversible platelet dysfunction. Ann Thorac Surg 205:175–181, 1987.
63. Van Oeveren W, Harder MP, Roozendaal KJ, et al: Aprotinin protects platelets against the initial effect of cardiopulmonary bypass. J Thorac Cardiovasc Surg 99:788–797, 1990.
64. Wachtfogel YT, Musial J, Jenkin B, et al: Loss of platelet α_2-adrenergic receptors during stimulated extracorporeal circulation: Prevention with prostaglandin E_1. J Clin Lab Med 5:601–607, 1985.
65. Walsh PN: Platelet-mediated coagulant protein interactions in hemostasis. Semin Hematol 22:178–186, 1985.
66. Wenger RK, Lukasiewicz H, Mikuta BS, et al: Loss of platelet fibrinogen receptors during clinical cardiopulmonary bypass. J Thorac Cardiovasc Surg 97:235–239, 1989.
67. Woodman RC, Harker LA: Bleeding complications associated with cardiopulmonary bypass. Blood 76:1680–1697, 1990.
68. Yardumian DA, Mackie IJ, Machin SJ: Laboratory investigation of platelet function: A review of methodology. J Clin Pathol 39:701–712, 1986.
69. Zilla P: Blood platelets and bypass [letter]. J Thorac Cardiovasc Surg 98:797–800, 1989.
70. Zilla P, Fasol R, Groscurth P, et al: Blood platelets in cardiopulmonary bypass operations. Recovery occurs after initial stimulation, rather than continual activation. J Thorac Cardiovasc Surg 97:379–388, 1989.

CHAPTER 6

Heparin-induced Thrombocytopenia and Thrombosis in Cardiovascular Surgery

HARRY L. MESSMORE, M.D.
GAURAV UPADHYAY, M.D.
SOFIA FARID, Ph.D.
RAMADEVI PARACHURI, M.D.
WILLIAM WEHRMACHER, M.D.
JOHN GODWIN, M.D.

All physicians who prescribe heparin in any form or by any route of administration should be aware of the syndromes of heparin-induced thrombocytopenia (HIT) and heparin-induced thrombocytopenia-thrombosis (HITT). The physician should monitor platelet counts frequently and observe the patient for any evidence of arterial or venous thromboembolism.[59,95,131] Although HIT occurs in only approximately 5% of patients receiving the drug for at least 5 days, the morbidity and mortality rates are so high that failure to diagnose it early and to treat it promptly results in disastrous outcome.[29,128] The majority of the cases encountered are medically and surgically treated adults, but the syndrome has been encountered during pregnancy and in the newborn.[44,117] One unexplained clinical observation is the infrequency of HIT and HITT in patients on hemodialysis who receive heparin over long periods.[56,66]

This chapter uses current literature and the authors' experience of the past 20 years to provide some understanding of the pathophysiology of HIT and HITT, along with guidelines that may be useful in their diagnosis and treatment.

DIAGNOSIS

The diagnosis of HIT depends on clinical criteria, with confirmation by specific laboratory tests. Any unexplained fall in platelet count or unexplained thromboembolism in a patient receiving heparin is sufficient reason to make a presumed clinical diagnosis of HIT (Table 1). It is not possible to select a platelet count above which the diagnosis should not be considered, nor is a platelet count below normal necessary for clinical diagnosis.[99,155] For example, many patients receive heparin in association with a surgical procedure such as cardiopulmonary bypass, which is almost universally associated with

TABLE 1.   Clinical and Laboratory Conditions that Correlate with Heparin-induced Thrombocytopenia (HIT) or HIT-Thrombosis Syndromes

Condition	Comment
Decrease in platelet count ≥ 30% from baseline level	Significant fall in platelets, even if in normal range, in a patient receiving heparin or low-molecular-weight heparin, with no other explanation evident
Platelet count below lower limit normal reference range (e.g., < 150,000)	Even mild thrombocytopenia in a patient receiving heparin or low-molecular-weight heparin, with no other explanation evident
Unexplained new arterial or venous thrombosis	Sudden onset of new thrombotic event in a patient receiving heparin or low-molecular-weight heparin, with no other explanation evident
Unexplained disseminated intravascular coagulation (DIC)	Onset of consumptive coagulopathy (DIC) ± hemorrhagic/thrombotic manifestations in a patient receiving heparin or low-molecular weight heparin, with no other explanation evident

thrombocytopenia, yet the diagnosis of HIT would not be considered unless the platelet count was lower than one would expect. However, if an unexplained thrombotic problem arises in a patient on heparin whose platelet count is at or near the expected level for his or her clinical state, a diagnosis of HIT must be strongly considered, and the heparin should be promptly stopped. Failure to monitor platelet counts and to assess the patient for any manifestation of thromboembolism or hemorrhage may result in a delay in diagnosis.[59,95,105,131]

Confirmation of Diagnosis

The diagnosis may be confirmed by laboratory testing or by observing a prompt rise in platelet count (within 1–7 days) after stopping the heparin in the absence of any other factor that could prompt such a rise. Some patients may have a positive laboratory test confirming the diagnosis, yet the platelet rise after discontinuance of heparin may be delayed up to 14–16 days. On the contrary, the platelet count may rise, yet the test may be negative. In either case, the probability that the patient has HIT is high, and heparin should not be given without consultation with a hematologist or other expert; use of alternative drugs should be carefully considered.

Laboratory testing for HIT has evolved over the past 20 years. The use of platelet counts and several tests based on the immune reactions in HIT serum are available for laboratory confirmation of the clinical diagnosis (Table 2). Details of some of these tests are discussed later, because the tests reflect pathophysiologic processes in the patient. If the patient has the immune-mediated type of HIT, there is usually a delay of 5 or more days after starting heparin before the platelet count begins to drop. If the platelet count decreases, another platelet count should be ordered immediately, and blood should be drawn

TABLE 2.   Laboratory Testing for Heparin-induced Thrombocytopenia

Test Method	Authors	Reference
Platelet aggregation	Fratantoni et al.	36
Platelet aggregation	Kelton et al.	68
Serotonin release	Sheridan et al.	109
ELISA (platelet IgG)	Howe et al.	62
ELISA (platelet factor 4–heparin)	Amiral et al.	4
Platelet activation	Greinacher et al.	43
Lumi-aggregometry	Stewart et al.	117

ELISA = enzyme-linked immunosorbent assay.

for one or more of the confirmatory tests. There is usually a delay of at least 4 hours before the result is available. In the meantime, heparin should be discontinued.

A "benign" form of HIT occurs earlier (1–2 days or less), is usually transient, and results in modest decrease in the platelet count. It is chemically mediated through an interaction of heparin with platelets.[39,59,130] This form of HIT should be suspected when the fall in platelet count is early and the additional laboratory tests are negative. However, the immune type of HIT may occur a few hours after heparin is started in patients who have received heparin previously, most commonly within the past 3 months.[59] For this reason, a careful history of drugs given in the past is needed when the patient is evaluated after a fall in platelet count. The history may reveal that heparin was given before. Prior heparin use may be suspected in a patient who has had thromboembolism or even major surgery, in which heparin is commonly used for prophylaxis or therapy.[28,56] In some patients heparin may have been given only to flush out vascular lines.[22,80,95,104]

The clinical decisions in the setting of early fall in platelet count can be difficult because one has to differentiate the benign form of HIT from an immune process due to prior exposure to heparin or from another cause of thrombocytopenia that is not yet apparent. When possible, it is prudent to consider alternative drugs if there is a prior history of heparin use, particularly within the past 3 months. The results of one or more of the laboratory tests for HIT are an important consideration in such patients. One such test is to use the patient's own platelet-rich plasma, adding heparin in a laboratory aggregometer and observing for platelet aggregation or activation. This test has been clinically useful before cardiopulmonary bypass surgery.[63,97] Whenever such a test is positive or when heparin has been used in the past, there is a strong risk for HIT, even if heparin was given only by subcutaneous route (minidose), as line flushes, or to coat in-line prosthetic or bypass devices.[22,58] Use of an alternative brand or type of standard heparin is of no avail, and testing of alternative standard heparin does not permit one to select a safe alternative.[15,16,20,42,47] If the tests for HIT are negative, it means only that heparin may be given with relative safety for purposes of a short surgical intervention. If the fall in platelet count is in fact due to immune HIT, an anamnestic immune response may occur with disastrous consequences in some patients.

Unfortunately, there is no highly sensitive and specific laboratory test for HIT; false-positive and false-negative results may be encountered despite extensive research to resolve this problem.[3–6,10,11,13,14,18,23,35,36,38,43,46–48,50,61–64,67–72,75,78,79,94,109,117,120,129,130,132,133] Some of these problems were recently summarized in an editorial by Kelton and Warkentin.[72]

PATHOPHYSIOLOGY

Much of what we believe to be the pathologic process in HIT and HITT is due to the generation of antibodies to a heparin complex, formed by the binding of heparin to one or more peptides, proteins, or glycoproteins on various cellular surfaces. The result is immune-mediated injury and destruction of platelets, endothelial cells, and possibly leukocytes.[4,6–8,11,21,25,38,46,47,50,60,61,70,78,79,117,118,120] These concepts began to evolve in the 1970s with reports by Babcock, Bell, Ansell, Towne, and others. Initially, the platelet-rich nature of the thrombi was emphasized by Towne et al. in their report of the "white clot" syndrome.[118] Isolation of an antibody of the IgG type in the 1970s and 1980s was followed by demonstration of IgA and IgM antibodies in the 1990s when more sophisticated methods evolved.[11] The antibodies are directed at heparin and the protein or peptide to which it is complexed, and the interaction of this antigenic complex with the antibody results in platelet and endothelial cell destruction.[7,8,11,25] In HIT, destruction of platelets appears to be induced by activation and aggregation; combined with endothelial cell injury, this process may be one explanation for the procoagulant state that occurs in some patients. The release of microparticles by platelets has been implicated in the thrombotic process of disorders associated with so-called "white" arterial and arteriolar thrombi. The microparticle

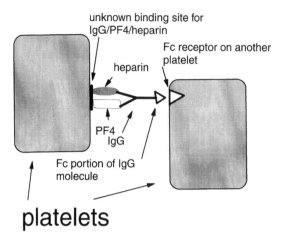

unknown binding site for
IgG/PF4/heparin

Fc receptor on another
platelet

heparin

PF4
IgG

Fc portion of IgG
molecule

platelets

FIGURE 1. A hypothetical mechanism for the binding of heparin complexes to platelets and the triggering of platelet activation. The IgG antibodies react with a complex of heparin and platelet factor 4 (PF4). This immune complex binds to an unknown site on the platelet surface. Alternatively, the actual immune reaction may start on the platelet surface when heparin binds to PF4 attached to the platelet. In either case, the Fc portion of the IgG antibody bound to the heparin–PF4 complex reacts with the Fc receptor on adjacent platelets and triggers platelet activation.

has phospholipid molecules that may be involved in the formation of prothrombinase, which converts prothrombin to thrombin.[73,84,134] HIT is unique among all other drug-induced thrombocytopenias in that acute thrombosis is regularly seen. Figure 1 summarizes proposed mechanisms.

The arterial thrombi are commonly formed on atherosclerotic plaques, suggesting an interaction of previously injured endothelium with activated platelets. There may be an interaction with other disorders known to be associated with thromboembolism, such as hereditary protein C deficiency, protein C activation disorders (factor V Leiden defect), and acquired disorders (e.g., antiphospholipid syndrome and lupus anticoagulant).[12,37,54,108,119] Livedo reticularis has been associated with HIT and HITT as well as with the antiphospholipid antibody syndrome (Sneddon's syndrome).

Venous thromboembolism is probably more common than arterial thrombosis, but arterial thrombosis is so dramatic that it is less likely to be overlooked than venous thrombosis. The spectrum of clinical disorders that one may encounter is represented in Table 3, but this list is no doubt incomplete.[59] Adrenal hemorrhage with acute adrenal insufficiency deserves special mention because it may be clinically inapparent at first.[19,33,83,107,115] Disseminated intravascular coagulation with hemorrhage or pure thrombocytopenia with hemorrhage also may occur. The apparent paradox of a fall in platelet count with thrombotic rather than hemorrhagic complications is analogous to the syndrome of thrombotic thrombocytopenic purpura.

Heparin resistance, the phenomenon of increased heparin requirement to maintain a therapeutic partial thromboplastin time (PTT) is also a well-known clinical sign of the onset of HIT. Heparin resistance is probably due to massive release of platelet factor 4. Alternatively or in association, the binding of released platelet factor 4 to the glycosaminoglycans on endothelial surfaces (heparan sulfate) reduces the ability of antithrombin III (AT III) to bind to the glycosaminoglycans and thus reduces the ability of AT III to neutralize factor Xa and thrombin. Thus, a need for escalation of the heparin dose later in the course of treatment should trigger a suspicion that HIT is developing.[9] Understanding these pathophysiologic processes provides clues to the prevention and management of such complications and their sequelae.[57]

MANAGEMENT OF HEPARIN-INDUCED THROMBOCYTOPENIA AND HEPARIN-INDUCED THROMBOCYTOPENIA–THROMBOSIS

The rapid progression of HIT and HITT can be modified by stopping all heparin. But how soon the process stops completely may be related not only to the absolute plasma

TABLE 3.   Adverse Events Secondary to Heparin-induced Thrombocytopenia

Fall in platelet count	**Venous thrombosis**
Significant fall (> 30%) that is otherwise unexplained	Superficial or deep venous thrombosis
Decrease to less than normal that is otherwise	Pulmonary embolism
unexplained	Cerebral sinus vein thrombosis
Decrease to < 100,00 that is otherwise unexplained	Adrenal vein hemorrhagic necrosis
Arterial thrombosis	**Intracardiac thrombosis**
Aorta	Arterial mural thrombosis
Iliac artery	Ventricular mural thrombosis
Lower extremity	Mechanical valve thrombosis
Upper extremity	**Vascular grafts or lines**
Renal artery	Coronary bypass vein graft thrombosis
Cerebral artery	Central venous line clot
Coronary artery	Dialysis shunt
Mesenteric artery	**Disseminated intravascular coagulation**
Livedo reticularis	Isolated
Spinal artery	Associated with thromboembolism

half-life of heparin in the patient, which may be extremely variable, but also to the possibility that circulating heparin-immune complexes may exist for a long time. In addition, the antibodies may be cross-reactive with other heparinoids and bind to endothelial cell-associated glycosaminoglycans, causing persistent endothelial cell injury or destruction.

It is mandatory to make certain that all sources of heparin are eliminated (e.g., arterial lines, flushes). Angiography, bypass pumps, hemodialysis, and intraaortic balloon pumps should be used without heparin, substituting another drug when necessary or feasible.

When no further acute anticoagulation is needed and long-term prophylaxis is desired, it is reasonable to start warfarin therapy. But if there is ongoing thrombosis (HITT), some substitute other than warfarin may be a better choice, because patients may require rapid anticoagulation and events may occur before adequate anticoagulation with warfarin.

Our proposed approach to therapy is based on our experience at the Loyola University and the Hines Veterans Affairs hospitals over the past 20 years and on published literature. Table 4 provides one method of addressing the management problems. The details of these various therapeutic modalities with the rationale for each are in the cited references.

It is important to consult with various specialists in hematology, vascular surgery, cardiology, and others as needed during the clinical evaluation of the problem. Supportive measures include the maintenance of vital systems while major adverse events are addressed. The lack of availability of an adequate substitute anticoagulant may necessitate the use of thrombolytic therapy or surgical intervention, such as a filter in the vena cava.[2]

Surgical removal of thrombi using direct arteriotomy with or without Fogarty catheter may be necessary. The consideration of a heparin substitute for postoperative anticoagulation is reasonable. Low-molecular-weight dextran and various experimental drugs are available for special protocols sanctioned by the Food and Drug Administration (Tables 4 and 5). The clinical utility versus clinical safety of some of these drugs is still being determined; for this reason, in certain situations the clinician-surgeon will opt to use heparin for short periods based on his or her clinical assessment of risks versus benefits.[96]

The rationale for therapy outlined in Table 4 is based on our understanding of the pathophysiology of HIT and HITT and clinical trials that have used various approaches. No prospective trial compares treatment with no treatment other than stopping heparin, but retrospective analysis of the outcome of stopping heparin plus use of warfarin and dextran may provide a means to determine whether a new treatment is efficacious and safe.[103,125,126] Altering the immune process by removing antibody (plasmapheresis) or by interfering with platelet aggregation has appeared to be useful in some early studies.

TABLE 4.   Treatment of Thrombotic Events Associated with Heparin-induced Thrombocytopenia

Intervention	Reference
1. Stop heparin	
2. Manage the thromboembolism	
Medical management	
Supportive therapy	
Anticoagulation	
Warfarin	
Dextran 40	15, 40
Heparinoid (ORG 10172)	24, 31, 35, 44, 73, 74, 87, 90, 123
Low-molecular-weight heparin	17, 74, 82, 86, 92, 98, 110, 121, 122, 131
Venom (ancrod)	30
Antithrombin drugs	
Hirudin	32, 51, 101, 102, 106, 124
Hirulog	
Hirugen	
Argatroban	77, 91
Thrombolytic therapy	27, 34, 93
Surgical management	
Arteriotomy-clot extraction	
Fogarty catheter extraction of clot	
Vena cava filter	
3. Antiplatelet agents	
Aspirin	26, 53, 65, 85, 88, 89, 113
Iloprost	54
Ticlopidine	53
4. Manage the immune process	
Plasmapheresis	84, 110
Intravenous gammaglobulin	41, 45
Immune adsorption—staphylococcus protein A column	

* In some cases, consider administration of protamine sulfate.

It is highly probable that newer antiplatelet drugs will be given in clinical trials. Newer antithrombotic agents are being cautiously tested. Whether low-molecular-weight heparin can be used in patients who have had HIT or HITT in the recent or remote past is highly controversial. Low-molecular-weight heparin may react with the patient's antibody in vitro, yet not cause thrombocytopenia.[72,74,131] More commonly, however, low-molecular-weight heparin will cause HIT or HITT in patients who have the syndrome with heparin and who have a positive antibody test with low-molecular-weight heparin. Rare patients develop the syndrome even when the test is negative with low-molecular-weight heparin and positive with regular heparin (see Table 4). The likelihood of HIT or HITT with heparinoids (see Table 4) is less, and cross-reaction in the in vitro test occurs uncommonly. Large studies have confirmed that in vivo cross-reaction is also less common. Efficacy in terms of antithrombotic effect and hazard in terms of bleeding may not be that much different from standard heparin except in surgical cases or cardiopulmonary bypass, in which bleeding may be problem because low-molecular-weight heparins are not completely neutralized by protamine sulfate or any other antidote.

Dextran 40 has been used because it does not interact with antibody and may even interfere with the formation of antibodies to the heparin–PF4 complex in vitro and in vivo.[1,2,15,114]

Nonheparin antithrombins, such as the natural and recombinant forms of hirudin and its analogs (Hirulog, Hirugen), may be useful substitutes, but they are still in clinical trials. A synthetic antithrombin (argatroban) is also being tested. Snake venom (ancrod) is useful but still experimental and may be associated with bleeding. Repeat use of ancrod may be impossible because of its antigenic potential. The low-molecular-weight heparins

TABLE 5.   Treatment Options for Cardiopulmonary Bypass in Heparin-induced Thrombocytopenia

Category I
No heparin for past 3 months
Current HIT testing negative, platelet count normal
Therapeutic options
  Standard heparin
    Limited to duration of the procedure; intraoperative monitoring of platelet count; platelet transfusion if unusual bleeding or thrombocytopenia.
  Experimental drugs
    Only if patient is enrolled in research protocol

Category II
Heparin in the past 3 months
Current HIT testing negative
Therapeutic options
  Experimental drugs
    Heparinoid (ORG 10172), ancrod, hirudin
  Heparin
    Surgeon's choice; especially in emergency, informed consent recommended; concurrent antiplatelet agent recommended
    Low-molecular-weight heparin

Category III
Heparin exposure—anytime
Current HIT testing positive
Therapeutic options
  Plasmapheresis or immune adsorption—repeat HIT testing. *If test is negative,* standard heparin may be used, limited to duration of procedure; intraoperative monitoring of platelet count; platelet transfusion if unusual bleeding or thrombocytopenia.
  Plasmapheresis or immune adsorption—repeat HIT testing. *If test is positive,* repeat plasmapheresis (3000 ml exchange) until test is negative; then use standard heparin as above.
    Experimental drug—heparinoid (ORG 10172), ancrod, hirudin
    Heparin or low-molecular-weight heparin—surgeon's choice in emergency. Informed consent recommended; concurrent antiplatelet agent recommended.

and heparinoids seem to be much less antigenic when used as primary therapy in patients who have never had heparin, but they can produce an anamnestic response in those who have had heparin in the past. The potential benefit of using antiplatelet drugs in conjunction with heparin for some indications, such as cardiopulmonary bypass surgery, is reasonably good if we can judge by a number of successful anecdotal reports (see Table 4).

TREATMENT OPTIONS FOR CARDIOPULMONARY BYPASS SURGERY

The cardiac surgeon faces one of the most difficult decisions about the clinical use of heparin in a patient who has or has had HIT or HITT. Some of the available options are listed in Table 5.

Several possible scenarios may influence decision making in this setting. The patient who has recently developed the syndrome is more likely to have severe thrombocytopenia, bleeding, or thrombosis, and unless it is an emergency, surgery should be postponed for 3–6 weeks. The antibody titer commonly falls to low levels within this period.[63]

When the HIT-HITT laboratory tests revert to negative, it is reasonable to proceed for a short surgical procedure, stopping the heparin and neutralizing with protamine sulfate as soon as possible.[63,96] It is also reasonable to add an antiplatelet drug in an attempt to blunt the in vivo reaction without greatly increasing the risk of hemorrhage. In considering experimental and alternative approaches, it may be valuable to consider plasmapheresis to remove the antibody, especially in urgent cases. This approach has been successful at our institutions, but a statistically significant result from a research study has not yet been reported.[84,100]

Gammaglobulin also may be useful, but it appears that some commercial brands may be better than others.[41,45] Whenever possible, the patient should be on a research protocol so that more definitive answers are obtained about the best choices among the various alternatives. Detailed informed consent with adequate documentation is part of most protocols, and we encourage this approach as part of nonprotocol case records as well.

It is apparent that additional studies are needed to help resolve critical questions about therapy of HIT and HITT.

Acknowledgments.   Loyola University Departments of Medicine, Surgery, and Pathology have generously supplied intramural research funds for laboratory and animal studies and clinical and laboratory support in the investigation of heparins, low-molecular-weight heparins, and experimental antithrombins. Drs. Roque Pifarré, Jawed Fareed, Jeanine Walenga, Michael Koza, and M.J. Seghatchian have provided clinical and laboratory expertise in the in vitro, animal, and human studies performed at the Loyola and Hines VA Hospitals over the past 20 years.

REFERENCES

1. Aburhama AF, Malik F, Boland JP: Heparin induced thrombocytopenia with thrombotic complications. W V Med J 88:95–100, 1992.
2. Aburhama AF, Boland JP, Wittsberger T: Diagnostic and therapeutic strategies of white clot syndrome. Am J Surg 162:175–179, 1991.
3. Adams J, Humphrey L, Zhang X, et al: Do patients with heparin induced thrombocytopenia syndrome have heparin-specific antibodies? J Vasc Surg 21:247–254, 1995.
4. Amiral J, Bridey F, Dreyfus M, et al: Platelet factor 4 complexed to heparin is the target for antibodies generated in heparin induced thrombocytopenia. Thromb Haemost 68:95–96, 1992.
5. Amiral J, Bridey F, Wof M, et al: Antibodies to macromolecular platelet factor 4–heparin complexes in heparin-induced thrombocytopenia: A study of 44 cases. Thromb Haemost 73:21–28, 1995.
6. Amiral J, Meyer D: Role du facteur plaquettaire 4 (PF4) dans les thrombpenies induites par l'heparine. Sang Thromb Vaiss 7:549–555, 1995.
7. Anderson GP: Insights into heparin-induced thrombocytopenia. Br J Haematol 80:504–508, 1992.
8. Anderson GP, van de Wenkel J, Anderson CL: Anti-GP 11b/111a (CD41) monoclonal antibody-induced platelet activation requires Fc receptor-dependent cell–cell interaction. Br J Haematol 7:75–83, 1991.
9. Ansell J, Deykin D: Heparin-induced thrombocytopenia and recurrent thromboembolism. Am J Hematol 8:325–332, 1980.
10. Arepally G, Reynolds C, Tomaski A, et al: Comparison of PF4/heparin ELISA assay with the ^{14}C-serotonin release assay in the diagnosis of heparin-induced thrombocytopenia. Am J Clin Pathol 104:648–654, 1995.
11. Aster RH: Heparin-induced thrombocytopenia and thrombosis. N Engl J Med 332:1374–1376, 1995.
12. Auger WR, Permpikul P, Moser KM: Lupus anticoagulant, heparin use, and thrombocytopenia in patients with chronic thromboembolic pulmonary hypertension. A preliminary report. Am J Med 90:392–396, 1995.
13. Babcock RB, Dumper CW, Scharfman WB: Heparin-induced immune thrombocytopenia. N Engl J Med 295:237–241, 1976.
14. Bachelot C, Saffroy R, Gandrille S, et al: Role of FcγRIIa gene polymorphism in platelet activation by monoclonal antibodies. Thromb Haemost 74:1557–1563, 1995.
15. Bell WR: Heparin-associated thrombocytopenia and thrombosis. J Lab Clin Med 111:600–605, 1988.
16. Bell WR, Royall RM: Heparin-associated thrombocytopenia: A comparison of three heparin preparations. N Engl J Med 303:902–907, 1980.
17. Berkowitz N, Beckman J: Heparin-induced thrombocytopenia [letter]. N Engl J Med 333:1006, 1995.
18. Beshkov LK, Warkentin TE, Hayward CP, et al: Heparin-induced thrombocytopenia and thrombosis: Clinical and laboratory studies. Br J Haematol 84:322–328, 1993.
19. Bleaser JF, Raska JE, Reckard KA, et al: Acute adrenal insufficiency secondary to heparin-induced thrombocytopenia-thrombosis syndrome. Med J Aust 157:192–193, 1992.
20. Blockmans D, Bounameaux H, Vermylen J, et al: Heparin-induced thrombocytopenia. Platelet aggregation studies in the presence of heparin fractions or semi-synthetic analogues of various molecular weights and anticoagulant activities. Thromb Haemost 55:90–93, 1986.
21. Brandt JT, Isenhart CE, Osborne JM, et al: On the role of platelet FcγRIIA phenotype in heparin induced thrombocytopenia. Thromb Haemost 74:1564–1572, 1995.
22. Brushwood DB: Hospital liable for allergic reaction to heparin used in injection flush. Am J Hosp Pharm 49:1491–1492, 1992.
23. Chong BH, Burgess J, Ismail F, et al: The clinical usefulness of the platelet aggregation test for the diagnosis of heparin-induced thrombocytopenia. Thromb Haemost 69:344–350, 1993.
24. Chong BH, Manani HN: Orgaran in heparin-induced thrombocytopenia. Haemostasis 22:85–91, 1992.
25. Cines DB, Tomaski A, Tannenbaum S: Immune endothelial-cell injury in heparin associated thrombocytopenia. N Engl J Med 316:581–589, 1987.

26. Cofrancesco E, Colombi M, Fowst C, et al: Heparin-induced platelet aggregation and its inhibition by antagonists of the thromboxane pathway. Thromb Res 42:867–868, 1986.

27. Coulon M, Goffette P, Dondelinger RF, et al: Local thrombolytic infusion in arterial ischemia of the upper limb: Mid-term results. Cardiovasc Interven Radiol 17:81–86, 1994.

28. Cummins D: Which patients undergoing cardiopulmonary bypass should be assessed for development of heparin-induced thrombocytopenia? Thromb Haemost 73:890–898, 1995.

29. Demasi R, Bode AP, Knupp C, et al: Heparin induced thrombocytopenia. Am Surg 60:26–29, 1994.

30. Demers C, Ginsberg J, Brill-Edwards P, et al: Rapid anticoagulation using ancrod for heparin-induced thrombocytopenia. Blood 78:2194–2197, 1991.

31. DeValk HW, Banga JD, Wester WJJ, et al: Comparison of subcutaneous Danaparoid with intravenous unfractionated heparin for treatment of venous thromboembolism. Ann Intern Med 123:1–9, 1995.

32. Edmunds LH: HIT, HITT and desulfatohirudin: Look before you leap [editorial]. Thorac Cardiovasc Surg 110:1–3, 1995.

33. Ernest D, Fisher M McD: Heparin-induced thrombocytopenia complicated by bilateral adrenal hemorrhage. Intens Care Med 17:238–240, 1991.

34. Fiessinger JN, Aiach M, Roncato M, et al: Critical ischemia during heparin induced thrombocytopenia, treatment by intraarterial streptokinase. Thromb Res 33:235–238, 1984.

35. Follea G, Hamandjian I, Irzeciak M, et al: Pentosan polysulphate associated thrombocytopenia. Thromb Res 42:413–418, 1986.

36. Frantantoni JC, Pollet R, Gralnick HR: Heparin induced thrombocytopenia: Confirmation of diagnosis with in vitro methods. Blood 45:395–401, 1997.

37. Gardyn J, Sorkin P, Kluger Y, et al: Heparin-induced thrombocytopenia and fatal thrombosis in a patient with activated protein C resistance. Am J Haematol 50:292–295, 1995.

38. Goad KE, Horne MK, Gralnick HR: Pentosan-induced thrombocytopenia: Support for an immune complex mechanism. Br J Haematol 88:803–808, 1994.

39. Gogstad A, Solum NO, Krutnes MB: Heparin binding platelet proteins demonstrated by crossed affinity immunoelectrophoresis. Br J Haematol 53:563–573, 1983.

40. Gouault-Heimanm MB, Huet Y, Adnot S, et al: Low molecular weight heparin fractions as an alternate therapy in heparin induced thrombocytopenia. Haemostasis 17:134–140, 1987.

41. Grau E, Linares M, Olaso M: Heparin induced thrombocytopenia—response to intravenous immunoglobulin in vivo and in vitro. Am J Hematol 39:312–313, 1992.

42. Green D, Martin GJ, Shoichet SH, et al: Thrombocytopenia in a prospective, randomized, double-blind trial of bovine and porcine heparin. Am J Med Sci 288:60–64, 1984.

43. Greinacher A, Amiral J, Dummel V, et al: Laboratory diagnosis of heparin-associated thrombocytopenia and comparison of platelet aggregation test, heparin-induced platelet aggregation test, and a platelet factor 4/heparin enzyme-linked immunosorbent assay. Transfusion 34:381–388, 1994.

44. Greinacher A, Eckhardt T, Mussman J, et al: Pregnancy complicated by heparin associated thrombocytopenia management by a prospective in vitro selected heparinoid (ORG 10172). Thromb Res 71:123–126, 1993.

45. Greinacher A, Lieberhoff V, Kiefel V, et al: Heparin associated thrombocytopenia: The effects of various intravenous IgG preparations on antibody mediated platelet activation—a possible new indication for high dose IV IgG. Thromb Haemost 71:641–645, 1994.

46. Greinacher A, Michels I, Liebenhoff U, et al: Heparin-associated thrombocytopenia: Immune complexes are attached to the platelet membrane by the negative charge of highly sulphated oligosaccharides. Br J Haematol 84:711–716, 1993.

47. Greinacher A, Michels I, Mueller-Eckhardt C: Heparin associated thrombocytopenia: The antibody is not heparin specific. Thromb Haemost 67:547–549, 1992.

48. Greinacher A, Michels I, Schafer M, et al: Heparin associated thrombocytopenia in a patient treated with polysulphated chondroitin sulphate: Evidence for immunological cross reaction between heparin and polysulphated glycosaminoglycans. Br J Haematol 81:252–254, 1992.

49. Greinacher A, Phillipen KH, Kemkis-Matthes B, et al: Heparin-associated thrombocytopenia type II in a patient with end-stage renal disease; successful anticoagulation with low-molecular-weight heparinoid ORG 10172 during haemodialysis. Nephrol Dial Transplant 8:1176–1177, 1993.

50. Greinacher A, Pötzsch B, Amiral J, et al: Heparin-associated thrombocytopenia: Isolation of the antibody and characterization of a multi-molecular PF-4 heparin complex as the major antigen. Thromb Haemost 71:247–251, 1994.

51. Greinacher A, Volpel H, Pötzsch B: A prospective study with r-hirudin (HBW023) in the treatment of heparin associated thrombocytopenia (HAT) type II [author's report—study in progress].

52. Gross AS, Thompson FI, Arzubiaga MC, et al: Heparin induced thrombocytopenia and thrombosis presenting with livedo reticularis. Int J Dermatol 32:276–279, 1993.

53. Gruel Y, Lermusiaux P, Lang M, et al: Usefulness of antiplatelet drugs in the management of heparin-associated thrombocytopenia and thrombosis. Ann Vasc Surg 5:552–555, 1991.

54. Gruel Y, Rupen A, Watier H, et al: Anticardiolipin antibodies in heparin associated thrombocytopenia. Thromb Res 67:601–606, 1992.

55. Hach-Wunderle V, Kainer K, Krug B, et al: Heparin associated thrombosis despite normal platelet counts. Lancet 344:469–470, 1994.
56. Hall AV, Clark WF, Parbtani A: Heparin induced thrombocytopenia in renal failure. Clin Nephrol 38:86–89, 1992.
57. Heck HA, Lutcher CL, Falls DG: Fatal thrombocytopenia coagulopathy after cardiopulmonary bypass: Clinico-pathologic correlations implicating heparin. South Med J 87:789–793, 1994.
58. Haeger PS, Backstrom JT: Heparin flushes and thrombocytopenia. Ann Intern Med 105:143, 1986.
59. Hirsh J, Raschke R, Warkentin T, et al: Heparin mechanism of action, pharmacokinetics, dosing considerations, monitoring, efficacy and safety. Chest 108(Suppl):258S–268S, 1995.
60. Hollander G, Bashevkin M, Feldman H, et al: Heparin-induced thrombotic thrombocytopenia. Chest 79:234–236, 1981.
61. Horne MK, Atkins BR: Platelet binding of IgG from patients with heparin induced thrombocytopenia. Blood 86(Suppl 1):Abst 2186, 1995.
62. Howe SG, Lynch DM: An enzyme-linked immunosorbent assay for the evaluation of thrombocytopenia induced by heparin. J Lab Clin Med 105:554–559, 1985.
63. Hussey CV, Bernhard VN, McLean M, et al: Heparin induced platelet aggregation: In vitro confirmation of thrombotic complications. Ann Clin Lab Sci 9:487–493, 1979.
64. Isenhart CE, Brandt JAT: Platelet aggregation studies for the diagnosis of heparin-induced thrombocytopenia. Am J Clin Pathol 99:324–330, 1993.
65. Kalangos A, Relland JYM, Massonet-Castel S, et al: Heparin-induced thrombocytopenia and thrombosis following open heart surgery. Eur J Cardio-Thorac Surg 8:199–203, 1994.
66. Kappers-Klunne M, Van Vliet H, Zietse R, et al: Presence of heparin dependent antibodies in patients on continuous intermittent hemodialysis. Blood 86(Suppl 1):Abst 3586, 1995.
67. Kelton JG: Heparin-induced thrombocytopenia. Haemostasis 16:173–186, 1986.
68. Kelton JG, Sheridan D, Brain H, et al: Clinical usefulness of testing for a heparin-dependent platelet aggregating factor in patients with suspected heparin-associated thrombocytopenia. J Lab Clin Med 103:606–612, 1984.
69. Kelton JG, Sheridan D, Santos A, et al: Heparin-induced thrombocytopenia: Laboratory studies. Blood 72:925–930, 1988.
70. Kelton JG, Sheridan D, Smith J, et al: Heparin induced thrombocytopenia: Heparin-IgG immune complexes bind to the platelet glycoprotein 1b [abstract]. Blood 68(Suppl):110a, 1986.
71. Kelton JG, Smith JW, Warkentin TE, et al: Immunoglobulin G from patients with heparin-induced thrombocytopenia binds to a complex of heparin and platelet factor 4. Blood 83:3232–3239, 1994.
72. Kelton JG, Warkentin TE: Diagnosis of heparin-induced thrombocytopenia. Still a journey, not yet a destination [editorial]. Am J Clin Pathol 104:611–613, 1995.
73. Kelton JG, Warkentin TE, Hayward CPM, et al: Calpain activity in patients with thrombotic thrombocytopenia purpura is associated with platelet microparticles. Blood 80:2246–2251, 1992.
74. Kikta MJ, Keller MP, Humphrey PW, et al: Can low molecular weight heparins and heparinoids be given safely to patients with heparin-induced thrombocytopenia syndrome? Surgery 114:705–710, 1993.
75. King DJ, Kelton JG: Heparin-associated thrombocytopenia. Ann Intern Med 100:535–540, 1984.
76. Kleinschmidt S, Seyfert UT: Heparin associated thrombocytopenia (HAT)—still a diagnostic and therapeutic problem in clinical practice. Angiology 46:37–44, 1995.
77. Koza MJ, Walenga JM, Terrell MR, et al: Thrombin inhibitor argatroban as anticoagulant in cardiopulmonary bypass surgery [abstract]. Blood 86(Suppl):88a, 1995.
78. Lane DA, Pejler G, Flynn AM, et al: Neutralization of heparin-related saccharides by histidine-rich glycoprotein and platelet factor 4. J Biol Chem 261:3980–3986, 1986.
79. Laroche J, Clofent-Sanchez G, Jallu V, et al: Further evidence that heparin-dependent thrombocytopenia may result from Fc receptor-mediated interactions. Nouv Rev Franc Hematol 34:111–121, 1992.
80. Laster JL, Nichols WK, Silver D: Thrombocytopenia associated with heparin-coated catheters in patients with heparin-associated antiplatelet antibodies. Arch Intern Med 149:2285–2287, 1989.
81. Lee DH, Warkentin TE, Hayward CPM, et al: The development and evaluation of a novel test for heparin induced thrombocytopenia. Blood 84(Suppl 1):188a, 1993.
82. Leroy J, Leclerc MH, Delahousse B, et al: Treatment of heparin-associated thrombocytopenia and thrombosis with low molecular weight heparin (CY 216). Semin Thromb Hemost 11:326–329, 1985.
83. Leschi JP, Golan-Brissoniere O, Coggia M, et al: Heparin-related thrombocytopenia and adrenal hemorrhagic necrosis following aortic surgery. Ann Vasc Surg 8:506–508, 1994.
84. Lewis BE, Rao RC, Robinson JA, et al: Early plasmapheresis reduces mortality in patients with heparin-induced thrombosis. Blood 86(Suppl 1):Abst 3666, 1995.
85. Long RW: Management of patient with heparin induced thrombocytopenia requiring cardiopulmonary bypass. J Thorac Cardiovasc Surg 89:950–951, 1985.
86. Luzzatto G, Cardiano I, Patrassi G, et al: Heparin induced thrombocytopenia: Discrepancies between the presence of IgG cross-reacting in vitro with Fraxiparine and its successful clinical use. Thromb Haemost 74:1604–1612, 1995.

87. Magnani HN: Heparin induced thrombocytopenia (HIT): An overview of 230 patients treated with organan (ORG 10172). Thromb Haemost 70:554–561, 1993.
88. Makhoul RG, Greenberg CS, McCann RL: Heparin-associated thrombocytopenia and thrombosis: A serious clinical problem and potential solution. J Vasc Surg 4:522–528, 1986.
89. Makhoul RG, McCann RL, Austin EH, et al: Management of patients with heparin-associated thrombocytopenia and thrombosis requiring cardiac surgery. Ann Thorac Surg 43:617–621, 1987.
90. Marshall LR, Cannell PR, Hermann RP: Successful use of APTT in monitoring of the anti-XA activity of the heparinoid Orgaran 10172 in a case of HITS requiring open heart surgery. Thromb Haemost 67:587, 1992.
91. Matsuo T, Kario K, Chikahira Y, et al: Treatment of heparin induced thrombocytopenia by use of argatroban, a synthetic thrombin inhibitor. Br J Haematol 82:627–628, 1992.
92. Maurin N, Biniek R, Heintz B, et al: Heparin induced thrombocytopenia and thrombosis with spinal ischemia—recovery of platelet count following a change to low molecular weight heparin. Intens Care Med 17:185–186, 1991.
93. Mehta DP, Yoder EL, Appel J, et al: Heparin induced thrombocytopenia and thrombosis: Reversal with streptokinase. A case report and review of literature. Am J Hematol 36:275–279, 1991.
94. Messmore HL, Nand S, Godwin J: Heparin-induced thrombocytopenia and platelet activation in cardiovascular surgery. In Pifarre R (ed): Anticoagulation, Hemostasis and Blood Preservation in Cardiovascular Surgery. Philadelphia, Hanley & Belfus, 1995, pp 185–188.
95. Moberg P, Geary V, Sheikh M: Heparin-induced thrombocytopenia: A possible complication of heparin-coated pulmonary artery catheters. J Cardiothorac Anesth 4:266–228, 1990.
96. Olinger GN, Hussey CV, Olive JA, et al: Cardiopulmonary bypass for patients with previously documented heparin-induced platelet aggregation. Thorac Cardiovasc Surg 87:673–677, 1984.
97. Ortel TL, Gocherman JP, Califf RM, et al: Parenteral anitcoagulation with the heparinoid Lomoparan (ORG 10172) in patients with heparin-induced thrombocytopenia and thrombosis. Thromb Haemost 67:292–296, 1992.
98. Patrassi GM, Luzzatto G: Heparin-induced thrombocytopenia with thrombosis of the aorta, iliac arteries and right axillary vein successfully treated by low molecular weight heparin. Acta Haematol 91:55–56, 1994.
99. Phelan BK: Heparin-associated thrombosis without thrombocytopenia. Ann Intern Med 99:637–638, 1983.
100. Raible M, Walenga H, Lewis BE, et al: Plasmapheresis successfully removes heparin-platelet factor 4 antibodies from patients with heparin induced thrombocytopenia. Blood 86(Suppl 1): Abstr 3613, 1995.
101. Riess KFC, Behr J, Potzsch KT, et al: Recombinant r-hirudin as a potential anticoagulant in open-heart surgery studies in a pig model. Thromb Haemost 69:Abstr 2728, 1993.
102. Riess KFC, Lower C, Seelig C, et al: Recombinant hirudin as a new anticoagulant during cardiac operations instead of heparin: Successful for aortic valve replacement n man. J Thorac Cardiovascular Surg 110:265–267, 1995.
103. Rizzoni WE, Miller K, Rich M, et al: Heparin-induced thrombocytopenia and thromboembolism in the postoperative period. Surgery 103:470–476, 1988.
104. Rama BN, Haake RE, Bander SJ, et al: Heparin flush associated thrombocytopenia-induced hemorrhage: A case report. Nebr Med J 76:392–394, 1991.
105. Schmitt BP, Adelman B: Heparin-associated thrombocytopenia: A critical review and pooled analysis. Am J Med Sci 305:208–215, 1992.
106. Schiele F, Vuellemenot A, Kramary P, et al: Use of recombinant hirudin as antithrombotic treatment in patient with heparin-induced thrombocytopenia. Am J Hematol 50:20–25, 1992.
107. Scully RE (ed): Case records of the Massachusetts General Hospital. Adrenal hemorrhage in a patient with heparin-induced thrombocytopenia and thrombosis. N Engl Med 321:1595–1603, 1989.
108. Shebata S, Harpel PC, Gharari A, et al: Autoantibodies to heparin from patients with antiphospholipid antibody syndrome inhibit formation of antithrombin III–thrombin complexes. Blood 83:2532–2540, 1994.
109. Sheridan D, Carter C, Kelton JG: A diagnostic test in heparin induced thrombocytopenia. Blood 67:27–30, 1986.
110. Shumate M: Heparin-induced thrombocytopenia [letter]. N Engl J Med 333:1006, 1995; and Warkentin T, Hirsh J, Kelton JG: Heparin induced thrombocytopenia [reply]. N Engl J Med 333:1007, 1995.
111. Reference deleted.
112. Silver D, Kapsch DN, Tsoi EKM: Heparin-induced thrombocytopenia, thrombosis and hemorrhage. Ann Surg 198:301–304, 1983.
113. Singer RL, Mannion JD, Bauer TL, et al: Complications from heparin-induced thrombocytopenia in patients undergoing cardiopulmonary bypass. Chest 104:1436–1440, 1993.
114. Sobel M, Adelman B, Greenfield LJ: Dextran reduces heparin mediated platelet aggregation. J Surg Res 40:382–387, 1986.
115. Souied F, Pourriat JL, Le Roux G, et al: Adrenal hemorrhage necrosis in heparin associated thrombocytopenia. Crit Care Med 19:297–299, 1991.
116. Spadone D, Clark F, James F, et al: Heparin-induced thrombocytopenia in the newborn. J Vasc Surg 15:306–312, 1992.

117. Stewart MW, Etches WS, Boshkov LK, et al: Heparin-induced thrombocytopenia: An improved method of detection based on lumi-aggregometry. Br J Haematol 91:173–177, 1995.
118. Towne JB, Bernhard VM, Hussey C, et al: White clot syndrome. Arch Surg 114:372–377, 1979.
119. Van Besien K, Hoffman R, Golechowski A: Pregnancy associated with lupus anticoagulant and heparin induced thrombocytopenia: Management with a low molecular weight heparinoid. Thromb Res 62:23–29, 1991.
120. Visentin GP, Ford SE, Scott JP, et al: Antibodies from patients with heparin-induced thrombocytopenia/thrombosis are specific for platelet factor 4 complexed with heparin or bound to endothelial cells. J Clin Invest 93:81–83, 1995.
121. Vitoux JF, Mattieu JF, Roncato M, et al: Heparin-associated thrombocytopenia. Treatment with low molecular weight heparin. Thromb Haemost 55:37–39, 1986.
122. Vitoux JF, Roncato M, Hourdebaigt P, et al: Heparin-induced thrombocytopenia and pentosan polysulphate: Treatment with a low molecular weight heparin despite in vitro platelet aggregation. Thromb Haemost 55:294–295, 1985.
123. Vun CM, Evans S, Chong BH: Cross-reactivity study of low molecular heparins and heparinoid in heparin-induced thrombocytopenia. Thromb Res 81:525–532, 1996.
124. Walenga JM, Bakhos M, Messmore ML, et al: Potential use of recombinant hirudin as an anticoagulant in a cardiopulmonary bypass model. Ann Thorac Surg 51:271–277, 1991.
125. Walls JT, Boley TM, Curtis JJ, et al: Heparin induced thrombocytopenia in patients undergoing intra-aortic balloon pumping after open-heart surgery. ASAIO J 38:M574–M576, 1992.
126. Walls JT, Curtis JJ, Silver D: Heparin induced thrombocytopenia in patients who undergo open heart surgery. Surgery 108:686–693, 1990.
127. Walls JT, Curtis JJ, Silver D: Heparin induced thrombocytopenia in open heart surgical patients: Sequelae of late recognition. Ann Thorac Surg 53:787–791, 1992.
128. Weismann RE, Tobin RW: Arterial embolism occurring systemic heparin therapy. AMA Arch Surg 76:219–226, 1958.
129. Warkentin TE, Hayward CP, Boshkov CK, et al: Sera from patients with heparin-induced thrombocytopenia generate platelet derived microparticles with procoagulant activity: An explanation for the thrombotic complications of heparin induced thrombocytopenia. Blood 84:3691–3699, 1994.
130. Warkentin TE, Kelton JG: Heparin-induced thrombocytopenia. Annu Rev Med 40:31–44, 1989.
131. Warkentin TE, Levine MN, Hirsh J, et al: Heparin-induced thrombocytopenia in patients treated with low-molecular-weight heparin or unfractionated heparin. N Engl J Med 332:1330–1335, 1995.
132. Warkentin TE, Hayward CPM, Smith CA, et al: Determinants of donor platelet variability when testing for heparin induced thrombocytopenia. J Lab Clin Med 120:371–379, 1992.
133. Wolf H, Nowack H, Wick G: Detection of antibodies interacting with glycosaminoglycan polysulphate in patients treated with heparin or other polysulphated glycosaminoglycans. Int Arch Allergy Appl Immunol 70:157–163, 1983.
134. Zwaal RFA, Comfurius P, Smeets E, et al: Platelet procoagulant activity and microvesicle formation. In Seghatchian MJ, Samama M, Hecker SP (eds): Hypercoagulable States. Boca Raton, FL, CRC Press, 1996, pp 29–36.

CHAPTER 7

Current Developments in Anticoagulant and Antithrombotic Agents

JAWED FAREED, Ph.D.
DEMETRA D. CALLAS, Ph.D.
DEBRA A. HOPPENSTEADT, M.S., M.T. (ASCP)
WALTER JESKE, Ph.D.
JEANINE M. WALENGA, Ph.D.
ROQUE PIFARRÉ, M.D.

The pathophysiology of thrombotic events is multicomponent and involves blood, the vascular system, and target sites. Figure 1 depicts the process of thrombogenesis. Initially, vascular injury results in localized alterations of vessels and subsequent activation of platelets. Activated cells mediate several direct or signal transduction-induced processes resulting in activation of platelets. Cellular activation also results in the release of various mediators that amplify vascular spasm and the coagulation process. Thus, anaphylatoxins (C_3a and C_5a), superoxide, leukotrienes (LTC4), thromboxane B_2 (TxB$_2$), serotonin, platelet factor 3 (PF3), platelet factor 4 (PF4), platelet-activating factor (PAF), endothelin-1, and numerous cytokines play a role in the overall pathophysiology of the thrombotic process. Drugs that target various sites of the activation process can be developed to control thrombotic events. Because of the coupled pathophysiology, a single drug may not be able to target these sites to produce therapeutic actions. Furthermore, many of the mediators produce localized actions at cellular and subcellular levels. The feedback amplification process also plays an important role. This understanding has led to the concept of polytherapy in the management of thrombotic disorders.

Venous insufficiency, blood plasma-related disorders, fibrinolytic deficit, and an imbalance of regulatory proteins result in activation of the hemostatic process. Postsurgical trauma, inflammation, and sepsis also can activate the hemostatic process, leading to venous thrombosis. The primary process in venous thrombosis is generation of thrombin. Thus, drugs targeting coagulation protease activation are useful in the treatment of venous disorders.[1] However, platelet and cellular activation contribute significantly to arterial thrombotic events; therefore, drugs targeting those sites are important in the management of arterial thrombosis and microangiopathic disorders.

During cardiovascular surgery, the hemostatic function is significantly modified by hemodilution, drugs, and other procedure-related alterations. In addition, large amounts of

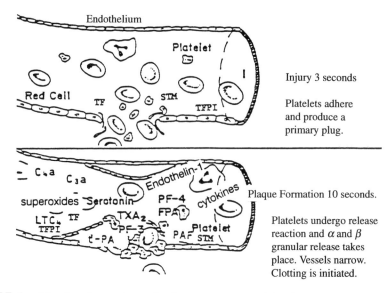

FIGURE 1. Blood and vascular activation processes resulting in thrombogenesis. Vascular damage, cell activation, and related products contribute to the development of thrombus and vascular constriction. Antithrombotic drugs can target single or multiple sites in the control of thrombogenesis.

thrombogenic material are generated. Thus, the use of anticoagulants requires special care and dosage optimization. The newer drugs may be of special value for cardiovascular surgery. In addition, some of these drugs may be useful for postsurgical prophylaxis.

The newer developments in antithrombotic drugs are rather significant. Many advanced techniques to develop antithrombotic drugs are used at present. Advances in biotechnology and separation techniques have also contributed to the development of newer antithrombotic drugs.[2-8] These drugs may prove to have a better efficacy in the control and treatment of thrombogenesis. Drugs and devices developed on the basis of the newer concepts can be classified into the groups listed below. The drugs marked with an asterisk may be useful in trauma patients, because their safety/efficacy index is claimed to be higher than conventional anticoagulants.

Heparin-related drugs
1. Low-molecular-weight heparins
2. Medium-molecular-weight heparins
3. High-molecular-weight heparins
4. Chemically modified heparins
5. Dermatans
6. Heparans*
7. Semisynthetic heparin derivatives (suleparoide)
8. Chemically synthesized antithrombotic oligosaccharides
9. Sulfated dextrans
10. Synthetic hypersulfated compounds
11. Polyanionic agents
12. Marine polysaccharides
13. Heparinoids (Lomoparan)
14. Thioxyloside derivatives

Antiplatelet drugs
1. (Ticlopidine)-related antiplatelet drugs

2. (Pletaal)-related phosphodiesterase inhibitors
3. (Iloprost) prostanoid modulators
4. Eicosanoids and related drugs
5. ω-3 Fatty acids and fish oil-related products
6. Antibodies targeting membrane glycoproteins
7. Peptides and proteins modulating platelet function

Endothelial lining modulators
1. Nucleic acid derivatives (defibrotide)
2. Sulfomucopolysaccharide mixtures
3. 1-Deamino-8-D-arginine vasopression (DDAVP) and related peptides
4. Growth factor-related peptides
5. Protein digests
6. Vitamins

Viscosity modulators
1. Synthetic and natural polymers
2. Pentoxifylline
3. Venoms, defibrinating agents (ancrod)
4. Polyelectrolytes

Biotechnology-based proteins
1. Tissue-type plasminogen activator (tPA) and mutants
2. Hirudin, mutants and fragments
3. Protein C and protein S
4. Thrombomodulin
5. Thrombomodulin—thrombin complex
6. Antithrombin III (AT III)
7. Antithrombin III–heparin complex
8. Recombinant heparin cofactor II
9. Glycoprotein-targeting proteins and peptides
10. Protease-specific inhibitors
11. Recombinant tissue factor pathway inhibitor

Synthetic antithrombin agents
1. Hirulogs
2. D-Me-Phe-Pro-Arg-derived antithrombotic drugs
3. Argatroban
4. Inogatran
5. Napsagatran
6. Borohydride derivatives

Synthetic and recombinant anti-Xa agents
1. DX 9065
2. Chemically synthesized agents
3. Antistatin oligosaccharides
4. Yagin
5. Peptides

Optimized polytherapy for trauma-induced thrombotic disorders
1. Heparin/antiplatelet drugs
2. Coumadin/antiplatelet drugs
3. Thrombolytic agents/heparin
4. Thrombolytic agents/antiplatelet drugs
5. Thrombolytic agents/hirudin and other thrombin inhibitors
6. Recombinant drug conjugates
7. Hirudin/antithrombotic agents
8. Hirudin/glycoprotein-targeting antibodies

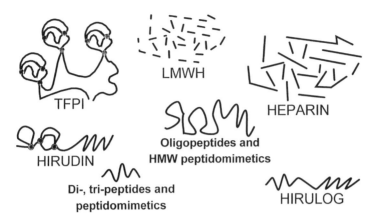

FIGURE 2.   Structural diversity in anticoagulant drugs, which include proteins, peptides, nucleic acids, carbohydrates, and synthetic heterocyclic agents.

Newer drug delivery systems and formulations
1. Oral
2. Ointments
3. Transdermal
4. Sustained release
6. Target-specific antithrombotic drugs (antibody-directed)
7. Catheters and devices capable of targeted drug delivery

Antithrombotic drugs represent a wide spectrum of natural, synthetic, semisynthetic and biotechnology-produced agents with marked differences in chemical composition, physicochemical properties, biochemical actions, and pharmacologic effects. Figure 2 depicts the molecular diversities in the structure of various classes of new anticoagulant drugs, including proteins, peptides, carbohydrates and synthetic oligosaccharides. In addition to structural heterogeneity, each of these agents also shows distinct functional properties.

The endogenous actions of the antithrombotic drugs are remarkably complex. It is no longer valid to assume that an antithrombotic drug must produce an anticoagulant action in blood that is similar to that of conventional heparin and oral anticoagulants. Many of the drugs in various categories produce no alteration of blood-clotting parameters, yet they are effective therapeutic agents because of their interactions with the various elements of the vasculature and other blood components. In addition, several of these agents require endogenous transformation to become active products. Therefore, it becomes important to rely on their pharmacodynamic actions rather than on their in vitro characteristics to assess potency or efficacy. Hematologic modulation plays a key role in their mediation of antithrombotic actions, involving red cells, white cells, platelets, and blood proteins. This is particularly true in trauma-induced thrombotic disorders, in which multiple processes are involved in thrombogenesis.

NEWER APPLICATIONS OF UNFRACTIONATED HEPARIN
Unfractionated heparin is used primarily as an anticoagulant for both therapeutic and surgical indications. Usually beef lung- and porcine mucosal-derived products are available. The unfractionated heparins recently have been used for the following additional therapeutic purposes:
1. Management of unstable angina
2. Adjuncts to chemotherapeutic agents

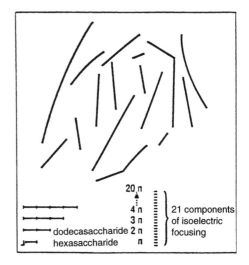

FIGURE 3.   Molecular heterogeneity in unfractionated heparin. In addition to compositional variation, heparin exhibits functional heterogeneity in terms of its interaction with endogenous proteins and cells. The antithrombotic and anticoagulant effects of heparin are based on its polypharmacologic actions.

3. Adjuncts to anti-inflammatory drugs
4. Modulatory agents for growth factors
5. Treatment of hemodynamic disorders

The unfractionated heparins are heterogeneous in nature (Fig. 3). Their molecular weight varies with their origin. The beef lung heparin preparations are usually of higher molecular weight than porcine mucosal heparin. However, the charge density and other characteristics, such as serpin affinity, are similar for both preparations. Several newer pharmacologic effects, independent of the anticoagulant effects, have been described, including glycosylation-mediated functional modulation of macromolecules, growth factor modulation, release of endothelial products, and interactions with various endogenous sites.

The heparins standardized by the United States Pharmacopoeia (USP) differ in overall anticoagulant responses because of their origin and structural make-up. Thus, such endogenous effects as the release of tissue factor pathway inhibitor and platelet receptor modulation are product-dependent. For this reason, a USP standardized product may not perform in an identical manner when used at a higher dosage for anticoagulation purposes.

Chemical modification of the unfractionated heparins, such as desulfation, deamination, and coupling with various agents, have resulted in products of a nonanticoagulant nature with selective actions on enzymes and cellular receptors. Thioxyloside derivatives also have been reported to produce oral antithrombotic actions in animal models. However, relatively larger dosages are needed to produce such effects. These heparin derivatives are currently under evaluation for such indications as sepsis, viral infections, and proliferative disorders.

NEW HEPARINS

Development of Low-Molecular-Weight Heparins

The development of low-molecular-weight heparins (LMWHs) has added a new dimension to the clinical management of thrombotic disorders. LMWHs have revolutionized the prophylaxis of postsurgical thrombosis.[9–11] More recently they have been used for the treatment of trauma-related thrombosis. In particular, their relative effects on platelets are minimal in comparison with heparin. Thus, LMWHs are of value in platelet-compromised patients. Several other agents, such as chemically synthesized analogs of heparin, nonheparin glycosaminoglycans (e.g., dermatan sulfate, heparan sulfate), and

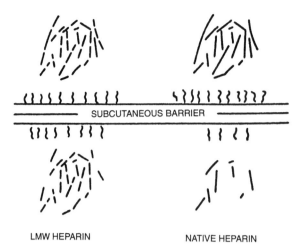

FIGURE 4. Bioavailability of heparin and low-molecular-weight heparin after subcutaneous administration. The subcutaneous barrier allows the absorption of only lower-molecular-weight components of heparin. This observation was one of the major factors in the development of LMWHs.

various other antithrombotic agents, have also become available for the management of thrombotic disorders. In the United States, however, most of these agents are in clinical trials and not yet available for general clinical use.

For the past few decades, heparin has been widely used for the prevention of postoperative thromboembolism.[12–14] However, several adverse side effects are associated with its use, such as bleeding, heparin-induced thrombocytopenia, heparin-induced thrombosis,[15,16] and osteoporosis.[17] In addition, the regimen of prophylactic heparin used in the prevention of deep venous thrombosis (DVT) is tedious, requiring 2–3 daily injections because of the limited bioavailability and short half-life of heparin when administered subcutaneously.

The many clinical problems associated with heparin led several investigators to study its structure and to identify its active component(s). The observation that only LMWHs are absorbed after subcutaneous administration has led to their clinical development. As shown in Figure 4, the bioavailability of LMWH is much greater than that of unfractionated heparin. Experimental studies revealed that the first LMWH had a subcutaneous bioavailability of about 90% compared with 15–25% for unfractionated heparin.[18] Furthermore, LMWHs exhibit a much longer biologic half-life than heparin.[5] Thus, LMWH preparations can be administered with a single daily injection, making them easy to use as a prophylactic agent. Eight LMWHs have already been approved for the prophylaxis of thrombosis in Europe. Several of these LMWHs are under clinical trials in the United States. One was approved in 1993 for use after orthopedic surgery for prophylaxis of DVT. It is expected that two other agents will be approved for clinical use in 1994.

Low-molecular-weight components in unfractionated heparins were identified long before the development of clinically effective agents. However, because of technologic problems, they were not made available for clinical use. The very first LMWH was obtained by a fractionation method.[19] However, this method yielded a limited amount of active product and was cost-prohibitive. During the past decade, different chemical and enzymatic processes have been developed to obtain LMWH from the parent unfractionated heparin (UFH). The depolymerization process for the production of LMWH is shown in Figure 5.

Table 1 lists some of the commercially available LMWHs. Fraxiparin was originally obtained by a fractionation method. However, it is now obtained by an optimized nitrous acid depolymerization.[20] Enoxaparin (Lovenox) is obtained by benzylation followed by alkaline depolymerization (ß-elimination). Enoxaparin, which contains a double-bond at the

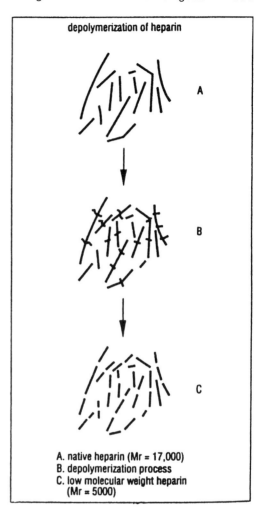

depolymerization of heparin

A

B

C

A. native heparin (Mr = 17,000)
B. depolymerization process
C. low molecular weight heparin
(Mr = 5000)

FIGURE 5. Manufacturing processes for low-molecular-weight heparins. Unfractionated heparin of porcine or bovine origin is depolymerized by chemical or enzymatic digestion in controlled conditions. The degree of depolymerization is adjusted to obtain low-molecular-weight heparins of varying weight.

reducing end, originally required the addition of large amounts of sodium bisulfite to prevent oxidation of the terminal groups.[1] A recent formulation that contains no sodium bisulfate is claimed to exhibit pharmacologic effects similar to the original product.[7,8] Fragmin is obtained by nitrous acid depolymerization followed by ion exchange chromatography. It markedly differs from the other LMWHs in physicochemical characteristics and pharmacologic profile.[1] Fluxum is obtained from beef mucosa by a peroxidative depolymerization process. This agent has been found to mediate some of its actions through non-AT III-mediated pathways.[5] Ardeparin, a product prepared by peroxidative digestion procedures with Hepar (KabiVitrum), has been developed by Wyeth Laboratories for clinical use. The Novo LMWH (Logiparin) is prepared by enzymatic digestion using *Flavobacterium heparinicum* heparinase. Logiparin also contains large amounts of sodium bisulfite as an antioxidant.[5] Innohep is also prepared by a heparinase digestion method and is identical to Logiparin.

Embolex NM is prepared by isoamyl nitrite digestion and is supplemented with dihydroergotamine. A monosubstance that does not contain dihydroergotamine also has been introduced. Reviparin (Clivarin), a product of Knoll Laboratories (Ludwigshafen, Germany), is also prepared by nitrous acid digestion. Bioparin, a LMWH from Bioiberica

TABLE 1. Currently Available Low-Molecular-Weight Heparins

Trade Name	Manufacturer/Supplier	Method of Preparation
Fraxiparin, Seleparin	Sanofi (Paris)	Fractionation, optimized nitrous acid depolymerization
Enoxaparin, Clexane Lovenox	Rhône Poulenc (Paris)	Benzylation followed by alkaline hydrolysis
Fragmin	Kabi (Stockholm)	Controlled nitrous acid depolymerization
Fluxum	Opocrin (Corlo, Italy)	Peroxidative cleavage
Ardeparin, Normiflo	Wyeth (Philadelphia)	Peroxidative cleavage
Logiparin	Novo (Copenhagen)	Heparinase digestion
Innohep	Leo (Copenhagen)	Heparinase digestion
Sandoparin, Certoparin	Sandoz AG (Nurnberg)	Isoamyl nitrate digestion
Reviparin, Clivarin	Knoll AG (Ludwigshafen, Germany)	Nitrous acid digestion
Boxol	Rovi (Madrid)	β-elimination or nitrous acid digestion
Miniparin	Syntex (Buenos Aires)	Nitrous acid digestion
Clivarin	Knoll (Ludwigshafen, Germany)	Controlled nitrous acid depolymerization followed by chromatographic purification

(Barcelona), is prepared by a β-elimination method. Boxol (Rovi Pharmaceutical, Madrid) is prepared by either β-elimination or nitrous acid digestion. Marked differences in the two different batches of this product have been observed. Miniparin, a product of Syntex Argentina, is prepared by a nitrous acid digestion method.

Recent studies have shown that the LMWHs obtained from each process exhibit chemical and pharmacological differences.[21–25] Such differences may influence clinical outcome, especially with the higher doses used for cardiovascular indications.

Low-Molecular-Weight Heparins in the Management of Thrombosis

In the past, LMWHs have been used for postsurgical prophylaxis of DVT. However, they are now also used in the treatment of preexisting events by both subcutaneous[14] and intravenous (Breddin, personal communication) administration.

Table 2 summarizes randomized studies in which LMWHs have been compared with unfractionated heparin in patients undergoing abdominal surgery. In two studies a significant decrease in DVT was observed in patients receiving LMWHs compared with unfractionated heparin.[26–29] Other studies found no statistical difference in efficacy of the two treatments.[12,30–36] Most studies found no significant difference between the observed bleeding effects of the LMWHs and unfractionated heparin. In all of these studies, LMWH was given as a single daily dose, whereas unfractionated heparin was administered 2 or 3 times daily. The results of these studies suggest that LMWHs are effective and well tolerated in patients undergoing general surgery. The primary advantage of LMWHs over heparin was the reduced number of injections per day.

Administration of LMWH has been the most extensively studied method of prophylaxis of DVT in orthopedic patients in recent years. Evidence that this treatment is both effective and safe is quickly accumulating.

Ten recent randomized trials using venography or ^{125}I fibrinogen uptake as the endpoint are summarized in Table 3. Four studies compared LMWH with dextran. Two of these studies found no significant difference between the LMWH and dextran groups. However, in the other two studies, LMWH was more effective than dextran. The different results are probably due to the different dosages selected for dextran as well as the difference in the dosages and composition of the LMWHs. Two other studies compared

TABLE 2.   Comparison between Unfractionated Heparin and Low-Molecular-Weight Heparin Efficacy in General Surgery in Recent Randomized Studies

Reference	LMWH	UFH	Incidence of Thrombosis		
			LMWH (%)	UFH (%)	p-Value
European Fraxiparin Group[28]	Fraxiparin 7500 AXa U/day	5000 IU 3 ×/day	2.8	4.5	< 0.05
Caen[31]	Fragmin 2500 AXa U/day	5000 IU 2 ×/day	3.1	3.7	NS
Bergqvist[26]	Fragmin 5000 AXa U/day	5000 IU 2 ×/day	5.0	9.2	< 0.05
Verardi[36]	Fluxum 4000 IU or 8000 AXa U/day	5000 IU 2 or 3 ×/day	3.2	6.3	NS
Kakkar[33]	Sandoz LMWH/DHE 1500 APTT U/day	UFH/DHE 5000 U 2 ×/day	11.4	11.0	NS
Hartl[32]	Fragmin 2500 AXa U/day	5000 IU 2 ×/day	7.9	8.1	NS
Samama[34]	Enoxaparin, 60 mg/day 40 mg 3 ×/day 20 mg day	5000 IU	2.9 2.9 3.8	3.8 2.7 7.6	NS NS NS
Baumgartner[30]	Sandoz LMWH/DHE 1500 APTT U/day	UFH/DHE 2500 IU 2 ×/day	3.1	3.7	NS

NS = nonsignificant, UFH = unfractionated heparin, LMWH = low-molecular-weight heparin.

TABLE 3.   Comparison between Low-Molecular-Weight Heparins and Control Group Efficacy in Patients Undergoing Hip Surgery

Reference	LMWH	Control Drug	Incidence of Deep Venous Thrombosis		
			LMWH (%)	Control (%)	p-Value
Matzsch[39]	Logiparan 35 AXa U/kg/day	Dextran 500 ml alt. day	23	37	NS
Pini[84]	Fluxum 7500 AXa U/2 ×/day	UFH 5000/3 ×/day	20	29	NS
Monreaul[41]	Fragmin 5000 AXa U/day	UFH 5000/3 ×/day	30	13.6	< 0.05
Planes[35]	Enoxaparin 40 mg/day	UFH 5000/3 ×/day	12.5	25	< 0.05
Eriksson[37]	Fragmin 2500 APTT U/2 ×/day	Dextran 500 ml alt. day	20	45	< 0.05
Matzsch[40]	Logiparan 35 AXa U/kg/day	Dextran 500 ml alt. day	28	39	NS
Sorensen[85]	Logiparan 50 IU/kg/day	Placebo/daily	27	39	NS
Borris[27]	Enoxaparin 40 mg/day	Dextran 60 mg/ml alt. day	6	21	< 0.05
Haas[29]	Sandoz LMWH/DHE 1500 APTT U/day	UFH/DHE 5000 U 2 ×/day	20.5	20.5	NS
Turpie[86]	Enoxaparin 30 mg/2 × /day	Placebo 2 ×/day	12	43	< 0.05

NS = nonsignificant, alt. = alternate, UFH = unfractionated heparin, LMWH = low-molecular-weight heparin.

LMWH with placebo. One study found a difference in the incidence of DVT, whereas the other did not.

Many surgeons and physicians around the world now appreciate that a large number of cases of venous thromboembolism, particularly after surgery, can be avoided by correct prophylaxis. With additional education and introduction of newer, more efficacious agents, it should become routine for all patients undergoing surgery to be assessed for risk of venous thrombosis and protected accordingly.

Of the many drugs used as prophylactic antithrombotic agents, heparin has the longest history as therapy for both DVT and pulmonary embolism (PE). Many studies have shown that in moderate- and high-risk patients, heparin can prevent postoperative DVT and PE.[9,37–43] With the introduction of LMWHs, these benefits can be obtained together with easier dosing and potentially less risk of bleeding. Many surgeons, however, still harbor fears and doubts about using thromboprophylaxis. One of the most common fears is bleeding. Some surgeons are not convinced that the benefits of prophylaxis outweigh the risks.

During the 1980s there have been great advances in our understanding of how heparinlike compounds work. LMWHs are less anticoagulant (in vitro clot-inhibiting) than heparin but retain antithrombotic (in vivo thrombosis-inhibiting) potential.[44–47] Thus the risk of bleeding is less with LMWHs than with heparin when they are used properly, particularly with patient-adjusted doses. However, minor wound bleeding after a successful operation is preferable to death from PE.

Each year over 1 million Americans require hospitalization for postsurgical and medical thromboembolic disorders. Approximately 10% of these patients develop serious PE. As a result, the National Institutes of Health called a consensus meeting in March 1986 to discuss the magnitude of thromboembolic disorders and the need for prophylactic therapy. The consensus conference identified the magnitude of the problem and made a strong recommendation to use prophylactic measures. Although the consensus meeting reviewed various pharmacologic and physical methods for the prophylaxis of thromboembolic disease, it specifically discussed the use of low-dose heparin and made the following recommendations:

1. Low-dose heparin can be used for the prophylaxis of DVT in general surgical patients (patients with medium risk).

2. Individualized dosages should be given to high-risk patients (trauma and orthopedic surgery).

3. None of the prophylactic regimens available in 1986 were considered optimal.

When these recommendations were made, only one LMWH was commercially available in France, and limited information was available in the United States. Today the LMWHs are commonly used in many European countries for prophylaxis of thromboembolic disorders in both surgical and medical patients. Several LMWHs are currently under evaluation in phase II and phase III trials in the United States.

Available clinical data suggest that LMWHs can be safely substituted for low-dose heparin. To validate this conclusion, several comparative trials of low-dose heparin and LMWHs are in progress throughout the world. In several European clinical trials, the efficacy of LMWHs in the prevention of postsurgical DVT has been proved, and LMWHs are considered the drug of choice for this indication.[26,33,48,49]

When used subcutaneously for prophylactic treatment, most LMWHs mediate their actions in a similar manner; however, their efficacy and tolerability profiles and the recommended doses differ markedly. Because of the differences among products, such practices as standardization by a single in vitro assay and assignment of a single International Nonproprietary Names (INN) designation are deemed invalid for LMWHs as a group. The individualized approach to all LMWHs has recently been adopted by the World Health Organization (WHO), Food and Drug Administration (FDA), and the Scientific and

Standardization Subcommittee of the International Society of Thrombosis and Hemostasis (ISTH). The recognition of the individuality of each of the LMWHs is extremely important to avoid excessively high or low doses of a given product. Dose-finding studies are essential and will have a major impact on the prophylactic and therapeutic acceptance of LMWHs.

Having satisfactorily passed their first step in clinical use, LMWHs are now being applied to other clinical settings. LMWHs are moving into the area of established DVT and therapeutic treatment of thrombosis. LMWHs may be therapeutic alternatives to heparin in some, but not all patients who develop heparin sensitivity or heparin-induced thrombocytopenia. At optimal dosages, the LMWHs clearly produce antithrombotic effects, but whether they have fewer adverse effects than standard heparin may vary with the product and is unproved for many. LMWHs have proved to be equally effective as heparin in general and orthopedic surgery.[8,32,33,43,50]

Based on data from several studies, it is proposed that in addition to their antithrombotic effects, the LMWH-mediated profibrinolytic effects may be responsible for therapeutic actions.[8,51,52] However, this claim requires verification in well-designed experimental and clinical studies.

More recently, LMWHs have been used for specific indications, such as percutaneous transluminal coronary angioplasty (PTCA), and as adjuncts to thrombolytic agents in treatment of disseminated intravascular coagulation (DIC) and hypercoagulable states. A recent study reported inhibition of cellular proliferation after experimental balloon angioplasty by LMWH in rabbits.[53] There are several other indications, such as treatment of cardiovascular disorders, for which they also may prove to be useful. LMWHs have been used in isolated areas as anticoagulants during cardiovascular bypass surgery. However, a relatively larger amount of LMWHs is needed to produce comparable anticoagulant responses. Furthermore, it is rather difficult to antagonize the effect of LMWHs with conventional use of protamine. Thus, their role in cardiovascular surgical indications requires additional clinical studies.

CURRENTLY USED ANTITHROMBOTIC AGENTS

For prophylaxis of medical and surgical thromboembolic disorders, several pharmacologic agents other than heparin and certain physical methods are currently in clinical use. Table 4 compares some of the newer antithrombotic drugs currently used for prophylaxis of postsurgical thrombosis.

Oral anticoagulants are often used for prophylaxis of thrombosis. Patient compliance is generally good, because one oral dosage is sufficient for the daily prophylaxis of thrombotic complications; however, the need for laboratory monitoring and dose adjustment are major drawbacks. Dextrans are generally administered intravenously. Prolonged usage of dextran, however, often results in hypervolemia, bleeding, and platelet dysfunction. Although aspirin is useful for prophylaxis of arterial thrombosis, it is of questionable value in the prophylaxis of venous thrombosis. Furthermore, it may cause bleeding or gastric ulcers. More recently, sequential compression devices have been used for the prophylaxis of postsurgical thrombosis. Their advantages include minor or no adverse effects, no pharmacologic manipulation, and activation of the patient's own physiologic systems. However, these devices are bulky, patient compliance is not as high as desired, and efficacy in high-risk patients is questionable.

GLYCOSAMINOGLYCAN-RELATED ANTITHROMBOTIC AGENTS

Both synthetic and natural analogs of various glycosaminoglycans have been developed for antithrombotic use. These agents work through interactions with serine protease inhibitors by releasing tissue factor pathway inhibitor (TFPI) from endogenous sites.

TABLE 4.   Comparison of Current Agents for Prophylaxis of Postsurgical
and Medical Thromboembolism

Agent	Advantages	Disadvantages
Heparin	Subcutaneous administration (2–3 doses)	Dose adjustment, bleeding, thrombocyto-penia
Low-molecular-weight heparin	Single, subcutaneous administration, sustained actions, outpatient use	Dose adjustment in high-risk patients, bleeding, products not readily interchangeable
Warfarin	Oral administration	Bleeding, delayed action, need for laboratory monitoring
Dextran	High efficacy	Hypervolemia, bleeding, cost, intravenous administration
Aspirin	Low cost, ease of administration	Questionable efficacy, bleeding
Compression devices	Few complications or side effects	Low compliance, rehabilitation, ineffective in high-risk patients

Heparin-related and Other Antithrombotic Agents

Several newer drugs to prevent thromboembolic disorders have been or are being de-veloped (Table 5). Most of these drugs are in their early phases of development, and it will take some time before their clinical efficacy is proved.

A very-low-molecular-weight heparin fraction (CY 222) has been developed for clin-ical trials. This agent produces its effects by multiple mechanisms. Pentasaccharides are synthetic materials with a structure based on the critical binding region of heparin to an-tithrombin. They function by inhibiting activated factor X, do not impair primary hemosta-sis, and have a high bioavailability. They exhibit no anticoagulant effects at antithrombotic doses. Attempts have also been made to produce ultra-LMWH preparations (MW < 3000 Da). One such preparation, CY 231, was developed by Sanofi (MW = 2400 Da).

TABLE 5.   Newer Pharmacologic Strategies for the Management of Thrombotic Disorders

Drug	Advantages	Disadvantages
Very low-molecular-weight heparins	Better bioavailability, promotes endogenous fibrinolysis	Polycomponent GAGs with poor bioavailability, mechanism of action is unknown
Pentasaccharide	Synthetic, well-defined antithrombotic agent	Cost, efficacy not yet proven
Dermatan sulfate and derivatives	No effect on platelets, do not require AT III	Polycomponent GAGs with poor bioavailability, mechanism of action is unknown
Heparan sulfate and derivatives	Modulate endogenous cellular and plasmatic functions independent of HC II and AT III	Poorly defined agents whose mecha-nism of action is unknown, poor bioavailability
Synthetic lactobionic acid derivatives	Synthetic, homogenous antithrombotic agents	Hypersulfated, may bind to endoge-nous sites
Depolymerized heparinoids	Contain mixtures of GAGs with multiple sites of action	Polycomponent drugs with several activities
Polydeoxyribonucleotide derivatives	DNA-derived agents with endogenous modulatory actions on blood/vascular cells	Mechanism of action is unknown, poor bioavailability via SC route
Synthetic peptides and related drugs	Specific inhibitors of thrombin and other proteases, good bioavailability	Short half-life, pharmacologic antagonist is unknown
Recombinant hirudin and related anticoagulants	Specific antithrombotic agents, extremely potent inhibitors	Highly specific inhibitors of thrombin, limited bioavailability

GAG = glycosaminoglycan, AT III = antithrombin III, HC II = heparin cofactor II, SC = subcutaneous.

Currently several dermatan sulfates are under development for the prophylaxis of venous thromboembolism. Although similar in structure to heparin, they have no effect on platelets. Furthermore, they are poorly absorbed after subcutaneous administration. Recently produced low-molecular-weight dermatans, however, are absorbed subcutaneously, unlike dermatan sulfate.

Heparan sulfates have been developed as prophylactic antithrombotic agents. They are not homogeneous and contain other chondroitin sulfates. They bind to antithrombin and heparin cofactor II, but to a lesser degree than heparin and are weakly anticoagulant. Thus, large doses of heparan are needed for effective antithrombotic treatment. Depolymerized heparans have better bioavailability than native heparans.

A synthetic hypersulfated lactobionic acid amide (Aprosulate) has been developed for prophylactic antithrombotic use. This agent produces its action via heparin cofactor II and by inhibiting protease generation. Its bioavailability is better than that of dermatan and heparan sulfates. However, Aprosulate exhibits heparin-induced thrombocytopenic effects and some teratogenetic potential. Thus, its use in clinical trials has been stopped.

Many other glycosaminoglycans are under development for the prophylaxis of thromboembolism. Some are mixtures of glycosaminoglycans with varying molecular weight profiles. Noteworthy are Lomoparan and Suleparoide, both of which are depolymerized heparan preparations. These agents exert their antithrombotic actions via unknown mechanisms; both, however, are clinically quite effective. Other agents, such as Hemoclar and Arteparon, are sulfated polymers of natural origin with antithrombotic activities. Although they have been in existence for many years, data about their prophylactic antithrombotic actions are not clear at this time.

Nonheparin Glycosaminoglycans

In addition to LMWHs, nonheparin glycosaminoglycan-derived products have also been developed as antithrombotic drugs. It is no longer believed that a sulfomucopolysaccharide of natural origin must exhibit some interaction with antithrombin to have effective antithrombotic properties. Several agents without this interaction have been found to produce therapeutic effects on the blood and vascular system.[51,54,55] Several mammalian glycosaminoglycan-derived drugs are currently used in Europe as antithrombotic, antilipemic and antiatherosclerotic agents.[56] These agents represent mixtures of native sulfomucopolysaccharides or their derivatives obtained by depolymerization and/or fractionation. At present, the chemistry and pharmacology of these drugs is not fully understood.

Table 6 lists several important issues in the development of glycosaminoglycans. Most currently available agents are mixtures of mammalian glycosaminoglycans obtained as side products or specific products during the manufacturing of heparin. Specific glycosaminoglycans can be obtained from various organs such as the spleen, pancreas, kidney, and skin. Fractionation and chemical depolymerization, along with extraction methods, have been used to obtain these agents in large quantities for clinical usage. Despite claims that some of the nonheparin glycosaminoglycans may be homogeneous, the molecular profile suggests that each is a polycomponent drug with structural and molecular heterogeneity that varies widely from product to product. Thus, concerns exist over reproducible

TABLE 6.   Important Issues in the Development of Glycosaminoglycans as Drugs

- Mixtures of glycosaminoglycans of natural origin (degree of heterogeneity; batch control)
- Mechanisms of therapeutic clinical effects
- Pharmacologic profiling in established models
- Standardization and cross-referencing
- Indications in various thrombotic conditions
- Clinical acceptance

batch-to-batch composition as well as product-to-product differences in mechanism of action and potency.

Because of compositional variations, the mechanisms of pharmacologic and clinical actions differ markedly. As with LMWHs, each product must be individually character-ized. The pharmacologic actions of nonheparin glycosaminoglycans are mediated by sev-eral endogenous interactions in which both humoral and cellular receptors are involved. In addition to plasmatic effects, these agents are capable of producing several cellular ac-tions. The measure of a single plasma parameter, therefore, cannot be a true reflection of the overall pharmacologic action.

The initial development of nonheparin glycosaminoglycans was mostly empirical; much of the needed pharmacologic information about their application was unavailable. These agents represent complex mixtures of linear polymers with varying endogenous in-teractions. Thus, their efficacy in the common pharmacokinetic models for antithrombotic effects and bleeding, their pharmacodynamics, and their biotransformation may differ in clinical reality. With the use of newer biochemical and pharmacologic screening methods, valid pharmacologic screening can be used to develop these nonheparin glycosaminogly-cans for specific clinical indications. A cautious approach should be taken in interpreting data from experimental models and extrapolating to the clinical setting. With these com-plex drugs, direct correlations like those used with the development of earlier drugs may not be possible in all situations.

Because of such complexities, the glycosaminoglycan-derived drugs cannot be stand-ardized as a single or multiple group. Each drug should be considered as a separate entity. Such issues as bioavailability and mechanism of action have been targeted by regulatory agencies for standardization of the new drugs. Several other issues, such as the clinical in-dications for use and route of administration, also should be considered.

When first developed, each of the glycosaminoglycan-derived drugs was accepted as a derivative of heparin. However, with an increase in our knowledge of their structure and functional activity, preliminary pharmacologic studies were carried out to determine the proper indications for their use. The glycosaminoglycan-derived drugs are generally used as antithrombotic agents; however, several other indications, such as atherosclerosis, stroke, hyperlipemia, and senile dementia are now under consideration.

Currently Available Nonheparin Glycosaminoglycans

A partial list of the available glycosaminoglycan-derived drugs is given in Table 7. Most of the agents in this list are currently in clinical development or actual usage. Several agents not yet in preclinical development are omitted. The listed agents are mainly of mammalian origin with the exception of SP 54 (Hemoclar), which is obtained from a plant. However, SP 54 is a hypersulfated pentosan polysulfate that is similar to the other sulfated glycosaminoglycans in its structural and functional characteristics.

ORG 10172 is a depolymerized mixture of heparans, dermatans, heparin, and other chondroitin sulfates. It has been developed under the commercial name of Lomoparan by Organon, Inc. (Oss, Netherlands). Currently Lomoparan is undergoing clinical trials for the prophylaxis of deep venous thrombosis after general and orthopedic surgery. It is also being used in the prevention of ischemic complications associated with stroke. Researchers claim that it has a better safety-to-efficacy ratio than heparin and produces minimal antihemostatic effects at antithrombotic doses.[57]

Suleparoide is a semisynthetic glycosaminoglycan that has been used for prophylaxis of both arterial and venous thrombosis.

MF 701 is the code name of a dermatan preparation currently under development by Mediolanum Laboratories of Milan. This heterogeneous mixture of dermatan sulfate is claimed to be of mammalian mucosal origin. Currently it is being developed for prophy-laxis against thrombosis after general and orthopedic surgery. Because its bioavailability

TABLE 7. Development of Glycosaminoglycan-derived Drugs

Drug	Composition	Status
ORG 10172	Depolymerized mixture of GAGs	Prophylactic antithrombotic drug—ongoing clinical trials
MF 701	Mixture of native and depolymerized dermatans	Prophylactic antithrombotic drug—ongoing clinical trials
Suleparoide	Semisynthetic GAG	Available for various indications
OP 435	Mixture of dermatans	Prophylactic antithrombotic—preclinical
OP 370	Low-molecular-weight dermatans	Prophylactic antithrombotic—preclinical
SP 54	Hypersulfated pentosan polysulfate	Prophylactic antithrombotic—preclinical
MPS	Depolymerized hypersulfated mixture of GAGS	Antithrombotic agents—developed for animal use
Sulfomucopolysaccharide mixtures	Mixture of GAGs	Clinically used

GAG = glycosaminoglycans.

via subcutaneous administration is rather limited, MF 701 is administered intramuscularly. Several clinical trials are ongoing.

OP 435, another dermatan preparation, is currently under development at Opocrin Laboratories (Corlo, Italy) for prophylactic antithrombotic usage in patients undergoing general surgery. OP 435 is extracted from bovine mucosa.

Several questions have been raised about the safety and efficacy of the higher-molecular-weight dermatans such as MF 701 and OP 435. Both agents exhibit limited bioavailability and thus have been administered in rather large dosages. Because of these concerns, low-molecular-weight dermatan preparations have been recently introduced. One such preparation is OP 370 (Desmin), currently under development by Alfa-Wasserman (Modena). This agent exhibits a much better bioavailability than high-molecular-weight dermatan sulfate and may also have a longer duration of action. Currently OP 370 is under development for prophylactic antithrombotic usage.

Hemoclar (SP 54 or pentosan polysulfate) is a linear cationic polymer from the beechwood tree that has been used for prophylaxis of deep venous thrombosis. It is under development by Bene Chemical (Munich). Because of its origin, Hemoclar can be obtained in relatively large quantities and may prove to be useful in various indications.

MPS is a mixture of mucopolysaccharides obtained from mammalian trachea. It is manufactured by Luitpold-Werk (Munich) for the treatment of joint diseases in both humans and horses. Data about the structure-activity relationship of MPS are limited. It may have various applications as an antithrombotic agent; additional pharmacologic studies may be needed for other indications.

The sulfated mucopolysaccharides (SMPSs) are a large class of drugs currently sold under various commercial names. They are noncharacterized glycosaminoglycans that contain dermatan, heparan, chondroitin sulfate, and other noncharacterized glycosaminoglycans. Although composition of the SMPSs does not differ markedly, each product is marketed for a specific indication. The mechanism of action and pharmacodynamics are not understood, and understanding of the pharmacology is limited.

In Italy six or seven mucopolysaccharide preparations are in clinical use (Table 8). Despite similar chemical composition, different companies offer these agents for different clinical indications.

Biologic Sources of Nonheparin Glycosaminoglycans

Table 9 lists various biological sources from which glycosaminoglycans are extracted. Although they can be obtained from various animal tissues (e.g., porcine, bovine,

TABLE 8. Commercially Available Sulfomucopolysaccharide Preparations

Brand Name	Indication
Ateroid (Crinos)	Senile dementia
Prisma (Alfa Wasserman)	Antilipemic agent
Vessel (Mediolanum)	Vascular disease
Mesoglycan	Antithrombotic agent
Others	Several indications

sheep), bovine tissues provide the most abundant source. In addition to mucosal tissue, organs such as the spleen, kidney, and pancreas also provide raw material for the isolation of various glycosaminoglycans. It is difficult to distinguish the products isolated from different species and tissues. However, the products of plant origin can be easily differentiated from the mammalian products on the basis of chemical structure. The pharmacopeial specifications for the current products are rather flexible and do not require molecular profiles or other chemical characterization studies. It may be necessary in the future to provide data about the molecular profile and chemical structure of glycosaminoglycan products.

Pharmacologic Aspects of Nonheparin Glycosaminoglycans

The pharmacologic aspects of various glycosaminoglycan derived drugs are shown in Table 10. In addition to molecular weight profile, several behavioral characteristics must be taken into account in the development of these agents. Bioavailability varies widely, depending mainly on molecular weight. For example, lower-molecular-weight glycosaminoglycans such as ORG 10172 and OP 370 are more readily bioavailable than MF 701 and OP 435. The duration of action of each of the glycosaminoglycans also varies according to molecular weight, with the lower-molecular-weight agents having a longer duration of action. The exact mechanism for the longer duration of action is not known.

Most of the currently available nonheparin glycosaminoglycans exhibit no significant interaction with antithrombin. If any activity is observed, it may be due primarily to contamination by heparin. Varying degrees of interaction with heparin cofactor II, however, have been observed. Native dermatans such as MF 701 and OP 435 produce a significant activation of heparin cofactor II, whereas the lower-molecular-weight derivatives have much weaker effects. This finding suggests that the activation of heparin cofactor II is most probably related to molecular weight.

TABLE 9. Sources of Natural Glycosaminoglycans

Source	Gylcosaminoglycan
Porcine tissues	
Mucosa	Dermatans
Skin	Dermatans
Trachea	Others
Bovine tissues	
Mucosa	Dermatan, sulfomucopolysaccharides
Skin	Dermatans
Spleen	Heparans
Pancreas	Heparins
Lungs	Heparin
Trachea	Mucopolysaccharides
Sheep tissues	?
Plants	SP 54

TABLE 10.   Pharmacologic Aspects of Various Glycosaminoglycan-derived Drugs

Drug	Bioavailability	Sustained Action	AT Dependence	HC II Dependence	Protamine Neutralization	TFPI Release
ORG 10172	++++	++	±	±	++	±
MF 701	+	++	±	+++	++	+
OP 435	+++	+	±	+++	+	+
OP 370	+++	++	±	++	+	+
SP 54	++	+	±	++	+	++
MPS	++	+	−	+	+	++

AT = antithrombin, HC II = heparin cofactor II, TFPI = tissue factor pathway inhibitor.

Almost all of the glycosaminoglycans show some degree of neutralization by protamine sulfate. However, in contrast to heparin, relatively higher amounts of both protamine sulfate and platelet factor 4 are needed.

Synthetic Analogs Of Nonheparin Glycosaminoglycans

With knowledge of various viral contaminants in natural products of livestock origin (e.g., BSE and foot-and-mouth virus), there is increasing fear that such products may be contaminated. Thus, some countries in Europe have barred bovine products completely. Thus many synthetic analogs of glycosaminoglycans are under development, including (1) heparin pentasaccharide, (2) sulfated lactobionic acid amides, and (3) sulfonated polyphenolic compounds. These agents have been shown to produce dose-dependent antithrombotic effects in animal models. Although similar to heparin, they exhibit markedly different antithrombotic effects. Thus, each agent is developed in a defined manner for certain indications; the overall process may have a major impact on approaches to the management of thrombosis.

Clinical Applications of Nonheparin Glycosaminoglycans

Despite basic unresolved pharmacologic issues, the development of glycosaminoglycans is progressing. Although the thrust is to develop an antithrombotic agent, the glycosaminoglycans also may be used as alternate treatments in conditions in which heparin may not be safe, especially heparin-induced thrombocytopenia and heparin-induced thrombosis-related syndromes. Table 11 lists the various clinical indications. Some of the newer indications include antiinflammatory and antiatherosclerotic applications, treatment of vascular disorders, topical agents for wound healing, and treatment of AIDS. Other indications may include senile dementia and cytoprotection in surgery or transplant. Several small-scale clinical trials have been done to study these different indications.[58–65]

Heparan sulfate has been studied in deep venous thrombosis, chronic venous insufficiency, and intermittent claudication.[58,60,61] Although the trials involved small numbers of patients, the results appear to be positive.

Dermatan sulfate also has been studied in several small-scale clinical trials.[62,63] Most recently a pilot study was completed using dermatan sulfate to control disseminated

TABLE 11.   Clinical Application of Glycosaminoglycan-derived Drugs

• Antithrombotic agent	• Topical agents for wound healing
• Antinflammatory agent	• Acquired immunodeficiency syndrome
• Antiatherosclerotic agent	• Senile dementia
• Vascular deficit	• Cytoprotective actions

TABLE 12.   Developmental Status of the Site-directed Thrombin Inhibitors

Agents	Chemical Nature	Developmental Status
Hirudin and analogs	Recombinant protein	Developed for both arterial and venous thrombosis
Hirulogs	Synthetic bifunctional oligopeptides	Several clinical studies are completed; additional studies are planned in various indications
Peptidomimetics	Synthetic heterocyclic derivatives (argatroban, inogatran, napsagatran)	Phase II clinical development in U.S.; used in Japan
Peptides and derivates	Peptide arginials (efegatran)	Phase II clinical development
Aptamers	DNA- and RNA-derived oligonucleotides with thrombin-binding domains (defibrotide)	Preclinical stage; limited animal data available
Plasma-derived antithrombin	Protein and recombinant equivalent products	AT III is currrently used; HC II is still in developmental status
Transition-state peptide analogs	Oligopeptides and synthetic organic agents (boronic acid derivatives)	Preclinical screening is being completed

AT III = antithrombin III, HC II = heparin cofactor II.

intravascular coagulation in patients with acute leukemia.[62] Other clinical trials of nonheparin glycosaminoglycans are also under way.

RECOMBINANT AND SYNTHETIC ANTITHROMBIN DRUGS

Thrombin plays a crucial role in the overall thrombotic events leading to both arterial and venous thrombosis.[66] In addition to the transformation of fibrinogen to fibrin, thrombin is thought to mediate the activation of platelets and macrophages and produces on-site vascular effects leading to ischemia and vascular contraction. Furthermore, it is also linked with cellular proliferation and related events that lead to restenosis. Thus, the development of agents that target only thrombin is an important approach to developing newer drugs for treatment of venous and arterial thrombosis. Table 12 lists the currently available thrombin inhibitors and their clinical development status.

One of the building blocks used to develop synthetic inhibitors is arginine with optimal C and/or N-terminal modifications. Many such agents have been found to be highly toxic because of inhibition of butyl cholinesterase.[67] The introduction of a COOH group on the carboxy terminal results in decreased affinity for butyl cholinesterase and therefore less toxicity. After further modifications an isomer called argatroban (MD805 or MCI9038) was generated as a selective reversible inhibitor of thrombin (Ki = 0.019 μM).[67] This compound also has a significant affinity for trypsin (Ki = 5.0 μM).[67] It inhibits thrombin directly and prevents it from acting in the coagulation and fibrinolytic system.[68–70] Argatroban is effective in preventing thrombus formation in various animal models at low concentrations (>1 μM).[67,70] It is being tested clinically for several indications.[71–74] Inogatran, another promising reversible peptidomimetic thrombin inhibitor with a molecular weight of 439 Da, is currently under development by Astra Hässle Ab (Sweden). Phase I clinical studies of this potent thrombin inhibitor (Ki = 15 nM) have been completed and indicate a half-life of about 1 hour.[75]

A series of tripeptide aldehydes containing arginine have been developed as the first reversible peptide thrombin inhibitors. The prototype compound is D-Phe-Pro-Arg-H (GYKI-14166),[76] a highly selective and potent inhibitor of thrombin that is, however, unstable in neutral aqueous solution, where it cyclizes and is inactivated. To prevent cyclization, a derivative was synthesized with a protective amino terminal t-butyloxycarbonyl (Boc) group: Boc-D-Phe-Pro-Arg-H (GYKI 14451).[77] This compound is more stable than its parent but is not as specific for thrombin; it also inhibits plasmin. To achieve

TABLE 13. Comparison of Recombinant Hirudin and Heparin

Recombinant Hirudin	Heparin
Monocomponent protein with single target (thrombin)	Polycomponent drug with multiple sites of action
Thrombin-mediated amplification of coagulation is affected only under certain conditions	Thrombin and factor Xa feedback amplification of clotting is affected; fibrinolysis and platelet function affected
No known interactions with endothelium other than blocking thrombin-thrombomodulation mediated activation of protein C	Significant interactions with endothelium; both physical and biochemical modulation of endothelial function
Shorter half-life via intravenous route	Short half-life via intravenous route
Functional bioavailability depends on structure of r-hirudin	Functional bioavailability is 20–30%; low-molecular-weight heparins are better absorbed
Endogenous factors (PF4, FVIII) do not alter antithrombotic action	Marked modulation by endogenous factors; several factors may alter the anticoagulant action
Relatively inert protein not altered by metabolic processes	Transformed by several enzyme systems and reduces anticoagulant actions
Information about cellular uptake and depo formation not presently known	Significant cellular uptake and depo formation

compounds that are both stable and specific for thrombin, a series of N-alkyl derivatives was synthesized with a basic amino terminus that promotes thrombin specificity. Of this series, the methyl derivative D-MePhe-Pro-Arg-H (GYKI 14766)[78–80] has been found to be as potent and as selective in its reversible inhibition of thrombin as the prototype aldehyde. The Ki for the aldehyde derivatives is around 0.1 μM. All three aldehydes are effective antithrombotics in various animal models. Efegatran (D-MePhe-Pro-Arg-H) was developed by Eli Lily and studied briefly in clinical trials for prevention of reocclusion during interventional cardiovascular procedures.

With the availability of molecular biology techniques, it has become possible to produce pharmaceutical quantities of the recombinant equivalent of hirudin, a potent antithrombin agent originally isolated from the medicinal leech, *Hirudo medicinalis*.[81] This 65-amino acid protein is much stronger in producing its anticoagulant effects than heparin. Furthermore, it does not require any endogenous factors. Table 13 compares recombinant hirudin (r-hirudin) and heparin.

From a practical perspective, r-hirudin will probably be compared with heparin, the dominant anticoagulant agent. However, because the mechanism of action of r-hirudin differs from that of heparin, one must be cautious in the applications of the new drug. As a monocomponent, single-acting drug, r-hirudin should offer certain advantages over heparin, which has many and varied activities. Although r-hirudin is a stronger antithrombin agent than heparin, the thrombin generation pathways in the coagulation cascade appear to be inhibited only under certain conditions. Thus, a much higher dose of r-hirudin than heparin may be needed for effective antithrombotic activity, because only one target site can be inhibited. By inhibiting thrombin, r-hirudin also may inhibit the bioregulatory actions of thrombin, such as protein C activation, release of tPA ,and cellular function. Such additional actions may have certain physiological effects beyond the anticoagulation response and must be addressed before r-hirudin is used clinically.

The half-life of r-hirudin, when given intravenously, is shorter than that of heparin, as measured by antithrombin assays. Because of the multiple activities associated with heparin, other pharmacologic effects remain, even when the antithrombin activity is no longer detectable. This should not be the case with r-hirudin, because thrombin inhibition is its only effect. The subcutaneous bioavailability of r-hirudin is low, somewhat similar to that of standard heparin. Because of its low bioavailability and short half-life, r-hirudin is unlikely to play an important role in prophylaxis. However, its short-term therapeutic role seems promising. Coupled with the fact that the bleeding effects are apparently minor, particularly compared with heparin, the efficacy-to-tolerance index of r-hirudin appears to be highly favorable.

Hirulog (Biogen), a synthetic analog of hirudin, has also been developed and tested in various clinical trials for anticoagulant indications.[82] A recent report described its use as an anticoagulant during angioplasty.[83] Hirulog is a completely synthetic analog with anticoagulant actions comparable to those of heparin. However, it requires no plasmatic factors for its anticoagulant actions. Currently, it is being evaluated for various indications, such as management of unstable angina and occlusive phenomena related to interventional cardiology.

Recombinant and synthetic antithrombin drugs may be extremely useful as alternate anticoagulants for heparin-compromised patients, because they do not produce many of the adverse effects (thrombocytopenia and white clot syndrome) associated with heparin.[87] However, their therapeutic efficacy in several other indications must be tested in parallel with heparin before any recommendations are made. Recent clinical trials of the direct antithrombin agents have provided some data about their adverse effects, including bleeding, rebound phenomena, and perturbation of the regulatory role of such proteases as activated protein C and thrombin.[88] Such effects may be due to nonoptimized dosage, drug interactions, or individual predisposing factors in tested populations. For proper development, additional clinical trials are warranted.

Several other developmental issues related to the use of thrombin inhibitors remain unresolved, including nonavailability of antagonists, potential generation of neutralizing antibodies after prolonged usage, and valid therapeutic monitoring. It must be emphasized that the new agents are not heparin and produce their anticoagulant effects by mechanisms that are quite distinct. Thus, each agent must be developed in a stepwise manner, using well-designed pharmacologic and ethical clinical trials.

Developmental Perspective for New Antithrombin Agents

Table 12 summarizes the current developmental status of various thrombin inhibitors. Site-directed antithrombin agents, such as recombinant hirudin, Hirulog, and synthetic tripeptides, are currently undergoing various phases of clinical trials. These agents were initially developed with the premise that sole targeting of thrombin may be the most important step in the development of anticoagulants and antithrombotic drugs to treat thrombotic and cardiovascular disorders.[89–92] It is nearly 5 years since these agents have undergone clinical trials. Hirudin and Hirulog have completed several phase II trials, whereas the peptide D-MePhe-Pro-Arg-H, marketed under the generic name efegatran sulfate, has recently entered a phase II trial. The trials have focused primarily on cardiovascular indications, such as pretreatment of ischemic heart disorders, anticoagulation during coronary angioplasty, treatment of postinterventional abrupt closure and late reocclusion (restenosis), and adjunct usage during thrombolysis. It is too early to suggest that the new agents have a definitive advantage over heparin. However, in heparin-compromised patients, they may be useful on a compassionate basis. Hirudin is relatively more expensive than heparin. The relative cost for the synthetic antithrombin agents may be lower than hirudin, but cost analysis is valid only after a comprehensive pharmacoeconomic analysis for specific prophylactic and therapeutic indications.

Several peptidomimetic antithrombin agents are also currently in clinical development for both cardiovascular and therapeutic indications, including argatroban (Mitsubishi, Japan), inogatran (Astra, Sweden), and napsagatran (Roche, Switzerland). The results of some of these clinical trials are expected later this year. In addition, many other antithrombin agents are in active preclinical development.

Of the various peptide-derived antithrombin agents, efegatran (Eli Lilly) is the only one that is currently developed for cardiovascular indications. Many other agents developed by different companies were initially investigated in various preclinical studies, but their clinical development was abandoned because of various problems.

Aptamers are DNA- and RNA-derived oligonucleotides with weaker anticoagulant effects. Although they are not developed for the purpose of anticoagulation, some of these agents show antithrombin actions in vitro. Defibrotide (Crinos, Italy), a mammalian DNA-derived product, has been used as an antiischemic drug, but its actions are not attributed solely to the inhibition of thrombin. Like heparin, defibrotide produces multiple pharmacologic effects on platelets, endothelial cells, and the release of tissue factor pathway inhibitor (TFPI).[93]

Many other synthetic and recombinant approaches have been used to develop antithrombin agents, including the transition-state analogs. Despite their potent antithrombin actions, these agents have not been pursued for clinical purposes because of undesirable toxic effects.

Most antithrombin agents have been designed and developed as specific inhibitors of thrombin. However, they also exhibit variable interactions with the serine protease network, including the fibrinolytic, kallikrein, and complement systems. Because thrombin belongs to the serine protease family of enzymes, as do most of the coagulation factors and fibrinolytic enzymes, development of an inhibitor with strong affinity for thrombin but no affinity for the other enzymes remains a challenge to the pharmaceutical industry. Aptamers, hirudin, and Hirulog inhibit only thrombin because they recognize and inhibit sites, other than the catalytic site, that are unique for thrombin. The other thrombin inhibitors, which are designed to bind to the catalytic site, also have weaker inhibitory activities against other enzymes. Thus, at high doses, they may interfere with the fibrinolytic system and activated protein C. This interaction may compromise the safety of patients, especially at high doses.

Some of the thrombin inhibitors also possess direct vasodilatory effects, independent of their activity on thrombin. These effects are believed to be mediated through metabolic products containing guanidino groups, which increase the generation of nitric oxide Depending on the specific indication for which the thrombin inhibitor is developed, this vascular effect may be desirable. In any case, it should be investigated and taken into account.

Since their introduction, most of the clinical indications for the new anticoagulants have been in cardiovascular intervention.[94] The initial focus was prevention of abrupt closure during coronary angioplasty.[91,92] The new agents also have been tested for prevention of both early and late reocclusion after PTCA. In addition, some of the thrombin inhibitors have been used for treatment of unstable angina. More recently, some agents have been tested for efficacy in stenting.

Despite several reports of the experimental use of antithrombin agents in cardiovascular surgery in animal models, only isolated reports in human studies are available.[95] The lack of an antagonist to neutralize their effects has raised concern.[96] Because no pharmacologic antagonists are available for hirudin or any of the other direct thrombin inhibitors, the management of precipitated hemorrhagic effects is problematic. Current strategies for hirudin reversal include administration of prothrombin complex concentrate to neutralize the circulating antithrombin agents or dialysis to remove the antithrombin agent from the blood. Strategies under development include production of mutant thrombin molecules that are devoid of clotting activity but retain a high affinity for antithrombin agents. Their use may saturate circulating levels of the antithrombin agents.

Thrombin inhibitors are attractive to both clinicians and surgeons as substitute anticoagulants, particularly in heparin-compromised patients. Several trials are currently in progress to test their efficacy in patients with HIT who require anticoagulation. Although thrombin inhibitors are potent anticoagulants and, unlike heparin, require no endogenous cofactors for their actions, their development as surgical anticoagulants has been rather slow because of the nonavailability of a pharmacologic antagonist. Only when such an antagonist is clinically validated will the new agents find their way into general surgical applications.

Interest in the use of thrombin inhibitors for prevention and treatment of deep venous thrombosis is growing.[95–98] A recent study by Eriksson et al. reported the successful use of r-hirudin in prophylaxis after orthopedic surgery. Unfractionated heparin (5000 IU, 3 times/day, subcutaneously) was compared with hirudin (15 mg, 3 time/day, subcutaneously). Hirudin was found to be superior. Several additional trials are currently being conducted on other antithrombin agents.

Current clinical trends also point to polypharmacologic approaches for the treatment and management of cardiovascular disorders. Combination modalities have used anticoagulants with other drug classes, such as antiplatelet and fibrinolytic agents. Although clinically developed thrombin inhibitors are reportedly specific for thrombin inhibition, they interact with other drugs. Antiplatelet drugs such as aspirin and ticlopidine have additive or synergistic effects when used in conjunction with thrombin inhibitors. Similar interactions would be expected when thrombin inhibitors are used with heparin and LMWHs or AT III concentrates. On the other hand, adjunct use of thrombin inhibitors with thrombolytic agents, depending on the dose, may result in facilitation of thrombolysis or, if the dose of thrombin inhibitor is high, in thrombolytic compromise. Some of these agents may also directly inhibit activated protein C or its formation by neutralizing thrombomodulin-bound thrombin.[99,100] Furthermore, thrombin inhibitors may neutralize the coagulant actions of factor VIIa and prothrombin complex concentrates. Therefore, the interactions of thrombin inhibitors must be well studied and taken into account when designing drug combination protocols for clinical applications.

The development of thrombin inhibitors has added a new dimension to the management of thrombotic and vascular disorders.[101–103] Although the major clinical indications for thrombin inhibitors include interventional cardiovascular procedures and prophylaxis of deep venous thrombosis, very little is known about their use for surgical and therapeutic anticoagulation. It is projected that many of the newer thrombin inhibitors, such as Hirulog and hirudin, will be developed as anticoagulants and may be substituted for heparin. Synthetic tripeptides with a broader serine protease inhibitory spectrum offer unique tools to control thrombogenesis at different levels and may prove to be more useful in chronic indications, including prophylaxis. However, the usefulness of various thrombin inhibitors in a given medical or surgical indication can be proved only in properly designed clinical trials.

Drug Interactions with Antithrombin Agents

Drug interactions play an important role in the overall safety and efficacy of antithrombin agents. In many indications, they are administered in conjunction with other agents such as antiplatelet drugs. Many of the patients are often on other medications. A systematic study of the interactions of antithrombins with other drugs is not available. However, it is feasible to develop a testing system for antithrombin agents before their interaction with other drugs is studied.

Unlike heparin, antithrombin drugs do not exhibit complex interactions, primarily because of their high specificity. Their actions can be readily predictable because of the known pharmacologic profile. However, dosage optimization in the presence of other anticoagulant or antithrombotic drugs is important. Antithrombin drugs are expected to augment the anticoagulant actions of oral anticoagulant drugs, which suppress the formation of functional forms of factors II, VII, IX, and X. In addition, they also augment the functional forms of protein C and S. In this setting, antithrombin drugs may inhibiting thrombomodulin-bound thrombin, which is needed for the activation of protein C. The consequences of this process are not known. In some clinical conditions, antithrombin drugs may augment the action of heparin and LMWH. Although no preclinical or clinical data are available, in vitro studies suggest that antithrombin agents may produce other additive or synergistic actions of the anticoagulant effects. Dosage adjustments may be required, depending on the dose of heparin, to optimize the therapeutic index of r-hirudin.

Most cardiovascular patients take aspirin for prophylactic or therapeutic reasons. Because thrombin plays a key role in the activation of platelets, antithrombin drugs are expected to produce an augmentation or synergism of the antiplatelet action of aspirin. This may be a complex situation that results in compromised hemostasis. The bleeding complications observed in the TIMI 9A and GUSTO II trials may be attributable to the use of aspirin. On the other hand, the interaction may also be of clinical benefit if the dose of both agents is optimized. Other agents that affect platelets, such as factor IIb/IIIa inhibitors and antagonists of adenosine diphosphate (ADP), are expected to have similar interactions with r-hirudin.

Some of the peptides and peptidomimetic antithrombin agents are capable of causing fibrinolytic compromise. Unlike these agents, r-hirudin does not directly inhibit such fibrinolytic enzymes as plasmin, plasminogen activators, and defibrase. However, it augments the anticoagulant actions of the fibrinogen/fibrin degradation products. Thus, r-hirudin is expected to augment thrombolytic efficacy and may prevent rethrombosis (reocclusion).

No other studies have reported additional drug interactions with antithrombin agents. However, such interactions are important and should be carefully investigated to optimize safety as well as efficacy.

Cost-Effective Considerations for New Antithrombin Agents

In the case of r-hirudin, cost considerations have been taken into account only for specific indications; a limited database is available at present. Currently, most of the indications for hirudin are the same as for unfractionated heparin or LMWHs. The cost analysis for various indications, therefore, must be based on site-specific indications, such as surgical anticoagulation, prophylaxis and treatment of deep venous thrombosis, and cardiovascular use. From the standpoint of production cost, r-hirudin is certainly more expensive than the heparins. However, for each of the specific indications, a comprehensive pharmacoeconomic analysis must take into account the dosage, nursing care, monitoring, and incidence of adverse reactions and clinical outcome. Such a comprehensive analysis may provide different cost values for hirudin and related drugs.

A cost analysis from a pharmacoeconomic substudy was reported recently in conjunction with the GUSTO IIb study (SCRIP No. 2115, 1996, p 23). Reimbursement was received from 50% of the treated patients. Estimating that 2 deaths and 7 myocardial infarctions can be prevented for each 1000 patients, the report computed that if the drug is priced at $500, the cost per year of life saved would be around $16,000. If the price of r-hirudin is $1000, the cost would be $32,000; at a price of $1500, the estimated cost would be around $48,000. The report concluded that a cost below $1500, therefore, may be considered cost-effective. The projected cost, however, is much higher than the cost for heparin and other synthetic antithrombotic agents. Whether the cost calculated on the basis of survival estimates is valid for such comparisons is questionable. If the mortality rates alone were used, then the drug would have to be priced at a much lower level to be cost-effective, with a price of $500 yielding a cost per year of life saved of $31,250. A cost-effectiveness analysis based on nonsignificant results, such as the one reported in the Gusto IIb substudy, may not be accurate; additional data are needed.

A cost analysis for the use of r-hirudin for prophylaxis of deep venous thrombosis after hip surgery can be based on the recent study by Erickson, in which r-hirudin was used in protocols comparable to those for LMWHs. The cost of r-hirudin was 3–5-fold higher than the current price for LMWH. However, if monitoring and other adverse outcomes are included in this analysis, the figures may be different. Similar analysis can be performed for prevention of deep venous thrombosis in other indications. Obviously further study is required.

ANTIPLATELET DRUGS IN DEVELOPMENT

Antiplatelet drugs such as aspirin and propionic acid derivatives have been conventionally used to manage platelet-mediated thrombotic disorders such as peripheral arterial occlusive disease, thrombotic stroke, and coronary artery disease. A newer generation of antiplatelet drugs, such as ticlopidine and clopidogrel, has been introduced for the management of stroke.[104] More recently, ticlopidine and clopidogrel were tested for other indications. Although both drugs are useful, they inhibit only certain activation processes. None of the newer agents can inhibit tissue factor- and thrombin-mediated activation of platelets. Direct thrombin inhibitors, such as hirudin,[105] may be useful in targeting tissue factor and coagulation activation processes in which platelet activation is mediated by thrombin. It is therefore clear that different sites of activation are independently responsible for activating platelets in platelet-related thrombotic events. For this reason, glycoprotein IIb/IIIa (GpIIb/IIIa) antagonists, thromboxane A_2 receptor blockers, thromboxane synthase inhibitors, synthetic cyclooxygenase inhibitors, prostacyclin analogs, and 5-HT$_2$ receptor blockers have been developed (Table 14).

Figure 6 illustrates the sites of platelet action of various anticoagulant and antithrombotic drugs. Different drugs, such as modulators of platelet receptors (GpIIb/IIIa, thromboxane B_2, ADP), cyclooxygenase inhibitors, and inhibitors of the thrombin-mediated function of platelets, have different sites of action.

Drugs that target the GpIIb/IIIa receptors are thought to act on the final common pathways for platelet activation by various activating processes.[106] The interaction of fibrinogen with GpIIb/IIIa sites is partly mediated by the arginine-glycine-aspartic acid (RGD) recognition site.[107] Several synthetic peptides and peptidomimetic agents have been developed to target this site in an effort to prevent activation of platelets.[108] Monoclonal antibodies, such as 7E3 (ReoPro),[109] have been clinically tested. ReoPro was recently approved by the Food and Drug Administration for prevention of restenosis after PTCA. A fragment (YM-337) of a humanized monoclonal antibody against the GpIIb/IIIa site has also been identified. The use of monoclonal antibodies as therapeutic agents may have limitations, such as immunogenicity, lack of reversibility, and nonavailability by subcutaneous or oral route. Thus, the development of analogs of RGD or modification of the RGD sequence is considered more practical, safe, and cost-effective.

Many of the drugs listed on Table 14 are currently undergoing clinical trials. Pharmacologic data for each of these drugs was obtained primarily in experimental settings that investigated only their effect on platelet function. Non–platelet-mediated effects on cells have not been taken into account during clinical development. It is conceivable that some of these effects may contribute to overall clinical outcome. Furthermore, little is known about the interactions of these agents with other drugs. For proper development, valid preclinical pharmacologic data about drug interactions may be crucial.

DEFIBROTIDE AND RELATED AGENTS

Aptamers are oligonucleotides (double- or single-stranded DNA or single-stranded RNA) that act directly on proteins to inhibit disease processes. Thirty-two such aptamers have been recently isolated as inhibitors of thrombin, with binding affinities in the range of 20–200 nM.[110] One of the most potent thrombin aptamers has been found to interact with thrombin's anion-binding exosite; it competes with substrates that interact with a specific site, such as fibrinogen and thrombin platelet receptors.[111,112] This aptamer recently was shown to reduce arterial platelet thrombus formation in an animal model and to inhibit clot-bound thrombin in an in vitro system.[113] Recently, researchers isolated a second pool

TABLE 14.   Antiplatelet Drugs in Development

Glycoprotein IIb/IIIa receptor antagonists	**Thromboxane synthase inhibitors**
7E3 (Centnocor/Lily)	Isbogrel/CV 4151 (Takeda)
YM 337 (Yamanouchi)	Y-20811 (Yoshitomi)
Integrelin (Cor Therapeutics)	Rolafagrel (Farmitalia Carlo Erba)
MK-383 (Merck)	RS-5186 (Sankyo)
MK-852 (Merck)	KB-3022/TO-192 (Kanebo)
DMP-728 (DuPont)	Camonagreal (Ferrer)
Bibou-104 (Boehringer Ingelheim)	DDTX-30 (Boehringer Ingelheim)
SC-49992 (Searle)	**Platelet cyclooxygenase inhibitors**
SC-52012 (Searle)	Kc-764 (Kyorin)
RO-44-9883 (Roche)	Thrombodipine (Alter)
TA-993 (Tanabe Seiyaku)	Trapidil (UCB)
SDZ-GPI-462 (Sandoz)	**Prostaglandin analogs**
Thromboxane A$_2$ receptor blockers	Ataprost (Ono)
Sulotroban (Boehringer Mannheim)	Taprostene (Gruenenthal)
Satigrel (Eisai)	Cicaprost (Schering AG)
Ridogrel (Janssen)	**5-HT$_2$ receptor blockers**
BAY-U-3405 (Bayer)	Kantanserine (Janssen)
S-1452 (Shinogi)	Sarprogrelate (Mitsubishi)
FK-070 (KDI-792)	Nexompamil (Knoll)
KT2-962 (Kotobuki)	CV-5197 (Takeda)
MED-27 (Medosan)	Irindalone (Lundbeck)
Vapiprost (Glaxo)	**New antiplatelet drugs**
AH-23848 (Glaxo)	Ticlopidine (Sanofi)
Eptaloprost (Schering AG)	Clopidogrel (Sanofi)
SQ-30741 (BMS)	Defibrotide (Crinos)
9 products (Japanese)	

of aptamers, with a different sequence composition from the first class and with modified bases, that has shown promising anticoagulant activities.[114] Another recent development was the isolation of two RNAs that bind thrombin with high affinity (Kd in the nM range). These oligonucleotides have been shown to inhibit fibrinogen clotting in an in vitro test.[115]

Defibrotide is a polydeoxyribonucleotide-derived drug from mammalian tissues such as lung and spleen. Like heparin, it is heterogeneous and composed of nucleic acid strands ranging in molecular weight from 2,000–30,000 Da.[101] The mean molecular weight of defibrotide is around 17,000. Figure 7 compares the heterogeneous nature of defibrotide and heparin. Like heparin, defibrotide is composed of several molecular components, whose molecular weight ranges from 2–50 kDa.

Despite the fact that defibrotide produces no systemic anticoagulant effects after intravenous injection, it produces dose- and time-dependent antithrombotic effects in a stasis-thrombosis model.[116] Defibrotide contains nucleotide sequences capable of producing direct antithrombin actions.[117] The antithrombotic mechanisms of defibrotide include endothelial modulation and increased release of cyclic adenosine monophosphate and tissue factor pathway inhibitor. Of greatest interest, it produces antithrombotic action with no systemic anticoagulant effects. It has therefore been used for the management of peripheral vascular disease and different microangiopathic disorders.

NEWER ANTICOAGULANTS AND ANTITHROMBOTICS IN INTERVENTIONAL CARDIOLOGY AND CARDIOVASCULAR SURGERY

Despite the dramatic development of newer anticoagulant and antithrombotic drugs, their application in cardiovascular surgery has been rather limited. On the other hand, many of these drugs have been used for the interventional cardiologic indications. (Table 15).

In interventional cardiology, LMWHs have been evaluated for the management of both acute and late reocclusion. In random studies, the LMWHs have been shown to be effective in the reduction of abrupt closure in angioplasty. LMWHs also have been useful

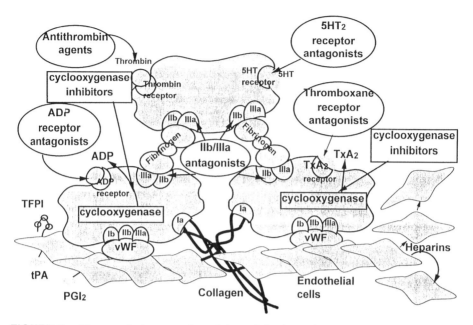

FIGURE 6.   Pharmacologic target sites of the antiplatelet actions of various anticoagulant and antithrombotic drugs. Receptors, enzymes, and other membrane sites are targeted by these drugs.

in stenting in both mono- and polytherapeutic approaches. The use of LMWHs as anticoagulants in cardiovascular surgical procedures has been rather limited. Because of lower anticoagulant activity and difficulties with neutralization, LMWHs may not be practical for this indication.

Viscosity and endothelial-lining modulators such as pentoxifylline (Trental) have no direct application in cardiologic or cardiovascular surgery. However, they may be used as adjunct drugs, especially in cardiac transplantation and artificial heart programs.

Antithombin agents such as hirudin can be effectively used as an alternate anticoagulant for surgical and cardiologic indications. Several studies have been carried out in

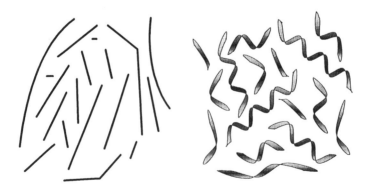

FIGURE 7.   Comparison of the molecular heterogeneity in unfractionated heparin and defibrotide. Both drugs are polycomponent and exhibit an apparent mean molecular weight of 15 kDa. Whereas heparin is composed of sulfated mucopolysaccharide chains, defibrotide is composed of single-stranded nucleic acid (DNA fragments). Both drugs produce polypharmacologic effects and target multiple sites in blood and vasculature.

TABLE 15.   Application of New Anticoagulant and Antithrombotic Drugs in Interventional Cardiology and Cardiovascular Surgery

Drugs	Interventional Cardiology	Cardiovascular Surgery
Low-molecular-weight heparins	Adjunct to thrombolytics; prevention of early and late reocclusion	Prophylaxis of postsurgical thromboembolism
Antiplatelet drugs	Prophylaxis for coronary syndromes; adjunct usage; prevention of early and late restenosis; stents	Prevention of graft reocclusion
Endothelial-lining modulators	Adjunct usage	Adjunct use with other drugs
Viscosity modulators	Adjunct usage	Adjunct use; may be useful in assist devices
Antithrombins	Anticoagulation during various procedures	Anticoagulation during various procedures
Thrombolytic agents	Myocardial infarction; dissolution of thrombotic lesions	Dissolution of occluded graft

angioplasty and atherectomy. Data about the use of these agents in open-heart surgery are limited, primarily because no antidote is available.

Thrombotic agents have been used extensively for the treatment of myocardial infarction. They are also used for the improvement of patency of occluded bypass grafts.

CONCLUSION

Recently, both pharmaceutical companies and academic researchers have made remarkable progress in the development of many newer anticoagulant and antithrombotic drugs. These developments are possible only as a result of newer technology, such as molecular biology, improved isolation methods, and newer synthetic organic chemistry methods. Newer drugs include LMWHs, hirudin, Hirulog, and many other synthetic antiplatelet agents.

The use of LMWH has added a new dimension to the management of venous thrombosis. Currently, LMWHs are undergoing trials for various cardiovascular indications, such as treatment of unstable angina and prevention of restenosis after PTCA. Although derived from heparin, the LMWHs exhibit different pharmacologic actions and individual behavior. Thus, unlike heparin, the agents are not interchangeable.

Nonheparin glycosaminoglycans, such as dermatan sulfate and heparan sulfate, have also been developed for various indications. However, convincing clinical evidence has not established their safety and efficacy. Mixtures of glycosaminoglycans, such as Lomoparan, have been tested extensively in the management of thrombosis; however, additional data are needed for clinical applications.

Recombinant and synthetic antithrombin agents, such as hirudin and Hirulog, are potentially useful alternatives for anticoagulation, which once was considered to be manageable solely by heparin. They are stronger than heparin and lack some of its adverse effects; therefore, they may be useful in acute anticoagulation protocols. Because recombinant and synthetic agents are markedly different from heparin, they do not produce some of its therapeutic effects. Thus, their clinical effects are not comparable to the clinical effects of heparin. Additional clinical trials are needed for validation of antithrombin agents in medical indications.

The remainder of the 1990s will witness further progress in anticoagulant and antithrombotic therapy. Many newer drugs will become available for the management of venous and arterial thrombosis. However, it should be kept in mind that conventional anticoagulants, such as heparin, and antiplatelet drugs, such as aspirin, have been remarkably useful, despite their limited indications. Newer information about their use, optimization of dosage for additional indications, and an understanding of their therapeutic effects represent an equally important area for additional clinical data and research.

REFERENCES

1. Fareed J: Antithrombotic drugs in vascular disorders: Newer developments and future perspectives. Minerva Angiol 17(2):41–47, 1992.
2. Fareed J, Walenga JM, Pifarre R: Newer approaches to the pharmacologic management of acute myocardial infarction. Card Surg State Art Rev 6:101–111, 1992.
3. Fareed J, Walenga JM, Pifarre R, et al: Some objective considerations for the neutralization of the anticoagulant actions of recombinant hirudin. Haemostasis 21:64–72, 1991.
4. Fareed J, Bacher P, Messmore HL, et al: Pharmacological modulation of fibrinolysis by antithrombotic and cardiovascular drugs. Prog Cardiovasc Dis 6:379–398, 1992.
5. Fareed J, Walenga JM, Hoppensteadt D, et al: Chemical and biochemical heterogeneity in low molecular weight heparins: Implications for clinical use and standardization. Semin Thromb Hemost 15:440–463, 1989.
6. Fareed J, Walenga JM, Racanelli A, et al: Validity of the newly established low molecular weight heparin standard in cross-referencing low molecular weight heparins. Haemostasis 18:33–47, 1988.
7. Fareed J, Walenga JM, Hoppensteadt D, Et al: Study on the in vitro and in vivo activities of seven low-molecular-weight heparins. Haemostasis 18:3–15, 1988.
8. Fareed J, Walenga JM, Lassen M, et al: Pharmacologic profile of a low molecular weight heparin (Enoxaparin): Experimental and clinical validation of the prophylactic antithrombotic effects. Acta Chirur Scand 556(Suppl):75–90, 1990.
9. Hull R, Raskob G, Pineo G: Subcutaneous low molecular weight heparin compared with continuous intravenous heparin in the treatment of proximal vein thrombosis. N Engl J Med 326:975–982, 1992.
10. Messmore HL: Clinical efficacy of heparin fractions: Issues and answers. CRC Clin Rev Clin Lab Sci 23:77–94, 1986.
11. Prandoni P, Lensing A, Buller H, et al: Comparison of subcutaneous standard low-molecular weight heparin with intravenous standard heparin in proximal deep-vein thrombosis. Lancet 339:441–445, 1992.
12. Hirsh J, Levine M: The development of low molecular weight heparins for clinical use. In Verstraete M, et al (eds): Thrombosis and Haemostasis. Leuven, Leuven University Press, 1987, pp 425–448.
13. Hull R, Delmore T, Carter C, et al: Adjusted subcutaneous heparin versus warfarin sodium in the long-term treatment of venous thrombosis. N Engl J Med 306:954–958, 1983.
14. Nieuwenhuis HK, Albada J, Banga JD, Sixma JJ: Identification of risk factor for bleeding during treatment of acute venous thrombolysis with heparin or low molecular weight heparin. Blood 78:2337–2343, 1991.
15. Kelton JG: Heparin induced thrombocytopenia. Haemostasis 16:173–186, 1986.
16. Silver D, Kapsch D, Tosi E: Heparin induced thrombocytopenia, thrombosis and haemorrhage. Ann Surg 198:301–305, 1983.
17. Griffith GC, Nichols G Jr, Asher JD, Flanagan B: Heparin osteoporosis. JAMA 193:85–88, 1965.
18. Bara L, Billaud E, Gramond G, et al: Comparative pharmacokinetics of low molecular weight heparin (PK 10169) and unfractionated heparin after intravenous and subcutaneous administration. Thromb Res 39:631–636, 1985.
19. Choay J, Petitou M, Lormeau JC, et al: Structure activity relationship in heparin A synthetic pentasaccharide with high affinity for antithrombin III and eliciting high anti-Xa activity. Biochem Biophys Res Comm 116:491-499, 1983.
20. Choay J, Lormeau JC, Petitou M, et al: Anti-Xa active heparin oligosaccharides. Thromb Res 18:573–578, 1980.
21. Atha DH, Stephens AW, Rimon A, Rosenberg RD: Sequence variation in heparin octasaccharides with high affinity for antithrombin III. Biochemistry 23:5801–5812, 1984.
22. Bianchini P, Osima B, Parma B, et al: Pharmacological activities of heparins obtained from different tissues: Enrichment of heparin fractions with high lipoprotein lipase, anti-hemolytic and anticoagulant activities by molecular seiving and antithrombin III affinity chromatography. J Pharmacol Exp Ther 220:406–410, 1982.
23. Fussi F, Federli G: Oligoheteropolysaccharides with heparin-like effects. Ger Offen 2:833–898, 1977.
24. Hook M, Bjork I, Hopwood J, Lindahl U: Anticoagulant activity of heparin: Separation of high activity and low activity heparin species by affinity chromatography on immobilized antithrombin. FEBS Lett 66:90–93, 1976.
25. Hurst RE, Poon M, Griffith MJ: Structure-activity relationships of heparin. J Clin Invest 72:1042–1045, 1983.
26. Bergqvist D, Mätzsch T, Burmark US, et al: Low molecular weight heparin given the evening before surgery compared with conventional low-dose heparin in prevention of thrombosis. Br J Surg 75:888-891, 1988.

27. Borris LC, Hauch O, Jorgensen LN, Lassen MR: Enoxaparin versus dextran 70 in the prevention of post-operative deep vein thrombosis after total hip replacement. A Danish multicenter study. Proceeding of the Danish Enoxaparin Symposium, Feb 3, 1990.
28. European Fraxiparin Study Group: Comparison of low molecular weight heparin and unfractionated heparin for the prevention of deep vein thrombosis is patients undergoing abdominal surgery. Br J Surg 75:1058–1063, 1988.
29. Haas S, Stemberger A, Fritsche HM, et al: Prophylaxis of deep vein thrombosis in high risk patients undergoing total hip replacement with low molecular weight heparin plus dihydroergotamine. Arzneimittel-Forschung 37:839–843, 1987.
30. Baumgartner A, Jacot N, Moser G, Krahenbuhl B: Prevention of postoperative deep vein thrombosis by one daily injection of low molecular weight heparin and dihydroergotamine. Vasa 18:152–156, 1989.
31. Caen JP: A randomized double-blind study between a low molecular weight heparin Kabi 2165 and standard heparin in the prevention of deep vein thrombosis in general surgery. A French multicenter trial. Thromb Haemost 59:216–220, 1988.
32. Hartl P, Brucke P, Dienstl E, Vinazzer H: Prophylaxis of thromboembolism in general surgery: Comparison between standard heparin and Fragmin. Thromb Res 57:577–584, 1990.
33. Kakkar W, Stringer MD, Hedges AR, et al: Fixed combinations of low molecular weight or unfractionated heparin plus dihydroergotamine in the prevention of postoperative deep vein thrombosis. Am J Surg 157:413–418, 1989.
34. Samama M, Combe-Tamazali S: Prevention of thromboembolic disease in general surgery with Enoxaparin. Br J Clin Pract 65:9–15, 1989.
35. Planes A, Vochelle N, Mazas F, et al: Prevention of postoperative venous thrombosis: A randomized trial comparing unfractionated heparin with low molecular weight heparin in patients undergoing total hip replacement. Thromb Haemost 60:407–410, 1988.
36. Verardi S, Casciani CU, Nicora E, et al: A multicentre study on LMW-heparin effectiveness in preventing postsurgical thrombosis. Int Angiol 7:19-24, 1988.
37. Eriksson BI, Zachrisson BE, Teger-Nilsson AC, Risberg B: Thrombosis prophylaxis with low molecular weight heparin in total hip replacement. Br J Surg 75:1053–1057, 1988.
38. Leyvraz PF, Richard J, Bachmann F, et al: Adjusted versus fixed subcutaneous heparin in the prevention of deep vein thrombosis after total hip replacement. N Engl J Med 309:954–958, 1983.
39. Matzsch T, Bergqvist D, Fredin H, Hedner U: Safety and efficacy of a low molecular weight heparin (Logiparin) versus dextran as prophylaxis against thrombosis after total hip replacement. Acta Chirur Scand 543:80–84, 1988.
40. Matzsch T, Bergqvist D, Fredin H, Hedner U: Low molecular weight heparin compared with dextran as prophylaxis against thrombosis after total hip replacement. Acta Chirur Scand 156:445–450, 1990.
41. Monreal M, Lafoz E, Navarro A, et al: A prospective double-blind trial of a low molecular weight heparin once daily compared with conventional low-dose heparin three times daily to prevent pulmonary embolism and venous thrombosis in patients with hip fracture. J Trauma 29:873–875, 1989.
42. Lindblad B: Prophylaxis of postoperative thromboembolism with low dose heparin alone or in combination with dyhydroergotamine A review. Acta Chirur Scand 154:31–42, 1988.
43. Verstraete M: Pharmacotherapeutic aspects of unfractionated and low molecular weight heparins. Drugs 40:498–530, 1990.
44. Holmer E, Mattson C, Nilsson S: Anticoagulant and antithrombotic effects of heparin and low molecular weight heparin fragments in rabbits. Thromb Res 25:475–485, 1982.
45. Ockelford PA, Carter CJ, Mitchell L, Hirsh J: Discordance between the anti-Xa activity and antithrombotic activities of an ultra-low molecular weight heparin fraction. Thromb Res 28:401–409, 1982.
46. Thomas DP, Merton RE, Gray E, Barrowcliffe TW: The relative antithrombotic effectiveness of heparin, in a low molecular weight heparin and a pentasaccharide fragment in an animal model. Thromb Haemost 61:204–207, 1989.
47. Walenga JM, Petitou M, Lormeau JC: Antithrombotic activity of a synthetic heparin pentasaccharide in a rabbit stasis thrombosis model using different thrombogenic challenges. Thromb Res 46:187–198, 1987.
48. Kakkar VV, Murray WJG: Efficacy and safety of low molecular weight heparin (CY 216) in preventing postoperative venous thrombo-embolism: A cooperative study. Br J Surg 72:786–791, 1985.
49. Levine MN, Hirsh J: An overview of clinical trials with low molecular weight heparin fractions. Acta Chirur Scand 154:73–39, 1988.
50. Koppenhagen K, Adolf J, Matthes M, et al: Low molecular weight heparin and prevention of postoperative thrombosis in abdominal surgery. Thromb Haemost 67:627–630, 1992.
51. Hoppensteadt D, Racanelli A, Walenga JM, Fareed J: Comparative antithrombotic and hemorrhagic effects of dermatan sulfate, heparan sulfate and heparin. Semin Thromb Hemost 15:378–385, 1989.
52. Bacher P, Welzel D, Iqbal O, et al: The thrombotic potency of LMW-heparin compared to urokinase in a rabbit jugular vein clot lysis model. Thromb Res 66:151–158, 1992.

53. Hanke H, Oberhoff M, Hanke S, et al: Inhibition of cellular proliferation after experimental balloon angioplasty by low molecular weight heparin. Circulation 85:1548–1556, 1992.
54. Bianchini P: Therapeutic potential of non-heparin glycosaminoglycans of natural origin. Semin Thromb Hemost 15:365–369, 1989.
55. Marcum JA, Rosenberg RD: Role of endothelial cell surface heparin-like polysaccharides. In Ofosu FA, Danishefsky I, Hirsh J (eds): Heparin and Related Polysaccharides: Structure and Activities. New York, New York Academy of Sciences, 1989, pp 81–94.
56. Sirtori CR: Pharmacology of sulfomucopolysaccharides in atherosclerosis prevention and treatment. In Ricci G, et al (eds): Selectivity and Risk-Benefit Assessment of Hyperlipidemia Drugs. New York, Raven Press, 1982, pp 189–194.
57. Fareed J, Hoppensteadt D, Jeske W, Walenga JM: An overview of non-heparin glycosaminoglycans as antithrombotic agents. In Poller L (ed): Blood Coagulation. New York, Churchill Livingstone, 1993.
58. Agrati AM, DeBartolo G, Palmieri G: Heparan sulfate: Efficacy and safety in patients with chronic venous insufficiency. Minerva Cardioangiol 39(10):395–400, 1991.
59. Caramelli L, Mirchioni R, Carini J: Effectiveness of short-term sulodexide treatment on peripheral vascular disease clinical manifestations. Rivista Europea per le Scienze Mediche e Farmacologiche 10(1):55–58, 1988.
60. Seccia M, Bellomini MG, Goletti O, et al: The prevention of postoperative deep venous thrombosis with heparan sulfate per os. A controlled clinical study vs. heparin calcium. Minerva Chirur 47(1-2):45–48, 1992.
61. Romeo S, Grasso A, Costanzo C: A controlled clinical experiment "within subjects" with heparan sulfate in intermittent claudication. Minerva Cardioangiol 39(9):345–352, 1991.
62. Cofrancesco E, Boschetti C, Leonardi P, Cortellaro M: Dermatan sulphate in acute leukaemia. Lancet 339:1177–1178, 1992
63. Lane DA, Ryan K, Ireland H, et al: Dermatan sulphate in haemodialysis. Lancet 339:334–335, 1992.
64. Rowlings PA, Mansberg R, Rozenberg MC, et al: The use of a low molecular weight heparinoid (ORG 10172) for extracorporeal procedures in patients with heparin dependent thrombocytopenia and thrombosis. Aust N Z J Med 21:52–54, 1991.
65. Bergqvist D, Kettunen K, Fredin H, et al: Thromboprophylaxis in patients with hip fractures A prospective, randomized, comparative study between Org 10172 and dextran 70. Surgery 109:617–622, 1991.
66. Fareed J, Walenga JM, Iyer L, et al: An objective perspective on recombinant hirudin A new anticoagulant and antithrombotic agent. Blood Coagul Fibrinol 2:135–147, 1991.
67. Hijikata-Okunomiya A, Okamoto S: A strategy for a rational approach to designing synthetic selective inhibitors. Semin Thromb Hemost 18:135–149, 1992.
68. Tamao Y, Yamamoto T, Kimumoto R, et al: Effect of a selective thrombin-inhibitor MCI-9038 on fibrinolysis in vitro and in vivo. Thromb Haemost 562:28–34, 1986.
69. Tamao Y, Yamamoto T, Hirata T, et al: Effect of argipidine (MD-805) on blood coagulation. Jpn Pharmacol Ther 14:869–874, 1986.
70. Maruyama I: Synthetic anticoagulants. Jpn J Clin Hematol 31:776–781, 1990.
71. Yonekawa Y, Handa H, Okamoto S, et al: Treatment of cerebral infarction in the acute stage with synthetic antithrombin MD805: Clinical study among multiple institutions. Arch Jpn Chir 55:711–726, 1986.
72. Kumon K, Tanaka K, Nakajima N, et al Anticoagulation with a synthetic thrombin inhibitor after cardiovascular surgery and for treatment of disseminated intravascular coagulation. Crit Care Med 12:1039–1043, 1984.
73. Oshiro T, Kanbayashi J, Kosaki G: Antithrombotic therapy of patient with peripheral arterial reconstruction-clinical study on MD805. Blood Vessel 14:216–218., 1983.
74. Matsuo T, Kario K, Kodama K, Okamoto S: Clinical applications of the synthetic thrombin inhibitor, Argatroban (MD-805). Semin Thromb Hemost 18:155–160, 1992.
75. Teger-Nilsson A, Eriksson U, Gustafsson D, et al: Phase I studies on Inogatran, a new selective thrombin inhibitor. J Am Coll Cardiol 117A–118A, 1995.
76. Bajusz S, Barabás E, Széll E, Bagdy D: Peptide aldehyde inhibitors of the fibrinogen-thrombin reaction. In Meienhofer J (ed): Peptides: Chemistry, Structure and Biology. Ann Arbor, MI, Ann Arbor Science Publishers, 1975, pp 603–608.
77. Bajusz S, Barabás E, Tolnay P, et al: Inhibition of thrombin and trypsin by tripeptide aldehydes. Int J Peptide Protein Res 12:217–221, 1978.
78. Bajusz S, Széll E, Bagdy D, et al: US Patent No. 4,703,036, 1987.
79. Bajusz S, Széll E, Bagdy D, et al: Highly active and selective anticoagulants D-Phe-Pro-Arg-H, a free tripeptide aldehyde prone to spontaneous inactivation, and its stable N-methyl derivative, D-MePhe-Pro-Arg-H. J Med Chem 33:1729-–1735, 1990.
80. Bagdy D, Barabás E, Bajusz S, Széll E: In vitro inhibition of blood coagulation by tripeptide aldehydes: A retrospective screening study focused on the stable D-MePhe-Pro-Arg-H-H_2SO_4. Thromb Hemost 67:325–330, 1992.

81. Markwardt F, Fink G, Kaiser B, et al: Pharmacological survey of recombinant hirudin. Pharmazie 43:202–207, 1988.
82. Maraganore JM, Bourdon P, Jablonski J, et al: Design and characterization of hirulogs: A novel class of bivalent peptide inhibitors of thrombin. Biochemistry 29:7095–7101, 1990.
83. Topol EJ, Bonan R, Jewitt D, et al: Use of a direct antithrombin, hirulog, in place of heparin during coronary angioplasty. Circulation 87:1622–1629, 1993.
84. Pini M, Tagliaferri A, Manotti C, et al: Low molecular weight heparin (Alfa LMWH) compared with unfractionated heparin in prevention of deep-vein thrombosis after hip fractures. Int Angiol 8:134–139, 1989.
85. Sorensen JV, Lassen MR, Borris LC, et al: Reduction of plasma levels of prothrombin fragments 1 and 2 during thrombophylaxis with a low-molecular-weight heparin. Blood Coagul Fibrinol 3:55–59, 1992.
86. Turpie AGG, Levine MN, Hirsh J, et al: A randomized controlled trial of low molecular weight heparin (Enoxaparin) to prevent deep vein thrombosis in patients undergoing elective hip surgery. N Engl J Med 315:925–929, 1987.
87. Lefkovits J, Topol EJ: Direct thrombin inhibitors in cardiovascular medicine. Circulation 90:1522–1536, 1994.
88. Theroux P, Lidon R: Anticoagulants and their use in acute ischemic syndromes. In Topol EJ (ed): Textbook of Interventional Cardiology. Philadelphia, W.B. Saunders, 1994.
89. Iyer L, Fareed J: Recombinant hirudin: a perspective. Exp Opin Invest Drugs 5:469–494, 1996.
90. Lefkovits J, Topol EJ: Direct thrombin inhibitors in cardiovascular medicine. Circulation 90:1522–1536, 1994.
91. Topol EJ, Bonan R, Jewitt D, et al: Use of a direct antithrombin, hirulog in place of heparin during coronary angioplasty. Circulation 87:1622–1629, 1993.
92. Topol EJ: Novel antithrombotic approaches to coronary artery disease. Am J Cardiol 76(6):27B–33B, 1995.
93. Fareed J, Callas DD: Pharmacological aspects of thrombin inhibitors: A developmental perspective. Vessels 1(4):15–24, 1995.
94. Resnekov L, Chediak J, Hirsh J, Lewis HD Jr: Antithrombotic agents in coronary artery disease. Chest 95(2):52S–72S, 1989.
95. Riess FC, Lower C, Seelig C, et al: Recombinant hirudin as a new anticoagulant during cardiac operations instead of heparin: successful for aortic valve replacement in man. J Thorac Cardiovasc Surg 110:265–267, 1995.
96. Edmunds LH: HIT, HITT and desulfatohirudin: look before you leap. J Thorac Cardiovasc Surg 110:1-3, 1995.
97. Ericksson BI, Lindbratt S, Toerholm C, et al: Recombinant hirudin, CGP 39393 15 mg (Reasc-Ciba) is the most effective and safe prophylaxis of thromboembolic complications in patients undergoing total hip replacement. Thromb Haemost 73:1093, 1995.
98. Ericksson BI, Lindbratt S, Toerholm C, Kalebo P: Prevention of deep vein thrombosis after total hip replacement: Direct thrombin inhibition with recombinant hirudin, CGP 39393. Lancet 347:635–639, 1996.
99. Callas DD, Fareed J: Direct inhibition of protein Ca by site directed thrombin inhibitors: Implications in anticoagulant and thrombolytic therapy. Thromb Res 78:457–460, 1995.
100. Callas DD, Iqbal O, Hoppensteadt D, Fareed J: Fibrinolytic compromise by synthetic and recombinant thrombin inhibitors. Implications in the management of thrombotic disorders. Clin Appl Thromb Hemost 1:114–124, 1995.
101. Verstraete M: Desirudin: Review of Its Pharmacology and Prospective Uses. Norwich, Royal Society of Medicne Press.
102. O'Donnell CJ, Ridker PM, Herbert PR, Hennekens CH: Antithrombotic therapy for acute myocardial infarction. J Am Coll Cardiol 25:23S–29S, 1995.
103. Herrmann JP, Serruys PW: Thrombin and antithrombotic therapy in interventional cardiology. Texas Heart Inst J 21:138–147, 1994.
104. Saltiel E, Ward A: Ticlopidine: A review of its pharmacodynamic and pharmacokinetic properties and therapeutic efficacy in platelet-dependent disease states. Drugs 34:222–262, 1987.
105. Walenga JM, Pifarre R, Fareed J: Recombinant hirudin as an antithrombotic agent. Drugs Future 15:267–270, 1990.
106. Pytele R, Pierschbacher MS, Ginsberg MH, et al: Platelet membrane glycoprotein IIb/IIIa: Member of a family of RGD specific adhesion receptors. Science 231:1559–1562, 1986.
107. Philips DR, Charo IF, Scarborough RM: GPIIb-IIIa: The responsive integrin. Cell 65:359—362, 1991.
108. Ruggeri ZM, Houghton RA, Russel SR, Zimmerman TS: Inhibition of platelet function with synthetic peptide designed to be high affinity antagonist of fibrinogen binding to platelets. Proc Natl Acad Sci USA 83:5708–5712, 1986.
109. Mickelson JK, Simpson PJ, Cronin M, et al: Antiplatelet antibody [7E3 f(ab')$_2$] prevents rethrombosis after recombinant tissue-type plasminogen activator-induced coronary artery thrombolysis in a canine model. Circulation 81:617–627, 1990.

110. Bock LC, Griffin LC, Latham JA, et al: Selection of single-stranded DNA molecules that bind and inhibit human thrombin. Nature 355:564–566, 1992.

111. Macaya RF, Schultze P, Smith FW, et al: Thrombin-binding DNA aptamer forms a unimolecular quadruplex structure in solution. Proc Natl Acad Sci USA 90:3745–3749, 1993.

112. Paborsky LR, McCurdy SN, Griffin LC, et al: The single-stranded DNA aptamer binding-site of human thrombin. J Biol Chem 268:20808, 1993.

113. Li WX, Kaplan AV, Grant GW, et al: A novel nucleotide-based thrombin inhibitor inhibits clot-bound thrombin and reduces arterial platelet thrombus formation. Blood 83:677–682, 1994.

114. Latham JA, Johnson R, Toole JJ: The application of a modified nucleotide in aptamer selection novel thrombin aptamers containing 5-(1-pentynyl)-2'-deoxyuridine. Nucl Acids Res 22:2817–2822, 1994.

115. Kubik MF, Stephens AW, Schneider D, et al: High-affinity RNA ligands to human α-thrombin. Nucl Acids Res 22:2619–2626, 1994.

116. Fareed J, Walenga JM, Hoppensteadt DA, et al: Pharmacologic profiling of defibrotide in experimental models. Semin Thromb Hemost 14:27–37, 1988.

117. Bracht F, Schror K: Isolation and identification of aptamers from defibrotide that act as thrombin antagonists in vitro. Biochem Biophys Res Com 200:933–937, 1994.

CHAPTER 8

Low-Molecular-Weight Heparin in the Prevention and Management of Deep Vein Thrombosis

SYLVIA HAAS, M.D.

Numerous publications have provided firm evidence that prophylaxis with low-dose unfractionated heparin (UFH) has contributed significantly to the reduction of thromboembolic complications in surgery. Without prophylaxis, the rate of deep vein thrombosis (DVT) is about 30% in patients undergoing general surgery and rises to 70% in orthopedic and trauma surgery. According to Collins et al.[12] and Clagett et al.,[10] heparin prevents at least 60% of DVT. Despite heparin prophylaxis, however, a relatively high incidence of DVT has still been observed in high-risk patients undergoing orthopedic or trauma surgery. In the meantime, various heparin fragments and fractions have become available for clinical use, and the question arises whether low-molecular-weight heparins (LMWHs) are equal or even superior to unfractionated heparin in preventing and treating thromboembolic complications. Because the antithrombotic activity of UFH and LMWH cannot be reduced simply to their anticoagulant effects but depends on multifactorial reactions, the pharmacologic mode of action of these compounds is briefly reviewed.

MODE OF ACTION OF UNFRACTIONATED HEPARIN

The main targets of the antithrombotic actions of heparin are antithrombin III (AT III)-mediated inhibition of various clotting factors (especially factors Xa and IIa) and release of tissue factor pathway inhibitor (TFPI), tissue plasminogen activator (tPA), and heparinlike substances from the endothelium. For primary prophylactic use, unfractionated heparin is given in low doses (5000 IE 2 or 3 times/day); the dosage cannot be increased because of the inherent risk of bleeding, which is due to inhibition of factor IIa (thrombin). This low-dose heparin (LDH) prophylaxis is recommended in general surgery (including gynecologic and urologic operations), orthopedic surgery, and trauma patients; however, fixed LDH prophylaxis is considered to be only moderately effective. Adjusting the heparin dosage by a coagulation assay is more effective but adds to management problems. The clinical use of unfractionated heparin is associated with several adverse side effects, such as bleeding and heparin-induced thrombocytopenia (HIT), and also requires at least twice-daily injections.

MODE OF ACTION OF LOW-MOLECULAR-WEIGHT HEPARIN

The above problems associated with the clinical use of UFH prompted research targeted at the identification of heparin derivatives with more favorable attributes. It was found that heparin fragments below 16–20 monosaccharides per heparin molecule (molecule weight < 5000 Da), while containing the specific pentasaccharide sequence essential for binding to AT III, are not long enough to permit binding to thrombin; they therefore inhibit only factor Xa.[3] LMWHs prolong the clotting time only moderately (indicating no thrombin inhibition) but are still capable of potentiating the inhibition of factor Xa; this raised the hope of dissociating the antithrombotic property (anti-Xa) from the anticoagulant property (inhibition of thrombin), which would avoid the hemorrhagic effects of UFH.[19] The rationale for this assumption is that it would be important to inhibit the cascade system at the earliest stage possible without altering normal hemostasis. Yin et al. have shown that 1 µg of AT III is capable of inhibiting 32 units of factor Xa, which in turn can inhibit the formation of 1600 units of factor IIa, whereas direct inhibition of this amount of factor IIa requires 1000 µg of AT III.[39] Recent studies have provided evidence that prevention of thrombosis cannot be attributed to the specific anti-Xa activity but rather to an interaction of LMWH fractions with the prothrombinase complex, thereby leading to an inhibition of thrombin generation (Fig. 1).

USE OF LOW-MOLECULAR-WEIGHT HEPARIN IN PREVENTION OF DEEP VEIN THROMBOSIS IN SURGERY

Although the substance- and dosage-related differences of UFH and LMWH prophylaxis shown in Table 1 do not support the assessment of efficacy by metaanalysis, this method may allow global orientation. The conclusions derived from previous metaanalyses comparing prophylaxis with UFH to placebo or LMWHs to UFH, respectively, are summarized in Table 2.

The statements of the metaanalyses performed by Nurmohamed et al.,[30] Lassen et al.,[23] and Leizorovicz et al.[25] agree with the assessment of the antithrombotic efficacy of LMWH prophylaxis vs. UFH prophylaxis provided by Haas et al. in 1993. This overview concluded that despite difficulties and concerns about general assessments, single daily injections of LMWH seem to be at least as efficacious as multiple daily doses of UFH. The most evident reduction of the relative risk has obviously been achieved in high-risk patients—that is, in patients who are still at high risk despite prophylaxis with UFH.[15] The

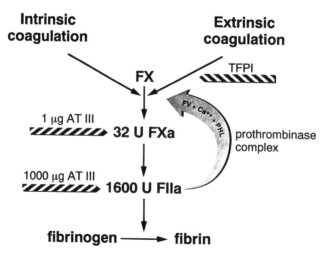

FIGURE 1.   Simplified graph of the amplification mechanism of the blood coagulation cascade.

TABLE 1.   Concerns about Assessment of Efficacy of Prophylaxis with Unfractionated and Low-Molecular-Weight Heparins by Metaanalysis

Unfractionated Heparin	Low-Molecular-Weight Heparin
Various fixed-dosage schedules 5,000 IU 2 or 3 times/day 7,500 IU 2 times/day	Heterogeneity of substances
Various adjusted-dosage schedules APTT-adjusted (2–5 sec above control) APTT, range not defined Thrombin-time, range not defined Time point of blood sampling different Different sensitivity of APTT reagents	Various fixed dosages
Combination of fixed and adjusted dosages	Body weight-adjusted doses
Start pre- or postoperatively	Various time intervals of administration
Combination of various doses with dihydroergotamine	

APTT = activated partial thromboplastin time.

great intertrial variations, however, have been observed not only with different preparations but also with each product in various trials. Table 3 and 4 summarize the variations in incidence of DVT in general surgery based on fibrinogen uptake test and in orthopedic surgery based on phlebography.

There are many reasons for the wide range of variation in frequencies of DVT in the heparin groups as well as in the LMWH groups. The substance- and dosage-related differences may account for this wide range to a significant degree, but study-related variations also may play a significant role. Bergqvist et al. analyzed potential reasons for interstudy variations in the frequency of postoperative DVT in their overview on the incidence of venous thromboembolism in medical and surgical patients.[5] For example, the distribution of risk factors and types of anesthesia may affect the study outcome, and geographic influences or fluctuations over time also may play a role. In addition, the variations in frequencies of DVT may be related to diagnostic differences, differences in general care of patients, cross-section of patient population, and differences in statistics.

In the meantime, LMWH has become the standard of care for prophylaxis in high-risk patients in several European countries. In France and Germany, low-dose heparin is no longer accepted by health authorities as a control in orthopedic patients. New prophylactic modalities must compete either with adjusted-dose heparin or LMWH in future trials. Although no specific recommendations have been given for the reference groups, it has become common practice in Europe to compare with single daily doses of LMWH.

TABLE 2.   Assessment of Antithrombotic Efficacy of Unfractionated Heparin and Low-Molecular-Weight Heparin by Metaanalysis

Unfractionated Heparin vs. Placebo or None	Low-Molecular-Weight Heparin vs. Unfractionated Heparin
Colditz et al., 1986[11] General surgery: reduction of DVT from 27% to 9.6%	Nurmohamed et al., 1991[30] General and orthopedic surgery: LMWH superior in high-risk patients
Clagett and Reisch, 1988[10] General surgery: reduction of DVT from 25.2 to 8.7%	Lassen, et al., 1991[23] General and orthopedic surgery: LMWH in general surgery more effective than UFH thrice daily, comparable to UFH twice daily; LMWH in orthopedic surgery more effective
Collins et al., 1988[12] General, orthopedic, and urologic surgery: reduction of DVT by 50%	Leizorovicz et al., 1992[25] General and orthopedic surgery: LMWH more efficacious than UFH

TABLE 3.   Variations in Incidences of Deep Venous Thrombosis in General Surgery

Drug	Low-Molecular-Weight Heparin			Unfractionated Heparin		
	x (%)	Min (%)	Max (%)	x (%)	Min (%)	Max (%)
LMWH$_1$	5.5	2.9	9.0	5.3	0	9.2
LMWH$_2$	2.7	2.5	2.8	6.0	4.5	7.5
LMWH$_3$	4.4	2.8	8.1	5.1	2.7	7.6
LMWH$_4$	9.1	6.9	11.4	10.8	7.9	13.2
LMWH$_5$	4.0	2.3	5.6	3.0	3.0	3.0
LMWH$_6$	5.2	4.6	5.8	7.0	4.2	9.8

USE OF LOW-MOLECULAR-WEIGHT HEPARIN IN PREVENTION OF DEEP VEIN THROMBOSIS IN INTERNAL MEDICINE

In internal medicine, pharmacologic prophylaxis of thromboembolism in bed-ridden patients who suffer from severe heart disease after apoplexia, malignancies, or hemi- or paraplegia is necessary when mobilization of the patient is not possible. The use of LMWH for this indication has been proved in various studies and is accepted by more and more clinicians.

In a double-blind study of 1,968 patients, Harenberg et al. compared the once-daily administration of 36 mg of nadroparin with the thrice-daily administration of 5,000 IU of UFH. For both prophylactic treatments an equally good antithrombotic efficacy was found, but the patients who received LMWH had fewer side effects and better compatibility. In the UFH group, bleeding, bruising, and pruritus occurred significantly more often; the plasma levels of triglycerides, cholesterol, glutamate oxaloacetate transaminase, and glutamate-pyruvate transaminase were significantly increased; the activated partial thromboplastin time (APTT) was significantly longer; and the AT III levels were significantly lower. In the nadroparin group, there was no incidence of thrombocytopenia, whereas in the UFH group there were four cases of thrombocyte readings of 40,000–80,000/mm^3.[18]

In a total of 885 patients, Lechler et al. compared the thrice-daily administration of UFH (443 patients) with single daily doses of 40 mg of enoxaparin, a LMWH (442 patients). No statistically significant difference was seen between the frequency of thromboembolic complications (1.4% for the UFH group and 0.2% for the enoxaparin group); however, the parameters of tolerance were significantly better in the LMWH group.[24]

A study of geriatric patients conducted by Bergmann et al. showed an equally good primary therapeutic efficacy of enoxaparin compared with UFH. Because of the low thrombus risk of these patients, the once-daily administration of 20 mg of enoxaparin was compared with twice-daily injections of 5,000 IU of UFH.[4] Dahan et al.[13] and Poniewierski et al.[31] had earlier proved the antithrombotic efficacy of dalteparin for a broad variety of indications in internal medicine.

The major advantage of enoxaparin in prophylaxis in internal medicine, apart from more comfortable follow-through due to the once-daily injection, is improved safety.

TABLE 4.   Variations in Incidences of Deep Venous Thrombosis in Orthopedic Surgery

Drug	Low-Molecular-Weight Heparin			Unfractionated Heparin		
	x (%)	Min (%)	Max (%)	x (%)	Min (%)	Max (%)
LMWH$_1$	14.9	4.9	30.0	20.6	10.0	42.0
LMWH$_2$	21.2	12.6	29.7	21.8	16.0	27.4
LMWH$_3$	15.9	12.5	19.4	24.1	23.2	25.0
LMWH$_4$	15.4	9.6	22.9	22.5	11.8	30.6

Heparin-induced urticaria should be reason enough to switch to LMWH. In patients with HIT, however, the heparinoid orgaran is the medication of choice.

Another possible use for LMWHs in internal medicine is the prophylaxis of arterial emboli due to chronic atrial fibrillation. However, results from clinical trials are preliminary.

USE OF LOW-MOLECULAR-WEIGHT HEPARIN IN TREATMENT OF DEEP VEIN THROMBOSIS

Treatment of acute DVT is aimed mainly at preventing recurrent venous thromboembolism. The classic regimen consists of an initial continuous intravenous administration of UFH followed by long-term oral anticoagulant therapy. In contrast to prophylaxis with low doses of heparin, therapeutic use aims at inhibiting thrombin and preventing further growth of fibrin thrombi due to the anticoagulant activity of heparin. In addition, the profibrinolytic effect of heparin may play a significant role in thrombus regression. To achieve this therapeutic aim, heparin is given in APTT-adjusted dosages, whereby a 1.5–2-fold increase in APTT is sought. The therapeutic range should be reached within the first 24 hours.

Although this therapeutic approach shows acceptable clinical results, certain modifications and simplifications are needed for the following reasons:

- The therapy does not always lead to the desired goal. Regression of the thrombus cannot be obtained for all patients, and thromboembolic recurrence (i.e., the occurrence of postthrombotic syndrome) cannot always be avoided.
- Even with strict laboratory controls, bleeding still occurs.
- The continuous infusion demands hospitalization.

It was therefore investigated whether LMWHs also could be used for the treatment of thrombosis. The investigation was two-directional: LMWH vs. UFH and intravenous route (for UFH) vs. subcutaneous injection (for LMWH). Subcutaneous injection was used because of the specific pharmacokinetic and pharmacodynamic properties of LMWHs.

In two studies Bratt et al. compared intravenous administration of the LMWH dalteparin with the intravenous administration of UHF. In the first study the original dose of 240 anti-Xa units/kg/12 hr was reduced to 120 anti-Xa units/kg/12 hr because of bleeding complications. In the dalteparin group no thrombus growth was diagnosed, whereas in the UFH group the frequency was 11%. According to the Marder score assessment, there was no difference between the two groups. The reduction of AT III was significantly stronger in the UFH group.[7,8]

Albada et al. compared intravenous infusions of dalteparin with intravenous infusions of UFH. The dosage was adjusted each time according to the anti-Xa activity in the plasma; for patients with no noticeable bleeding risk, the target plasma level was 0.4–0.9 anti-Xa units/ml; for patients with a high risk of bleeding, the target level was 0.3–0.6 anti-Xa units/ml. The therapeutic success rate, determined by repeated ventilation and perfusion scintigraphy, was the same for both groups. The frequency of bleeding complications was relatively high for both groups: 38.5% in the dalteparin group and 48.9% in the UFH group.[2]

The use of twice-daily subcutaneous injections of LMWH instead of intravenous infusions of UFH was investigated in various studies. The therapeutic success in all studies was phlebographically controlled; the endpoint was thrombus regression as measured by the Arnesen or Marder score system. The second phlebography as done usually between the fifth and seventh day of therapy. Twice-daily administration of LMWH provided results at least equal to the results of intravenous infusions of UFH.[9,16,17,29,32] In a further study, the twice-daily subcutaneous injection of 1 mg/kg of enoxaparin was compared with the intravenous administration of UFH. There was no difference in the recurrence of DVT or in the frequency of bleeding complications.[34]

Subcutaneous injection of nadroparin was compared with intravenous administration of UFH in a randomized multicenter study. An APTT 1.5–2-fold longer than normal was sought in the UFH group. Nadroparin, 255 anti-Xa units/kg body weight, was injected subcutaneously twice daily. The phlebographically proven thrombus regression was significantly better in the nadroparin group than in the UFH-group; compatibility was equally good for both groups.[1]

In 1992 Prandoni et al. reported the results of their randomized study of patients with clinically symptomatic proximal thrombi, in which a body weight-stratified dosage regimen of subcutaneously administered nadroparin was compared with APTT-adjusted doses of intravenous injections of UFH. The patients in the nadroparin group were divided into three groups according to body weight: patients weighing < 55 kg received 12,500 anti-Xa units; patients weighing 55–88 kg, 15,000 anti-Xa units; and patients weighing > 80 kg, 17,500 anti-Xa units. The daily dose was divided into two injections. Symptomatic recurrent deep vein thrombus or pulmonary embolism was chosen as the primary endpoint to judge the efficacy of the treatment; the second endpoint was changes in the phlebographic and scintigraphic results on the tenth day compared with the first day. The frequency of the objectively proven thromboembolic recurrences did not differ significantly between the two groups (UFH, 14%; nadroparin, 7%); clinically manifest bleedings occurred in both groups with the same frequency (UFH, 3.5%; nadroparin, 1%). Six months later, a control examination revealed that in the meanwhile, 12 patients treated with UFH and 6 patients treated with nadroparin had died. The reason for this difference, however, may be that in the UFH group the cause of death was more often carcinoma.[33]

Nadroparin was also investigated for use in treating pulmonary embolisms. Théry et al. compared various body weight-related, subcutaneous dosages of nadroparin (400, 600, and 900 anti-Xa units/kg/24 hr) with intravenous infusions of UFH. The treatment with the two higher dosages of nadroparin was stopped because of bleeding complications. The study proved that the lowest dose of nadroparin was as efficient and as compatible as infusions with UFH.[36]

In a double-blind multicenter study, the efficacy and safety of the LMWH logiparin was tested. Hull et al. compared once-daily subcutaneous injection of body weight-related doses of logiparin (175 anti-Xa-E IU/kg) with intravenously administered UFH. For the daily adjusted dose of UFH, a 1.5–2.5-fold increase in APTT compared with the original value was sought. Only patients with a phlebographically proven proximal thrombus were accepted. Endpoints were defined as increased thrombus growth, thromboembolic recurrence, minor or major bleedings, thrombocytopenia, and death. In the LMWH group only 2.8% of patients displayed a thromboembolic recurrence, whereas the UFH group had a recurrence rate of 6.9%. The frequency of major bleedings during the initial therapy was 0.5% in the LMWH group and 5.0% in the UFH group. However, major bleedings increased to 2.3% in the LMWH group after patients were given oral anticoagulants, whereas this increase occurred in none of the UFH patients. In the logiparin group 4.7% of patients died compared with 9.6% of the UFH group.[20]

In a pilot study of 25 patients, Kirchmaier et al. proved the efficacy and compatibility of certoparin for treating deep vein thrombus in the leg. They discovered a definite thrombus regression correlated with duration of treatment.[21] A controlled, randomized study comparing subcutaneously and intravenously administered certoparin with intravenous infusions of UFH is in its final stage.

To summarize the results of these studies, in treatment of DVT the initial intravenous administration of UFH can be replaced by subcutaneous injections of LMWH. This conclusion is supported by several metaanalyses of the therapeutic use of LMWH.[25,35,37] In an updated metaanalysis of results from 20 randomized controlled clinical studies comparing LMWH with UFH, Leizorovicz provided evidence of statistically significant reductions in mortality, major hemorrhage, and thrombus extension with use of LMWH. A nonsignificant trend, also in favor of LMWH, was observed for recurrence of venous thromboembolic events. The results of this metaanalysis show that LMWHs seem to have a higher benefit/risk ratio than UFH in the treatment of DVT.[26] However, some questions have to be answered by future trials. The first question concerns the optimal duration of the initial treatment phase. Most physicians start treatment with either unfractionated heparin or LMWH, and it is common practice to switch to oral anticoagulants soon afterward. The results of some clinical trials suggest, however, that prolongation of the initial phase with either UFH or LMWH may be beneficial in significantly reducing the thrombus size because of the profibrinolytic potential of these compounds. This question has attracted the attention of several research groups, because previous preclinical experiments have shown that the profibrinolytic effect of LMWH seems to be increased compared with UFH.

Based on their improved pharmacodynamic profile (higher bioavailability, increased tissue factor pathway inhibitor release, stronger thrombin generation inhibition, less effect on platelets and other cells, delayed antithrombotic effects, more selective binding to target sites, enhanced endothelial modulatory actions), LMWHs were injected subcutaneously in most clinical studies. However, the optimal interval of administration (once or twice per day) is still debatable, the optimal dosage is as yet unknown, and the question of the lowest dose of LMWH still effective in treating established DVT remains unanswered.

Treatment with UFH leads to a wide scattering of APTT response and, therefore, requires regular laboratory monitoring. Because LMWHs catalyze thrombin inhibition by AT III to a lesser extent than UFH, they induce a weaker prolongation of the thrombin clotting time and APTT. The decreased ability of LMWH to prolong APTT is inversely correlated with its anti Xa/anti IIa ratio. In addition, other factors may account for the low sensitivity of APTT in monitoring LMWH. For example, factor Xa bound to phospholipids in the prothrombinase complex is partly protected from inactivation by the AT III–heparin complex. After parenteral administration, the clearance of heparin chains of any LMWH preparation varies with its molecular weight: the longer chains supporting both anti-Xa and Anti-IIa activities are cleared twice as fast as the shorter chains supporting only the anti-Xa activity. These pharmacologic properties account for the low sensitivity of APTT in monitoring LMWH therapy, even when the circulating anti-Xa activity is high. They also indicate that neither anti-Xa nor anti-IIa activity reflects the entire spectrum of the complex pharmacologic activities of LMWH. It was recently proposed to quantify the pharmacologic effects of LMWHs by measuring the area under the curve of thrombin generation tests. This approach is attractive but requires further validation.[6] At present, the only tests available for monitoring LMWH therapy measure anti-Xa activity in plasma. Plasma anti-Xa activity generated by a given dose of LMWH is more predictable than for UFH. Therefore, interpatient variability is far less pronounced for LMWHs; thus less frequent dose adjustments are required.

Several pharmacologic properties may account for the more predictable effects of LMWH compared with UFH. The nonspecific binding of heparin to plasma proteins and its interaction with endothelial cells and macrophages are more pronounced for UFH than for LMWH. However, because of its half-life, accumulation of LMWH should be excluded for each substance separately, particularly in patients suffering from renal insufficiency. If monitoring is required in this particular situation, the question arises as to what test to use: should anti-Xa activity be measured by chromogenic or chronometric assays? However, based on the multifactorial pharmacologic profile of LMWHs, it remains questionable whether any laboratory parameter can reflect their antithrombotic activity.

Another question concerns the efficacy of LMWH in preventing the postthrombotic sequelae of swelling, skin alterations, and ulceration. To answer this question, long-term follow-up studies using objective phlebodynamometric tests are needed. Furthermore, long-term investigations should focus on the evaluation of mortality rate. The results of several studies provide evidence that overall mortality and mortality in cancer patients were significantly reduced by LMWH.[20,27,35] Whether these differences in mortality indicate a true effect of LMWHs remains to be determined.

Several studies have evaluated the home administration of LMWH in the treatment of DVT. The investigators concluded that many patients with acute proximal DVT can be treated safely and effectively at home with LMWH adjusted for the patient's weight.[22,28] However, it seems too early to recommend this approach as standard treatment. Koopman and coworkers claim that three potential hazards must be recognized. First, because the clinical diagnosis is unreliable, the presence of disease should be confirmed objectively in every patient to avoid unnecessary treatment. Second, risk factors must be assessed adequately to explain the possible cause of thrombosis. Finally, care outside the hospital increases pressure on community facilities to provide proper anticoagulant therapy, and they need to be prepared for this task.[22]

Despite the questions that should be answered by future trials, treatment of DVT with LMWH offers many advantages compared with UFH, especially since some of the questions also apply for heparin or have been answered only by the empirical use of UFH for more than three decades.

DISCUSSION

The availability of various LMWH preparations has raised the question of whether their antithrombotic efficacy is equal to or better than that of UFH. However, finding an answer is hampered by the fact that LMWHs show greater chemical and biologic heterogeneity than UFH. Indeed, LMWHs were recommended for prophylaxis in high-risk patients by the European Consensus Statement in 1991, but this statement also points to the individuality of the different compounds: "Fixed dose low molecular weight heparins and one heparinoid are currently the most effective prophylaxis. However, the efficacy and safety of each product need to be documented separately."[14]

Without doubt, LMWH now plays a pivotal role in prevention of thromboembolic complications in high-risk surgical patients; however, an important question is whether to start prophylaxis pre- or postoperatively. The European Consensus Statement recommended that "prophylaxis should preferably be started before operation." Recent evidence, however, indicates that postoperative commencement of prophylaxis is also effective.

In addition, some trials provide evidence that the safety profile of LMWH seems to be superior to that of UFH. In particular, the hemorrhagic profile for bleeding episodes favored the use of LMWH in orthopedic patients. Also, HIT seems to occur less frequently with prophylaxis with LMWH compared with UFH. Warkentin et al. obtained daily platelet counts in 665 patients in a randomized, double-blind clinical trial comparing UFH with LMWH as prophylaxis after hip surgery. HIT occurred in 9 of 332 patients (2.7%) who received UFH and in none of the 333 patients who received enoxaparin (p = 0.0018). Eight of the 9 patients with HIT also had one or more thrombotic events, of which venous thrombi occurred in 7 patients and arterial thrombosis in 1 patient. A subgroup analysis of 387 patients revealed a significantly higher frequency of heparin-dependent IgG antibodies among patients who received UFH than among those who received enoxaparin (7.8% vs. 2.2%). The authors concluded that HIT, associated thrombotic events, and heparin-dependent IgG antibodies are more common in patients treated with UFH than in those treated with LMWH.[38]

Thus, LMWHs have a number of potential and demonstrated clinical advantages over UFH. The potential advantage is the reduced hemorrhagic-to-antithrombotic ratio of LMWH in experimental animals. The demonstrated advantages of LMWHs are their greater bioavailability at lower doses, longer half-life, and more predictable anticoagulant response when administered in fixed doses. These properties allow LMWHs to be administered once daily and without laboratory monitoring. Recent evidence also suggests that the incidence of HIT is lower with LMWH than with UFH. These advantages of LMWH over UFH provide an excellent basis for their widespread use in the prevention and management of DVT.

REFERENCES

1. A Collaborative European Multicentre Study: A randomised trial of subcutaneous low molecular weight heparin (CY 216) compared with intravenous unfractionated heparin in the treatment of deep vein thrombosis. Thromb Haemost 65:251–256, 1991.
2. Albada J, Niewenhuis HK, Sixma JJ: Treatment of acute venous thromboembolism with low molecular weight heparin (Fragmin). Results of a double-blind randomized study. Circulation 80:935–940, 1993.
3. Barrowcliffe TW, Johnson EA, Eggleton CA, et al: Anticoagulant activities of high and low molecular weight heparin fractions. Br J Haematol 41:573–583, 1979.
4. Bergmann JF, for the Geriatric Enoxaparin Study Group: Prevention of venous thromboembolism in elderly medical in-patients: A double blind comparative study of unfractionated heparin (2 x 5000 IU) and enoxaparin (20 mg) [abstract]. Ann Hematol 68(Suppl II):183, 1994.
5. Bergqvist D, Lindblad D: Incidence of venous thromboembolism in medical and surgical patients. In Bergqvist D, Comerota AJ, Nicolaides AN, Scurr JH (eds): Prevention of Venous Thromboembolism. London, Med Orion, 1994, pp 3–15.
6. Boneu B: Low molecular weight heparin therapy: Is monitoring needed? Thromb Haemost 72:330–334, 1994.
7. Bratt G, Törnebohm E, Granqvist S, et al: A comparison between low molecular weight heparin (Kabi 2165) and standard heparin in the intravenous treatment of deep venous thrombosis. Thromb Haemost 54:813–817, 1985.
8. Bratt G, Törnebohm E, Lockner D, Bergstrom KL: A human pharmacological study comparing conventional heparin and a low molecular weight heparin fragment. Thromb Haemost 53:208–211, 1985.
9. Bratt G, Aberg W, Johansson M, et al: Two daily subcutaneous injections of Fragmin as compared with intravenous standard heparin in treatment of deep venous thrombosis (DVT). Thromb Haemost 64:506–510, 1990.
10. Clagett P, Reisch J: Prevention of venous thromboembolism in general surgical patients: Results of meta-analysis. Ann Surg 208:227–240, 1988.
11. Colditz G, Tuden R, Oster G: Rates of venous thrombosis after general surgery: Combined results of randomised clinical trials. Lancet 19:143–146, 1986.
12. Collins R, Scrimgeour A, Yusuf S, Peto R: Reduction in fatal pulmonary embolism and venous thrombosis by perioperative administration of subcutaneous heparin. N Engl J Med 318:1162–1172, 1988.
13. Dahan D, Houlbert D, Caulin C, et al: Prevention of deep vein thrombosis in elderly patients by a low molecular weight heparin—a randomised double-blind trial. Haemostasis 16:159–164, 1986.
14. European Consensus Statement: Prevention of thromboembolism. In Bergqvist D, Comerota AJ, Nicolaides AN, Scurr JH (eds): Prevention of Venous Thromboembolism. London, Med Orion, 1994, pp 445–456.
15. Haas S, Haas P: Efficacy of low molecular weight heparins: An overview. Semin Thromb Hemost 19(Suppl 1):101–105, 1993.
16. Handeland GF, Abildgard U, Holm HA, Arnesen KE: Dose adjusted heparin in treatment of deep venous thrombosis: A comparison of unfractionated and low molecular weight heparin. Eur J Clin Pharmacol 39:107–112, 1990.
17. Harenberg J, Kuck K, Bratsch H, et al: Therapeutic application of subcutaneous low molecular weight heparin in acute venous thrombosis. Haemostasis 20:205–219, 1990.
18. Harenberg J, Roebruck P, Heene DL, and the HESIM-group: Subcutaneous low molecular mass heparin (lmm) against unfractionated (UF) heparin for prophylaxis of thromboembolism in medical patients [abstract]. Ann Hematol 68(Suppl II):51, 1994.
19. Holmer E, Kurachi K, Söderström G: The molecular-weight dependence of the rate-enhancing effect of heparin on the inhibition of thrombin, factor Xa, factor IXa, factor XIa, factor XIIa and kallikrein by antithrombin. Biochem J 193:395–400, 1981.
20. Hull RD, Raskob GE, Pineo GF, et al: Subcutaneous low-molecular weight heparin compared with continuous intravenous heparin in the treatment of proximal vein thrombosis. N Engl J Med 326:975–982, 1992.
21. Kirchmaier CM, Lindhoff-Last E, Rübesam D, et al: Regression of deep vein thrombosis by i.v. administration of a low molecular weight heparin: Results of a pilot study. Thromb Res 73:337–348, 1994.
22. Koopman MMW, Prandoni P, Piovella F, et al: Treatment of venous thrombosis with intravenous unfractionated heparin administered in the hospital as compared with subcutaneous low-molecular-weight heparin administered at home. N Engl J Med 334:682–687, 1996.
23. Lassen M, Borris L, Christiansen H, et al: Clinical trials with low molecular weight heparins in the prevention of postoperative thromboembolic complications: A meta-analysis. Semin Thromb Hemost 17(Suppl 3):284–290, 1991.
24. Lechler E, Schramm W, Flosbach CW, and the PRIME-Study-Group: A randomised, multicentre double blind study investigating the efficacy and safety of the low molecular weight heparin enoxaparin versus unfractionated heparin in the prevention of thromboembolism in immobilised medical patients [abstract]. Ann Hematol 68(Suppl II):52, 1994.
25. Leizorovicz A, Haugh M, Chapuis F, et al: Low molecular weight heparin in prevention of perioperative thrombosis. BMJ 307:913–920, 1992.

26. Leizorovicz A, Simonneau G, Decousus H, Boissel JP: Comparison of efficacy of low-molecular weight heparins and unfractionated heparin in initial treatment of deep vein thrombosis: A meta-analysis. BMJ 309:299–304, 1994.
27. Leizorovicz A: Comparison of efficacy of low-molecular weight heparins and unfractionated heparin in initial treatment of deep vein thrombosis: An updated meta-analysis. Drugs 1996.
28. Levine M, Gent M, Hirsh J, et al: A comparison of low-molecular-weight heparin administered primarily at home with unfractionated heparin administered in the hospital for proximal deep-vein thrombosis. N Engl J Med 334:677–681, 1996.
29. Lopaciuk S, Meissner AJ, Filipecki S, et al: Subcutaneous low molecular weight heparin versus subcutaneous unfractionated heparin in the treatment of deep vein thrombosis: A Polish multicenter trial. Thromb Haemostas 68:14–18, 1992.
30. Nurmohamed MT, Rosendaal FR, Büller HR, et al: Low molecular weight heparin versus standard heparin in general and orthopaedic surgery: A meta-analysis. Lancet 340:152–156, 1991.
31. Poniewierski M, Barthels M, Kuhn M, Poliwoda H: Über die Wirksamkeit niedermolekularen Heparins (Fragmin) in der Thromboembolieprophylaxe bei internistischen Patienten: Eine randomisierte Doppelblindstudie. Med Klin 83:241–245, 1988.
32. Prandoni P, Vigo N, Ruol A: Treatment of deep venous thrombosis by fixed doses of a low molecular weight heparin (CY 216). Haemostasis 20(Suppl):220–233, 1990.
33. Prandoni P, Lensing AW, Büller HR, et al: Comparison of subcutaneous low-molecular-weight heparin with intravenous standard heparin in proximal deep-vein thrombosis. Lancet 339:441–445, 1992.
34. Simonneau G, Charbonnier B, Decousus H, et al: Subcutaneous low molecular weight heparin compared with continuous intravenous unfractionated heparin in the treatment of proximal deep vein thrombosis. Arch Intern Med 153:1541–1546, 1993.
35. Siragusa S, Cosmi B, Puovella F, et al: Low-molecular-weight heparins and unfractionated heparin in the treatment of patients with acute venous thromboembolism: Results of a meta-analysis. Am J Med 100:269–277, 1966.
36. Théry C, Simonneau G, Meyer G, et al: Randomized trial of subcutaneous low-molecular-weight heparin CY 216 (Fraxiparine) compared with intravenous unfractionated heparin in the curative treatment of submassive pulmonary embolism. A dose-ranging study. Circulation 85:1380–1388, 1992.
37. Volteas SK, Kalodiki E, Nicolaides AN: Low molecular weight heparins in the initial treatment of deep vein thrombosis. Int Angiol 15:67–74, 1996.
38. Warkentin TE, Levine MN, Hirsh J, et al: Heparin-induced thrombocytopenia in patients treated with low-molecular-weight heparin or unfractionated heparin. N Engl J Med 332:1330–1335, 1995.
39. Yin ET: Effect of heparin on the neutralization of factor Xa and thrombin by the plasma alpha-II globulin inhibitor. Thromb Diathes Haemorrh 33:43–50, 1975.

CHAPTER 9

Use of Low-Molecular-Weight Heparin in Cardiac Surgery

S. MASSONNET CASTEL, M.D.
N. D'ATTELLIS, M.D.
A. CARPENTIER, M.D., Ph.D.

Low-molecular-weight heparins (LMWHs), first described 20 years ago, are obtained by depolymerization of unfractionated heparin. Substitution of LMWH for unfractionated heparin decreases the incidence of heparin-induced thrombocytopenia (HIT) and may be associated with a lower hemorrhagic risk.[1,6]

Cardiac surgery requiring cardiopulmonary bypass (CPB) necessitates a high level of anticoagulation to keep the extracorporeal circuit (ECC) free of blood clots. However, high levels of heparin often result in increased postoperative bleeding, which also may be due to the altered coagulation profile created by CPB (activation of fibrinolysis, inhibition of platelet function, and vascular dysfunction). In fact, it is well documented that unfractionated heparin is a cause of thrombocytopenia and platelet dysfunction.[10,25] The use of LMWH during cardiac surgery with CPB is thus a possible alternative to heparin for anticoagulation therapy.

LMWHs are already commonly used instead of unfractionated heparin for the postsurgical prophylaxis of thromboembolism and as a therapeutic antithrombotic drug.[5,12] LMWHs appear to interfere less with platelet function and may be associated with less bleeding than unfractionated heparin, but not at higher doses. At present, the importance and usefulness of LMWHs and their therapeutic role in the management of arterial thromboembolic diseases are well established. In addition, LMWHs can limit the proliferation of smooth muscle cells and seem to be more effective than the combination of aspirin and dipyridamole.[8] However, although LMWHs appear to be effective and safe anticoagulants during CPB, they have two major disadvantages: (1) the effective dose is difficult to define, and (2) neutralization with protamine sulfate is not very effective. Several authors, including ourselves, have demonstrated the need for neutralization of LMWHs because of increased postoperative bleeding problems.[7,13] The use of protamine to neutralize heparin after CPB can also be associated with side effects, such as anaphylactic and allergic reactions, hypotension, pulmonary hypertension, respiratory compromise, and shock.

This chapter describes a study performed at our institution to evaluate (1) the effective and safe dose of LMWH for patients undergoing CPB and (2) in vitro and in vivo neutralization of LMWH by protamine sulfate.[23] Previously our laboratory evaluated the use of LMWH during CPB in sheep.[2] The results of this study permitted us to perform a randomized, double-blind study with humans undergoing cardiac surgery with CPB.[22]

MATERIALS AND METHODS

In Vivo Study

Patient Selection and Monitoring.   Twenty-three patients undergoing elective cardiac surgery were enrolled in the study (15 women, 8 men); the mean age was 44 years (range: 15–64 years). The following procedures were performed: 12 isolated valve replacements, 5 double valve replacements, 4 coronary artery bypass grafts, and 2 repairs of congenital heart defects. The average CPB time was 95 minutes (range: 30–165 minutes).

Methods.   For safety reasons, two CPB circuits were set up for the first 4 patients. The first CPB circuit with two filters was anticoagulated with the LMWH enoxaparin; the second was anticoagulated with unfractionated heparin. Most patients participated in an autologous blood donation program; when predonation was not possible, normovolemic hemodilution was performed.

Anticoagulation Management.   All doses were calculated according to body surface area (BSA). In the first trial, for safety reasons, patients received decreasing doses of enoxaparin that ranged from 160 to 80 mg/m^2. The final dose of 80 mg/m^2 BSA/hr was based on the results of this trial. In a second trial, the total dose of enoxaparin varied from 70–80 mg/m^2 BSA/hr, with the addition of 10 mg to the CPB prime for each unit of blood. In patient 1 the drug was administered hourly, with intravenous infusion beginning immediately before CPB; in patients 2–10, one-half of the dose was administered by bolus injection, with continuous intravenous infusion of the remaining half; and in the remaining 5 patients, the entire dose was administered by continuous intravenous infusion. When postoperative bleeding was judged to be profuse, neutralization was performed with doses of protamine ranging from 50–100 mg/m^2.

Laboratory Monitoring.   LMWHs inhibit factor Xa and the generation of thrombin. Anticoagulation was monitored by multiple tests, including anti-Xa activity, anti-IIa activity, activated partial thromboplastin time (APTT), platelet count, fibrinogen level (using the Von Class chronometric method), and euglobulin lysis time. Tests were performed systematically at the following times: (1) before injection of enoxaparin, (2) every 5 minutes during CPB, (3) on completion of CPB (with complete clotting studies), and (4) every hour thereafter until the tested parameters had normalized. Protamine was administered between 20 and 120 minutes after completion of bypass if bleeding was thought to be excessive. Postoperative bleeding, defined as blood loss > 500 ml in the first hour or > 900 ml during the first 24 hours, was observed in some patients. Similar clotting studies were performed 20 minutes after the injection of protamine sulfate.

In Vitro Study

Materials
- Standard unfractionated heparin at a concentration of 5000 IU/ml (Fournier Laboratories)
- Enoxaparin (PK 10169, Bellon Pharmuka) at a concentration of 115 IU anti-Xa/mg, 28 IU anti-IIa, and 50 USP/mg
- Protamine sulfate (Choay) at a concentration of 1000 IU antiheparin/ml (1000 IU = 10 mg)
- Plasma obtained by two successive centrifugations of pooled donor blood 900 gm for 7 minutes, followed by 2500 gm for 20 minutes.

Methods.   Samples of normal human plasma were prepared with PK 10169 to obtain concentrations of 10, 20, 30, 40 and 50 mg/ml. Similar samples were prepared with unfractionated heparin at concentrations of 0.25, 0.5, 0.75, and 1 IU/ml, corresponding, respectively, to 1.5, 3, 4.5, and 6.1 mg/ml. Neutralization of samples was achieved by addition of protamine sulfate to aliquots of each sample in gravimetric ratios of 1:1, 1.5:1, and 2:1. For example, 1:1 neutralization of 10 µg of enoxaparin was obtained by addition of 10 μg of protamine. Protamine control samples were prepared by addition of the same dose of protamine to plasma without addition of PK. Each of the above samples was evaluated by titration of anti-Xa and anti-IIa activity as well as by thrombin time and APTT.

Anti-Xa activity was determined using chromogenic substrate CBS 3139 and purified factor Xa (Stago Labs). This method was adapted to the ISAMAT and GILFORD 3500 programs by automatization of the technique described by Teien.[28] Anti-IIa activity was titrated, using chromogenic substrate S 2238 with a technique adapted to the ISAMAT and GILFORD programs according to the method described by Lie Larsen.[20] Thrombin times were assessed with two reagents, Thrombozyme (Stago Labs) and human thrombin (Ortho Labs) at a concentration of 1 IU/ml to obtain a control of 22 ± 2 sec. Tests were performed manually by the classic method, combining 0.2 ml of reagent and 0.2 ml of the sample to be tested. Activated partial thromboplastin time was also assessed with two reagents, Pathromtin (Behring Labs) and Diacellin (Diamed Labs), according to the techniques advised by the manufacturer.

RESULTS

In Vivo Study

For the 23 surgical patients, the duration of CPB varied from 30 to 165 minutes, and the total dose of enoxaparin ranged from 105 to 267 mg. This wide range in total dose is related to great differences in body surface area and duration of CPB and hypothermia. No clotting was observed in the circuit in any of the patients; however, postoperative bleeding during the first 24 hours after CPB was significant. The anti-Xa and anti-IIa activity titers also varied widely at completion of bypass. In 11 patients protamine sulfate could be avoided, despite abnormal postoperative bleeding in three (Table 1). The same 3 patients also demonstrated the highest titers of anti-IIa activity and received a larger total dose of LMWH.

The 6 patients who received protamine sulfate had been given a continuous intravenous infusion of enoxaparin and had the highest antithrombin activity. In 3 patients with

TABLE 1. Patients Not Receiving Protamine

Patient	Total Dose Enoxaparin (mg)	Duration of Bypass (min)	Anti-XA Activity	Anti-IIa Activity (UI)	TT (Control: 24 sec)	APTT (Control: 35 sec)	Bleeding Time	
							First Hour	At 24 Hr
1*	150	60	2.26	0.2	> 120	85	40	310
4†	80	115	0.86	0.11	> 120	140	190	440
5†	80	45	3.14	0.33	> 120	360	200	830
8†	105	95	0.4	0.07	> 120	300	300	860
10†	120	60	0.37	0	120	270	250	520
11‡	215	105	1.3	0.9	> 120	240	300	1220
12‡	173	85	1.8	0.85	> 120	124	600	2470
13‡	167	100	1.5	0.48	> 120	150	350	1560
14‡	132	120	0.79	0.31	60	80	50	700
16‡	190	140	1.08	0.44	26	100	140	1200
17‡	115	120	1.29	0.46	120	110	150	1250

TT = thrombin time, APTT= activated partial thromboplastin time.
* Bolus injection.
† Intravenous infusion.
‡ Bolus injection + infusion.

TABLE 2. Patients Receiving Protamine

Patient	Total Dose PK10169 (mg)	Total Dose Protamine	Anti-Xa Activity Before	Anti-Xa Activity After	Anti-IIa Activity Before	Anti-IIa Activity After	APTT (Control: 35 sec) Before	APTT (Control: 35 sec) After	Bleeding (ml) Before	Bleeding (ml) After	Total at 24 hr
2*	170	135	1.6	0.9	0.49	0.05	90		540	1460	2000
3*	125	250 (150 + 100)‡	3	2.17	0.32	0	360	120	600	480	1020
9*	205	125	1.49	0.9	0.82	0.14	238	140	600	2120	2720
15†	105	150	0.8	0.75	0.4	0.25	120	70	450	150	600
6†	267	130	1.3	1.2	0.69	0	360	110	550	300	850
7†	135	150	3.8	1.82	0.9	0	240	120	0	490	490

APTT = activated partial thromboplastin time.
* Protamine given to correct bleeding.
† Protamine given systemically upon completion of bypass.
‡ Second dose of 100 mg given when no effect noted from first dose.

"abnormally profuse" bleeding, protamine was only partially effective; blood loss in the first 24 hours after surgery was > 1000 ml (patients 2, 3, and 9; Table 2). The other 3 patients received prophylactic protamine at the same dose customarily used in similar circumstances for unfractionated heparin. No abnormal bleeding was observed in these patients.

The biologic parameters investigated demonstrated a dissociation between the reversal of anti-IIa and anti-Xa activity, which paralleled the results of the in vitro study. In fact, correction of anti-Xa activity reached a maximum of only 50% (Figs. 1 and 2). Fibrinogen, platelets, and euglobulin clot lysis were no different from the usual values obtained with unfractionated heparin.

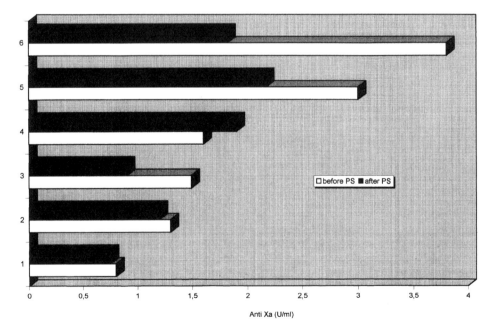

FIGURE 1.   Effect of protamine on anti-Xa in the six patients receiving protamine.

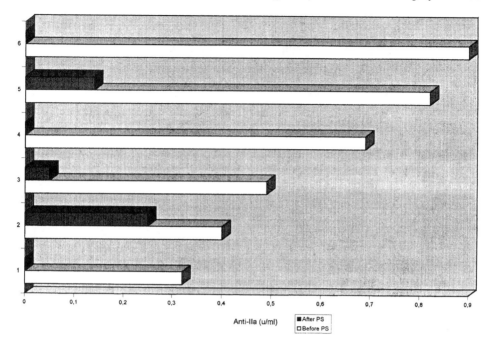

FIGURE 2. Effect of protamine on anti-IIa in the six patients receiving protamine.

In Vitro Study

Anti-Xa and anti-IIa activities expressed in international units of standard unfractionated heparin were neutralized with protamine/heparin gravimetric ratios of 1.6 and 1.3, respectively. Thrombin times were also corrected by protamine, with complete correction achieved at a ratio of 1.6. The APTT was corrected completely by a dose of protamine that was nearly double the dose of heparin. In patients receiving PK 10169, there was a clear dissociation between the neutralization of anti-Xa and anti-IIa activities. Whereas the anti-IIa activity was rapidly and completely neutralized at a protamine/PK gravimetric ratio of about 1, the anti-Xa activity was only partially (40%) inhibited at the same ratio. Even at a ratio of 2:1, anti-Xa inhibition was incomplete (60%) and remained so at even higher doses.

At such doses, protamine sulfate alone has no effect on the substrate or enzymatic activity. Despite the persistence of anti-Xa activity, thrombin time was totally corrected as soon as anti-IIa activity was reversed. However, incomplete reversal of the APTT was observed only for doses of PK > 10 μg; at this level, protamine sulfate alone prolongs APTT. Above 30 μg of protamine, only APTT was significantly prolonged.

Furthermore, considerably more LMWH than heparin is necessary to prolong APTT in the same proportions: 30 μg of PK 10169 has the same activity as 0.5 U of heparin (2.89 mg) on APTT prolongation. Finally, the anticoagulant effect of enoxaparin is reversed by protamine sulfate with approximately 2 times the dose of PK at doses ≤ 10 μg of PK. At doses above 10 μg, total neutralization is never obtained, because the effect of protamine alone at these doses is to prolong APTT.

DISCUSSION

LMWHs can be used as anticoagulants during cardiac surgery. Although few authors have described concomitant reversal of anti-IIa and anti-Xa activity for standard heparin, our in vitro results agree with reports in the literature about the unfractionated molecule.

Protamine sulfate corrects both thrombin time and APTT. This finding is logical and supports the clinical use of protamine sulfate in such circumstances.[20] However, because protamine can alter coagulation,[16] high doses should be avoided.

The apparent paradox in this study is that protamine sulfate behaves differently with respect to LMWH, as demonstrated by the dissociation between its neutralization of anti-IIa and anti-Xa activity. Although this dissociation has already been described,[24] we have found only one report during in vitro neutralization.[13]

Despite the small number of patients studied, the differences noted in vivo are in accordance with the in vitro findings. Thrombin time and anti-IIa activity were corrected under conditions comparable to those found with unfractionated heparin. However, APTT remained more prolonged than after conventional CPB with heparin; this result cannot be explained.

The different behavior of protamine with regard to heparin and enoxaparin can be related to the size of the anticoagulant molecule. Inactivation of the large unfractionated heparin molecule is probably easier than inactivation of the small enoxaparin molecule.

At this point, at least two hypotheses can be proposed: (1) protamine sulfate binds more easily to a long-chain molecule than to a short-chain molecule, and (2) LMWH may induce in vivo the appearance of protamine resistant anti-Xa and anticoagulant activity. The second theory has already been suggested by Kraemer et al. and Thomas et al. for other heparin analogs.[19,29] The difficulties that we noted in vivo with neutralization of enoxaparin seem to support the second hypothesis. Other studies have shown that heparins containing low-molecular-weight components tend to resist protamine neutralization.[26]

The relationship between anti-Xa and anti-IIa activity and blood loss is not evident. However, patients receiving a larger total dose of PK had higher anti-IIa plasma levels and more pronounced postoperative bleeding. The small number of patients studied does not allow any further conclusions; all other statements would be only speculative.

From a practical point of view, the difficulty observed with reversal of anti-Xa activity may constitute a clinical drawback to the use of LMWH. This difficulty was demonstrated by the excessive bleeding that persisted after protamine administration in two of our patients. In such circumstances, it seems necessary either to find a new antidote or to increase the dose of protamine, which in itself has disadvantages.[17] In any case, the partial reversal of LMWH activity must be considered in evaluating an otherwise appealing anticoagulant agent.[14]

Various models and multiple animal studies[18,30] have shown no difference in efficacy of anticoagulation, as measured by deposits in the CPB pumpline filter. However, blood oozing from incised surfaces (sternum and muscles at femoral cutdown sites) is much more pronounced and longer lasting with LMWH than with heparin. In these studies protamine sulfate did not reverse all of the effects of the LMWH.

Although our study demonstrates that the use of LMWH is possible during cardiac surgery requirng CPB, we recommend that its use be reserved for patients suffering from heparin allergy (HIT).[22] HIT is seen in approximately 5% of all patients receiving heparin.[15] When CPB is necessary, the use of LMWH may permit CPB without serious consequences, provided that the LMWH does not cross-react with the HIT antibody.[9,16,21] In such cases differents types of LMWH can be used: Clivarin, Fragmin, and Tedelparine.[3,4,11]

Despite the lack of serious complications, postoperative bleeding was greater with LMWH than with conventional unfractionated heparin. The antithrombotic role of LMWHs is well established, but bleeding and only partial neutralization by protamine are major drawbacks to its routine use. Furthermore, LMWHs do not decrease the severe alterations in coagulation profile produced by CPB and, consequently, do not decrease homologous blood transfusions. Thus, the advantages of LMWH are lost when one considers postoperative bleeding and the only partial neutralization by protamine.

Anticoagulation Protocol

Anticoagulation Management during CPB. Enoxaparin, 75 mg/m^2 BSA, is administred as a single intravenous bolus injection. An additional 10 mg is added to the CPB circuit with each unit of transfused blood. Aortic cannulation should be performed when the level of anti-Xa activity is > 1 IU/ml. Monitoring of anticoagulation by activated clotting time (ACT) is acceptable only if the duration of CPB is < 60 minutes; otherwise, anti-Xa activity should be controlled. When anti-Xa activity is < 1.4 IU/ml, enoxaparin should be added at a dose of 40 mg/m^2 BSA/hr. During CPB a circulating level of 1.5 IU anti-Xa activity is adequate. As for neutralization of enoxaparin, the dose of protamine is calculated as two times the dose of enoxaparin in mg.

Postoperative Management. Eight hours after CPB enoxaparin is administered as a subcutaneous injection. The dose varies according to the procedure performed:

- 1.5 mg/kg/24 hr for valve surgery
- 1 mg/kg/24 hr for coronary artery bypass surgery

The dose should be divided into two daily injections. The level of anticoagulation is assessed by monitoring anti-Xa activity; the first control should be performed 6 hours after administration. The level of anti-Xa activity required for patients who have undergone coronary artery bypass surgery is 0.4–0.5 IU. Antiplatelet therapy with aspirin is started 24 hours after surgery. This combination therapy should be continued for at least 1 week, after which low-dose aspirin (150 mg/day) is continued indefinitely for the prevention of graft occlusion. The level of anti-Xa activity required for patients who have undergone heart valve surgery is 0.6–0.8 IU. Patients are then started on oral Coumadin, and the LMWH is stopped when Coumadin takes effect.

CONCLUSION

The introduction of newer heparins has added another dimension to the medical and surgical management of thrombotic disorders. Enoxaparin can be used as an anticoagulant during CPB, and its partial neutralization by protamine has permitted its use during cardiac surgery. However, the only partial reversal of LMWH activity by protamine must be considered as a possible risk factor for increased postoperative bleeding.

LMWHs have been widely accepted in the management of various clinical situations, but their use during CPB is limited. Although standard unfractionated heparin remains the anticoagulant of choice for cardiac surgery, LMWHs offer a safe and effective alternative for cases in which unfractionated heparin cannot be used.

REFERENCES

1. Aiach M, Michaud A, Ballian JL, et al: A new molecular weight heparin derivative. In vitro and in vivo studies. Thromb Res 31:611–621, 1983.
2. Aiach M, Dreyfus G, Michaud A, et al: Low molecular weight heparin derivatives in experimental extracorporeal circulation. Haemostasis 14:325–332, 1984.
3. Altes A, Martino R, Gari M, et al: Heparin-induced thrombocytopenia and heart operation: Management with Tedelparin. Ann Thorac Surg 59:508–509, 1995.
4. Bagge L, Holmer E, Wahlberg T, et al: Fragmin vs heparin for anticoagulation during in vitro recycling of human blood in cardiopulmonary by-pass circuits : Dose dependence and mechanisms of clotting. Blood Coag Fibrinol 5:273–280, 1994.
5. Bergqvist D, Burmark US, Frisell J, et al: Prospective double-blind comparison between Fragmin and conventional low-dose heparin: Thromboprophylactic effect and bleeding complications. Haemostasis 16:11–18, 1986.
6. Cade JF, Buchanan MR, Boneu B, et al: A comparaison of the antithrombotic and haemorrhagic effects of low molecular weight heparin fractions: The influence of the method of preparation. Thromb Res 35:613–625, 1984.
7. Carter CJ, Kelton JG, Hirsh J, et al: The relationship between the haemorrhagic and antithrombotic properties of low molecular weight heparin in rabbits. Blood 59:1239–1245, 1982.
8. Edmonson RA, Cohen AT, Das SK, et al: Low-molecular weight heparin versus aspirin and dipyridamol after femoropopliteal by-pass grafting. Lancet 344:914–918, 1994.

9. Goualt-Heillmann M, Hufty Y, Contant G, et al: Cardiopulmonary by-pass with low molecular weight heparin fraction. Lancet 11:1374, 1983.

10. Green D: Heparin-induced thrombocytopenia. Med J Aust 144:HS37–HS39, 1986.

11. Heller W, Wendel HP: Clivarin and other LMWHS in an ex vivo cardiopulmonary by-pass model. Blood Coag Fibrinol 451:545–554, 1993.

12. Hirsh J: From unfractionated heparins to low molecular weight heparins. Acta Chir Scand 556:42–50, 1990.

13. Holmer E, Soderstrom G: Neutralization of unfractionated heparin and a low molecular weight (LMW) heparin fragment by protamine [abstract]. Int Thromb Haemost 50:103, 1983.

14. Kakkar VV, Murray W: Efficacy and safety of low-molecular weight heparin (CY 216) in preventing postoperative venous thromboembolism: A cooperative study. Br J Surg 72 :766–791, 1985.

15. Kalangos A, Relland J, Massonnet-Castel S, et al: Heparin-induced thrombocytopenia and thrombosis following open-heart surgery. Eur J Cardiothorac Surg 8:199–203, 1994.

16. Kitani T, Nagarajan SC, Shangerge JN: Effect of protamine on heparin-antithrombin III complexes. In vitro studies. Part 1. Thromb Res 17:367–374, 1980.

17. Kitani T, Nagarajan SC, Shangerge JN: Effect of protamine on heparin-antithrombin III complexes. In vitro studies. Part II. Thromb Res 17:375–382, 1980.

18. Koza MS, Messmore HL, Wallock ME, et al: LMWHs in an ex vivo cardiopulmonary by-pass model. Blood Coag Fibrinol 4(Suppl 1):545–554, 1993.

19. Kraemer PM: Heparin releases heparin sulfate from the cell surface. Biochem Biophysi Res Commun 78:31–840, 1977.

20. Lie Larsen M, Abilgaard U, Teien AN, Gjesdal K: Assay of plasma heparin using thrombin and the chromogenic substrate H-D-Phe-Pip-Arg-pNA (S 2238). Thromb Res 13:285, 1978.

21. Massonnet-Castel S, Fabiani JN, Couetil JP, et al: Thrombose de la veine cave inférieure et embolie pulmonaire compliquant un traitement par héparine standard utilisation d'une CEC sous enoxaparin. J Mal Vasc 12:138–140, 1987.

22. Massonnet-Castel S, Pelissier E, Dreyfus G, et al: Low molecular weight heparin in extra-corporeal circulation. Lancet 1(8387):1182–1184, 1984.

23. Massonnet -Castel S, Pelissier E, Bara L, et al: Partial reversal of low molecular weight heparin (PK 10169) anti-Xa. Activity by protamine sulfate: In vitro and in vivo study during cardiac surgery with extra corporeal circulation. Haemostasis 1:659, 1986.

24. Ockelford P, Carter CJ, Mitchell L, Hirsh J: Discordance between the anti-Xa activity and the antithrombotic activity of an ultra low molecular weight heparin fraction. Thromb Res 28:401–409, 1982.

25. Olinger GN, Hussey CU, Olive JA, Malik MJ: Cardiopulmonary by-pass for patients with previously documented heparin induced platelet aggregation. J Thorac Cardiovasc Surg 87:673–677, 1984.

26. Racanelli A, Hoppensterdt DA, Fareed J: In vitro protamine neutralization profiles of heparins differing in source and molecular weight. Semin Thromb Hemost 15:386–389, 1989.

27. Sobel M, Adelman B, Szenrpary S, et al: Surgical management of heparin-associated thrombocytopenia. J Vasc Surg 8:395–401, 1988.

28. Teien AN, Lie M, Abilgaard U: Assay of heparin in plasma using a chromogenic substrate for activated factor X. Thromb Res 8:413, 1976.

29. Thomas DP: Annotation: Heparin, low molecular weight heparin and heparin analogues. Br J Hematol 58:385–390, 1984.

30. Walenga J, Koza M, Pifarre R: Potential use of new thrombin inhibitors and low molecular weight heparins as anticoagulants in cardiopulmonary by-pass surgery. In Pifarre R (ed): Anticoagulation, Hemostasis, and Blood Preservsation in Cardiovascular Surgery. Philadelphia, Hanley & Belfus, 1993, pp 343-352.

CHAPTER 10

The Development of Hirudin as an Antithrombotic Drug

FRITZ MARKWARDT, M.D., Ph.D.

HISTORICAL BACKGROUND

The medicinal leech (*Hirudo medicinalis*) contains a substance with anticoagulant properties that the leech uses to maintain the fluidity of its victim's blood.[27] At the beginning of the 20th century anticoagulant extracts prepared from leeches were given the name hirudin. These preparations contained minute amounts of the active substance, their chemical nature was unknown, and the concepts of the anticoagulant mechanism were erroneous. Nevertheless, until the discovery of heparin, it was the only means of preventing the blood from clotting in the presence of calcium ions.

Over a century has passed since the anticoagulant properties of hirudin were identified. Attempts to isolate the anticoagulant agent and to characterize its site of action were successful after protein chemistry was developed and after the biochemistry of blood coagulation had been elucidated. In the late 1950s we succeeded in isolating the anticoagulant agent produced by the peripharyngeal glands of medicinal leeches. It was characterized as a specific tight-binding thrombin inhibitor with a polypeptide structure containing 65 amino acids and having a molecular weight of about 7000 Da.[38,39,62]

In the following years procedures of isolation and purification were developed, the amino acid analysis of hirudin was completed, and the primary structure of the thrombin inhibitor was established.[2,59,62,85] An update on hirudin was published in 1970.[41] In the 1980s the complete secondary and tertiary structure of hirudin and of a family of structurally related isoproteins, with 85% amino acid sequence homology, was described.[13,34,74]

The isolation of the pure substance and the clarification of its mode of action contributed substantially to its use in biochemical and pharmacologic investigations in hemostasis. Since that time, hirudin preparations have been used for hemostatic diagnosis and research.[40,43]

Experimental pharmacological studies showed that, because of its pronounced and specific antithrombin effect, hirudin is an antithrombotic agent of high quality. Clinicopharmacologic studies corroborated the specific pharmacodynamic and pharmacokinetic properties of hirudin found in animal experiments.[3,40,42,52,55] The historical background of hirudin isolation as well as the individual steps of its biochemical and pharmacologic characterization have been described in several reviews.[43–45]

Although the introduction of hirudin into clinical medicine represented significant progress in the prophylaxis and therapy of thrombosis, its clinical use remained limited to a few pilot studies. Because hirudin had to be isolated from medicinal leeches, it was not available in adequate amounts for therapeutic purposes.

The past decade has witnessed explosive developments in the pharmacology of hirudin, made possible by recent breakthroughs in biotechnology. Because of the simple protein nature of hirudin, it was relatively easy to clone the gene for its expression; cloning, in turn, led to the design of recombinant hirudins and to their production on a large scale.[37]

Several structural variants of native hirudin were produced by recombinant DNA technologies, including point mutations and N-terminal modifications. This process led to new insights into structure-activity relationships of the thrombin inhibitor, and the understanding of this unique and promising miniprotein has grown steadily. As a result, clinical use became possible.

Based on previous experience with native hirudin, we began a pharmacotoxicologic profile of recombinant hirudin. Extensive studies with recombinant hirudin in experimental animals confirmed not only its antithrombotic efficiency, but also its outstanding tolerance. Clinical pilot studies confirmed that hirudin is well tolerated and causes antithrombotic effects in humans.[49,51,53,56,57]

In the following years development focused on recombinant hirudin, which was responsible for the comeback of the most potent natural inhibitor of thrombin and its increasing popularity as a clinical anticoagulant. Comprehensive reviews of recombinant hirudin have been previously published.[17,46–49,84]

LABORATORY EVALUATION

Hirudin has an unusual asymmetry of structural elements, consisting of a compact, hydrophobic core region in the amino-terminal half of the molecule, which contains alternating polar and nonpolar segments and all three disulfide bonds, and a more extended and extremely hydrophilic carboxy-terminal region.

The natural and recombinant hirudins are multimeric under physiologic conditions but become monomeric when interacting with thrombin under equilibrium-binding conditions. Hirudin inactivates thrombin by forming a 1:1 stoichiometric complex, which is stable throughout the physiologic pH range. The tight and essentially irreversible binding of hirudin to thrombin is achieved by a number of ionic and hydrophobic interactions. The dissociation equilibrium constant (k_i), found to be 20 fM for the complex formed by human thrombin and natural hirudin, indicates that hirudin is to date the most potent thrombin inhibitor known (Fig. 1).

Although native hirudin and recombinant variants have the same mechanism of action, there are differences in the individual pharmacologic properties of the numerous hirudin preparations. The recombinant molecules described to date lack the sulfate group on Tyr 63 and are thus called desulfated hirudins. Their anticoagulant activity in clotting assays is as high as that of native hirudin. However, the complex of thrombin with desulfated hirudin shows a tenfold increased k_i value compared with native hirudin. Therefore, the use of recombinant hirudins requires an exact definition of the preparation, including detailed information about its structure. At present recombinant products of the structure shown in Figure 2 are available for preclinical and clinical use.

```
     ┌──────┐ ┌────────┐
VVYTDCTESGQNLCLCEGSNVCGQGNKCILGSDGEKNQCVTGEGTPKPQSHNDGDFEEIPEEYLQ
              └────────┘

(CGP 39 393, Ciba-Geigy, Switzerland)

     ┌──────┐ ┌──────┐
LTYTDCTESGQNLCLCEGSNVCGQGNKCILGSDGEKNQCVTGEGTPKPQSHNDGDFEEIPEEYLQ
              └──────┘

(HBW 023, Hoechst-Behring, Germany)
```

FIGURE 1.   Primary structure of recombinant hirudins in clinical development. Amino acids are in the single-letter code.

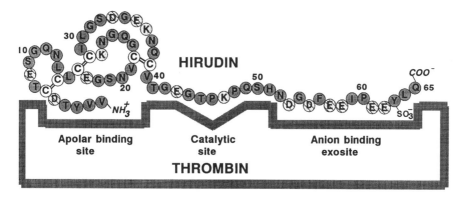

FIGURE 2. Scheme of the hirudin–thrombin interaction. The carboxyl tail of hirudin (residues 50–65) wraps around thrombin along the fibrinogen secondary binding site (anion-binding exosite) and is anchored there through ionic and hydrophobic interactions. The hydrophobic core region occupies the active site region opposite the fibrinogen-binding cleft, whereas the three N-terminal residues interact with the apolar binding site of thrombin by nonpolar contacts.

Influence on the Hemostatic System

Thrombin has a central position in the coagulation system and mediates several non-hemostatic cellular events. Therefore, in the equimolar, noncovalent thrombin–hirudin complex, all of the biologic functions of thrombin are blocked, including its effects on vascular endothelium and other cells (Fig. 3).

Hirudin prevents not only fibrinogen clotting but also other thrombin-catalyzed hemostatic reactions, such as activation of clotting factors V, VIII, and XIII and thrombin-induced platelet activation. Therefore, by instantaneous inhibition of the initially small amount of thrombin generated after activation of the coagulation system, the positive feedback triggered

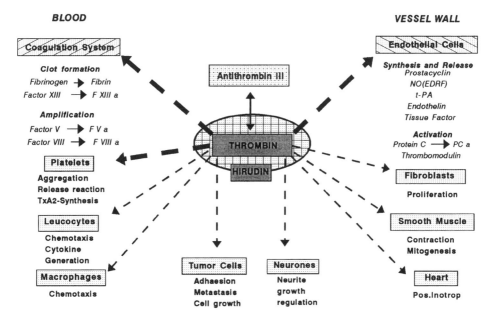

FIGURE 3.   Inhibition of haemostatic and cellular effects of thrombin by hirudin.

by prothrombin activation, which normally leads to accelerated generation of thrombin, is prevented and thrombin generation is delayed. Furthermore, thrombin complexed with hirudin does not react with plasma antithrombin III. Moreover, the thrombin-induced stabilization of platelet aggregates by fibrinogen clotting and cross-linking fibrin is inhibited by hirudin. Thus, hirudins influence the common laboratory coagulation tests, whether coagulation is induced by the intrinsic (activated partial thromboplastin time [APTT]) or extrinsic (prothrombin time [PT]) route or directly by thrombin (thrombin time [TT]). Depending on the hirudin concentration in blood, coagulation is retarded or completely inhibited.

After complexing with hirudin, thrombin loses its effect on platelets; i.e., thrombin-induced platelet release reaction and aggregation are prevented in hirudinized blood. Because the affinity of thrombin for its receptors at the platelet cell membrane is higher than for the substrate fibrinogen, it appears that higher concentrations of hirudin are necessary for the inhibition of platelet activation than for inhibition of clotting.[20,29]

The influence of hirudin on the thrombin reaction with vascular endothelium is of special interest. Hirudin inhibits the thrombin-induced synthesis and release of some mediators. The binding of thrombin to thrombomodulin may result in reduced activation of protein C.[20,33]

After complexing with hirudin, thrombin loses its cellular nonhemostatic effects, such as proliferation of fibroblasts and contraction and mitogenesis of smooth muscle and nerve cells. Hirudin inhibits the vasoconstrictor action of thrombin in deendothelialized vessels and may therefore inhibit thrombogenesis.[22,50]

Diagnostic Use

The large-scale production of hirudin by recombinant technologies provided a useful instrument for thrombin-related research. The use of hirudin as a laboratory tool helps to unravel the physiologic role of thrombin and to detect and characterize thrombin-dependent biologic and biochemical processes. Furthermore, its specific inhibition of thrombin provides a unique opportunity for development of novel thrombin-dependent test systems.

Standardization.   The calibration of the biologic activity of hirudin preparations has been a major concern. The estimation of hirudin activity is based on the essential fact that one molecule of hirudin complexes with one molecule of enzyme via a fast and specific reaction. Hence the titration of hirudin with thrombin is possible, and the potency of hirudin is expressed in antithrombin units (ATU). One ATU is the amount of hirudin that neutralizes one international unit (IU) of thrombin. One microgram of pure hirudin inhibits about 5 μg of human thrombin. Pure hirudin contains approximately 10,000–15,000 ATU/mg of protein. The findings of a collaborative study suggest that a high quality standard for alpha-thrombin may be important in the standardization of hirudin.[30,60]

The first and most simple method for quantification of hirudin was thrombin titration. Aliquots of a thrombin solution calibrated with a thrombin standard are added to a mixture of hirudin and either fibrinogen or citrated plasma. The amount of hirudin, expressed in arbitrary units, corresponds to the amount of thrombin used minus the amount required to initiate clotting. This somewhat crude assay has subsequently been modified by several groups.[41] Aminolytic assays also can be used to measure hirudin. A constant volume of standardized thrombin solution is mixed with a sample containing hirudin. After the addition of chromogenic peptide substrate, residual thrombin activity is determined spectrophotometrically. Concentration is calculated from either the residual thrombin activity or a calibration curve.[23]

Determination of Thrombin and Prothrombin.   By reversing the simple procedure of hirudin titration, thrombin concentrations can be measured by a defined quantity of standardized hirudin. The prothrombin content in blood and plasma is determined after the transformation of prothrombin into thrombin.[41] Disturbances in prothrombin activation—for example, in hemophilia—can be detected with the so-called hirudin tolerance test. By the inhibition of thrombin initially generated after activation of the coagulation system by a small amount of hirudin, the positive feedback of thrombin for prothrombin activation is prevented and the clotting time is prolonged.

Discrimination between Thrombin and Other Plasma Proteinases.   Because hirudin is highly specific in its action against thrombin, it may be used in conjunction with chromogenic substrates to discriminate between actions mediated by thrombin, its precursors, cofactors, and effectors and actions of other enzyme systems. Hirudin also is used to differentiate between thrombin and enzymes with thrombinlike effects. For example, the clotting activity of the complex of staphylocoagulase with the N-terminal fragment prothrombin and of proteases isolated from snake venoms (e.g., batroxobin) is not blocked by hirudin.

Testing Thrombin-induced Cell and Corpuscle Functions.   After complexing with hirudin, thrombin loses its cellular nonhemostatic effects. Therefore, hirudin was used in studies of thrombin-binding to membrane receptors of platelets, endothelial cells, leukocytes, fibroblasts, and malignant cells. Because of its special mechanism of action, hirudin is sometimes superior to other coagulation inhibitors in the investigation of thrombin effects on cells. Citrate, which chelates calcium, actually changes the state of the blood sample, because native calcium levels cannot be reestablished and calcium is necessary for proper platelet functions and cellular events. The use of hirudin as an anticoagulant allows cytochemical tests in the presence of calcium ions.

Hirudin has been used in a large number of experiments to clarify different problems of platelet function. Hirudin has no effect on platelet reactions caused by agents other than thrombin, such as adenosine diphosphate (ADP), collagen, arachidonic acid, and platelet-activating factor (PAF). The response of platelets to aggregating substances in hirudinized plasma differs from the response in citrated plasma, especially with regard to serotonin release and the formation of thromboxane.[20,29]

Blood Stabilization.   From 1 ml of human plasma, approximately 100–150 IU of thrombin may be generated by activation with thromboplastin. The inhibition of this amount of thrombin requires 100–150 ATU of hirudin. An uncoagulable state in human blood is reached at concentrations of more than 100 ATU or 10 µg of hirudin/ml of blood.

PRECLINICAL EVALUATION

Gene technology made it possible to provide sufficient quantities of hirudin for extensive preclinical studies. We began a pharmacologic profile of the recombinant products. These and subsequent studies by other researchers show that the pharmacodynamic and pharmacokinetic properties of recombinant hirudins are similar to those of native hirudin.

Tolerance and Pharmacokinetics

Apart from its anticoagulant effect, the hirudins are pharmacodynamically inert and well tolerated in vivo. Intravenous injection of up to 250 mg/kg in laboratory animals leads to no perceptible functional or morphologic changes and no effects on the cardiovascular system. After long-term treatment no hirudin-related histopathologic, hematologic, or biochemical changes could be found. No antibody formation was detected.[51,52]

The pharmacokinetic behavior of recombinant hirudin can be described best by an open two-compartment model with first-order kinetics. After the intravenous bolus injection of hirudins in experimental animals, values of 10–15 minutes for the distribution and 60 minutes for the elimination half-life were obtained. After subcutaneous administration, peak plasma levels were reached after 1–2 hours, and bioavailability was calculated at 70–80%. There is some absorption of hirudins after intratracheal instillation. Rectal or intraduodenal administration does not lead to detectable plasma levels. Hirudin does not seem to pass the blood-brain barrier, but there is a slight transfer through the placenta.

The hirudins are distributed into the extracellular space and are predominantly excreted in the urine. The percentage of the dose that was renally excreted in unmodified form differed in various species. In dogs hirudin was almost completely eliminated via glomeru-lar filtration, whereas in baboons the renal excretion amounted to approximately 40%, in pigs to 20%, and in rats to 10%. Anephretic animals exhibited longer duration of activity than normal animals, suggesting that the kidney is a major route of elimination. Special studies have shown that a portion of hirudin is metabolized during elimination in the kidney. The hirudin–thrombin complex, formed in small amounts after the administration of hirudin, can be eliminated by proteolytic degradation in the liver and kidney.[24]

Experimental hemodialysis demonstrates that the hirudin plasma level can be diminished to undetectable values. The elimination rate of hirudin from the circulation via dialysis depends on the pore size of the hemodialyzer membrane. For example, using a membrane with a cut-off point of 15 kD, the half-life was 6–8 hours. Using a high flux capillary hemodialyzer, the hirudin plasma level diminished within a short time.[63]

Hirudin elimination from blood can be retarded by coupling it to biomacromolecules or other high-molecular-weight carriers. For example, the application of dextran or poly-ethylene glycol-bound hirudin (PEG-hirudin) resulted in a long-lasting level.[16,58]

Antithrombotic Effects

The efficacy of hirudin in preventing venous and arterial thrombosis was demonstrated in various animal models in which the pathologic mechanism corresponded significantly with the pathologic mechanisms of thromboembolic disorders in humans. The antithrombotic effect was affirmed by prevention both of venous thrombosis in the venous stasis model, in which thrombus formation occurs in static, hypercoagulable blood, and of arterial thrombosis induced by vessel wall lesions.[53]

The action of hirudin in disseminated intravascular coagulation (DIC) has repeatedly been demonstrated in animal experiments. Diffuse activation of the clotting system was induced either by infusion of active coagulation factors or by inducing a septicemia-like syndrome with infusion of an endotoxin. When hirudin was given, the previously induced changes in the clotting system, which are typical of consumption coagulopathy and circulatory disturbances, were less pronounced, and the number of fibrin deposits in the organs investigated was significantly reduced.

The efficiency of hirudin in preventing clot formation on artificial surfaces was confirmed by experiments in which materials of varying degrees of thrombogenicity were placed in blood flowing through an extracorporeal circuit. The development of occlusive thrombi, as measured by occlusion time, was prevented. Furthermore, hirudin was successfully used for anticoagulation in experimental hemodialysis. After the administration of hirudin, no fibrin deposits were found in the dialyzer; platelet counts and fibrinogen level remained unchanged.

In light of the possible clinical indications, the effect of hirudin on arterial reocclusion after experimental thrombolysis and angioplasty was studied. The formation of occlusive arterial thrombi in the femoral and the carotid arteries was initiated by damage to the endothelium and the consequent stasis. Within a relatively short time after thrombolysis or angioplasty, a thrombotic reocclusion of the arteries occurred. In a dose-dependent manner injection of hirudin reduced the incidence of reocclusion or prolonged the time until reocclusion occurred.[32]

The experimental models show different dose-response relationships. In general, the outstanding efficacy of hirudin and its analogs became obvious in cases of thrombosis in which thrombin was initially formed by diffuse intrinsic or extrinsic activation of the coagulation pathway. Stasis-induced venous thrombosis and disseminated microthrombosis are most sensitive. Comparatively higher doses are required in arterial thrombosis and extracorporeal shunt thrombosis, in which platelets play a role. These differences may be explained by the finding that inhibition of the thrombin–platelet reaction requires higher concentrations than inhibition of the thrombin–fibrinogen reaction (Fig. 4).

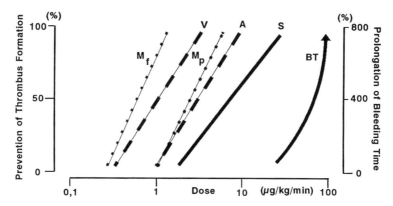

FIGURE 4. Dose-effect relationship of hirudin on experimental thrombosis and bleeding time in rats. V = venous thrombosis; A = arterial thrombosis; M_f = microthrombosis, fibrin deposits; M_p = microthrombosis, platelet aggregates; S = arteriovenous shunt thrombosis; BT = bleeding time.

Antihemostatic Effects

Because of its potent anticoagulant nature, it is not surprising that hirudin increases bleeding time. In preclinical studies, however, prolongation of bleeding time was found only with doses higher than those required for achieving the antithrombotic effect. Thus it may be assumed that in normal individuals with no hemostatic deficit the inhibitors at therapeutic levels produce no effect on bleeding. The reason may be that hirudin does not affect the ADP- and collagen-induced platelet response and does not prevent platelets from adhering to the subendothelium.

Despite the pharmacologic characteristics of hirudin, it is desirable to have a special antidote available for the instant neutralization of unexpected anticoagulant and bleeding effects, particularly when antithrombotic therapy is combined with fibrinolytic treatment or antiplatelet agents. Animal models confirmed that noncoagulant forms of thrombin—namely τ-thrombin, thrombin–α_2-macroglobulin complexes, and acylated thrombin and meizothrombin—act as hirudin antagonists in blood circulation without detectable effects on the coagulation system. But these antidotes cannot yet be used in patients because they have not yet been approved.[6,12,18] Furthermore, the thrombinlike enzyme batroxobin can act as a hemostatic agent after hirudin treatment. The fibrinogen coagulant effect of batroxobin is not inhibited by hirudin.[54]

CLINICAL EVALUATION

In light of the results of preclinical studies, we postulated that the genetically engineered hirudins have several advantages as antithrombotic agents and are very useful in the prophylaxis and therapy of thrombosis. Based on our experience with native hirudin, we began clinicopharmacologic investigations of the genetically engineered products in 1988.[56,57] These studies were completed after pharmaceutical companies had produced clinical-grade material.[10,21,36,64,71,82] Therefore, clinical trials are needed to look for special indications and appropriate dosages.[31,49]

Because of its quantifiable effects on the commonly used laboratory clotting tests, it is possible to monitor the plasma concentration of hirudin and thus to measure its pharmacokinetic behavior. For monitoring the functional anticoagulant effect of hirudin, the clot-based assays are superior to immunologic and chromogenic substrate assays because they evaluate the actual functionality of the anticoagulant. This point is important in the clinical setting, in which the anticoagulant effects of hirudin are the only parameter of value. From a practical standpoint, the routinely used partial thromboplastin time (PTT) and thrombin time (TT) assays are suitable. Because PTT is used to monitor heparin therapy, it was chosen in most comparative studies. However, the large interindividual variability of PTT and the lack of a linear dose-effect ratio limit its value for reliable monitoring of the anticoagulant effect of hirudin. Therefore, the ecarin clotting time (ECT) was evaluated under conditions that allow conclusions about the clinical reliability of hirudin.[70]

Tolerance

The aim of phase I studies performed on healthy human volunteers was to assess the tolerability of hirudin and to obtain ex vivo data about its effects on different coagulation values and pharmacokinetic parameters. In general, healthy volunteers tolerated therapeutic doses of hirudin from 0.5–1.0 mg/kg, administered subcutaneously and intravenously, with no adverse effects. No significant changes were observed in blood pressure and heart rate. Clinical chemistry tests and hematologic values remained unaffected.

Because hirudin does not interact with other blood constituents, hirudin-specific antibodies were not found in human sera after treatment with hirudin. Studies in humans have shown no immune or allergic reactions.[11,49] In one phase I study specific antibodies directed against hirudin appeared in 1 of 263 volunteers. Hirudin thus may be characterized as a weak immunogen, and the risk of allergenicity appears to be low.

Like all potent anticoagulants currently available, recombinant hirudin has the potential to cause unwanted bleeding. In healthy human volunteers no signs of bleeding tendencies have been observed at therapeutic doses. Clinical trials have shown that the risk of severe hemorrhage was strongly associated with high blood levels of hirudin. Therefore, complications can be expected, because even severe overdosage may not be detected or hirudin may be given with heparin and other antiplatelet medications. In particular, additional precautions may be required when hirudin is used with invasive procedures or fibrinolytic treatment in patients with a predisposition to abnormal bleeding.

The rapid clearance of hirudin by the kidneys provides adequate management of the hemostatic system in cases of overdosage and bleeding. When elimination is impaired—for example, in patients with renal malfunction—the circulating hirudin can be removed by methods such as hemodialysis. Dialyzers with high-flux membranes easily penetrated by hirudin should be used. Furthermore, the administration of prohemostatic agents, such as prothrombin complex concentrates, are useful in antagonizing the anticoagulant effects of hirudin. They produce antagonism by generating thrombin, which can form an inactive complex with the circulating hirudin.[11,18]

Currently the use of hirudin, particularly postoperatively, is tempered by the absence of an effective antidote, such as vitamin K and protamine sulfate for reversal of the biologic effects of coumarin and heparin, respectively. The availability of an antagonist to hirudin is essential for instant neutralization of antithrombotic action.

Pharmacokinetics

The effect of the thrombin inhibitors in vivo depends decisively on their blood level. Blood not only transports the drugs; it is also the site of their action. Investigations of the pharmacokinetics, especially of the time course of blood and plasma levels, are prerequisites for starting clinical trials.

Pharmacokinetic data about hirudin from evaluation of its blood level and urinary excretion in phase I studies have shown that hirudin is distributed into the extracellular space and eliminated with a half life of 60–100 minutes. With subcutaneous administration peak plasma levels were reached after 1–2 hours. The area-under-the-curve (AUC) values correspond to an absorption rate of 75%. Of special interest is the blood level of hirudin after repeated subcutaneous injection, which allowed the maintenance of a relatively constant level over an extended period.

A large percentage of hirudin is eliminated in active form through the kidneys by glomerular filtration.[28] The high recovery of active hirudin in urine identified renal excretion as the predominant route of clearance. In patients suffering from chronic renal malfunctions the elimination phase was prolonged. Renal clearance of hirudin was significantly and linearly correlated with creatinine clearance. In bilateral nephrectomized patients, hirudin showed an apparent half-life of approximately 10 days, indicating that it was stable in blood and not metabolized in the liver.[69] With intact renal function, a PEG–hirudin, administered subcutaneously, produces a constant blood level over a long period.[16]

Potential Indications

The introduction of hirudin into clinical medicine led to fundamental questions. Clinical trials of the efficacy of hirudins as antithrombotic agents are faced with the problem that no other specific, directly acting thrombin inhibitor is available for comparison. Therefore, a comparison of hirudin and heparin contributes to the clear characterization of hirudin before its introduction into clinical medicine. The characteristics of hirudin that are especially useful in therapy are listed in Table 1.

Compared with heparin, hirudin has the advantage of not requiring the presence of endogenous cofactors, such as antithrombin III (AT III). Furthermore, hirudins are not bound or inactivated by platelet factors or other proteins acting as antiheparin substances. Hirudin has no influence on platelet function and no direct or immune-mediated platelet-activating activity. Moreover, hirudin is able to block thrombin bound to a thrombus, where it is inaccessible to inhibition by AT III or heparin–AT III complex. Therefore, the growth of a preexistent thrombus can be prevented. In addition, the direct and specific mode of action of hirudin may result in an absence of the side effects of heparin not associated with its anticoagulant properties, such as lipolysis. These differences between hirudin and heparin led to the use of clinical situations in which qualitative or quantitative defects of heparin cofactor (AT III) or heparin-induced thrombocytopenia (HIT) present a risk.

In view of the results of pharmacologic studies, hirudin appears to be beneficial in the management of the following conditions:

- Disseminated intravascular coagulation (DIC)
- Postoperative venous thrombosis (DVT)
- Rethrombosis after thrombolysis or percutaneous transluminal coronary angioplasty (PTCA)
- Anticoagulation in hemodialysis and extracorporeal circulation.

In addition, hirudin is recommended as the drug of choice in interventional cardiology, especially in coronary artery bypass graft surgery and heart transplantation, and may be used as an adjunct drug to enhance the antithrombotic properties of thrombolytic agents. A promising field of application may be the coating of artificial devices to provide

TABLE 1.   Pharmacologic Characteristics of Recombinant Hirudins

- Potent anticoagulant that does not require any endogenous cofactors
- Pharmacodynamically inert, with only one target (thrombin)
- No effects on blood cells (platelets), plasma proteins, or enzymes
- Weak immunogen
- Extracellular distribution, dose-dependent biologic half-life
- High bioavailability after subcutaneous administration
- Stable in blood
- Renal excretion in predominant active (unchanged) form
- Minor endogenous modulation (kidney); not metabolized in the liver
- No deposition in organs
- No bleeding complications at antithrombotically active dosages
- Quality control and monitoring of therapy by measurement of thrombin time (TT) or partial thromboplastin time (PTT)

a nonthrombogenic surface in catheters, tubings, membranes, extracorporeal pumps, and hemodialysis units.

Clinical Trials

The present state of development of hirudin justifies phase II and III studies to promote its future clinical use. Further clinical studies scrutinized potential indications.

Disseminated Intravascular Coagulation.   Controlled clinical studies in comparable groups of patients are complicated by the etiologic diversity and diagnostic difficulties of DIC. Therefore, only a few pilot studies have focused on this indication.[5,75,83] Clinical reports provide the only data about a small number of patients in whom an effect could be expected after a short period of treatment, particularly patients suffering from chronic DIC. After subcutaneous injection of 0.1 mg/kg at 8-hour intervals, changes in blood indicative of consumption coagulopathy (such as a decrease in fibrinogen level and platelet counts and the appearance of fibrin monomer and plasma hemoglobulin) were prevented or reduced. The same dose resulted in normalization of the enhanced values of thrombin–antithrombin complexes, F_{1+2} cleavage products, and D-dimers, which are indicators of the activated clotting system.

Venous Thrombosis.   Hirudin may be ideally suited for the use as a postoperative prophylactic agent. Because of its ability to inhibit clot-bound thrombin, hirudin has the potential to prevent a thrombus formation at relatively low systemic anticoagulating doses. It is also possible that such doses would be effective if initiated even 2 or 3 days after the thrombogenic stimulus in patients who are at particularly high risk of bleeding.

Thrombin inhibitors have been evaluated in a small number of trials for the prevention of venous thromboembolism.[14,15,73,76] Results of an open pilot study of the curative treatment of acute venous thromboembolism showed that the prophylactic effect of hirudin at doses of 15 or 20 mg twice daily compares favorably with previous results with standard and low-molecular-weight heparin. Preliminary testing of hirudin for the prevention of deep venous thrombosis after major orthopedic surgery has been completed. In patients undergoing elective hip replacement, hirudin was administered subcutaneously twice daily, beginning immediately before surgery and continued for a mean of 11 days postoperatively. In a large study comparing ascending doses of recombinant hirudin with heparin in the prevention of DVT in patients undergoing elective hip prosthesis surgery, hirudin was highly effective in reducing both total and proximal DVT. Such data indicate that hirudin has a significant potential in the prevention of deep vein thrombosis.

Coronary Ischemic Syndromes.   The central role of thrombosis in the pathogenesis of acute myocardial infarction, unstable angina, and complications after angioplasty has led to intense interest in developing hirudin as an antithrombotic agent for the management of coronary ischemic syndromes. Similarly, as an adjunct to thrombolytic therapy in acute myocardial infarction, in treatment of unstable angina, and in support of coronary angioplasty, hirudin appeared to improve indexes of coronary reperfusion and patency. Initial results with clinical endpoints, including death and myocardial infarction, appear to favor hirudin over heparin.

Based on the results from the phase I and II trials, a number of major, multicenter phase III trials were organized, such as the Global Use of Strategies to Open Occluded Arteries (GUSTO), Hirudin for Improvement of Thrombolysis (HIT), Thrombolysis in Myocardial Infarction (TIMI), Hirudin in a European Restenosis Prevention Trial Versus Heparin Treatment in PTCA Patients (HELVETICA), Organization to Assess Strategies for Ischemic Syndromes (OASIS), and the first American Study of Infarct Survival (ASIS 1). These trials will compare the balance of risks and benefits of aspirin (ASA) and hirudin in patients with myocardial infarction who do not receive thrombolytic therapy (Table 2).[7,26]

Unstable Angina.   Several pilot studies in acute coronary ischemia demonstrate that hirudin may be more effective than heparin in the management of acute unstable

TABLE 2.   Clinical Trials with Recombinant Hirudin in Coronary Syndromes

Study	Year	(Ref)	Design	Monitoring
PTCA	1993	(4)	Dose ranging	Clinical efficacy MI
UA	1994	(80)	R, HC 4 dose groups	Angiography
TIMI-5	1994	(8,9)	R, HC Dose ranging	Reperfusion, reocclusion
TIMI-6	1995	(35)	R, HC 3 dose groups	MI, mortality, lethality
TIMI-9a	1994	(1)	R, HC	Clinical efficacy
TIMI-9b	OG		R, HC	Mortality
HIT I	1993	(67)	Dose ranging	Safety observations
HIT II	1995	(86)	Dose ranging	MI, reperfusion
HIT-III	1994	(68)	R, HC	Trial stopped Safety observations
HIT-IIIb	OG		R, HC 2 dose groups	MI
HIT-IV	OG		R, HC	Mortality and reinfarction
HIT-SK	1996	(65)	R, HC Dose ranging	Patency rates
HELVETICA	1994 1995	(77) (78, 79)	R, HC	Early complications Restenosis
GUSTO-2a	1994	(26)	R, HC	MI, mortality
GUSTO-2b	OG		R, HC	Mortality and reinfarction
OASIS	1996	(19)	R, HC, ASA	UA, MI, mortality
ASIS 1	1995	(72)	R, HC, ASA Comparison	MI, mortality

OG = ongoing; R = randomized; HC = heparin control; ASA = acetylsalicylic acid; MI = myocardial infarction; UA = unstable angina; PTCA = percutaneous transluminal coronary angiography.

angina. The results from phase II clinical trials are encouraging. Patients treated with hirudin consistently showed greater improvement than patients treated with heparin in angiographic parameters.[7]

In a double-blind, randomized, large-scale trial, patients with recent-onset angina, worsening angina, or angina at rest began treatment before PTCA with heparin or hirudin. Quantitative coronary angiography was performed immediately before and after PTCA and again 6 months later. The incidence of early major adverse cardiac events was significantly reduced by the regimen that incorporated subcutaneous hirudin for three days.[4,23,82]

The efficacy data indicate that the hirudin has great potential, particularly in the initial management of patients with acute unstable angina and non-Q-wave infarction. It was concluded that hirudin suppresses thrombus growth within coronary arteries, thus enhancing endogenous thrombolysis. However, there is much to learn about the mechanism of action, optimal dose, and optimal concomitant therapy in the management of acute coronary ischemia. Dose-finding studies should be performed to determine safe regimens of hirudins for large-scale trials with important clinical outcomes.[18,80,88]

Myocardial Infarction.   The value of hirudin as adjunct therapy to thrombolytic agents in acute myocardial infarction has been assessed in major trials. The aim is to inhibit clot-bound thrombin and thrombin that may be released from the fibrin network of a thrombus during thrombolysis. Release of enzymatically active thrombin is assumed to account for the early reocclusion of coronary vessels after primary successful thrombolysis.[1,8,9,25,35,65,68,72]

In studies of the improvement of thrombolysis, escalating doses of hirudin were used. Hirudin was given simultaneously with tissue-type plasminogen activator (tPA) or streptokinase in an accelerated dosage regimen. Patency seemed to be improved by doses of 0.15 mg/kg each hour, with a decreased incidence of reocclusion and a lower incidence of in-hospital death and reinfarction compared with heparin. Hirudin has also been associated with a stable level of anticoagulation and an acceptable hemorrhagic complication rate when given in carefully chosen doses.

The phase II Hirudin for the Improvement of Thrombolysis (HIT III) study compared recombinant hirudin with heparin in a randomized, double-blind trial in patients with acute myocardial infarction. Death or reinfarction was the primary endpoint. The trial was stopped after an increased rate of intra- and non-intracranial bleeding was observed in hirudin-treated groups.

Recent clinical reports suggest that there is a narrower window of safety with recombinant hirudin than initially thought, particularly when it is used in conjunction with thrombolytic agents and aspirin in patients with acute myocardial infarction. In view of the observation that infusion of hirudin at a dose of 0.1 mg/kg/h appears to be as effective as higher doses in both unstable angina and myocardial infarction, reformulated trials (TIMI 9 and GUSTO II) using lower doses of hirudin have now started and should allow testing of whether the initial favorable results observed in pilot trials will translate into improved clinical outcome, with an acceptable safety profile, for patients with acute myocardial infarction or unstable angina or patients undergoing angioplasty.

Coronary Angioplasty.   Occluding thrombi in arteries, particularly in coronary vessels, may develop from previously existing arteriosclerotic stenosis that persists after intravascular lysis or angioplasty and thus predisposes the vessels to rethrombosis. Hirudin is more effective than heparin in inhibiting thrombin bound on subendothelial extracellular matrix. Thus hirudin is expected to be more effective than heparin in preventing thrombotic coronary reocclusion after PTCA.

The merits of hirudin, relative to heparin, were evaluated in clinical trials in patients undergoing elective balloon coronary angioplasty.[4,73,78,79,86,87] A pilot trial of hirudin during coronary angioplasty has shown that hirudin has a more favorable anticoagulant profile than heparin. The administration of hirudin reduced thrombotic complications after PTCA and resulted in complete perfusion with fewer acute cardiac complications than heparin. Periprocedural complications (myocardial infarction and emergency bypass procedures) were observed in only 1.4% of hirudin-treated patients compared with 4% of heparin-treated patients. Overall, patients treated with hirudin tended to show a greater improvement than patients receiving heparin in terms of primary efficacy variable (average cross-sectional area) as well as minimal cross-sectional area, minimal luminal diameter, and percentage of diameter stenosis.

Heparin-induced Thrombocytopenia.   Thrombocytopenia is a common adverse effect of heparin therapy. Heparin can induce antibodies that interact with platelets and endothelial cells, thus causing thrombocytopenia and thromboembolic complications. Patients with heparin-induced thrombocytopenia (HIT) need effective parenteral anticoagulation. Therefore, it is important to determine whether hirudin is a successful anticoagulant in patients with heparin-induced allergy.[66] Furthermore, it may be demonstrated that regular use of hirudin as an anticoagulant, along with dialyzers impermeable to hirudin, provides good results in hemodialysis treatment of HIT.

Hemodialysis.   The renal excretion of hirudin is of special importance, particularly in connection with its clinical use in hemodialysis. Therefore, clinical studies were designed to determine the blood level course after impaired renal function. The AUC-levels of hirudin, which represent the portion of the administered dose remaining in the organism, are higher in patients with nephropathy than in healthy volunteers. Correspondingly, the elimination half-lives of hirudin are many times longer in such patients, and the administration of hirudin requires individually adjusted dosages. Furthermore, the elimination of hirudin from the circulation via dialysis depends on the pore size of the hemodialyzer membrane. In case of overdoses, dialyzers with high-flux membranes that may easily be penetrated by hirudin should be used.[69,81]

CONCLUSION

The progress in molecular biology and biotechnology has stimulated growing interest in hirudin, the most potent known natural inhibitor of thrombin. This development led to the design of recombinant forms and analogs of the miniprotein and to an understanding of its structure and function.

The biologic properties of hirudin combined with its ready availability make it well suited for use as an anticoagulant agent. The pharmacologic profile showed that, as a specific thrombin inhibitor, hirudin is an antithrombotic drug of high quality and allows a new approach to prophylaxis and treatment of thromboembolic diseases of both arterial and venous origin.

Information about the clinical efficacy of hirudin, obtained from phase II and III studies, favors the introduction of recombinant hirudin into clinical medicine. Its use should lead to a decisive progress in the therapy of thrombosis, especially in diseases in which thrombin plays a crucial role.

REFERENCES

1. Antman EM for the TIMI 9A investigators: Hirudin in acute myocardial infarction. Safety report from the Thrombolysis and Thrombin Inhibition in Myocardial Infarction (TIMI) 9A trial. Circulation 90:1624–1630, 1994.
2. Bagdy D, Barabas E, Graf L, et al: Hirudin. In Lorand L (ed): Methods in Enzymology, Vol. 45: Proteolytic Enzymes. New York, Academic Press, 1976, pp 669–678.
3. Bichler J, Fichtl B, Siebeck M, Fritz H: Pharmacokinetics and pharmacodynamics of hirudin in man after single subcutaneous and intravenous bolus administration. Arzneimittelforschung 38:704–710, 1988.
4. Bos van den AA, Deckers JW, Heyndrickx GR, et al: Safety and efficacy of recombinant hirudin (CGP 39 393) versus heparin in patients with stable angina undergoing coronary angioplasty. Circulation 88:2058–2066, 1993.
5. Breddin HK, Markwardt F: Clinical experience with hirudin in disseminated intravascular coagulation. Thromb Haemost 69:1299, 1903.
6. Brüggener E, Walsmann P, Markwardt F: Neutralization of hirudin anticoagulant action by DIP-thrombin. Pharmazie 44:648–649, 1989.
7. Cannon CP, Braunwald E: Hirudin: Initial results in acute myocardial infarction, unstable angina and angioplasty. J Am Coll Cardiol 25(Suppl 7):30–37, 1995.
8. Cannon CP, McCabe CH, Henry TD, et al: Hirudin reduces reocclusion compared to heparin following thrombolysis in acute myocardial infarction: Results of the TIMI 5 trial [abstract]. J Am Coll Cardiol 21:136A, 1993.
9. Cannon CP, McCabe CH, Henry TD, et al, for the TIMI 5 investigators: A pilot trial of recombinant desulfatohirudin compared with heparin in conjunction with tissue-type plasminogen activator and aspirin for acute myocardial infarction: Results of the Thrombolysis in Myocardial Infarction (TIMI) trial. J Am Coll Cardiol 23:993–1003, 1994.
10. Cardot JM, Lefevre GY, Godbillon JA: Pharmacokinetics of rec-hirudin in healthy volunteers after intravenous administration. J Pharmacokinet Biopharm 22:147–156, 1994.
11. Close P, Bichler J, Kerry R, et al, on behalf of the European Hirudin in Thrombosis group (HIT group): Weak allergenicity of recombinant hirudin CGP 39393 in immunocompetent volunteers. Coron Art Dis 5:943–949, 1994.
12. Diehl KH, Römisch J, Hein B, et al: Investigation of activated prothrombin complex concentrate as potential hirudin antidote in animal models. Haemostasis 25:182–192, 1995.
13. Dodt J, Müller HP, Seemüller U, Chang JY: The complete amino acid sequence of hirudin, a thrombin specific inhibitor. FEBS Lett 165:180–183, 1984.
14. Eriksson BI, Kälebo P, Ekman S, et al: Direct thrombin inhibition with rec-hirudin (CGP 39393) as prophylaxis of thromboembolic complications after total hip replacement. Thromb Haemost 72:227–231, 1994.
15. Eriksson BI, Kälebo P, Ekman S, et al: Effective prevention of thromboembolic complications after total hip replacement with three different doses of recombinant hirudin, CGP 39393 (Revasc), Ciba, compared to unfractionated heparin. Circulation 90:386–388, 1994.

16. Esslinger HU, Dübbers K, Müller-Peltzer H: First data on safety and anticoagulant activity after single i.v. and s.c. PEG-hirudin administration in healthy volunteers. Thromb Haemost 73:2109, 1995.

17. Fareed J, Walenga JM, Hoppensteadt D, Pifarre R: Developmental perspectives for recombinant hirudin as an antithrombotic agent. Biol Clin Hematol 11:143–152, 1989.

18. Fareed J, Walenga JM, Hoppenstaedt D, et al: Neutralization of recombinant hirudin. Some practical considerations. Semin Thromb Hemost 17:137–144, 1991.

19. Flather M for the Organisation to Assess Strategies for Ischemic Syndromes (OASIS): Recombinant hirudin in the treatment of patients with unstable angina pectoris: Preliminary results of the OASIS pilot study. Ann Hematol 72(Suppl 1):A91, 1996.

20. Glusa E, Markwardt F: Platelet functions in recombinant hirudin-anticoagulated blood. Hemostasis 20:112–118, 1990.

21. Glusa E, Schenk J, Breddin K, et al: Studies in human pharmacology of recombinant hirudin. Thromb Res 65:118, 1992.

22. Glusa E, Markwardt F: Studies on thrombin-induced endothelium-dependent vascular effects. Biomed Biochim Acta 47:623–630, 1988.

23. Griesbach U, Stürzebecher J, Markwardt F: Assay of hirudin in plasma using a chromogenic thrombin substrate. Thromb Res 37:347–350, 1985.

24. Grötsch H, Hropot M, Bergscheid G, et al: Pharmacokinetic investigation of the α-human thrombin-hirudin complex in Rhesus monkeys. Thromb Res 66:271–275, 1992.

25. GUSTO Investigators: An international randomised trial comparing four thrombolytic strategies for acute myocardial infarction. N Engl J Med 329:673–682, 1993.

26. GUSTO IIa Investigators (Global Use of Strategies to Open Occluded Coronary Arteries): Randomised trial of intravenous heparin versus recombinant hirudin for acute coronary syndromes. Circulation 90:1631–1637, 1994.

27. Haycraft JB: On the action of secretion obtained from the medicinal leech on the coagulation of the blood. Proc R Soc Lond 36:478–487, 1884.

28. Henschen A, Markwardt F, Walsmann P: Identification by HPLC analysis of the unaltered forms of hirudin and desulfated hirudin after kidney passage [abstract]. Thromb Res 7(Suppl):37, 1987.

29. Hoffmann A, Markwardt F: Inhibition of thrombin platelet reaction by hirudin. Haemostasis 14:164–169, 1984.

30. Iyer L, Fareed J: Determination of specific activity of recombinant hirudin using a thrombin titration method. Thromb Res 78:259–263, 1995.

31. Johnson PH: Hirudin: Clinical potential of a thrombin inhibitor. Annu Rev Med 45:165–177, 1994.

32. Kaiser B, Simon A, Markwardt F: Antithrombotic effects of recombinant hirudin in experimental angioplasty and intravascular thrombolysis. Thromb Haemost 63:44–47, 1990.

33. Klöcking HP, Hoffman A, Markwardt F: Influence of hirudin on the thrombin-induced release of tissue plasminogen activator from isolated perfused pig ear. Folia Haematol 115:110–120, 1988.

34. Konno S, Fenton II JW, Villaneuva GB: Analysis of the secondary structure of hirudin and the mechanism of its interaction with thrombin. Arch Biochem Biophys 267:158–166, 1988.

35. Lee LV, McCabe CH, Antman EM, et al, for the TIMI 6 investigators: Initial experience with hirudin and streptokinase in acute myocardial infarction: Results of the thrombolysis in myocardial infarction (TIMI) 6 trial. J Am Coll Cardiol 75:7–13, 1995.

36. Marbet GA, Verstraete M, Kienast J, et al: Clinical pharmacology of intravenously administered recombinant hirudin (CGP) in healthy volunteers. J Cardiovasc Pharmacol 22:2015–2032, 1993.

37. Märki WE, Grossenbacher H, Grütter MG, et al: Recombinant hirudin: Genetic engineering and structure analysis. Semin Thromb Hemost 17:88–93, 1991.

38. Markwardt F: Untersuchungen über den Mechanismus der blut-gerinnungshemmenden Wirkung des Hirudins. Naunyn Schmiedeberg's Arch Exp Pathol Pharmacol 229:389–399, 1956.

39. Markwardt F: Die Isolierung und chemische Charakterisierung des Hirudins. Hoppe Seylers Z Physiol Chem 308:147–156, 1957.

40. Markwardt F: Versuche zur pharmakologischen Charakterisierung des Hirudins. Naunyn Schmiedeberg's Arch Exp Pathol Pharmacol 234:516–529, 1958.

41. Markwardt F: Hirudin as an inhibitor of thrombin. In Colowick SP, Kaplan NO (eds) Methods in Enzymology, vol. 9: Proteolytic Enzymes. New York, Academic Press, 1970, pp 924–932.

42. Markwardt F: Pharmacology of hirudin: One hundred years after the first report of the anticoagulant agent. Biomed Biochim Acta 44:1007–1013, 1985.

43. Markwardt F: Biochemistry and pharmacology of hirudin. In Pirkle H, Markland FS Jr (eds): Hemostasis and Animal Venoms. New York, Dekker, 1988, pp 255–269.

44. Markwardt F: The comeback of hirudin—an old-established anticoagulant agent. Folia Haematol 115:10–23, 1988.

45. Markwardt F: Development of hirudin as an antithrombotic agent. Semin Thromb Hemost 15:269–282, 1989.

46. Markwardt F: Past, present and future of hirudin. Haemostasis 21(Suppl 1):11–26, 1991.

47. Markwardt F: Hirudin and derivatives as anticoagulant agents. Thromb Haemost 66:141–152, 1991.

48. Markwardt F: Hirudin: The promising antithrombotic. Cardiovascular Drug Reviews 10:211–232, 1992.
49. Markwardt F: The development of hirudin as an antithrombotic drug. Thromb Res 74:1–23, 1994.
50. Markwardt F Jr, Franke T, Glusa E, Nilius B: Pharmacological modification of mechanical and electrical responses of frog heart to thrombin. Naunyn-Schmiedebergs Arch Pharmacol 341:341–346, 1990.
51. Markwardt F, Fink E, Kaiser B, et al: Pharmacological survey of recombinant hirudin. Pharmazie 43:202–207, 1988.
52. Markwardt F, Hauptmann J, Nowak G, et al: Pharmacological studies on the antithrombotic action of hirudin in experimental animals. Thromb Haemost 47:226–229, 1982.
53. Markwardt F, Kaiser B, Nowak G: Studies on antithrombotic effects of recombinant hirudin. Thromb Res 54:377–388, 1989.
54. Markwardt F, Kaiser B, Richter M: Haemostypic effects of batroxobin with regard to hirudin treatment. Thromb Res 68:475–482, 1992.
55. Markwardt F, Nowak G, Stürzebecher J, et al: Pharmacokinetics and anticoagulant effect of hirudin in man. Thromb Haemost 52:160–163, 1984.
56. Markwardt F, Nowak G, Stürzebecher J, et al: Clinico-pharmacological studies with recombinant hirudin. Thromb Res 52:393–400, 1988.
57. Markwardt F, Nowak G, Stürzebecher J: Clinical pharmacology of recombinant hirudin. Haemostasis 21(Suppl 1):133–136, 1991.
58. Markwardt F, Richter M, Walsmann P, et al: Preparation of dextran-bound recombinant hirudin and its pharmacokinetic behaviour. Biomed Biochim Acta 49:1103–1108, 1990.
59. Markwardt F, Schäfer G, Töpfer H, Walsmann P: Die Isolierung des Hirudins aus medizinischen Blutegeln. Pharmazie 22:239–241, 1967.
60. Markwardt F, Stürzebecher J, Walsmann P: The hirudin standard. Thromb Res 59:395–400, 1990.
61. Markwardt F, Walsmann P: Die Reaktion zwischen Hirudin und Thrombin. Hoppe Seylers Z Physiol Chem 312:85–98, 1958.
62. Markwardt F, Walsmann P: Reindarstellung und Analyse des Thrombin-Inhibitors Hirudin. Hoppe Seylers Z Physiol Chem 348:1381–1386, 1967.
63. Markwardt F, Nowak G, Bucha E: Hirudin as anticoagulant in experimental haemodialysis. Haemostasis 21(Suppl 1):149–155, 1991.
64. Meyer BH, Luus HG, Müller FO, et al: The pharmacology of recombinant hirudin, a new anticoagulant. South Afr Med J 78:268–270, 1990.
65. Molhock GP, Laarman GJ, Lok DJA, et al: Effects of recombinant hirudin on early, complete and sustained coronary patency in patients with acute myocardial infarction treated with streptokinase (final results on the HIT-SK study). Ann Hematol 72(Suppl 1):A91, 1996.
66. Nand S: Hirudin therapy for heparin-associated thrombocytopenia and deep venous thrombosis. Am J Hematol 43:310–311, 1993.
67. Neuhaus KL, von Essen R, Niederer W, et al: r-Hirudin and front-loaded alteplase in acute myocardial infarction: results of the HIT (hirudin for Improvement of Thrombolysis) study [abstract]. Eur Heart 14(Suppl):106, 1993.
68. Neuhaus KL, von Essen R, Tebbe U, et al: Safety observations from the pilot phase of the randomised r-hirudin for improvement of thrombolysis (HIT III) study. Circulation 90:1638–1642, 1994.
69. Nowak G, Bucha E, Göock T, et al: Pharmacology of r-hirudin in renal impairment. Thromb Res 66:707–715, 1992.
70. Nowak G, Bucha E: A new method for therapeutical monitoring of hirudin. Thromb Haemost 69:1306, 1993.
71. Nurmohamed MT, Knipscheer HC, Buller HR, Cate JW: Ten: An open study to investigate the biological efficacy of repeated subcutaneous applications of r-hirudin (CGP 39393) in healthy volunteers. Thromb Haemost 65:640, 1991.
72. O'Donnell CJ, Ridker PM, Hebert PR, Hennekens CH: Antithrombotic therapy for acute myocardial infarction. J Am Coll Cardiol 26(Suppl 7):23–29, 1995.
73. Parent F, Bridey F, Dreyfus M, et al: Treatment of severe venous thrombo-embolism with intravenous hirudin (HBW 023): An open pilot study. Thromb Haemostas 70:386–388, 1993.
74. Rydel TJ, Tulinsky A, Bode W, Huber R: Refined structure of the hirudin-thrombin complex. J Mol Biol 20:583–601, 1991.
75. Saito M, Asakura H, Jokaji H, et al: Recombinant hirudin for the treatment of disseminated intravascular coagulation in patients with haematological malignancy. Blood Coag Fibrinolysis 6:60–64, 1995.
76. Schiele F, Vuillemenot A, Kramarz P, et al: A pilot study of subcutaneous recombinant hirudin (HBW 023) in the treatment of deep vein thrombosis. Thromb Haemost 71:558–562, 1994.
77. Serruys PW, Deckers JW, Close P, on behalf of the HELVETICA study group: A double-blind, randomised heparin controlled trial evaluating acute and longterm efficacy of r-hirudin (CGP 39393) in patients undergoing coronary angioplasty. Circulation 90:1624–1630, 1994.
78. Serruys PW, Fox KA, Herman JPR, et al, HELVETICA investigators: Recombinant hirudin (CGP 39393) reduces the incidence of major adverse cardiac events, reported within the first 96 hours post angioplasty in unstable patients (Braunwald classification) pretreated by heparin [abstract]. J Am Coll Cardiol 23:90A, 1995.

79. Serruys PW, Herman JP, Simon R, et al: A comparison of hirudin with heparin in the prevention of restenosis after coronary angioplasty, HELVETICA investigators. N Engl J Med 333:757–763, 1995.

80. Topol EJ, Fuster V, Harrington RA, et al: Recombinant hirudin for unstable angina pectoris: A multicentre, randomized angiographic trial. Circulation 89:1557–1566, 1994.

81. Vanholder RC, Camez AA, Veis MM, et al: Recombinant hirudin: A specific thrombin inhibiting anticoagulant for hemodialysis. Kidney Int 45:1754–1759, 1994.

82. Verstraete M, Nurmohamed M, Kienast J, et al, on behalf of the European Hirudin in Thrombosis group: Biologic effects of recombinant hirudin (CGP 39393) in human volunteers. J Am Coll Cardiol 22:1080–1088, 1993.

83. Vogel G, Markwardt F: Preliminary clinical reports on the antithrombotic action of hirudin. Thromb Res 7(Suppl):42, 1987.

84. Walenga JM, Piffare R, Fareed J: Recombinant hirudin as antithrombotic agent. Drugs Future 15:267–280, 1990.

85. Walsmann P, Markwardt F: On the isolation of the thrombin inhibitor hirudin. Thromb Res 40:563–570, 1985.

86. Zeymer U, von Essen R, Tebbe U, et al: Recombinant hirudin and front-loaded alteplase in acute myocardial infarction. Results of a pilot study: HIT I (Hirudin for the Improvement of Thrombolysis). Eur Heart J 16(Suppl D):22–27, 1995.

87. Zeymer U, von Essen R, Tebbe U, et al: Frequency of "optimal anticoagulation" for acute myocardial infarction after thrombolysis with front loaded recombinant tissue type plasminogen activator and consecutive therapy with recombinant hirudin (HBV 023). J Am Cardiol 76:997–1001, 1995.

88. Zoldhely P, Webster MWI, Furster V, et al: Recombinant hirudin in patients with chronic, stable coronary artery disease: Safety, half-life, and effect on coagulation parameters. Circulation 88:2015–2021, 1993.

CHAPTER 11

Pharmacologic Considerations in the Development of Hirudin and Its Derivatives for Cardiovascular Indications

VOLKER ESCHENFELDER, M.D., Ph.D.

Thrombotic and thromboembolic occlusions of diseased vessels lead to both acute life-threatening complications and chronic cardiovascular disability.[23,29,56,71] Knowledge of the molecular mechanisms involved in the thrombogenic process that play a key role in the pathophysiology of thrombotic and vascular disorders has aided in the discovery and development of potent and selective therapeutic strategies.[17,30,44,75] Although the past decade has witnessed remarkable progress in the diagnosis and clinical management of cardiovascular disease, it remains an important cause of morbidity and mortality.[23,29] Thus, treatment and prevention of thromboembolic disorders and their sequelae are important health priorities. Although heparin remained the surgical anticoagulant of choice, its use involves certain problems (Table 1). Because of the necessity of neutralizing the anticoagulant actions of heparin and its adverse hemodynamic effects, an alternative anticoagulant is needed. In addition, heparin-induced thrombocytopenia is a serious adverse event, leading to white clot syndrome.

Thrombin plays a pivotal role in the intricate balance between hemostasis and thrombosis.[13,21,48,57] It is a trypsinlike serum protease with multiple actions on the hemostatic system. Its generation is the final result of activation of both intrinsic and extrinsic coagulation pathways. Both free and clot-bound thrombin proteolytically cleave fibrinogen and activate factor XIII, thus allowing stabilization and propagation of the hemostatic plug. Furthermore, thrombin amplifies its own production in a positive feedback loop by activating coagulation factors V and VIII.

Under physiologic conditions the procoagulant and prothrombotic actions of thrombin are controlled by two counterregulatory mechanisms. First, antithrombin III (AT III) binds to and inactivates circulating free thrombin. Second, in combination with the cell surface protein thrombomodulin, thrombin loses its clotting action; protein C is transformed into protein Ca, which in turn complexes with plasma factor protein S to inactivate factors Va and VIIa, thus locally down-regulating the generation of thrombin.[4,21]

This balance between pro- and anticoagulant mechanisms controls the local generation of thrombin, preventing it from becoming a pathophysiologic, clinically relevant

TABLE 1.   Limitations of Heparin

• Unpredictable dose response	• Cofactor (antithrombin-III) dependent
• Need for close laboratory monitoring	• Major bleeding effects
• Limited activity against clot-bound thrombin	• Allergic reactions
• Multiple inhibitory sites	• Narrow benefit/risk ratio

process. Besides its involvement in coagulation, thrombin acts on many different cells. Agents that control the action or generation of this enzyme, therefore, have gained considerable attention.

LIMITATIONS OF CURRENT ANTITHROMBOTICS

Currently, unfractionated heparin is used for a wide range of thrombotic disorders, including acute coronary syndromes.[32] It is the only anticoagulant that can be used for cardiovascular surgical procedure at present.

The antithrombotic action of heparin depends essentially on the presence of endogenous coagulation inhibitor factors, AT III and heparin cofactor II (HCII).[61] Because of their heterogeneous mixture, not all heparin molecules have the capacity to potentiate the action of antithrombin. Only one-third of the chains constituting the heparin molecules possess a pentasaccharide sequence, which is required to bind to AT III. Furthermore, to inhibit thrombin, the pentasaccharide moiety must exist in a chain of at least octa/decasaccharide units. The HCII-mediated inactivation of thrombin requires higher concentrations of heparin. In addition to the ill-defined structure of heparin and its indirect efficacy, which depends on cofactors, several other limitations may decrease its therapeutic value. Heparin can be inactivated by heparinase and platelet factor IV, both of which are released by activated platelets.[46] Heparin also interacts with platelets, especially the higher-weight moieties, leading to impairment of platelet aggregation. This effect is assumed to induce bleeding complications. Binding to vitronectin, fibronectin, and other plasma proteins limits the amount of heparin available and decreases its anticoagulant effect. Some of these plasma proteins are acute-phase reactants and may significantly influence bioavailability and resistance in patients with acute illness or acute thrombosis. The clearance of heparin is nonlinear and dose-dependent, resulting in unpredictive variations in bioavailability that may lead to under- or overdosing of patients, regardless of extensive monitoring.

Most important, however, is the inability of the heparin–AT III complex to inactivate thrombin already bound to clots. The protected status of clot-bound thrombin is the major drawback to heparin use, because clot-bound thrombin can act as an ongoing source of thrombogenesis at sites of pathologic thrombus formation. This limitation of standard heparin therapy probably underlies many clinical failures, such as reocclusion after coronary thrombolysis or the so-called rebound phenomenon after discontinuation of heparin therapy in patients with unstable angina.

Because of the substantial limitations of available therapy, there is a significant need for improvement in antithrombotic agents for the prophylaxis and treatment of thrombotic disorders. Understanding the mechanisms through which thrombin mediates its various activities and the structural requirements for these actions provided the basis for strategies to modulate thrombin's action. The goal of many current antithrombotic strategies is to block thrombin activity or to prevent its generation.

DIRECT THROMBIN INHIBITORS

One possibility of controlling the thrombogenic effects of thrombin is to interact directly with the enzyme, thereby preventing its interaction with its substrates in an AT III- and HCII-independent fashion. Several synthetic and recombinant inhibitors of thrombin are currently the target of developing an alternate to heparin. The family of directly acting

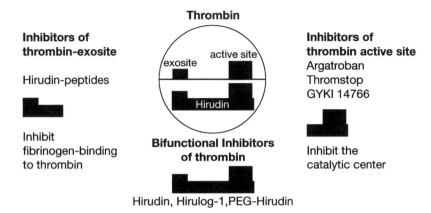

FIGURE 1.   Thrombin inhibitors and receptor-antagonists.

thrombin inhibitors include (1) natural and recombinant hirudins,[2,31,51] (2) the synthetic hirudin fragments hirugen and hirulog,[49,50,57] (3) a chemically modified polyethylene glycol-coupled recombinant hirudin (PEG-hirudin),[18,20,41,62] (4) low-molecular-weight inhibitors that bind to the active site of thrombin,[37,58,69] and (5) the recently described aptamers (Fig. 1).[45,47] Although all of these inhibitors bind directly to thrombin, their sites of interaction are different.

Hirudin is the most potent direct thrombin inhibitor. Figure 2 compares natural hirudin and its recombinant variant, rHV2-lys 47. The amino terminus of hirudin interacts with the apolar binding site of thrombin, whereas the carboxy terminus, which is highly acidic, interacts with the binding exosite for fibrinogen recognition.[68] Because hirudin recognizes two different exosites on thrombin rather than its catalytic site, it is a highly specific inhibitor of thrombin.[36,68]

Based on knowledge of the interaction of hirudin with thrombin and x-ray diffraction of the structure of the carboxy terminus of hirudin, a series of C-terminal peptide fragments of hirudin has been synthesized.[49] Hirugen, the first of these fragments, is a dodecapeptide

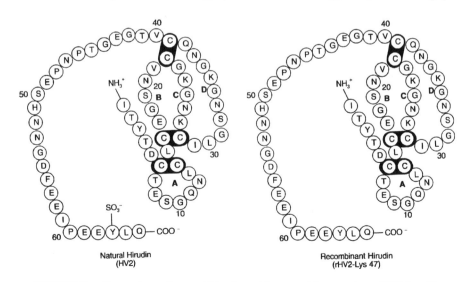

FIGURE 2.   Comparison of natural hirudin and its recombinant variant, rHV2-lys 47.

consisting of residues 53 to 64.[49] Hirugen blocks the anion-binding exosite of thrombin, thereby preventing access to fibrinogen, platelets, and other physiologic substrates; fibrinogen cleavage; and subsequent fibrin clot formation.[52] The active site of thrombin remains unaffected by hirudin, leading to thrombin-mediated hydrolysis of low-molecular-weight substrates.

Coupling of hirugenlike compounds to peptides that are specific for inhibition of the catalytic site of thrombin (D-Phe-Pro-Arg) converted hirugen from a weak competitive inhibitor of thrombin to a specific bivalent inhibitor of thrombin termed hirulog.[38,50,72,76] Like hirudin, the chimeric molecule hirulog inhibits thrombin by binding to both the catalytic site and the anion recognition site. However, catalytic site inhibition by hirulog is transient because, once complexed, thrombin proteolytically cleaves the Arg-Pro bond on the amino terminal extension, thereby converting hirulog to a weaker hirudinlike inhibitor.[59,66] Noncleavable hirulog derivatives have been developed to counteract this problem.[40] Recently, there has been a report of a novel synthetic thrombin inhibitor composed of 19 amino acids, in which recognition sequences for the catalytic and primary exosite-binding domains of thrombin have been linked by a transition-state analog.[73] When compared with hirulog, this agent is claimed to be superior at inhibiting platelet aggregation and venous thrombosis in a rat model.[73]

An interesting chimeric molecule described more recently consists of a tripeptide sequence found in adhesive proteins coupled to residues of hirudin.[14] The chimeric molecule is able to inhibit platelet adhesion to surfaces as well as inactive thrombin. The implications of this type of structuring are that thrombin inactivation can be targeted to specific cells trapped in thrombi. In a novel approach to target a thrombin inhibitor to the surface of a clot, hirudin was covalently linked to a fibrin-specific monoclonal antibody.[6] This chimeric agent was shown to be more effective than hirudin alone in preventing platelet deposition and clot formation in vitro and in an in vivo model of arteriovenous shunt.

Several recombinant variants are currently undergoing clinical trials for treatment and prophylaxis of thrombi in medical and interventional cardiology. A short half-life, which is their common attribute, may be advisable for acute treatment of thromboembolic events. However, most of the clinical situations in which antithrombotic drugs are indicated require more prolonged half-life, particularly in prevention of vascular events in atherosclerotic disease, which represents the bulk of indications for which antithrombotic drugs are sought. An additional reason for seeking prolonged half-life is that it allows better adjustment of drug level if there is considerable interindividual variation in metabolism of the drug.

Although hirudin is an effective anticoagulant, it is short-lived and may exhibit immunogenic behavior. To provide effective anticoagulant prophylaxis or long-term treatment of venous thrombosis, two subcutaneous injections per day of recombinant hirudin (r-hirudin) are necessary, as demonstrated by APTT.[15,16,51,75] In light of the pharmacokinetics of r-hirudin, broad long-term use is questionable. Consequently, r-hirudin has been bound to dextran in an attempt to prolong its biologic half-life.[60] This nonspecific binding, however, was associated with considerable loss of specific activity compared with free r-hirudin. Albumin also has been linked specifically to the carboxy terminus of hirudin to prolong its half-life without impairing its antithrombin activity. The albumin-hirudin conjugate has not yet been tested in vivo.

POLYETHYLENE GLYCOL-COUPLED HIRUDIN

Thus, the objective was to design and to synthesize a highly potent and specific thrombin inhibitor with improved pharmacodynamics and pharmacokinetics. A known method[47] for prolongation of action is conjugation to synthetic polymers such as polyethylene glycol (PEG). The advantage of PEG and monomethoxypolyethylene glycol as a carrier polymer is based on the fact that it is nontoxic, nonantigenic, and available in a wide range of molecular weights. PEG-bound proteins are reported to show altered properties, such as improved solubility, increased resistance to proteolytic degradation, and a longer half-life.[47]

TABLE 2. Physiochemical Characteristics of PEG-Hirudin vs. r-Hirudin

	r-Hirudin	PEG-Hirudin
Structure	Single chain polypeptide	Polyethylene glycol coupled monocomponent protein
Protein	65 aminoacids Tyr 63 desulphated	65 aminoacids Tyr 63 desulphated
Molecular weight	~ 7.000 Dalton	~ 17.000 Dalton
Polyethylene glycol content	—	1.7 mg PEG/mg rm-hirudin
Specific activity	~ 12.000 ATU	~12.000 ATU/mg protein
Isoelectric point	3.7	4.0

More recently, specific site-directed coupling of PEG to a specially designed stabler mutant of r-hirudin has been reported.[41,62] This modification resulted in a molecular weight increase from 7 to 17 kD, which prevents extravasation and retards renal elimination, substantially increasing biologic half-life without loss of activity and selectivity[8,18,20,62] (Table 2). Furthermore, the PEG-hirudin metabolite differs from the metabolite of hirudin, suggesting different renal metabolism of the two agents.[18,20,27] Like r-hirudin, PEG-hirudin is composed of a single polypeptide chain of 65 amino acids with three disulfide bridges and a molecular weight of the desulphated protein part of about 7,000. The anticoagulant properties of PEG-hirudin are comparable to the parent hirudin molecule; however, the pharmacokinetic profile differs significantly.[62]

Extensive profiling of PEG-hirudin has been carried out to establish similarities and differences in the biochemical and pharmacologic profiles of other direct thrombin inhibitors. The in vitro inhibitory activity of PEG-hirudin is highly selective for α-thrombin over a wide range of other serine proteases, including the digestive enzymes trypsin and chymotrypsin and other enzymes of the coagulation and fibrinolytic system (Table 3). PEG-hirudin and r-hirudin did not inhibit the amidolytic activity of the serine protease plasmin, trypsin, chymotrypsin, and factor Xa in concentrations up to 7 μg/L.[62]

IN VITRO STUDIES

Compared on the basis of protein contents, PEG-hirudin and r-hirudin revealed similar inhibitory activity in both a clotting assay and chromogenic assay (S-2238) with EC_{100} values (prolongation of thrombin-induced clotting time by 100%) of 161 and 176 μg/L and IC_{50} values of 34.5 and 30.7 μg/L, respectively.[62]

Thrombus-bound thrombin is reported to catalyze the deposition of new fibrin on the preformed thrombus, thus inducing rapid thrombus growth.[45,58,74] There is also considerable evidence that arterial thrombus formation is resistant to treatment with unfractionated heparin.[33,58,61] Like r-hirudin, PEG-hirudin seems to overcome this limitation, possibly because of its ability to antagonize not only soluble thrombin but also thrombin associated with fibrin or clot fragment.[35] PEG-hirudin and unfractionated heparin were similar in their ability to inhibit fluid-phase thrombin. Thrombin bound to fibrin was equally inhibited by

TABLE 3. Selectivity of PEG-Hirudin in Vitro

	Amidolytic Activity IC_{50} (mol/L)				
	Thrombin	Trypsin	Chymotrypsin	Plasmin	Factor Xa
r-Hirudin	4.4×10^{-9}	$> 10^{-6}$	$> 10^{-6}$	$> 10^{-6}$	$> 10^{-6}$
HL 20 (Hir-Mutein)	1.4×10^{-9}	$> 10^{-6}$	$> 10^{-6}$	$> 10^{-6}$	$> 10^{-6}$
Hirulog-1	1.9×10^{-7}	$> 10^{-6}$	$> 10^{-6}$	$> 10^{-6}$	$> 10^{-6}$
PEG-Hirudin	1.6×10^{-9}	$> 10^{-6}$	$> 10^{-6}$	$> 10^{-6}$	$> 10^{-6}$

TABLE 4.   Activity of PEG-Hirudin in Vitro

	Thrombin Time EC$_{100}$ (mol/L)	Thrombin-induced Platelet Aggregation IC$_{50}$ (mol/L)
r-Hirudin	2.2×10^{-8}	2.4×10^{-9}
HL 20 (Hir-Mutein)	3.2×10^{-8}	2.6×10^{-9}
Hirulog-1	1.1×10^{-7}	3.2×10^{-8}
PEG-Hirudin	2.0×10^{-8}	2.8×10^{-9}

PEG-hirudin and r-hirudin, whereas unfractionated heparin (UFH) showed significantly lower inhibitory effects.[35]

The results of platelet function studies with PEG-hirudin as the anticoagulant also agreed with the results obtained with r-hirudin. PEG-hirudin has no effect on platelet aggregation induced by agents other than thrombin, such as ADP and collagen.[39] PEG-hirudin and r-hirudin inhibited platelet aggregation induced by thrombin (150 NIH U/L) with IC$_{50}$ values of 19.3 and 16.6 μg/L, respectively, but had no influence on aggregation induced by U-46619 (0.5 μmol/L) and platelet activating factor (0.1 μmol/L) (Table 4).

Platelets are also reported to play an important role in the resistance to fibrinolytic therapy in both delaying reperfusion and mediating reocclusion. Ex vivo and in vivo evidence suggests that platelet-rich thrombi are particularly resistant to thrombolysis. Patients whose coronary arteries fail to reperfuse with thrombolytic therapy have thrombi that are generally rich in platelets. Comparative studies with UFH and PEG-hirudin showed that heparin induces a dose-dependent increase in platelet retention to the clot. In contrast, the retention of platelets to fibrin clots are not modified by hirudin or PEG-hirudin.[39,44] Fareed et al. investigated the influence of PEG-hirudin on recombinant tissue factor-mediated activation of platelet in native whole blood.[54] When whole blood was collected in PEG-hirudin (10 μg/ml), inhibition of platelet activation, as measured by flow cytometry, was complete.

IN VIVO STUDIES

In vitro findings on the activity and selectivity of PEG-hirudin were supported by recent publications.[7,8,28,34,63] clearly demonstrating that r-hirudin can be modified to exhibit in vivo sustained anticoagulant actions. Using various experimental models of venous and arterial thrombosis, the relative efficacy of PEG-hirudin has been compared with that of UFH[34] and PEG-hirudin.[64]

In rats, rabbits, dogs, and primates, PEG-hirudin proved to have a considerably longer terminal half-life than r-hirudin and hirulog as indicated by the antithrombin activity in plasma.[8,20,25,28,63,70,77] The duration of action of PEG-hirudin was more pronounced after subcutaneous administration than after intravenous injection. Subcutaneous injection of 4,000 U/kg body weight in dogs resulted in an increase in antithrombin activity up to a maximal plasma level of 10 U/ml 8 hours after administration.

The antithrombotic activity of PEG-hirudin, determined in a rat model of arteriovenous shunt was found to be equivalent to that of r-hirudin when measured 5 minutes after intravenous administration. There was no effect 1 hour after intravenous injection of 0.5 mg/kg body weight of r-hirudin, whereas PEG-hirudin exhibited similar antithrombotic efficacy to 5 minutes after administration. The antithrombotic effect was still present 6 hours after administration.

Based on the reduced renal elimination of PEG-hirudin, sustained plasma levels were maintained throughout the experimental period in most animal models. Consequently, the doses required for inhibition of venous and arterial thrombus generation were significantly lower than for r-hirudin and other inhibitors, such as hirulog-1 and UFH. ED$_{15}$ values were

0.25 mg/kg in a rat model of arteriovenous shunt with PEG-hirudin and corresponding values of 1.51 mg/kg for r-hirudin. To calculate the duration of action in arterial thrombosis of PEG-hirudin and r-hirudin, their antithrombotic effects were measured 5, 60, and 180 minutes after administration. Equipotent doses of PEG-hirudin and r-hirudin (0.464 and 2.15 mg/kg body weight, respectively) produced a 66% and 64% prolongation of arteriovenous shunt patency at 5 minutes, respectively. The effect of PEG-hirudin was 78% at 60 minutes and 37% at 180 minutes. The effect of r-hirudin fell to 21% by 60 minutes. In a rat model of electrically induced arterial thrombosis and a rabbit model of stasis-induced thrombosis, the EC_{50} values were 0.16 and 0.08 mg/kg body weight with PEG-hirudin, respectively; corresponding values with r-hirudin were 0.52 and 0.16 mg/kg body weight, respectively.[34]

Cofactor-independent direct thrombin inhibitors as comedication to thrombolytic therapy have been found to improve reperfusion and reduce the incidence of early reclusion better than heparin.[3,43,53] However, all direct thrombin inhibitors presently under clinical evaluation are short-lived, with the potential to cause rebound effects after cessation of infusion.[24] Recent experiments indicate that early reclusion after thrombolyses can be successfully reduced by concomitant treatment with the long-acting PEG-hirudin without negatively interacting with the hemostatic system.[63] During and after thrombolysis induced by a recombinant tissue plasminogen activator (r-tPA) in the carotid arteries of dogs, the animals received concomitant treatment of PEG-hirudin (infusion of 40 µg/kg body weight/hr), UFH (intravenous bolus of 100 U/kg body weight plus infusion of 100 U/kg body weight/hr), or physiologic saline. In the PEG-hirudin group, the incidence of reperfusion increased up to 100%, whereas reperfusion time was reduced to 39 ± 6 minutes compared with control groups (74 ± 15 minutes). In control animals the vessel rapidly reoccluded within 26 minutes after termination of r-tPA therapy but remained at a sustained level for the observation period of 4 hours in the PEG-hirudin group. The modulating effects of UFH were marginal for both the incidence of reperfusion and the improvement of carotid artery blood flow after reperfusion. However, buccal bleeding time and buccal blood loss were elevated in the UFH-treated dogs.

In a dog model of stenosed locally injured artery,[39] PEG-hirudin effectively reduced the frequency of platelet-dependent thrombus formation. Cyclic blood flow reductions (CRFs), the result of both local platelet accumulation and local thrombin generation, were induced in the left anterior descending artery of mongrel dogs by mechanical injury to the endothelium combined with critical stenosis. Maximum reduction of CRFs by 61% was already reached at a moderate dose of PEG-hirudin (bolus of 0.15 mg/kg body weight plus infusion of 0.08 mg/kg body weight/hr) without negative influence on primary hemostasis.

Chronic infusion of r-hirudin also reduced neointimal thickening after injury in a porcine coronary model.[67] PEG-hirudin administered early and in doses (1 mg/kg body weight intravenous bolus plus 0.1 mg/kg body weight/hr intravenously for 5 days) sufficient to maintain the activated clotting time (ACT) at 200 seconds decreased the mean neointimal thickness by 0.27 mm, a difference that would be angiographically detectable and clinically relevant. Similar results were reported by Hammerschmidt et al., who showed that short-term and longer-term treatment with PEG-hirudin were more effective than intravenous UFH in decreasing intimal thickening and changes in the vascular wall area.[28]

The efficacy and safety of r-hirudin coupled to PEG were evaluated after bolus intracardial injection in a canine model of cardiopulmonary bypass (CPB). In this dose-ranging study, PEG-hirudin was found to have similar safety and efficacy to r-hirudin with the advantage of bolus-only administration in CPB. Blood loss was less than with heparin but greater than with r-hirudin.[70]

Laux et al. showed that PEG-hirudin has a high antithrombotic efficacy and sustained antithrombotic activity in an experimental model of venous thrombosis compared with hirudin.[42] From the close correlation between antithrombin activity and the antithrombotic effect, the authors conclude that the difference in antithrombotic efficacy is due to the different kinetic behavior of both compounds.

The effectiveness of PEG-hirudin and r-hirudin in preventing growth of established thrombi was compared in a rabbit model of jugular vein thrombosis leading to venous thrombosis and pulmonary embolism. At doses equivalent in prolonging APTT, r-hirudin was twice as effective as standard heparin.[8] If PEG-hirudin was given to rats before thromboplastin injection, thrombosis was totally inhibited.[8,62] At equivalent antithrombotic doses, heparin caused a 2-fold longer prolongation of the bleeding time and a significantly greater increase in APTT than hirudin.

PEG-hirudin has also been shown to be effective in a rabbit model of disseminated intravascular coagulate (DIC).[77] When PEG-hirudin in a single dose of 1 mg/kg body weight was given simultaneously with the second endotoxin injection, the decreases in platelet count, AT III, protein C, plasminogen, antiplasmin, and fibrin monomers were less pronounced. The combined effect of all these alterations strongly points in the direction of a favorable influence of PEG-hirudin on the course of DIC. Of interest, 6 hours after intravenous injection of PEG-hirudin, its full effect on the thrombin time was still detectable. This was apparently due to a longer half-life in the circulation of PEG-hirudin than of natural hirudin.

A comparison of the antithrombotic and antihemostasis activities of UFH and PEG-hirudin in a mouse model of thrombin-induced pulmonary thromboembolism clearly demonstrated that both UFH and PEG-hirudin, given intravenously before thrombin, protected mice dose-dependently from thrombin-induced death.[25] On a weight basis PEG-hirudin was more potent (bovine thrombin, 1,000 U/kg intravenously = 9.16% mortality rate; IC_{50} for PEG-hirudin = 0.10 mg/kg; IC_{50} for UFH = 0.55 mg/kg) and produced less impairment of blood clotting test than UFH. At doses equipotent in protecting against mortality, the prolongation of the APTT was significantly increased with UFH compared with PEG-hirudin.

In the initial clinical studies PEG-hirudin[18,19,27] was administered to 75 healthy volunteers as a single intravenous (0.03–0.3 mg/kg body weight) (Table 5) and subcutaneous (0.05–0.6 mg/kg body weight) dose (Table 6), as once-daily subcutaneous (0.2–0.4 mg/kg body weight) injections for 5 days, as a combined single intravenous (0.3 mg/kg body weight) and multiple subcutaneous (0.3 mg/kg body weight) regimen with once-daily subcutaneous injections for 3 days or by intravenous infusion (0.01–0.2 mg/kg body weight). Anticoagulant effects and plasma levels of PEG-hirudin, measured by standard clotting assays and a chromogenic substrate method (S-2238), revealed a single intravenous bolus injection of 0.2 mg/kg body weight to be the maximal anticoagulant dose for healthy volunteers. Ten minutes after injection, the APTT showed a mean 3.2-fold prolongation compared with pretreatment values (Fig. 3). Because of the lower plasma clearance compared with r-hirudin, APTT was still 1.9-fold prolonged 4 hours after dosing. The single

TABLE 5.   Pharmacokinetic Parameters for Intravenously Administered PEG-Hirudin (LU 57291) and r-Hirudin (LU 52369)

Parameter	Symbol	Dimension	Parameter Value (mean ± SD)	
			PEG-Hirudin	**r-Hirudin**
Volume of distribution (central compartment)	V_C	[L/kg]	0.048 ± 0.01	0.041 ± 0.01
Volume of distribution (steady state)	V_{SS}	[L/kg]	0.16 ± 0.15	0.13 ± 0.03
Terminal half-life	$t_{1/2}$	[h]	12.0 (median)	1.5 ± 0.9
Total clearance	CL	[ml/hr/kg]	21 ± 18	108 ± 29
Recovery of activity in urine	f_e	[% of dose]	46 ± 15	54 ± 21

TABLE 6. Pharmacokinetic Parameters for Subcutaneously Administered PEG-Hirudin
(LU 57291) and r-Hirudin (LU 52369)

Parameter	Symbol	Dimension	Parameter Value (mean ± SD)	
			PEG-Hirudin	**r-Hirudin**
Peak plasma concentration (normalized to a subcutaneous dose of 1 mg/kg)	C_{max}	[ng/ml]	1010 ± 610	1533 ± 139
Time of C_{max}	T_{max}	[h]	21 ± 11	1 – 6
Recovery of activity in urine	f_e	[% of dose]	30 ± 12	42 ± 14
Bioavailability	f	[% of dose]	54 – 64*	88 ± 18

* Determined after subcutaneous 0.6 mg/kg body weight.

subcutaneous injection of r-hirudin showed a more rapid onset of APTT prolongation compared with PEG-hirudin; however, steady-state APTT levels of about 1.5-fold of baseline lasted more than 20 hr after 0.4 and 0.5 mg doses of PEG-hirudin/kg body weight but only about 7 hr after r-hirudin. With multiple subcutaneous doses of 0.4 mg/kg body weight, a 2-fold prolongation of mean APTT was seen until 24 hr after the last administration. A 2-fold prolongation of APTT was again reached at 6 hr after the start of an infusion of 0.02 mg/kg body weight/hr. Combined administration of single intravenous multiple subcutaneous doses of 0.3 mg/kg showed high antithrombin activity. However, the responsiveness obtained with APTT was less than expected. PEG-hirudin was well tolerated without immunoallergic side effects. Because of its prolonged anticoagulant activity, PEG-hirudin is promising for once-daily subcutaneous dosing. In contrast, r-hirudin has to be administered 2–3 times daily to achieve anticoagulant effects that are comparable to heparin. Because of its relatively rapid elimination from the central compartment, PEG-hirudin also may be well suited for intravenous injection or for low-dose continuous infusion. The clinical aspects of the pharmacodynamics and pharmacokinetics of PEG-hirudin therapy are described in Table 7. PEG-hirudin has distinct pharmacodynamic actions by inhibiting catalytic and receptor-mediated thrombin action. Because of weaker effects on platelets at antithrombotic dosages, it does not cause bleeding. No serious side effects or immunogenic responses have been reported at optimized dosages. PEG-hirudin exhibits higher

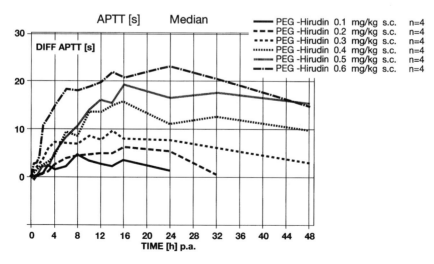

FIGURE 3. Single dose subcutaneous administration.

TABLE 7.   Clinical Aspects of PEG-Hirudin Therapy

Pharmacodynamics
• Direct inhibition of catalytic and receptor-mediated thrombin activities
• No unwanted effects on platelets
• Limited bleeding complications at antithrombotically effective doses
• No side effects after acute or chronic administration
• So far no evidence of immunogenicity after short-term application
Pharmacokinetics
• High bioavailability after subcutaneous administration
• Distribution in extracellular space
• No accumulation in organs
• Renal excretion of unmodified molecule
• Long biologic half-life, especially at subcutaneous injection

bioavailability after subcutaneous administration and is mainly distributed in extracellular spaces. There is no evidence of accumulation in organs, and PEG-hirudin is excreted without metabolic transformation. It also exhibits a prolonged half-life after subcutaneous and intravenous administration. These properties of PEG-hirudin make it an extremely useful antithrombotic and anticoagulant agent for prophylactic and therapeutic indications.

DRUG INTERACTIONS

Current clinical trends point to polypharmacologic approaches in the treatment and management of cardiovascular disorders. Combination modalities of anticoagulants with other drug classes, such as antiplatelets and fibrinolytics, have been used.[5,7] However, systematic studies of the interactions of antithrombin agents with other drugs are not available. Because thrombin plays a key role in the activation of platelets, thrombin inhibitors such as hirudin and its derivatives are expected to produce augmentation or synergism of the antiplatelet actions of aspirin.[7] Thus, the bleeding complications observed in recent trials[12,26,53] may be attributable to the concomitant use of aspirin. This theory is supported by a recent report[8] that the interaction of PEG-hirudin and aspirin in healthy volunteers resulted in prolongation of the bleeding time, which was not correlated with any platelet function test or any coagulation parameters.

In addition, clinical experience with r-hirudin and first results from clinical pharmacology studies of PEG-hirudin suggest that renal clearance is important for the elimination of this class of direct thrombin inhibitors. Thus, advanced age or renal dysfunction also may be associated with reduced PEG-hirudin elimination, higher plasma concentrations and consequently an increased risk of bleeding.

Similar interactions would be expected if PEG-hirudin was used with heparin and low-molecular-weight heparin or AT III concentrates.[5,63] Although the actions of PEG-hirudin are readily predictable, dosage adjustments in the presence of other anticoagulants and antithrombotic drugs may be required to optimize its therapeutic index.

On the other hand, adjunct usage of PEG-hirudin with thrombolytic agents, depending on the dose, may result in facilitation of thrombolysis or, if the PEG-hirudin dose is high, in thrombolytic compromise.[9] In addition, PEG-hirudin also may directly inhibit activation or formation of protein C by neutralizing thrombomodulin-bound thrombin.[11] The consequences of this process are not known. Unlike many direct thrombin inhibitors, PEG-hirudin does not produce direct inhibition of fibrinolytic enzymes such as plasmin and plasminogen activators. However, it does augment the anticoagulant actions of fibrinogen/fibrin degradation products and may cause rethrombosis (reocclusion).

Because of the complex nature of thrombotic disorders, the impact of drug interactions in various disorders has to be carefully assessed. Therefore, it is imperative that the interactions of thrombin inhibitors in general and of PEG-hirudin in particular are given much thought in designing drug combination protocols for clinical applications.

NEUTRALIZATION OF PEG-HIRUDIN

A major concern in the use of long-acting direct thrombin inhibitors such as PEG-hirudin is the risk of bleeding associated with the potential effect of the drug on hemostasis, particularly when antithrombotic therapy is combined with invasive procedures, fibrinolytic treatment, or predisposition to abnormal bleeding. Availability of an antagonist to PEG-hirudin is essential for instant neutralization of the antithrombotic action.

The neutralization pattern of PEG-hirudin by endogenous factors was studied to determine a method for antagonizing PEG-hirudin. These data suggest that like r-hirudin, endogenous modulators of platelet factor IV or human factor VIII produce no effect on the in vivo anticoagulant action of PEG-hirudin.

Studies were also performed to compare the neutralization effect of PEG-hirudin by agents that can be exogenously added to a system. Protamine, γ-thrombin, factor VIIa, and prothrombin complexes were evaluated. None of these agents altered the anticoagulant action of PEG-hirudin, except for a slight influence by factor VIIa and prothrombin complex.

Like all potent antithrombotic drugs, PEG-hirudin has the potential to cause undesirable bleeding. The antagonism of clinically used PEG-hirudin, therefore, may be necessary, especially in terms of its long-lasting effect. At present, no specific antidote can be recommended. Possible antidotes to PEG-hirudin, such as chemicals and genetechnologically modified thrombin derivatives, and meisothrombin, that are not prothrombotic but still bind to thrombin need careful preclinical and clinical evaluation. When bleeding becomes clinically relevant, such approaches as the use of platelet-rich packs, prothrombin complexes, and 1-deamino-8-D-arginine vasopressin (DDAVP), may be used to neutralize bleeding. In addition, the noncoagulation form of thrombin also may be useful in reversing the hemorrhagic effects of PEG-hirudin.[10]

A mutant derivative of human prothrombin, in which active-site aspartate at position 419 is replaced by an asparagine, has been designed, expressed in recombinant Chinese hamster ovary cells, and purified to homogeneity. D419N-prothrombin was converted to the related molecules D419N-meizothrombin and D419-thrombin. In vitro and in vivo studies confirmed that both products act as a hirudin antagonist in blood circulation without detectable effects on the coagulation system.[22]

IMMUNOLOGIC RESPONSE OF PEG-HIRUDIN

The covalent attachment of PEG to proteins is a widely used modification to extend circulating life times in vivo and to reduce or suppress the immunogenicity of the underlying native protein.[1] Compared with r-hirudin, PEG-hirudin has a theoretically minor potential to elicit immunologic response or allergic reactions in humans. First studies in immunocompetent healthy volunteers as well as in patients with unstable angina have shown that after repeated administration of PEG-hirudin the risk of allergenicity was minimized, with no sign of sensitization.[18,19,27]

MONITORING OF PEG-HIRUDIN

Among the various methods that can be used for monitoring of antithrombin agents, including PEG-hirudin, APTT has been widely applied. However, APTT has limited sensitivity, and different reagents produce a wide variety of results. The APTT test also can be influenced by several endogenous factors leading to a relatively broad intraindividual variation. Furthermore, the APTT response is nonlinear and already reaches saturation at therapeutic plasma concentrations. This widely used parameter for dose adjustments thus bears the risk of considerable overdosage, as shown in recent clinical trials with r-hirudin.[24,26,53,57] The Heptest time that measures both antifactor Xa and antithrombin activities has limited sensitivity to thrombin inhibitors. In interventional cardiovascular procedures, the ACT has proven to be quite useful, as supported by a recent report.[3,26] More recently, the ecarin clotting time (ECT) has been proposed as a highly specific and sensitive test to measure the anticoagulant effects of PEG-hirudin. The test shows a close, linear relationship with PEG-hirudin plasma concentration, even in the presence of heparin or oral anticoagulants. This assay is fast and highly reproducible, allowing bedside monitoring of blood levels of hirudin and its derivatives more reliably than APTT.[55,56]

FUTURE CONSIDERATIONS

The development of direct thrombin inhibitors has opened new perspectives in the control of the thrombotic process and added a new dimension to the management of vascular and thrombotic disorders. Although the major clinical indications for these agents include interventional cardiovascular procedures and prophylaxis of deep venous thrombosis, little is known of their use for surgical and therapeutic anticoagulation. PEG-hirudin may be a valuable drug when both short- and long-term treatment and prophylaxis of thrombotic disorders is required. In coming years, the usefulness of PEG-hirudin will be evaluated in the given medical and surgical indications, including unstable angina, peripheral bypass surgery, and heparin-induced thrombocytopenia. Furthermore, PEG-hirudin may be incorporated with biomaterials and formulated for depot delivery. PEG-hirudin, therefore, provides a wide spectrum of anticoagulation that can be developed for multiple indications to control thrombosis and related pathophysiologic events. If the apparent advantages of PEG-hirudin can be effectively shown, PEG-hirudin may become the drug of choice, probably not for general use, but for certain indications.

REFERENCES

1. Abuchowski A, McCoy JR, Palczuk NC, et al: Effect of covalent attachment of polyethylene-glycol on immunogenicity and circulating life of bovine liver catalase. J Biol Chem 252(11):3582–3586, 1977
2. Adams SL: The medicinal leech: Historical perspectives. Semin Thromb Hemost 15:261–264, 1989.
3. Antmann EM: Hirudin in acute myocardial infarction: Safety report from the thrombolysis and thrombin inhibition in myocardial infarction (TIMI) 9A trial. Circulation 90:1624–1630, 1994.
4. Berliner LJ: Thrombin structure and function. New York, Plenum Press, 1992.
5. Biemond BJ, Levi M, Nurmohamed MT, Buller HR, ten Cate JW: Additive effect of the combined administration of low molecular weight heparin and recombinant hirudin on thrombus growth in a rabbit jugular vein thrombosis model. Thromb Hemost 73:277–380, 1994.
6. Bode C, Mehwald P, Peter K, et al: Enhanced antithrombotic potency of fibrin-targeted recombinant hirudin in a non-human primate model [abstract]. Ann Hematol I:A52, 1995.
7. Breddin HK, Radziwon P, Eschenfelder V, et al: PEG-hirudin and acetylsalicylic acid show a strong interaction on bleeding time [abstract]. Ann Hematol I:A52, 1996.
8. Bucha E, Kossemehl A, Nowak G: Animal experimental studies on the pharmacokinetics of PEG-hirudin [abstract]. Ann Hematol I:A55, 1996.
9. Butler KD, Dolan SK, Talbot MD, Wallis RB: Factor VIII and DDAVP reverse the effect of desulfato hirudin (CGP 39393) in bleeding in the rat. Blood Coagul Fibrinol 4:459–464, 1993.
10. Callas DD, Iqbal O, Hoppensteadt D, Fareed J: Fibrinolytic compromise by synthesis and recombinant thrombin inhibitors. Implications in the management of thrombolytic disorders. Clin Appl Thromb Hemost 1:114–124, 1995.
11. Callas DD, Fareed J: Direct inhibition of protein Ca by site directed thrombin inhibitors: Implications in anticoagulant and thrombolytic therapy. Thromb Res 78:457–460, 1995.
12. Cannon CP, Braunwald E, Hirudin: Initial results in acute myocardial infarction, unstable angina and angioplasty. J Am Coll Cardiol 25(7):305–375, 1995.
13. Chesebro JH, Zoldehelyi P, Badimon P, Fuster V: Role of thrombin in arterial thrombosis: Implications for therapy. Thromb Haemost 66:1–5, 1991.
14. Church FC, Phillips JE, Woods JL: Chimeric antithrombin peptide. J Biol Chem 266:11975–11979, 1991.
15. Eriksson BI, Lindbratt S, Thoerholm C, et al: Recombinant hirudin, CGP 29292 15 mg (Revasc-Ciba), is the most effective and safe prophylaxis of thromboembolic complications in patients undergoing total hip replacement. Thromb Haemost 73:1093, 1995.
16. Eriksson BI, Ekmann ST, Kalebo P, et al: Prevention of deep-vein thrombosis after total hip replacement: Direct thrombin inhibition with recombinant hirudin, CGP 39393. Lancet 347:635–639, 1996.
17. Esmon CT: The regulation of natural anticoagulant pathways. Science 235:1348–1352, 1987.
18. Esslinger HU, Haas S, Lassmann A, et al: Phase I results on PEG-hirudin (Lu 57291), a safe and effective anticoagulant with prolonged activity [abstract]. Thromb Haemostasis 73:1452, 1995.

19. Esslinger H-U, Greger G, Lassman A, Maurer R: General tolerability and effects on clotting parameters after single i.v. and s.c. bolus administration of recombinant hirudin (LU 52369) in man [abstract]. Thromb Hemost 65:1291, 1991.
20. Fareed J, Walenga JM, Hoppensteadt D, et al: Comparative pharmacodynamics/pharmacokinetics of recombinant hirudin and its PEG-coupled derivatives in primates [abstract]. Thromb Haemost 65:1286, 1991.
21. Fenton JW II: Regulation of thrombin generation and functions. Semin Thromb Hemost 14:234–240, 1988.
22. Fischer B, Schlokat U, Mitterer A, Dorner F: Rational design recombinant preparation in vivo and in vitro characterization of human prothrombin-derived hirudin antagonists. Ann Hematol I:A5, 1996.
23. Fuster V, Verstraete M: Thrombosis in Cardiovascular Disorders. Philadelphia, W.B. Saunders, 1992.
24. Gold HK, Torres FW, Gorabedian HD, et al: Evidence for a rebound coagulation phenomenon after cessation of a 4-hour infusion of a specific thrombin inhibitor in patients with unstable angina pectoris. J Am Coll Cardiol 21:1039–1047, 1993.
25. Gresele P, Nasimi M, Nenci GG: Comparison between PEG-hirudin (PEG-hir) and unfractionated heparin (UFH) in a thrombin-induced pulmonary thromboembolism model in mice. Haemostasis 24:259, 1994.
26. Gusto II investigators randomized trial of intravenous heparin versus recombinant hirudin for acute coronary syndromes. Circulation 90:1631–1637, 1994.
27. Haas S, Esslinger HU, Stemberger A, et al: Placebo-controlled trial on the anticoagulant effects of PEG-hirudin (LU 57291) as intravenous infusion in health volunteers [abstract]. Ann Haematol IA:45, 1995.
28. Hammerschmidt S, Unterberg C, Bruch C, et al: Reduction of neointimal proliferation after coronary angioplasty using PEG-coupled hirudin in mini-pigs. Z Kardiol 84:231, 1995.
29. Harker LA, Mann KG: Thrombosis and fibrinolysis. In Fuster V, Verstraete M (eds): Thrombosis in Cardiovascular Disorders. Philadelphia, W.B. Saunders, 1992, pp 1–16.
30. Hauptmann J, Markwardt F: Pharmacologic aspects of the development of selective thrombin inhibitors as anticoagulants. Semin Thromb Hemost 18:200–217, 1992.
31. Haycraft JB: On the action of a secretion from the medicinal leech on the coagulation of blood. Proc R Soc 36:478–487, 1984.
32. Hirsh J: Heparin. N Engl J Med 324:1565–1574, 1991.
33. Hogg PJ, Jackson CM: Fibrin monomer protects thrombin from inactivation by heparin-antithrombin III: Implications for heparin efficacy. Proc Natl Acad Sci USA 86:3619–3623, 1989.
34. Hornberger W, Rübsamen K, Schweden J: Prolonged antithrombotic activity of a new polyethylene-glycol-coupled hirudin (LU 57291) in two rat thrombin models. Ann Hematol 66:Suppl 1, 1993.
35. Ioria A, Agnelli G, Leone M, et al: Hirudin and PEG-hirudin inhibit clot-bound thrombin more efficaciously than heparin [abstract]. Ann Hematol 66:Suppl 1, A19, 1993.
36. Ito R, Phaneauf MF, Lo Gerfo FW: Thrombin inhibition by covalently bound hirudin. Blood Coag Fibrinol 2:77–81, 1991.
37. Kelly AB, Maraganore JM, Bourdon P, et al: Antithrombotic effects of synthetic peptides targeting different functional domains of thrombin. Proc Natl Acad Sci USA 89:6040–6044, 1992.
38. Kettner C, Shaw E: D-phe-Pro-ArgCH$_2$Cl-a selective affinity label for thrombin. Thromb Res 14:969–973, 1979.
39. Kirchengast M, Rubsamen K: Prevention by PEG-hirudin of platelet dependent thrombus formation in the stenosed locally injured canine coronary artery [abstract]. J Invas Cardiol 7(c):9, 1995.
40. Kline T, Hammond C, Bourdon P, et al: Hirulog peptides with Scissile bond replacements resistant to thrombin cleavage. Biochem Biophys Res Commun 177:1049–1055, 1991.
41. Kurfurst MM: Detection and molecular weight determination of polyethylene glycol-modified hirudin by staining after sodium dececyl sulfate polyacrylamide gel electrophoresis. Ann Biochem 200:244–248, 1992.
42. Laux V, Schweden J, Maurer R, et al: Antithrombotic effect of a new polyethylene-glycol-coupled hirudin (LU 57291) in a venous thrombosis model in the rabbit. Correlation with anti-factor IIa activity in plasma [abstract]. Ann Hematol 66:Suppl 1, 27, 1993.
43. Lee LV: Initial experience with hirudin and streptokinase in acute myocardial infarction: Results of the thrombolysis in myocardial infarction (TIMI) 6 trial. Am J Cardiol 75:7–13, 1995.
44. Lefkovitis J, Topol EJ: Direct thrombin inhibitors in cardiovascular medicine. Circulation 90:1522–1535, 1994.
45. Li WX, Kaplan AV, Grant GW, et al: A novel nucleotide-based thrombin inhibitor inhibits clot-bound thrombin and reduces arterial platelet thrombus formation. Blood 83:677–682, 1994.
46. Loscalzo J, Melnick B, Handin R: The interaction of platelet factor 4 and glycosaminoglycans. Arch Biochem Biophys 240:446–455, 1985.
47. Macaya RF, Schultz P, Smith FW, et al: Thrombin-binding DNA aptamer forms a unimolecular quadruplex structure in solution. Proc Natl Acad Sci USA 90:3745–3749, 1993.
48. Magnusson S: Thrombin and prothrombin. Enzyme 3:277–321, 1971.
49. Maraganore JM, Chao B, Joseph ML, et al: Anticoagulant activity of synthetic hirudin fragments. J Biol Chem 264:8692–8698, 1989.
50. Maraganore JM, Bourdon P, Jablonski J, Ramachandran KL: Design and characterization of hirulogs: A novel class of bivalent peptide inhibitors of thrombin. Biochemistry 29:7095–7101, 1990.

51. Markwardt F: Development of hirudin as an antithrombotic agent. Semin Thromb Hemost 15:269–282, 1989.
52. Naski MC, Fenton JW, Maraganore JM, et al: The COOH-terminal domain of hirudin: An exosite-directed competitive inhibitor of the action of alpha-thrombin in fibrinogen. J Biol Chem 265:13484–13489, 1990.
53. Neuhaus KL, Essen RV, Tebber U, et al: Safety observations from the pilot phase of the randomized r-hirudin for improvement of thrombolysis (HITT-III) study. Circulation 90:1638–1640, 1994.
54. Norlund M, Koza M, Eschenfelder V, Fareed J: The effect of recombinant hirudin and its polyethyleneglycol-coupled derivative (PEG-hirudin) on tissue factor activation of human platelets as studied by flow cytometric analysis. Blood 84(Suppl 1):689, 1994.
55. Nowak G, Bucha E: Quantitative determination of hirudin in blood and body fluids. Semin Thromb 22:197–202, 1996.
56. O'Donnell CJ, Ridker RM, Herbert PR, Hennekens CH: Antithrombotic therapy for acute myocardial infarction. J Am Coll Cardiol 25:235–295, 1995.
57. Okamoto S, Hijikata A: Potent inhibition of thrombin by the newly synthesized arginine derivate no. 805: The importance of stereostructure of its hydrophobic carboxamide portion. Biochem Biophys Res Commun 101:440, 1981.
58. Powers JC, Kam CM: Synthetic substrates and inhibitors of thrombin. In Berliner LJ (ed): Thrombin: Structure and Function. New York, Plenum Press, 1992, pp 117–158.
59. Qui X, Padmanabhan KP, Carperos VE, et al: Structure of the hirulog 3–thrombin complex and nature of the S'subsites of substrates and inhibitors. Biochemistry 31:11689–11697, 1992.
60. Richter M, Walsmann P, Markwardt F: Plasma level of dextran-r-hirudin. Pharmazie 44:73:1989.
61. Rosenberg RD: The heparin-antithrombin system: A natural anticoagulation mechanism. In Colman RW, Hirsh J, Marder VJ, Salzman EW (eds): Hemostasis and Thrombosis: Basic Principles and Clinical Practice. Philadelphia, J.B. Lippincott, 1987, pp 1373–1392.
62. Rübsamen K, Hornberger W, Schweden J, Kurfurst M: Pharmacological characteristics of a long acting polyethylene glycol-coupled recombinant hirudin. Thromb Haemost 65:1291, 1991.
63. Rübsamen K, Hornberger W: Prevention of early reocclusion after thrombolysis of copper coil-induced thrombin in the canine carotid artery: Comparison of PEG-hirudin and unfractionated heparin. Thromb Haemost 76:105–110, 1996.
64. Rübsamen K, Hornberger W, Laux V, et al: Antithrombotic efficacy of the polyethylene-glycol-coupled hirudin mutein LU 57291 in experimentally induced venous and arterial thrombosis. Thromb Haemost 69:2717, 1993.
65. Rübsamen K, Hornberger W, Ruf A, Bode C: The ecarin clotting time, a rapid and simple coagulation assay for monitoring hirudin and PEG-hirudin in blood. Ann Hematol 72:Suppl 1, A56, 1996.
66. Skrzypczak-Jankin E, Carperos VE, Ravickandran KG, et al: Structure of the hirugen and hirulog-a complexes of alpha-thrombin. J Mol Biol 221:1379–1393, 1991.
67. Srivatsa SS, Edwards WD, Simari RD, et al: Chronic hirudin infusion reduces neointimal thickening after injury in a porcine coronary model. J Am Coll Cardiol 25:302A, 1995.
68. Stone SR, Maraganore JM: Hirudin interactions with thrombin. In Berliner JF (ed): Thrombin: Structure and Function. New York, Plenum Press, 1992, pp 219–256.
69. Tapparelli C, Metternich R, Ehrhardt C, Cook NS: Synthetic low-molecular weight thrombin inhibitors: Molecular design and pharmacological profile. Trends Pharmacol Sci 14:366–376, 1993.
70. Terrell MR, Koza MJ, Walenga JM, et al: PEG-hirudin as an anticoagulant in cardiopulmonary bypass [abstract]. Ann Hematol 1:A45, 1995.
71. Theroux P, Lidon R: Anticoagulants and their use in acute ischemic syndromes. In Topol EJ (ed): Interventional Cardiology. Philadelphia, W.B. Saunders, 1994, pp 23–45.
72. Theroux P, Perez-Villa F, Waters D, et al: Randomized double-blind comparison of two doses of hirulog with heparin as adjunctive therapy to streptokinase to promote early patency of the intaret-related artery in acute myocardial infarction. Circulation 91:2132–2139, 1995.
73. Vlasuk G, Vallar PL, Weinhouse MI, et al: A novel inhibitor of thrombin containing multiple recognition sequences linked by α-heto amide transition state. Circulation 90(4 Pt. 2):I348, 1994.
74. Weitz JL, Huboda M, Massel D, et al: Clot-bound thrombin is protected from inhibition by heparin-antithrombin but is susceptible to inactivation by antithrombin III-independent inhibitors. J Clin Invest 86:385–391, 1990.
75. Weitz JL, Hirsh J: Antithrombins: Their potential as antithrombotic agents. Annu Rev Med 43:9–16, 1992.
76. Witting JL, Bourdon P, Brezniak DV, et al: Thrombin-specific inhibition by and slow cleavage of hirulog-1. Biochem J 283(Pt 3): 737–743, 1992.
77. Zawilska K, Zozulinska M, Turowiecka Z, et al: The effect of a long-acting recombinant hirudin (PEG-hirudin) on experimental DIC in rabbits. Thromb Haemost 69:500, 1993.

CHAPTER 12

Hirudin as an Anticoagulant in Cardiopulmonary Bypass

JEANINE M. WALENGA, Ph.D.
ROQUE PIFARRÉ, M.D.

Leeches have commonly been used in the practice of bloodletting to remove bad humors from the body since the Stone Age. By the late 1800s bloodsucking was used to treat all kinds of maladies, and leeches nearly became extinct. In 1884 John Haycraft demonstrated that leech salivary secretion possessed an active anticoagulant.[3] This material was named hirudin by Karl Jacoby in 1904. After years of failed attempts by various investigators, Fritz Markwardt finally succeeded in isolating hirudin from medicinal leeches (*Hirudo medicinalis*) in 1955.[7] He subsequently showed that hirudin produced its anticoagulant effect through highly specific inhibition of thrombin.[8]

Hirudin is a single-chain polypeptide of 65 amino acids (7000 Da) that currently is prepared in recombinant (r) form by expression from vectors such as *Escherichia coli, Saccharomyces cerevisiae,* and *Bacillus subtilis*. Several variants have been characterized. Natural hirudins are mixtures of hirudin variants, but r-hirudins are homogeneous.[10] Recombinant hirudins have a 3–5-fold more potent antithrombin activity than heparin.[5] They have no interaction with platelets or heparin antibodies and no fibrinolytic or antithrombotic activity other than thrombin inhibition.

Recombinant hirudin forms a 1:1 stoichiometric complex with thrombin via strong and high affinity binding (Ki 50 pM/L).[6] It exhibits a predictable relationship between pharmacokinetics and pharmacodynamics with a desirable therapeutic index.[4] In humans, it has an elimination half-life of about 1 hour, distributes to an extracellular fluid compartment, and has a relatively uniform pattern of distribution in fat, brain, heart, liver, lungs, spleen, skeletal muscles, and pancreas. Up to 70–90% is eliminated unchanged by the kidneys after intravenous administration. Recombinant hirudin is presently in clinical trials as an antithrombotic agent in myocardial infarction, unstable angina, and percutaneous transluminal coronary angioplasty (PTCA). Phase I and phase II clinical trials were encouraging. However, the GUSTO IIa, HIT-III, and TIMI-9A trials reported an increased incidence of intracranial bleeding.[1,2,9] New trials are being configured with lower doses. Iyer and Fareed[5] have reviewed the current status of r-hirudin.

Peptide inhibitors against serine proteases have been under development and have been studied for their application to hemostatic abnormalities for many years. The primary enzyme of the coagulation system in terms of kinetics of activity is thrombin. Thrombin is also the final product of the activated coagulation cascade; it acts directly on fibrinogen to convert it to clottable fibrin. It is, therefore, reasonable to consider specific thrombin inhibitors as anticoagulants, particularly in situations that result in a major insult to blood, such as cardiopulmonary bypass (CPB) (foreign surfaces, membrane oxygenators, filters, roller pumps, changes in fluid dynamics), and thus create an optimal setting for thrombosis to occur.

Specific thrombin inhibitors such as r-hirudin have the following major advantages over heparin:

1. They are composed of pure material of one chemical structure.

2. They function by a single mechanism of action (thrombin inhibition) as opposed to multiple sites of activity for heparin (coagulation enzymes, platelets, fibrinolysis).

3. They exhibit no dependence on antithrombin III (AT III) or other cofactors for expression of activity.

4. They are relatively inert and therefore not altered by metabolic processes.

5. There may be no need to neutralize anticoagulant activity because of their very short half-life.

6. No platelet (or heparin-induced thrombocytopenia) interactions other than thrombin activation inhibition are known to occur.

A further consideration is the growing need to identify an alternative anticoagulant for patients intolerant to heparin who require cardiovascular procedures, (e.g., angioplasty, atherectomy, thrombolysis), cardiac surgery, or treatment for angina. Heparin-induced thrombocytopenia can be an unfortunate clinical complication of heparin treatment, resulting in loss of limb or life. Clearly, a drug such as r-hirudin, which has limited platelet interactions, holds promise for such patients.

MATERIAL AND METHODS

Male mongrel dogs (average weight: 28 kg) were anesthetized with pentobarbital (30 mg/kg intravenously), intubated, and ventilated to 3 cm peak end-expiratory pressure (PEEP). Vascular access lines were established in the left femoral vein and artery (for blood collection) and the right femoral vein (for drug infusion) by indwelling catheters. A drip injection of lactated Ringer's solution was established.

After median sternotomy the heart was suspended in a pericardial cradle with purse-string sutures placed in the ascending aorta and right atrial appendage for CPB cannulation. CPB at 38°C was immediately established with cannulation through the right atrial appendage and ascending aorta (70 ml/kg/min flow; 55–70 mmHg mean arterial pressure), using a Travenol roller pump (Travenol Labs, Ann Arbor, MI) and a previously unused variable prime Cobe membrane lung blood oxygenator (VPCML) (Cobe, Lakewood, CO) with previously unused surgical grade Tygon S-50-HL tubing (venous outflow tubing: 3/8" inside diameter; arterial inflow tubing: 1/4" inside diameter) and EC-3840 sterile 40-μm Pall blood filters (Biomedical Products, East Hills, NY). The priming volume of the circuit was 1000 ml. CPB was continued for 1 hour (38° C) followed by a 2-hour postoperative observation period.

After the pericardial cradle was in place, a single bolus of r-hirudin (Ciba Pharmaceuticals, Horsham, UK, or Knoll AG, Ludwigshafen, Germany) was administered by intracardiac injection directly into the right atrial space. For the bolus-only animals, a bolus dose of 1.0 mg/kg was administered immediately before going on pump, and at 30 minutes on pump, a second bolus was administered (n = 10). For the bolus-plus animals, a bolus of 1.0 mg/kg was administered immediately before going on pump with an infusion initiated at 0.21 ml/min for a dose of 0.75 mg/kg/hr (n = 5), 1.50 mg/kg/hr (n = 5), or 2.25 mg/kg/hr (n = 5). A 1.0-mg/kg bolus dose of r-hirudin (≈15 μg/ml circulating plasma concentration) was chosen based on the fact that this dose should give approximately the same anticoagulant response as about 3 mg/kg (≈ 40 μg/ml: ≈ 5 U/ml) of heparin, the usual clinical dose at our institution. Recombinant hirudin was obtained in powdered form and reconstituted in saline to a stock concentration of 10.0 mg/ml immediately before use.

A heparin control group consisted of dogs anticoagulated with 2.5 mg/kg heparin, which was supplemented to maintain the ACT response at 350 seconds (n = 6). The choice of the heparin dose (2.5 mg/kg) was based on pilot studies in the same canine model of CPB. This dose was found to be the lowest dose that would eliminate serious fibrin deposits in the pump line filter. This minimal effective dose made it possible to obtain information that would be lost if an "overdose" of heparin was used. The fact that it is lower than the usual clinical dose is most likely due to the differences between human and canine physiology and to a lesser degree of surgical manipulation in the canine model compared with clinical surgery.

Blood pressure and heart rate were continually monitored in the anesthetized dogs. Hemodynamic values (cardiac index and systemic vascular resistance) and blood gases were periodically measured with an indwelling Swan-Ganz catheter, using the thermodilution technique. Blood samples were periodically collected for immediate analysis of hematocrit (manual method), platelet count (manual method read by one person), fibrinogen (Clauss technique; Dade, Miami, FL), and celite activated clotting time (ACT) (Hemochron; International Technidyne, Metuchen, NJ). Dog pooled plasma (300 mg/dl = normal) was used to construct a calibration curve for the fibrinogen assay. The template bleeding time test was performed on the gingiva of the dogs (Simplate; Organon Teknika, Durham, NC). An in-house chromogenic substrate anti-factor IIa (thrombin) kinetic rate assay, specific for measuring the inhibition of thrombin, was performed on citrated plasma aliquots, stored at 4° C until frozen (–70° C) for analysis on the following day. All clotting assays were performed on Fibrometers. The chromogenic assay was performed on the ACL 300+ (Instrumentation Laboratory, Lexington, MA).

For assessment of efficacy, pump line filters were collected, washed with 1.0 L of saline, and dried by forced air for 10 minutes immediately after the dog was removed from pump. Deposits (clots) in the pump filters were measured by the Folin-Ciocalteu phenol fibrinogen/protein assay.

For assessment of safety, blood loss was measured by weight of aspirated blood collected from the chest cavity during the 2-hour postoperative observation period. Intraoperative blood loss was measured but not strictly evaluated because the results would reflect surgical manipulation and not anticoagulation alone. All surgical incision sites (sternum, catheter sites) were observed for oozing of blood. The abdominal cavity was explored for bleeding and clotting. All dogs were euthanized with supersaturated potassium chloride after the observation period.

No change in operating technique was made throughout the study. A certified clinical perfusionist ran the CPB pump, monitored the vital functions of the dog, and assisted the surgeon. These studies were conducted in the Animal Research Facilities of Hines, Veterans Administration Hospital (Hines, IL), which is accredited by the American Association for the Accreditation of Laboratory Animal Care (AAALAC) in compliance with the National Institutes of Health *Guide for the Care and Use of Laboratory Animals*. The protocol for this study was approved by the joint Animal Care Committee of Loyola/Hines.

Data are represented as a mean ± one standard error of the mean (SE). Statistical analysis was performed using the ANOVA program from the Primer of Biostatistics (McGraw-Hill) IBM-PC compatible package.

RESULTS AND DISCUSSION

Cardiopulmonary Bypass Model

The protein deposits measured on the filters from the pump line showed a significantly elevated level ($p < 0.01$) in the r-hirudin bolus-only group (126 ± 37 mg) compared with the heparin controls (22 ± 3 mg for heparin) (mean ± SE) (Fig. 1). Definite individual

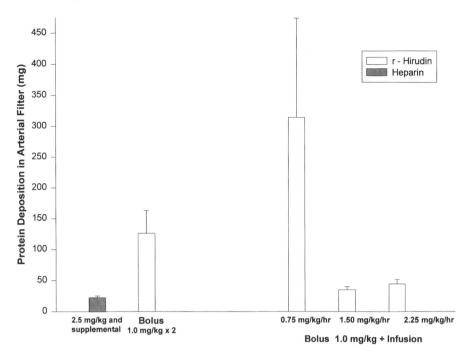

FIGURE 1.   Protein analysis of arterial line filters after CPB with r-hirudin (n = 10/bolus-only group; n =5/bolus-plus groups) or heparin (n = 6) as a measure of anticoagulant efficacy in dogs.

sensitivities to the dose of r-hirudin were observed (see large SE). The lowest dosed infusion group (1.0 mg/kg + 0.75 mg/kg/hr) also had significantly elevated filter deposits (314 ± 160 mg; p < 0.05). The two other infusion dosing groups showed equivalent levels of 35–44 mg, which were not significantly different from the heparin control group. The deposits were generally platelet rather than fibrin in nature. These data, as an indication of anticoagulation efficacy, suggest that bolus-only dosing of r-hirudin is not sufficient and that, although bolus-plus infusion is more effective, the minimal dose is about 1.0 mg/kg + 1.0 mg/kg/hr.

Blood loss into the chest cavity during the 2-hour postoperative period revealed no significant difference between the bolus-only and three r-hirudin infusion groups (Fig. 2). The values ranged from 6.5–10 gm/kg with no significant difference from the heparin group (11.3 ± 3.5 mg/kg). There was no trend of enhanced blood loss with increasing dose of r-hirudin. Moreover, there was less oozing of blood from surgical incision sites in all r-hirudin-treated animals compared with heparin-treated animals. These data suggest that r-hirudin may have a wide therapeutic index such that excessive bleeding may not occur at higher blood anticoagulation levels.

The bleeding time test was significantly (p < 0.05) more prolonged with heparin (856 ± 44 sec) than with bolus-only r-hirudin (540 ± 59 sec) at 5 minutes on CPB. The bleeding time results gave the same value after the second r-hirudin bolus (Fig. 3) and were similar for the bolus-plus regimens and the bolus-only dosing. There was, however, a dose-dependent effect of r-hirudin based on the infusion dose. All values were the same as for the heparin group at 2 hours after CPB. After CPB the bleeding time test was near normal for both heparin (reversed with protamine) and r-hirudin (natural elimination; short half-life). The lesser effect on the bleeding time test by r-hirudin than by heparin may be due to lesser inhibition of platelet function by r-hirudin.

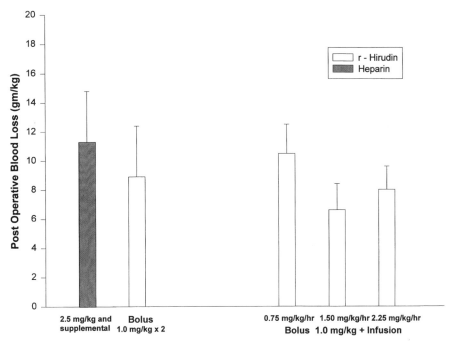

FIGURE 2.   Blood loss during 2-hour observation period after CPB with r-hirudin (n = 10/bolus-only group; n = 5/bolus-plus groups) or heparin (n = 6) as a measure of anticoagulant safety in dogs.

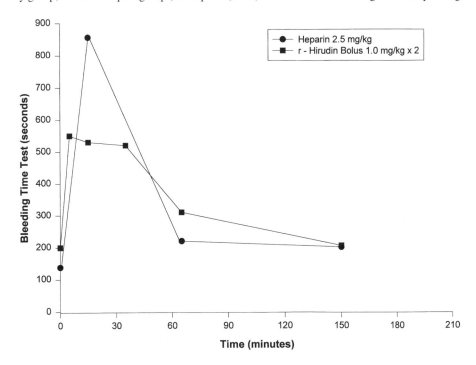

FIGURE 3.   Template bleeding time test performed on the gingiva of anesthetized dogs before, during, and after CPB with r-hirudin or heparin.

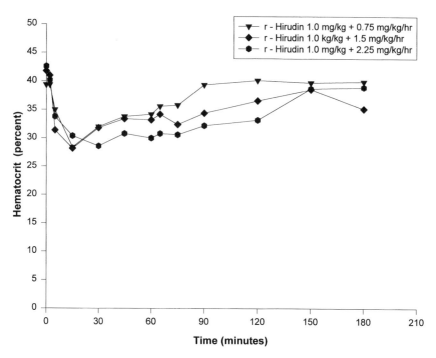

FIGURE 4.   Hematocrit levels during CPB for three doses of bolus plus infusion of r-hirudin as anticoagulant (n = 5/group).

The hematocrit showed an equivalent response in all four r-hirudin dosing groups. There was a decrease of about 30% due to hemodilution from a baseline average of 43% down to 30% hematocrit at 30 minutes on pump (Fig. 4). Within 30 minutes following CPB, the hematocrit rose to about 35% and reached near pre-operative levels by two hours post-CPB in all r-hirudin groups. The hematocrit of the heparin group tended to remain lower than baseline at two hours post-CPB.

With both r-hirudin and heparin, platelet counts decreased on pump because of hemodilution and remained lower than baseline until 2 hours postoperatively (Fig. 5). The average decrease for the four r-hirudin groups was 35% at 30 minutes on CPB. The four dosing groups of r-hirudin reacted similarly. Compared with the heparin group, the r-hirudin groups tended to show a slight increase in platelet count after CPB, whereas the platelet count in the heparin group did not increase after CPB.

The fibrinogen levels followed a similar pattern as the hematocrit and platelet count (Fig. 6). In the lowest dosed r-hirudin infusion group (1.0 mg/kg + 0.75 mg/kg/hr), a drop in fibrinogen was observed from 237 ± 45 mg/dl to an average of 116 ± 16 mg/dl (49% decrease) during CPB with a rise to an average of 181 ± 7 mg/dl after CPB (25% decrease from baseline). The two higher-dosed r-hirudin infusion groups showed a more marked decrease in fibrinogen, responding with an average decrease in fibrinogen of 70% (from an average of 230 mg/dl at baseline to an average of 60 mg/dl during CPB). A gradual rise after CPB to an average of 115 mg/dl at 30 minutes (50% decrease from baseline) and an average of 135 mg/dl at 2 hours (40% decrease from baseline) was observed. There was no significant difference in response between the four r-hirudin groups. As observed with hematocrit and platelet count, the heparin group showed a 45% decrease in fibrinogen, with no increase after CPB. The apparently higher drop in fibrinogen in the r-hirudin groups was dose-dependent. Most likely there was a false decrease in fibrinogen protein

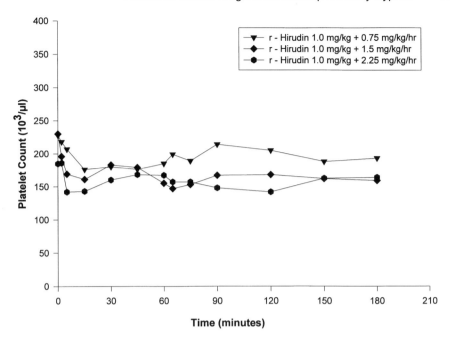

FIGURE 5.   Platelet counts during CPB for three doses of bolus plus infusion of r-hirudin as anticoagulant (n = 5/group).

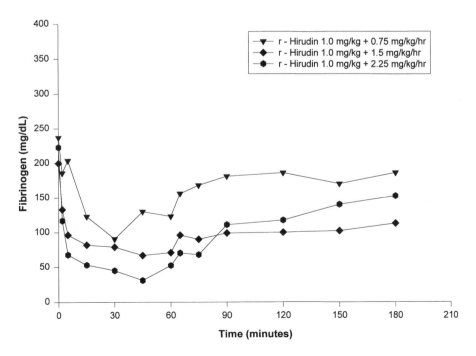

FIGURE 6.   Fibrinogen levels during CPB for three doses of bolus plus infusion of r-hirudin as anticoagulant (n = 5/group)

levels since r-hirudin, a thrombin inhibitor, interferes in the clot-based assay used to measure fibrinogen.

Hemodynamic values were continually monitored with a Swan-Ganz catheter for systemic vascular resistance (SVR) and cardiac index (CI). All r-hirudin-treated animals were stable during and after CPB, requiring less fluid replacement and support after CPB than the heparin-treated animals. There were no unexpected adverse hemodynamic effects. Generally, the SVR was maintained at 4000 dynes × sec × cm^{-5} for the r-hirudin groups throughout the perioperative period. The SVR of the heparin group was 3000 after CPB and gradually rose to 4000 (baseline value) by 2 hours after CPB. The CI was steady in both r-hirudin and heparin groups at 2.8 L/min/body surface area (BSA) throughout the perioperative period. All animals survived until euthanized.

The ACT results reveal a dose-response effect of r-hirudin and a higher response than the 350-second heparin response of heparin (Fig. 7A). Because the mechanism of action of r-hirudin is different from that of heparin, one should not expect the same ACT prolongation of time to clot at adequate anticoagulation levels. In other words, no magic ACT number corresponds to an adequate level of anticoagulation, regardless of the anticoagulant drug used. The way in which the anticoagulant effect is produced is related to a given time-to-clot value.

The short half-life of r-hirudin was obvious in the bolus-only group; after only 30 minutes on CPB, the ACT had dropped from 800 to 200 seconds. The poor anticoagulation reflected in the high filter deposits (Fig. 1) correlates with the low circulating levels of r-hirudin administered by the bolus-only regimen. The low infusion dose gave approximately an ACT response of 500 seconds during CPB (88 seconds = baseline average), and the two higher infusion doses give a response > 800 seconds (Fig. 7B). Because of the sensitivity of the ACT, no endpoint was reached during the pump run for the two higher doses. At 30 minutes after the infusion of r-hirudin was terminated (at the end of CPB), the ACT values were 131 ± 14, 260 ± 88, and 373 ± 177 seconds for the three increasing infusion doses. By 2 hours after CPB the ACT values were 107 ± 7, 162 ± 50, and 157 ± 38 seconds, respectively. There were no significant differences among the three dosing groups at any point.

The chromogenic anti-factor IIa assay revealed the short half-life of r-hirudin and stronger activity for r-hirudin than for heparin (Fig. 8A). Recombinant hirudin inhibits clotting by blocking thrombin, whereas heparin blocks not only thrombin and factor Xa, but also multiple other coagulation factors and platelet functions. Heparin also affects fibrinolysis and vascular endothelium. Thus, the single-targeted r-hirudin requires higher anti-factor IIa activity to achieve the same anticoagulant effect as the multiple-targeted heparin.

Recombinant hirudin showed a clear dose-response effect for anti-factor IIa activity (Fig. 8B). The two lower infusion doses showed a peak response from the bolus and a plateau at about one-half of the activity level of the bolus during CPB. Baseline was reached about 1 hour after CPB. For the highest infusion dose, the blood activity level began increasing after 30 minutes on pump because of the infusion and reached the bolus activity level at 60 minutes on pump. There was a loss of activity during the initial 30-minute pump time until the infusion took effect. Immediately after termination of the infusion (after CPB), the anti-factor IIa activity rapidly decreased to low levels within 30 minutes. However, this level of activity persisted up to 2 hours after CPB. There was a significant difference (p < 0.05) in response between the higher-dosed infusion group and the two lower-dosed infusion groups from 15 minutes on pump to 30 minutes after pump.

SUMMARY

The above study in a dog model of CPB evaluated the utility of r-hirudin as an anticoagulant to be used with extracorporeal circulation during cardiac surgery. Recombinant

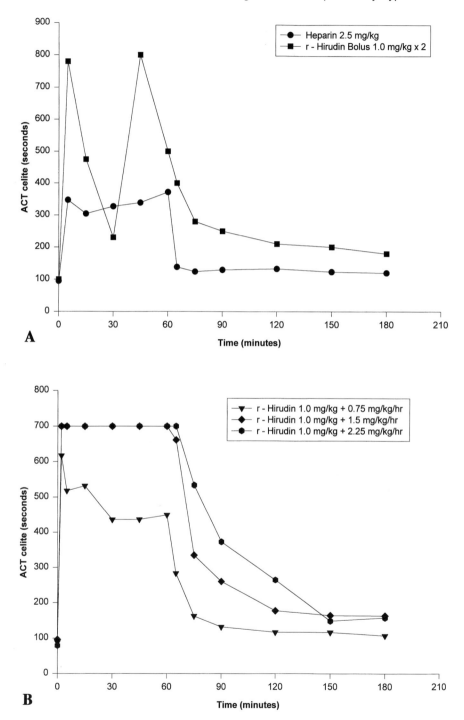

FIGURE 7. Celite activated clotting time (ACT) during the CPB perioperative period for *(A)* heparin (n = 6) vs. bolus-dosed r-hirudin (n = 10) as anticoagulant and *(B)* three doses of bolus plus infusion of r-hirudin as anticoagulant (n = 5/group).

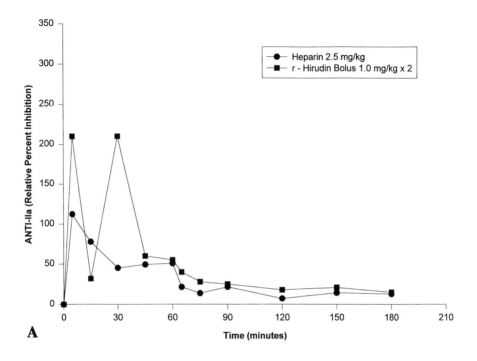

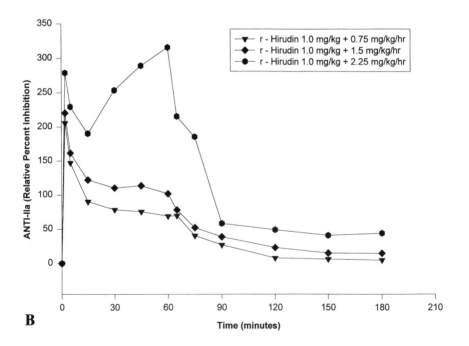

FIGURE 8.   Anti-factor IIa response during the CPB perioperative period for *(A)* heparin (n = 6) vs. bolus-dosed r-hirudin (n = 10) as anticoagulant and *(B)* three doses of bolus plus infusion of r-hirudin as anticoagulant (n = 5/group).

hirudin was well tolerated at all doses in all animals. In general, one could not distinguish animals treated with r-hirudin from animals treated with heparin with the following exceptions. Recombinant hirudin, when properly dosed, gave a more predictable anticoagulant response than heparin, with definitely less blood oozing from surgical incisions and greater hemodynamic stability after CPB. Hematocrit, platelet count, and fibrinogen tended to have a better recovery in the r-hirudin groups, and the bleeding time was less affected by r-hirudin.

A bolus-only administration, as used clinically for heparin, resulted in a marked "seesaw" effect of anticoagulation. For r-hirudin, the possibility of underdosing is too great by using a bolus-only approach. A bolus-plus infusion regimen was studied because of the short half-life of r-hirudin and the critical need for complete and continual anticoagulant protection during surgery. A bolus of 1.0 mg/kg with an infusion of about 1.0 mg/kg/hr or higher provided adequate anticoagulation in the canine model. An infusion of 0.75 mg/kg/hr was too low, as judged by enhanced filter deposits of clot-like substances, and an infusion of 2.25 mg/kg/hr was too high, as judged by the prolonged plasma activity (ACT and anti-factor IIa levels) after CPB. The infusion doses seem adequate to maintain a high drug concentration on pump and to allow rapid loss of activity after the infusion is terminated. The bolus dose, however, could probably be increased slightly (perhaps to 1.5 mg/kg) to avoid the fall in activity during the first 10 minutes on pump. This approach may decrease the filter deposits but should not prolong drug circulation after CPB. The safety index (bleeding) appeared to be rather large; higher doses of r-hirudin prolonged the time to clot of all assays but did not lead to increasing blood loss or oozing of blood from incision sites of the animals.

The ACT whole-blood clotting assay (celite-activated) is routinely used to monitor heparinization during CPB. This assay was incorporated to evaluate the feasibility of using the same system for r-hirudin. Although the ACT was too sensitive to detect blood levels of r-hirudin for the two higher (more effective) dosing groups during CPB, the ACT could be used to detect an underdose during surgery. In addition, it easily monitored postoperative blood levels of r-hirudin. Other clot-based assays (prothrombin time, activated partial thromboplastin time, thrombin clotting time), using whole blood or plasma, typically were too sensitive to measure the high level of activity (data not shown). The anti-factor IIa chromogenic assay revealed the strong, dose-dependent effect by r-hirudin. Unfortunately this is not a bedside assay.

At present there is no antagonist for r-hirudin comparable to protamine for heparin. Adequate dosing, therefore, must allow effective anticoagulation during CPB as well as elimination of antithrombin activity within 60 minutes postoperatively. Based on the above data, there appears to be no general necessity to have a pharmacologic agent or mechanical means to neutralize the anticoagulant effect of r-hirudin after CPB, provided that the dosing was adequate and regulated through the ACT or other blood assay. Because of its short half-life, r-hirudin is cleared rapidly from blood filtered through the kidneys, appearing in the urine (data not shown). If a higher-than-optimal dose of r-hirudin is used, or if kidney function is abnormal, the time-to-clot parameters will be prolonged, alerting the surgeon to the overdose. Yet because of the apparently wide safety index of r-hirudin, as shown in the dog model, a dramatic increase in blood loss would not be expected.

The study has limitations. It is not known precisely how the dog model compares with humans. In addition, the dog model used normothermic rather than hypothermic surgery, all animals were healthy, and no intense surgical manipulation was used (e.g., coronary artery bypass grafting with cardioplegia). Thus, although r-hirudin worked well in this model, it remains to be proved how unhealthy humans will respond.

The study shows that r-hirudin can be used with efficacy and safety in a dog model of CPB. This finding is clinically important because it indicates that alternatives to heparin are available for patients who have developed heparin-induced thrombocytopenia, who are allergic to protamine sulfate, or who have low levels of AT III. In addition, patients with the heparin rebound phenomenon, patients with platelet dysfunction, or patients who bleed excessively from heparin may better tolerate r-hirudin as an anticoagulant during cardiac surgery.

REFERENCES

1. Antman EM, for the TIMI 9A Investigators: Hirudin in myocardial infarction. Safety report from the thrombolysis and thrombin inhibition in myocardial infarction (TIMI) 9A trial. Circulation 90:1624–1630, 1994.
2. GUSTO IIA Investigators: Randomized trial of intravenous heparin versus recombinant hirudin for acute coronary syndromes. Circulation 90:1631–1637, 1994.
3. Haycraft JB: On the action of a secretion obtained from the medicinal leech on the coagulation of the blood. Proc Royal Soc Lond 36:478–487, 1884.
4. Iyer L: Pharmacokinetics and Pharmacodynamics of Recombinant Hirudin. Doctoral dissertation, Loyola University Chicago, 1995.
5. Iyer L, Fareed J. Recombinant hirudin: A perspective. Exp Opin Invest Drugs 5:469–494, 1996.
6. Markwardt F, Walsmann P: Die reaktion zwischen hirudin und thrombin. Hoppe-Seyler's Z Physiol Chem 312:85–98, 1958.
7. Markwardt F, Walsmann P. Reindarstellung und analyse des thrombin inhibitors hirudin. Hoppe-Seyler's Z Physiol Chem 348:1381-1386, 1967.
8. Markwardt F: Hirudin as an inhibitor of thrombin. Meth Enzymol 19:924–932, 1970.
9. Neuhaus K-L, Essen RV, Tebbe U, et al: Safety observations from the pilot phase of the randomized r-hirudin for improvement of thrombolysis (HIT-III) study. Circulation 90:1638–1642, 1994.
10. Rydel TJ, Ravichandran KG, Tulinsky A, et al:The structure of a complex of recombinant hirudin and human α-thrombin. Science 249:277-280, 1990.

CHAPTER 13

PEG-Hirudin Anticoagulation in Cardiopulmonary Bypass

JEANINE M. WALENGA, Ph.D.
MICHAEL J. KOZA, B.S., M.T. (ASCP)
MARK R. TERRELL, M.D.
ROQUE PIFARRÉ, M.D.

Cardiovascular disease is currently the major health risk in Western countries. In the United States it accounts for over 900,000 deaths annually, whereas cancer accounts for over 500,000 deaths annually.[6] Coronary heart disease (CHD) is the leading cause of death in adults. Diet control, exercise, change in lifestyle, and prescribed medication are used to reduce or control the disease. However, certain patients require more aggressive corrective measures, which may entail use of the cardiopulmonary bypass (CPB) pump for coronary artery graft placement. Technical advances have made this one of the more common operations performed today. The number of coronary artery bypass graft procedures in the U.S. more than tripled between 1991 and 1994.[1] The number of patients undergoing cardiac surgery in the U.S. is increasing yearly, including the number of patients needing first, second, and third reoperations as lifespan increases. Other indications for surgery with CPB include correction of congenital deficiencies, heart valve replacements, and heart/lung transplants.

During cardiac surgery with CPB it is necessary to use a high level of anticoagulation to keep the extracorporeal circuit free of blood clots. Heparin has been the only anticoagulant of choice for this indication. Disadvantages of heparin include variations in potency from lot to lot and in patient sensitivies. Heparin may also cause thrombocytopenia, arterial thrombosis, osteoporosis, platelet dysfunction, and severe bleeding. In addition, heparin rebound may cause postoperative bleeding, and in patients with a deficiency of the plasma inhibitor antithrombin III (AT III), heparin is ineffective. Furthermore, the use of protamine to neutralize heparin after CPB may be associated with side effects such as hypotension, anaphylaxis, respiratory compromise, and shock. The search for an alternative anticoagulant has not been completely successful.

Peptide inhibitors of serine proteases have been studied for application to hemostatic abnormalities for many years. The primary enzyme of the coagulation system in terms of kinetics of activity is thrombin. Thrombin is also the final product of the activated coagulation cascade, which directly acts on fibrinogen to convert it to fibrin (clot). It is, therefore, reasonable to consider specific thrombin inhibitors as anticoagulants, particularly for cases in which a major insult to blood—as in CPB (foreign surfaces, membrane oxygenators, filters, roller pumps, changes in fluid dynamics)—creates an optimal setting for thrombosis. The major advantages of specific thrombin inhibitors over heparin include:

- Purity of chemical structure and consistent lot-to-lot preparations
- Single mechanism of action as opposed to multiple sites of action for heparin (coagulation enzymes, platelets, fibrinolysis)
- No dependence on AT III or other plasma cofactors for expression of activity
- Limited platelet interactions (particularly advantageous for patients with heparin-induced thrombocytopenia)
- Used as alternative anticoagulants in patients in whom heparin is contraindicated
- Inhibition of bound and soluble thrombin
- Inhibition of thrombin-mediated platelet activation
- No inhibition by plasma proteins

Recent studies have focused on the development of alternative anticoagulants to replace heparin in cardiac surgery using CPB.[3,8,9] Hirudin, one of the first thrombin inhibitors, has been targeted for development as an antithrombotic drug since its isolation from the leech by Marwardt in 1957.[5] Biotechnology has made available the large quantitites needed for continued development. Early studies demonstrated that hirudin is an effective anticoagulant. Its use, however, was limited by its short half-life; hirudin could not be optimally administered as a single bolus in CPB.[2,8] PEG-hirudin is a variant of hirudin coupled to two molecules of polyethyleneglycol-5000 (molecular weight: 17,000 daltons); its half-life is 2–6-fold longer (depending on the animal model),[4,7] but it selectively inhibits thrombin with a similar potency.[4] We performed a single-bolus study to evaluate PEG-hirudin as an anticoagulant in cardiac surgery using CPB.

MATERIAL AND METHODS

Male mongrel dogs with a mean weight of 28 kg were sedated with xylazine (1.0 mg/kg intramuscularly) and anesthetized with pentobarbital (30 mg/kg intravenously). They were intubated and ventilated to a peak end-expiratory pressure of 2.5 cm on a Harvard ventilator (Harvard Apparatus, South Natick, MA). Vascular access lines were established in the left femoral vein and artery (for blood collection) and in the right femoral vein (for drug infusion) by indwelling catheters. Also established was a drip injection of lactated Ringer's solution.

After median sternotomy and pericardiotomy, the heart was suspended in a pericardial cradle with pursestring sutures placed in the ascending aorta and right atrial appendage. CPB was established with cannulation through the right atrial appendage and ascending aorta (70 ml/kg/min flow; 50–65 mmHg mean arterial pressure) using a Travenol roller pump (Travenol Labs, Inc., Ann Arbor, MI) and a variable prime Cobe membrane lung/ blood oxygenator (VPCML) (Cobe, Lakewood, CO) with surgical grade Tygon S-50-HL tubing (Norton Performance Plastics, Akron, OH; venous outflow tubing, $^3/_8$" inside diameter; arterial inflow tubing, $^1/_4$" inside diameter) and EC-3840 40-μm blood filters (Pall, East Hills, NY). The priming volume of the circuit was 1000 ml of lactated Ringer's solution. CPB was continued for 120 min. (mean temperature: 38°C), followed by a 120-minute postoperative observation period. The same surgical team was used for all experiments.

PEG-hirudin, 10,000 ATU/mg (Knoll AG, Ludwigshafen, Germany; lot 280100), was obtained in powdered form and reconstituted in saline to a stock concentration of 10.0 mg/ml immediately before use. Immediately before cannulation for CPB, PEG-hirudin was administered by single intracardiac injection directly into the right atrial space. The following dosing regimens were used: 0.75 mg/kg (n = 6), 1.00 mg/kg (n = 6), and 1.50 mg/kg (n = 6). Heparin bolus (2.5 mg/kg) was used in control animals (n = 4). Intravenous bolus injections of heparin were administered to maintain the activated clotting time (ACT) above 350 seconds during CPB, and protamine sulfate, 2.5 mg/kg, was used to reverse heparin after CPB.

Blood pressure and heart rate were continually monitored in the anesthetized dogs. Blood gases were periodically measured to ensure proper ventilation, and blood samples were periodically collected for immediate analysis of the following factors: hematocrit (manual method), platelet count (manual method read by one person), fibrinogen (Clauss technique; Dade, Miami, FL; performed on the Fibrometer), template bleeding time test on the buccal mucosa of the dog's upper lip (Simplate II; Organon Teknika, Durham, NC), and celite ACT (Hemochron; International Technidyne, Metuchen, NJ). Dog pooled plasma (300 mg/dl = normal) was used to construct a calibration curve for the fibrinogen assay.

Citrated plasma aliquots were maintained at 4°C until frozen (–70°C) for analysis on the following day. An in-house chromogenic substrate anti-factor IIa (thrombin) kinetic rate assay, specific for measuring the inhibition of thrombin, was also used. The results of the anti-IIa assay were reported as relative percent of thrombin inhibition based on the percent of inhibition of reagent thrombin and the dilution factor of the test sample. The chromogenic assay was performed on an ACL 300+ (Instrumentation Laboratory, Lexington, MA).

For assessment of efficacy, pump line filters were collected, washed with 1.0 L saline, and dried by forced air for 10 minutes immediately after the animal was removed from the pump. Deposits (clots) in the pump filters were measured by the Folin-Ciocalteu phenol fibrinogen/protein assay.

For assessment of safety, blood loss was measured by weight of aspirated blood collected from the chest cavity during the 120-minute postoperative observation period. Intraoperative blood loss was not used as a major endpoint, because variables other than the anticoagulant drug may contribute to blood loss. All incision sites (sternum, catheter sites) were observed perioperatively for oozing of blood. The abdominal cavity was explored for bleeding and clotting. All animals were sacrificed with supersaturated potassium chloride after the observation period.

These studies were conducted in the Animal Research Facilities of Hines Veterans Administration Hospital (Hines, IL), which is accredited by the American Association for the Accreditation of Laboratory Animal Care (AAALAC) in compliance with the National Institutes of Health *Guide for the Care and Use of Laboratory Animals.*

Statistical significance was determined by analysis of variance using the IBC compatible program Primer of Biostatistics (McGraw-Hill, New York). Results are represented as a mean ± 1 standard error of the mean; $p < 0.05$ was considered significant.

RESULTS

Postoperative blood loss (2 hours after CPB) was 14.0 ± 3.6 gm/kg for the 0.75 mg/kg dose, 16.2 ± 2.3 gm/kg for the 1.0 mg/kg dose, and 15.7 ± 2.6 gm/kg for the 1.5 mg/kg dose (Fig. 1). Compared with 9.7 ± 2.2 gm/kg for heparin, there was no significant difference between any treatment group and controls, although the trend for blood loss was higher for PEG-hirudin. There was no dose-dependent effect of PEG-hirudin on postoperative blood loss. There was less oozing of blood from surgical sites and an overall dry surgical field for PEG-hirudin compared with heparin.

Filter deposits were 37.5 ± 9.3, 17.5 ± 3.5, and 12.5 ± 2.0 mg, respectively, for the three PEG-hirudin doses of 0.75, 1.0, and 1.5 mg/kg (Fig. 2). A dose-dependent trend of anticoagulant efficacy by PEG-hirudin was observed. The 0.75 mg/kg dose of PEG-hirudin tended to provide less effective anticoagulation. However, in comparison with 11.3 ± 5.7 mg for heparin, there was no statistically significant difference between any treatment groups.

The celite ACT showed a dose-dependent effect, with the 1.5 mg/kg dose of PEG-hirudin exceeding the linear limits of the assay (> 700 seconds) throughout CPB (Fig. 3). The 1.0 mg/kg dose peaked at about 650 seconds during the first 60 minutes on pump and fell to about 350 seconds during the second 60 minutes on pump. The 0.75 mg/kg dose was similar in response to the 1.0 mg/kg dose, with slightly lower ACT values (peak = 600

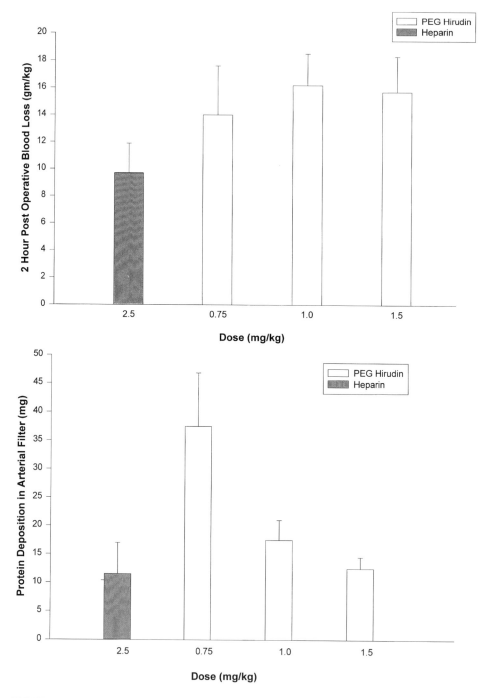

FIGURE 1 *(top).*   Blood loss from the thoracic cavity determined over the first 2 postoperative hours in a dog model of CPB.
FIGURE 2 *(bottom).*   Anticoagulant efficacy as determined by protein analysis of the arterial line filter. For both figures: pump time = 120 minutes (normothermic); results represent a mean ± SEM. There was no significant difference between groups (n = 6/group for PEG-hirudin; n = 4 for heparin).

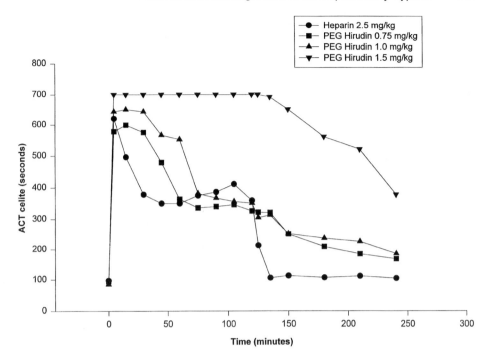

FIGURE 3.   Celite activated clotting time (ACT) values in a dog model during the 120-minute CPB period (normothermic) and during the 2-hour postoperative observation period. PEG-hirudin or heparin was administered as a single bolus immediately before cannulation for CPB; supplemental boluses of heparin were given to maintain the ACT > 350 seconds. Protamine sulfate was used to reverse heparin at termination of CPB. Results represent a mean of n = 6/group for PEG-hirudin and n = 4 for heparin.

seconds vs. 650 seconds) for the first 30 minutes on CPB. ACT values fell to about 325 seconds for the last 90 minutes on CPB. After termination of CPB the ACT for the 1.5 mg/kg dose slowly decreased to 378 seconds 2 hours postoperatively (baseline = 93 seconds). ACT values for the 1.0 and 0.75 mg/kg doses showed some decrease in activity after CPB to about 175 seconds by 2 hours postoperatively. The ACT for the heparin group immediately peaked at 600 seconds, rapidly fell to a plateau of about 400 seconds on CPB, and was maintained at that level with supplemental boluses of heparin. Baseline ACT values (mean = 105 seconds) returned after protamine neutralization of heparin (p < 0 .05 vs. all PEG-hirudin doses studied).

The chromogenic anti-IIa assay (Fig. 4), specific for PEG-hirudin quantitation in plasma, showed a dose-dependent effect of PEG-hirudin (p < 0.05 between PEG-hirudin doses). For all doses a rapid decline in activity was observed 30 minutes after CPB was initiated, with only a small loss of activity during the next 90 minutes on pump. At 2 hours after CPB, circulating dose-dependent drug levels remained. The 1.5 mg/kg dose peaked at 300% relative inhibition of thrombin (3-fold dilution required of plasma) and plateaued at 150% relative inhibition of thrombin. After terminating CPB, plasma levels slowly fell to 50% thrombin inhibition levels 2 hours later. The 1.0 mg/kg dose plateaued at 90% inhibition levels on pump and slowly fell after CPB to 35% inhibition 2 hours later. The 0.75 mg/kg dose plateaued at 65% inhibition on pump and slowly fell to 35% inhibition 2 hours after CPB. Heparin plateaued at 100% inhibition on pump and returned to 0% (baseline) after protamine neutralization (p < 0.05 vs. all PEG-hirudin doses studied).

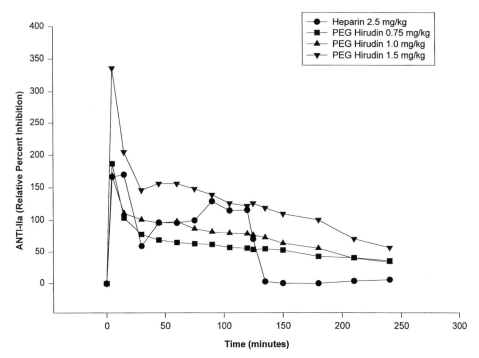

FIGURE 4.   Anti-IIa assay values in a dog model during the 120-minute CPB period (normothermic) and during the 2-hour postoperative observation period. PEG-hirudin or heparin was administered as a single bolus immediately before cannulation for CPB; supplemental boluses of heparin were given to maintain the ACT > 350 seconds. Protamine sulfate was used to reverse heparin at termination of CPB. Results represent a mean of n= 6/group for PEG hirudin and n = 4 for heparin.

Hematocrit (Fig. 5) and platelet count (Fig. 6) were not affected differently by treatment with PEG-hirudin or heparin. Hemodilution on CPB accounted for the observed decreases.

The fibrinogen levels (Fig. 7) appeared to be lower in the PEG-hirudin groups than in the heparin group. Because PEG-hirudin is a thrombin inhibitor, it interferes in the fibrinogen assay, which is a clot-based thrombin assay, producing falsely low levels of fibrinogen. Thus the actual protein content most likely was similar to that observed in the heparin group. The decrease in fibrinogen levels paralleled the anti-IIa assay results.

The bleeding time test (Fig. 8) showed a dose-dependent prolongation by PEG-hirudin. Heparin typically gives bleeding time values of > 900 seconds on CPB and returns to normal after protamine neutralization. The PEG-hirudin levels were less affected (peak on CPB = 538 ± 39 seconds for 0.75 mg/kg; 460 ± 76 seconds for 1.00 mg/kg; 709 ± 79 seconds for 1.50 mg/kg). The bleeding time values decreased 15 minutes after CPB, paralleling the drug levels. By 2 hours after CPB, the values were still slightly above normal for the 0.75 and 1.00 mg/kg groups (176 ± 12 seconds, 157 ± 15 seconds, respectively, vs. 111 seconds mean baseline) but even more elevated for the 1.50 mg/kg group (307 ± 22 seconds).

Other blood level monitors (prothrombin time, activated partial thromboplastin time, thrombin time, and Heptest on whole blood and plasma) were prolonged during PEG-hirudin anticoagulation with CPB but were too sensitive to be used for monitoring during CPB. Heart rate and blood pressure were stable in all but two animals. The decrease in heart rate and increase in blood pressure observed after intracardiac injection of PEG-hirudin (1.5 and 3.0 mg/kg) immediately self-corrected.

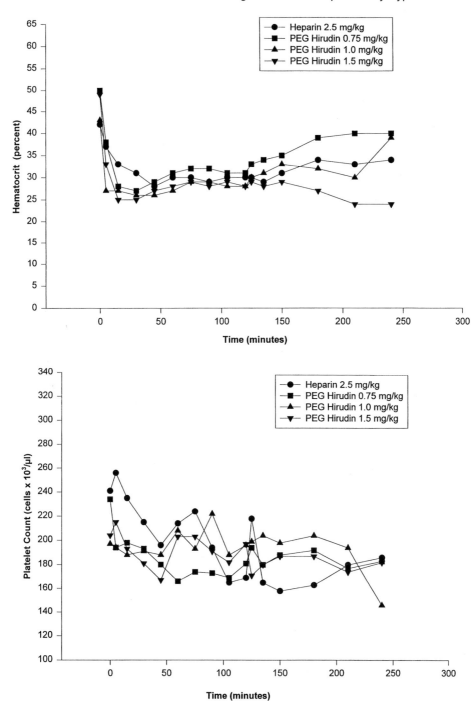

FIGURE 5 *(top).*   Hematocrit values.
FIGURE 6 *(bottom).*   Platelet count values. For both figures, values were assessed during the 120-minute CPB period and during the 2-hour postoperative observation period in a dog model (normothermic). Results represent a mean for n = 6/group for PEG-hirudin and n = 4 for heparin.

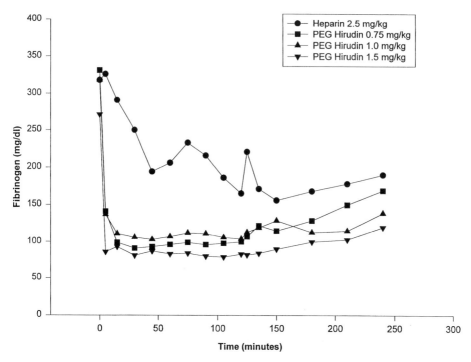

FIGURE 7. Fibrinogen values during the 120-minute CPB period and during the 2-hour postoperative observation period in a dog model (normothermic). Results represent a mean for n = 6/group for PEG-hirudin and n = 4 for heparin. The decrease in the PEG-hirudin groups reflects interference by the thrombin inhibitor in the fibrinogen assay.

DISCUSSION

This study was performed in a normal dog model (normothermic) of CPB as a first approach to evaluate the efficacy of PEG-hirudin as an anticoagulant for use with the extracorporeal circulation during cardiac surgery. A single bolus to the heart, as is used clinically with heparin, was the administration regimen. A dose-ranging study was performed.

The anticoagulant safety for all doses of PEG-hirudin studied, as determined by the 2-hour postoperative blood loss, was not significantly different from that obtained with heparin. There was no dose-dependent blood loss effect for PEG-hirudin. There was, however, a trend for higher blood loss in all PEG-hirudin groups than in the heparin group. But no oozing of blood from surgical incision sites was observed in the PEG-hirudin treated dogs (in contrast to the heparin-treated dogs), and there was a drier surgical field for PEG-hirudin treated than heparin-treated animals. These observations corresponded with the bleeding time test, which was less prolonged for PEG-hirudin than for heparin during CPB. In an additional study (n = 3), a 3.0 mg/kg dose of PEG-hirudin revealed no higher blood loss than the 1.5 mg/kg dose.

The anticoagulant efficacy, as determined by filter protein deposits (clots), appeared to be dose-dependent. The slightly higher deposits observed with the 0.75 mg/kg dose were not significantly different from the heparin response, although this finding indicates that a higher dose may be more efficacious. This response was largely due to an elevated filter deposit of 85 mg in one animal in the 0.75 mg/kg group. Filters obtained from heparin/human surgeries were at times found to have deposits up to 45 mg of protein. Thus, the 0.75 mg/kg PEG-hirudin dose may be effective. Nevertheless, a 0.50 mg/kg single bolus of PEG-hirudin (data not shown) had significantly higher filter clot deposits (425 ±

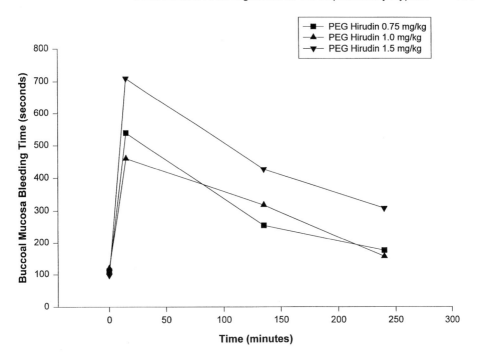

FIGURE 8.   Bleeding time results performed on the gingiva of the dogs during and after the 120-minute CPB period (normothermic). Results represent a mean of n = 6/group.

25 mg vs. 11 ± 6 mg for heparin; $p < 0.001$). The 1.0 and 1.5 mg/kg doses gave the same degree of clot deposit that was found in the heparin group.

The celite ACT, as used clinically for heparin, gave a useful dose-dependent response for PEG-hirudin. These data revealed individual animal sensitivities to anticoagulation with PEG-hirudin (e.g., ACT response of 300 to > 700 seconds for the same dose). Anticoagulation by the 0.75 mg/kg dose gave an ACT response that rapidly decreased to < 400 seconds within about 60 minutes on CPB. The higher dose of 1.50 mg/kg produced an elevated ACT response of > 700 seconds for the entire 2-hour CPB run, with elimination of PEG-hirudin beginning only after CPB was terminated. The ACT response, which seemed to correspond to adequate anticoagulation, was 650 seconds as achieved with 1.0 mg/kg PEG-hirudin during the initial 60 minutes on CPB. Taking the filter deposits into consideration along with the ACT response, the 1.0 and 1.5 mg/kg doses of PEG-hirudin, which gave filter deposits more similar to heparin, had ACT values ≥ 650 seconds as the initial response on CPB. The 0.75 mg/kg dose, which had ACT values closer to heparin during CPB, had higher filter clot deposits, indicating that the ACT for PEG-hirudin should be higher than it is for heparin to achieve good anticoagulation. New anticoagulants that have a mechanism different from heparin cannot be treated like heparin. ACT levels in relation to adequate anticoagulation need to be redefined for each new drug.

The chromogenic anti-IIa assay was also used to quantitate PEG-hirudin plasma levels. A clear dose-response was observed with plateau plasma levels averaging 100 and 200% relative thrombin inhibition (twice the maximum assay response determined with diluted plasma) during CPB. In comparison with the filter deposit data, plasma levels of ≥ 100% relative thrombin inhibition by PEG-hirudin were better for maintaining anticoagulation during CPB.

The single intracardiac bolus of PEG-hirudin was sufficient to anticoagulate for a 2-hour pump run. Even though the circulating drug level greatly decreased after 30 minutes on CBP, no rebolusing was needed. An initial high plasma level of activity was important to protect the blood during its first pass through the CPB circuit. This effect was obtained with the doses studied. However, lowering the dose caused a more rapid loss of activity during CPB, and increasing the dose prolonged the elimination time of PEG-hirudin. As shown by the ACT and anti-IIa assays, the 1.0 mg/kg dose did not lose activity as quickly as the 0.75 mg/kg dose, nor did it retain elevated values for an extended period after CPB termination, as the 1.5 mg/kg dose did. Thus, 1.0 mg/kg seemed to be the better dose in this animal model as studied by single bolus administration. Because there is no antagonist for PEG-hirudin, the elimination pattern is important.

In summary, in this first study of PEG-hirudin as an anticoagulant for cardiac surgery with CPB, effective anticoagulation without overdosing was obtained in a normal dog model at a dose of 1.0 mg/kg given as a single bolus. The response was generally similar to that of heparin with the exception of ACT values at 650 seconds (vs. 400 seconds for heparin) and an extended half-life after CPB, as observed by extended ACT, anti-IIa and bleeding time test values. Although PEG-hirudin remained in circulation after CPB, it did not lead to excessive blood loss or oozing in the dogs. The responses to anticoagulation varied among the animals. A single intracardiac bolus injection appeared adequate to maintain a plane of anticoagulation during a 2-hour pump run. Whether a high-plateau ACT level (i.e., $\geq$ 650 seconds) needs to be maintained throughout CPB or whether only the first 30–60 minutes are critical needs to be investigated. Infusion administration or rebolusing with PEG-hirudin during surgery may be considered to optimize maintenance of the target ACT/anti-IIa range without prolonged postoperative circulating levels.

This study in a normal dog model shows the potential usefulness of PEG-hirudin as an anticoagulant in CPB. Further studies are warranted to define optimal dosing regimens, effects of PEG-hirudin anticoagulation under hypothermia with full surgical technique, and perhaps effects in other species to predict a safe human dosing regimen.

Acknowledgment.   The authors express their gratitude to Yelena Khenkina and Scott Asselmeier for technical help with the animal model and Nick King, CCP, for expertise on CPB perfusion and help with the animal model.

REFERENCES

1. Annual Report of the National Data Base of the Society of Thoracic Surgeons, Chicago, IL, January 5, 1996.
2. Bakhos M, Walenga JM, Pifarré R, et al: Hirudin as an alternative anticoagulant to heparin in cardiopulmonary bypass. Surg Forum 41:289–291, 1990.
3. Chomiak PN, Walenga JM, Koza MJ, et al: Investigation of a thrombin inhibitor peptide as an alternative to heparin in cardiopulmonary bypass surgery. Circulation 88(Pt 2):407–412, 1993.
4. Fareed J, Walenga JM, Hoppensteadt D, et al: Comparative pharmacodynamics/pharmacokinetics of recombinant hirudin and its PEG-coupled derivatives in primates. Thromb Haemost 65:1286, 1991.
5. Markwardt F, Hauptmann J, Nowak G, et al: Pharmacological studies on the antithrombotic action of hirudin in experimental animals. Thromb Haemost 47:226–229, 1982.
6. National Center for Health Statistics and American Heart Association, 1991.
7. Rübsamen K, Hornberger W, Schweden J, Kurfürst M: Pharmacological characteristics of a long acting polyethyleneglycol-coupled recombinant hirudin (LU 56471). Thromb Haemost 65:571, 1991.
8. Walenga JM, Bakhos M, Messmore HL, et al: Potential use of recombinant hirudin as an anticoagulant in a cardiopulmonary bypass model. Ann Thorac Surg 51:271–277, 1991.
9. Walenga JM, Koza MJ, Park SJ, et al: Evaluation of CGP 39393 as the anticoagulant in cardiopulmonary bypass surgery in a dog model. Ann Thorac Surg 58:1685–1689, 1994.

Recombinant Hirudin as an Anticoagulant during Cardiac Surgery

FRIEDRICH-CHRISTIAN RIESS, M.D.
BERND POETZSCH, M.D.
GERT MUELLER-BERGHAUS, M.D.

Contact of flowing blood with the components of the heart-lung machine during cardiopulmonary bypass (CPB) leads to rapid activation of the clotting cascade. Therefore, high doses of unfractionated heparin are routinely used in CPB to avoid pump occlusion. However, the use of heparin by itself is associated with a number of adverse reactions, particularly bleeding, which occurs in about 5% of patients.[89] Bleeding complications are due in part to a direct inhibitory effect of heparin on platelets and to prolonged systemic anticoagulation, which is caused by reappearance of active heparin in the bloodstream 1–5 hours after adequate neutralization with protamine.[46]

In addition, heparin is contraindicated in patients with immune-mediated heparin-induced thrombocytopenia (HIT). HIT is characterized by the development of heparin-related and platelet-activating IgG-associated autoantibodies,[14,30,47,87] which are independent of both dose and route of administration.[45] As a result of intravascular platelet activation, within 5 or more days after beginning heparin therapy patients with HIT usually develop consumptive thrombocytopenia with platelet counts below 100×10^9/L or below 50% of the platelet value before the onset of heparin treatment.[7,41,74] Clinically, however, patients with HIT are at high risk of developing life-threatening arterial and venous thrombosis, which may result in myocardial infarction, stroke, and limb ischemia,[5,15,16,59,75] as the result of intravascular platelet aggregation.[15,74] Several laboratory tests[3,29,73] facilitate the diagnosis of HIT, but presently there is no reliable method to predict which patients are predisposed to develop HIT.[74] HIT is associated with high mortality rates of 23–29%.[41,44] Bleeding is rarely a problem in HIT, even in the immediate postoperative period. Moreover, another 5% of these patients develop adverse reactions to the heparin antagonist protamine.[82] Thus, although heparin has been useful in facilitating CPB and is at present the only anticoagulant in worldwide use for CPB, it is not the ideal anticoagulant for CPB.

Of interest, hirudin was the first drug to be used as an anticoagulant in hemodialysis in an animal model and in humans at the beginning of this century.[1] Hirudin is an anticoagulant naturally present in the salivary secretion of the leech (*Hirudo medicinalis*).[33] Its anticoagulation potency was first described by Haycraft[34] in 1884, and it was isolated and characterized as a direct thrombin inhibitor in the 1950s by Markwardt.[48,49] Recombinant (r) hirudin, which is genetically expressed in *Escherichia coli* bacteria and yeast (*Saccharomyces cerevisiae*), is now available for clinical use. Compared with native hirudin, all of the recombinant versions lack the sulphate on the tyrosine 63 residue.[54,78] The anticoagulant activity of r-hirudin, however, is identical to the 7,000-Da native protein.[52,69,78]

Recombinant hirudin forms a tight 1:1 complex with thrombin and thereby occupies the putative fibrinogen-binding site and blocks the catalytic site of thrombin.[21,32,77] As a result, all of the thrombin-catalyzed reactions, such as conversion of fibrinogen to fibrin, activation of factors V, VIII, XIII, and thrombin-induced platelet activation, are diminished. Several in vitro studies have shown that r-hirudin is 3–5-fold more potent than heparin, as determined by the activated partial thromboplastin time (APTT) and chromogenic anti-FIIa-assays.[6,84] This finding may explain the greater antithrombotic potency of r-hirudin in various animal models.[35,36,43,67] In this respect, the ability of r-hirudin to neutralize not only free but also clot-bound thrombin may be of particular importance. The data obtained in the animal model are supported by recently published data of a double-blind, randomized, large-scale trial in patients scheduled for coronary angioplasty.[72] The test group received r-hirudin, which was given as a bolus followed by an intravenous infusion for 24 hours, whereas the control group was treated with heparin. The incidence of early (< 196 hours after the beginning of treatment) major adverse cardiac events was significantly reduced (p < 0.01) in the hirudin-treated group.[72]

These experimental and clinical data prompted us to postulate that r-hirudin could be a useful alternative to heparin in cardiac surgery. To test this possibility, we performed two series of experiments using a porcine model of CPB[54,62] to determine whether successful CPB could be achieved with r-hirudin, and if so, to determine whether its use had any potential benefit over the more convential heparin treatment. In addition, we studied the potential use of hemofiltration to achieve rapid and safe elimination of r-hirudin from the circulation.[65]

Based on experiences obtained in the animal model, we were able to perform cardiac operations successfully in 5 patients suffering from HIT using r-hirudin as an anticoagulant during CPB instead of heparin.[63,64,66]

PIG MODEL OF CARDIOPULMONARY BYPASS

Animals. The pig was used as an animal model because of the similarity of its heart to the human heart.[38] The minipigs are especially suitable for animal experimentation because they are easy to keep, reach maturity quickly, and are big enough for catheterization, intubation, and adequate blood samples.[42] Moreover, pigs appear to be a good model for the study of anticoagulation, because platelet response in pigs approximates that in humans and initial proliferative lesions in pigs resemble those in humans.[43,71]

Experimental Design. Eighteen fully grown, 18-month-old Goettingen minipigs were anesthetized and ventilated.[62] After median sternotomy CPB was initiated with a flow rate of 70 ml/kg of body weight/min. A membrane oxygenator (VP-CML, Cobe Laboratories, Lakewood, CO) and an arterial filter (AF 10/40; pore size: 40 μm; American Bentley, Irvine, CA) were used. The body temperature was lowered to 27.9 ± 1.1°C (26–30°C), and the ascending aorta was cross-clamped. After the heart had been arrested by 10 ml/kg of a cold (4° C) crystalloid cardioplegic solution,[11] standard surgical procedures were performed during the phase of cardiac arrest lasting 30.6 ± 1.5 min (28–34 min). After rewarming, the heart was resuscitated and deaired. Reperfusion was continued to a total bypass time of 65.8 ± 4.2 min (60–74 min). At the end of CPB neither heparin nor r-hirudin was antagonized or removed. After a further 2-hour observation period, the animals were sacrificed with an intravenous injection of 20 ml of saturated potassium chloride solution.

Anticoagulation Protocols. The animals were randomly divided into three groups and treated by three different anticoagulation protocols (Fig. 1). Animals of group A (controls, n = 6) received a standard regimen of an initial intravenous bolus injection of

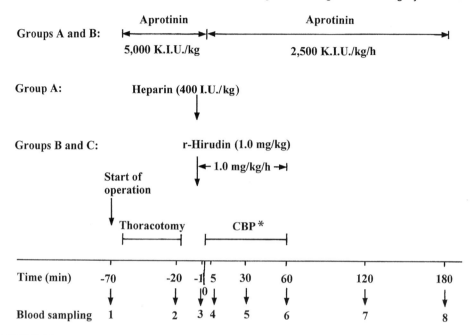

FIGURE 1. Experimental study using the pig model to compare the anticoagulatory effects of r-hirudin with heparin during cardiopulmonary bypass (CPB). The various groups were defined as follows: animals in group A were given a single injection of heparin before CPB, whereas animals in groups B and C were given a bolus of r-hirudin before CPB followed by a continuous infusion during CPB. In addition to heparin or r-hirudin, animals in groups A and B were treated with high doses of aprotinin during CPB. * Group A received 4.0 IU/ml of heparin in the priming solution, and groups B and C received 5.0 μg/ml of r-hirudin. In groups A and B, 5000 KIU/kg of aprotinin was added to the priming solution.

400 IU/kg of heparin (Hoffmann-La Roche, Basel, Switzerland) five minutes before the start of CPB, and 4 IU/ml of heparin was added to the priming solution. To lower the intraoperative and postoperative risk of bleeding,[19,20,27,28,68] a short infusion of 5,000 kallikrein inhibitor units (KIU)/kg of aprotinin (Antagosan, Behringwerke AG, Marburg, Germany) was initiated after tracheostomy and continued until the start of CPB. An infusion of 2,500 KIU/kg/hr of aprotinin was administered from the beginning of CPB until the end of the experiment. In addition, 5,000 KIU/kg of aprotinin was added to the priming solution. Animals of group B (n = 5) received an initial intravenous bolus (1.0 mg/kg) of r-hirudin (HBW 023, Behringwerke AG, Marburg, Germany) five minutes before the start of CPB, followed by an infusion of 1.0 mg/kg/hr until the end of CPB. R-hirudin (5.0 μg/ml) was added to the priming solution. Aprotinin was administered to group B as well as to group A. The animals of group C (n = 7) received the same r-hirudin regimen as group B but with saline instead of aprotinin.

Surgical Procedures. The ascending aorta and the left atrium were opened in the same manner as for aortic or mitral valve replacement, which actually was not performed. The left ventricle was opened at the apex by a 3-cm myotomy. All incisions were closed by continuous 5-0 sutures during cardiac arrest. The bleeding tendency during and after open heart surgery was low in all three groups. Only 15–25 ml of blood was collected from the pericardial cavity in the 2-hour period after CPB with no statistically significant difference among the three groups. All surgical procedures were carried out with no problems in all three groups. In particular, there was no oozing of blood from the cut tissues (skin, sternum, ventricular muscle) during the entire operation in any animal.

TABLE 1.   Tissue Bleeding in Histologic Examination in the Minipig Model of CPB*

Group	n	Number of Animals with Organ Tissue Bleeding				
		0	1	2	3	4–12
A Heparin/aprotinin[†]	6	0	3	2	1	0
B r-Hirudin/aprotinin[†]	5	3	2	0	0	0
C r-Hirudin/saline	7	5	0	0	2	0

* Investigated organs: brain, eyes, lung, right atrium, left ventricle, liver, spleen, pancreas, kidneys, adrenal glands, gut, and urinary bladder.
[†] The difference between group A and group B was statistically significant (p < 0.05).

Autopsy and Histology.   The abdomen, both pleural cavities, and the skull were opened and inspected for bleeding and clot formation. Subepicardial hemorrhages were found to be more pronounced in the heparin/aprotinin group than in the r-hirudin/aprotinin and r-hirudin/saline groups. Confluent petechial hemorrhages of the pericardium were found only in animals of the heparin/aprotinin group. In each animal samples were taken from 12 different organs (brain, eyes, lungs, right atrium, left ventricle, liver, spleen, pancreas, kidneys, adrenal glands, gut, and urinary bladder). From each organ four specimens were taken, coded, and sent to a pathologist. Two sections (measuring 1 cm by 1 cm) from each organ were stained with hematoxylin and eosin and completely investigated. No thrombi or tissue bleedings were macroscopically visible in any of the animals except for the petechial hemorrhages in the subepicardium and pericardium. However, a statistically significant (p < 0.05) higher amount of tissue bleedings were found in group A (heparin/aprotinin) than in group B (r-hirudin/aprotinin) (Table 1). These findings may be explained by the better preserved platelet function in animals treated with r-hirudin.

Monitoring of r-Hirudin Plasma Concentration.   Plasma concentrations of r-hirudin were measured with an anti-FIIa assay. Five minutes after the initial bolus injection, plasma levels of r-hirudin reached concentrations between 4.2 and 10.4 µg/ml (mean: 6.7 ± 2.5 µg/ml) in group B animals and between 4.4 and 7.2 µg/ml (mean : 5.7 ± 0.9 µg/ml) in group C animals. Values remained constant during the r-hirudin infusion and decreased in each animal after the end of the hirudin infusion (Fig. 2A). There was no statistically significant difference in r-hirudin plasma concentration between the r-hirudin/aprotinin and r-hirudin/saline groups, indicating that plasma concentrations of r-hirudin were not influenced by aprotinin.

Monitoring of Anticoagulation by APTT and Activated Clotting Time.   Administering either r-hirudin or heparin led to an increase in APTT values (Behringwerke AG, Marburg, Germany) in all animals from 15–25 seconds at baseline to > 120 seconds (Fig. 2B). One and two hours after CPB the APTT values were approximately 40 seconds in the r-hirudin/aprotinin and r-hirudin/saline groups, whereas the APTT values in the heparin/aprotinin group were > 120 seconds until the end of the experiment. These differences were statistically significant (p < 0.05 and p < 0.01, respectively). At the end of the r-hirudin infusion, the APTT and activated clotting time (ACT) did not reach the initial values within the 2-hour observation period. In contrast to these findings, Walenga and coworkers reported that in the dog model all coagulation variables had returned to low levels within 30 minutes after the end of the r-hirudin infusion, but that some anti-FIIa-activity persisted as long as 2 hours after CPB.[86] This may be explained by a higher glomerular filtration rate of r-hirudin in dogs (about 95%).[55] The administration of both heparin and aprotinin prolonged ACT, as measured in whole blood (Hemochron; International Technidyne, Edison, NJ), from values of approximately 100 seconds to > 2,000 seconds (Fig. 2C). The ACT values decreased after the end of r-hirudin infusion during the 2-hour-period after CPB to mean values of approximately 400 seconds in all three groups, with no statistically significant difference.

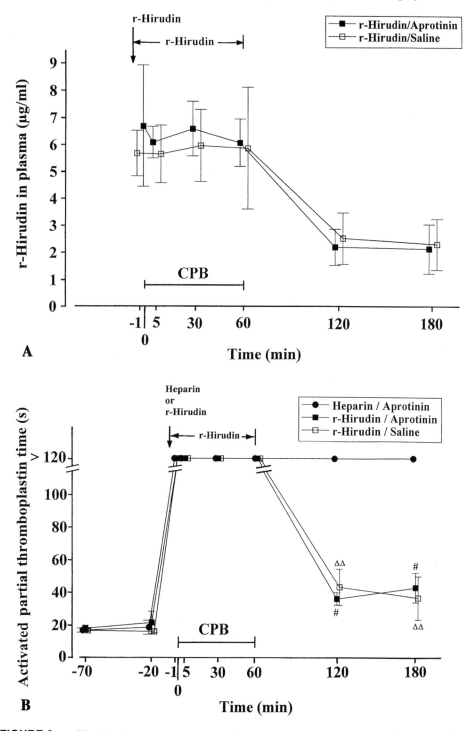

FIGURE 2. r-Hirudin plasma concentration *(A)* and activated partial thromboplastin time *(B)* before, during, and after CPB in pigs treated with heparin/aprotinin, r-hirudin/aprotinin, and r-hirudin/saline. *(Figure continued on next page.)*

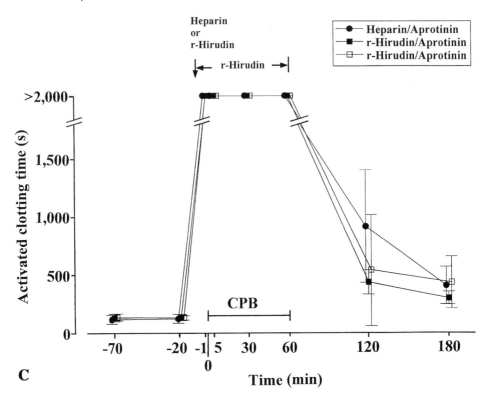

FIGURE 2 *(Continued).*   *C,* Activated clotting time before, during, and after CPB in pigs treated with heparin/aprotinin, r-hirudin/aprotinin, and r-hirudin/saline. Statistically significant differences among the three groups were determined by the exact version of the Wilcoxon-Mann-Whitney two-sample test. All values are expressed as mean ± standard deviation. # = heparin/aprotinin vs. r-hirudin/aprotinin groups; Δ = heparin/aprotinin vs. r-hirudin/saline groups. One or two marks indicate $p < 0.05$ or $p < 0.01$, respectively.

Platelet Count and Platelet Function.   There was no statistically significant difference in the changes in platelet counts between the heparin/aprotinin-treated and the r-hirudin/aprotinin-treated pigs (Fig. 3). The abrupt drop at the start of CPB is caused by hemodilution; the values do not indicate either bleeding or intravascular coagulation. Platelet aggregation was measured with a dual channel automated platelet aggregometer (LAbor, Ahrensburg, Germany) as follows: 180 µl of platelet-rich plasma (with platelet count adjusted to 100,000 µl) was placed into a plastic cuvette and stirred at 1,000 rpm at 37° C, and aggregation was initiated by adding 20 µl of aggregating agents. ADP (Sigma Chemical, München, Germany) and collagen (Hormon Chemie, München, Germany) were used. ADP was used in three different final concentrations of 0.5, 2.5, and 5.0 µM, respectively, and collagen was used in final concentrations of 1.0 and 2.0 µg/ml, respectively. The ADP- and collagen-induced platelet aggregation remained normal after administration of r-hirudin and before CPB, supporting the in vitro finding that r-hirudin does not influence platelet function.[10,23,25,26,50] After a CPB time of 60 minutes, the ADP- and collagen-induced platelet aggregation was found to be superior (statistically significant, $p < 0.01$ and $p < 0.05$) in animals treated with r-hirudin/aprotinin or r-hirudin/saline in comparison to animals treated with heparin/aprotinin (Fig. 4).

Cardiopulmonary Bypass.   Clot formation could not be detected in the heart-lung machine (HLM) during or after CPB in any animal of the three groups. This finding correlates

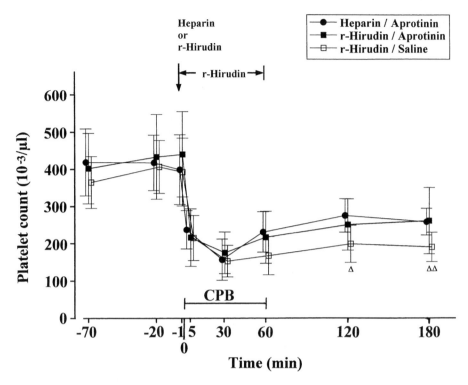

FIGURE 3.   Change in platelet count before, during, and after CPB in pigs. Statistically significant differences among the groups were determined by the exact version of the Wilcoxon-Mann-Whitney two-sample test. All values are expressed as mean ± standard deviation. Δ = heparin/aprotinin vs. r-hirudin/saline groups. One or two marks indicate $p < 0.05$ or $p < 0.01$, respectively.

with the observation that the inlet pressure of the oxygenator remained constant during the entire pump-time in all animals. The pressure varied between 140–400 mmHg, according to the flow rate of CPB and the size of the arterial cannula. There was no statistically significant difference among the three groups. The filter membranes of the cardiotomy reservoir and the arterial filter were fixed in glutaraldehyde (2%), then coded and sent to a pathologist for examination. Two 1 cm by 1 cm pieces from each membrane were completely examined. Scans of the filter membranes with an electronmicroscope showed red cells with no fibrin deposits in animals treated with r-hirudin/saline and r-hirudin/aprotinin (Fig. 5A). In contrast, small blood clots consisting of red cells and fibrin strands could be detected in all filter membranes from animals treated with heparin (Fig. 5B). These results demonstrate that the r-hirudin regimen used in our experiments was adequate to inhibit completely thrombin formation in minipigs. This result contrasts with the findings of Walenga et al.,[85,86] who used the same bolus dose of r-hirudin (1 mg/kg) but an infusion of 0.75 mg/kg/hr in the dog model of CPB and found a higher amount of protein deposits in the HLM filter membranes of r-hirudin-treated animals than in the filter membranes of dogs treated with heparin. However, when an infusion regimen of 1.5 mg/kg or higher was used, there were no differences in clot deposit from heparin-treated animals. Another explanation for this finding may be different pharmacokinetics in the two species. In particular, in our pig experiments r-hirudin plasma concentrations as high as 6 µg/ml could be measured as a result of the slow renal excretion of only 20% in pigs[52] compared with 95% in dogs.[55]

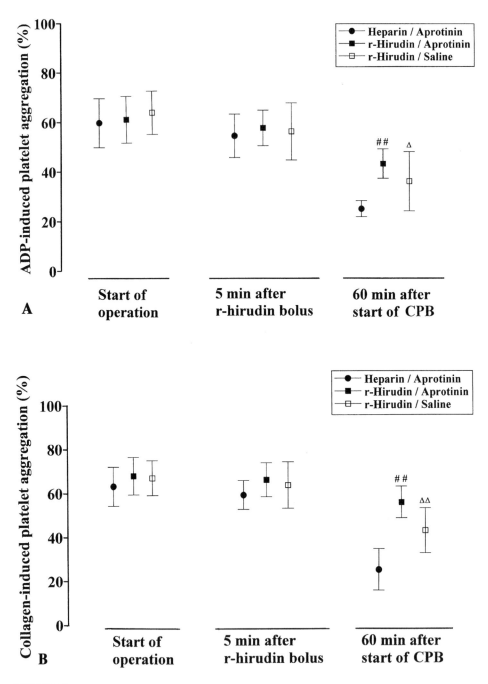

FIGURE 4. Platelet aggregation in heparin/aprotinin-, r-hirudin/aprotinin-, and r-hirudin/saline-treated pigs induced by adenosine diphosphate *(A)* or collagen *(B)*. Statistically differences among the three groups were determined by the exact version of the Wilcoxon- Mann-Whitney two-sample test. All values are expressed as mean ± standard deviation. # = heparin/aprotinin vs. r-hirudin/aprotinin groups; Δ = heparin/aprotinin vs. r-hirudin/saline groups. One or two marks indicate p < 0.05 or p < 0.01, respectively.

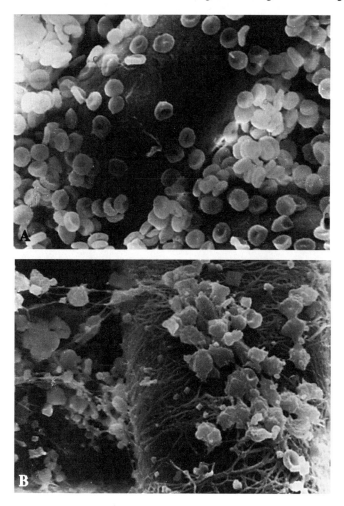

FIGURE 5.   Scanning electronmicrographs of oxygenator membranes. CPB was carried out for 1 hour with r-hirudin *(A)* or heparin *(B)* anticoagulation.

HEMOFILTRATION STUDY IN THE PIG MODEL

   The Question of an Antidote.   Presently no antidote is clinically available to reverse the anticoagulatory effect of r-hirudin. There may be no need to neutralize the anticoagulant activity in patients with normal renal function because of the short half-life of r-hirudin in humans (1–4 hr).[52] However, in case of accidental overdosing or other emergency situations, rapid reversal of the anticoagulant effect may be necessary. Theoretically, reversal could be achieved by the administration of a specific antidote, by enhancing the rate of endogenous thrombin production, or by removal of r-hirudin. Nowak and Bucha[57] have demonstrated that meizothrombin, an intermediate of the prothrombin activation pathway that binds to hirudin but possesses only moderate procoagulant activity, is an effective antidote. To date, however, meizothrombin is not available for clinical use, and it is not clear whether the administration of meizothrombin, which can be rapidly activated to thrombin, will cause thrombotic complications. Desmopressin and recombinant factor VII have been shown to reduce the bleeding time after administration of high doses of r-hirudin in rats by

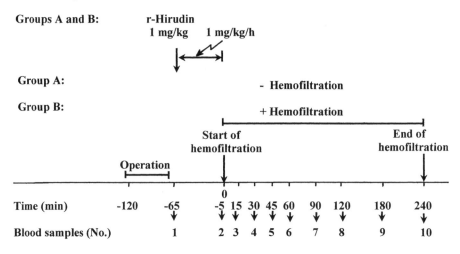

FIGURE 6.   Experimental hemofiltration study using the nephrectomized pig after application of r-hirudin as a bolus injection and infusion therapy. Pigs in group B were hemofiltered for 4 hours. Pigs in group A served as controls and were not hemofiltered.

enhancing the amount of thrombin formation.[13,39] The use of desmopressin, however, is associated with loss of sodium and tachycardia and is therefore restricted in patients undergoing cardiac operations. Because r-hirudin has been reported to penetrate the cellulose acetate filter membrane of a capillary dialyzer[12] with a cut-off point of 50,000 Da, we examined whether hemofiltration might be useful in removing r-hirudin from the circulation in emergency situations. The study was conducted on nephrectomized pigs.[65]

Experimental Design.   Eight fully grown, 18-month-old Goettingen minipigs were anesthetized and ventilated. Hemofiltration catheters were put into the right carotid artery and the internal jugular vein. Functional bilateral nephrectomy was performed by median laparotomy, which was carried out with no problems in all animals. A bolus intravenous injection of r-hirudin (1 mg/kg) was administered to all animals, followed by an intravenous infusion of 1 mg/kg/hr. The animals were randomly divided and treated according to one of two protocols (Fig. 6). Pigs of group A (controls, n = 4) were not hemofiltered, and an electrolyte solution of 150 ml/hr was substituted. In animals of group B (n = 4) the extracorporeal circuit containing a hemofilter (Haemoflow F 60 S, Fresenius AG, Bad Homburg, Germany) was connected to the catheters and arteriovenous hemofiltration was initiated. The flow through the hemofilter was adjusted between 50– 140 ml/min to yield 4 L of hemofiltrate each hour over a total of 4 hours. Volume substitution was performed according to the central venous blood pressure, measured continuously in the right atrium. Blood samples and probes of the hemofiltration fluid were taken at defined time points (Fig. 6). After a hemofiltration period, lasting a maximum of 4 hours, the animals were sacrificed with an intravenous injection of 20 ml of saturated protassium chloride solution, and an autopsy was performed on each animal.

R-Hirudin Plasma Concentrations and APTT.   A total r-hirudin dose of 2 mg/kg was administered intravenously in combined bolus-infusion therapy in the 4 animals of group B with a mean body weight of 32.5 ± 3.1 kg (28.3–35.5 kg). The mean total amount of r-hirudin was 64.9 ± 5.4 mg (56.6–71.0 mg) (Table 2). From this total amount a mean of 44.0 ± 9.3 mg (30.7–53.9 mg) or 68.0 ± 15.8 % (45–80%) was removed by hemofiltration that was continued for 183.8 ± 58.5 minutes (105–240 min). The amount of r-hirudin in the hemofiltration fluid was determined by the method of Griessbach et al.[31] A mean of 12.5 ± 4.8 L of an electrolyte solution was substituted on the basis of right arterial pressures,

TABLE 2. Hemofiltration in the Minipig Model After Administration
of a Total r-Hirudin Dose of 2 mg/kg

| | Animal Number | | | | |
	1	2	3	4	Mean ± SD
Total amount of administered r-hirudin (mg)	71.0	56.6	68.0	64.0	64.9 ± 5.4
Total time of hemofiltration (min)	240	150	105	240	183.8 ± 58.5
Total amount of r-hirudin in hemofiltrate (mg)	53.9	40.1	30.7	51.3	44.0 ± 9.3
Flow through hemofilter (ml/min)	100–140	50–70	60–100	120–140	—
First clots in hemofiltration circuit (min)	30	110	60	140	85 ± 42.7
APTT baseline prior to r-hirudin (sec)	15.4	15.7	15.3	16.3	15.7 ± 0.4
APTT at start of hemofiltration (sec)	> 200	> 200	> 200	> 200	—
APTT at end of hemofiltration (sec)	25.6	26.7	30.4	24.3	26.8 ± 2.3

APTT = activated partial thromboplastin time.

which ranged from 4–7 mmHg. The mean APTT values in both groups were about 16 seconds before administration of r-hirudin, increased rapidly to values over 200 seconds after bolus application of r-hirudin, and remained at this level in the animals of group A until the end of the experiment (Fig. 7A). In contrast, a rapid decrease of APTT values to a mean of 34.5 ± 5.9 seconds after 60 minutes and 26.8 ± 2.3 seconds after 240 minutes could be observed directly after the beginning of hemofiltration. The plasma concentration of r-hirudin correlated well with the rapid decrease of APTT values. In animals of group B, a mean r-hirudin plasma concentration of 7.95 ± 1.28 µg/ml was measured at the beginning of hemofiltration. After 30 minutes of hemofiltration the free r-hirudin plasma concentration was 4.46 ± 1.01 µg/ml and after 240 minutes 1.53 ± 0.31 µg/ml. In contrast, the r-hirudin plasma concentration in animals that were not hemofiltrated (group A) was 8.64 ± 0.26 µg/ml and remained almost constant during the comparable 240-minute period (Fig. 7B).

Platelet Count.   An immediate decrease of platelets as a result of the r-hirudin administration could not be observed in either group. The number of platelets in animals of group B decreased to about 80% and 60% of the initial values after 60 minutes and 240 minutes of hemofiltration, respectively, obviously because of activation by the artificial surfaces of the hemofiltration circuit.[22] In group A the number of platelets decreased only to 80% of the initial values in a comparable 240-minute period without hemofiltration.

Hemofiltration Circuit.   As a result of the removal of r-hirudin and the decreasing r-hirudin plasma levels, the first clots in the hemofiltration system were observed in a time period ranging from 30 to 140 minutes after the start of hemofiltration. Within this range the free r-hirudin plasma concentrations measured between 25% and 50% of the initial concentrations, indicating that the artificial surfaces of the extracorporeal circuit require higher doses of r-hirudin than the doses needed for prevention of venous thrombosis.[10,12,51] The pressure prior to the hemofilter was 70–130 mmHg at the beginning of hemofiltration and increased to values > 400 mmHg (0.6 kp/cm²) after 60–95 minutes in 3 of 4 animals of group B, obviously because of clot formations. After hemofiltration was completed, clot formations were detected in hemofilters and blood filters in all experiments. No macroscopical clots were observed in any of the animals, and no hint of cardiopulmonary embolism with right heart insufficiency could be observed. Nevertheless, in one animal a very small, nonadherent thrombus was detected in a capillary vessel of the lung in the histologic examination and may have been an embolus rising from the hemofilter circuit as a result of decreasing r-hirudin plasma concentrations. One should consider this fact when using hemofiltration for r-hirudin removal in humans, because a sudden decrease of the r-hirudin plasma level may lead to thromboembolic complications. In all other histologic examinations no thromboembolic complications were observed.

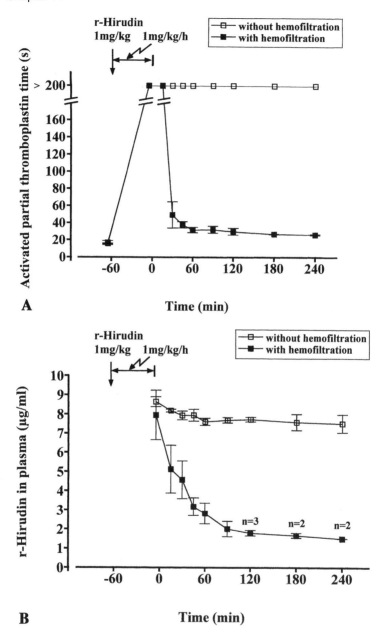

FIGURE 7.   Course of the activated partial thromboplastin time *(A)* and the free r-hirudin concentration *(B)* in nephrectomized pigs treated with r-hirudin, followed by 4-hour hemofiltration (group B). Four animals were not hemofiltered and served as controls (group A).

FIRST EXPERIENCES IN PATIENTS

Characteristics of Study Patients.   Five patients (2 men, 3 women; age: 69–78 years; weight: 54–66 kg) were admitted from other hospitals with the diagnosis of coronary heart disease (patients 1, 4, and 5) or aortic valve stenosis (patients 2 and 3) (Table 3). All patients had a clinical history of HIT, which was confirmed by a positive heparin-induced platelet

TABLE 3. Clinical Data for Patients Treated with r-Hirudin and CPB

	Patient Number				
	1	2	3	4	5
Sex	F	F	M	M	F
Age (years)	72	72	73	78	69
Weight (kg)	54	58	66	58	65
Confirmation of HIT	HIPAA	HIPAA	HIPAA	HIPAA	HIPAA
Preoperative hemoglobin (g/dl)	12.1	12.7	11.6	12.4	10.9
Creatinine (mg/dl)	1.0	0.9	0.9	1.7	1.1
Bilirubin (mg/dl)	0.4	0.7	1.1	2.1	0.3
Medical history	Calcification of ascending aorta	Deep pelvic thrombosis		Deep pelvic thrombosis, right heart failure	Generalized atherosclerosis with bilateral carotid artery stenosis
Indication for surgery	CAD	AS	AS	CAD, post-infarction VSD	CAD

HIT = heparin-induced thrombocytopenia, HIPAA = heparin-induced platelet aggregation assay, CAD = coronary artery disease, AS = aortic stenosis, VSD = ventricular septal defect.

aggregation assay (HIPAA). Because none of the patients received heparin in the preoperative period, platelet counts were in the range of $124–171 \times 10^9$/L. On admission patients 2 and 4 were taking coumarin for anticoagulation, because both had a medical history of deep pelvic thrombosis during an acute episode of HIT. In patient 2 oral anticoagulation was stopped 3 days before surgery, and anticoagulation with r-hirudin was initiated by administration of a single bolus (0.2 mg/kg), followed by an APTT-adjusted regimen starting with an infusion of 0.1 mg/kg/hr of r-hirudin. APTT values between 60–80 seconds and r-hirudin plasma levels of 1.0–1.5 µg/ml were defined as target ranges. To keep the APTT within this target range, we had to reduce the r-hirudin infusion to < 1.0 mg/kg/hr in the course of 3 days. This underlines the necessity of adjusted APTT control during r-hirudin therapy to avoid accumulation and bleeding complications, as described in TIMI 9A[4] and GUSTO IIa[79] studies, which were not APTT-adjusted.[17] Patient 2 responded well to the preoperative intravenous r-hirudin therapy, and no bleeding complications were observed. In patient 4 the operation had to be performed urgently because of life-threatening and progradient right-heart failure caused by a postinfarction ventricular septal defect (VSD) with a shunt volume of 70%. Therefore, oral anticoagulation could not be stopped before surgery, and the patient showed an international normalized ratio (INR) of 3.6 at the beginning of CPB. The patient also showed signs of congestion with impaired liver (bilirubin: 2.1 mg/dl) and kidney (creatinine: 1.7 mg/dl) function.

Intraoperative Management and Surgical Procedures.   Standard monitoring of cardiac surgery was performed, including measurement of arterial and central venous blood pressures, electrocardiography, pulse oximetry, capnography, urine output, and rectal and nasopharyngeal temperatures. After intubation a controlled positive pressure ventilation (FiO_2: 0.35–0.5) was initiated. Anesthesia was maintained with an intravenous infusion of propofol and sufentanyl and a single bolus injection of pancuronium bromide. A capillary membrane oxygenator (BARD 5701 or Cobe Optime) was used in all cases. The priming solution of CPB (1450–2000 ml) contained lactated Ringer's solution, mannitol (15%), and sodium bicarbonate. Because of the low hemoglobin value in 4 patients (see Table 3), packed red cells were added to the priming solution (Table 4). Standard CPB was established with a flow rate of 2.3–3.1 L/min/m², which was reduced in case of hypothermia.

Because of severe ascending aortic calcification, the coronary revascularization technique had to be modified in patient 1 to avoid calcareous embolization from manipulation

TABLE 4.   Intraoperative Data from Patients Treated with r-Hirudin and CPB

	Patient Number				
	1	2	3	4	5
Surgical procedures	CABG (1 × LIMA + 2 × RIMA)	AVR (bioprosthesis)	AVR (bioprosthesis)	CABG VSD closure (1 × LIMA + 2 × SVG)	CABG (1 × LIMA + 2 × SVG)
CPB time (min)	180	83	100	127	116
Aortic cross-clamp time (min)	0	60	83	82	76
Circulatory arrest (min)	12	0	0	0	0
Rectal temperature (°C)	20	33	37	37	37
Cardioplegia (ml/kg)	0	17	27	24	19
CPB flow (L/min/m^2)	1.3–3.3	2.3–3.2	2.4–3.1	2.3–3.0	2.3–2.7
Δp oxygenator (mmHg)	70–110	70–101	60–84	87–129	100–142
Pressure before arterial filter (mmHg)	135–260	200–271	218–270	180–220	150–220
Red cells into priming solution (ml)	600	200	200	0	200
Transfusion of red cells during surgery (ml)	800	400	200	400	200
Blood loss, end of CPB to end of surgery (ml)	700	100	300	750	300

CABG = coronary artery bypass grafting, LIMA = left internal mammary artery, RIMA = right internal mammary artery, SVG = saphenous vein graft, AVR = aortic valve replacement, VSD = ventricular septal defect.

of the ascending aorta.[64] We used both internal mammary arteries (IMAs) in combination with saphenous vein grafts (SVG). The bypass surgery was performed on the fibrillating heart in deep hypothermia without cross-clamping. Although this regimen required a perfusion time of 180 minutes, including a 12-minute period of circulatory arrest, we encountered no problems related to anticoagulation with r-hirudin.

In patients 2 and 3, an aortic valve replacement with bioprostheses was conducted in mild hypothermia (33° C) and normothermia (37° C) with cardioplegic cardiac arrest.[63,66] In patient 4 bypass surgery was performed in normothermia (37° C), using the left IMA and two saphenous vein grafts. A postinfarction VSD was closed by direct sutures after opening the right ventricle. In patient 5 we performed bypass surgery in normothermia (37° C) with one left IMA and three vein grafts (see Table 4).

All operations were carried out without problems. No oozing of blood from the cut tissues (skin, sternum, myocardium, ascending aorta, right atrium), no thromboembolic complications, and no allergic reactions were observed.

The Δp of the oxygenator and the pressure prior to the arterial filter was constant during CPB, according to the flow rates (see Table 4). All components of the HLM, including oxygenator, cardiotomy reservoir, filters, and tubing, remained free of clots. Cardiopulmonary status was stable, and all patients came off the pump without requiring cardiotonic drug support. During and after operations ECG and enzyme analysis showed no signs of myocardial ischemia, thus indicating effective anticoagulation.

R-Hirudin Anticoagulation and Monitoring during CPB.   To be prepared for a sudden drop in APTT or ecarin clotting time (ECT) and to avoid accumulation of r-hirudin during infusion therapy, we chose an r-hirudin bolus regimen during CPB.[51] Because we expected a long perfusion time in patient 1, including circulatory arrest, we used a relatively high initial r-hirudin bolus (patient: 0.93 mg/kg, CPB: 0.46 mg/kg) (Fig. 8), which had proved to be a safe and effective dosage in the pig model[62] and in one clinical case.[60] In the

following four clinical cases we reduced the r-hirudin dosage to obtain plasma concentrations of 2.0–3.5 µg/ml, which proved to be sufficient for effective anticoagulation during
CPB (Figs. 9–12). After median sternotomy the patients received an initial intravenous
bolus of r-hirudin 10–15 minutes before the start of CPB. Additional boluses during CPB

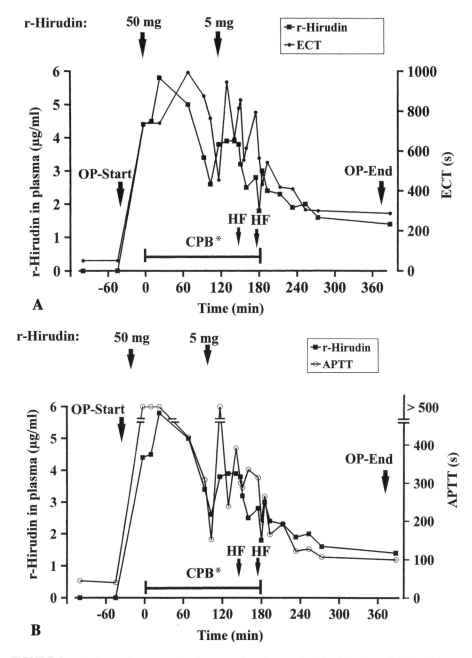

FIGURE 8.   Anticoagulation monitoring in patient 1 treated with r-hirudin and CPB. Change of
ecarin clotting time *(A)* and activated partial thromboplastin time *(B)* in relation to r-hirudin plasma concentration before, during, and after CPB. * 25 mg r-hirudin (0.46 mg/kg) added to priming solution.

were necessary to keep the r-hirudin plasma concentration above 2.0 µg/ml (Table 5). Patients 1 and 4 were treated with aprotinin in addition to r-hirudin anticoagulation. In both patients, 2 Mio KIU of aprotinin were added to the priming solution and 500,000 KIU/hr were administered during CPB. We used aprotinin because we expected an intensified bleeding tendency caused by great wound areas after bilateral IMA preparation, platelet

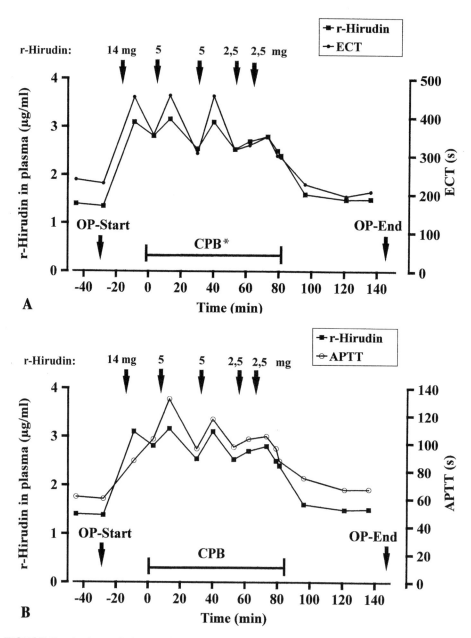

FIGURE 9. Anticoagulation monitoring in patient 2 treated with r-hirudin and CPB. Change of ecarin clotting time *(A)* and activated partial thromboplastin time *(B)* in relation to r-hirudin plasma concentration before, during, and after CPB. *5 mg r-hirudin (0.09 mg/kg) added to priming solution.

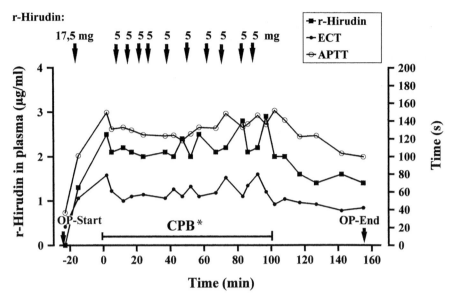

FIGURE 10.   Anticoagulation monitoring in patient 3 treated with r-hirudin and CPB. Change of ecarin clotting time and activated partial thromboplastin time in relation to r-hirudin plasma concentration before, during, and after CPB. *14 mg r-hirudin (0.21 mg/kg) added to priming solution.

damage due to long perfusion time and deep hypothermia[80] (patient 1), and full coumarin therapy as well as right ventriculotomy (patient 4). Numerous studies have proved that aprotinin reduces the risk of bleeding significantly in cardiac surgical patients.[19,20,27,28,68] The demand for intraoperative transfusion of red cells was highest in patient 1 (800 ml), probably because of the 180-minute perfusion time, the larger wounds following bilateral IMA preparation, and perhaps the high plasma concentration of r-hirudin up to 6 µg/ml (see Table 4). The postoperative bleeding in patient 3 was a surgical retrosternal hemorrhage unrelated to the anticoagulatory medication. Despite the coumarin therapy (INR: 3.6), patient 4 had no increased demand of packed red cells, and all wounds were without signs of bleeding.

In view of our results, we propose that a r-hirudin level of 2–3.5 µg/ml does not increase intraoperative bleeding. The intraoperative need for r-hirudin and the resulting r-hirudin plasma concentrations were different in the five patients (see Table 5), as described in animal experiments by Kaiser and coworkers.[40] The highest dosage of r-hirudin was used in patient 3 (12.4 µg/min of CPB).

Among the tools to monitor the anticoagulant activity of r-hirudin, APTT is considered the most suitable test because it is reliable, simple, and inexpensive.[9,36] Some experimental studies[53,81] reported statistical differences in the r-hirudin–dependent prolongation of APTT with different commercial assays. Like heparin measurements, the extent of APTT prolongation with r-hirudin is highly variable among individuals. With different assays the extent of APTT prolongation becomes less at higher concentrations of hirudin.[58] The addition of 350–600 ng r-hirudin/ml blood resulted in a large overlap in APTT ranges, whereas in the therapeutic range there was a linear response to hirudin concentration. The APTT values showed a dose-dependent increase with doses of 0.06–0.15 mg/kg/hr.[83] At concentrations of r-hirudin > 2.5 µg/ml, however, the APTT loses its linearity. Therefore, we used the ECT to monitor r-hirudin plasma levels during CPB (see Figs. 8–12).[56] Ecarin, an extract from the snake *Echis carinatus*, converts prothrombin to thrombin in the absence of any cofactor. In the presence of the direct thrombin inhibitor r-hirudin, the ECT is prolonged. The ECT is assessed in whole blood; the technique is simple and the results show linearity even at plasma concentrations of hirudin > 2.5 µg/ml. This makes the ECT superior to ACT and APTT methods. In our clinical experience, the correlation between ECT and APTT values and r-hirudin plasma concentration (patients 1, 2, 3, and 5) demonstrates that ECT and APTT are reliable indices of the free r-hirudin plasma concentration,[10,35,60,63,77] and that APTT and ECT can be used to monitor anticoagulant regimen during CPB (see Figs. 8–10, 12). In patient 4, r-hirudin plasma levels between 2.0–3.2 µg/ml corresponded to ECT values > 250 seconds and APTT values > 350 seconds (see Fig. 11). This lack of correlation may be due to the use of coumarin.

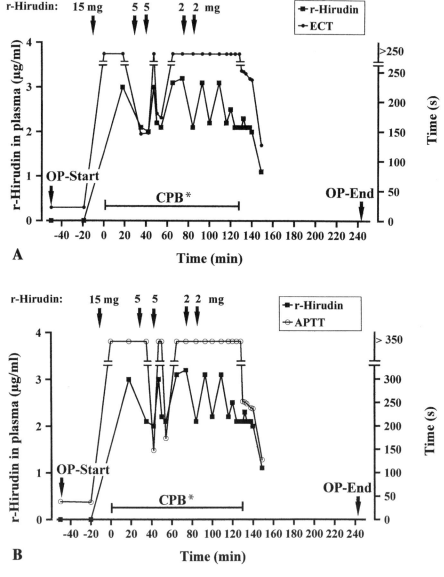

FIGURE 11.   Anticoagulation monitoring in patient 4 treated with r-hirudin and CPB. Change of ecarin clotting time *(A)* and activated partial thromboplastin time *(B)* in relation to r-hirudin plasma concentration before, during, and after CPB. *12 mg r-hirudin (0.21 mg/kg) added to priming solution.

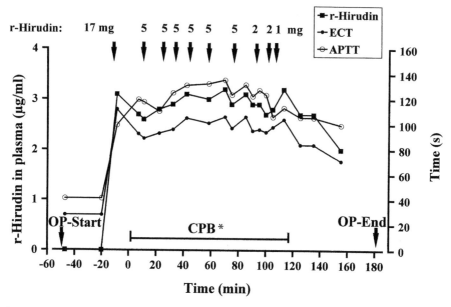

FIGURE 12. Anticoagulation monitoring in patient 5 treated with r-hirudin and CPB. Change of ecarin clotting time and activated partial thromboplastin time in relation to r-hirudin plasma concentration before, during, and after CPB. *13 mg r-hirudin (0.20 mg/kg) added to priming solution.

To determine the plasma concentration of r-hirudin, the thrombin activity was measured with an anti-FIIa-assay. The plasma concentration of r-hirudin was kept within 1.8–5.8 µg/ml in the first patient (see Fig. 8) and between 2.0–3.7 in the other 4 patients (see Figs. 9–12) throughout CPB. Because of the normal renal function and the short half-life of r-hirudin, the plasma concentration decreased rapidly during CPB, requiring 1–10 additional boluses of r-hirudin to provide a stable plasma concentration (see Table 5). The total amount of r-hirudin needed to keep plasma levels within 2.0–3.7 µg/ml during CPB varied between 5.6–12.4 µg/min of CPB, which provided sufficient anticoagulation.

TABLE 5. Anticoagulation Regimen in Patients Treated with r-Hirudin and CPB

	Patient Number				
	1	2	3	4	5
Preoperative anticoagulation	None	Coumarin ▼ r-Hirudin IV	None	Coumarin	None
r-Hirudin in HLM priming (mg/kg)	0.46	0.09	0.21	0.21	0.20
r-Hirudin initial bolus (mg/kg)	0.93	0.16	0.27	0.26	0.26
Number of additional r-hirudin boluses during CPB	1	4	10	4	9
Total amount of r-hirudin (µg/min of CPB)	8.2	6.0	12.4	5.6	8.6
Postoperative anticoagulation	r-Hirudin SC till 9th post-operative day ▼ Coumarin	r-Hirudin IV till 6th post-operative day ▼ Coumarin	r-Hirudin IV till 3rd post-operative day ▼ Coumarin	r-Hirudin IV till 3rd post-operative day ▼ Coumarin	r-Hirudin IV till 2nd post-operative day ▼ ASA

HLM = heart-lung machine, IV = intravenous, SC = subcutaneous, ASA = acetylsalicylic acid.

After the cessation of r-hirudin treatment at the end of CPB, plasma levels decreased continuously; therefore, no reversal or removal of r-hirudin was necessary. In patient 1 two periods of hemofiltration (Hemoflow F 60 S, High Flux; Fresenius, Bad Homburg, Germany), lasting 10 and 5 minutes, respectively, were performed during the final 30 minutes of CPB to speed the elimination of r-hirudin (see Fig. 8). This procedure decreased the r-hirudin plasma level from 3.2 to 1.8 µg/ml. The increase in plasma concentration at the end of hemofiltration and CPB can be explained by volume substitution with blood that contained r-hirudin from the filling volume of the HLM and was not treated by the cell-saver.

The first clots were observed when the plasma concentration of r-hirudin fell below 1.8 µg/ml. Despite prolonged ECT and APTT values, there was no increase in bleeding tendency, as demonstrated by the fact that blood loss from the end of CPB to the end of the operation amounted to only 100–750 ml (see Table 4). Because of preoperative coumarin therapy in patient 4, a total of 1,800 ml of fresh frozen plasma was administered after CPB to normalize coagulation. Because of dilution and CPB-mediated trauma, the platelet count decreased from preoperative values of $124–271 \times 10^9$/L to values of $38–156 \times 10^9$/L at the end of CPB.

The anticoagulant efficacy of the r-hirudin regimen used in all five patients was further demonstrated by assessment of the prothrombin fragment 1.2 as a marker for thrombin generation and by determination of the plasma concentration of the thrombin–antithrombin complex as a marker of thrombin inactivation. The linear increase in plasma concentration of the prothrombin fragment 1.2 during CPB indicates continuous thrombin generation. The plasma concentration of the thrombin–antithrombin complex, however, remained low (mean concentration at end of CPB: 11.4 µg/L) in all five patients, indicating that the generated thrombin is rapidly and effectively inactivated by r-hirudin.[61]

Platelet Preservation.   CPB has been associated with significant thrombocytopenia and platelet dysfunction. A decline of 30–50% in platelet count[37,70] and a decrease in platelet function occur immediately after initiation of CPB because of dilution of blood with priming solutions, interactions between platelets and foreign surfaces, and abnormal shear stresses, which lead to release of granular contents.[88,90] However, as the bypass continues, some platelets become detached, leaving a fragmented membrane, and therefore are not fully functional. Rapid platelet consumption is the most conspicuous event at the beginning of CPB.[90] Zilla reported platelet stimulation in the first minutes of CPB, primarily during the initial phase of cardiopulmonary bypass, and observed that platelets seem to recover during the later course of CPB, probably because of drastically decreased aggregability. Wenger et al.[88] showed the loss of platelet fibrinogen receptors and verified the presence of platelet membrane fragments. The cardiopulmonary suction system is a major source of hemolysis and may further decrease platelet numbers directly by trauma. Filtration further reduces platelet numbers by removing aggregates and platelet debris.[22] As a result, thrombocytopenia and poor platelet function cause poor clot formation and prolonged bleeding time after CPB. The defect may be induced also by the thrombin generated during surgery.[37] Furthermore, Stass and coworkers demonstrated that protamine sulfate significantly inhibits platelet aggregation.[76]

Most nonsurgical hemorrhages during or after CPB are thought to be secondary to platelet dysfunction, with or without hyperfibrinolysis.[24] Therefore the preservation of platelet count and function is important to the prevention of bleeding and reoperation. Prophylactic attempts have been aimed at modification of the surfaces and at pharmacologic inhibition of platelet reaction. Efforts have made to modify the platelet surface with drugs (e.g., dipyridamole, sulfinpyrazone, prostacyclin).[8] The modest reaction in platelet consumption in experimental bypass models[18] was followed by a long-lasting inhibition with some hemorrhagic side effects and lowering of arterial pressure. None of these protocols are really satisfactory for the preservation of platelet function.

On the basis of our experimental and clinical experience, we propose that r-hirudin is more successful in preventing the deterioration of platelet function than heparin. The more pronounced drops in platelet count in patient 1 (up to 25 % of the initial value) and patient 4 (up to 31 % of the initial value) may be explained by a perfusion time of 180 minutes and deep hypothermia (20° C)[80] in patient 1 and by intensive use of coronary suction while searching the VSD in patient 4.[22]

As a result of CPB-mediated trauma, ADP- and collagen-induced platelet function decreased during CPB in all patients except patient 3 (Fig. 13). ADP- and collagen-induced

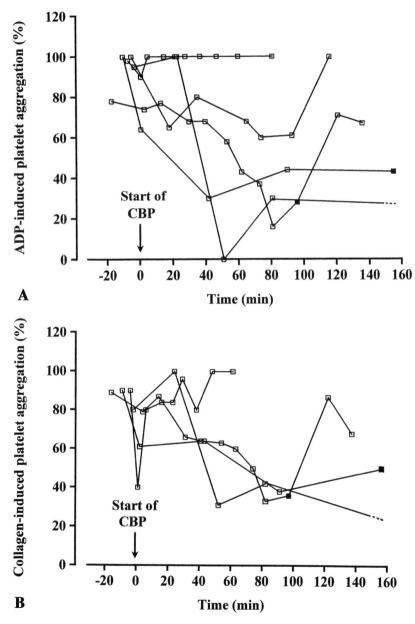

FIGURE 13.   Adenosine diphosphate-induced *(A)* (n = 5) and collagen-induced *(B)* (n = 4) platelet aggregation before, during, and after CPB and r-hirudin anticoagulation. For details of method, see the pig model of CPB. ■ = Platelet function at end of CPB.

TABLE 6. Postoperative Data for Patients Treated with r-Hirudin and CPB

	Patient Number				
	1	2	3	4	5
Total fluid loss from thorax drainages (ml)	1270	480	1950*	1080	1320
Transfusion of red cells (ml)	400	400	1000	200	600
Hospitalization (days)	24†	13	12	18	11
Anti-r-hirudin antibodies on 24th postoperative day	Yes	No	No	No	No
Anti-r-hirudin antibodies 6 months postoperatively	No	No	No	No	No

* Fluid loss from thorax drainages was 1220 ml until surgical reexploration and 730 ml after surgical reexploration.
† The first patient was hospitalized until the end of the study at the 24th postoperative day to allow close monitoring. Patients 2, 3, 4, and 5 were discharged before the end of the study, and final assessment was performed by ambulatory examination.

platelet aggregation were relatively well preserved after a CPB-time of 60 minutes. The deep decrease in ADP-induced platelet aggregation to zero in patient 1 was obviously caused by deep hypothermia.[80] Because of a technical defect, collagen-induced platelet aggregation could be determined in only 4 patients.

Postoperative Management and Follow-up. Postoperative anticoagulation was achieved by subcutanous r-hirudin therapy in patient 1 and the intravenous application of r-hirudin in the other four patients with an APTT target range of 60–80 seconds. Between the second and ninth postoperative days, r-hirudin therapy was stopped; coumarin therapy was begun in patients 1–4 and acetyl-salicylic-acid therapy in patient 5 (see Table 5). The postoperative course until the twenty-fourth day was uneventful; in particular, no anticoagulation-related bleeding or thromboembolic complications and no allergic reactions were observed. In patient 3 surgical reexploration was performed 6 hours postoperatively because of prolonged bleeding from the thoracic wound drains (200 ml/hr) (Table 6). Surgical retrosternal bleeding was found intraoperatively and coagulated by diathermia. The APTT at this time was 80 seconds (normal = 35 seconds), and clotting was observed in the thorax drains. The later postoperative course of this patient was uneventful.

Although patient 5 showed generalized atherosclerosis, including bilateral carotid artery stenosis, no thromboembolic complications—in particular, no myocardial or cerebral ischemia—were observed, despite relatively low APTT values (around 45 seconds) for several hours. This observation underlines the fact that the antithrombotic potential of r-hirudin was efficient. Agnelli and coworkers observed sustained antithrombotic activity and inhibition of clot growth with hirudin therapy even after plasma clearance.[2] In one patient who was treated for 9 days with intravenous r-hirudin, anti-r-hirudin antibodies were found in the plasma sample taken on the twenty-fourth postoperative day. A control sample taken 6 months later revealed that the antibodies had completely disappeared (see Table 6).

CONCLUSIONS AND FUTURE PERSPECTIVES

Current clinical and experimental data demonstrate that r-hirudin can be used as an anticoagulant during CPB surgery. At the dosage that we used, r-hirudin was as effective as heparin. Plasma concentrations during CPB were successfully monitored with the ecarin-clotting time. None of the five patients experienced thrombotic problems during CPB or increased postoperative bleeding due to hemostatic problems. These results support the impression that there is no pronounced intraoperative or postoperative bleeding in r-hirudin-treated patients compared with heparin-treated patients. Further clinical studies are needed to determine whether r-hirudin is indeed superior to heparin with respect to postoperative bleeding and platelet damage. Furthermore, it is important to determine whether r-hirudin in combination with other anticoagulants—in particular, antiplatelet agents—can improve the clinical outcome of patients undergoing CPB surgery.

Acknowledgments.   We are grateful to N. Bleese and D. Kupke for their advice; to A. Greinacher and H. Völpel for their cooperation in performing the clinical study; to B. Hein for the histologic examinations; to R. Rössing for the electronmicroscopic scans; to D. Neuhaus and K. Jäger for perfusion and for assistance in the animal experimentations; to G. Hollnick for perfusion in clinical trials and for help with the figures; to K. Madlener and R. Bader for assistance; to C. Löwer and J. Kormann for anesthesia; and to P. Schlizio for skillful secretarial assistance. The work reported in this chapter was supported in part by the state of Hessen and Behringwerke AG, Marburg, Germany.

REFERENCES

1. Abel JJ, Rowntree LG, Turner BB: On the removal of diffusible substances from the circulating blood of living animals by dialysis. J Pharmacol Exp Ther 5:275–316, 1913.
2. Agnelli G, Renga C, Weitz JI, et al: Sustained antithrombotic activity of hirudin after its plasma clearance: Comparison with heparin. Blood 80:960–965, 1992.
3. Amiral J, Bridey F, Dreyfus M, et al: Platelet factor 4 complexed to heparin is the target for antibodies generated in heparin-induced thrombocytopenia. Thromb Haemost 68:95–96, 1992.
4. Antman EM, et al: Hirudin in acute myocardial infarction. Circulation 90:1624–1630, 1994.
5. Arthur CK, Isbister JP, Aspery EM: The heparin induced thrombosis-thrombocytopenia syndrome (HITTS): A review. Pathology 17:82–86, 1985.
6. Bara L, Block MF, Samama MM: A comparative study of r-hirudin and standard heparin in the wessler model. Thromb Res 68:162–174, 1992.
7. Bell WR: Heparin-associated thrombocytopenia and thrombosis. J Lab Clin Med 111:600–605, 1988.
8. Bernabei A, Gikakis N, Kowalska MA, et al: Iloprost and echistatin protect platelets during simulated extracorporeal circulation. Ann Thorac Surg 59:149–153, 1995.
9. Bichler J, Fichtl B, Siebeck M, Fritz H: Pharmacokinetics and pharmaco-dynamics of hirudin in man after single subcutaneous and intravenous bolus administration. Arzneim Forsch/Drug Res 38:704–710, 1988.
10. Bichler J, Gemmerli R, Fritz H: Studies for revealing a possible sensitization to hirudin after repeated intravenous injections in baboons. Thromb Res 61:39–51, 1991.
11. Bleese N, Döring V, Kalmar P, et al: Intraoperative myocardial protection by cardioplegia in hypothermia. J Thorac Cardiovasc Surg 75:405–413, 1978.
12. Bucha E, Markwardt F, Nowak G: Hirudin in haemodialysis. Thromb Res 60:445–455, 1990.
13. Butler KD, Dolan SL, Talbot MD, Wallis RB: Factor VII and DDAVP reverse the effect of recombinant desulphatohirudin (CGB 39393) on bleeding in the rat. Blood Coag Fibrin 4:459–464, 1993.
14. Carreras LO: Thrombosis and thrombocytopenia induced by heparin. Scand J Haematol 25 (Suppl 36):66–80, 1980.
15. Chang JY: White clot syndrome associated with heparin-induced thrombocytopenia: a review of 23 cases. Heart Lung 16:403–407, 1987.
16. Chong BH, Berndt MC: Heparin-induced thrombocytopenia. Blut 58:53–57, 1989.
17. Conrad KA: Clinical pharmacology and drug safety: Lessons from hirudin. Clin Pharmacol Ther 58:123–126, 1995.
18. Coppe D, Sobel M, Seamans L, et al: Preservation of platelet function and number by prostacyclin during cardiopulmonary bypass. J Thorac Cardiovasc Surg 81:274–278, 1981.
19. Cosgrove DM III, Heric B, Lytle BW, et al.: Aprotinin therapy for reoperative myocardial revascularization: a placebo- controlled study. Ann Thorac Surg 54:1031–1038, 1992.
20. Dietrich W, Barankay A, Hahnel C, Richter JA: High-dose aprotinin in cardiac surgery: three years experience in 1,784 patients. J Cardiothorac Vasc Anesth 6:324–27, 1992.
21. Dodt J, Dohlet S, Schmitz T et al: Distinct binding sites of Ala[48]-hirudin on α-thrombin. J Biol Chem 265:713–718, 1990.
22. Edmunds LH Jr, Saxena NC, Hillyer P, Wilson TJ: Relationship between platelet count and cardiotomy suction return. Ann Thorac Surg 25:306–310, 1978.
23. Fareed D, Pifarre R, Walenga JM, Fareed J: Effect of recombinant hirudin and heparin on human platelet aggregation. Fed Proc 3:A308, 1949.
24. Friedenberg WR, Myers WO, Plotka ED, et al: Platelet dysfunction associated with cardiopulmonary bypass. Ann Thorac Surg 25:298–305, 1978.
25. Glusa E, Urban U: Studies in platelet functions in hirudin plasma. Folia Haematol 115:88–93, 1988.

26. Glusa E, Markwardt F: Platelet functions in recombinant hirudin-anticoagulated blood. Haemostasis 20:112–18, 1990.
27. Goldstein DJ, DeRosa CM, Mongero LB, et al: Safety and efficacy of aprotinin under conditions of deep hypothermia and circulatory arrest. J Thorac Cardiovasc Surg 110:1615–22, 1995.
28. Green D, Sanders J, Eiken M, et al: Recombinant aprotinin in coronary artery bypass graft operations. J Thorac Cardiovasc Surg 110:963–970, 1995.
29. Greinacher A, Michels I, Kiefel V, Mueller-Eckhardt C: A rapid and sensitive test for diagnosing heparin-associated thrombocytopenia. Thromb Haemost 66:734–736, 1991.
30. Greinacher A: Heparin-associated thrombocytopenia. Biomed Prog 7:53–56, 1994.
31. Griessbach U, Stürzebecher J, Markwardt F: Assay of hirudin in plasma using a chromogenic thrombin substrate. Thromb Res 37:347–350, 1985.
32. Grütter MG, Priestle JP, Rahuel J, et al: Crystal structure of the thrombin-hirudin complex: a novel mode of serine protease inhibition. EMBO J 9: 2361–2365, 1990.
33. Haas G: Dialysieren des strömenden Blutes am Lebenden. Klin Wochenschr 4:13–14, 1924.
34. Haycraft JB: On the action of a secretion obtained from the medicinal leech on the coagulation of blood. Proc R Soc Lond 36:478–483, 1884.
35. Heras M, Chesebro JH, Penny WJ, et al: Effects of thrombin inhibition on the development of acute platelet-thrombus deposition during angioplasty in pigs. Circulation 79:657–665, 1989.
36. Heras M, Chesebro JH, Webster MWI, et al: Hirudin, heparin and placebo during deep arterial injury in the pig. Circulation 82:1476–1484, 1990.
37. Hope AF, Heyns AduP, Lötter MG, et al: Kinetics and sites of sequestration of indium 111-labeled human platelets during cardiopulmonary bypass. J Thorac Cardiovasc Surg 81:880–886, 1981.
38. Horneffer PJ, Gott VL, Gardner TJ: Swine as a cardiac surgical model. In Umbleson ME (ed): Swine in Biomedical Research, vol 1. New York, Plenum Press, 1986, pp 321–325.
39. Ibbotson SH, Grant PJ, Kerry R, et al: The influence of infusions of 1-desamino-8-d-arginine vasopressin (DDAVP) in vivo on the anticoagulant effect of r-hirudin. Thromb Haemost 65:64–66, 1991.
40. Kaiser B, Simon A, Markwardt F: Antithrombotic effects of recombinant hirudin in experimental angioplasty and intravascular thrombolysis. Thromb Haemostas 63:44–47, 1990.
41. King DJ, Kelton JG: Heparin-induced thrombocytopenia. Ann Intern Med 100:535–540, 1984.
42. Köstering H, Mast WP, Kaethner T, et al: Blood coagulation studies in domestic pigs (Hanover breed) and minipigs (Goettingen breed). Lab Animals 17:346–349, 1983.
43. Lam JYT, Chesebro JH, Steele PM, et al: Antithrombotic therapy for deep arterial injury by angioplasty. Circulation 84:814–820, 1991.
44. Laster JL, Cikrit D, Walker N, Silver D: The heparin-induced thrombocytopenia syndrome: An update. Surg 102:763–770, 1987.
45. Laster JL, Nichols WK, Silver D: Thrombocytopenia associated with heparin-coated catheters in patients with heparin-associated antiplatelet antibodies. Arch Intern Med 149:2285–2287, 1989.
46. Levy JH: Anaphylactic Reactions in Anesthesia and Intensive Care, 2nd ed. Boston, Butterworth-Heinemann, 1992.
47. Lynch DM, Howe SE: Heparin-associated thrombocytopenia: antibody binding specifity to platelet antigens. Blood 66:1176–1181, 1985.
48. Markwardt F: Untersuchungen über Hirudin. Naturwissenschaften 42:537–538, 1955.
49. Markwardt F: Die Isolierung und chemische Charakterisierung des Hirudins. Hoppe Seylers Z Physiol Chem 308:147–156, 1957.
50. Markwardt F, Hoffmann A, Stürzenbecher J: Influence of thrombin inhibitors on the thrombin-induced activation of human blood platelets. Haemostasis 13:227–233, 1983.
51. Markwardt F, Fink G, Kaiser B, et al: Pharmacological survey of recombinant hirudin. Pharmazie 43:202–207, 1988.
52. Markwardt F: The development of hirudin as an antithrombotic drug. Thromb Res 74:1–23, 1994.
53. Monreal M, Monreal L, de Gopegui RR, et al: Effects of two different doses of Hirudin on APTT, determined with eight different reagents. Thromb Haemost 73:219–22, 1995.
54. Müller-Berghaus G, Riess FC, Pötzsch B, Nowak G: Hirudin update. In Neri Serneri GG, Gensini GF, Abbate R, Prisco D (eds): Thrombosis: An Update. Florence, Scientific Press, 1992, pp 133– 147.
55. Nowak G, Markwardt F, Fink E: Pharmacokinetic studies with recombinant hirudin in dogs. Folia Haematol 115:70–74, 1988.
56. Nowak G, Bucha E: A new method for the therapeutical monitoring of r-hirudin. Haemostasis 69 (6):A2736, 1993.
57. Nowak G, Bucha E: Prothrombin conversion intermediate effectively neutralizes toxic levels of hirudin. Thromb Res 80:317–325, 1995.
58. Nurmohamed MT, Berckmans RJ, Morrien-Salomons WM, et al: Monitoring anticoagulant therapy by activated partial thromboplastin time: Hirudin assessment. Thromb Haemost 72:685–692, 1994.
59. Ortel TL, Gockerman JP, Califf RM, et al: Parenteral anticoagulation with the heparinoid Lomoparan (ORG 10172) in patients with heparin induced thrombocytopenia and thrombosis. Thromb Haemost 67:292–296, 1992.

60. Pötzsch B, Iversen S, Riess FC, et al: Recombinant hirudin as an anticoagulant in open-heart surgery: A case report. Ann Hematol 68(Suppl II):A53, 1994.
61. Pötzsch B, Riess FC, Völpel H, et al: Recombinant hirudin as anticoagulant during open-heart surgery [abstract]. Thromb Haemost 73:1456, 1995.
62. Riess FC, Pötzsch B, Behr I, et al: Recombinant hirudin as an anticoagulant during cardiac operations: Experiments in a pig model. Eur J Cardiothorac Surg, 1996 [in press].
63. Riess FC, Löwer C, Seelig C, et al: Recombinant hirudin as a new anticoagulant during cardiac operations instead of heparin: Successful for aortic valve replacement in man. J Thorac Cardiovasc Surgery 110:265–267, 1995.
64. Riess FC, Pötzsch B, Bader R, et al: A case report on the use of recombinant hirudin as an anticoagulant for cardiopulmonary bypass in open-heart surgery. Eur J Cardiothorac Surg 10:386–388, 1996.
65. Riess FC, Pötzsch B, Jäger K, et al: Elimination of recombinant hirudin by hemofiltration in the pig model. Isr J Med Sci, 1996 [in press].
66. Riess FC, Pötzsch B, Bleese N, et al: Recombinant hirudin as an anticoagulant for cardiac surgery instead of heparin: First clinical experiences [abstract]. Thorac Cardiovasc Surg 44:173, 1996.
67. Rigel DF, Olson RW, Lappe RW: Comparison of hirudin and heparin as adjuncts to streptokinase thrombolysis in a canine model of coronary thrombosis. Circ Res 72:1091–1102, 1993.
68. Royston D, Bidstrup BP, Taylor KM, Sabsford RN: Effect of aprotinin on need for blood transfusion after repeat open-heart surgery. Lancet 2:1289–1291, 1987.
69. Rydel TJ, Tulinsky A, Bode W, Huber R: Defined structure of the hirudin-thrombin complex. J Mol Biol 20:583–601, 1991.
70. Salzman EW: Blood platelets and extracorporeal circulation transfusion. Transfusion 3:274–277, 1963.
71. Schwartz RS, Murphy IG, Edwards WD, et al: Restenosis after balloon angioplasty: A practical proliferative model in porcine coronary arteries. Circulation 82:2190–2200, 1990.
72. Serruys PW, Deckers JW, Close P, et al, on behalf of the HELVETICA study investigators: A comparison of hirudin with heparin in the prevention of restenosis after coronary angioplasty. N Engl J Med 333:757–763, 1995.
73. Sheridan D, Carter C, Kelton JG: A diagnostic test for heparin-induced thrombocytopenia. Blood 67:27–30, 1986.
74. Shulman NR, Reid DM: Platelet immunology in hemostasis and thrombosis. In Colman RW, Hirsh J, Marder VJ, Salzman EW (eds): Basic Principles and Clinical Practice, 3rd ed. Philadelphia, J.B. Lippincott, pp 414–468, 1994.
75. Singer RL, Mannion JD, Bauer TL, et al: Complications from heparin-induced thrombocytopenia in patients undergoing cardiopulmonary bypass. Chest 104:1436–1440, 1993.
76. Stass SA, Bishop CF, Fosburg RG, et al: Platelets as affected by cardiopulmonary bypass [abstract]. Am J Clin Pathol 66:459, 1976.
77. Stone SR, Hofsteenge J: Kinetics of the inhibition of thrombin by hirudin. Biochemistry 25:4622–4628, 1986.
78. Stringer KA, Lindenfeld JA: Hirudins: Antithrombin anticoagulants. Ann Pharmacother 26:1535–1540, 1992.
79. The Global Use of Strategies to Open Occluded Coronary Arteries (GUSTO) IIa Investigators: Randomized trial of intravenous heparin versus recombinant hirudin for acute coronary syndromes. Circulation 90:1631–1637, 1994.
80. Tonz M, Mihaljevic T, von Segesser LK, et al: Normothermia versus hypothermia during cardiopulmonary bypass: a randomized controlled trial. Ann Thorac Surg 59:137–143, 1995.
81. Tripodi A, Chantarangkul V, Arbini AA, et al: Effects of hirudin on activated partial thromboplastin time determined with ten different reagents. Thromb Haemost 70:286–288, 1993.
82. Umlas J, Taff RH, Garvin G, Sevierk R: Anticoagulant monitoring and neutralization during open heart surgery—a rapid method for measuring heparin and calculating safe reduced protamine doses. Analg 62:1095–1099, 1983.
83. Verstrate M, Nurmohamed M, Kienast J, et al: Biological effects of recombinant hirudin CGP 39393 in human volunteers. J Am Coll Cardiol 22:1080–1088, 1993.
84. Walenga JM, Pifarre R, Fareed J: Recombinant hirudin as antithrombotic agent. Drugs Future 15:267–280, 1990.
85. Walenga JM, Bakhos M, Messmore HL, et al: Potential use of recombinant hirudin as an anticoagulant in a cardiopulmonary bypass model. Ann Thorac Surg 51:271–277, 1991.
86. Walenga JM, Koza MJ, Park SJ, et al: Evaluation of CGP 39393 as the anticoagulant in cardiopulmonary bypass operation in a dog model. Ann Thorac Surg 58:1685–1689, 1994.
87. Warketin TE, Kelton JG: Heparin-induced thrombocytopenia. Prog Hemost Thromb 10:1–34, 1991.
88. Wenger RK, Lukasiewicz H, Mikuta BS, et al: Loss of platelet fibrinogen receptors during clinical cardiopulmonary bypass. J Thorac Cardiovasc Surg 97:235–239, 1989.
89. Woodman RC, Harker LA: Bleeding complications associated with cardiopulmonary bypass. Blood 76:1680–1697, 1990.
90. Zilla P, Fasol R, Groscurth P, et al: Blood platelets in cardiopulmonary bypass operations. J Thorac Cardiovasc Surg 97:379–388, 1989.

CHAPTER 15

Argatroban in the Management of Patients with Heparin-induced Thrombocytopenia and Heparin-induced Thrombocytopenia and Thrombosis Syndrome

BRUCE E. LEWIS, M.D.
JEANINE M. WALENGA, Ph.D.
ROQUE PIFARRÉ, M.D.
JAWED FAREED, Ph.D.

The clinical diagnoses of heparin-induced thrombocytopenia (HIT) and heparin-induced thrombocytopenia and thrombosis syndrome (HITTS) have become more recognized in clinical medicine over the past decade. Both syndromes are thought to be immune-mediated through HIT antibody. The spectrum of disease associated with HIT antibody ranges from the relatively benign thrombocytopenia seen with HIT to the devastating thrombotic occlusions associated with HITTS.[1] The probability of progression from HIT to HITTS appears to be approximately 35%.[2,3,4] HITTS is more common in diabetics, but other clinical markers that suggest a risk of progression from HIT to HITTS are unknown.

The pathophysiology of HIT and HITTS is much better characterized than the clinical markers of risk.[5–12] The thrombocytopenia that marks the disease process in patients with HIT antibody is secondary to platelet activation and subsequent platelet destruction and consumption. Platelet activation results from a complex interaction between platelets, platelet factor 4, heparin, and HIT antibody. The HIT antibody combines with heparin and platelet factor 4 in a precise stoichiometric relationship. This relationship occurs on the platelet membrane in proximity with an Fc receptor. The platelet Fc receptor then undergoes a structural shift, resulting in activation of the platelet. The platelet releases platelet-activating factor, adenosine diphosphate (ADP), thromboxane A_2, fibrinogen, and platelet factor 4, all of which promote local thrombotic events.

HIT antibody is manufactured in certain patients after exposure to heparin. The HIT antibody is usually expressed 5–14 days after heparin exposure. However, patients who have had previous heparin exposures probably have an anamnestic response and may redevelop HIT antibody much more rapidly on repeat exposures than on the initial exposure. Patients may also express thrombotic occlusions later than 14 days because the initial thrombus may remain nonocclusive, progressing to complete occlusion weeks after HIT antibody has been expressed. HIT antibody is generally believed to diminish over a 3-month period. However, our group has encountered patients who remain positive for HIT antibody (as detected by the enzyme-linked immunosorbent assay [ELISA]) more than 1 year after presentation. The clinical implication for patients who remain HIT antibody-positive is not known. However, the numerous intrinsic heparins and heparanoids present in the human body theoretically could interact with HIT antibody and promote thrombosis.[13]

The HIT antibody recognizes not only epitopes on the platelet membrane but also endothelial cell epitopes that share the platelet membrane epitope sequences.[14,15] The precise mechanism of the endothelial cell–HIT antibody interaction and the contribution of that interaction to thrombosis are not known. Clinical observations suggest that thrombotic complications associated with HIT antibody occur at sites of endothelial damage.[16–18] The shared recognition by HIT antibody of both platelet and endothelial cell epitopes may explain the catastrophic thrombosis seen in these syndromes.

DIAGNOSIS

The gold standard for diagnosis of patients with HIT antibody remains the clinical impression. The hallmark of the diagnosis is heparin exposure followed by thrombocytopenia. The distinction between HIT and HITTS is the presence of new thrombosis after heparin therapy. Patients who are treated with heparin for preexisting thrombus are not diagnosed with HITTS unless thrombocytopenia develops after heparin exposure and a new thrombus is identified during the course of thrombocytopenia. Like patients with HITTS, however, patients who develop thrombocytopenia while taking heparin as treatment for a thrombus require alternative anticoagulants.

Mild thrombocytopenia is frequently seen within 24 hours of heparin exposure and is best labeled a type I response.[19–21] Generally type I thrombocytopenic response is not associated with a thrombotic propensity unless the patient has had previous heparin exposure. Type II thrombocytopenic response, which is associated with HIT antibody, is usually recognized 5–14 days after heparin exposure. A 30% reduction in platelet count from baseline should alert the managing physician to a high probability of HIT antibody in the patient on heparin.[22] In contrast to type I response, type II response has a high probability of thrombus formation. Heparin should be discontinued, and alternative anticoagulation should be initiated. The platelet count should be frequently measured (as often as every 12 hours) for the next 48 hours. Patients with HIT antibody often express a continued decline in platelet count over the next 24 hours, despite discontinuation of heparin. Platelet count begins to recover in most patients at 3–4 days after heparin is discontinued.

The clinical criteria associated with confirmation of HIT vary from author to author. The following criteria serve as generally accepted guidelines to establish a clinical diagnosis of HIT:[23]

1. Thrombocytopenia that follows heparin administration by 5–14 days
2. Reduction in platelet count to less than 100,000 or 50% of baseline
3. Recovery of platelet count after discontinuation of heparin
4. Absence of clinical thrombosis associated with heparin administration
5. Exclusion of other causes of thrombocytopenia

The clinical diagnosis of HITTS can be established by using the same criteria, except that thrombosis is present after initiation of heparin therapy. Patients who develop thrombocytopenia while taking heparin for treatment of a known thrombus are generally diagnosed with HIT. However, the clinical risk to such patients is probably much higher than to a patient who has HIT without thrombosis because of the underlying thrombus.

Many laboratory tests can be applied to patients suspected of having HIT antibody. Platelet aggregometry, serotonin release tests, and ELISA tests have been advocated for confirmation of the diagnosis when HIT antibody is suspected.[24–26] These tests share a common theme of high specificity but low sensitivity. A positive result in a patient with thrombocytopenia while taking heparin can be considered as confirmation of the presence of HIT antibody. A negative test does not exclude the presence of HIT antibody. Sequential testing over a 3–4 day period can increase the diagnostic yield, because antigen excess (heparin-platelet factor 4) can yield a false-negative result. A battery of tests consisting of multiple laboratory examinations may also increase the diagnostic yield.[27]

Each of the tests has limitations. Few medical centers have the capability to perform serotonin release assays, which require handling of radioactive materials. ELISA kits are expensive and difficult to obtain. Large series with ELISA testing are forthcoming, but the precise optical density that is necessary to confirm or refute the presence of HIT antibody is not known. The interpretation of results may therefore require refinement. Platelet aggregometry depends on interpretation of a percentage of platelet aggregation. Furthermore, methods of platelet aggregation testing vary among institutions and lack standardization. The major limitation of the tests remains poor sensitivity, which may reflect the heterogeneity of the HIT antibody. The two most important principles to remember in diagnosing patients with HIT antibody are as follows:

1. The gold standard for diagnosing HIT antibodies remains the clinical impression.
2. A positive HIT antibody test is confirmatory, but a negative test does not exclude the diagnosis.

A positive HIT antibody test should prompt a careful clinical search for sites of thrombus. Our group has reported approximately 2.5 thrombotic events per patient testing positive for HIT antibody.[4] Clinicians should have a low threshold for work-up of deep venous thrombosis, pulmonary embolism, acute myocardial infarction, stroke, acute arterial insufficiency, and ischemic bowel. Doppler scans and/or venography, ventilation-perfusion scans and/or pulmonary arteriography, cardiac enzymes, electrocardiography and/or cardiac catheterization, computed tomographic (CT) scans and/or angiography, mesenteric angiography, and arteriography should be considered for any clinical event suggestive of a local thrombotic event. Early diagnosis of thrombotic events may direct therapeutic strategies and prevent the devastating consequences of occlusion.

MANAGEMENT

The management of patients diagnosed with HIT antibody continues to evolve. The major distinction is between patients with and without thrombosis, and strategies vary with the wide spectrum of clinical severity. Some principles, however, are uniform for all patients with HIT antibody. The first step is to stop the administration of heparin immediately. Because heparin is ubiquitous in hospitalized patients, an exhaustive search for sources in catheter flushes, subcutaneous prophylaxis, and even indwelling catheters is warranted.[28–32] Swan-Ganz catheters are frequently heparin-coated and may need to be replaced. Arrow catheters are not heparin-coated and can be reliably substituted for indwelling heparin-coated catheters.

The managing physician should resist the temptation to treat thrombocytopenia unless significant clinical bleeding is observed. Transfused platelets are deposited within sites of existing thrombi and perpetuate their growth. Minor bleeding is common in patients with HIT antibody, but major bleeding is infrequent. The most significant clinical problem is clearly thrombosis, which platelet transfusions will only worsen. Patients with HIT but no thrombosis may appear clinically well, but they remain a high-risk group, with 30–40% progressing to thrombosis during hospitalization.[2–4] Furthermore, a subgroup will not present with thrombotic complications until after discharge. Late thrombotic events may represent progression of subclinical thrombosis not detected during the initial thrombocytopenic event. Warkentin screened patients with sequential venography after hip surgery and found subclinical venous thrombus in over 80% of patients thought to have HIT antibody.[36] Data from our institution suggest that patients with HIT who develop thrombotic events frequently express multiple thrombotic events[4] and have a high incidence of death, amputation, stroke, deep venous thrombosis, and bowel infarction.[1,4,37,38] Such observations suggest that prophylactic anticoagulation is justified in patients with HIT antibody but no clinical evidence of thrombosis.

Patients with HIT antibody and thrombosis have clear indications for anticoagulation. The reported mortality rate is 20-35%.[1,4,37,38] Much of the mortality is related to the complications of thrombotic occlusion. Acute and chronic morbidity is also quite high. Amputation, deep venous thrombosis and postphlebitic syndrome, stroke with long-term neurologic impairment, mesenteric infarction and its consequent nutritional handicaps, myocardial infarction with associated heart failure, and renal arterial thrombus with chronic renal failure may contribute to the dismal long-term outcome. Treatment and prevention of these events are clinically justified.

Numerous anticoagulants have been considered for the treatment of HIT antibody. The first was the traditional oral anticoagulant, warfarin.[1] Warfarin, however, has several disadvantages. The time required to establish therapeutic levels is prolonged, and the patient is left at risk for thrombosis during the period of warfarinization. A second, more worrisome problem is the paradoxic thrombosis observed in patients who receive large doses of warfarin. This phenomenon is probably related to the short half-life of protein C. Rapid initiation of warfarin without thrombin inhibition can selectively deplete protein C, tipping the scales of the coagulation cascade toward coagulation and away from anticoagulation and thus promoting thrombus formation and propagation. The Canadian HIT registry and our local data include multiple cases of overwhelming thrombosis attributed to warfarin therapy in the absence of a thrombin inhibitor.

Many clinicians now advocate the use of intravenous anticoagulation during the time therapy is initiated. Maintenance of a therapeutic anticoagulant effect during initiation of warfarin should prevent the paradoxic thrombosis seen with initiation of unopposed warfarin therapy. The problem with this recommendation is that no intravenous alternative to heparin is approved in the United States.

Previous investigations have used ORG 10172 (Orgaron) and recombinant hirudin to treat patients with HIT antibody.[37] The results suggest that thrombotic events and mortality can be reduced in patients with HIT antibody. ORG 10172, however, presents clinical problems of laboratory monitoring for many centers that do not routinely measure factor 10a. ORG 10172 poses the additional concern of cross-reactivity with HIT antibody.[37,39] Finally, ORG 10172 has had little impact on 30-day mortality rates.

Argatroban is a direct thrombin inhibitor with no in vitro cross-reactivity with HIT antibody.[39,40] The molecular basis for its anticoagulant effect is a direct, reversible binding to the catalytic site of thrombin. The small molecular size (approximately 500 Da) of argatroban offers significant advantage over other direct thrombin inhibitors (recombinant hirudin and hirulog are much larger molecules). The smaller size of argatroban allows improved penetration of both fibrin-bound and clot-bound thrombin. In vitro measurement of argatroban's anticoagulant activity shows only a twofold reduction of activity in clot-bound thrombin compared with a 100–1000-fold reduction with hirulog and recombinant hirudin. The improved retention of anticoagulant activity against clot-bound thrombin allows more effective treatment of thrombosis at clinically tolerated blood levels of argatroban. Stated differently, argatroban can penetrate clot-bound thrombin with levels of anticoagulation that are not associated with an unacceptable frequency of spontaneous hemorrhage.

A further theoretic advantage of argatroban is in vitro evidence of its activity in HIT blood.[41] Platelet activation can be experimentally eliminated with argatroban. No data suggest a similar phenomenon with the other thrombin inhibitors.

Argatroban is an L-arginine derivative metabolized in the liver to three identified metabolites: M-1, M-2, and M-3. M-3 is thought to produce nitric oxide, which may offer local vasodilating properties. M-1 may have mild anticoagulant properties. M-2 is thought to be inert. The half-life of argatroban is 20–30 minutes. The half-life of M-1 is considerably longer. Argatroban is eliminated through the kidney. Therefore, patients with hepatic dysfunction or renal insufficiency and patients treated with other medications that are metabolized in the liver require more frequent laboratory monitoring of anticoagulation levels. Such patients also may require downward dose adjustments in argatroban infusion rates.

The initial experience with argatroban for the treatment of patients with HIT antibody is encouraging. The drug is administered intravenously in doses of 2–10 μg/kg/min. The activated partial thromboplastin time (APTT) can be used to monitor the anticoagulant activity of argatroban. The target APTT varies with the patient's clinical condition, but generally it should reflect the level of anticoagulation that a physician would select to treat a similar thrombotic site with heparin. Prophylactic argatroban should be titrated to an APTT of $1^1/_2$–2 times the control value. Therapeutic doses should probably be titrated to higher levels of 2–$2^1/_2$ times the control value. Once laboratory monitoring has confirmed a stable APTT with argatroban therapy, it can be performed once daily. The initial monitoring of APTT should be performed 2–3 times daily until the target APTT is achieved. The APTT should be repeated 2–4 hours after dose adjustments.

The most common negative consequence of treatment with argatroban is bleeding. Previous reports suggest that approximately 50% of patients with HIT antibody experience some bleeding. Most have been hospitalized for procedures such as cardiac or orthopedic surgery or have prolonged medical courses preceding the identification of HIT antibody; therefore, they have multiple fresh surgical wounds and puncture sites. Such patients also have a high prevalence of stress-related gastric erosions. The overall result is a tendency to minor bleeding from surgical wounds and mucosal surfaces. Care must be taken to monitor wounds and gastrointestinal bleeding. Gastrointestinal bleeding should be prophylaxed with Carafate or antacids. Cimetidine should be avoided because of a pharmacologic interaction with argatroban. Further care must be taken to monitor hemoglobin and laboratory probes of level of anticoagulation.

Patients treated with argatroban experience frequent episodes of minor bleeding. Trace microscopic hematuria, hemoccult-positive stools, epistaxis at nasogastric tube insertion sites, and minor bleeding at surgical wounds have been seen. However, the incidence of clinically significant bleeding that requires transfusions is < 5%.

The other side effects of argatroban are minor. Nausea, diarrhea, constipation, dizziness, and headache have been infrequently reported. Patients tolerate treatment with argatroban quite well. In addition, argatroban has no in vitro or in vivo ability to complex with HIT antibody. Therefore, patients with HIT antibody do not require platelet activation testing before administration of argatroban.

The outcome analysis of patients with HIT antibody who receive argatroban therapy can be divided into 2 groups: treatment of patients with HITTS and treatment of patients with HIT. Patients with HITTS historically have carried a 30-day mortality rate of approximately 30%. Treatment with Orgaron has been associated with a reduction in death secondary to thrombosis, but the 30-day mortality rate approaches 30%. Preliminary evidence suggests that argatroban-treated patients show a 30-day mortality rate of approximately 15%. The probability of developing a new site of thrombosis on argatroban is < 10% compared with a probability of 35–40% with traditional therapy. Such markedly improved outcomes in patients with HITTS justify the risk of minor bleeding associated with argatroban therapy.

The mortality rate of patients with HIT has not been well documented in the literature. Patients who have HIT and a positive HIT antibody test carry a mortality rate of

20–30%. Many deaths are related to the development of new thrombotic events. The probability of developing a new thrombotic event in this group of patients is 35–40%. Strong consideration, therefore, should be given to anticoagulation with argatroban. The mortality rate in argatroban-treated patients with HIT is 15%, and the probability of new thrombosis is < 10%. Patients with HIT and a low risk of bleeding, therefore, should be considered for prophylaxis with argatroban.

Argatroban is generally used to bridge the gap of anticoagulation until therapeutic levels of warfarin can be established. The duration of argatroban treatment varies with the clinical condition of the patient and requirements for invasive or surgical procedures. Warfarin administration is generally deferred until surgical procedures have been completed. Warfarin is initiated at low doses while argatroban is at therapeutic levels and only after argatroban has been infused for at least 48 hours. The delay is necessary to avoid the paradoxic thrombosis associated with warfarin administration in patients with HIT antibody. Initial low doses of warfarin are also recommended to avoid the paradoxic thrombosis seen with warfarin. Furthermore, patients with HIT antibody are frequently quite ill and nutritionally depleted; therefore, they are often highly sensitive to administration of the vitamin K antagonist, warfarin.

The recommendation for conversion of argatroban to warfarin is somewhat obscured by the effect of argatroban on the prothrombin time (PT). Argatroban has a linear effect on PT that makes interpretation of the warfarin effect difficult. One should measure the baseline PT after the steady-state level of argatroban has been achieved. The desired therapeutic PT for warfarin should then be determined. The difference between the desired PT with warfarin and the control (normal) PT can be added to the steady-state argatroban PT to establish the PT for warfarin plus argatroban. Warfarin dosing can then be adjusted to the warfarin-plus-argatroban PT. When this level is approached, the patient can weaned from argatroban. The warfarin-plus-argatroban PT should not exceed 30 seconds.

The treatment of patients with HIT antibody will continue to evolve. Thrombin inhibition with argatroban offers the first viable alternative for treatment of these critically ill patients. Currently, argatroban offers a reliable therapeutic option that can be easily monitored with conventional laboratory parameters. Treatment with argatroban does not require testing for cross-reactivity with HIT antibody before initiation of therapy. Evidence supports the safety of argatroban in treatment of patients with HIT antibody.

REFERENCES

1. King DE, Kelton JG: Heparin-induced thrombocytopenia. Ann Intern Med 100:535–540, 1984.
2. Warkentin TE, Kelton JG: Heparin and Platelets. Hematol Oncol Clin North Am 4:243–264, 1990.
3. Walls JT, Curtis JJ, Silver D, Boley TM: Heparin-induced thrombocytopenia in patients who undergo open heart surgery. Surgery 108:686–693, 1990.
4. Wallis DE, Lewis BE, Pifarré R, Scanlon PJ: Active surveillance for heparin-induced thrombocytopenia on thromboembolism. Chest 106:1205, 1994.
5. Adelman B, Sobel M, Fujimura Y, et al: Heparin-associated thrombocytopenia; observations on the mechanism of platelet aggregation. J Lab Clin Med 113:204–210, 1989.
6. Kelton JG, Sheridan D, Santos A, et al: Heparin-induced thrombocytopenia: Laboratory studies. Blood 72:925-930, 1988.
7. Chong BH, Castaldi PA, Berndt M: Heparin-induced thrombocytopenia: effects of rabbit IgG and FAB and FC fragments on antibody-heparin-platelet interaction. Thromb Res 55:291-295, 1989.
8. Kelton JG, Smith IW, Warkentin TE, et al: Immunoglobulin G from patients with heparin-induced thrombocytopenia binds to a complex of heparin and platelet factor 4. Blood 83:3232-3239, 1994.
9. Greinacher A, Poetzsch B, Amiral J, et al: Heparin-associated thrombocytopenia: Isolation of the antibody and characterization of a multimolecular PF4-heparin complex as the major antigen. Thromb Haemost 71:247–251, 1994.
10. Visentin GP, Ford SE, Scott JP, Aster RH: Antibodies from patients with heparin-induced thrombocytopenia/thrombosis are specific for platelet factor 4 complexes with heparin or heparin bound endothelial cells. J Clin Invest 93:81–88, 1994.
11. Gueinadheu A, Liebenhoff U, Kiefel V, et al: Heparin-associated thrombocytopenia: The effects of various intravenous IgG preparations on antibody mediated platelet activation. A possible new indication for high dose IV IgG. Thromb Haemost 71:641–645, 1994.

12. Amiral J, Bridey E, Dreyfus M, et al: Platelet factor 4 complexed to heparin is the target for antibodies generated in heparin-induced thrombocytopenia. Thromb Haemost 68:95–96, 1992.
13. Greinacher A, Michels I, Mueller-Eckhardt C: Heparin associated thrombocytopenia: The antibody is not heparin specific. Thromb Haemost 67:547–549, 1992.
14. Visentin GP, Ford SE, Scott JP, Aster RH: Antibodies from patients with heparin-induced thrombocytopenia/thrombosis are specific for platelet factor 4 complexes with heparin or heparin bound endothelial cells. J Clin Invest 93:81–88. 1994.
15. Cines DB, Tomaski A, Tannenbaum S: Immune endothelial cell injury in heparin-associated thrombocytopenia. N Engl J Med 316:581–589, 1987.
16. Lefemine AA: Complications of heparin-induced thrombocytopenia. Am Surg 48:202, 1982.
17. Makhoul RG, Greenberg CS, McCann RL: Heparin-associated thrombocytopenia and thrombosis: A serious clinical problem and potential solution. J Vasc Surg 4:522, 1986.
18. Krueger SK, Andres E, Weinand E: Thrombolysis in heparin-induced thrombocytopenia [letter]. Ann Intern Med 103:159, 1985.
19. Darvey MG, Landeu H: Effect of injected heparin on platelet levels in man. J Clin Path 21:55, 1968.
20. Heiden D, Mielke CH, Rodvieu R: Impairment by heparin of primary haemostasis and platelet 5-hyroxytryptamine release. Br J Haematol 36:427, 1977.
21. Heinrich D, Gorg T, Schultz M: Effects of unfractionated and fractionated heparin on platelet function. Haemostasis 18(Suppl):48, 1988.
22. Singer RL, Mannion JD, Bauer TL, et al: Complications from heparin-induced thrombocytopenia in patients undergoing cardiopulmonary bypass. Chest 102(2):73S, 1992.
23. Aburahma AF, Malik FS, Boland JP: Heparin-induced thrombocytopenia with thrombotic complications. W Va Med J 88(3):95–100, 1992.
24. Chong BH, Grace CS, Rozenberg MC: Heparin-induced thrombocytopenia: effect of heparin-platelet antibody on platelets. Br J Haematol 49:531–540, 1981.
25. Sheridan D, Carter C, Kelton JG: A diagnostic test for heparin-induced thrombocytopenia. Blood 67:27–30, 1986.
26. Greinacher J, Amiral J, Dummel AM, et al: Laboratory diagnosis of heparin-associated thrombocytopenia and comparison of platelet aggregation test, heparin-induced platelet activation test and platelet factor 4/heparin enzyme-linked immunosorbent assay. Transfusion 34:381–385, 1994.
27. Arepally G, Reynolds C, Tomaski A, et al: Comparison of PF4/heparin Elisa assay with the 14C-serotonin release assay in the diagnosis of heparin-induced thrombocytopenia. Am J Clin Pathol 104:648–654, 1995.
28. Potter C, Gill JC, Scott, McFarland JG: Heparin-induced thrombocytopenia in a child. J Pediatr 121:135–138, 1992.
29. Klemp V, Bisler H: Case report: Acute infra renal aortic occlusion and leg vein thrombosis in heparin-induced thrombocytopenia. Vasa Suppl 33:289–290, 1991.
30. Lester J, Elfrink R, Silver D: Response to heparin of patients with heparin-associated antibodies. J Vasc Surg 9:677–681, 1989.
31. Rizzoni WE, Miller K, Rick M, Lotze MT: Heparin-induced thrombocytopenia and thromboembolism in the postoperative period. Surgery 103:470–476, 1988.
32. Laster J, Silver D: Heparin-coated catheters and heparin-induced thrombocytopenia. J Vasc Surg 7:667, 1988.
33. Walls JT, Boley TM, Curtis JJ, Silver D: Heparin-induced thrombocytopenia in patients undergoing intra-aortic balloon pumping after open heart surgery. ASAIO J 38:M574–M576, 1992.
34. Walls JT, Curtis JJ, Silver D, et al: Heparin-induced thrombocytopenia in open heart surgical patients; sequelae of late recognition. Ann Thorac Surg 53:787–791, 1992.
35. Boshkov LK, Warkentin TE, Hayward CP, et al: Heparin-induced thrombocytopenia and thrombosis: Clinical and laboratory studies. Br J Haematol 84:322–328, 1993.
36. Warkentin TE, Levine MN, Hirsh J, et al: Heparin-induced thrombocytopenia in patients treated with low-molecular-weight heparin or unfractionated heparin. N Engl J Med 332:1330-1335, 1995.
37. Magnani HN. Heparin-induced thrombocytopenia (HIT): An overview of 230 patients treated with Organon (Org 10172). Thromb Hemost 70:554–561, 1993.
38. Aburahma AF, Boland JP, Witsberger T: Diagnostic and therapeutic strategies of white clot syndrome. Am J Surg 162:175–179, 1991.
39. Walenga JM, Koza MJ, Lewis BE, Pifarré R: Relative heparin-induced thrombocytopenia potential of low molecular weight heparins and new antithrombotic agents. Clin Appl Thromb Hemost 2:S1-S27, 1996.
40. Blockmans D, Bounameaux H, Vermylen J, Verstraete M: Heparin-induced thrombocytopenia platelet aggregation studies in the presence of heparin fractions or semi-synthetic analogues of various molecular weights and anticoagulant activities. Thromb Haemost 55:90-93, 1986.
41. Matsuo T, Yamada T, Yamanashi T, Ryo R: Anticoagulant therapy with MD805 of hemodialysis patients with heparin-induced thrombocytopenia. Thromb Res 58:663–666, 1990.

CHAPTER 16

The Preclinical and Clinical Pharmacology of Novastan (Argatroban)

RICHARD P. SCHWARZ, JR., Ph.D.

THROMBIN: MECHANISMS OF ACTION

The procoagulant and prothrombotic actions of thrombin are numerous.[1] Thrombin catalyzes the transformation of soluble fibrinogen into fibrin monomers I and II and activates factor XIII to XIIIa to cross-link fibrin into a stable, insoluble clot. It promotes and amplifies clot formation by activating factor V to Va and generating additional thrombin via the prothrombinase complex and activates factor VIII in the intrinsic coagulation pathway. It is also one of the most potent agents for platelet activation, adhesion, and aggregation. Thrombin causes vasodilation in vessels with an intact, undamaged endothelium via release of prostacyclin and nitric oxide; however, in vessels with a damaged endothelium, it acts as a vasoconstrictor, at least in part due to the release of endothelin-1.[2] In addition to these precoagulant and prothrombotic actions, thrombin activates two counter-regulatory systems. First, thrombin binds to thrombomodulin on the endothelium, activating protein C, which together with factor S inactivates factors Va and VIIIa. Second, thrombin stimulates the release of tissue plasminogen activator (tPA) and plasminogen activator inhibitor type 1 (PAI-1), both of which are involved in the regulation of endogenous thrombolysis.[2]

The currently available thrombin-inhibiting agents can be classified as indirect and direct thrombin inhibitors. The indirect thrombin inhibitors either (1) inhibit the formation or activity of factors in the coagulation cascade involved in the production of thrombin or (2) require an endogenous cofactor, such as antithrombin III (AT III), to exert their thrombin-inhibitory actions. The direct thrombin inhibitors, also called site-directed thrombin inhibitors, exert their inhibitory action via interaction with one or more of the three functional domains (sites) on the thrombin molecule.

INDIRECT THROMBIN INHIBITORS

Unfractionated Heparin

The intravenous agent heparin is a heterogeneous mixture of polysaccharide chains (mean molecular weight = 15,000; range = 3,000–30,000).[3] Its anticoagulant and antithrombotic actions are principally attributable to its catalytic enhancement of the inhibitory actions of AT III on thrombin. Heparin reversibly binds to and induces a conformational change in AT III, enhancing the binding of AT III to thrombin with result-ant thrombin inhibition. In addition, heparin catalyzes the inhibition of thrombin by hep-arin cofactor II, as well as the inhibition of factor Xa by AT III. Furthermore, the heparin–AT III complex inactivates factors IX, X, XI, and XII and the tissue factor VIIa complex in the coagulation cascade.[4,5] Thus, heparin may be considered as an indirect, re-versible inhibitor of both thrombin activity and thrombin formation. Although in wide-spread clinical use, the drug has several well-recognized, significant limitations.

First, poor predictability of drug effect with administered dose often results in under-anticoagulation (therapeutic failure) or overanticoagulation (bleeding risk).[3] Estimates of the incidence of hemorrhagic complications and bleeding vary with the mode of adminis-tration—from 1–7% for patients receiving continuous intravenous infusion and from 8–14% for patients administered repeat bolus injections.[3,6,7]

A second limitation, in part related to the poor dose-effect relationship, is the fre-quently observed phenomenon of heparin resistance, in which failure to achieve clinically efficacious APTT levels is encountered despite administration of significant doses. The un-derlying causes of heparin resistance may include (1) a functional abnormality or familial deficiency of AT III;[8] (2) the inability of the heparin—AT III complex to access and inacti-vate clot-bound thrombin, probably due to the large molecular mass of the heparin—AT III complex;[9] (3) the protective effects of both fibrin monomers[10] (in the case of thrombin) and the prothrombinase complex[11] (in the case of factor Xa) in preventing inactivation of these prothrombotic systems; and (4) the action of heparinases and the release of platelet factor IV from activated platelets, which interferes with the binding of heparin to AT III.[12]

Third, as many as 10% of patients receiving heparin show the paradoxical response of heparin-induced thrombocytopenia (HIT),[13] in which clinically significant reductions in platelet count are observed approximately 3–15 days after initiation of heparin and which cannot be reasonably attributed to other, intercurrent conditions. The incidence of HIT is higher with bovine lung heparin than with heparin derived from porcine mucosal sources.[14] The thrombocytopenia is believed to be caused by heparin-dependent IgG anti-bodies, which recognize a complex of heparin with platelet factor IV and activate platelets through their Fc receptors.[15,16] In approximately 0.5% of patients receiving hep-arin, the clinical syndrome of heparin-induced thrombocytopenia and thrombosis (HITT) is reported, marked by the recognition of a potentially debilitating or life-threatening arterial thrombosis,[17] with a reported combined mortality and major morbidity rate of 25–37%.[18,19]

Low-Molecular-Weight Heparins and Heparinoids

The limitations of heparin have led to the development of the low-molecular-weight heparin (LMWH) agents, which are produced by enzymatic or chemical fragmentation of the heparin molecule, and the heparinoids, which are composed of synthetic sulfated poly-mers or naturally occurring glycosaminoglycans. The mean molecular weights of the LMWH agents and the heparinoids range from 4500–6500, with a broad range of variation in individual preparations.[20]

Like heparin, the LMWH agents and heparinoids possess a binding site for the AT III complex but have fewer thrombin binding sites than the parent molecule. This results in (1) enhanced capacity for inhibition of factor Xa by the bound AT III complex, and (2) di-minished ability for inactivating thrombin (factor IIa). The ratio of these two effects depends on the proportion of short to long polysaccharide chains in the individual prep-aration. The ratio (anti-Xa/anti-IIa) activity ranges from 2.7 for enoxaparin to 20.0 for lomoparin.[20]

Compared with heparin, the LMWH agents and heparinoids possess the advantages of (1) longer pharmacokinetic half-life; (2) better subcutaneous absorption and bioavail-ability; (3) less binding to plasma proteins; (4) greater access to and inhibition of factor Xa in the prothrombinase complex; and (5) reduced potential for HIT and HITT, although both remain a significant concern.[21–23] These advantages have led to extensive clinical investigation of these agents for the prophylaxis and treatment of venous thrombosis as well as the treatment of unstable angina and non-Q wave MI. Once- or twice-daily administration is possible, with significantly less monitoring than with heparin.

Warfarin

The oral anticoagulant warfarin and the related Coumarin agents exert their antithrombotic effects by blocking the formation of γ-carboxylglutamic acid (Gla) residues, which are generated via the vitamin K-dependent γ-carboxylation of glutamic acids in the liver. The Gla residues are essential to the functioning of a number of factors in the coagulation cascade, including factors II, VII, IX, and X, prothrombin, protein C, and protein S.

Because warfarin acts by inhibiting the de novo synthesis of factors that are essential to the functioning of the intrinsic and extrinsic coagulation pathways, it has a relatively slow onset of action and requires prolonged dosing (3–4 days) before a consistent antithrombotic effect is achieved. In addition, actions are not easily reversible after cessation of therapy.[1] Warfarin is highly protein-bound and has a relatively long pharmacokinetic half-life (≈35 hours); considerable individual variation in response requires close monitoring to avoid the risk of bleeding.[1,5] The antithrombotic actions of the drug are influenced by dietary levels of vitamin K and enhanced by agents that either inhibit the metabolic clearance of warfarin (e.g., sulfinpyrazone, cimetidine, amiodarone) or increase the metabolic clearance of vitamin K-dependent factors (e.g., cephalosporins, fibrates.)[1]

DIRECT THROMBIN INHIBITORS

The limitations of the indirect thrombin inhibitors have prompted efforts focused on the discovery and development of site-directed (i.e., direct) thrombin inhibitors,[24] the molecular properties of which permit their interaction with one or more of the functional domains of the thrombin molecule with resultant thrombin inhibition.

Molecular Characteristics

The molecular characteristics of the direct thrombin inhibitors may be presented in terms of properties that distinguish their mechanism of action from that of heparin and, in some cases, from each other. These characteristics, which offer the potential for antithrombotic efficacy that is superior to that of heparin and minimal risk of bleeding, include:
- Selectivity for interacting with the functional domains of thrombin
- Fast vs. slow thrombin inhibition
- Reversible vs. irreversible thrombin inhibition
- Large vs. small molecular weight
- Ability (potency) to inhibit clot-bound thrombin

Selectivity for Interacting with the Functional Domains of Thrombin

The catalytic site, the anion-binding exosite, and the apolar region are the three functional domains of the thrombin molecule that interact with the direct thrombin inhibitors.[2] The catalytic site, as the name implies, is the active site of thrombin, containing the catalytic triad (serine/histidine/aspartic acid); it has a basic specificity pocket that binds to arginine and lysine side-chains of some of the site-directed thrombin inhibitors. The small-molecule direct thrombin inhibitors, such as argatroban, interact with this site at the serine and the basic pocket, along with an adjacent hydrophobic site (apolar region). The anion-binding exosite (also known as the substrate recognition site) is located on a region of the thrombin molecule distant from the catalytic site and is the binding site for hirudin and hirulog. It is comprised of multiple basic amino acids that permit it to form ionic bonds with the carboxyl terminal of some of the direct thrombin inhibitors, such as hirudin. The apolar region is located near the catalytic site. It binds via hydrophobic inter-action with the amino-terminal region of some of the direct thrombin inhibitors (hirudin and hirulog) as well as with hydrophobic groups of argatroban.

Thus, the small-molecule direct thrombin inhibitors, such as argatroban, inhibit thrombin by selectively interacting with the catalytic site and apolar region, whereas hirudin's thrombin-inhibitory actions involve interactions with the anion-binding exosite and apolar region, thereby indirectly blocking access of substrates to the active site do-mains of thrombin.

In addition to these three sites, which are important for the actions of the direct thrombin inhibitors, the fibrin-binding exosite, a region distinct from the anion-binding exosite, is the functional domain that permits the binding of thrombin to fibrin (i.e., clot-bound thrombin), whereas the heparin-binding site is involved in the binding of the hep-arin–AT III complex to thrombin.

Fast vs. Slow Thrombin Inhibition

Hirudin binds to and inhibits the thrombin molecule in a two-stage process. The first (and rate-limiting) step involves the electrostatic binding of the C-terminus of hirudin to the anion-binding exosite; the second step involves the binding of the N-ter-minus residues of hirudin to the apolar region.[25] The basic specificity pocket at the cat-alytic site of thrombin, responsible for its enzymatic specificity in cleaving substrates at arginine residues, is not occupied by hirudin. The association constant for hirudin's binding to thrombin (k_a) is 1.4×10^{-8}/M-sec.[26] The small-molecule direct thrombin in-hibitor, argatroban, binds rapidly to thrombin at the catalytic site and apolar region at a diffusion controlled rate.[24]

The two-stage (i.e., "slow") inhibition of thrombin by hirudin may result in a disad-vantage relative to argatroban with respect to antithrombotic efficacy. Experimental evi-dence indicates that the activation of thrombin may be characterized as occurring in "pulse" or "burst" events, which are highly localized spatially and of short duration. The antithrombotic efficacy of thrombin inhibitors, it is assumed, requires rapid, complete inhibition of the high local concentrations of thrombin present at the physiologic sites of thrombotic events.[27-30] Whether the rapid k_a of argatroban compared with hirudin trans-lates into a clinical advantage must await antithrombotic efficacy results from clinical trials.

Reversible vs. Irreversible Thrombin Inhibition

In addition to its slowness, the binding of hirudin to thrombin is essentially irre-versible (dissociation constant, $k_d = 3.2 \times 10^5$/sec);[26] Argatroban, however, is fully re-versible.[24] These differences in binding properties of the agents may be significant in two ways. First, the rapid dissociation of argatroban may lead to a more rapid return of the clinical laboratory coagulation markers (APTT, activated clotting time [ACT]) to premedication values on cessation of medication. Second, the reversibility of thrombin inhibition by argatroban may be associated with a greater propensity for induction of a hypercoagulable state when the medication is terminated without tapering of dosage (the so-called rebound effect; see below), particularly in disease states such as unstable angina.

Large vs. Small Molecular Weight

Hirudin is a 65-amino acid protein with a molecular weight of ≈ 7000[31] and is pro-duced by the relatively complex and expensive methods of recombinant technology. Argatroban (molecular weight = 508)[32] is a synthetic small molecule produced by rela-tively simple manufacturing techniques, with the potential for substantial cost advantages compared with hirudin.

Ability (Potency) to Inhibit Clot-Bound Thrombin

Experimental data from several laboratories[9,33–35] have indicated that the small-molecule direct thrombin inhibitors, such as argatroban, offer the potential to be more effective than heparin and perhaps hirudin in terms of ability to inhibit thrombin that is both bound to and incorporated within the clot matrix. This potential is discussed in greater detail below. Thus, argatroban differs from hirudin in terms of its small molecular size, its selective, fast, noncovalent, and reversible inhibition of the catalytic site of thrombin, and its apparently greater potency for inhibiting clot-bound thrombin.

ARGATROBAN: PRECLINICAL PHARMACOLOGY

Argatroban—molecular formula: $C_{23}H_{36}N_6O_5S \cdot H_2O$; chemical name: (2R,4R)-4-methyl-1-[N^2-[(RS)-3-methyl-1,2,3,4-tetrahydro-8-quinolinesulfonyl-L-arginyl]-2-pyperidinecarboxylic acid hydrate]—is a small-molecule (molecular weight: 508 Da) derived from the amino acid L-arginine[32] (Fig. 1).

Argatroban is a 64:36 mixture of 21-(R) and 21-(S) diastereoisomers, with the latter being approximately twice as potent as the former in an in vitro coagulation assay. However, the 21-(S) form is much less soluble than the 21-(R) form, suggesting that the mixture of the two requires a smaller volume than the 21-(S) form to deliver a therapeutic dose.[36]

Animal Models of Arterial and Venous Thrombosis

The thrombin-inhibitory actions of argatroban have been demonstrated in a variety of in-vitro and in-vivo pharmacologic studies. Green et al. demonstrated that argatroban (1.0 μM) doubled the thrombin clotting time in the presence of calcium, with the same 2-fold increase evident at 0.1 μM in the absence of calcium. Over the same concentration range, argatroban doubled the prothrombin time (PT) and the APTT.[37]

The in vitro tPA- or urokinase-induced lysis of human plasma clots was accelerated by 70% with an argatroban concentration of 0.3 μM, with a similar effect observed on rabbit plasma clots.[38] This same study also showed that the formation of both factor XIIIa and cross-linked fibrin was inhibited by argatroban.

Berry et al.[39] investigated the antithrombotic activity of argatroban in three rodent models of arterial and venous thrombosis as well as the bleeding potential in the rat model

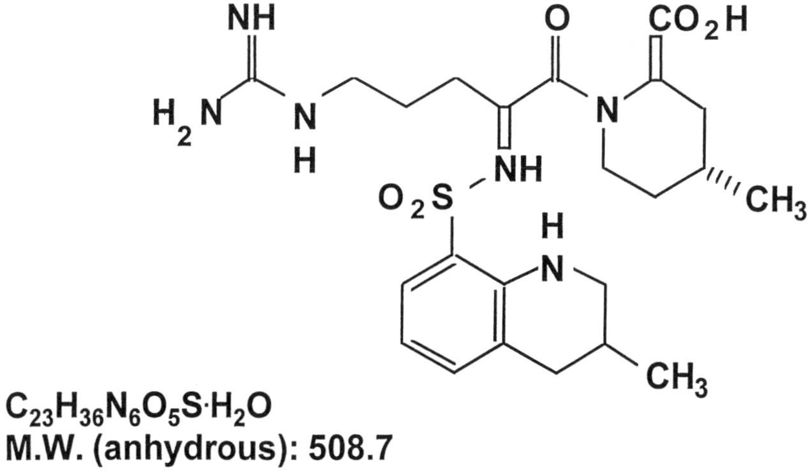

$C_{23}H_{36}N_6O_5S \cdot H_2O$
M.W. (anhydrous): 508.7

FIGURE 1.   Chemical structure of argatroban (Novastan); chemical name: (2R,4R)-4-methyl-1-[N^2-[(RS)-3-methyl-1,2,3,4-tetrahydro-8-quinolinesulfonyl-L-arginyl]-2-pyperidinecarboxylic acid hydrate].

of tail transection bleeding time. In the rat model of venous thrombosis induced by thromboplastin followed by stasis of the abdominal vena cava, similar median effective doses (ED_{50}), defined as the dose that reduced thrombus weight by 50% compared with that in control animals, were observed with continuous intravenous infusions of argatroban ($ED_{50} = 1.5\mu g/kg/min$) as with heparin ($ED_{50} = 1.2 \mu g/kg/min$). In the rat model of arteriovenous shunt model, the ED_{50} was 6.0 $\mu g/kg/min$ for argatroban and 3.0 $\mu g/kg/min$ for heparin when both were administered by continuous intravenous infusion.

When an occlusive arterial thrombus was induced by electrical stimulation of the left carotid artery, argatroban, at a continuous intravenous infusion dose of 20.0 $\mu g/kg/min$, produced a 111% increase in the duration of postlesion vessel patency, similar to that observed for heparin. However, these antithrombotic effects were observed with only small increases in APTT for argatroban, whereas even subthreshold doses of heparin produced statistically significant, 7-fold increases in APTT. Continuous intravenous infusions of both argatroban and heparin produced dose-dependent increases in rodent tail transection bleeding time; however, the dose of argatroban that doubled the bleeding time (ED_{100}) was 5 times greater than the dose of heparin (11 $\mu g/kg/min$ vs. 2.2 $\mu g/kg/min$).

The results by Berry et al.[39] suggest that argatroban achieves an in vivo antithrombotic efficacy equivalent to that of heparin, with a lower degree of systemic anticoagulation and lower hemorrhagic potential than that observed for heparin.

Thrombin has different vasomotor effects in the intact vs. the damaged endothelium, producing nitric oxide-mediated vasodilation in vessels with intact endothelia and endothelin-mediated vasoconstriction in vessels with damaged endothelia.[2] Winn et al.[40] showed that argatroban inhibits thrombin-induced vasodilation ($ED_{50} = 0.3 \mu M$) in isolated canine coronary arteries with undamaged endothelia. However, in coronary arteries in which the endothelium was damaged by mechanical abrasion, argatroban reduced thrombin-induced vasoconstriction to approximately 20% of the maximal value.

In a rodent model of pulmonary thromboembolism, Kumada et al.[41] demonstrated that argatroban was effective in AT III-deficient animals (produced by administration of anti-AT III antibodies); heparin, however, was inactive. This finding substantiates the lack of dependence of argatroban on this heparin cofactor.

Enhancement of Thrombolysis and Prevention of Reocclusion

Argatroban also has been shown to enhance the clot-lysing activity of thrombolytic agents while decreasing the potential for reocclusion after restoration of occluded vessel patency. Nishiyama et al.,[42] using a guinea pig model of femoral artery thrombosis, showed that argatroban, when co-administered with tPA, (1) reduced the time to vessel reopening; (2) increased the duration of vessel reflow; and (3) decreased the frequency of 24-hour reocclusion. Mellott[43] and coworkers showed that argatroban shortens the time to lysis achieved with tPA and prevents reocclusion after blood flow restoration in a canine model of femoral artery thrombosis. Jang et al.[44] investigated the comparative effects of argatroban and heparin on tPA-induced thrombolysis in a rabbit model of femoral artery thrombosis, demonstrating that argatroban significantly (1) increased the magnitude of blood reflow and (2) reduced the time in which blood reflow was achieved. In two separate studies using the same conscious canine model of coronary artery thrombosis, Fitzgerald and coworkers[45,46] provided evidence that argatroban accelerated thrombolysis produced by tPA and delayed reocclusion in a dose-dependent manner. Heparin, however, did not prevent reocclusion at a dose that elevated the APTT 10-fold.

Other Animal Models of Acute Coronary Syndromes

A comparative study of argatroban and abciximab or monoclonal antibody-directed 7E3-(Fab')$_2$, a glycoprotein IIb/IIIa (platelet fibrinogen receptor)-blocking agent, was performed in dogs with fibrin-rich thrombi produced by denuding and tightly constricting the coronary arteries.[47] Argatroban and abciximab had generally similar reductions in lysis time; abciximab was slightly superior in preventing reocclusion. However, the addition of aspirin to argatroban produced results slightly better than those achieved with abciximab.

In an open-chest canine model of unstable angina, both argatroban and heparin were equally efficacious in abolishing cyclic flow reductions (CFRs) caused by formation and dislodgement of platelet-rich, fibrin-poor thrombi.[48]

Inhibitory Effects on Soluble and Clot-Bound Thrombin

Berry et al.[33] compared the inhibitory potencies of argatroban, hirudin, and heparin for soluble thrombin vs. clot-bound thrombin. Argatroban showed virtually no reduction in potency for clot-bound thrombin compared with soluble thrombin; however, both hirudin and heparin showed a thousand-fold loss in inhibitory potency for clot-bound thrombin compared with soluble thrombin. Reductions in inhibitory potency against clot-bound thrombin for hirudin and heparin were also observed in other studies,[9,34,35] although the magnitude of the shifts was less than that reported by Berry et al.[33] One explanation for the reduction in the inhibitory potency of hirudin and heparin for clot-bound thrombin may be that thrombin, which is incorporated into clots, has a reduced binding capacity for large molecules such as hirudin and heparin (molecular weights ≈7,000 and 12,000, respectively) because of steric constraints imposed on thrombin when bound to fibrin. In addition, the cross-linked fibrin matrix may reduce the accessibility of thrombin, which is embedded in the clot by larger molecules. The clinical significance of these observed reductions in potency must await the results of clinical trials of both large and small direct thrombin inhibitors.

Pharmacokinetics of Argatroban in Animals

The pharmacokinetics, metabolism, and elimination of argatroban have been investigated in rabbits and dogs.[49] Radiolabeled drug was cleared from the plasma in a biphasic manner, with α and β elimination half-lives of 3–6 and 26–36 minutes, respectively. Although radiolabeled product was recovered from both urine and feces 24 hours after intravenous infusion, the majority of the drug was fecally excreted, indicating hepatic metabolism and biliary excretion.

Comparative Preclinical Pharmacology of Heparin, Hirudin, and Argatroban

Table 1 is a compilation derived in most part from the comprehensive work by Fareed and Callas[24,50] but incorporating other studies as well. Conclusions include the following:

- Argatroban, unlike heparin and hirudin, is a synthetic, small molecule thrombin inhibitor.
- Argatroban and hirudin, unlike heparin, are direct inhibitors of thrombin.
- Argatroban is a fast, reversible, direct thrombin inhibitor that is selective for the catalytic site/apolar region of thrombin; hirudin is a slow, essentially irreversible, direct thrombin inhibitor that interacts with several of the functional domains of thrombin.
- Heparin and hirudin are more potent on a molar basis than argatroban for the inhibition of soluble thrombin; however, argatroban, unlike hirudin and heparin, shows essentially no reduction in potency for inhibiting clot-bound thrombin compared with soluble thrombin.
- Argatroban and hirudin have substantial in vivo antithrombotic efficacy, somewhat greater than that for heparin.
- Argatroban has a lower in vivo hemorrhagic potential than either heparin or hirudin.

TABLE 1.   Comparative Pharmacology of Heparin, Hirudin and Argatroban

	Heparin	Hirudin	Argatroban
Class	Mucopolysaccharide	65 AA polypeptide	Small molecule
Molecular weight	$\cong$ 12 kd (plus AT III)	$\cong$ 7000 d	508.7
Potency (μM)[1]	0.06	0.01	29.0
Direct thrombin inhibitor?	No	Yes	Yes
Thrombin binding sites[2]	Heparin-AT III	ABE, CS, AR	CS
Fast vs. slow inhibition (k_a)	Fast	Slow	Fast
Binding affinity for thrombin	++	+++	+
Reversibility of inhibition (k_d)	Reversible	Irreversible	Reversible
Effect on global coagulation tests			
APTT	+++	+++	++
PT	+	+++	++
TT	+++	+++	+
Inhibition of clot-bound thrombin	0	+	+++
In vivo antithrombotic efficacy[3]	++	+++	+++
In vivo hemorrhagic potential[4]	+++	+++	++
In vitro inhibition of protein C	0	0	0
In vitro inhibition of thrombolytic enzymes	0	0	0
In vivo inhibition of thrombolysis[5]	0	0	0

[1] 50% inhibition of maximal extrinsic activation of thrombin
[2] ABE = anion binding exosite; CS = catalytic site; AR = apolar region
[3] Wessler rabbit model
[4] Rabbit ear bleeding model
[5] Rabbit FEIBA model (factor eight inhibitor bypass activator)
Effects: 0 = none; + = minor; ++ = moderate; +++ = major

- Argatroban, hirudin, and heparin have no in vitro inhibitory effects on the formation or activity of activated protein C or endogenous thrombolytic enzymes, nor do any of these agents cause in vivo inhibition or thrombolysis (i.e., fibrinolytic compromise).

ARGATROBAN PHASE I CLINICAL PHARMACOLOGY
The clinical pharmacologic profile of argatroban has been investigated in phase I studies, which addressed the following:
- Pharmacodynamics of argatroban compared with heparin in respect to the commonly used clinical monitoring parameters, APTT and ACT
- Effects (s) of renal impairment, age, and gender on argatroban pharmacodynamics
- Metabolism and elimination
- Safety of argatroban administration via bolus injection and continuous intravenous infusion

Pharmacodynamics of Argatroban Compared with Heparin
Table 2 shows the effects of argatroban and heparin in 36 normal subjects (18 treated with argatroban and 18 with heparin). For APTT, argatroban showed a slowly increasing dose-response effect, with an 8-fold increase in dose (30 to 240 μg/kg) resulting in only a 2-fold increase in APTT (43 ± 1 to 82 ± 4 sec). Heparin, however, shows a pronounced, rapidly rising effect on APTT, with a 2-fold increase in dose (15 to 30 IU/kg) increasing the APTT by 395% (68 ± 6 to 269 ± 40 sec). Doses higher than 30 IU/kg are above the limit of detection (> 400). Generally, similar relationships between dose and ACT level were observed for both argatroban and heparin.

TABLE 2. Pharmacodynamics of Single Bolus Injections of Argatroban and Heparin in Normal Subjects

Activated Partial Thromboplastin Time (APTT)					
Argatroban			Heparin		
Dose (µg/kg)	N	APTT (sec)	Dose (IU/kg)	N	APTT (sec)
30	18	43 ± 1	15	15	68 ± 6
60	18	52 ± 2	30	18	269 ± 40
120	18	68 ± 8	60	18	> 400
240	18	82 ± 4	120	12	> 400
Activated Clotting Time (ACT, Hemotec)					
Argatroban			Heparin		
Dose (µg/kg)	N	ACT (sec)	Dose (IU/kg)	N	ACT (sec)
30	18	152 ± 5	15	15	127 ± 2
60	18	185 ± 6	30	18	142 ± 2
120	18	209 ± 7	60	18	173 ± 4
240	18	261 ± 10	120	12	243 ± 7

All values are mean ± SEM

The dose-response effects of continuous intravenous infusions of argatroban on APTT and Hemotec ACT in 9 normal subjects are shown in Table 3. Over a 32-fold escalation in dose (1.25 to 40.0 µg/kg/min), APTT increased by only a factor of 2.2 (54 ± 3 to 119 ± 5) and ACT by only a factor of 1.8 (163 ± 8 to 294 ± 9). Although there are missing data points, particularly at the two highest doses studied, it is clear that argatroban's pharmacodynamic effects on APTT and ACT show little variation over a broad range of doses.

Figure 2 compares the effects of argatroban and heparin on APTT. Over a 2-fold increase in dose, heparin displays a steep dose-response curve, with substantial variability in APTT at each dose. Argatroban, however, displays a gently-rising, predictable response over an 8-fold range in infusion dose.

Figure 3 compares the time course of a combined bolus and continuous intravenous infusion regimen (4 hours' duration) for argatroban (250 µg/kg bolus and 10 µg/kg/min infusion) and heparin (125 U/kg bolus and 0.3 U/kg/min infusion) on Hemotec ACT. Both drugs achieve rapid improvements in ACT over baseline values. Argatroban maintained the ACT values at steady levels for 4 hours; the response with heparin, however, decreased

TABLE 3. Dose-Response Effects of Argatroban on APTT and Hemotec ACT for Continuous Intravenous Infusions of 1.25 to 40.0 µg/kg/min

Infusion Dose (µg/kg/min)	APTT (sec)		ACT (sec)	
	N	Mean ± SEM	N	Mean ± SEM
1.25	9	54 ± 3	7	163 ± 8
2.5	8	62 ± 4	9	180 ± 5
5.0	6	71 ± 7	9	215 ± 7
10.0	8	88 ± 7	9	262 ± 10
15.0	6	86 ± 4	8	224 ± 7
20.0	6	92 ± 5	8	239 ± 9
30.0	4	105 ± 4	8	266 ± 9
40.0	5	119 ± 5	7	294 ± 9

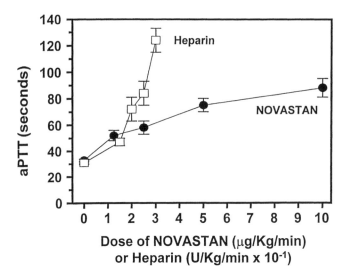

FIGURE 2.   Pharmacodynamic effects of continuous infusions of heparin (*squares*) and arga-troban (*circles*) on activated partial thromboplastin time (APTT) in normal subjects. The doses used were: argatroban—1.25, 2.5, 5.0, and 10.0 µg/kg/min; heparin—15, 20, 25, and 30 IU/kg/min.

during the infusion, probably as a result of the release of platelet factor IV from activated platelets, which interferes with the binding of heparin to AT III. When the infusion was discontinued at 4 hours, the argatroban ACT levels showed a rapid return to predrug values, approaching near-normal levels within 1–2 hours.

Effects of Renal Impairment, Age, and Gender

Recent large-scale clinical trials of the direct thrombin inhibitor hirudin have reported an increased risk for bleeding events in patients with an APTT > 90 seconds, particularly

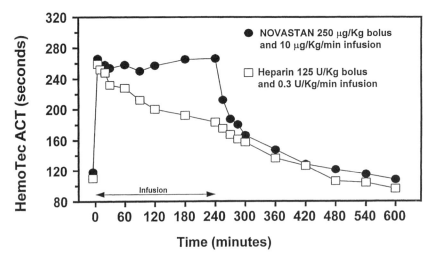

FIGURE 3.   Comparative effects of combined bolus injection/continuous infusion of heparin (*squares*) and argatroban (*circles*) on Hemotec-activated clotting time (ACT) in normal subjects.

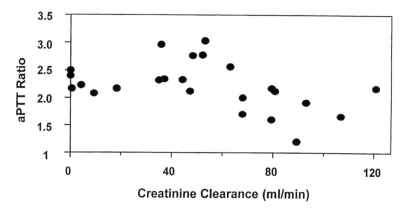

FIGURE 4.   Relationship between creatinine clearance and steady state APTT ratio in normal subjects and renally impaired patients receiving a continuous intravenous infusion of argatroban (5.0 mg/kg/minute). Steady state was defined as four hours following the initiation of the infusion. There is only a mild effect of the level of renal function on steady-state APTT levels (correlation coefficient, $r^2 = 0.176$, $p = 0.04$).

in elderly patients, patients with low body weight (especially female patients), and patients with renal impairment.

To assess the potential effects of renal impairment on the pharmacodynamics of argatroban, a study was performed in 24 normal subjects and patients with varying degrees of renal function, from subjects with normal and near-normal renal function (creatinine clearance, Cl_{cr} of ≥ 90 ml/min) to patients with severely impaired renal function ($Cl_{cr} < 29$ ml/min). All subjects and patients received a continuous intravenous infusion of argatroban, 5.0 μg/kg/min for 4 hours.

Figure 4 displays the steady-state APTT ratio (the ratio of APTT after 4 hours of argatroban administration to APTT before drug administration) vs. the Cl_{cr} for each subject and patient. The mild effect of the level of renal impairment on the levels of APTT (correlation coefficient, $r^2 = 0.176$, $p = 0.04$) indicates little potential for underdosing or overdosing in patients with widely varying degrees of renal function.

Another study was performed to determine the effects of age and gender on argatroban pharmacokinetics and pharmacodynamics. Four cohorts of 10 patients each (40 total) were studied: young men (n = 10) and young women (n = 10), 18–45 years old, and elderly men (n = 10) and elderly women (n = 10), 65–80 years old. All were administered a continuous intravenous infusion of argatroban, 2.5 μg/kg/min for 4 hours, and a bolus of 125 μg/kg.

Figure 5 depicts steady-state APTT levels (4 hours after initiation of the infusion). No difference can be seen in the four cohorts, with APTT levels ranging from 50 ± 3 in the elderly female cohort to 62 ± 3 in the young male cohort. No significant effects of age and/or gender are apparent. In fact, the highest APTT levels are found in the young males and the lowest APTT levels in the elderly females, the opposite of what would be expected if increasing age, female gender, and low body weight were determinants for increased APTT level with argatroban.

Figure 6 presents the APTT pharmacodynamic half-life data for the four cohorts, with the APTT pharmacodynamic half-life defined as the time required for the APTT to fall to 50% of maximal value after cessation of the argatroban infusion. As with the steady-state APTT levels, no significant effects of age or gender are apparent. The pharmacodynamic half-life is approximately 20–25 minutes, which closely parallels the pharmacokinetic half-life of 24 ± 2 minutes reported previously in a study in 6 normal subjects.[51]

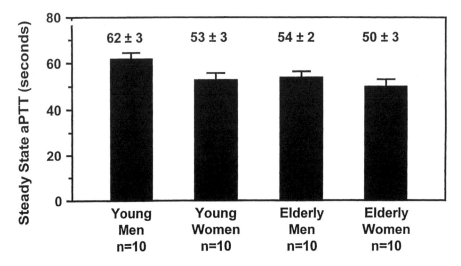

FIGURE 5.   Steady-state APTT levels for four cohorts of normal subjects (stratified by age and gender) receiving a continuous intravenous infusion of argatroban (2.5 mg/kg/minute). No effect of age or gender is apparent.

Metabolism and Elimination

A study in normal subjects reported that argatroban is hepatically metabolized.[52] The main route of metabolism in humans is the same as in laboratory animals; that is, hydroxylation and aromatization of the 3-methyltetrahydroquinoline ring. Unchanged drug excreted in the urine amounted to 23% within the first 24 hours after dosing, and fecal excretion of unchanged drug amounted to 12% within the first 24 hours.

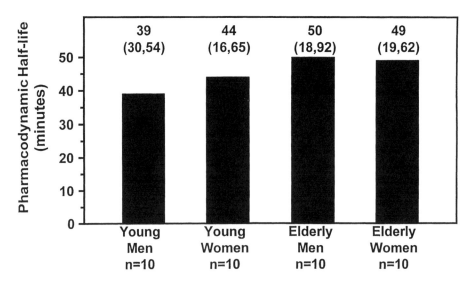

FIGURE 6.   APTT pharmacodynamic half-life for four cohorts of normal subjects (stratified by age and gender) receiving a continuous intravenous infusion of argatroban (2.5 mg/kg/minute). The pharmacodynamic half-life was defined as the time required for the APTT level to fall to 50% of maximal value following cessation of a 4-hour infusion. No effect of age or gender is apparent.

TABLE 4.   Adverse Events Observed during the Administration
of Argatroban and Heparin in Phase I Studies

	Number of Occurrences of Each Adverse Event (%)	
Adverse Event	Argatroban (110 Subjects)	Heparin (36 Subjects)
Headache	20 (18.2)	4 (11.1)
Dizziness	9 (8.2)	2 (5.6)
Pain	7 (6.4)	3 (8.3)
Rash	7 (6.4)	2 (5.6)
Injection site reaction	2 (1.8)	1 (2.8)
Nausea	2 (1.8)	2 (5.6)
Asthenia	2 (1.8)	0 (0.0)

Phase I Clinical Safety Studies

Adverse events observed during the phase I clinical pharmacologic studies in the United States for subjects receiving argatroban (n = 110) and heparin (n = 36) are presented in Table 4. No significant differences were reported in the frequency of the observed adverse events with argatroban and heparin administration. The most frequently reported adverse event was headache (18.2% with argatroban, 11.1% with heparin; p = NS). None of the adverse events were serious in nature, and all resolved without adverse sequelae. No relationship between the frequency of observed adverse events and dose of argatroban was evident over the infusion dose range of 1.25–40.0 µg/kg/min.

Advanced Clinical Development and Potential Clinical Uses

The clinical development program for argatroban in North America is focused on investigating the safety and efficacy of the agent in three multicenter controlled clinical trials involving two potential clinical indications:
- Adjuvant therapy to thrombolytic agents in patients with AMI
- Anticoagulant and antithrombotic therapy in patients with HIT and HITTS

ADJUVANT THERAPY TO THROMBOLYTIC AGENTS IN ACUTE MYOCARDIAL INFARCTION

Background and Rationale

The acute coronary syndromes of AMI, non-Q wave MI, and unstable angina result from an abrupt fissure or rupture of an unstable atheromatous plaque in a coronary artery, with exposure of circulating hemostatic components to the thrombogenic plaque core and formation of an overlying thrombus that can partially or completely block flow in the myocardial region distal to the occlusion. Clinical manifestations depend on the magnitude and duration of occlusion, the contractile tone of the occluded vessel, and the energy demands of the myocardium supplied by the occluded vessel. They include:
- **Unstable angina**—new, accelerated, or changing pattern of ischemic chest pain, including pain at rest, in the absence of detectable myocardial necrosis. It is diagnosed by the appearance of chest pain greater than 30 minutes in duration and a nondiagnostic ECG.
- **Non-Q wave MI**—coronary insufficiency of a duration long enough (usually 30–60 minutes) to cause a relatively small amount of myocardial necrosis. Permanent changes in the ECG (Q-waves) are not detectable. Diagnosis is made on the basis of ST segment depression and ST-T abnormalities.

• **AMI (also called Q-wave MI)**—coronary insufficiency of longer duration (usually > 60 minutes) that results in substantial myocardial necrosis, as evidenced by the development of Q-waves on the ECG. Its diagnostic features are ST segment elevation, T-wave changes, and left bundle-branch block.

During the 1980s, the development and testing of thrombolytic agents such as tPA (recombinant tissue plasminogen activator), streptokinase, and anisoylated plasminogen streptokinase activator complex (APSAC) for the management of AMI have provided incontrovertible proof of the ability of these agents to reduce 1-month post-MI mortality by approximately 20–30%.[53] In addition, it is now widely accepted that the reduction in mortality directly depends on (1) shortening the time between the onset of symptoms of AMI and the administration of the thrombolytic agent and (2) achievement of reperfusion of the culprit coronary artery that is immediate (within 60–90 minutes of attempted thrombolysis), complete (TIMI flow 3), and sustained (without intermittent reperfusion or reocclusion).[53]

Results of the GUSTO trial[54,55] indicate a modest (1% absolute; 14% relative) but significant reduction in mortality with the use of accelerated tPA and heparin compared with streptokinase and heparin. However, even the most successful strategies and regimens cannot be expected to produce immediate and complete reperfusion without reocclusion in more than one-fourth to one-third of patients.[53]

The past few years have brought heightened interest in the potential of direct thrombin inhibitors as adjunctive therapy to thrombolytic treatment in AMI. Plaque rupture and clot formation and extension are dynamic processes with a delicate balance between prothrombotic forces (that cause platelet aggregation and thrombogenesis) and factors (both endogenous and exogenous) that enhance thrombolysis. The balance between thrombogenesis and thrombolysis affects the rate of clot formation and dissolution and therefore the duration and extent of coronary insufficiency. Inhibition of thrombin may (1) shift the balance from thrombogenesis to thrombolysis, thus facilitating the achievement of earlier and more complete reperfusion, and (2) prevent thrombus extension, thus preventing reocclusion.[56]

In pilot studies with both tPA[57] and streptokinase,[58] hirudin has shown the potential to be as safe as heparin in terms of bleeding risk and to increase the percentage of patients who achieve rapid, complete, and sustained reperfusion of the culprit coronary artery. However, three large-scale trials of hirudin were terminated prematurely in 1994 because of increased bleeding risk.[59–61] The trials were restarted at a substantially reduced dose of hirudin in an attempt to mitigate untoward effects.[62]

In addition, a study by Théroux et al.,[63] assessing the comparative efficacy of hirulog and heparin to improve the coronary artery patency rate achieved with streptokinase, showed that a low dose of hirulog significantly enhanced the thrombolytic efficacy of streptokinase compared with heparin, whereas a higher dose was less effective than the lower dose. Although the reasons for the lesser efficacy at a higher dose of hirulog are not established, it is possible that higher doses of thrombin inhibitors block the formation or inhibit the activity of activated protein C, with a resultant compromise in the functioning of this anticoagulant pathway. This theory suggests that an excessive degree of thrombin inhibition, in addition to increasing the bleeding risk, may compromise the efficacy of thrombolytic agents.

Argatroban, as well as other direct thrombin inhibitors, has been investigated in pilot studies in patients with unstable angina/non-Q wave MI. In one study with argatroban, Gold et al.[64] reported that cessation of intravenous therapy was associated with rebound thrombin generation (as measured by levels of plasma thrombin–antithrombin complex [TAT]), and with an early dose-related recurrence of unstable angina. This phenomenon of rebound coagulation activation is perhaps best described as a hypercoagulable state, evident on abrupt termination of a thrombin inhibitor, that decreases thrombin activity (as measured by fibrinotide A [FPA] formation) but not thrombin generation (as measured by the formation of either TAT or polypeptide fragment–F1.2). The reactivation of angina has also been reported 5–15 hours after termination of heparin therapy.[65]

Two publications[66,67] have questioned the interpretation of the findings with argatroban by Gold et al., because (1) the influence of heparin administered within 4 hours of argatroban therapy may have confounded the analysis; (2) no decrease in plasma TAT concentration was observed during the argatroban infusion, calling into question whether the TAT increase after cessation of argatroban therapy is artifactual; and (3) no elevation in plasma FPA was observed after cessation of therapy, as would be expected in a hypercoagulable state.

However, it remains to be established whether argatroban and other direct thrombin inhibitors offer a favorable clinical profile in unstable angina and non-Q wave MI. Potential reasons for a lack of efficacy include (1) the possibility that the reversible nature of some of the direct thrombin inhibitors may cause the induction of a hypercoagulable state unless the dose is tapered rather than terminated abruptly, and (2) the possibility that the underlying pathophysiologic processes in unstable angina/non-Q wave Mi may not involve the same degree of thrombin generation and fibrin formation as other acute coronary syndromes, such as AMI.[68] The results of the GUSTO IIb trial provide evidence that the utility of hirudin in unstable angina and non-Q wave MI is marginally superior to heparin.[69]

Phase II Clinical Program in Acute Myocardial Infarction

In North and South America, two phase II, multicenter, randomized, blinded, controlled clinical trials were initiated during 1995 to assess the efficacy and safety of argatroban as adjunctive therapy to thrombolytic agents in the treatment of AMI. The Argatroban in Myocardial Infarction (AMI) Study (Pierre Théroux, M.D., Montreal Heart Institute, principal investigator) is enrolling approximately 750 patients with a diagnosis of AMI within the first 6 hours of onset of symptoms. All patients will receive aspirin and streptokinase and will be randomized to receive either high-dose argatroban (3.0 μg/kg/min), low-dose argatroban (1.0 μg/kg/min), or placebo for 48–72 hours. The dose of argatroban is to be titrated downward if the APTT exceeds 90 seconds. Patients will be followed for 30 days to assess the incidence of death, AMI, recurrent angina, need for coronary revascularization procedures (percutaneous transluminal coronary angioplasty or coronary artery bypass grafting), and new-onset congestive heart failure (CHF). In a substudy of approximately 120 patients, patency of the culprit coronary artery will be assessed angiographically at 90 and 120 minutes after initiation of therapy.

A second trial, the Myocardial Infarction with Novastan and tPA (MINT) Study (I. K. Jang, M.D., Harvard Medical School/Massachusetts General Hospital, principal investigator) will enroll approximately 120 patients with the same diagnosis of AMI as in the AMI trial. All patients will receive aspirin and accelerated tPA and will be randomized to one of three groups: (1) high-dose argatroban (3.0 μg/kg/min); (2) low-dose argatroban (1.0 μg/kg/min); or (3) heparin for 48–72 hours. As in the AMI study, patency of the culprit coronary artery will be assessed angiographically at 90 and 120 minutes after initiation of therapy.

It is projected that the results of the AMI and MINT trials will be available in mid to late 1996. If the results warrant, a larger phase III trial will assess the efficacy and safety of argatroban and thrombolytic therapy in improving outcome in patients with AMI.

ANTICOAGULANT AND ANTITHROMBOTIC THERAPY IN PATIENTS WITH HEPARIN-INDUCED THROMBOCYTOPENIA AND THROMBOCYTOPENIA/THROMBOSIS

Background and Rationale

HIT and HITT involve a paradoxical response to heparin administration, in which clinically significant reductions in platelet count are observed approximately 3–15 days after initiation of heparin, which normalize with discontinuation of the drug and cannot be reasonably attributed to other intercurrent conditions. The clinical condition of HIT is observed in as many as 10% of patients receiving heparin.[13] In approximately 0.5% of patients receiving heparin, the clinical syndrome of HITT is reported,[17] marked by the recognition of a potentially debilitating or life-threatening arterial thrombosis, with a reported mortality and major morbidity rate of 25–37%.[18,19]

At present, no agent available in the United States is indicated for the treatment of this serious and potentially life-threatening disorder; in Canada, ancrod (the defibrinogenating agent derived from the Malaysian pit viper)[70] is approved for this indication. However, ancrod has several notable limitations, including slow onset of action and difficulties in monitoring its therapeutic effect as well as the production and supply restrictions inherent in a natural product.[71]

Phase III Clinical Program in Heparin-induced Thrombocytopenia and Thrombocytopenia/Thrombosis

In North America, a phase III, multicenter trial was initiated in 1995 to assess the safety and efficacy of argatroban in patients with HIT or HITT. The study (ARG-911; Bruce Lewis, M.D., Loyola University Medical School, principal investigator) is an open, historical-control study of argatroban in approximately 300 patients with HIT or HITT. Because of widespread concern that randomization to a placebo control group was ethically untenable in this patient population, a design was chosen in which prospectively treated patients (up to 14 days of argatroban at a dose of 2.0 to 10.0 μg/kg/min) will be matched with historical controls collected at the participating clinical centers. The endpoint for the study is the 1-month incidence of new thrombosis, limb amputation, or death. The results are expected to be available during the first half of 1997.

SUMMARY

Because of the unsatisfactory properties of heparin, recent research and development efforts have focused on direct thrombin inhibitors. Novastan (argatroban) is a small-molecule direct thrombin inhibitor that reversibly binds to the catalytic site of the thrombin molecule.

Argatroban possesses molecular properties that may prove beneficial compared with heparin. These properties include:

1. **Selectivity.** Argatroban binds to the catalytic site on the thrombin molecule.

2. **Reversibility.** Argatroban binding to thrombin is reversible in contrast to hirudin binding, which is essentially irreversible. Reversibility may improve controllability of anticoagulant therapy in the intensive care setting.

3. **Speed.** Argatroban rapidly binds to the catalytic site of thrombin, whereas hirudin binding occurs in a two-stage process that may be overwhelmed by the burstlike activation of thrombin.

4. **Low molecular weight.** Argatroban is a synthetic small molecule with the potential for substantial cost advantages compared with hirudin, which is produced by the relatively complex and expensive methods of recombinant technology.

5. **Ability to inhibit clot-bound thrombin.** Argatroban has been shown in experimental studies to have equivalent potency with both clot-bound and soluble thrombin, whereas larger structures, such as heparin or hirudin, have reduced or essentially no activity against clot-bound thrombin.

The clinical pharmacologic properties of argatroban are related to its reversible binding and short half-life and offer the potential for rapid achievement of therapeutic antithrombotic efficacy as well as rapid restoration of hemostatic systems to normal with discontinuation of the infusion. The fine level of control possible with argatroban may make over- and underanticoagulation less likely.

REFERENCES

1. Théroux P, Lidon R-M: Anticoagulants and their use in acute ischemic syndromes. In Topol EJ (ed): A Textbook of Interventional Cardiology. Philadelphia, W.B. Saunders, 1994, p 23.
2. Lefkovits J, Topol EJ: Direct thrombin inhibitors in cardiovascular medicine. Circulation 90:1522, 1994.
3. Hirsch J: Heparin. N Engl J Med 324:1565, 1991.
4. Rosenberg RD: The heparin-antithrombin system: A natural anticoagulant mechanism. In Colman RW, Hirsch J, Marder VJ, et al: (eds): Hemostasis and Thrombosis: Principles and Clinical Practice, 2nd ed. Philadelphia, J.B. Lippincott, 1987, p 1373.
5. Hirsh J, Dalen JE, Deykin D, et al: Oral anticoagulation: Mechanism of action, clinical effectiveness, and optimal therapeutic range. Chest 102:312S, 1992.
6. Glazier RL, Crowell EB: Randomized prospective trial of continuous vs. intermittent heparin therapy. JAMA 236:1365, 1976.
7. Salzman EW, Deykin K, Shapiro RM, et al: Management of heparin therapy. N Engl J Med 292:1046, 1975.
8. Marcianek E, Gockerman JP: Heparin-induced decrease in circulating antithrombin-III. Lancet 2:581, 1977.
9. Weitz JI, Huboda M, Massel D, et al: Clot-bound thrombin protected from inhibition by heparin-antithrombin III but is susceptible to inactivation by antithrombin III-independent inhibitors. J Clin Invest 86:385, 1990.
10. Hogg PJ, Jackson CM: Fibrin monomer protects thrombin from inactivation by heparin–antithrombin III: Implications for heparin efficacy. Proc Natl Acad Sci USA 86:3619, 1989.
11. Teifel JM, Rosenberg RD: Protection of factor Xa from neutralization by the heparin–antithrombin complex. J Clin Invest 71:1383, 1983.
12. Loscalzo J, Melnick B, Handin RI: The interaction of platelet factor 4 and glycosaminoglycans. Arch Biochem Biophys 240:446, 1985.
13. Greinacher A: Antigen generation in heparin-associated thrombocytopenia: The nonimmunologic type and the immunologic type are closely linked in their pathogenesis. Semin Thromb Hemost 21:106, 1995.
14. Bell WR, Tomasulo PA, Alving BM, et al: Thrombocytopenia occurring during the administration of heparin: A prospective study in 52 patients. Ann Intern Med 85:155, 1976.
15. Visentin GP, Ford SE, Scott JP, et al: antibodies from patients with heparin-induced thrombocytopenia/thrombosis are specific for platelet factor a completed with heparin or bound to endothelial cells. J Clin Invest 93:81, 1994.
16. Kelton JG, Sheridan D, Brain M, et al: Clinical usefulness of testing for a heparin-dependent platelet aggregating factor in patients with suspected heparin-associated thrombocytopenia. J Lab Clin Med 103:606, 1984.
17. Weissman RE, Tobin RW: Arterial embolism occurring during systemic heparin therapy. Arch Surg 76:219, 1958.
18. Wallis DE, Lewis BE, Pifarré R, et al: Active surveillance for heparin-induced thrombocytopenia and thromboembolism. Am Coll Chest Phys, 1994.
19. Magnani HN: Heparin-induced thrombocytopenia (HIT): An overview of 230 patients treated with Orgaran (Org 10172). Thromb Haemost 70:554, 1993.
20. Hirsh J, Levine MN: Low molecular weight heparin. Blood 79:1, 1992.
21. Bara L, Billaud E, Gramond G, et al: Comparative pharmacokinetics of low molecular weight (PK 10169) and unfractionated heparin after intravenous and subcutaneous administration. Thromb Res 39:631, 1985.
22. Handeland GF, Abidgaard GF, Holm U, et al: Dose-adjusted heparin treatment of deep vein thrombosis: A comparison of unfractionated and low molecular weight heparin. Eur J Clin Pharmacol 39:107, 1990.
23. Aster R: Heparin-induced thrombocytopenia and thrombosis. N Engl J Med 332:1374, 1995.
24. Callas D, Fareed J: Comparative pharmacology of site directed antithrombin agents. Implication in drug development. Thromb Haemos 74:473, 1995.
25. Stone SR, Betz A, Parry MAA, et al: Molecular basis for the inhibition of thrombin by hirudin. In Claeson G, et al (eds): The Design of Synthetic Inhibitors of Thrombin. New York, Plenum Press, 1993, p 35.
26. Braun PJ, Dennis S, Hofsteenge J, et al: use of site-directed mutagenesis to investigate the basis for the specificity of hirudin. Biochemistry 27:6517, 1988.
27. Jackson CM: Mechanisms of prothrombin activation. In Colman RW, Hirsh J, Marder VJ, et al (eds): Hemostasis and Thrombosis, 2nd ed. Philadelphia, J.B. Lippincott, 1987, p 1373.
28. Naski MC, Shafer JA: A kinetic model for the α-thrombin-catalyzed conversion of plasma levels of fibrinogen to fibrin in the presence of antithrombin III. J Biol Chem 266:13003, 1991.
29. Lawson JH, Kalafatis M, Stram S, et al: A model for the tissue factor pathway to thrombin. J Biol Chem 269:23357, 1994.
30. Jones KC, et al: A model for the tissue factor pathway to thrombin. J Biol Chem 269:23367, 1994.
31. Dodt J, Müller H-P, Seemüller U, et al: The complete amino acid sequence of hirudin, a thrombin specific inhibitor. FEBS Lett 165:180, 1984.
32. Bush LR: Argatroban, a selective, potent thrombin inhibitor. Card Drug Rev 9:247, 1991.

33. Berry CN, Giradot C, Lecoffre C, et al: Effects of the synthetic thrombin inhibitor argatroban on fibrin- or clot-incorporated thrombin: Comparison with heparin and recombinant hirudin. Thromb Haemost 72:381, 1994.
34. Gast A, Tschopp TB, Schmid G, et al: Inhibition of clot-bound and free (fluid-phase thrombin) by a novel synthetic thrombin inhibitor (Ro 46-6240), recombinant hirudin and heparin in human plasma. Blood Coag Fibrinol 5:879, 1994.
35. Mirshahi M, Soria J, Soria C, et al: Evaluation of the inhibition by heparin and hirudin of coagulation activation during r-tPA-induced thrombolysis. Blood 74:1025, 1989.
36. Rawson TE, VanGorp KA, Yang J, et al: Separation of 21-(R)- and 21-(S)-argatroban: Solubility and activity of the individual diastereoisomers. J Pharm Sci 82:672, 1993.
37. Green D, Ts´ao C, Reynolds N, et al: Ín vitro studies of a new synthetic thrombin inhibitor. Thromb Res 37:145, 1985.
38. Tamao Y, Yamamoto T, Kikumoto R, et al: Effect of a selective thrombin inhibitor MCI-9038 on fibrinolysis in vitro and in vivo. Thromb Haemost 56:28, 1986.
39. Berry CH, Girard D, Lochot S, et al: Antithrombotic actions of argatroban in rat models of venous, 'mixed' and arterial thrombosis, and its effects on the tail transection bleeding time. Br J Pharm 113:1209, 1994.
40. Winn MJ, Jain K, Ku DD: Argatroban and inhibition of the vasomotor actions of thrombin. J Card Pharm 22:754, 1993.
41. Kumada T, Abiko Y: Comparative study on heparin and a synthetic thrombin inhibitor no. 805 (MD-805) in experimental antithrombin deficient animals. Thromb Res 24:285, 1981.
42. Nishiyama H, Umemura K, Saniabadi AR, et al: Enhancement of thrombolytic efficacy of tissue-type plasminogen activator by adjuvants in the guinea pig thrombosis model. Eur J Pharm 264:191, 1994.
43. Mellott MJ, Connelly TM, York SJ, et al: Prevention of reocclusion by MCI-9038, a thrombin inhibitor, following t-PA induced thrombolysis in a canine model of femoreal arterial arterial thrombosis. Thromb Haemost 64:526, 1990.
44. Jang I-K, Gold HK, Leinbach RC, et al: In vivo thrombin inhibition enhances and sustains arterial recanalization with recombinant tissue plasminogen activator. Circ Res 67:1552, 1990.
45. Fitzgerald DJ, FitzGerald GA: Role of thrombin and thromboxane A_2 in reocclusion following coronary thrombolysis with tissue plasminogen activator. Proc Natl Acad Sci USA 86:7585, 1989.
46. Fitzgerald DJ, Wright F, FitzGerald GA: Increased thromboxane biosynthesis during coronary thrombolysis. Evidence that platelet activation and thromboxane A_2 modulate the response to tissue type plasminogen activator in vivo. Circ Res 65:83, 1989.
47. Yasuda T, Gold HK, Yaoita H, et al: Comparative effects of aspirin, a synthetic thrombin inhibitor and a monoclonal antiplatelet glycoprotein IIb/IIIa antibody on coronary artery reperfusion, reocclusion and bleeding with recombinant tissue type plasminogen activator in a canine preparation. J Am Coll Cardiol 16:714, 1990.
48. Eidt JF, Allison P, Noble S, et al: Thrombin is an important mediator of platelet aggregation in stenosed canine coronary arteries with endothelial injury. J Clin Invest 84:18, 1989.
49. Iida S, Komatsu T, Hirano T, et al: Pharmacokinetic studies of argipidine (MD-805) in dogs and rabbits. Blood or plasma level profile, metabolism, excretion and accumulation after single or consecutive intravenous administration of argipidine. Oyo Yakuri 32:1117, 1986.
50. Callas DD, Hoppensteadt D, Fareed J, et al: Comparative studies on the anticoagulant and protease generation inhibitory actions of newly developed site-directed thrombin inhibitory drugs. Sem in Thromb and Hemost 21:177, 1995.
51. Clarke RJ, Mayo G, FitzGerald GA, et al: Combined administration of aspirin and a specific thrombin inhibitor in man. Circulation 83:1510, 1991.
52. Izawa O, Katsuki M, Komatsu T, et al: Pharmacokinetics studies of argatroban (MD-805) in human concentrations of argatroban and its metabolites in plasma, urine and feces during and after drip intravenous infusion. Jap Pharm Ther 14:251, 1986.
53. Topol EJ: Thrombolytic intervention. In Topol EJ (ed): A Textbook of Interventional Cardiology. Philadelphia, W.B. Saunders, 1994, p 68.
54. The GUSTO Investigators: An international randomized trial comparing four thrombolytic strategies for acute myocardial infarction. N Engl J Med 329:673, 1993.
55. The GUSTO Angiographic Investigators: The effects of tissue plasminogen activator, streptokinase, or both on coronary-artery patency, ventricular function, and survival after acute myocardial infarction. N Engl J Med 329:1615, 1993.
56. Becker RC: Improving the efficacy and stability of coronary reperfusion following thrombolysis: Exploring the thrombin hypothesis. J Thromb Thrombolysis 1:133, 1995.
57. Cannon CP, McCabe CH, Henry TD, et al: A pilot trial of recombinant desulfatohirudin compared with heparin in conjunction with tissue-type plasminogen activator and aspirin for acute myocardial infarction: Results of the thrombolysis and myocardial infarction (TIMI) 5 trial. J Am Coll Cardiol 23:993, 1994.
58. Lee LV, for the TIMI 6 Investigators: Initial experience with hirudin and streptokinase in acute myocardial infarction: Results of the thrombolysis in myocardial infarction (TIMI) 6 trial. Am J Cardiol 75:7, 1995.

59. Antman EM, for the TIMI 9A investigators: Hirudin in acute myocardial infarction: Safety report from the thrombolysis and thrombin inhibition in myocardial infarction (TIMI) 9A trial. Circulation 90:1624, 1994.
60. GUSTO IIa Investigators: Randomized trial of intravenous heparin versus recombinant hirudin for acute coronary syndromes. Circulation 90:1631, 1994.
61. Neuhaus K-L, Essen R, Tebbe U, et al: Safety observations from the pilot phase of the randomized r-hirudin for improvement of thrombolysis (HIT-III) Study: A study of the Arbeitsgemeinschaft Leitender Kardiologischer Krankenhausärzte (ALKK). Circulation 90:1638, 1994.
62. Sobel BE: Intracranial bleeding, fibrinolysis, and anticoagulation: Causal connections and clinical implications. Circulation 90:2147, 1994.
63. Théroux P, Perez-Villa F, Waters D, et al: Randomized double-blind comparison of two doses of hirulog with heparin as adjunctive therapy to streptokinase to promote early patency of the infarct-related artery in acute myocardial infarction. Circulation 91:2132, 1995.
64. Gold HK, Torres FW, Garabedian HD, et al: Evidence for a rebound coagulation phenomenon after cessation of a 4-hour infusion of a specific thrombin inhibitor in patients with unstable angina pectoris. J Am Coll Cardiol 21:1039, 1993.
65. Théroux P, Waters D, Lam J, et al: Reactivation of unstable angina following discontinuation of heparin. N Engl J Med 327:141, 1992.
66. Willerson JT, Casscells W: Thrombin inhibitors in unstable angina: Rebound or continuation of angina after argatroban withdrawal? J Am Coll Cardiol 21:1048, 1993.
67. Zoldhelyi P, Bichler J, Owen WG, et al: Persistent thrombin generation in humans during specific thrombin inhibition with hirudin. Circulation 90:2671, 1994.
68. Becker RC, Bovill EG, Corrao JM, et al: Dynamic nature of thrombin generation, fibrin formation, and platelet activation in unstable angina and non-Q-wave myocardial infarction. J Thromb Thrombolysis 2:57, 1995.
69. Topol E: Oral presentation. 45th Annual Scientific Session of the American College of Cardiology Meeting in Orlando, FL, 1996.
70. Demers C, Ginsberg JS, Brill-Edwards P, et al: Rapid anticoagulation using ancrod for heparin-induced thrombocytopenia. Blood 78:2194, 1991.
71. Lewis BE, Leya FS, Wallis D, et al: Failure of ancrod in the treatment of heparin-induced arterial thrombosis. Can J Cardiol 10:559, 1994.

CHAPTER 17

Experimental Evaluation of Argatroban for Cardiopulmonary Bypass

JEANINE M. WALENGA, Ph.D.
MICHAEL J. KOZA, B.S., M.T. (ASCP)
MARK R. TERRELL, M.D.
VASSYL LONCHYNA, M.D.
JOSEPH ARCIDI, M.D.
ROQUE PIFARRÉ, M.D.

There is a growing need to identify an alternative anticoagulant for patients intolerant of heparin who require invasive cardiovascular procedures (e.g., angioplasty, atherectomy, thrombolysis), treatment for angina, or cardiac surgery. The disadvantages of heparin include lot-to-lot potency variations, individual patient sensitivities, platelet dysfunction, and excessive bleeding. Antithrombin III deficiency renders heparin ineffective, heparin rebound may cause postoperative bleeding, and anaphylactic shock as a side effect of protamine has been reported. Heparin-induced thrombocytopenia (HIT) can be a severe clinical complication, resulting in loss of limb or life. Thrombin inhibitors are gaining acceptance as anticoagulants as their clinical trials progress. Because they have a chemical structure different from heparin and limited interactions with platelets, they hold promise as alternative anticoagulants.

Several different drugs have been considered for cardiopulmonary bypass (CPB) in cardiac surgery. Low-molecular-weight (LMW) heparins have been used with limited success. For various reasons LMW heparin is not the drug of choice for cardiac surgery. LMW heparins provide safe and effective antithrombotic prophylaxis by single daily subcutaneous injection. However, when a strong anticoagulant effect is needed for a short, defined period, LMW heparin may not be potent enough. Moreover, the pharmacokinetic characteristics of LMW heparins do not lend themselves to this indication.[12] The half-life is longer than heparin's and protamine only partially reverses the anticoagulant and bleeding effects. Serious postoperative bleeding has occurred in CPB,[6,9,10] and there have also been reports of thrombosis during cardiac surgery with LMW heparin.[1,9] Moreover, in patients with HIT, LMW heparin is not the drug of choice, because a positive platelet aggregation response can be obtained.[4,15]

Organon 10172 is a heparinoid that has also been used in CPB. It is a mixture of heparan sulfate, dermatan sulfate, chondroitin sulfate, and LMW heparin with a predominant antifactor-Xa activity. Because its activity is long-lasting, a high degree of postoperative bleeding has been experienced after cardiac surgery.[5,8] Protamine sulfate only partially neutralizes Organon 10172, and no other antagonist is available.

Ancrod, a defibrinogenating agent, has also been used in cardiac surgery for patients with HIT. Ancrod treatment is begun 24–48 hours before surgery to achieve fibrinogen levels of 20–70 mg/dl. The soluble fibrin formed by ancrod cleavage of the fibrinogen molecule is degraded by plasmin. Thus, fibrin deposition and clot formation are prevented by endogenous fibrinolysis. Thrombosis may occur if the native fibrinolytic activity is abnormally low, if antifibrinolytic agents such as epsilon amino caproic acid are present, or if the rate of fibrin formation is greater than the rate of fibrin degradation. Ancrod also has been associated with marked postoperative bleeding.[3] Reversal of ancrod is accomplished by termination of infusion or use of cryoprecipitate for a more rapid increase of fibrinogen levels. Antivenom is available, but its use is associated with severe allergic reactions.

Synthetic and recombinant thrombin inhibitors have the potential for anticoagulation in cardiac surgery with CPB.[12] One synthetic agent, argatroban (Novastan), is a specific thrombin inhibitor derived from L-arginine. It is a small molecule (532 Da) that binds reversibly to thrombin and has a half-life of about 30 minutes in normal humans. Since 1993 argatroban has been in clinical use in Japan for treatment of chronic arterial obstruction. Pilot clinical studies have shown its potential as an effective anticoagulant in HIT, unstable angina, percutaneous transluminal coronary angioplasty (PTCA), peripheral artery disease, cerebral thrombosis, disseminated intravascular coagulation (DIC), and hemodialysis.

Argatroban is currently under clinical trial to assess its anticoagulant efficacy in patients with HIT-induced thrombosis or acute myocardial infarction (as an adjunct to thrombolytic therapy) and in PTCA in patients with HIT. Argatroban has previously been tested in one study of extracorporeal circulation in dogs in 1983.[7] The authors stated that a dose of 3 mg/kg was used to perform extracorporeal circulation for 1 hour 15 minutes, with a bubble oxygenator and roller pump at room temperature. The hydroxyethyl starch added to the system, however, may have augmented the anticoagulant effect of argatroban. Moreover, the animals were not thoroughly examined for thrombosis formation to establish clearly the efficacy of the chosen dose. We have thus undertaken a more thorough dose-ranging evaluation of argatroban as an anticoagulant alternative to heparin in the model of cardiac surgery using CPB. The same model was previously used to study the other thrombin inhibitors recombinant hirudin,[13] DuP 714,[2] and PEG-hirudin.[14]

MATERIAL AND METHODS

Argatroban

Aqueous-based argatroban (lot no. 270I0694) in 500-ml bottles was used for most studies. Ethanol-based argatroban (lot no. 349I0894) was used for dogs no. 26 and higher. In the initial studies, CPB was performed under normothermic conditions with a 1.5-hour pump run to study increasing doses administered by pump prime, bolus to the animal, or infusion during CPB. Our previous experience indicated that infusion of short-acting drugs is necessary to avoid thrombosis during CPB.[11] Therefore, the first argatroban studies analyzed bolus and infusion because of the 30-minute half-life found in volunteer studies. Because of the maximal concentration at which the drug was soluble, a large volume of argatroban was required. Thus argatroban in aqueous solution was added to the pump as priming solution before placing the animal on CPB to avoid further volume overload. Lactated Ringer's solution made up the remainder of the pump volume.

After the initial dose-finding observations, CPB under hypothermic conditions for 2.5 hours with a total pump run of 4 hours was used to study argatroban (aqueous solution) dosed by pump prime plus bolus to the animal. Using the same experimental set-up, several dose preparations were subsequently evaluated. Argatroban diluted in dextrose in water (D5W) was added to the pump as priming solution before placing the animal on

CPB, and argatroban (ethanol-based) diluted in lactated Ringer's solution was also studied. In both cases, lactated Ringer's solution made up the remainder of the pump volume.

Cardiopulmonary Bypass Model

The model chosen for the study was a simplified version of the clinical surgical procedure, used to screen new drugs for their potential candidacy as anticoagulants in the setting of CPB. Full operating technique (graft placement) and adjunct agents (cardioplegia) or devices (cell saver) were not used.

Male mongrel dogs (average weight of 28 kg) were sedated with xylazine (1 mg/kg intramuscularly) followed by anesthesia with pentobarbital (30 mg/kg intravenously). After intubation and preparation of incision sites, dogs were ventilated to 2.5 cm of positive end-expiratory pressure (PEEP) with a Harvard ventilator. Vascular (femoral) access lines were established. After median sternotomy and pericardiotomy, the heart was suspended in a pericardial cradle with pursestring sutures placed in the ascending aorta and right atrial appendage for cannulation. CPB was established with cannulation through the right atrial appendage and ascending aorta (70 ml/kg/min flow; 55–70 mmHg mean arterial pressure) using a Travenol roller pump (Travenol Labs, Ann Arbor, MI) and a variable prime Cobe membrane lung-blood oxygenator (VPCML) (Cobe, Lakewood, CO) with surgical grade Tygon S-50-HL tubing (venous outflow tubing with inside diameter of $3/8$ inch, arterial inflow tubing with inside diameter of $1/4$ inch) and EC-3840 sterile 40-μm Pall blood filters. The priming volume of the circuit was 1000 ml.

Blood pressure and heart rate were continuously monitored. Periodic blood gases were measured to guide adjustments in the bypass circuit, ventilator, and bicarbonate administration. Blood samples were collected periodically.

For assessment of efficacy, pump line filters were collected, washed with 1.0 L of saline, and dried by forced air for 10 minutes immediately after the dog was removed from pump. Deposits (clots) in the pump filters were measured by the Folin-Ciocalteu phenol fibrinogen/protein assay. Microscopic examination of selected filters was also performed by a pathologist (blinded to study doses).

All raw tissue surfaces at incision sites (sternum, catheter insertion) were observed for bleeding during the entire perioperative period. For assessment of safety, blood loss was measured by weight of aspirated blood collected from the chest cavity during the 120-minute postoperative observation period, and the abdominal cavity was explored for bleeding and clotting. Intraoperative blood loss was not used as a hard end-point, because too many variables other than the anticoagulant could relate to bleeding.

Tissue samples of the adrenal glands were placed in formalin for histologic examination by a pathologist (blinded to study doses). Brains were grossly examined after sacrifice for hemorrhagic or thrombotic events. All dogs were euthenized with supersaturated potassium chloride after the observation period.

All studies were conducted in the Animal Research Facilities of Hines, Veterans Administration Hospital (Hines, IL), which is accredited by the American Association for the Accreditation of Laboratory Animal Care (AAALAC) in compliance with the National Institute of Health *Guide for the Care and Use of Laboratory Animals*.

Statistical Analysis

Statistical analysis was performed using the ANOVA program from the Primer of Biostatistics (McGraw-Hill) IBM-PC compatible package; $p < 0.05$ was considered significant.

RESULTS

A wide total dose range of 2–30 mg/kg was given by various administration regimens. Tables 1 and 2 summarize the dosing regimens for each dog.

TABLE 1. $1\frac{1}{2}$-Hour Cardiopulmonary Bypass (Normothermic)

Dog No.	Pump Prime (mg/kg)	Bolus (mg/kg)	Infusion (mg/kg/hr)	**Total Bolus Dose (mg/kg)**	**Total Dose (mg/kg)**	**Filter Deposit (mg)**	**Blood Loss (ml/kg)**
		Dose					
			Phase I				
10	0.1	1.0	1.2	1.1	2.33	220	12.5
2	0.2	1.0	2.4	1.2	3.61	26	6.3
3	0.2	1.5	3.6	1.7	5.26	24	8.6
4	0.2	2.0	4.8	2.2	7.01	18	8.3
5	0.4	3.0	7.2	3.4	10.53	5	1.7
6	0.4	3.0	7.2	3.4	10.55	16	7.0
7	0.4	3.0	7.2	3.4	10.54	20	—
			Phase II				
8	3.0	3.0	7.2	6.0	13.2	15	4.0
9	3.0	3.0	7.2	6.0	13.2	100	11.0
11	4.0	4.0	7.2	8.0	15.2	25	4.8
12	5.0	5.0	7.2	10.0	17.2	42	5.6
13	6.0	6.0	7.2	12.0	19.2	45	13.4
14	18.0	6.0	7.2	24.0	31.2	45	8.0
			Phase III				
17	12.0	—	—		12.0	120	10.8
18	18.0	—	—		18.0	25	9.8
19	18.0	—	—		18.0	30	1.9
15	24.0	—	—		24.0	25	12.1
16	24.0	—	—		24.0	20	4.1

Figure 1 shows the measured 2-hour postoperative blood loss from the thoracic cavity over the dose range of 2–30 mg/kg. Because of the dose-finding nature of the study, single animals were used per dose regimen unless otherwise indicated. The loading bolus constituted 25–50% of the total dose administered over the CPB period, depending on the size of the infusion. There were no significant differences in blood loss among the doses and no trend in blood loss per dose. Hypothermia was associated with more blood loss than normothermia. No argatroban-treated dogs showed the type of oozing of blood from incision sites at any time intraoperatively or postoperatively as has been observed with heparin in this model.

Figure 2 shows the results of the analysis of protein deposition in the arterial line filters, a measure of anticoagulation efficacy. For the dog that received the lowest dose (2 mg/kg of argatroban), protein analysis of fibrin deposition showed a high, significantly elevated amount of fibrin/platelets (220 mg; $p < 0.05$). One dog that received a total dose of 13 mg/kg by bolus plus infusion (6.0 mg/kg + 7.2 mg/kg/hr) also had elevated filter deposits (100 mg), and another dog that received a dose of 12 mg/kg of argatroban as a pump prime only had a significant elevation in clot deposit (120 mg). For the other dogs that received total doses of 2–30 mg/kg, there was no significant difference in filter deposition among the doses.

Microscopic evaluation of the filters revealed that the deposits were largely composed of platelets. The filters from the dog experiments were at least as clean the filters used in humans treated with heparin when the deposits were 45 mg or less.

Histologic examination of the adrenal glands revealed microthrombi in several dogs that received the lower doses of argatroban (i.e., ≤ 12 mg/kg by pump prime only or ≤ 10 mg/kg by bolus, pump prime + infusion) (Table 3). No gross hemorrhages or thromboses were found in the brains.

TABLE 2. 4-Hour Cardiopulmonary Bypass (Hypothermic)

Dog No.	Dose Pump Prime (mg/kg)	Bolus (mg/kg)	Total Bolus Dose (mg/kg)	Pump Time (hrs)	Temperature/ Time	Filter Deposit (mg)	Blood Loss (ml/kg)
			Phase IV				
20	16.0	2.0	18.0	3.0	27° C/1 hr	20	10.9
21	16.0	2.0	18.0	3.0	27° C/1.5 hr	40	11.9
22	16.0	2.0	18.0	4.0	25° C/2.5 hr	40	18.8
23	16.0	2.0	18.0	4.0	25° C/2.5 hr	30	15.9
24	25.0	5.0	30.0	4.0	25° C/2.5 hr	40	11.9
25	25.0	5.0	30.0	4.0	25° C/2.5 hr	20	20.4
			Phase V Ethanol Preparation				
26	25.0	5.0	30.0	4.0	25° C/2.5 hr	20	13.6
27	25.0	5.0	30.0[*1]	4.0	25° C/2.5 hr	25	14.3
28	25.0	5.0	30.0[*2]	4.0	25° C/2.5 hr	10	20.7
29	25.0	5.0	30.0[*3,†]	4.0	25° C/2.5 hr	25	8.9
30	45.0	5.0	50.0[†]	4.0	25° C/2.5 hr	15	14.4

* Bolus to maintain activated clotting time > 800 sec during CPB:
[1] 1.0×1 mg/kg   [2] 1.0×2 mg/kg   [3] 1.0×4 mg/kg
† Argatroban in Ringer's not D5W (2.5 mg/ml).

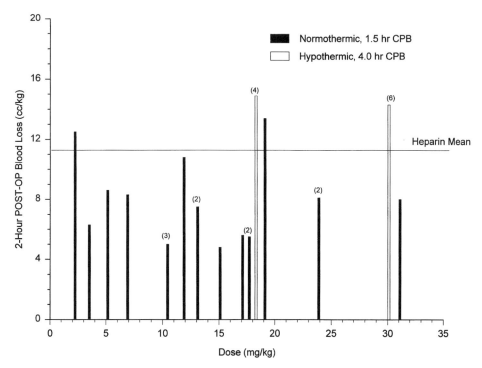

FIGURE 1. Blood loss measured during the 2-hour postoperative observation period is shown for the dose range of argatroban studied. Data bars represent values for individual animals unless indicated as a mean for n=2–6 animals. The heparin mean was obtained from 10 dogs administered 2.5 mg/kg supplemented to maintain the initial celite ACT response during CPB.

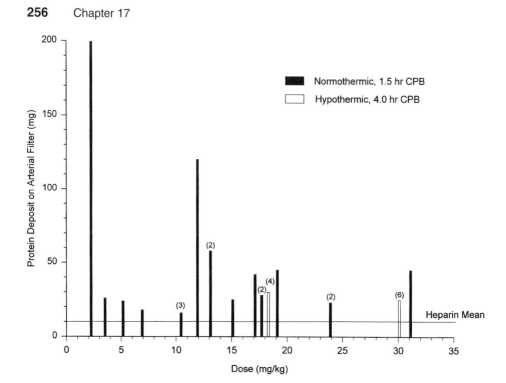

FIGURE 2.   Levels of protein/clot deposits quantitated on the arterial line filter are shown for the dose range of argatroban studied. Data bars represent values for individual animals unless indicated as a mean for n=2–6 animals. The heparin mean was obtained from 10 dogs administered 2.5 mg/kg supplemented to maintain the initial celite ACT response during CPB.

Sporadic clot formation was visibly observed in the oxygenator or blood lines for individual animals at total doses of 17 mg/kg and below (normothermic). Dogs that were anticoagulated by pump prime only (normothermic) showed visible clotting even at doses as high as 24 mg/kg (see Table 3). Dogs undergoing hypothermic CPB also had sporadic visible clotting at total doses of 16 and 25 mg/kg (given as bolus plus pump prime for a 4-hour CPB run). The clots observed in the suction trap, oxygenator, and arterial lines during and immediately after CPB were considered critical. The clots observed at termination of postoperative observation (at time of sacrifice) were probably due to consumption of the argatroban after CPB (external to the animal), and unrelated to in vivo thrombosis. Likely underlying factors are the short half-life of argatroban and/or thrombin generation in the pump or pump lines after the run had been terminated. Based on these data, the minimal dose of argatroban for CPB was > 13 mg/kg total dose given as bolus, pump prime, and infusion (not pump prime only). Among the dosing regimens studied, the > 13 mg/kg total dose consisted of a total bolus of 6.0 mg/kg with an infusion of 7.2 mg/kg/hr.

The celite activated clotting time (ACT) is typically used to measure the anticoagulant effects of heparin in human surgeries. ACT data from selected dogs treated with argatroban for CPB are shown in Figures 3 (with infusion) and 4 (no infusion). There was a dose-dependent effect based on the total bolus/pump prime dose with some exceptions. The regimen consisting of 3.0 mg/kg + 7.2 mg/kg/hr + 0.4 mg/kg prime gave a higher ACT response than expected. Peaking ACT levels were observed twice in the dog treated with 5.0 mg/kg + 7.2 mg/kg/hr + 5.0 mg/kg prime during the period when steady state should have existed. For the three lower-dosed animals in Figure 3 and the lowest-dosed animal in Figure 4, clots were detected during CPB. For the > 13 mg/kg total doses, with

TABLE 3. Perioperative Observations

Dog No.	Argatroban Dose			Clotting	Adrenal Thrombi	Bleeding
	Bolus (mg/kg)	Infusion (mg/kg/hr)	Pump Prime (mg/kg)			
1.5-Hour Cardiopulmonary Bypass (Normothermic)						
10	1.0	1.2	2.5	Clot in arterial line after CPB; clots in chest and suction trap after termination; high filter deposits	X	
2	1.0	2.4	5.0	Clot in oxygenator 30 min after bolus	X	
3	1.5	3.6	5.0	Clot in arterial line after CPB	X	
4	2.0	4.8	5.0	Clot in suction trap after CPB; clots in chest after termination		
6	3.0	7.2	10.0	Clots in chest after temination	X	
7	3.0	7.2	10.0	Clot in oxygenator	X	
9	3.0	7.2	3.0	High filter deposits	X	
11	4.0	7.2	4.0	Clot in suction trap after termination		
12	5.0	7.2	5.0	Clots in chest after termination		
17			12.0	Clot in arterial line after CPB; high filter deposits	X	
18			18.0	Clot in suction trap after CPB		
19			18.0	Clot in suctioin trap after CPB		
16			24.0	Clot in suction trap after CPB and termination		
4.0-Hour Cardiopulmonary Bypass (Hypothermic)						
22	2.0		16.0	Increased blood loss		Higher than average postoperative blood loss
23	2.0		16.0	Clots in chest after termination		Higher than average postoperative blood loss
24	5.0		25.0	Clots in chest after termination		
25	5.0		25.0			Higher than average postoperative blood loss
26	5.0		25.0	Clots in chest after CPB and termination		
28	5.0		25.0	Clot in suction trap after termination		Higher than average postoperative blood loss
30	5.0		45.0	Bleeding from tracheal tube; oozing from chest; high intraoperative blood loss		Higher than average postoperative blood loss

which no clotting was detected during CPB, the ACT was 500 seconds or higher. Argatroban doses that held the ACTs to > 700 seconds during CPB seemed optimal to avoid all possible clot formation. At the end of CPB when the infusion was terminated, the ACT values began to decrease.

With the split route of administration of the initial bolus (to pump vs. to animal), there was a difference in the kinetics of the anticoagulant response (Figure 4). If low ACT levels were obtained during the pump run (12.0 mg/kg prime), clotting became evident somewhere in the model. It was critical to obtain elevated ACT levels (at least 700 sec) at the onset of CPB to avoid clotting. However, at the critical argatroban level (i.e., > 13 mg/kg) the ACT levels after either the 1.5-hour normothermic or 4.0-hour hypothermic CPB remained significantly elevated over baseline.

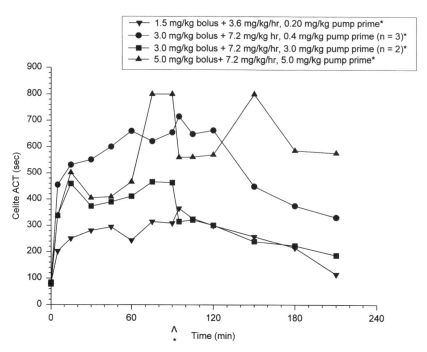

FIGURE 3.   Celite activated clotting time (ACT) values are shown for a selected dosing range of bolus + pump prime + infusion of argatroban. Time off pump is indicated by ^ (*1.5 hour CPB normothermic). Animals represented by the three lower doses had some form of clotting during CPB.

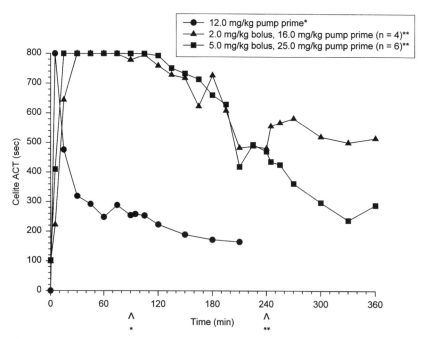

FIGURE 4.   Celite activated clotting time (ACT) values are shown for a selected dosing range of bolus + pump prime or pump prime only of argatroban. Time off pump is indicated by ^ (*1.5 hour CPB normothermic; **4.0 hour CPB hypothermic). Only the animal dosed with 12.0 mg/kg prime had clotting during CPB.

The hypothermic dogs showed a longer prolongation of clotting time by ACT, because of the extended half-life of the drug from slower metabolism. As the dog was rewarmed before coming off pump, the elimination rate of argatroban was accelerated, and a more rapid change toward normal was measured in many of the clotting parameters. Close inspection of the data, however, revealed some remaining activity during the 2-hour postoperative period at all doses that provided anticoagulation. Argatroban was not reversed with protamine after surgery; no antidote is currently available. The infusion of argatroban was terminated at the end of surgery.

Figures 5 and 6 show the anti-IIa (thrombin) activity, as measured by the chromogenic method. Activity levels that held > 150 relative percent of inhibition (of the thrombin in the assay system) during the entire CPB run corresponded to proper anticoagulation with no clotting problems during CPB. Baseline values (0% inhibition) were not obtained by 2 hours after CPB with any dose > 10 mg/kg, except when a pump-prime-only dose was used.

One dog, purposely overdosed at 50 mg/kg as an initial bolus, showed no increase in postoperative blood loss from the chest cavity; however, intraoperative blood loss and oozing at the incision sites were greater than in the lower-dosed dogs. This response was the same as we had seen in our heparin dog studies. In addition, there was blood near the tracheal tube during and after CPB. Two hours after surgery, at time of sacrifice, the ACT had not decreased.

Thrombin–antithrombin (TAT) complex is a measure of activated coagulation (ELISA assay; Behring, San Jose, CA). At the dose range evaluated, with samples taken after 30 minutes on the heart-lung machine when the animal should have been well anticoagulated, the TAT levels were higher than normal at total doses ≤ 15 mg/kg of argatroban, indicating ongoing generation of thrombin (Fig. 7). There seemed to be a critical total dose of 18 mg/kg at which a low (normal) level of TAT complex in the plasmas was measured (normal dog level = 9.0 ± 3.0 µg/L). For doses < 18 mg/kg TAT levels averaged 30.5 ± 3.1 µg/L, whereas at doses ≥ 18 mg/kg TAT levels averaged 3.84 ± 0.61 µg/L (mean ± SEM).

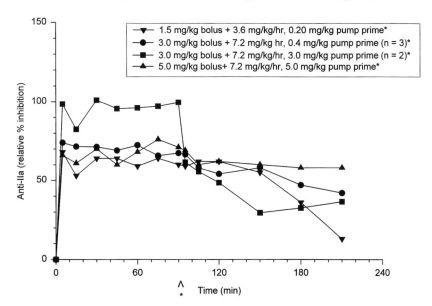

FIGURE 5.   Anti-IIa values are shown for selected dosing range of bolus + pump prime + infusion of argatroban. Time off pump is indicated by ^ (*1.5 hour CPB normothermic). Animals represented by the three lower doses had some form of clotting during CPB.

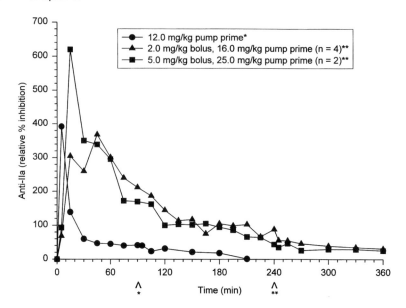

FIGURE 6.   Anti-IIa values are shown for a selected dosing range of bolus + pump prime or pump prime only of argatroban. Time off pump is indicated by ^ (*1.5 hour CPB normothermic; **4.0 hour CPB hypothermic). Only the animal dosed with 12.0 mg/kg prime had clotting during CPB.

Values nearly equal to baseline levels were achieved with a 15–30-mg/kg total dose of argatroban. This finding supports a critical dose of > 13 mg/kg for initial bolusing, as suggested by the visible clots found and the filter analyses. There was a wide scatter in the TAT data at lower doses, but when the animals were fully anticoagulated, the data became

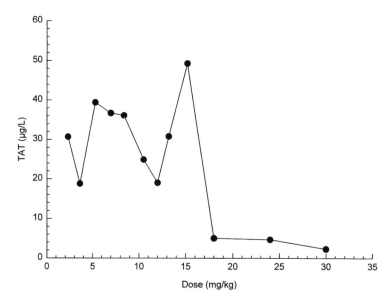

FIGURE 7.   Thrombin-antithrombin levels are shown for total doses of argatroban administered at the start of CPB (i.e., bolus [mg/kg] ± pump prime [mg/kg] ± infusion [mg/kg]). Data points represent from 1–6 animals.

very reproducible. Of interest, no animal gave TAT levels ≥ 100 µg/L, as would be expected with poor anticoagulation.

There were no differences in the hematocrit among the different doses and no differences in platelet counts, except for the pump-prime-only group, which tended to show lower platelet counts throughout the perioperative period compared with the infusion group. This finding may be explained by adherence of platelets to the pump lines during the first pass of blood through the circuit. Argatroban had no effect on respiration, heart rate, and blood gases, which were monitored throughout the experiment.

The bleeding time tests in the anesthetized dogs, as measured by a Simplate device and performed on the gingiva, were longest with the highest doses. But these data did not correlate with postoperative blood loss from the chest or oozing from the incision sites, neither of which was dose-dependent. Bleeding times lowered but remained elevated 2 hours postoperatively.

The dosing studies also demonstrated the following: (1) argatroban is an effective anticoagulant under hypothermic (25° C) conditions; (2) an ethanolic preparation of argatroban behaved like an aqueous-based preparation; and (3) argatroban was equally effective diluted in Ringer's lactate or dextrose in water.

CONCLUSION

The animal model of CPB used in the dosing studies was intended to serve simply as a means to screen argatroban as a potential anticoagulant in CPB. The studies were a first approach to determining a dose of argatroban for CPB. Full surgical manipulation, as in coronary artery grafting, was not used. The following conclusions can be made:

1. There was less intraoperative bleeding with argatroban than with heparin. Postoperative blood loss was, on average, similar with both drugs, but with argatroban it was not dose-dependent over a wide dose range of 2–30 mg/kg. Compared with heparin, little to no oozing of blood from incision sites was observed in argatroban-treated animals.

2. Based on the clot/protein deposits and microscopic examination of the arterial line filters, perioperative observations of the surgical field, and histologic examination of adrenal glands, total doses of argatroban > 2 mg/kg were needed to avoid serious thrombosis during CPB. However, there was obvious intersubject variation, and occasional animals had clots in the surgical field during CPB at doses up to 13 mg/kg (6.0 mg/kg bolus). Thus, a dose > 13 mg/kg (bolus plus infusion over 4.0 hours) was needed to achieve anticoagulation.

3. The studied doses were effective for 1.5- and 4.0-hour CPB runs at the level at which adequate anticoagulation was achieved (> 13 mg/kg).

4. Blood clotting in the chest or suction trap 2 hours after CPB was observed in many animals. This finding may be related to thrombin generation and argatroban consumption ex vivo without consequence in vivo, but it has implications if blood salvage is to be used.

5. Based on thrombin–antithrombin complex levels, the dose that produced effective anticoagulation without completely inhibiting coagulation activation was between 15 and 20 mg/kg. This dose could be given by combination of pump prime, bolus and infusion for a 4-hour surgical period. A dose of 30 mg/kg completely shut down thrombin generation and TAT formation.

6. An initial high bolus is critical to protect against clotting. In the first minutes on CPB there must be full anticoagulation. Intermittent small boluses can be given throughout the surgical period, if desired. Using the drug as pump prime only is not recommended, because the animal/patient is not protected before the blood actually circulates to the pump.

7. The celite ACT was used to monitor argatroban activity during surgery. ACT times > 700 seconds correlated with no clot formation and low TAT values.

8. Under hypothermic conditions argatroban gave a more potent anticoagulant response (ACT) and slower elimination than under normothermic conditions. Rewarming enhanced drug elimination. Thus physiologic metabolism of argatroban was temperature-dependent. Blood loss tended to be higher with hypothermia, although results were inconsistent.

9. As determined by ACT, anti-IIa, bleeding time, and clot-based assays, argatroban at total doses > 10 mg/kg remained in circulation for more than 2 hours postoperatively. The half-life of argatroban was more prolonged in dogs on CPB than in normal dogs. Thus, because higher doses are needed to avoid thrombosis (doses > 13 mg/kg to avoid sporadic blood clotting), an antidote for rapid elimination of argatroban after CPB is needed.

10. Hematologic parameters (platelets, hematocrit, complete blood count) revealed no abnormal response to argatroban. Blood pressure, heart rate, body temperature, and respiration were unaffected. Fibrinogen levels were falsely decreased in the presence of argatroban as an assay artifact due to the drug.

11. The aqueous and ethanol preparations of argatroban behaved similarly. Solubility of the drug precluded the use of high concentrations, but Ringer's lactate (pump prime) or dextrose in water can be used effectively as diluent.

In conclusion, initial studies in a normal dog model demonstrated that argatroban may be a candidate alternative drug for cardiopulmonary bypass. This finding is encouraging, particularly for patients with HIT. Like the Japanese study, our data also show that a dose of 3 mg/kg allows CPB. However, by using more sophisticated examinations such as adrenal histologies, arterial line filter protein deposit measurements, and TAT measurements, we were able to determine that 3 mg/kg is associated with thrombosis. Our study better defines a higher dose as more effective for CPB; however, bleeding risk and antidote become important considerations. Further studies on the pharamcokinetics of the relatively high doses of argatroban needed to avoid thrombosis during CPB, as well as optimal dosing regimens, are warranted, with particular attention to the elimination pattern. An antagonist may be necessary for rapid elimination of argatroban after CPB. Evaluation in a CPB model of a different species also may be useful in the event of interspecies variations in pharmacokinetic response. Finally, how the normal dog model relates to an unhealthy human is not known.

Acknowledgments. The authors express their gratitude to the following people who helped make these studies possible: Areta Kowal-Vern, M.D. for tissue histologies; Raoul Fresco, M.D., for microscopic analysis of filters; and Nicolas King, CCP, for perfusion during surgery.

REFERENCES

1. Altés A, Rodrigo M, Gari M, et al: Heparin-induced thrombocytopenia and heart operation: Management with tedelparin. Ann Thorac Surg 59:508–509, 1995.
2. Chomiak PN, Walenga JM, Koza MJ, et al: Investigation of a thrombin inhibitor peptide as an alternative to heparin in cardiopulmonary bypass surgery. Circulation 88(Pt 2):407–412, 1993.
3. Demers C, Ginsberg JS, Brill-Edwards P: Rapid anticoagulation using ancrod for heparin-induced thrombocytopenia. Blood 78:2194–2197, 1991.
4. Greinacher A, Feigl M, Mueller-Eckhardt C: Crossreactivity studies between sera of patients with heparin associated thrombocytopenia and a new low molecular weight heparin reviparin. Thromb Haemost 72:644–645, 1994.
5. Magnani HN: Heparin-induced thrombocytopenia (HIT): An overview of 230 patients treated with orgaran (Org 10172). Thromb Haemost 70:554–561, 1993.
6. Massonnet-Castel S, Pelissier E, Dreyfuss G, et al: Low-molecular-weight heparin in extracorporeal circulation. Lancet 8387:1182–1183, 1984.
7. Matsukura H, Uzawa S, Takeda H, Tanabe T: Experimental extracorporeal circulation with a synthetic thrombin inhibitor, MD-805, without heparin. J Jpn Assoc Thorac Surg 31:1377–1382, 1983.
8. Ortel TL, Gockerman JP, Califf RM, et al: Parenteral anticoagulation with the heparinoid Lomoparan (Org 10172) in patients with heparin induced thrombocytopenia and thrombosis. Thromb Haemost 67(3):292–296, 1992.

9. Robitaille D, Leclerc JR, Laberge R, et al: Cardiopulmonary bypass with a low-molecular-weight heparin fraction (enoxaparin) in a patient with a history of heparin-associated thrombocytopenia. J Thorac Cardiovasc Surg 103:597–599, 1992.
10. Roussi JH, Houbouyan LL, Goguel AF: Use of low-molecular-weight heparin in heparin-induced thrombocytopenia with thrombotic complications. Lancet:1183, 1984.
11. Walenga JM, Bakhos M, Messmore HL, et al: Potential use of recombinant hirudin as an anticoagulant in a cardiopulmonary bypass model. Ann Thorac Surg 51:271–277, 1991.
12. Walenga JM, Koza MJ, Pifarré R: Potential use of new thrombin inhibitors and low molecular weight heparins as anticoagulants in cardiopulmonary bypass surgery. In Pifarré R (ed): Anticoagulation, Hemostasis, and Blood Preservation in Cardiovascular Surgery. Hanley & Belfus, Inc., Philadelphia, 1993, pp 343–352.
13. Walenga JM, Koza MJ, Park SJ, et al: Evaluation of CGP 39393 as the anticoagulant in cardiopulmonary bypass surgery in a dog model. Ann Thorac Surg 58:1685-1689, 1994.
14. Walenga JM, Terrell MR, Koza MJ, et al: PEG-hirudin as anticoagulant in cardiopulmonary bypass. Blood 84 (Suppl 1):72a, 1994.
15. Walenga JM, Koza MJ, Lewis BE, Pifarré R: Relative heparin-induced thrombocytopenic potential of low molecular weight heparins and new antithrombotic agents. Clin Appl Thromb Hemost 2 (Suppl 1):S21-S27, 1996.

CHAPTER 18

Efegatran: A New Cardiovascular Anticoagulant

GERALD F. SMITH, Ph.D., J.D.
DONETTA GIFFORD-MOORE, B.S.
TRELIA J. CRAFT, B.S.
NICKOLAY CHIRGADZE, Ph.D.
KENNETH J. RUTERBORIES, B.S., M.S.
TERRY D. LINDSTROM, Ph.D.
JULIE H. SATTERWHITE, Ph.D.

Thrombin is the serine protease, ultimately produced during the cascade of blood coagulation factor activation steps,[42] that proteolytically activates plasma fibrinogen and thereby causes and controls fibrin formation.[22,89] Thrombin is also the most potent agonist[50] for platelet aggregation. These two properties enable thrombin to perform its key dual role during thrombus formation,[58,114] in which thrombin mediates blood coagulation (fibrin formation) and platelet activation events, including platelet recruitment in thrombogenesis.[1,52] Fibrin formation is a major element of thrombus formation, even in high shear circumstances (arterial thrombosis), as shown by the success of fibrinolytic agents in myocardial infarction, by the success of warfarin in preventing reinfarction,[96] and by the success of heparin in preventing infarction in unstable angina.[107] Therefore, the potential exists for a direct-acting thrombin inhibitor to interfere dually with both elements (fibrin formation and thrombin-induced platelet aggregation) of cardiovascular thrombotic disease and to produce antithrombotic therapeutic index results different from those of the indirect anticoagulants warfarin and heparin and the platelet antagonists.[101]

Drug research[34,100,103] has produced direct-acting thrombin inhibitors with antithrombotic activity in models pertinent to both arterial and venous thrombosis[4,7,54,82] and to extracorporeal circulation (e.g., cardiopulmonary bypass during cardiac surgery).[33,115–117] Such direct-acting thrombin inhibitors are believed to offer potential mechanistic and clinical advantages over heparin.[30,86,104,108] Presently, the direct thrombin inhibitors hirudin,[49,110] Hirulog,[41,83,109] argatroban,[79,102] and efegatran[87,88] are undergoing clinical evaluation in patients with cardiovascular thrombotic diseases[86,104] and venous thrombosis.[39]

This chapter describes the new direct thrombin inhibitor efegatran (LY294468), N-methyl-D-phenylalanyl-L-prolyl-L-arginal, as a potentially useful new anticoagulant antithrombotic agent, including preclinical biochemistry and pharmacology as well as preliminary results from phase I and phase II clinical studies.

265

DISCOVERY OF EFEGATRAN

The quest for useful organic-molecule thrombin inhibitors dates back to the mid 1960s, motivated by the fact that the term coronary thrombosis had been nearly synonymous with the term myocardial infarction.[66] Through the mid 1970s the laboratories of Geratz,[45] Markwardt,[64] and Okamoto[61] synthesized large numbers of thrombin inhibitors. Compounds from these early efforts did not produce successful anticoagulant products (the exception may be argatroban, an older arginine derivative still being evaluated in clinical testing),[46,79] largely because of the difficulty in demonstrating antithrombotic activity in animal models. A breakthrough occurred when Bajusz synthesized D-Phe-Pro-Arginals at the Hungarian Institute for Drug Research in the mid 1970s. These tripeptide arginals were an early example of rational drug design. Biophysical and biochemical studies suggested that the interaction of human fibrinogen with thrombin involved specific binding with the fibrinogen A-chain sequence, . . Phe_8 . . $Val_{16}Arg_{17}$ . ., in which the contorted Phe_8 and Val_{16} residues are in close proximity and bind adjacent hydrophobic sites, fitting the Arg_{17} into the thrombin ionic pocket as a scissile bond residue.[21,67] Bajusz produced molecules with the D-Phe-Pro-Arg sequence,[11,12] which were intended to compete with the Phe_8 . . $Val_{16}Arg_{17}$ . . interaction, and included C-terminal aldehyde groups. The aldehyde groups, in turn, were intended to produce a transitional intermediate bonding with the thrombin active site Ser_{195}. These intended interactions do occur, as illustrated by x-ray diffraction analysis of the crystal complex between efegatran and human thrombin.

We considered Bajusz's tripeptide arginals as a breakthrough because of our evaluation of BOC-D-Phe-Pro-Arginal (LY178207) in a rat model of arterial thrombosis for response to warfarin.[92] Although warfarin reduced the arterial thrombogenic response in dose-dependent fashion (and in correlation with reduction of blood concentrations of vitamin K-dependent factors[92]), warfarin was able to prevent thrombosis completely only at a dose of LD_{100} continued for 7 days. Heparin was ineffective in the arterial model through intravenous infusions and injections, even though acute bleeding was produced.[90,91] In contrast, LY178207 completely prevented thrombosis at an intravenous dose of 1 mg/kg/hr, and when infusion doses were raised by 16-fold, no bleeding and no toxicity were observed.[90] This tripeptide arginal clearly demonstrated a unique advantage in therapeutic index over both warfarin and heparin in the same thrombosis model and, therefore, offered large potential for anticoagulant drug discovery. Some of the most potent arginals demonstrated properties that precluded development as pharmaceutical agents (e.g., LY178207 lacked sufficient selectivity to spare the fibrinolytic proteases).[10,13,14,94] However, efegatran, the N-methyl derivative synthesized by Bajusz, has shown promise for development as a new anticoagulant antithrombotic.[10,54,90,94]

PRECLINICAL STUDIES

Materials

Human and bovine thrombin (lots HT 390, HT660, HT740, and BT300) was purchased from Enzyme Research Laboratories (South Bend, IN). Other enzymes for inhibition studies were human plasmin from Boehringer Mannheim (Indianapolis, IN); human factors $IXa\alpha$, $IXa\beta$, Xa XIa, and XIIa, and plasma kallikrein from Enzyme Research Laboratories; bovine trypsin from Worthington Biochemicals (St. Louis); recombinant native tissue plasminogen activator (ntPA) (single-chain activity) from American Diagnostica (New York); and streptokinase (SK) from Hoechst Pharmaceuticals (Newark, NJ). Urokinase was purchased from Leo Pharmaceuticals (Copenhagen), and coagulation reagents Actin, thromboplastin, and human plasma were purchased from Dade (Miami). Hirudin (10,000 antithrombin units/mg), purchased from American Diagnostica, included native hirudin (lot 6077/126) and recombinant hirudin (lot HHF060188). Trasylol was purchased from Miles (West Haven, CT); H-D-Phe-Pro-Arg-chloromethyl ketone (PPACK), from Calbiochem (San Diego, CA); chromogenic para-nitroanilide peptide protease substrates, from KabiVitrum (Franklin, OH) or Midwest Biotech (Fishers, IN); and hirudin-related peptide (54-65), from Midwest Biotech.

Methods

Chemistry. Peptide arginals were synthesized by solution-phase peptide synthesis using standard procedures:[13,85] Boc-D-Phe-Pro-Arg-H H_2SO_4 (LY178207). Efegatran, D-MePhe-Pro-Arg-H H2SO4 (LY294468), was batch no. 910320-33.

Enzyme Inhibition Kinetics. Enzyme inhibition kinetics were performed in 96-well polystyrene plates, and rates of reaction were determined from hydrolysis rates of appropriate p-nitroanilide substrates at 405 nm, using a Thermomax plate reader from Molecular Devices (San Francisco).[90] The same protocol was followed for all enzymes studied: 50 μl buffer in each well, followed by 25 μl of inhibitor solution and 25 μl of enzyme. Within 2 minutes 150 μl of chromogenic substrate was added to start the enzymatic reactions. The rates of benzoyl-Phe-Val-Arg-p-NA hydrolysis provide a linear relationship with human thrombin such that free thrombin can be quantitated in reaction mixtures. Data were analyzed directly as rates by the Softmax program to produce [free enzyme] calculations for tight-binding Kass determinations. Thrombin concentrations were converted to molar concentrations from the molecular weights of 37,000 for human thrombin and 39,000 for bovine thrombin.[43] The thrombin preparations were homogeneous according to sodium dodecylsulfate-polyacrylamide gel electrophoresis (SDS/PAGE), and titrations with p-nitrophenyl guanidinobenzoate[31] supported the purity of the preparations. Kinetics using other proteases were performed with the same methods, using appropriate substrates.

Coagulation Studies. Coagulation studies were performed with a CoAScreener (American LABor, Raleigh, NC).[92]

Plasma Clot Lysis Tests. Plasma clot lysis tests were performed with radio-labeled human fibrinogen.[90]

Pharmacokinetics Methods. The plasma pharmacokinetics of efegatran in rats and dogs after intravenous bolus administration or continuous infusion were determined using stereospecific high-performance liquid chromatography (HPLC). Peptidyl arginine aldehydes are known to exist in aqueous media as an equilibrium mixture of physical forms (including aldehyde hydrate, free aldehyde, and epimeric cyclic hemiaminals), none of which is stable to reequilibration on isolation in solution[37,105,106] (Fig. 1). Efegatran was derivatized with 2,4-dinitrophenylhydrazine (DNPH) after extraction from plasma to stabilize the compound in a single physical form and to introduce a highly absorbent chromophore. In addition, the resulting DNPH hydrazone prevents epimerization of efegatran to DLD-efegatran, its inactive N-methyl-D-phenylalanyl-L-prolyl-D-arginal isomer. Plasma was mixed with pH 6 buffer containing internal standard and then rapidly extracted with a solid-phase extraction column. After washing the extraction column with aqueous and organic solvents, the analytes were eluted and derivatized with DNPH. The reaction mixture was passed through a silica gel extraction column and then washed with methanol to remove residual DNPH and reaction byproducts. The efegatran and DLD-efegatran derivatives were then eluted and analyzed by reverse-phase HPLC with ultraviolet detection at 360 nm. Radioactivity concentrations were determined with liquid scintillation counting. The pharmacokinetic parameters of efegatran and plasma radioactivity were calculated with model-independent kinetic analysis. The pharmacokinetic parameters of blood radioactivity in rats were determined by Nedler-Mead nonlinear iterative estimation.[111]

X-Ray Crystallography. *Crystallization.* Thrombin–efegatran complex crystals acceptable for x-ray analysis were grown by vapor diffusion from 6 mg/ml of human thrombin (lot HT660) solution in 25 mM of sodium phosphate buffer (pH = 7.5) with 375 mM of sodium chloride. Also added were 10–15% PEG3500, 200 mM of magnesium

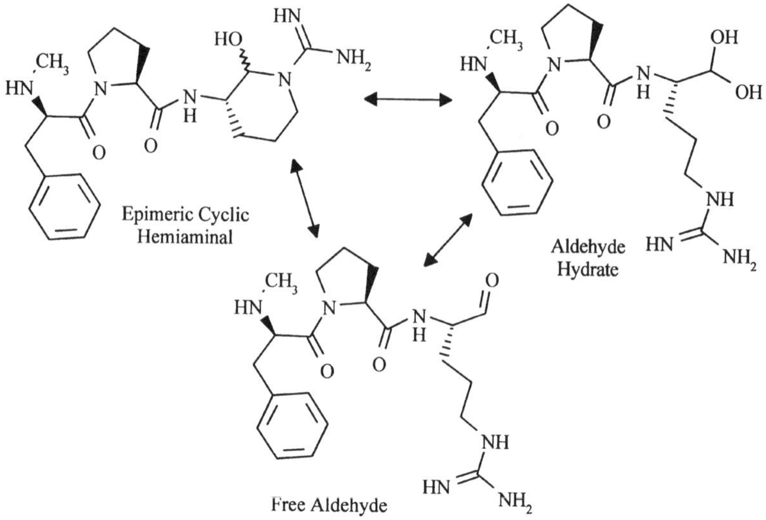

FIGURE 1.   Physical forms of efegatran.

chloride, and 100 mM of sodium acetate (pH = 4.5) at 4°C. The inhibitor efegatran and hirudin-derived peptide (54-65) were 3 and 2 times in excess, respectively. The linear dimensions of the crystals were approximately $0.2 \times 0.2 \times 0.3$ mm. The crystals belong to the orthorhombic space group $P2_12_12$ with the unit cell constants, a = 108.1 Å, b = 80.7 Å, c = 45.8 Å. The asymmetric unit contains one human α-thrombin molecule (Mr = 36 kD), one hirudin-related peptide (54-65) molecule (Mr = 1,254), and one efegatran molecule bound in the active site.

   Data Collection.   X-ray intensity data were collected at room temperature from single crystals by oscillation technique using the R-AXIS II system.[84] A Fuji imaging plate detector was used with conventional rotating anode x-ray generator. The number of unique reflections with I > σ was 16,563 with R_{merge} 7.1%. These reflections present 60% of the theoretically possible observations for the space resolution 2.0 Å.

   Structure Solution and Refinement.   Crystal structures were solved by the molecular replacement method.[32] A search model was constructed from a bovine thrombin structure provided by Dr. Brian Edwards of Wayne State University. The orientation and position of this model in the new unit cell were determined with the X-PLOR package program.[2] Refinements were made with the PROLSQ program[53]; inspection and manual correction were done with the interactive graphic FRODO program.[59] The final model includes 2518 nonhydrogen atoms. The crystallographic R-factor was 19.4% at 2.0 Å resolution. Standard deviations from ideal values for bond lengths, interbond angle distances, and planarities were 0.016, 0.035, and 0.039 Å, respectively. Generally, electron densities of all parts of the structure are well defined; exceptions are the five N-terminal amino acid residues, for which positions remain tentative.

PRECLINICAL PHARMACOLOGY

Thrombin Inhibition

   Molecular Structure of the Efegatran–Thrombin Complex.   The interaction of efegatran with human thrombin is illustrated by the x-ray crystallographic result in Figure 2. Crystals were obtained with the efegatran–thrombin complex by use of a hirugen-like peptide co-complex. The x-ray crystallographic structure shows that the P3, P2, and

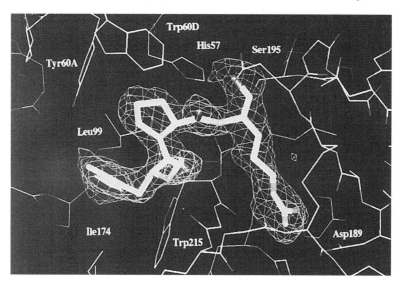

FIGURE 2. X-ray crystal structure of the efegatran–human thrombin complex. This view depicts the active site region of the complex x-ray crystal structure solved at 2.0-A resolution. A reversible covalent bond is formed between the efegatran aldehyde carbonyl carbon and the hydroxyl oxygen of the catalytic Ser_{195} of thrombin. The arginal residue of efegatran fits into the specificity pocket with its guanidinium group hydrogen bonded to Asp_{189}. The proline ring fits into a hydrophobic pocket defined by His_{57}, Tyr_{60A}, Trp_{60D}, and Leu_{99}. A third point of interaction is a hydrophobic region formed by residues Leu_{99}, Trp_{215}, and Ile_{174}.

P1 elements of efegatran do indeed interact with the fibrinogen-analogous S3, S2, and S1 sites in thrombin. The P3 N-methyl-D-Phe group of efegatran fits into a hydrophobic pocket defined by Trp_{215}, Ile_{174}, and Leu_{99}; the P2 proline group fits into a hydrophobic pocket defined by Leu_{99}, His_{57}, Trp_{60D}, and Tyr_{60A}; and the P1 arginine side chain fits into the specificity pocket for ionic guanidinium interaction with Asp_{189}. The crystallographic data prove that the hemiacetal bond forms between the aldehydic carbonyl carbon atom and the oxygen of Ser_{195}. Figure 2 shows the hemiacetal carbon-oxygen bond from well-defined electron densities with a bond length of 1.5 Å. The binding of efegatran to thrombin, therefore, should serve functionally to compete with the Phe_8 . . $Val_{15}Arg_{16}$-binding surface in fibrinogen to produce anticoagulation. The added binding strength of the reversible hemiacetal bond formation at Ser_{195} is consistent with the tight-binding reversible thrombin inhibition observed with efegatran.[90]

Equilibrium Kass from Inhibition Kinetics.   The thrombin inhibition properties of efegatran were evaluated using hydrolysis kinetics with the chromogenic substrate Bz-Phe-Val-Arg-pNA, which has been successful in predicting anticoagulant activity for thrombin inhibitors. To generate a cumulative database of potential thrombin inhibitors that includes tight-binding inhibitors, we used the concept of the apparent association constant (Kass).[74,81,90,119] Assuming a bimolecular reaction between the inhibitor (I) and thrombin (E):

$$E + I = EI$$
and
$$\text{apparent Kass} = [EI]/[E][I] = [E_{bound}]/[E_{free}][I^O - E_{bound}]$$

To determine the Kass values from the above equation, the free thrombin (E_{free}) was measured from rates of hydrolysis in inhibited reactions; bound thrombin (E_{bound}) was calculated by subtraction from the initial thrombin concentration; and [I] was calculated by subtracting $[E_{bound}]$ from the initial inhibitor concentration $[I^O]$. Such calculations were used to determine the apparent Kass, in triplicate, at each inhibitor concentration, and the values were averaged over the inhibitor range in which enzyme inhibition is 20–80%. The Kass values so obtained generally agree within a standard deviation of < 25%. Alternatively, the Kass is determined graphically with a linearized solution for the Morrison general equation[70] for tight-binding inhibition, as shown by Henderson[51,120] and Beith,[17] and written below in terms of Kass:

$$a = E_{free}/E^O; \text{ and } 1 - a = \text{fraction of } E_{bound};$$
$$\text{apparent Kass} = [E_{bound}]/[E_{free}][I^O - E_{bound}]$$
$$= E^O[1 - a]/[a][E^O] \times [I^O - (1 - a)E^O]$$

which reduces to the linear equation:

$$I^O/1 - a = 1/\text{apparent Kass}[a] + E^O$$

where plots of $I^O/1 - a$ vs. $1/[a]$ yield 1/appKass as the slope of a straight line. Competitive inhibition produces a relationship between apparent Kass and substrate concentration[18,71,99,121] such that

$$\text{Kass} = [\text{apparent Kass}] [1 + S^O/Km]$$

and the slope of a plot of 1/[apparent Kass] vs. $[1 + S^O/Km]$ or vs. $[S^O/Km]$ yields 1/Kass values corrected for substrate dependence. Figure 3 illustrates the dependence of a graphically determined set of apparent efegatran Kass values on the concentration of Bz-Phe-Val-Arg-pNA and shows that efegatran behaves as a competitive, reversible, tight-binding thrombin inhibitor.

Algebraically determined apparent Kass values (n = 4 sets) corrected for substrate concentration dependence produced for efegatran:

$$\text{Kass} = 24.3 \pm 3.0 \times 10^8 \text{ l/mole with human thrombin; and}$$
$$\text{Kass} = 12.6 \pm 4.0 \times 10^8 \text{ l/mole with bovine thrombin}$$

The fact that efegatran forms a transition-state, intermediate structure with thrombin suggests that there should be a slower "on-rate" (with reference to the final transition-state

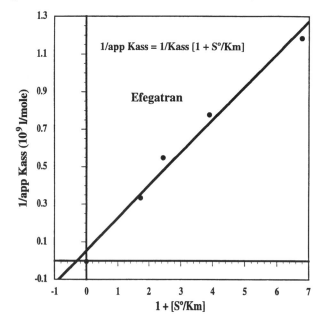

FIGURE 3. Dependence of appKass on substrate concentration—appKass values for efegatran determined with 2.5 nM human thrombin and plotted as 1/app Kass vs. 1 + S^O/Km. Km was determined as 62.7 µM under these conditions. Concentrations of Bz-PheValArg-pNA were 45, 90, 180, and 360 µM. Linear fit was $R^2 = 0.984$.

TABLE 1.   Inhibition of Human Coagulation System Serine Proteases by Efegatran
(Apparent Kass Values, L/mole × 10^6)

	n	Thrombin	Factor Xa	Factor IXaα	Factor IXaβ	Factor XIa	Factor XIIa	Kallikrein	r-aPC
Efegatran	3	668± 174	0.346 ± 0.019	0.052 ± 0.026	0.04 ± 0.0	0.558 ± 0.176	0.150 ± 0.024	0.161 ± 0.081	1.497 ± 0.107
r-Hirudin	3	1000–2000	0.000	0.00	0.00	0.00	0.000	0.000	0.000
Trasylol	3	0.000 ± 0.0	0.004 ± 0.002	0.016 ± 0.003		0.954 ± 0.221	0.006 ± 0.002	12.200 ± 0.0	1.573 ± 0.254
		$E^0 = 5.91$ nM $(S^0 = 0.196$ nM)	$E^0 = 1.34$ nM $(S^0 = 0.182$ nM)	$E^0 = 0.77$ nM $(S^0 = 0.342$ nM)	$E^0 = 0.77$ nM $(S^0 = 0.342$ nM)	$E^0 = 1.15$ nM $(S^0 = 0.398$ nM)	$E^0 = 10.01$ nM $(S^0 = 0.19$–0.25 nM)	$E^0 = 2.9$ nM $(S^0 = 0.8$ nM)	$E^0 = 2.9$ nM $(S^0 = 0.175$ nM)

Apparent Kass values for serine proteases determined from amidase hydrolysis rate inhibition. One substrate concentration (given) was used for each appropriate amide substrate. Each enzyme concentration is given. (n) shows the number of times such determinations were performed, with the resulting mean value given ± standard deviation. For hirudin, the nonthrombin values were not statistically different from zero. Chromogenic substrates were thrombin/BzPheValArgpNA; IXaα/factor X at 6 nm with 0.02 MCa^{2+} and CbzArgProArgpNA; IXaβ included 50 nM PC/PS (1:1) vesicles; Xa/BzIleGluGlyArgpNA; XIa/pyroGluProArgpNA; XIIa/HDPProPheArgpNA; kallikrein/HDPProPhe ArgpNA; aPC/GluClyArgpNA. Thrombin Kass value for LY178207 was 40 × 10^8 1/mole.

intermediate) compared to the rate of thrombin binding with non–transition-state inhibitors.[71,72] Product vs. time curves show that, although substantial amounts of thrombin are rapidly inhibited, efegatran reaches equilibrium with thrombin within minutes, in agreement with similar studies using a different substrate.[15] Incubation of efegatran with thrombin longer than the 2 minutes of the kinetic protocol did not produce different Kass values, indicating that the approach to equilibrium binding was substantially complete during that period. Equilibria considerations with efegatran are also complicated by the fact that the molecule appears to exist in a variety of solution forms (cyclic aminals and hydrates); the aldehyde form represents only a few percent of the population.[14] The practical consequences of reaching tight-binding equilibrium more slowly than with a diffusion-limited process are highly speculative; comparing inhibitors with similar affinity, the former produce slower on-rate and slower off-rate. Beith[19] suggests that slower rates may be more efficient in controlling coagulation proteases. Speculation that efegatran should inhibit thrombin-induced platelet aggregation at concentrations larger than its Ki value[62] are not consistent with the potent antiaggregation activity shown in vitro[9] and ex vivo.[54] Hirudin is considered ideal[77,100] in the sense of both tight binding and fast binding, with a second-order rate constant of association with thrombin of about 10^7 l/mole-sec; therefore, direct comparison with hirudin activities should address the practical value of efegatran's anticoagulant thrombin inhibition. The Kass values for hirudin (native or recombinant) inhibition of thrombin in the system described above are about 3–5-fold more potent than the Kass values for efegatran. Anticlotting activities are compared below.

Anticoagulant Protease Selectivity

The selectivity of efegatran toward nonthrombin proteases of the human coagulation system was evaluated by determining apparent Kass values for each human clotting factor protease with an appropriate chromogenic substrate. Table 1 provides Kass values at a single substrate concentration for thrombin, factors Xa, IXaα, IXaβ, XIa, and XIIa, plasma kallikrein, and activated protein C (aPC). Trasylol (aprotinin) provides a pertinent comparison, not only as a basic reference protease inhibitor, but also because it is frequently used in cardiovascular patients during surgery[20,63,76] in large intravenous doses. The toleration of Trasylol in cardiovascular patients can be useful in estimating the toleration of serine protease inhibition from other agents similarly administered.

Table 1 shows that efegatran inhibits thrombin much more potently than it inhibits the nonthrombin proteases of the human coagulation system. The selectivity for thrombin over other enzymes is presented below as ratios of the inhibition effects from the Kass values in Table 1:

Efegatran Selectivity Ratios* for Thrombin/Coagulation Factor Inhibition

Xa	IXaα	IXaβ	XIa	XIIa	Kallikrein	aPC
2,200	13,400	16,700	1,340	3,340	6,680	450

* Ratio of thrombin appKass values to protease appKass value.

The apparent Kass values of 0.3×10^6 l/mole and 0.5×10^6 l/mole with factors Xa and XIa, respectively, suggest that efegatran may show some inhibitory effect at concentrations of approximately 3 or 2 μM, but these effects should not be expected to be substantial (and do not appear to be important), given the effects of efegatran on activated partial thromboplastin time (APTT) and prothrombin time (PT) (see below). Apparent Kass values with factors IXaα, IXaβ, and XIIa and plasma kallikrein suggest that no anticoagulant effects by efegatran are mediated through these proteases. These data suggest that efegatran should produce plasma anticoagulant effects largely (possibly solely) by the inhibition of thrombin. The broad-spectrum inhibitor Trasylol inhibited plasma kallikrein (appKass ~ 12×10^6 l/mole) and factor XIa (appKass ~ 1×10^6 l/mole) with little effect on other enzymes. Both of these activities are consistent with the prolongations in APTT and ACT reported with Trasylol in vitro and ex vivo during its use in cardiac surgery and cardiopulmonary bypass.[40,73] The apparent Kass value (1.5×10^6 l/mole) for efegatran with aPC is the largest among the nonthrombin coagulation proteases. Similar efegatran inhibition of aPC has been reported by others,[26,30,68] raising the question of the practical consequences to be expected with this level of interaction. Efegatran has demonstrated antithrombotic efficacy in numerous preclinical thrombosis models but has not yet demonstrated any preclinical or clinical effects that suggest interference with aPC. Of interest, Trasylol shows the same ability to inhibit aPC (Kass value ~ 1×10^6 l/mole) as efegatran, in agreement with Callas and Fareed.[26,30] Because Trasylol is so frequently used in cardiovascular patients (at doses producing large blood concentrations), clinical experience suggests that it does not demonstrate effects attributable to aPC inhibition. In fact, when clinical data with Trasylol in a large number of patients were analyzed specifically to search for thrombogenic effects (hypothetically from the inhibition of plasmin), no prothrombotic effects could be found.[63] The DLD-epimer of efegatran, which can slowly form in solution (see below), had no detectable inhibitory activity toward thrombin or the other proteases in Table 1.

From the selectivity properties of efegatran shown in Table 1, we conclude that efegatran, like hirudin (which shows essentially no ability to inhibit nonthrombin proteases), should mediate anticoagulation effects in the various coagulation assays exclusively through interference with thrombin functions.

Anticoagulant Activity and Selectivity

The effects of efegatran as a human plasma anticoagulant are illustrated by the concentration vs. clotting time curves of Figure 4. The effects on thrombin time (TT) are nonlinear and reach maximal prolongation (> 300 sec) at a plasma concentration of about 200 ng/ml. The effects on APTT and PT are linear through plasma concentrations of 3 μg/ml. For quantitative comparison of efegatran and hirudin, we determined the concentrations that would prolong each coagulation assay by twofold (Table 2).

Given that the Ki for hirudin is in the fM range,[99] it is remarkable that efegatran (33 nM to double the TT) was nearly as potent as recombinant hirudin (18 nM) and native hirudin (16 nM) in the inhibition of thrombin in the TT assay. Moreover, hirudin

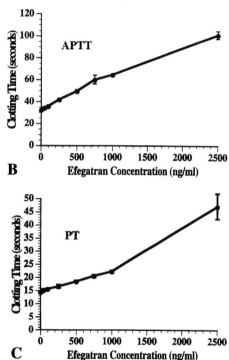

FIGURE 4. Anticoagulant effects of efegatran in human plasma. Efegatran was added to the various coagulation assays immediately before the final reagent addition. Ordinates show time to clotting. Final assay concentrations of efegatran (ng/ml) are given on the abcissa. Thrombin was lot HT740. Standard deviations (n = 3) are shown as range bars. *A*, Thrombin time (TT). *B*, Activated partial thromboplastin time (APTT). *C*, Prothrombin time (PT).

TABLE 2. Inhibition of Human Thrombin Clotting Activity

	Human Thrombin Affinity	**Concentration for Twofold Prolongation of Plasmin Thrombin Time (TT)**	
		(ng/ml)	(nM)
Efegatran	Kass = 2.4 × 10⁹ 1/mole	19 ± 2	33
n-Hirudin	Ki ~ fM*	109 ± 4	16
r-Hirudin	Ki ~ fM*	126 ± 17	18

Thrombin time assays were performed in human plasma with extrapolations of anticoagulant effects to determine concentrations of each thrombin inhibitor required to prolong the TT by twofold. n = 3 (± standard deviation). Control TT was 33 seconds.

* From Stone SR, Hofsteenge J: Kinetics of the inhibition of thrombin by hirudin. Biochemistry 25:4622–4628, 1986, with permission.

is described as the ideal thrombin inhibitor, with small Ki and fast rate of binding.[77,100] However, because the TT assay protocol involves adding thrombin (16 nM final concentration) to plasma containing the inhibitor and the substrate (fibrinogen), the similar anti-TT potencies of efegatran and hirudin are evidence that any "slow-binding" kinetic effects during hemiacetal bond formation may be of no practical consequence in the direct inhibition of human thrombin clotting activity compared with the rate of inhibition by hirudin.

Selectivity Toward Activated Partial Thromboplastin Time

Efegatran and hirudin are quite distinct in their effects on APTT. Efegatran is required at about 1 µg/ml (~1,800 µM) to prolong the APTT by twofold. This finding was not unexpected for two reasons: (1) the amounts of thrombin generated[25,69] in the APTT and PT assays are larger than the amounts used in TT protocols, and (2) efegatran produces anticoagulant effects solely by thrombin inhibition. The functional anticoagulant selectivity for efegatran can be estimated by the ratio of the concentrations that prolong by twofold the APTT. The APTT/TT effect ratio is about 55 (Table 3).

Unexpectedly, hirudin (native or recombinant) produced twofold prolongations of APTT at very low concentrations (40–49 nM), which were near the concentrations needed to prolong the TT by twofold and thus produce APTT/TT effect ratios of 2–3, much different from the anticoagulant selectivity of efegatran.

These data suggest that although both agents are direct-acting inhibitors of thrombin, efegatran and hirudin act differently on the APTT pathway, possibly by inhibiting a different APTT element in addition to thrombin or possibly by affecting thrombin-mediated functions differently in the APTT pathway. The data from Table 1 show that hirudin inhibits none of the nonthrombin coagulation factors in the APTT pathway and, therefore, do not explain the APTT mechanistic distinction between efegatran and hirudin. The functional, and therefore mechanistic, anticoagulant difference between hirudin and efegatran is apparently confined to the APTT pathway. A possible explanation is that hirudin may be more effective in interfering with the feedback activation of factor VIII as a thrombin substrate. Such an explanation could result from the large mechanistic differences in how the two compounds directly interfere with the active site function of thrombin. Hirudin binds thrombin at multiple distal sites (which may interfere with thrombin binding to many types of substrates[44]) and positions its N-terminus in an antiparallel orientation near the active serine of thrombin.[48] In contrast, efegatran binds the P3, P2, and P1 sites in the thrombin-binding pocket in a parallel orientation and forms a reversible hemiacetal bond with the active serine (see Fig. 1), without necessarily competing with other thrombin substrates that initially bind to distal sites.

The differences in APTT/TT effect ratios have a practical result: when efegatran is increased in dose or concentration, whether in preclinical testing or clinical evaluation, the

TABLE 3.   Human Plasma Anticoagulation

	Concentration Required for Twofold Prolongation		
	Prothrombin Time	Activated Partial Thromboplastin Time	Ratio of APTT/TT*
Efegatran	1360 ng/ml (2360 nM)	1050 ng/ml (1820 nM)	55
n-Hirudin	1800 ng/ml (260 nM)	280 ng/ml (40 nM)	2.5
r-Hirudin	3600 ng/ml (510 nM)	340 ng/ml (49 nM)	2.7

Coagulation assays were performed with human plasma, extrapolating the anticoagulant effects to determine concentrations (ng/ml) of the thrombin inhibitors to prolong each assay by twofold. n = 3 (± standard deviation < 20%). Control APTT was 32 seconds; control PT was 18 seconds.
* Ratios of APTT/TT effects were calculated by dividing the above APTT values by the TT values from Table 2.

TT values initially are prolonged, with no effect on the APTT; only at higher concentrations or doses is the APTT substantially prolonged. On the other hand, increasing doses or concentrations of hirudin should produce effects on the APTT at concentrations much closer (relative to efegatran) to doses that substantially prolong the TT.[24,52] Whether such anticoagulant differences are important in defining clinical efficacy or safety must await the results of clinical testing.

Platelet Aggregation Inhibition and Selectivity

Efegatran has been shown to be a potent inhibitor of thrombin-induced platelet aggregation in vitro[9,27,60] and in vivo.[6,54] In fact, doses and concentrations of efegatran that are not high enough to produce anticoagulant responses have produced interference with thrombin-induced platelet aggregation.[6,7,9,54] In contrast, efegatran has essentially no ability to interfere with platelet aggregation induced by nonthrombin agonists, such as collagen, arachidonic acid, and adenosine diphosphate (ADP).[6,54,60] A platelet antagonist selectivity may be important in the pharmacology of efegatran: thrombin-mediated activation and recruitment of platelets during thrombogenesis[114] could be antagonized, whereas aggregation mechanisms from nonthrombin stimulants would be spared. If the nonthrombin platelet aggregation pathways not antagonized by efegatran are important to physiologic hemostasis, this selectivity may produce a favorable therapeutic index for efegatran in clinical testing, especially compared with platelet antagonists that do not discriminate among platelet aggregation mechanisms.

Anticoagulant Selectivity and Antithrombotic Activity of Efegatran in Preclinical Studies

Efegatran was evaluated for antithrombotic activity by constant infusion dosing in a canine model of coronary artery thrombosis.[54,122] Figure 5 shows the in vivo effects of efegatran on TT in the canine model,[54] including a dose-dependent increase in TT and a corresponding dose-dependent increase in antithrombotic effect (the increase in time to thrombotic occlusion after electric injury to the coronary artery).

After each 2-hour intravenous infusion was stopped, the TT values returned toward control and thrombosis occurred. Plasma concentrations of efegatran could be measured by correlation with TT or by HPLC, and the resulting half-life in dogs was about 35 minutes.[78] The TT effects in Figure 4 correlated with antithrombotic activity for efegatran. Indeed, thrombosis did not occur in this protocol until the TT returned to a range between 50–100 seconds (about 2.5–5-fold) greater than the TT control.

The APTT effects from the efegatran studies in dogs[54] are shown in Figure 6. There was no correlation between the APTT and antithrombotic effects of efegatran. The APTT was not measurably prolonged at the two lowest doses (0.25 and 0.5 mg/kg/hr), although both doses were effective in prolonging time to thrombosis and produced marked TT effects (see Fig. 5). The APTT was gradually prolonged at higher doses and reached approximately twofold prolongation at a dose of 2.0–4.0 mg/kg/hr. This dose is 8–16-fold larger than the minimal antithrombotic dose. (Preliminary clinical data suggest that efegatran produces twofold APTT prolongations at about 0.8 mg/kg/hr).

The large in vitro APTT/TT effect ratio for efegatran in human plasma was also found in dog plasma studies in vitro. Therefore, the large APTT/TT effect ratios were reproduced in vivo (see Figs. 5 and 6). Studies with efegatran in rats, with arterial and venous protocols,[47,82,94] also noted that antithrombotic activity was produced at doses that did not cause substantial prolongation of the APTT. A number of studies have shown the antithrombotic activity of efegatran, at low doses, in various animal species.[4,7,14] Two attributes may distinguish efegatran from other thrombin inhibitors and other types of anticoagulants in clinical experimentation: (1) its anticoagulant selectivity profile has an

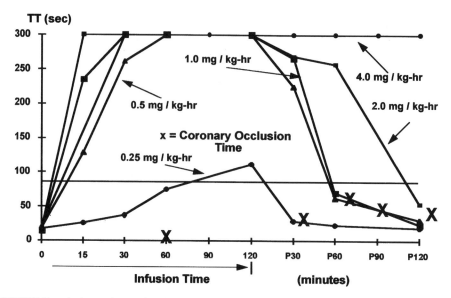

FIGURE 5. Anticoagulant and antithrombotic effects of efegatran in dogs. Data composite of dose response (intravenous infusion) studies in a canine model of coronary artery thrombosis. Plasma thrombin time (TT) values plotted vs. time during two-hour infusions. Approximate mean occlusion times for each dose group are illustrated by X symbols. The control group occluded about 60 minutes after electric injury. (From Smith GF, Craft TJ, Gifford-Moore DS, et al: A family of arginal thrombin inhibitors related to efegatran. Semin Thromb Hemost 22:173–183, 1996, with permission.)

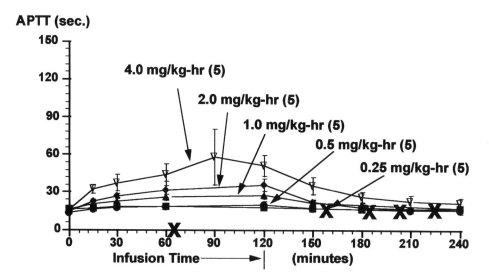

FIGURE 6. Anticoagulant and antithrombotic effects of efegatran in dogs. Data composite of dose response (intravenous infusion) studies in a canine model of coronary artery thrombosis. Plasma activated partial thromboplastin time (APTT) values plotted during two-hour infusions. Approximate mean occlusion times for each dose group are illustrated by X symbols. The control group occluded about 60 minutes after electric injury. (From Smith GF, Craft TJ, Gifford-Moore DS, et al: A family of arginal thrombin inhibitors related to efegatran. Semin Thromb Hemost 22:173–183, 1996, with permission.)

APTT/TT effect ratio much larger than that of hirudin, and (2) in certain protocols efegatran appears to produce antithrombotic effects without requiring perturbation of the APTT.

Bleeding Time and Bleeding in Preclinical Studies

The thrombosis and thrombolysis models used to evaluate efegatran have produced data suggesting that the doses required to produce antithrombotic effects do not substantially prolong bleeding time measurements.[54,57,122] In a rabbit model, Badgy et al.[8] infused large doses of efegatran that resulted in major increases in APTT and noted that bleeding time was minimally prolonged. On an acute basis, efegatran has not shown bleeding effects in many different animal models,[6,8,14] suggesting the possibility of a favorable therapeutic index.

Selectivity Toward the Fibrinolytic System

Necessary selectivity toward the fibrinolytic system requires that useful thrombin inhibitors should not interfere with endogenous or therapeutic fibrinolysis. Because transition-state types of thrombin inhibitors have a large potential to interfere with the proteases of the fibrinolytic system,[16,28,36] we attempted to evaluate thoroughly the ability of efegatran to spare both endogenous and therapeutic fibrinolysis. In vitro, we assessed the ability to spare the enzymes of the fibrinolytic system and plasma clot fibrinolysis induced by plasminogen activators. In vivo, efegatran was evaluated as an antireocclusive antithrombotic adjunct during thrombolysis with ntPA[57] and streptokinase.[55] The ability of efegatran to inhibit the amidolytic activities of plasmin, urokinase (UK), and ntPA is shown in Table 4. Comparative data are included for the antithrombotic prototype tripeptide arginal (LY178207), PPACK (a chloromethylketone with similar amino acid sequence), and the cardiovascular surgery adjunct, Trasylol.

Efegatran demonstrated plasmin Kass values about 200-fold less than Trasylol, with small effects on UK and ntPA. PPACK, an agent widely accepted as a highly selective thrombin inhibitor, showed the largest inhibitory effect on ntPA. Trasylol does not inhibit ntPA or UK. The data in Table 4 generally agree with similar comparative studies by others[16,29,30] but suggest substantially more selectivity for efegatran than reported by Maryanoff et al.[62,68] The respective selectivity ratios of efegatran for thrombin and fibrinolytic proteases, based on a comparison of appKass values, are shown below. Larger ratio values indicate higher selectivity:

TABLE 4. Inhibition of Human Fibrinolytic System Proteases
(Apparent Kass Values, L/mole $\times 10^6$)

	(n)	Plasmin	n-Tissue-type Plasminogen Activator	Urokinase
LY178207	7	4.85 ± 0.68	0.87 ± 0.23	0.32 ± 0.03
Efegatran	9	1.53 ± 0.21	0.05 ± 0.01	0.06 ± 0.00
r-Hirudin	3	0.00	0.00	0.000
Trasylol	3	163.00 ± 58.4	0.00 ± 0.00	0.01 ± 0.00
PPACK	3	0.22 ± 0.01	3.12 ± 1.21	0.20 ± 0.02
		$E^O = 3.4$ nM ($S^O = 0.500$ nM)	$E^O = 1.2$ nM ($S^O = 0.816$ nM)	$E^O = 0.37$ nM ($S^O = 0.300$ nM)

Apparent Kass values for serine proteases determined from amidase hydrolysis rate inhibition. One substrate concentration (given) was used for each appropriate amide substrate. Each enzyme concentration is given. (n) shows the number of times such determinations were performed, with the resulting mean value given ± standard deviation. For hirudin, the values were not statistically different from zero. Substrates were plasmin/HDValLeuLyspNA; nt-PA/HDIleProArgpNA; urokinase/pyroGluGlyArgpNA.

Selectivity Ratos* for Thrombin/Fibrinolytic Protease Inhibition

Compound	Thrombin/tPA	Thrombin/Plasmin	Thrombin/Urokinase
LY178207	46	8	125
Efegatran	13,360	450	11,130

tPA = Tissue-type plasminogen activator.
* Ratio of thrombin appKass value/protease appKass value.

The ratio values show marked improvement in selectivity for efegatran over LY178207 and, together with the Kass values from Table 4, suggest that efegatran may be sufficiently selective to spare fibrinolytic processes.

Efegatran was further studied in vitro for the ability to spare human plasma clot fibrinolysis (1) by using low plasminogen activator concentrations, intended to be relevant to basal-like levels of tPA and UK, and (2) by using therapeutically relevant activator concentrations of ntPA, UK, and streptokinase (SK), intended to reflect the potential use of efegatran as an adjunct to thrombolysis. Table 5 shows the IC_{50} effect concentrations toward "basal-like" concentrations of the activators (12 ng/ml of ntPA and 50 IU/ml of UK).

The prototype arginal LY178207 interfered with fibrinolysis induced by tPA and UK (IC_{50} values of 2 µg/ml and 6 µg/ml, respectively). In contrast, efegatran did not interfere with low-concentration UK or SK and produced an IC_{50} value of about 10 µg/ml with the low-concentration ntPA. Both PPACK (a compound typically described as a "selective" thrombin inhibitor) and Trasylol strongly inhibited clot fibrinolysis by all three plasminogen activators, demonstrating low IC_{50} concentrations. Table 6 gives the plasma clot lysis results using plasminogen activator concentrations approximating therapeutic levels (500 ng/ml ntPA, 1000 U/ml UK and SK). Efegatran showed no measurable interference with SK- or UK-mediated fibrinolysis and produced IC_{50} effects in ntPA-mediated lysis at high concentrations (42 µg/ml). In contrast, PPACK and Trasylol interfered with clot lysis in all three activator systems. The arginal LY178207 interfered with large-concentration ntPA at 11 µg/ml.

The blood concentrations of efegatran (LY294468) during successful antithrombotic testing in the canine coronary thrombosis model[54] were in the range of 0.6 –2.0 µg/ml. At antithrombotic concentrations, therefore, efegatran should spare the endogenous fibrinolytic proteases. The collective in vitro data also suggest that efegatran should be sufficiently sparing of fibrinolysis to be useful adjunctively during thrombolytic treatments with tPA, SK, or UK. Jackson et al.[57] tested efegatran in the canine coronary thrombolysis

TABLE 5.   Plasma Clot Fibrinolysis—Low Levels of Plasminogen Activators

Test Compound Added to Activator	IC_{50} Values (µg/ml)		
	n-Tissue-type Plasminogen Activator	Streptokinase	Urokinase
LY178207	1.9	∞	5.7
Efegatran	9.6	∞	∞
Hirudin	∞	∞	∞
PPACK	0.3	3.4	1.6
Trasylol	5.6	0.8	3.2

Human plasma clots containing ^{125}I-fibrinogen were overlaid with n-tissue-type plasminogen activator (12 ng/ml), streptokinase (50 IU/ml), or urokinase (50 IU/ml). Test compounds in a range of concentrations were added to activator solutions. Fibrinolysis was measured as soluble radioactivity. IC_{50} values were determined from extrapolations from n = 3 tests and are shown as mean values (standard deviation < 15%).
∞ No measurable inhibition of lysis.

TABLE 6.   Plasma Clot Lysis—Therapeutic Levels of Plasminogen Activators

Test Compound Added to Activator	IC$_{50}$ Values (μg/ml)		
	n-Tissue-type Plasminogen Activator	Streptokinase	Urokinase
LY178207	11	∞	∞
Efegatran	42	∞	∞
Hirudin	∞	∞	∞
PPACK	0.3	50	6.6
Trasylol	9.0	18.3	9.4

Human plasma clots containing ^{125}I-fibrinogen were overlaid with n-tissue-type plasminogen activator (500 ng/ml), streptokinase (1000 IU/ml), or urokinase (1000 IU/ml). Test compounds in a range of concentrations were added to activator solutions. Fibrinolysis was measured as soluble radioactivity. IC$_{50}$ values were determined from extrapolations from n = 3 tests and are shown as mean values (standard deviation < 15%). ∞ No measurable inhibition of lysis.

model in which a sufficient dose of ntPA was administered to effect thrombolysis. They found that efegatran was effective in prolonging or preventing thrombotic reocclusion at 0.5 and 1.0 mg/kg/hr. In contrast, the prototype arginal LY178207 failed to prolong or to prevent reocclusion and appeared to shorten the reocclusion time, which can be attributed to interference with plasmin and tPA during thrombolysis and during the reocclusion period. The in vivo selectivity testing, therefore, was in perfect agreement with the selectivity predicted from the in vitro studies.

Important for the clinical expectations of efegatran, a clinically relevant dose of heparin (80 U/kg injection + 30 U/kg/hr infusion) failed to prolong thrombotic reocclusion in this protocol.[57] The failure of heparin as a thrombolytic adjunct can be attributed to its poor antithrombotic mechanism in the context of arterial thrombosis[52,101] and also may involve the inhibition of plasmin by the ATIII-heparin pathway at high concentrations of heparin.[93] Jackson et al.[55] found that efegatran was also successfully administered adjunctively with SK in the canine thrombolysis model. Not only was the thrombotic reocclusion time prolonged, but also the time to thrombolytic reperfusion was shortened. Therefore, the in vitro and in vivo evaluation of efegatran supports its selectivity requirements for sparing of endogenous fibrinolysis and for potential adjunctive use with thrombolytic therapy.

Selectivity Note.   Tables 4, 5, and 6, as well as the in vivo tests results,[55,57] suggest that the thrombin/ntPA Kass ratio (or the absolute ntPA Kass values) allows a better prediction of in vivo selectivity than the thrombin/plasmin Kass ratios (or the absolute plasmin Kass values). Clinical data support this idea. Large doses of Trasylol (a potent plasmin inhibitor not capable of inhibiting ntPA) are given successfully in conjunction with heparin to surgical patients at risk of thrombosis without apparent prothrombotic (antifibrinolytic) effects.[20,63,76] Also, large doses of Trasylol have been used to reverse the increases in bleeding time caused by combination treatment with tPA and aspirin in a canine thrombolysis model.[44] The poor IC$_{50}$ plasma clot fibrinolysis values for the prototype arginal LY178207 and correlative poor selectivity in vivo can be attributed to the combination of moderate plasmin Kass values and moderate tPA Kass values. Favorable IC$_{50}$ clot lysis values found in vitro for efegatran and the favorable in vivo effects of efegatran can be attributed to its lack of interference with the plasminogen activators.

Selectivity Toward Trypsin and Tissue Kallikrein

Efegatran is an inhibitor of trypsin amidolytic activity, with about the same potency as Trasylol, according to the Kass values in Table 7. The potential effects of trypsin inhibition during the use of efegatran in vivo, at the doses expected to be required for antithrombotic efficacy, are not known. The clinical experience with Trasylol[20,63,76] has not yet

TABLE 7.   Inhibition of Trypsin and Tissue Kallikrein (Apparent Kass Values, L/mole × 106)

	(n)	Bovine Trypsin	Porcine Tissue Kallikrein
LY178207	7	75.2 ± 28.5	0.00 ± 0.00
Efegatran	9	100.1 ± 30.8	0.00 ± 0.00
r-Hirudin	2	0.045*	
Trasylol	3	94.6 ± 10.2	35.9 ± 14.4
PPACK	3	551.7 ± 169.9	0.00 ± 0.00
		$E^O = 1.43$ nM $(S^O = 0.18$ nM$)$	$E^O = 7.44$ nM $(S^O = 0.15$ nM$)$

Apparent Kass values for serine proteases determined from amidase hydrolysis rate inhibition. One substrate concentration (given) was used for each appropriate amide substrate. Each enzyme concentration is given. (n) shows the number of times such determinations were performed, with the resulting mean value given ± standard deviation. Substrates were trypsin/BzPheValArgpNA; tissue kallikrein/HDValLeuArgpNA.
* Mean of n =2, range: 0.055–0.035.

shown effects attributable to trypsin inhibition. Parenteral administration of Trasylol or any other trypsin inhibitor (such as efegatran) may add only a small additional concentration of trypsin inhibition to the > 10 μM concentration of broad-acting serine protease inhibitors already present in plasma.[35] Efegatran did not show inhibition of tissue kallikrein, whereas Trasylol (as expected) was a potent kallikrein inhibitor.

PRECLINICAL DISPOSITION AND METABOLISM

Pharmacokinetics

Rats.   In rats administered a 1-mg/kg intravenous dose of efegatran, the plasma concentration was 2970 ng/ml three minutes after injection and decreased monoexponentially, with a half-life of 24 minutes (Fig. 7 and Table 8). The area under the curve (AUC),

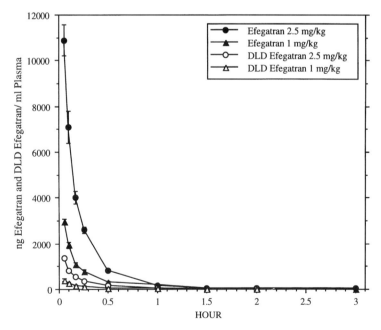

FIGURE 7.   Efegatran and DLD-efegatran plasma concentrations in rats (n = 4) given 1 and 2.5 mg/kg intravenous doses of efegatran.

TABLE 8. Pharmacokinetics of Efegatran and Radioactivity in Rats and Dogs Given Intravenous Doses of Efegatran or ^{14}C-Efegatran

	C_{max} (ng/ml)	Tmax (min)	Half-life α (min)	β (min)	Cl (L/hr•kg)	V (L/kg)	AUC (ng•hr/ml)
Rat							
1 mg/kg	2,970	3	24	—	1.18	0.67	850
2.5 mg/kg	10,900	3	13	—	0.98	0.30	2,545
1 mg/kg*	1,410	2	7	10.5	0.42	0.62	2,860
3 mg/kg*	4,900	2	8	5.8	0.72	0.51	8,140
10 mg/kg*	16,900	2	11	3.4	0.95	0.44	11,750
1 mg/kg/hr	844†	—	—	—	—	—	286,900
Dog							
1 mg/kg	4,250	3	34	—	0.56	0.45	1,830
2 mg/kg							
^{14}C	8,970	5	15	104	0.11	16.1	19,545
Efegatran	9,700	5	34	—	0.41	0.34	4,895
0.5 mg/kg/hr	1,050†	—	—	1.6	0.46	1.08	368,400
1 mg/kg/hr	3,140†	—	—	2.1	0.52	1.53	1,005,200

* Pharmacokinetics of blood radioactivity after intravenous doses of ^{14}C-efegatran.
† Mean steady-state efegatran plasma concentration.

volume of distribution, and systemic clearance of efegatran were 850 ng/hr/ml, 0.67 L/kg, and 1.18 l/hr/kg, respectively. With a 2.5-mg/kg intravenous dose, the plasma concentration was 10,900 ng/ml three minutes after injection and decreased monoexponentially, with a half-life of 13 minutes. The AUC, volume of distribution, and systemic clearance of efegatran were 2545 ng/hr/ml, 0.30 L/kg, and 0.98 L/hr/kg, respectively. The 2.5-fold increase in dose resulted in a 3.7-fold increase in the 3-minute plasma concentration and a 3-fold increase in AUC, indicating good proportionality of dose and systemic exposure to efegatran; systemic clearance was not appreciably affected. The inactive isomer, DLD-efegatran, formed by chemical inversion of the arginal chiral center (see below), accounted for 12–13% of the total efegatran plus DLD-efegatran concentrations throughout the postdosing interval.

Rats were continuously infused with 1 mg/kg/hr of efegatran into the femoral vein for 2 weeks and blood was collected via a jugular vein cannula at selected intervals during and after the infusion. Efegatran plasma concentrations were 700 ng/ml three hours after dose initiation, increasing to 970 ng/ml at 48 hours (Fig. 8). Efegatran concentrations generally remained within a standard deviation of the 48-hour mean value, with no accumulation through the remaining dose interval. The range of the observed steady-state efegatran concentrations was accurately predicted using the clearance values obtained from the 1- and 2.5-mg/kg intravenous bolus data. DLD-efegatran plasma concentrations observed during the infusion were 16% of the drug present during the infusion. No efegatran was detected 24 hours after dose cessation.

Male and female rats were administered a 1-, 3-, or 10-mg/kg intravenous dose of ^{14}C-efegatran. The whole blood radioactivity concentrations two minutes after injection increased in proportion to dose; concentrations were 1410, 4900, and 16900 ng equivalents/ml, respectively (see Table 8). The AUC values for the 1- and 3-mg/kg doses were proportional. However, the AUC value for the 10 mg/kg dose was only 4-fold greater than that of the 1-mg/kg dose. The whole blood radioactivity volume of distribution did not change appreciably across the 1–10 mg/kg dose range, whereas the α-phase half-life and whole blood clearance increased slightly with dose. The terminal elimination half-lives of residual plasma radioactivity ranged from 3.4–10.5 hours and decreased with increasing dose.[111]

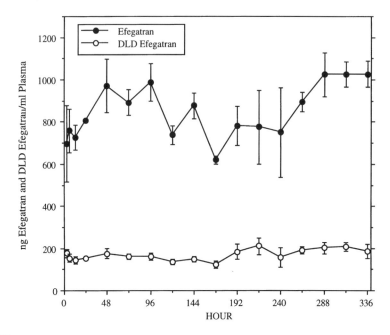

FIGURE 8.   Efegatran and DLD-efegatran plasma concentrations in rats during a 1 mg/kg/hr infusion with efegatran (n = 4).

Dogs.   In dogs given a 1-mg/kg intravenous dose of efegatran, the plasma concentration was 4250 ng/ml three minutes after injection and decreased monoexponentially, with a mean harmonic half-life of 34 minutes (see Table 8). The mean volume of distribution and systemic clearance values were 0.45 L/kg and 0.56 L/hr-kg, respectively. Continuous infusion with 0.5- and 1.5-mg/kg/hr of efegatran for 336 hours produced steady-state plasma concentrations by 2 and 24 hours, respectively (Fig. 9). The steady-state efegatran concentrations agreed well with those predicted by the single intravenous bolus systemic clearance values. After the infusion was stopped, the elimination of efegatran from plasma followed biphasic kinetics, with terminal half-lives of 1.6 and 2.1 hours for the 0.5- and 1.5-mg/kg/hr doses, respectively (Fig. 10). The $AUC_{(0-\infty)}$ and mean steady-state plasma concentrations were proportional to dose, and the clearance values and volumes of distribution were similar for both doses (see Table 8). DLD-efegatran plasma concentrations observed with continuous infusion were approximately 14% of the drug present during the infusion for both doses.

In dogs given a 2-mg/kg intravenous dose of ^{14}C-efegatran, the plasma radioactivity concentration was 8970 ng ^{14}C-equivalents/ml five minutes after injection and declined with an initial 15-minute half-life, followed by a 103-hour terminal elimination half-life. The terminal plasma radioactivity concentrations were below 80 ng ^{14}C-equivalents/ml and less than 1% of the 5-minute plasma radioactivity concentration. The blood radioactivity concentration five minutes after injection was 4780 ng ^{14}C-equivalents/ml and was eliminated according to biphasic kinetics, with initial and terminal half-lives of 16 minutes and 87 hours, respectively. Plasma-to-blood radioactivity ratios were 1.8–1.9 five minutes to 1 hour after dosing and decreased to 1.1 at 12 hours. These ratios indicate that circulating drug is contained mainly in the plasma for 1 hour; thereafter, compound-related material is increasingly associated with the cellular component of blood. Efegatran plasma concentrations 5 minutes after injection were 9700 ng/ml and declined with a 34-minute

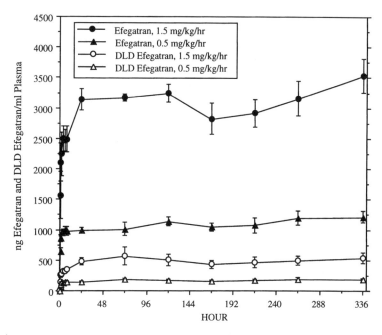

FIGURE 9. Efegatran and DLD plasma concentrations in dogs *during* 0.5 and 1.5 mg/kg/hr infusions with efegatran (n = 4).

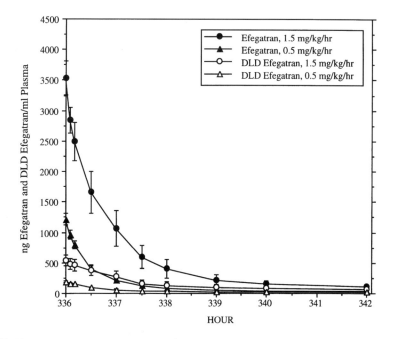

FIGURE 10. Efegatran and DLD plasma concentrations in dogs *after* 0.5 and 1.5 mg mg/kg/hr infusions with efegatran (n = 4)

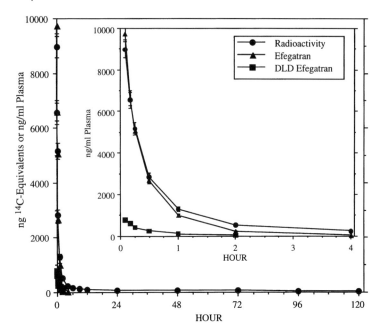

FIGURE 11.   Plasma concentrations of radioactivity, efegatran, and DLD-efegatran in dogs (n = 4) given a 2 mg/kg intravenous dose of ^{14}C-proline-labeled efegatran.

half-life (Fig. 11). The volume of distribution was 0.34 L/kg, and systemic clearance was 0.41 L/hr-kg (see Table 8). Efegatran accounted for 85% of the plasma radioactivity during the initial 4 hours after dosing. Thereafter, efegatran was not detected, even though drug-related material was present at low concentrations through 120 hours. DLD-efegatran was 8% of the total efegatran plus DLD-efegatran observed.

Thrombin Time Assay vs. High-Performance Liquid Chromotagraphy.   The plasma concentrations determined by HPLC analysis are equivalent to the concentrations determined by a thrombin time plasma bioassay for plasma samples obtained from dogs given a 1-mg/kg intravenous dose of efegatran. The results of the two assays are compared in Figure 12, which demonstrates that the correlation between the two procedures is excellent (r^2 = 0.966). Thus the HPLC assay measures the pharmacologically active thrombin inhibitor. Other drug-related material present in plasma has little if any thrombin inhibitory activity.

Metabolism

Efegatran metabolites have been evaluated in rat urine and bile and dog urine after intravenous doses of ^{14}C-efegatran. Analysis by HPLC with tandem mass spectrometry (LC-MS/MS) showed that rat urine contained primarily efegatran (41%) and DLD-efegatran (9%), with small amounts of efegatran acid and efegatran alcohol (Fig. 13). In contrast, rat bile contained only efegatran and DLD-efegatran. Dog urine contained mainly efegatran (25%) and some DLD-efegatran (5%); efegatran acid and alcohol were not observed. A diketopiperazine, a degradation product of efegatran formed by amidolysis of the prolyl-arginal bond and subsequent intramolecular reaction, was identified by LC-MS/MS analysis in rat and dog urine. This intramolecular cyclization is particularly facile in dipeptides in which one amino acid residue is of the L-configuration and the other is of the D-configuration.[23] It is not presently known whether this diketopiperazine is formed in vivo or is an artifact of the analytical procedure.

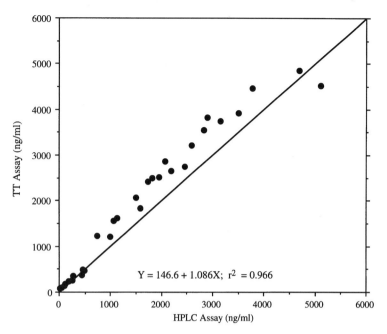

FIGURE 12. Efegatran plasma concentrations in dogs given a 1-mg/kg intravenous dose of efegatran (n = 4), determined by HPLC and thrombin time assay.

Four major drug-related compounds observed in rat (50%) and dog (70%) urine were identified as efegatran-urea adducts (Fig. 14). The identification was confirmed by matching the LC-MS/MS product ion mass spectra of the HPLC peaks in urine to the LC-MS/MS product ion mass spectra of HPLC peaks with the same parent mass ion and the same chromatographic retention time in an efegatran plus urea mixture. Aldehydes interact with ammonia derivatives to form an equilibrium between reactants and a hemiaminal adduct that, upon removal of water, forms an imine.[97] However, in urine the reaction would not go to completion, and the product would be the hemiaminal adduct. The efegatran-urea adduct has an additional chiral center forming a diastereomeric pair for efegatran and for DLD-efegatran, thus yielding four compounds separable by HPLC. These adducts were also formed by incubating efegatran in control rat and dog urine in vitro, suggesting that the efegatran-urea adducts are not enzymatically formed metabolites but rather are formed in the urine after clearance by the kidney. Rat bile does not contain these efegatran-urea adducts.

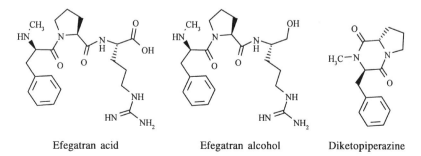

Efegatran acid   Efegatran alcohol   Diketopiperazine

FIGURE 13. Efegatran metabolites as evaluated by HPLC with tandem mass spectrometry in rat and dog urine after intravenous doses of ^{14}C-efegatran.

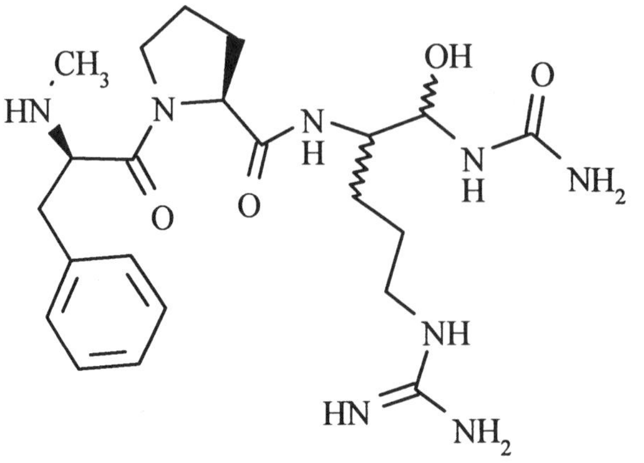

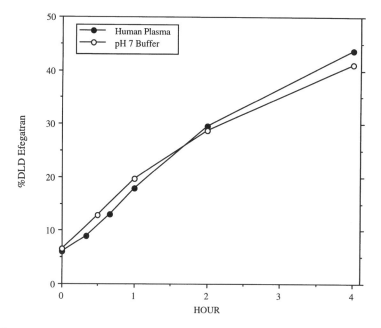

FIGURE 14. Proposed structure of efegatran-urea adduct.

Isomerization

Inversion of efegatran to DLD-efegatran represents an inactivation pathway (see above), and the rate of inversion may affect the pharmacologic efficacy during dose administration. The inversion was examined in vitro by incubating efegatran in human plasma and various pH buffers at 37° C, then determining the percent of DLD-efegatran at selected intervals. In plasma, the DLD-efegatran concentration was initially 6%, increasing to 30% after 2 hours and 44% after 4 hours (Fig. 15). The inversion rate was linear during the first 2 hours of incubation having a rate of approximately 12% per hour, and thereafter, decreased to about 7% per hour. The decrease in inversion with time suggests that at some time beyond 4 hours the efegatran and DLD efegatran concentrations would reach a 50/50 equilibrium mixture.

FIGURE 15. Percent of DLD-efegatran in human plasma and pH-7 sodium phosphate buffer incubated at 37°C.

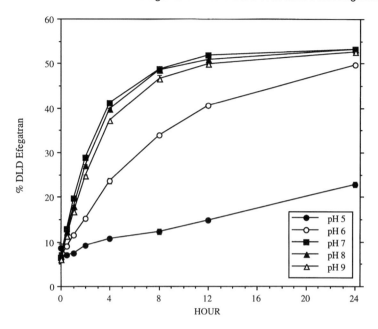

FIGURE 16.   Percent of DLD-efegatran in pH-5–9 sodium phosphate buffers at 37° C.

The inversion of efegatran to DLD-efegatran in sodium phosphate buffer at 37° C is pH-dependent (Fig. 16). The percent of DLD-efegatran in pH-5 buffer was initially 7%, increasing to 11% at 4 hours and 23% at 24 hours. At pH 7, the initial DLD-efegatran concentration was 7%, increasing to 41% at 4 hours and to 53% at 24 hours. The inversion rate in pH-7 sodium phosphate buffer during the initial 4 hours paralleled the rate observed in human plasma (see Fig. 15). Aldehydes in aqueous solution exist as keto-enol tautomers of mostly aldehyde (keto form) in equilibrium with a small amount of a corresponding enol.[98] Efegatran-enol serves as the intermediate between the active DLL isomer and the inactive DLD isomer of efegatran (Fig. 17). Tomori et al. observed this pH-dependent inversion with peptidyl arginals.[105,106] Leupeptin, another peptidyl arginal, was also prone to inversion on contact with silica gel during chromatography.[37] This suggests that the inversion of efegatran to DLD-efegatran is a pH-dependent chemical process rather than an enzyme-mediated reaction.

Protein Binding

The ex vivo and in vitro binding of ^{14}C-efegatran to serum proteins, as determined by equilibrium dialysis at 37° C, is not substantial.[112,113] Only 18% of the radioactivity was bound to proteins in serum obtained from rats five minutes after a 1-mg/kg intravenous dose of ^{14}C-efegatran. In vitro protein binding of ^{14}C-efegatran in rat serum at concentrations of 10, 100, and 1000 ng/ml was 55, 50, and 27%, respectively. In vitro protein binding of ^{14}C-efegatran in dog serum at 1000 ng/ml was 32%.

Excretion

The pattern of excretion of radioactivity by rats and dogs after intravenous administration of ^{14}C-efegatran is similar. During a 96-hour observation period, rats given a 5-mg/kg intravenous dose of ^{14}C-efegatran excreted about 1.5 times more radioactivity in the urine than the feces. In the initial 24 hours after dosing, 49% of the dose was recovered in urine and 18% in feces. Within 96 hours after dosing, 53% of the radioactivity

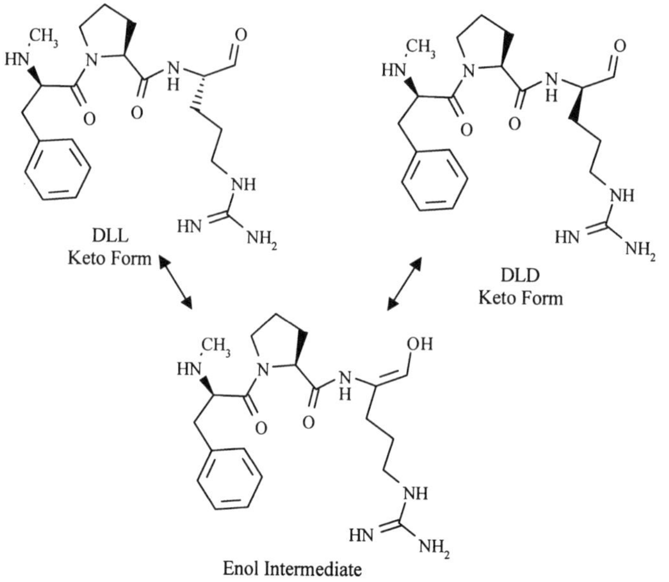

FIGURE 17.   Chemical inversion of the efegatran arginal chiral center.

was recovered in urine and 35% in feces; 6% remained in the rat. Bile duct-cannulated rats excreted 28% of a 5-mg/kg intravenous dose of ^{14}C-efegatran in the bile within 72 hours. After a 2-mg/kg intravenous dose of ^{14}C-efegatran to dogs, 36% of the radioactivity was recovered in the urine within 24 hours, increasing to 40% at 120 hours after dosing. The feces contained 15% of the dose at 24 hours and 39% at 120 hours after injection. The incomplete excretion of radioactivity by rats and dogs is consistent with the pharmacokinetic results that show a long terminal elimination half-life associated with low plasma radioactivity concentrations.

Conclusions

Preclinical studies demonstrate that efegatran is rapidly eliminated from plasma after intravenous administration, although low levels of drug-related material persist after efegatran is no longer detectable. There is excellent agreement between efegatran plasma concentrations determined by HPLC and thrombin time plasma bioassays; metabolites of efegatran appear to have little or no thrombin inhibitory activity. Efegatran-related material is not completely excreted during intervals up to 120 hours after dosing. Continuous infusion to dogs and rats results in predictable steady-state efegatran plasma concentrations with little or no accumulation. Very low amounts of efegatran metabolites have been observed in rat urine and bile and dog urine. In addition, the inactive isomer DLD-efegatran, is observed in plasma after administration of efegatran but does not exceed approximately 16% of the total efegatran and DLD-efegatran measured. Protein binding of efegatran is low in rat and dog serum and increases at lower concentrations.

CLINICAL STUDIES

Materials and Methods

Phase I Dose Escalation Studies.   The tolerability, anticoagulant activity, and pharmacokinetics of efegatran were assessed in two placebo-controlled, dose-escalation studies with intravenous infusion of 15 minutes' duration, and longer term intravenous infusions of duration ranging from 4–48 hours. The study subjects were healthy men aged 18–35 years and within 15% of normal body weight based on height. They had a normal physical examination and screening tests. All study subjects were admitted to Guy's Drug Research Unit (GDRU) in London. The experimental protocols were reviewed and approved by the Ethics Committee of Guy's Hospital. All studies were conducted in a single-subject blind fashion.

A total of 63 volunteers participated in the studies, with 40 receiving 15-minute intravenous infusions (0.01–0.3 mg/kg) and 23 receiving prolonged intravenous infusions of 0.21, 0.42, 0.63, or 0.84 mg/kg/hr for 4 hours, 0.42 and 0.63 mg/kg/hr for 12 or 24 hours, or 0.63 mg/kg/hr for 48 hours. In each of these studies dose escalation occurred in a sequential manner and only after evaluations of tolerability and pharmacodynamic responses to previous dose levels were made.

After administration of efegatran or placebo, subjects were monitored closely within GDRU for at least 24 hours, then returned at 5–7 days after their final admission for follow-up evaluations. The general tolerability of efegatran was assessed by collection of clinical data related to adverse events in combination with data obtained from physical examinations before and after exposure to efegatran or placebo. Bleeding risk associated with exposure to efegatran or placebo was assessed by measurement of Simplate II bleeding times, by urinalysis with microscopy, and by fecal occult blood assessment. The pharmacodynamic effect of efegatran was assessed in terms of its anticoagulant effects by measurement in citrated plasma samples (1:10 v/v 3.8% sodium citrate) of TT and APTT. Blood samples were also drawn for the measurement of plasma concentrations of efegatran.

Assays for Coagulation and Hemostasis. Coagulation time assays were performed with a MCA Bio/Data coagulometer. APTT assays were performed with a platelet factor 3 reagent containing micronised silica (Auto-APTT, Organon Teknika, Oklahoma City, OK). TT assays were performed using a bovine thrombin (Diagnostic Reagents, Ltd, Thames, UK) solution (3 U/ml) containing 0.45% sodium chloride and 0.0125 M calcium chloride. The final concentration of thrombin in the TT assay was adjusted to provide a control time of 12–14 seconds. Bleeding times were performed before adminstration of efegatran or placebo, at the end of the infusion, and at the end of the experimental protocol. Template bleeding times were measured using a Simplate II device with a sphygmomanometer cuff inflated to 40 mmHg.[68] The "normal" reference range for bleeding time was 2–10 minutes, with values greater than 15 minutes considered to be of potential clinical significance.

Assay for Efegatran Plasma Concentrations. Plasma concentrations of efegatran were determined by HPLC. This assay was sensitive and specific, with a sensitivity of 20 ng/ml and linearity over a range of 20–1550 ng/ml. Intra- and inter-day variabilities, tested at 20, 120, 400 and 1400 ng/ml, were less than 15% and 10% for the 20 ng/ml and 120–1400 ng/ml controls, respectively.

Phase II Unstable Angina Study. The safety, anticoagulant effect, and anti-ischemic activity of efegatran were also assessed in a study of 102 patients with unstable angina conducted in the Netherlands. Patients with unstable angina (defined as ischemic chest pain at rest or on minimal exertion) accompanied by dynamic ST segment and/or T-wave EKG changes were randomized to receive a 48-hour intravenous infusion of either efegatran or heparin. The dosage levels of efegatran were 0.105 mg/kg/hr (n = 10), 0.32 mg/kg/hr (n = 24), 0.63 mg/kg/hr (n = 6), or 0.84 mg/kg/hr (n =24). Patients randomized to heparin therapy received a 5,000-IU bolus followed by an infusion of 1,000 IU/hr (adjusted for an APTT range of 2–2.5 times baseline). All patients also received aspirin at a dose of at least 80 mg/day; intravenous nitroglycerin, beta-blockers, calcium antagonists, and other antianginal therapies were used as clinically indicated. Patients were monitored until hospital discharge or 7 days (whichever occurred first).

Results

Phase I Studies.   Efegatran was well tolerated at all doses administered. No subject experienced a serious life-threatening event during the studies. Mild events, such as headache or dizziness, occurred infrequently. None of the event patterns could be consistently attributed to efegatran; indeed, the majority occurred with similar frequency in treatment and placebo groups. Mild sporadic elevations of hepatic enzymes (alanine transaminase and/or aspartate transaminase) were detected in some subjects during the studies. None of the elevations were of clinical significance, all resolved within the course of the study, and there was no apparent dose-response relationship to efegatran.

Pharmacokinetics.   Plasma concentrations of efegatran reached 85% of steady-state values at approximately 2 hours after starting the intravenous infusions. Mean plasma concentrations for each dose of efegatran during the 4-hour infusion are shown in Figure 18. During prolonged infusions, concentrations were maintained for up to 48 hours without accumulation. Upon stopping the infusion, efegatran concentrations declined in a biphasic fashion, with substantial elimination of the drug occurring during the first phase (i.e., the distribution phase).

Systemic exposure, expressed as the area under the plasma concentration vs. time curve, increased in a linear fashion with increasing dose (Fig. 19), indicating that no saturable disposition processes exist over the dosage range studied. Indeed, systemic plasma clearance was rapid, averaging 0.383 L/hr/kg, and remained independent of the rate and duration of infusion (15 minutes to 48 hours). Efegatran is distributed into slowly equilibrating tissues during constant-rate infusion. Although not statistically significant, the volume of distribution at steady state (V_{ss}), which takes into account the distribution and elimination phases of the compound, appeared to increase with increasing duration of infusion ranging from 4 hours to 48 hours. The overall V_{ss} value averaged 0.46 L/kg. The volume of distribution of the elimination phase (V_{β}) for the 15-minute infusions averaged 0.36 L/kg. If distribution between various tissues in the peripheral compartment is at an equilibrium, V_{β} should be much larger than V_{ss}. The fact that V_{ss}, which was obtained during constant-rate infusions of 4–48 hours' duration, is considerably larger than V_{β}, which was obtained during 15-minute infusions, provides further evidence of a peripheral compartment of tissues into which the drug distributes, thus taking a long time to reach equilibrium. The combination of a larger volume of distribution with longer-term infusions

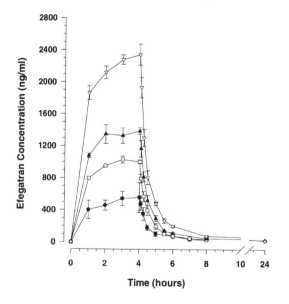

FIGURE 18.   Efegatran concentrations as a function of time in normal volunteers after a 4-hour intravenous infusion. The doses are represented by: (●) 0.21 mg/kg/hr, n = 3; (□) 0.42 mg/kg/hr, n = 4; (▲) 0.63 mg/kg/hr, n = 4; and (▽) 0.84 mg/kg/hr, n = 5. Each point represents the mean ± SEM of the number of individuals studied.

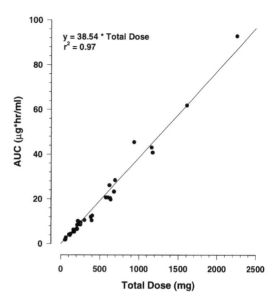

FIGURE 19. Correlation of area under the plasma concentration curve versus time curve with total dose in normal volunteers (n = 31).

and a clearance that was consistent for infusion durations ranging from 15 minutes to 48 hours resulted in a longer terminal half-life ($t_{1/2}$) of 2.5 hours with steady-state infusions compared with a 35-minute $t_{1/2}$ after 15-minute infusions. During long-term infusions, however, the majority of efegatran elimination (82%) was associated with events defined by the distribution phase, which had a harmonic mean $t_{1/2}$ of 18 minutes. These data suggest that the majority of efegatran elimination after termination of the infusion is rapid. Therefore, both the time to reach steady-state concentrations and the elimination $t_{1/2}$ are more heavily influenced by the rate of distribution than by the rate of elimination of efegatran.

Anticoagulant Activity. The pharmacodynamic effects of efegatran in healthy volunteers and in patients with unstable angina have been previously presented by Jackson et al.[56] The results of their analyses are repeated in this chapter. Intravenous administration of efegatran produced a dose-dependent prolongation of coagulation times, assessed by measurement of TT and/or APTT. For 15-minute intravenous infusions of efegatran, a dosage level of approximately 0.025 mg/kg was required to double the TT value. TT was a specific and extremely sensitive measure of the anticoagulant activity of efegatran. The upper limit of quantification for TT (120 seconds for the automated method chosen) was exceeded at doses above 0.1 mg/kg, making interpretation of the anticoagulant effect of efegatran, in terms of TT prolongation, more difficult. At higher doses of efegatran (0.225–0.3 mg/kg), APTT was prolonged in a dose-dependent fashion. Immediately after termination of the 15-minute infusion of 0.3 mg/kg, APTT prolongation ranged from 175–238% of baseline. The offset of anticoagulant effect (measured by prolongation of APTT) after cessation of drug infusion was rapid, with a pharmacologic $t_{1/2}$ for efegatran of approximately 30 minutes. This study demonstrated that the approximate ratio of the dose of efegatran required to produce an APTT prolongation of 200% of baseline to the dose required to produce a TT prolongation of 200% of baseline was 12:1.

Prolonged intravenous administration of efegatran produced dose-related anticoagulant activity with no accumulation of effect. For all infusion rates except 0.21 mg/kg/hr, the TT was prolonged beyond the 120-second limit of the automated technique used. Dose-related prolongations of APTT were observed (Fig. 20). On termination of drug infusion, the disappearance of the anticoagulant effect was rapid. The average time for

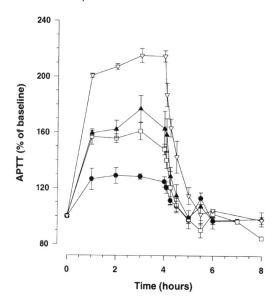

FIGURE 20. Prolongation of activated partial thromboplastin time (APTT) in normal volunteers by increasing doses of efegatran. The doses are represented by: (●) 0.21 mg/kg/hr, n = 3; (□) 0.42 mg/kg/hr, n = 4; (▲) 0.63 mg/kg/hr, n = 4; and (▽) 0.84 mg/kg/hr, n = 5. Each point represents the mean ± SEM of the number of individuals studied. (Redrawn from Jackson CV et al: Preclinical and clinical pharmacology of efegatran. Clin Appl Thromb Hemost 22:258–267, 1996, with permission from Lippincott-Raven Publishers.)

APTT to return to baseline (± 5%) was 60 minutes, regardless of the rate or duration of infusion. The anticoagulant effect of efegatran, measured by APTT prolongation as a percentage of baseline values, correlated in a linear fashion ($p < 0.001$) with the rate of infusion, regardless of the duration of infusion (Fig. 21). At each rate of infusion an increase in plasma concentration of efegatran was accompanied by a prolongation of the APTT (Fig. 22), indicating that no saturable processes exist in the relationship between efegatran plasma concentration and prolongation of APTT over the range of infusion rates tested.

Effects on Hemostasis. Efegatran administration in healthy men was not associated with any clinically significant evidence of bleeding as assessed by physical examination, urinalysis, and measurements of fecal occult blood. No clinically significant dose-related

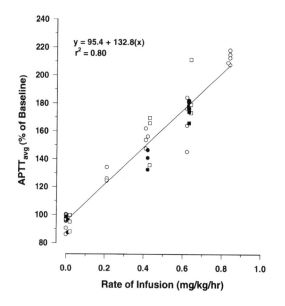

$y = 95.4 + 132.8(x)$
$r^2 = 0.80$

FIGURE 21. Linear dose-response relationship produced by efegatran in normal volunteers when comparing activated partial thromboplastin time (APTT) at steady state vs. the rate of drug infusion. The different infusion times were: (O) 4 hours, (●) 12 hours, (□) 24 hours, and (■) 48 hours. Each point represents the average APTT value for the respective rate of infusion. (Redrawn from Jackson CV et al: Preclinical and clinical pharmacology of efegatran. Clin Appl Thromb Hemost 22:258–267, 1996, with permission from Lippincott-Raven Publishers.)

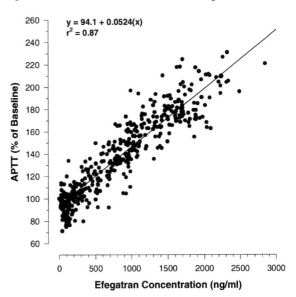

FIGURE 22. Linear relationship between changes in activated partial thromboplastin time (APTT) as a function of circulating plasma concentrations of efegatran at all doses studied in normal volunteers. Data points represent all observations made during efegatran infusion and the washout period from 31 volunteers. (Redrawn from Jackson CV et al: Preclinical and clinical pharmacology of efegatran. Clin Appl Thromb Hemost 22: 258–267, 1996, with permission from Lippincott-Raven Publishers.)

changes in hematology or blood chemistry parameters were observed. Template bleeding time was used as a surrogate assessment of bleeding risk. Bleeding times fell within the reference range for the method of 2–10 minutes, regardless of the dose level or duration of infusion. In a few individuals sporadic prolonged bleeding time measurements were recorded, without clear evidence of a dose-response relationship to efegatran. In no individual was a prolonged bleeding time associated with any clinically significant bleeding episode. All prolonged bleeding times measured during efegatran infusion had returned to baseline by follow-up assessment at 6 hours after termination of infusion.

Phase II Unstable Angina Study.   All dose levels of efegatran were clinically well tolerated. No clinically significant prolongation of bleeding time, as measured by the Ivy or Simplate methods, was observed. One patient receiving efegatran required a 2-unit packed-cell transfusion after a hematoma associated with cardiac catheterization. Efegatran infusions produced rapid-onset, dose-dependent prolongations of APTT with no accumulation of anticoagulant effect over time and a rapid return to baseline activity after termination of infusion (Fig. 23). No rebound coagulation phenomenon was observed. The clotting data are reflective of highly stable plasma concentrations of efegatran in these patients (Fig. 24).

With respect to clinical outcomes at 7 days, one death occured in the group receiving efegatran. Myocardial infarction occurred in 4 of 85 patients receiving efegatran and in 3 of 17 receiving heparin. Revascularisation procedures (percutaneous transluminal coronary angioplasty or coronary artery bypass grafting) were performed in 5 of 85 patients receiving efegatran, whereas none of the 17 patients receiving heparin underwent such procedures. The final data analysis for this study is incomplete.

In summary, efegatran has demonstrated dose-dependent pharmacokinetics and anticoagulant activity in humans. The pharmacokinetic/pharmacodynamic model developed from clinical trials conducted in healthy volunteers appears to be predictive of the effects observed in patients with unstable angina. Approximately 85% of steady-state concentrations can be achieved 2 hours after starting a constant-rate infusion. Steady state can be achieved more rapidly with the addition of a loading dose (data not discussed in this chapter). The offset of anticoagulant activity is rapid, with APTT values returning to baseline approximately 60 minutes after termination of the intravenous infusion. Ongoing phase II

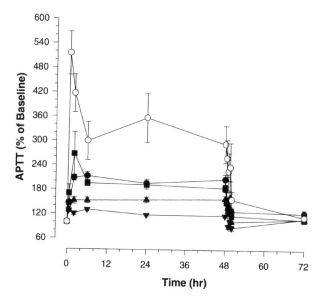

FIGURE 23. Activated partial thromboplastin time (APTT) as a function of time and dose in patients with unstable angina receiving 48-hour infusions of efegatran or heparin. The dose groups for efegatran are: (▼) 0.105 mg/kg/hr, n = 10; (▲) 0.32 mg/kg/hr, n = 24; (■) 0.64 mg/kg/hr, n = 26; and (●) 0.84 mg/kg/hr, n = 24. The heparin group is denoted by (O) 5000 IU bolus + 1000 IU/hr infusion, n = 17. Each point represents the mean ± SEM of the number of individuals in each group (n). (Redrawn from Jackson CV et al: Preclinical and clinical pharmacology of efegatran. Clin Appl Thromb Hemost 22:258–267, 1996, with permission from Lippincott-Raven Publishers.)

clinical trials in patients with unstable angina and acute myocardial infarction will be evaluated to determine whether efegatran can provide benefit with an improved therapeutic index as an antithrombotic anticoagulant.

EFEGATRAN AS A NEW ANTITHROMBOTIC THROMBIN INHIBITOR

There is a recognized need for replacement of warfarin and heparin as anticoagulant, antithrombotic agents, because neither is ideal with respect to therapeutic index and predictability.[3,30,38,41,86,104,108] Thrombin inhibitors offer effects different from the total hemostatic depression provided by warfarin[92] and from the catalytic indirect thrombin inactivation provided by heparin.[75,95] Moreover, the direct inhibition of thrombin-induced platelet aggregation is highly selective, because aggregation by other agonists (e.g., collagen, ADP) is not inhibited,[5,54,60] and may provide control over thrombus formation while leaving the hemostatic system intact. This, in turn, may explain the lack of acute bleeding generally observed with testing of thrombin inhibitors in animal models of thrombosis.[118]

As a new thrombin inhibitor, efegatran has shown mechanistic distinctions from other anticoagulant agents. The compound binds at the active site of thrombin, forming a reversible hemiacetal bond at Ser_{195}, which contributes largely[90] to tight-binding, reversible competitive thrombin inhibition. The difference in empirical anticoagulant selectivity between efegatran and hirudin is manifested by large differences in their respective APTT/TT effect ratios. The underlying anticoagulant mechanistic differences between efegatran and hirudin cannot be explained by differential inhibition of the contact pathway serine proteases but appear to be confined to the APTT pathway, possibly involving different inhibitory effects on the thrombin feedback activation of factor VIII. With the exception of trypsin, efegatran shows good selectivity with respect to nonthrombin serine

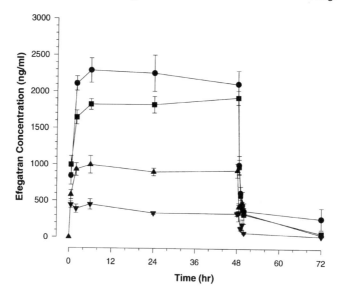

FIGURE 24.   Plasma efegatran concentrations as a function of time in patients with unstable angina during 48-hour infusions of efegatran. Increasing rates of infusion of efegatran are denoted by: (▼) 0.105 mg/kg/hr, n = 10; (▲) 0.32 mg/kg/hr, n = 24; (■) 0.64 mg/kg/hr, n = 26; and (●) 0.84 mg/kg/hr, n = 24. Each point represents the mean ± SEM of the number of individuals in each group (n). (Redrawn from Jackson CV et al: Preclinical and clinical pharmacology of efegatran. Clin Appl Thromb Hemost 22:258–267, 1996, with permission from Lippincott-Raven Publishers.)

proteases. Studies of selectivity regarding the fibrinolytic system suggest that efegatran may be useful as an antithrombotic adjunct to thrombolytic therapy with tPA, UK, or SK and may spare endogenous fibrinolysis. Antithrombotic effects in a number of animal species occur at low infusion doses and appear to correlate with effects on thrombin time. The animal studies suggest that efegatran can produce antithrombotic effects in some protocols without necessarily perturbing the APTT, an attribute which may be unique among anticoagulants. Preliminary pharmacokinetic calculations, using plasma concentrations derived from TT effects in dog models of thrombosis, suggest that plasma half-life values for efegatran range from 35–45 minutes.

Preclinical disposition studies demonstrate that efegatran is rapidly eliminated from plasma, with low levels of drug-related material persisting after efegatran is no longer detectable. Efegatran-related material is not completely excreted as long as 120 hours after dosing. Efegatran plasma concentrations determined by HPLC agree well with concentrations derived from thrombin time plasma bioassays. Continuous infusion to dogs and rats results in predictable steady-state plasma concentrations with little or no accumulation. Very low amounts of efegatran metabolites have been observed in rat urine and bile and in dog urine. Such metabolites appear to have little or no thrombin inhibitory activity. The inactive isomer DLD-efegatran is observed in plasma after administration of efegatran but does not exceed approximately 16% of the total efegatran and DLD-efegatran measured. Efegatran shows low protein binding in rat and dog serum.

Efegatran has been evaluated in phase I clinical studies and is being tested in phase II protocols in patients with unstable angina[87,88] and acute myocardial infarction. Intravenous infusions produced predictable and stable anticoagulant activities that reached steady state within about two hours, with no accumulation of effect, through doses of 0.84 mg/kg/hr. The effects on APTT were linear and returned rapidly to baseline on termination of the infusions, with the APTT effect disappearing with a half-life of 35 minutes. This property should allow rapid withdrawal of anticoagulant effect without the need for an antidote. The APTT effect correlated highly with efegatran plasma concentration. The intravenous half-life in humans[80] was 35 minutes $(t_{1/2}\alpha)$, in excellent agreement with the preclinical disposition studies, and clearance from plasma was rapid (0.4 L/hr/kg). The pharmacokinetic/ pharmacodynamic model developed from clinical trials in healthy volunteers appears to be predictive of the effects in patients with unstable angina. Approximately 85% of steady-state concentrations can be achieved two hours after starting a constant-rate infusion. The 35-minute half-life should represent a useful range for such an anticoagulant compound, especially for prospective parenteral use, with the safety advantage of rapid reversal of effect on stopping the infusion dose or following injection. Efegatran has behaved as a potent anticoagulant with linear phamacokinetics and linear APTT effects. No clinically significant prolongations in bleeding times were recorded in any patient treated with efegatran (through doses of 0.84 mg/kg/hr). The APTT effect was dose-dependent and predictable, with no APTT overshoot (in contrast to treatments with heparin). Ongoing phase II clinical trials in patients with unstable angina and acute myocardial infarction will be evaluated to determine whether efegatran can provide benefit with an improved therapeutic index.

REFERENCES

1. Adams GA, Brown SJ, McIntire LV, et al: Kinetics of platelet adhesion and thrombus growth. Blood 62:69–74, 1983.
2. Axel TB: X-PLOR Version 3.1 A System for X-Ray Crystallography and NMR. New Haven, CT, Yale University Press, 1992.
3. Amerena J, Mashford ML, Wallace S: Adverse effects of anticoagulants. Adverse Drug React Acute Poison Rev 9:1–36, 1990.
4. Bacher P, Walenga JM, Iqbal O, et al: The antithrombotic and anticoagulant effects of a synthetic tripeptide and recombinant hirudin in various animal models. Thromb Res 71:251–263, 1993.
5. Bagdy D, Bararas D, Bajusz S, Szell E: In vitro inhibition of blood coagulation by tripeptide aldehydes: A retrospective study focused on the stable D-MePhe-Pro-Arg-H-H2SO4. Thromb Haemost 67:325–330, 1992.
6. Bagdy D, Barabas E, Szabo G, et al: In vivo anticoagulant and antiplatelet effect of D-Phe-Pro-Arg-H and D-MePhe-Pro-Arg-H. Thromb Haemost 67:357–365, 1992.
7. Bagdy D, Szabo G, Barabas E, Bajusz S: Inhibition by D-MePhe-Pro-Arg-H (GYKI-14766) of thrombus growth in experimental models of thrombosis. Thromb Haemost 68:125–129, 1992.
8. Bagdy D, Szabo G, Barabas E: An experimental approach to estimate the efficacy and tolerability of a synthetic direct thrombin tnhibitor, D-MePhe-Pro-Arg-H, efegatran sulfate (GYKI-14766). Thromb Haemost 73:1307, 1995.
9. Bagdy D, Barabas E, Bajusz S, Szell E: In vitro inhibition of blood coagulation by tripeptide aldehydes: A retrospective screening study focused on the stable D-MePHE-Pro-Arg-H.H2SO4. Thromb Haemost 67:325–330, 1992.
10. Bagdy D, Szabo G, Barabas E, Bajusz S: Inhibition by D-MePhe-Pro-Arg-H (GYKI-14766) of thrombus growth in experimental models of thrombosis. Thromb Haemost 68:125–129, 1992.
11. Bajusz S, Barabas E, Tolnay P, et al: Inhibition of thrombin and trypsin by tripeptide aldehydes. Int J Peptide Protein Res 12:217–221, 1978.
12. Bajusz S, Barabas E, Szell E, Bagdy D: Peptide aldehyde inhibitors of the fibrinogen-thrombin reaction. In Walter K, Meinenhofer J (eds): Peptides: Chemistry, Structure and Biology. Ann Arbor Science, Ann Arbor, MI, 1975, pp 603–668.
13. Bajusz S, Szell E, Badgy D, et al: Highly active and selective anticoagulants: D-Phe-Pro-Arg-H, a free tripeptide aldehyde prone to spontaneous inactivation, and its stable N-methyl derivative, D-MePhe-Pro-Arg-H. J Med Chem 33:1729–1735, 1990.
14. Bajusz S: Chemistry and biology of the peptide anticoagulant D-MePhe-Pro-Arg-H (GYKI-14766). Adv Exp Med Biol 340:91–108, 1993.
15. Bakonyi A, Kovacs L, Duong H T, Aranyi P: Biochemical effect and kinetics of thrombin inhibition by GYKI-14766. Acta Physiol Hung 82:29–36, 1994.
16. Barabas E, Szell E, Bajusz S: Screening for fibrinolysis inhibitory effect of synthetic thrombin inhibitors. Blood Coagul Fibrinol 4:243–248, 1993.
17. Bieth JG: Pathophysiological interpretation of kinetic constants of protease inhibitors. Bull Eur Physiopathol Respir 16:183–195, 1980.

18. Bieth JG: Pathophysiological interpretation of kinetic constants of protease inhibitors. Bull Eur Physiopathol Respir 16:183–195, 1980.
19. Bieth JG: In vivo significance of kinetic constants of macromolecular proteinase inhibitors. Adv Exp Med Biol 167:97–109, 1984.
20. Bidstrup B, Royston D, Sapsford RN, Taylor KM: Reduction in blood loss and blood use after cardiopulmonary bypass with high dose aprotinin (Trasylol). J Thorac Cardiovasc Surg 97:364–372, 1989.
21. Blomback B, Hessel B, Hogg D, Claesson G: Substrate specificity of thrombin on proteins and synthetic substrates. In Lundblad RL (ed): Chemistry and Biology of Thrombin. Ann Arbor Science, Ann Arbor, MI, 1977, pp 275–285.
22. Blomback B, Hessel B, Hogg D, Therkildsen L: A two-step fibrinogen-fibrin transition in blood coagulation. Nature 275:501–505, 1978.
23. Bodansky M, Martinez J: Protection of functional groups in peptide synthesis. In Gross E, Meienhoffer J (eds): The Peptides: Analysis, Synthesis, Biology. New York, Academic Press, 1983, p 121.
24. Brill-Edwards P, Ryn-McKenna JV, Cai L, et al: Prevention of thrombus growth by antithrombin III-dependent and two direct thrombin inhibitors in rabbits: Implications for antithrombotic therapy. Thromb Haemost 68:424–427, 1992.
25. Brinkhous KM, Dombrose FA: Partial thromboplastin time. In Schmidt RM (ed): Hematology, Boca Raton, FL, CRC Press, 1980, pp 221–246, 1980.
26. Callas D, Fareed J: Direct inhibition of protein Ca by site directed thrombin inhibitors: Implications in anticoagulant and thrombolytic therapy. Thromb Res 78:457–460, 1995.
27. Callas DD, Hoppensteadt D, Fareed J: Comparative studies on the anticoagulant and protease generation inhibitory actions of newly developed site-directed thrombin inhibitory drugs: Efegatran, argatroban, hirulog, and hirudin. Semin Thromb Hemost 21:177–183, 1995.
28. Callas D, Bacher P, Iqbal O, et al: Fibrinolytic compromise by simultaneous administration of site-directed inhibitors of thrombin. Thromb Res 74:193–205, 1994.
29. Callas DD, Iqbal O, Hoppensteadt D, Fareed J: Fibrinolytic compromise by synthetic and recombinant thrombin inhibitors: Implications in the treatment of thrombotic disorders. Clin Appl Thromb Hemost 1:114–124, 1995.
30. Callas D, Fareed J: Comparative pharmacology of site directed antithrombin agents: Implication in drug development. Thromb Haemost 74: 473–481, 1995.
31. Chase T, Shaw E: p-Nitrophenyl-p'-guanidinobenzoate HCl: A new active site titrant for trypsin. Biochem Biophys Res Comm 29:508, 1967.
32. Chirgadze NY, Clawson D, Gesellchen PD, et al: The x-ray structure at 2.2A resolution of a ternary complex containing human alpha-thrombin, a hirudin peptide (54-65) and an active site inhibitor. Presented at the American Crystallographic Association Meeting, August 9–14, Pittsburgh, PA, 1992.
33. Chomiak PN, Walenga JM, Koza MJ, et al: Investigation of a thrombin inhibitor peptide as an alternative to heparin in cardiopulmonary bypass surgery. Circulation 88:407–412, 1993.
34. Claeson G: Synthetic peptides and peptidomimetics as substrates and inhibitors of thrombin and other proteases in the blood coagulation system. Blood Coag Fibrinol 5:411–436, 1994.
35. Colman RW, Marder VJ, Salzman EW, Hirsh J: Overview of hemostasis. In Colman RW, Marder VJ, Salzman EW, Hirsh J (eds): Hemostasis and Thrombosis: Basic Principles and Clinical Practice, 3rd ed. Philadelphia, J.B. Lippincott, 1994, pp 3–18,.
36. Das J, Kimball SD: Thrombin active site inhibitors. Bioorg Med Chem 3:999–1007, 1995.
37. Dsino Y, Domrno Y, Miyazaki H, Ishii S: Semisynthesis of 14C-labeled leupeptin. Chem Pharm Bull 30. 2319–2325, 1982.
38. Estes JW: The fate of heparin in the body. Current Ther Res 18: 45–65, 1975.
39. Eriksson BI, Kalebo P, Dykman S, et al: The most effective and safe prophylaxis of thromboembolic complications in patients undergoing total hip replacement with recombinant hirudin, Revasc, (CGP 39393), Ciba. Circulation 92(Suppl 1):I-686, 1995.
40. Fareed JW, Hoppensteadt D, Koza MJ, et al: Pharmacokinetics of aprotinin and its relevance to antifibrinolytic and other biologic effects. In Pifarre R (ed): Blood Conservation with Aprotinin. Philadelphia, Hanley & Belfus, 1995, pp 131–149.
41. Fuchs J, Cannon CP, and the TIMI 7 Investigators: Hirulog in the treatment of unstable angina—Results of the Thrombin Inhibition in Myocardial Ischemia (TIMI) 7 Trial. Circulation 92:727–733, 1995.
42. Fenton JW: Regulation of thrombin generation and functions. Semin Thromb Hemost 14: 234–240, 1988.
43. Fenton JW, Fasco MJ, Stackrow AB, et al: Production, evaluation and properties of alpha-thrombin. J Biol Chem 252: 3587–3597, 1977.
44. Garabedian HD, Gold HK, Leinbach RC, et al: Bleeding time prolongation and bleeding during infusion of recombinant tissue-type plasminogen activator in dogs: Potentation by aspirin and reversal with aprotinin. J Am Coll Cardiol 17: 1213–1222, 1991.
45. Geratz D, Tidwell RA: Current concepts of action of synthetic thrombin inhibitors. Haemostasis 7:170, 1987.

46. Gold HK, Torres FW, Garabedian HD, et al: Evidence for a rebound coagulation phenomenon after cessation of a 4-hour infusion of a specific thrombin inhibitor in patients with unstable angina pectoris. J Am Coll Cardiol 21:1039–1047, 1993.
47. Green DJ, Ford AJ, Longridge DJ: The effects of orally administered D-MePhe-Pro-Arg-H (GYKI-14766) on thrombin-induced thrombocytopenia and disseminated microthrombosis in rats. Br J Pharmacol 107(Suppl):411P, 1992.
48. Grutter MG, Priestle R, Grossenbacher H, et al: Crystal structure of the thrombin-hirudin complex: A novel mode of serine protease inhibition. EMBO J 9:2361–2365, 1990.
49. The GUSTO IIa Investigators: Randomized trial of intravenous heparin versus recombinant hirudin for acute coronary syndromes. Circulation 90:1631–1637, 1994.
50. Harmon JT, Jamieson GA: Activation of platelets by alpha-thrombin is a receptor-mediated event. J Biol Chem 261:15928–15933, 1986.
51. Henderson PJF: A linear equation that describes the steady-state kinetics of enzymes and subcellular particles interacting with tightly bound inhibitors. Biochem J 127:321–333, 1972.
52. Heras M, Chesebro JH, Penny WJ, et al: Effects of thrombin inhibition on the development of acute platelet-thrombus deposit or during angioplasty in pigs: heparin vs. hirudin, a specific thrombin inhibitor. Circulation 79:657–665, 1989.
53. Hendrickson WA, Konnert JH: In Srinivasan R (ed): Biomolecular Structure, Function, Conformation, and Evaluation, vol 1. Pergamon, Oxford, 1981, pp 43–57.
54. Jackson CV, Crowe VG, Frank JD, et al: Pharmacological assessment of the antithrombotic activity of the peptide thrombin inhibitor, D-methyl-phenylalanyl-prolyl-arginal (GYKI-14766), in a canine model of coronary artery thrombosis. J Pharmacol Exp Ther 261:546–552, 1992.
55. Jackson CV, Crowe VG, Bailey BD, Wilson HC: Conjunctive therapy with the thrombin inhibitor, LY294468, and aspirinSK produced enhanced antireocclusive activity when used in a canine model of streptokinase-induced coronary thrombolysis. Pharmacologist 35:207, 1993
56. Jackson CV, Satterwhite, J, Roberts E: Preclinical and clinical pharmacology of efegatran (LY294468): A novel antithrombin for the treatment of acute coronary syndromes. Clin Appl Thrombos Hemost 22:258–267, 1996.
57. Jackson CV, HC Wilson, VG Crowe, et al: Reversible tripeptide thrombin inhibitors as adjunctive agents to coronary thrombolysis: A comparison to heparin in a canine model of coronary artery thrombosis. J Cardiovasc Pharmacol 21:587–594, 1993.
58. Jang IJ, Gold HK, Ziskind AA, et al: Prevention of platelet-rich arterial thrombosis by selective thrombin inhibition. Circulation 81:219–225, 1990.
59. Jones TA: FRODO: A graphics fitting program for macromolecules. In Sayre E (ed): Computational Crystallography. Oxford, Clarendon Press, 1982, p 303.
60. Kaiser B, Koza M, Shankey T V, et al: Modulation of r-tissue factor and arachidonic acid induced platelet activation in whole blood by various thrombin inhibitors. Thromb Haemost 73:1308, 1995.
61. Kikumoto R, Tamao Y, Tezuka T, et al: Selective inhibition of thrombin by (2R,4R)-4-methyl-[N2-[3-methyl 1,2,3,4-tetrahydro-8-quinolinyl)sulfonyl]-L-arinyl) 2-peperidinecarboxylic acid. Biochemistry 23: 85–90, 1984.
62. Kimball SD: Challenges in the development of orally bioavailable thrombin active site inhibitors. Blood Coag Fibrinol 6:511–519, 1995.
63. Levy JH, Pifarre R, Schaff HV, et al: A multicenter, double-blind, placebo-controlled trial of aprotinin for reducing blood loss and the requirement for donor-blood transfusion in patients undergoing repeat coronary artery bypass graftting. Circulation 92:2236–2244, 1995.
64. Markwardt F, Hauptmann J: Synthetic thrombin inhibitors as anticoagulants: Pharmacological aspects. Adv Exp Med Biol 340:143–171, 1993.
65. Maryanoff BE, Qiu X, Padmanabhan KP, et al: Molecular basis for the inhibition of human alpha-thrombin by the macrocyclic peptide cyclotheonamide A. Proc Natl Acad Sci 90: 8048–8052, 1993.
66. Meade TW, Chakrabarti R, Haines AP, et al: Haemostatic function and cardiovascular death: Early results of a prospective study. Lancet 1(8177):1050–1054, 1980.
67. Meinwald YC. Martinelli RV, van Nispen JW, Scheraga HA: Size of the Aa fibrinogen-like peptide that contacts the active site of thrombin. Biochemistry 19:3820–3830, 1980.
68. Mielke CH, International Committee on Communications: Measurement of the bleeding time. Thrombo Haemost 52:210, 1984.
69. Monkhouse FC: Thrombin generation. In Kazal LA, Grannis GF, Tocantins LM (eds): Blood Coagulation, Hemorrhage, and Thrombosis. New York, Grune & Stratton, 1964, pp 187–189.
70. Morrison JF: Kinetics of the reversible inhibition of enzymze-catalysed reactions by tight-binding inhibitors. Biochim Biophys Acta 185:269–286, 1969.
71. Morrison JF: The slow-binding and slow, tight-binding inhibition of enzyme-catalyzed reactions. Trends Biochem Sci 7:102–105, 1982.
72. Morrison JF, Walsh CT: The behavior and significance of slow-binding enzyme inhibitors. Adv Enzymol 61: 201–301, 1988.

73. Najman DM, Walenga JM, Fareed J, Pifarre R: Effects of aprotinin on anticoagulant monitoring: Implications in cardiovascular surgery. Ann Thorac Surg 55:662–666, 1993.
74. Neubauer BL, Best, LK, Goode RL, et al: Anticoagulant and inhibitory effects on the lymphatic metastasis of the PAIII prostatic adenocarcinoma in male rats by recombinant DNA-derived hirudin (rHV2). Cell Pharmacol 1:113–119, 1994.
75. Rosenberg RD: Chemistry of the hemostatic system and its relationship to the action of heparin. Fed Proc 36:10–18, 1977.
76. Royston D, Bidstrup B, Taylor KM, Sapsford, RN: Effect of aprotinin on need for blood transfusion after repeat open-heart surgery. Lancet 2:1289–1291, 1987.
77. Rupin A, Mennecier P, de Nanteuil G, et al: A screening procedure to evaluate the anticoagulant activity and the kinetic behaviour of direct thrombin inhibitors. Thromb Res 78:217–225, 1995.
78. Ruterbories KJ, Hanssen BR, Lindstrom TD: Proceedings of the Fourth North American ISSX Meeting. Ball Harbour, FL, 1992, p 204.
79. Sakamoto S, Hirase T, Suzuki S, et al: Inhibitory effect of argatroban on thrombin-antithrombin III complex after percutaneous transluminal coronary angioplasty. Thromb Haemost 74:801–802, 1995.
80. Satterwhite J, Roberts A, Lachno R, et al: Pharmacokinetics (PK) and anticoagulant activity (AA) of Efegatran (E), a direct thrombin Iinhibitor. Pharmacol Res 11:S428, 1994.
81. Schacht AL, Chirgadze N, Clawson D, et al: N- substituted glycines as replacements for proline in tripeptide aldehyde thrombin inhibitors. Bioorg Med Chem Letters 5:2529–2534, 1995.
82. Schumacher WA, Steinbacher TE, Heran CL, et al: Comparison of thrombin active site and exosite inhibitors and heparin in experimental models of arterial and venous thrombosis and bleeding. J Pharmacol Exp Ther 267:1237–1242, 1993.
83. Sharma GVRK, Lapsley DE, Vita JA, et al: Safety and efficacy of Hirulog in patients with unstable angina. Circulation 86 (Suppl I):386, 1992.
84. Shibata A: Diffraction data collection with R-Axis II, an x-ray detecting system using imaging plate. Rigaku J 7:28–32, 1990.
85. Shuman RT, Rothenberger RB, Campbell CS, et al: Highly selective thrombin inhibitors. J Med Chem 36:314–319, 1992.
86. Simoons ML, Deckers JW: New directions in anticoagulant and antiplatelet treatment. Br Heart J 74:337–340, 1995.
87. Simoons M, Lenderink T, Scheffer M, et al: Efegatran, a new direct thrombin inhibitor: Safety and dose response in patients with unstable angina. Circulation 90:I231, 1994.
88. Simoons M, van Miltenburg A, Scheffer MG, et al: Anticoagulant properties of efegatran, a direct thrombin inhibitor in patients with unstable angina. Eur Heart J 15:120, 1994.
89. Smith GF: Fibrinogen as the specific substrate. In Machovich R (ed): The Thrombin. Boca Raton, FL , CRC Press, 1984, pp 55–83.
90. Smith GF, Craft TJ, Gifford-Moore DS, et al: A family of arginal thrombin inhibitors related to Efegatran. Semin Thromb Hemost 22:173–183, 1996.
91. Smith GF, Sundboom JL, Best K, et al: heparin, Boc-Phe-Pro-arginal, and warfarin (fibrin antagonists) inhibit metastasis in an in vivo model [abstract]. Biochemistry 70:198, 1987.
92. Smith GF, Neubauer BL, Sundboom JL, et al: Correlation of the in vivo anticoagulant, antithrombotic, and antimetastatic efficacy of warfarin in the rat. Thromb Res 150:163–174, 1988.
93. Smith GF, Sundboom JL: Heparin and protease inhibition. II: The role of heparin in the ATIII inactivation of thrombin, plasmin, and trypsin. Thromb Res 22:115–133, 1981.
94. Smith GF, Shuman RT, Gesellchen PD, et al: A new family of thrombin inhibitors with improved specificity and favorable therapeutic index. Circulation 84:II-579, 1991.
95. Smith GF, Sundboom JL: Heparin and protease inhibition. II: The role of heparin in the ATIII inactivation of thrombin, plasmin, and trypsin. Thromb Res 22:115–133, 1981.
96. Smith P, Arnesen H, Holme I: The effect of warfarin on mortality and reinfarction after myocardial infarction. N Engl J Med 323:147–152, 1990.
97. Solomons TWG: Organic Chemistry, 2nd ed. New York, John Wiley & Sons, 1980, p 711.
98. Solomons TWG: Organic Chemistry, 2nd ed. New York, John Wiley & Sons, 1980, p 722.
99. Stone SR, Hofsteenge J: Kinetics of the inhibition of thrombin by hirudin. Biochemistry 25:4622–4628, 1986.
100. Stone, SR, Tapparelli C: Thrombin inhibitors as antithrombotic agensts: The importance of rapid inhibition. J Enzyme Inhibit 9:3–15, 1995.
101. Stein B, Fuster V, Halperin JL, Chesebro JH: Antithrombotic therapy in cardiac disease: An emerging approach based on pathogenesis and risk. Circulation 80:1501–1513, 1989.
102. Tabata H, Mizuno K, Miyamoto A, et al: The effect of a new thrombin inhibitor (argatroban) in the prevention of reocclusion after reperfusion therapy in patients with acute myocardial infarction. Circulation 86(Suppl I): I-260, 1992.
103. Tapparelli C, Metternich R, Ehrhardt C, Cook N S: Synthetic low-molecular-weight thrombin inhibitors: Molecular design and pharmacological profile. Trends Pharmacol Sci 14: 366–376, 1993.

104. Tcheng JE: Enhancing safety and outcomes with the newer antithrombotic and antiplatelet agents. Am Heart J 130:673–679, 1995.
105. Tomori E, Szell E, Barabas E: High performance liquid chromatography of a new tripeptide aldehyde (GYKI-14766): Correlation between structure and activity. Chromatographia 19:437–442, 1984
106. Tamori E, Szell E, Barabas E: Equilibrium structures of the Arg-aldehyde moiety upon HPLC of peptides.Chromatographia 27:228, 1989.
107. Theroux P, Ouimet H, McCans J, et al: Aspirin, heparin, or both to treat acute unstable angina. N Engl J Med 319:1105–1111, 1988.
108. Topol EJ: Novel antithrombotic approaches to coronary artery disease. Am J Cardiol 75:27B–33B, 1995.
109. Topol EJ, Bonan R, Jewitt D, et al: Use of a direct antithrombin, Hirulog, in place of heparin during coronary angioplasty. Circulation 87:1622–1629, 1993.
110. Topol EJ, Fuster V, Califf RM, et al: Recombinant hirudin for unstable angina pectoris: A multicenter, randomized angiographic trial. Circulation 87:1557–1566, 1994.
111. Vereczkey L, Valko I, Laszlo L, et al: Hungarian Institute for Drug Research, 1991, unpublished results.
112. Vereczkey L, Valko I, Laszlo L, et al: Hungarian Institute for Drug Research, 1991, unpublished results.
113. Vereczkey L, Valko I: Hungarian Institute for Drug Research, 1992, unpublished results.
114. Wagner WR, Hubbell JA: Local thrombin synthesis and fibrin formation in an in vitro thrombosis model result in platelet recruitment and thrombus stabilization on collagen in heparinized blood. J Lab Clin Med 116: 636–650, 1990.
115. Walenga JM, Koza MJ, Park SJ, et al: Evaluation of CGP 39393 as the anticoagulant in cardiopulmonary bypass operation in a dog model. Ann Thorac Surg 58:1685–1689, 1994.
116. Walenga JM, Bakhos M, Messmore HL, et al: Comparison of recombinant hirudin and heparin as an anticoagulant in a cardiopulmonary bypass model. Blood Coagul Fibrinol 2:105–111, 1991.
117. Walenga JM, Bakhos M, Messmore HL, Fareed J, Pifarre R: Potential use of recombinant hirudin as an anticoagulant in a cardiopulmonary bypass model. Ann Thorac Surg 51:271–277, 1991.
118. Wallis RB: Inhibition of thrombin, a key step in thrombosis. Drugs Today 25:597–605, 1989.
119. Wiley MR, Schacht AL, Coffman WJ, et al: Serine protease selectivity of the thrombin inhibitor D-Phe-Pro-Agmatine and its homologs. Bioorg Med Chem Lett 5:2835–2840, 1995.
120. Williams JW, JF Morrison: The kinetics of reversible tight-binding inhibition. Methods Enzymol 63:437–467, 1979.
121. Williams JW, Morrison JF: The kinetics of reversible tight-binding inhibition. Methods Enzymol 63:437–467, 1979.
122. Wilson H, Frank J, Crowe V, et al: Anticoagulant and antithrombotic efficacy of the novel thrombin inhibitor D-methyl-Phg-Pro-Arginal, in a canine model of coronary thrombosis. Arteriosclerosis 11:1586A, 1991.

CHAPTER 19

Argatroban as an Anticoagulant for Coronary Procedures in Patients with HIT Antibody

BRUCE E. LEWIS, M.D., FACC
SARAH A. JOHNSON, M.D., FACC
ERIC D. GRASSMAN, M.D., Ph.D., FACC
LAURA L. WRONA, R.N., CCRC

Our institution has examined the feasibility and safety of anticoagulation with argatroban during coronary interventions in patients with the antibody for heparin-induced thrombocytopenia (HIT). Argatroban was selected for anticoagulation because previous work suggested that heparin-induced platelet aggregation is inhibited in a dose-dependent manner when HIT serum is incubated with argatroban.[1] Other work proves that argatroban has no structural resemblance to heparin and therefore does not cross-react with HIT antibody.[2] The final property of argatroban that led to its use for anticoagulation during coronary procedures was the observation that the laboratory tests commonly used to measure activated clotting time (ACT) provide reliable indices of anticoagulation levels.[3] Previous work in patients without HIT antibody suggested that an argatroban dosing regimen of 150 µg/kg bolus and 10 µg/kg/min infusion did not provide sufficient anticoagulation for percutaneous transluminal coronary angioplasty (PTCA).[4]

Our group, therefore, applied an elevated dose of argatroban to coronary interventions in patients documented to have HIT antibody. Outcomes were assessed by using the ACT as laboratory evidence of adequate anticoagulation during the procedure. Angiographic success provided clinical evidence of adequate anticoagulation. Laboratory success was defined as the ability to maintain an ACT of more than 300 seconds throughout the procedure. Angiographic success was defined as reduction in postprocedural minimal luminal diameter to less than 50% and absence of thrombotic complications during the procedure. Angiographic measurements were made with quantitative computer analysis (QCA). Clinical success was defined as angiographic success and absence of periprocedural myocardial infarction, death, cerebrovascular accident, and acute closure. Safety was assessed by recording the need for blood transfusion, evidence of major clinical bleeding, or identification of a significant groin hematoma.

Patients with known HIT antibody and symptomatic coronary artery disease (CAD) were included in the evaluation. Symptomatic CAD was confirmed with evidence of reversible ischemia on noninvasive testing and a visual estimate of > 70% diameter narrowing by coronary angiogaphy. QCA measurements were not made until the procedures were completed. QCA measurements were made by an independent angiographer. Patients with traditional contraindications to anticoagulation were not treated until the contraindication had resolved.

Baseline laboratory values were recorded for the patients. Platelet aggregation testing with platelet-rich plasma was performed by a modified method of Chong to document the presence of HIT antibody.[5] An abnormal result, defined as platelet aggregation in excess of 20%, was recorded in the data as positive. When multiple tests were performed, a positive result was recorded if any test showed > 20% aggregation. ACTs were performed on the HemoTec ACT machine (Medtronic, Parker, CO). Results of Hemochron ACT have been inconsistent when applied to measurement of argatroban-induced anticoagulation. Therefore, the report of ACT results was limited to HemoTec ACT.

Our treatment strategy was somewhat conservative. Patients with active heparin-induced thrombocytopenia and thrombosis syndrome (HITTS), combined with unstable coronary syndromes, were given an intravenous infusion of argatroban (2–10 µg/kg/min) to stabilize the coronary lesion before being taken to the cardiac catheterization laboratory. Intravenous argatroban was directed by the activated partial thromboplastin time (APTT), with a target value of 50–70 seconds. Platelet counts were allowed to return toward normal while the patient remained on the argatroban infusion before initiation of the interventional procedure. This strategy was used in an attempt to reduce the increased complications associated with treatment of unstable coronary lesions. The conservative approach was also adopted in an attempt to reduce the potential for bleeding associated with periprocedural thrombocytopenia. All patients received pretreatment with 325 mg/day of aspirin, which was started at least 24 hours before the procedure.

Another goal of the conservative approach was to limit deep wall injury. The presumed "hypercoagulable state" associated with the HIT antibody may represent a clinical state susceptible to acute thrombotic closure after balloon injury. Therefore, every attempt was made to avoid deep medial wall injury. Balloon sizes were selected not to exceed a balloon-to-vessel wall diameter of 1 to 1. In procedures involving rotational atherectomy, burr sizes were selected not to exceed a burr-to-vessel wall ratio of 0.7. High-pressure balloon inflation was used after stent deployment, but the selected balloon size did not exceed the diameter of the vessel wall when the balloon was inflated to high pressure.

The initial patient was treated after a constant infusion of argatroban had been titrated to maintain the ACT between 300 and 450 seconds. The ACT values were selected to exceed 300 seconds, because previous data with heparin in angioplasty suggest that ACT values above 300 seconds are associated with a low incidence of thrombotic closure.[6] The remaining patients were given a 0.35 mg/kg bolus followed by a constant infusion of 20–40 µg/kg/min. The ACT was checked 10 minutes after the bolus injection to ensure an ACT of 300–450 seconds. The constant infusion was started immediately after the bolus injection and maintained for the duration of the procedure. ACTs were measured every 30 minutes throughout the argatroban infusion and 10 minutes after dose changes. Argatroban infusion rates were adjusted by the operator based on the ACT value. The argatroban infusion was stopped when the procedure was completed. ACTs were measured hourly after the procedure. Sheaths were removed when the ACT was below 175 seconds.

The demographic data of patients treated at our institution are presented in Table 1. The patients are similar to the usual patients treated percutaneously in the cardiac catheterization laboratory. The average age was 66 years. Ten patients were male; five patients were female. The coronary indication for the procedure was stable angina in three procedures,

TABLE 1. Preprocedural Data

	Patient Number							
	1	2	3*	4	5*	6	7	8
Age (yrs)	65	50	75	52	75	64	70	67
Sex	Female	Male	Female	Female	Female	Female	Male	Male
Indication for procedure	Unstable angina	Angina	Unstable angina	Acute MI	Acute MI	Unstable angina	Acute MI	Acute MI
Indication for argatroban	History of HITTS	HITTS	HITTS	History of HIT	History of HITTS	History of HITTS	HITTS	History of HITTS

	9	10	11	12	13	14	15
Age (yrs)	73	70	70	74	81	71	71
Sex	Male	Male	Male	Male	Male	Male	Male
Indication for procedure	Unstable angina	Acute MI	Acute MI	Acute MI	Angina	Acute MI	Acute MI
Indication for argatroban	History of HITTS	HIT	HIT	HITTS	History of HIT	HITTS	HITTS

MI = myocardial infarction; HIT = heparin-induced thrombocytopenia; HITTS = heparin-induced thrombocytopenia and thrombosis syndrome.
* Interventions performed on different vessels of the same patient at different settings.

unstable angina in four procedures, and acute myocardial infarction in eight procedures. The clinical HIT antibody syndrome was active HIT in two procedures, active HITTS in six procedures, history of HIT in two procedures, and history of HITTS in five procedures.

The laboratory data for patients with HIT antibody are reported in Tables 2 and 3. At least one abnormal platelet aggregation test for HIT antibody was recorded in each patient. The average platelet count at the time of the procedure was 222,000 per mm^3; values varied between 82,00 per mm^3 and 321,000 per mm^3. The average baseline HemoTec ACT was 141 seconds; values varied between 106 and 176 seconds. The average HemoTec ACT after the initial argatroban bolus was 382 seconds; values ranged from 301 to 479 seconds. The initial ACT after argatroban bolus was > 1000 seconds in two procedures when the ACT was measured with a Hemochron machine. The average ACT during argatroban infusion was 445 seconds; values varied between 337 seconds and 609 seconds.

Each category of interventional device has been used in the treatment of 18 coronary lesions in the 15 procedures. Angioplasty was performed on 9 lesions, atherectomy

TABLE 2. Preprocedural Laboratory Testing

	Patient Number							
	1	2	3	4	5	6	7	8
Heparin-induced platelet aggregation test*	+	+	+	+	+	+	+	+
Platelet count†	233 k	268 k	82 k	269 k	112 k	220 k	321 k	240 k

	9	10	11	12	13	14	15
Heparin-induced platelet aggregation test*	+	+	+	+	+	+	+
Platelet count†	194 k	252 k	252 k	269 k	193 k	261 k	261 k

+ = Abnormal platelet aggregation.
* All patients had preprocedural laboratory confirmation of abnormal platelet aggregation.
† Platelet counts were recorded within the 24 hours preceding coronary intervention. No procedure was initiated until the platelet count had spontaneously recovered to > 50,000 per mm^3.

TABLE 3. Procedural Argatroban and Activated Clotting Time Data

	Patient Number							
	1	2	3	4	5	6	7	8
Baseline ACT (sec)	NP	163	132	129	176	106	159	106
Bolus dose (mg)	NP	35	19	18	19	28	36	26
ACT after bolus (sec)	NP	367	429	354	479	301	382	382
Infusion rate (μg/kg/min)	15	20	20	40	20	40	30	30
ACT after infusion (sec)	337	609	429	429	433	341	369	369
	9	10	11	12	13	14	15	
Baseline ACT (sec)	158	NP	NP	127	125	136	136	
Bolus dose (mg)	24	28	28	26	23	27	27	
ACT after bolus (sec)	309	893*	1018*	331	506	420	422	
Infusion rate (μg/kg/min)	30	20	30	30	30	30	30	
ACT after infusion (sec)	392	546	369	511	663	492	472	

NP = not performed.
* Hemochron ACT. All other values are HemoTec ACTs.

was performed on 3 lesions, and stent implant was performed on 6 lesions (Table 4). Five lesions were type A, 7 lesions were type B, and 6 lesions were complex type C lesions by ACC/AHA criteria.[7] Five vessels had angiographic evidence of thrombus within the lesion. The average preprocedural stenosis was 69%. The average postprocedural stenosis was 18%.

Angiographic success was therefore recorded for all 18 coronary lesions treated. Clinical success was seen in 17 of 18 lesions. One patient suffered a periprocedural myocardial infarction secondary to coronary dissection and was successfully treated with stent implant. No patient suffered periprocedural death, cerebrovascular accident, or acute closure. No patient suffered a major bleed or required blood transfusion. One patient with a 5-cm segment of thrombosed vein graft required adjuvant thrombolytic therapy with 30 mg of intragraft tissue-type plasminogen activator to establish graft patency before balloon dilation of a distal anastomotic stenosis.

Laboratory evidence supporting the adequacy of anticoagulation with the argatroban dosing regimen for coronary interventions used in this series is reported in Figures 1 and 2 and Table 3. Procedural ACTs of > 300 seconds reflect adequate anticoagulation.[6] The initial bolus of 350 μg/kg of argatroban provided an average initial procedural ACT of 393 seconds; values varied between 301 and 479 seconds (Fig. 2 and Table 3). The maintenance dose of argatroban was titrated using ACT measurements to a dose between 15 and 40 μg/kg/min. The titrated maintenance dose of argatroban yielded procedural ACTs between 309 seconds and 609 seconds from 10 minutes after initiation of the infusion until the conclusion of the procedure (Fig. 1). The average ACT during the maintenance infusion was 431 seconds. The average ACT was 427 seconds when the highest and lowest ACTs were discarded from the data pool. Argatroban infusion rates between 15 and 40 μg/kg/min provided reliable and consistent levels of anticoagulation.

The postprocedural ACT data are shown in Figure 2, which demonstrates the behavior of the ACT after discontinuation of the argatroban infusion. In all cases except one, the ACT reached a level approximating baseline within 180 minutes of discontinuing the drug. The patient who had a delayed return to baseline was extremely ill at the time of her initial procedure and required dopamine drip, mechanical ventilation, and intensive care monitoring. Of interest, when she returned for a second interventional procedure, ACT returned to baseline within the expected period.

TABLE 4. Procedural Data for Individual Coronary Lesions and Vessels

| | **Patient Number** | | | | | | | | |
	1			2	3	4	5	6	
Vessel	CX	OM1	PL	RCA	LAD	LAD-SVG	RCA	CX	PDA
Lesion type*	B2	C	C	A	C	C	B2	C	B
Thrombus	+	–	–	–	+	+	–	–	–
Preprocedural stenosis	62%	82%	50%	56%	67%	100%	58%	78%	59%
Postprocedural stenosis	9%	32%	28%	38%	27%	1%	12%	38%	20%
Angiographic success	Y	Y	Y	Y	Y	Y	Y	Y	Y
Complication	N	N	N	N	N	N	N	N	N
Procedural success	Y	Y	Y	Y	Y	Y	Y	Y	Y

	7	8	9	10	11	12	13	14	15
Vessel	AnCx	OM-SVG	OM-SVG	OM	RCA	OM1	LAD	RRA	LRA
Lesion type*	A	C	B	A	A	B2	B2	A	B2
Thrombus	+	–	+	–	–	–	–	–	–
Preprocedural stenosis	60%	64%	75%	70%	80%	75%	90%	80%	85%
Postprocedural stenosis	12%	13%	0%	15%	0%	35%	10%	20%	0%
Angiographic success	Y	Y	Y	Y	Y	Y	Y	Y	Y
Complication	N	N	N	N	N	N	N	N	N
Procedural success	Y	Y	Y	Y	Y	Y	Y	Y	Y

CX = circumflex, AnCx = anomalous circumflex, OM = obtuse marginal, PL = posterolateral branch, RCA = right coronary artery, LAD = left anterior descending, SVG = saphenous vein graft, PDA = posterior descending artery.
* According to ACC/AHA criteria.

DISCUSSION

Patients who acquire the coronary syndromes associated with HIT antibody and subsequently require anticoagulation for vascular procedures have previously been left with few treatment options. Rechallenge with heparin in patients who acquire HIT antibody is considered to carry extreme risk for reactivation of the HIT-driven thrombotic process. One alternative, ORG 10172, has been approved for use in Europe. However, ORG 10172 carries significant clinical problems, which include both lack of a quick, reliable method for laboratory monitoring of procedural levels of anticoagulation and prolonged postprocedural period of anticoagulation secondary to a long half-life. Furthermore, ORG 10172 has cross-reactivity with HIT antibody and must be tested in vitro before administration.[7] A second alternative is low-molecular-weight heparin, which also cross-reacts with HIT antibody.[8] Rapid measurement of levels of anticoagulation with low-molecular-weight is not possible.

Our data suggest that conventional laboratory monitoring with the HemoTec ACT reflects adequate procedural levels of anticoagulation and documents a rapidly diminished anticoagulant effect after the procedure. Furthermore, the laboratory data during the argatroban infusion, combined with the clinical success of the procedures, strongly support the

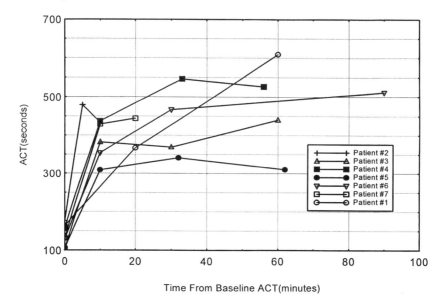

FIGURE 1. Response of activated clotting time (ACT) to constant infusion of argatroban during coronary interventions. Baselines ACTs are recorded at time 0. The first ACT point after the baseline ACT represents the first ACT value drawn 10 minutes after initiation of the argatroban infusion. The remainder of the points represent the steady state maintained with constant argatroban infusion. ACT values remain within a fairly narrow range.

use of argatroban during coronary interventions in patients with HITTS. The strategy of using 350 µg/kg as a bolus infusion of argatroban consistently provided an ACT value of > 300 seconds, which is considered to be a safe anticoagulation level for coronary interventions.[6] Adequate anticoagulation was maintained by a continuing infusion rate between 15 and 40 µg/kg/min. The lower-dose infusions were associated with low therapeutic ACT values but did not fall below the minimum safety standard of 300 seconds by ACT. Our ACT data also show that the anticoagulant effect of argatroban rapidly diminishes after the procedure. The patients were allowed to have an ACT value below 175 seconds before arterial sheaths were removed. This practice was associated with no postprocedural hematomas or bleeding. The ACT, therefore, appears to ensure a safe measure of anticoagulation for postprocedural manipulations such as sheath removal.

The HemoTec ACT is ideal for monitoring argatroban during vascular procedures because it provides "point of service" access. Therefore, laboratory results can be obtained rapidly, and dose adjustments reflect the current state of anticoagulation. The HemoTec ACT is available in most cardiac catheterization laboratories, and most teams have experience in the interpretation of ACTs and subsequent management decisions. The ability to measure anticoagulation levels of argatroban with the ACT machine should simplify the learning curve when argatroban is substituted for heparin.

One concern about percutaneous coronary interventions in patients with HITTS is the endothelial damage associated with balloon injury, atherectomy, and stenting.[9–11] The observations of some investigators suggest that HIT antibody reacts not only with platelets but also with endothelial cells.[12–14] Clinicians have long noted that thrombotic events in patients with HIT antibody frequently occur at the site of vascular injury.[14–16] Such in vitro and clinical observations raise some concern about an exaggerated potential for thrombosis at the site of therapeutic injury associated with percutaneous interventional techniques. Thrombosis at the site of coronary interventions is one mechanism for

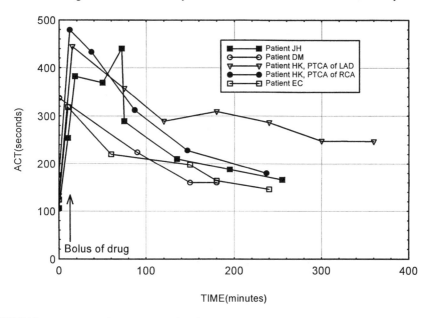

FIGURE 2.   Response of activated clotting time (ACT) to a 350 µg/kg bolus of argatroban and the decline in ACT after discontinuation of the infusion. The procedural ACTs are omitted from the figure. The ACTs recorded after the bolus represent the decline in the level of anticoagulation after argatroban is stopped in individual patients. Note that the duration of anticoagulation is prolonged after discontinuation of the procedure compared with percutaneous transluminal coronary angioplasty (PTCA) of the right coronary artery (RCA). The PTCA of the left anterior descending (LAD) artery was performed when the patient was quite ill in the intensive care unit. The PTCA of the RCA was performed on an outpatient basis, and the ACT declined normally.

acute coronary closure, which can result in myocardial infarction or death. This reasoning led to a conservative approach to treatment and limitation of treatment of patients with truly life-threatening lesions. The conservative approach was also adopted for the procedural strategy of using smaller device sizes to limit deep wall injury in individual interventions. "Bigger is better" may not apply to this subset of patients.

Our experience has looked at argatroban as a sole agent for the percutaneous treatment of coronary artery disease in patients with known HIT antibody. We have not added adjuvant therapies such as glycoprotein IIB/IIA inhibitors to the treatment because our initial goal was to establish the efficacy of the thrombin inhibitor argatroban for treatment of such patients. Theoretically, the addition of IIb/IIIA inhibitors and the subsequent suppression of platelet activation should provide an improved margin of safety in this group of patients at high risk for acute thrombotic closure.

The successful percutaneous endovascular treatment of clinically significant coronary lesions represents a major advance in therapeutic options for patients known to have HIT antibody. Although only 18 coronary lesions were treated, the absence of complications related to anticoagulation in any of the treated lesions is encouraging. Future efforts to document further the safety and efficacy of argatroban anticoagulation during coronary interventions will be made by extending the investigation to other centers. The infrequency of patients with HITTS who require coronary intervention, combined with the lack of an approved alternative treatment for HITTS, dictates use of a registry format for data collection to establish safety and efficacy. Future work must also be directed toward establishing the safety and efficacy of argatroban anticoagulation during open heart surgery.

REFERENCES

1. Matsuo T, Yamanda T, Yamanashi J, Ryo R: Anticoagulant therapy with MD 805 of hemodialysis patients with heparin-induced thrombocytopenia. Thromb Res 58:663–666, 1990.
2. Walenga JM, Koza MJ, Pifarre R: Comparative studies of heparin analogues, recombinant TFPI, and thrombin inhibitors devoid of heparin-induced thrombocytopenia response[abstract]. Thromb Haemost 73:970, 1995.
3. Lewis BE, Laffaldano R, McKiernan T, et al: Report of successful use of argatroban as an alternative anticoagulant drug during coronary stent implantation in a patient with heparin-induced thrombocytopenia and thrombosis syndrome. Cathet Cardiovasc Diag 38:206–209, 1996.
4. Data on file with Texas Biotechnology Corporation. Printed with permission of Texas Biotechnology Corporation.
5. Chong BH, Grace CS, Rozenberg MC: Heparin-induced thrombocytopenia: Effect of heparin platelet antibody on platelets. Br J Haematol 49:531–540, 1981.
6. Daugherty KG, Marsh KC, Edelman SK, et al: Relationship between procedural activated clotting time and in-hospital post-PTCA outcome [abstract]. Circulation 82:111–189, 1990.
7. Magnani HN: Heparin-induced thrombocytopenia (HIT): An overview of 230 patients treated with Organon (ORG 10172). Thromb Hemost 70:554–561, 1993.
8. LeRoy J, LeClerc MH, Delahouse B, et al: Treatment of heparin-associated thrombocytopenia and thrombosis with low molecular weight heparin. Semin Thromb Hemost 11:326–329, 1985.
9. Ellis SG, Vandormael MG, Cowley MJ, et al: Coronary morphologic and clinical determinants of procedural outcome with angioplasty for multivessel coronary disease. Implications for patient selection. Circulation 82:1193–1202, 1990.
10. Gravanis MB, Roubin GS: Histologic phenomena at the site of coronary angioplasty. Br Heart J 20:477–485, 1987.
11. Potkin BN, Roberts WC: Effects of coronary angioplasty on atherosclerotic plaques and relation of plaque composition and arterial size to outcome. Am J Cardiol 62:41–50, 1988.
12. Fourier JL, Stankowiak C, Lablanche JM: Histopathology after rotational angioplasty of peripheral arteries in human beings [abstract]. J Am Coll Cardiol 11:109, 1988.
13. Visentin GP, Ford SE, Scott JP, Aster RH: Antibodies from patients with heparin-induced thrombocytopenia/thrombosis are specific for platelet factor 4 complexes with heparin or heparin bound endothelial cells. J Clin Invest 93:81–88, 1994.
14. Cines DB, Tomaski A, Tannenbaum E: Immune endothelial cell injury in heparin-associated thrombocytopenia. N Engl J Med 316:581–589, 1987.
15. Krueger SK, Adres E, Weinard E: Thrombolysis in heparin-induced thrombocytopenia with thrombosis. Ann Intern med 103:159, 1985.
16. Lefemine AA: Complications of heparin-induced thrombocytopenia. Am Surg 48:202–206, 1982.

CHAPTER 20

Antithrombin Agents in the Management of Heparin-induced Thrombocytopenia

MICHAEL J. KOZA, B.S., M.T. (ASCP)
BRUCE E. LEWIS, M.D., FACC
JEANINE M. WALENGA, Ph.D.
ROQUE PIFARRÉ, M.D.
JAWED FAREED, Ph.D.

HEPARIN-INDUCED THROMBOCYTOPENIA SYNDROME

Heparin-induced thrombocytopenia (HIT) represents a disease spectrum triggered by an immune response to heparin. The cause of thrombocytopenia probably relates to activation of platelets and their rapid consumption. There are several current theories regarding the mechanism of action in HIT. One theory is that heparin binds to platelets, triggering a neoantigen on the platelet surface that is responsible for the production of HIT antibodies.[6] Another proposed mechanism is based on the development of an antibody to the heparin–platelet factor 4 (PF4) complex, which is either bound to the complex on the platelet surface[2] or first binds to the heparin-PF4 complex in plasma, then to the platelet surface.[29] Some, but not all platelet reactions, have been mediated via an FcγRII receptor on the platelet.[7,13] This antibody was found not to be heparin-specific, because it reacted with several highly sulfated materials.[11,38] IgG isotypes IgG_1, IgG_2, and IgG_3, as well as IgM (which provides an early signal) and IgA antibodies (which occur both early and late), have been identified in patients with HIT.[30]

Clinical HIT with or without thrombosis can appear despite the absence of exogenous heparin for other reasons. The body manufactures numerous endogenous heparins and heparinoids that cross-react with the HIT antibody. These endogenous materials may interact with the HIT antibody and drive thrombosis. The clearance of exogenous heparin in patients with HIT antibody is probably delayed. Exogenous heparin can then remain complexed to the antibody and not be eliminated at the usual rate. Moreover, traditional commercial heparin preparations are composed of a heterogeneous mixture of heparin chains. The heparin molecules range in size from 2,000–30,000 Da. The HIT antibody response, like heparin, is heterogeneous. Thus the heterogeneous nature of the HIT antibody and its interactions, combined with the wide variability of commercial heparin preparations and endogenous heparins, may explain the wide spectrum of clinical manifestations in patients who develop HIT antibody.

The mildest clinical response of HIT is the isolated presence of antibody without either thrombocytopenia or thrombosis. A significant percentage of patients develop HIT antibody in response to heparin; however, the actual number of patients with HIT antibody without overt thrombocytopenia and thrombosis is unknown. An isolated positive HIT antibody response without clinical expression can probably be explained pathophysiologically. Thrombocytopenia may be relative but not absolute. For example, if the suggested 30% reduction in platelets is considered sufficient to diagnose HIT, platelet counts reduced only 30% from a high normal baseline would remain normal and, therefore, would not be labeled as thrombocytopenia.

The time required to develop HIT antibody from the initial heparin exposure appears to be at least 5 days but may be much longer. However, patients who have had previous heparin exposures may develop thrombocytopenia in less than 5 days. Other patients present with thrombocytopenia even later than 14 days. The economic pressure to shorten hospital stays can obscure the diagnosis in many patients. Such patients may develop and recover from the thrombocytopenia and develop an unsuspected thrombosis in the outpatient setting. Like other antibody responses, such as the response to hepatitis B, the HIT antibody response probably varies in an individual patient. Patients with multiple heparin exposures may have "memory" and thus be able to develop an accelerated antibody response. The duration of antibody production in individual patients is also variable. The antibody response is thought to be short-lived, in most patients ranging from weeks to months, but we have seen patients who remain HIT antibody-positive for longer than one year. This subset of patients may represent the HIT analog of chronic active hepatitis. Patients who are HIT antibody-positive only may be simply caught in a clinical window in which antibody titers are very low or very high and therefore not in a proper stoichiometric relationship with heparin and PF4 to activate platelets.

The most dramatic clinical expression of HIT is HIT antibody-driven thrombosis (HITTS). Thrombosis can occur anywhere throughout the venous and arterial circulation. Previous reports suggested that arterial thrombosis was more common than venous thrombosis.[21] However, more recent reports document a higher frequency of venous thrombosis than arterial thrombosis.[39] Microthrombi or clinically insignificant thrombi are probably formed in many patients with HIT, but often not in locations that result in clinically expressed adverse events. Indeed, Warkentin's work supports this concept by noting that a high percentage of patients with HIT antibody had lower extremity venous thromboses detected only by study-driven screening venography despite an absence of symptoms for deep venous thrombosis (DVT).[40] Very few patients without detected HIT antibody had the small thrombi.

Data from multiple institutions suggest that the presence of HIT antibody is a marker that predicts future clinically significant thrombotic events.[21] Patients with documentation of HIT antibody have a 35% probability of developing a clinically significant thrombosis during hospitalization.[39] Patients with a clinical thrombosis carry a reported mortality rate of 25–30%,[39] with amputation in up to 25% of patients, mesenteric infarction in up to 15%, myocardial infarction in up to 20%, and cerebral infarction in up to 10%. DVT with chronic venous insufficiency and pulmonary embolism is also seen with regularity. The morbidity and mortality associated with HITTS justifies aggressive treatment.

CURRENT CLINICAL MANAGEMENT

Initial Steps

The initial step in the clinical management of HIT is to establish the link between heparin and thrombocytopenia. One must exclude the other causes of thrombocytopenia, which make up a long differential diagnosis. One must also consider that thrombocytopenia is a type 1 reaction to heparin and thus represents no threat to the patient. Most clinicians define

TABLE 1.   Clinical Diagnosis of Heparin-induced Thrombocytopenia

1. Thrombocytopenia after heparin exposure; platelet count < 100,000/μl or a 50% decrease from baseline
2. Heparin exposure before thrombocytopenia ≥ 5 days
3. Reasonable exclusion of other causes of thrombocytopenia

thrombocytopenia in HIT as a platelet count of less than 100,000/μl or a decrease in platelet count to 50% of baseline. However, the level of thrombocytopenia required to suspect the diagnosis is probably different from the level required to establish the diagnosis. The diagnosis of HIT should be based on clinical criteria and not on laboratory testing (Table 1).

If the diagnosis of HIT is reasonable, the patient should be managed as though he or she has an allergy to heparin (Table 2). The physician should immediately discontinue all heparin administration. The ubiquitous nature of heparin in hospitalized patients requires a meticulous search to eliminate all exogenous, often unrecognized, sources of heparin. Common sources of exogenous heparin include intravenous heparin, subcutaneous heparin, and heparin flushes routinely prescribed to maintain catheter patency. Another common, but poorly recognized source of heparin, is the heparin-coated catheter. For example, 80% of Baxter Swan-Ganz catheters are heparin-coated. If the heparin status of a catheter is unknown, the catheter should be removed and replaced with a catheter known not to contain a heparin coating.

Despite the devastating consequences of the HIT antibody, the diagnosis of HIT is not made promptly in many hospitals. The average time from a 50% reduction in platelet count to recognition and discontinuation of heparin is 4 days. Intense education of nursing staff, ancillary staff, house staff, and attending physicians can reduce time to recognition of the syndrome to less than 2 days. Educational efforts should be directed at areas in the hospital associated with frequent heparin use, such as cardiovascular surgery, coronary care, orthopedic surgery, and intensive care units.

Postoperative cardiac patients represent a special group because most of them have platelet counts of 100,000–150,000/μl on postoperative day one. We, therefore, make the diagnosis of HIT only when the platelet count is reduced by 50% from the count on postoperative day one. However, a 20–30% reduction in the platelet count from the postoperative day-one baseline prompts suspicion of HIT or HITTS and the immediate discontinuance of all heparin. One must be careful to exclude postoperative platelet consumption processes such as unrecognized hematoma formation or bleeding, because treatment with anticoagulants in such patients would worsen their clinical condition. Patients with HIT who also develop thrombosis and who had not previously been known to have thrombus are then diagnosed with HITTS.

The high probability of thrombosis in patients with clinical evidence of HIT antibody should prompt a vigorous search for both venous and arterial thrombosis. All clinical symptoms or physical signs should be evaluated with appropriate diagnostic testing. Local swelling, erythema or pain, and blue digits require Doppler testing or venography.

TABLE 2.   Current Treatment of Heparin-induced Thrombocytopenia and Thrombosis

- Discontinue *all* heparin
- Plasmapheresis × 3
- Immunoglobulin therapy
- Pharmacologic agents
  Dextran
  Warfarin
  Aspirin
  Thrombolytics

Dyspnea should prompt ventilation-perfusion (V/Q) scanning. Subtle neurologic symptoms should prompt cerebral arteriography. A commonly overlooked syndrome in such patients is mesenteric ischemia. Patients with unexplained acidosis and elevated white blood cell (WBC) counts should undergo mesenteric angiography or diagnostic laparotomy or laparoscopy. Patients who have undergone coronary artery bypass have a high frequency of venous graft closure.[1,39] Coronary angiography with consideration of percutaneous transluminal coronary angioplasty (PTCA) with direct thrombin inhibitors should be considered in all patients with symptoms of postoperative coronary insufficiency.

The gold standard for diagnosis remains the clinical impression. Management decisions should not be influenced by negative laboratory tests for HIT antibody, because platelet aggregation testing using platelet-rich plasma, serotonin-release testing, and enzyme-linked immunosorbent assays (ELISA) have significant false-negative rates. Conversely, these tests rarely give false-positive results; therefore, a positive test nearly always confirms the diagnosis of HIT antibody.

The improved survival of patients with HITTS who are treated with early plasmapheresis compared with historic controls not treated with plasmapheresis[16,26] prompts the use of plasmapheresis in our patients (see Table 2).[23] Patients who are HIT antibody-positive are retested after each plasmapheresis treatment. Plasmapheresis is performed daily until a negative HIT antibody test is obtained. Patients who remain positive after three consecutive plasmapheresis treatments are also given immunoglobulin therapy.

Continued Anticoagulation

Unfortunately, early discontinuation of heparin does not appear to effect the rate of thrombotic events, although early recognition may improve mortality rates.[39] Of patients with HIT, 35% develop thrombosis and 85% have subclinical thrombus, whether heparin is discontinued early or late. Thus, prophylaxis against thrombosis may be beneficial. Many explanations account for the development of clinical thrombosis despite absence of clinical evidence of thrombosis at the time heparin is discontinued. Thrombus may be small and therefore unrecognized at the time heparin is discontinued. The discontinuation of heparin not only removes the stimulus for HIT antibody production but also eliminates the usual treatment for thrombus. Untreated thrombus will continue to propagate and eventually becomes a clinically significant thrombotic event.

To date, attempts at treatment of HITTS have involved clinically available drugs such as warfarin and dextran (see Table 2). These agents are of limited value in the initial treatment of HIT. For example, tachyphylaxis to the anticoagulant properties of dextran is seen within 48–72 hours of continuous administration. Dextran also carries the risk of anaphylaxis. Warfarin requires a loading period of 48–72 hours, during which patients are without anticoagulant protection. Warfarin's mechanism of action also includes a nonspecific inhibition of the naturally occurring anticoagulant protein C. Protein C activity can be dramatically reduced during warfarin administration, resulting in a balance of the coagulation cascade that favors a prothrombotic state. Patients given warfarin thus represent a double paradox. They are prothrombotic secondary to HIT antibody produced in response to heparin, and they are prothrombotic secondary to a reduction in protein C activity due to the anticoagulant warfarin.

The demonstrated lack of platelet activation in vitro with aspirin and HIT serum has led to our addition of aspirin to the warfarin. Aspirin is usually started after platelets have recovered to at least 100,000/µl (see Table 2). Patients who have limb-threatening or life-threatening thrombosis are treated with selective thrombolytic infusion.[8,9,27] Patients treated with thrombolytic infusions are monitored in an intensive care setting. Postoperative patients are treated with a lower dose of selective thrombolytic infusions (urokinase, 30,000–60,000 U/hr). Patients who are not postoperative are treated with higher-dose infusions (urokinase, 50,000–200,000 U/hr). Fibrinogen levels are monitored every eight hours to maintain levels at 200 mg/dl. Thrombolytic infusions are discontinued or decreased when significant clinical bleeding is observed. The selective infusions are continued until angiographic evidence of complete resolution of thrombus is found.

Selective thrombolytic infusion has been more successful than surgical thrombectomy. The endothelial damage that occurs with thrombectomy, combined with the involvement of endothelial cells observed with HIT antibody, may explain the limited success of surgical thrombectomy. However, surgical thrombectomy remains a reasonable therapy in patients who have dire clinical circumstances and cannot afford the time required for selective thrombolytic infusions.

ANTITHROMBIN ALTERNATIVES

Alternative fast-acting anticoagulants have been sought for treatment of thrombosis in patients with HIT. Unfortunately, the alternatives have been less than optimal because of high bleeding risk, slow onset of activity, poor efficacy, and lack of an antidote. Thus the field is open for further development of alternative anticoagulants. Several new antithrombin agents in development hold promise for use in patients with HIT. The synthetic or biotechnology-derived thrombin inhibitors—hirudin, hirulog, efegatran, and argatroban—are currently in phase II and III development. Polyethylene (PEG)-coupled hirudin and Inogatran are in phase I development (Table 3).

The currently available site-directed thrombin inhibitors represent a diverse class of proteins, peptides, synthetic organic agents, and their derivatives. Thus, these agents have a wide degree of chemical and functional heterogeneity. Although all thrombin inhibitors have anticoagulant properties, the mechanisms of their actions differ significantly among each other and also in comparison with heparin. Each antithrombin agent is unique in its characteristics, including specificity, rate of thrombin inhibition, and hemodynamic effects. In addition, some are reversible and others are nonreversible inhibitors with different binding sites on the thrombin molecule.

Thrombin plays a crucial role in thrombotic events leading to both arterial and venous thrombosis. However, the anticoagulant effects of thrombin inhibitors depend not only on inhibition of thrombin but also on the ability to inhibit generation of thrombin. Furthermore, besides the transformation of fibrinogen to fibrin, thrombin mediates the activation of platelets and macrophages and produces vascular effects leading to ischemia and vascular contraction. Thrombin is also linked with cellular proliferation and restenosis. Thus, inhibition of thrombin inhibits its bioregulatory actions, which may have physiologic effects beyond the anticoagulation response.

With the availability of molecular biology techniques, it has become possible to produce pharmaceutical quantities of a recombinant (r) equivalent of hirudin, the first antithrombin agent originally isolated from the medicinal leech, *Hirudo medicinalis*.[18] Hirudin is a 65-amino acid protein and a much stronger anticoagulant than heparin. It does not require any endogenous factors to produce its effects. Recombinant hirudin is under development by several companies (Ciba, Hoechst, Knoll).

TABLE 3. Thrombin Inhibitors

Agent		Chemical Nature	Developmental Status
Hirudin and related variants; PEG-hirudin	Revasc	Recombinant analogs of natural hirudin	Various clinical phases of development
Hirulogs		Synthetic oligopeptides	Phase II clinical studies
Peptides	Argatroban (Novastan) Efegatran Inogatran	Synthetic heterocyclic and modified amino acid derivatives; peptide arginals and boronic acid derivatives	Phase I and II clinical studies; argatroban used clinically in Japan
Aptamers		DNA- and RNA-derived oligonucleotides	Preclinical stage

Because the mechanism of action of r-hirudin differs from that of heparin, one must be cautious in the applications of this new agent. Recombinant hirudin is a monocomponent, single-acting drug, whereas heparin has many and varied activities. Although r-hirudin is a stronger antithrombin agent than heparin, the thrombin generation pathways in the coagulation cascade appear to be inhibited only under certain conditions. As a result, a very high dose of r-hirudin is needed for effective antithrombotic activity, because only one target site can be inhibited. Thus, excessive bleeding can be associated with its use. Because of the multiple activities associated with heparin, other pharmacologic effects remain even after its antithrombin activity is no longer detectable. This does not seem to be the case with r-hirudin.

Recombinant hirudin has a relatively short half-life when given intravenously. The subcutaneous bioavailability of r-hirudin is low, being somewhat similar to that of standard heparin. Based on this and the short half-life, it is unlikely that r-hirudin will have an important role in prophylaxis. However, the PEG-hirudin has an exaggerated half-life and could be potentially useful.

A synthetic analogue of hirudin, hirulog (Biogen, Cambridge, MA) has also been developed.[17] Hirulog has a bivalent structure whereby the C-terminal portion of hirudin (thrombin anion-binding exosite recognition moiety) is coupled to a D-Phe-Pro-Arg sequence (thrombin active-site inhibitory moiety) via a Gly_4 linker region. A recent report has described its use as an anticoagulant during angioplasty.[33] Hirulog has also been evaluated in the management of unstable angina and occlusive phenomena related to interventional cardiology.

Argatroban (MD805 or MCI9038) is a selective reversible peptide inhibitor of thrombin derived from arginine. It is effective in preventing thrombus formation, as shown in animal models at low concentrations (< 1 μM) as well as in several clinical thrombotic conditions.[19] It is being tested clinically for thrombotic indications, in particular HIT, disseminated intravascular coagulation (DIC), and stroke. Argatroban (Novastan, Texas Biotechnology Corp., Houston, Texas) is currently available under investigational protocol in the United States for treatment of patients with HIT and HITTS and, therefore, represents the most practical option at this time.

To achieve compounds that are both stable and specific for thrombin, a series of N-alkyl derivatives has been synthesized (a basic amino terminus promotes thrombin specificity).[3] From this series the methyl derivative, D-MePhe-Pro-Arg-H (GYKI 14766), has been found to be a potent and selective reversible inhibitor of thrombin. Under the name efegatran, this agent is being developed by Eli Lilly for prevention of reocclusion during interventional cardiovascular procedures.

Another promising low-molecular-weight (439 Da), reversible peptidomimetic thrombin inhibitor, Inogatran, is currently being developed by Astra Hässle Ab (Sweden). Its half-life is about 1 hour.[31] Phase I clinical studies have been completed.

Recombinant and synthetic antithrombin drugs may be extremely useful as alternate anticoagulants for heparin-compromised patients, because they do not produce many of heparin's adverse effects (thrombocytopenia and white clot syndrome).[15] Thrombin inhibitors have no structural similarity to heparin and therefore do not cross-react with the HIT antibody. The thrombin inhibitors show no activity by any HIT-positive serum in the platelet aggregation assay (Fig. 1). Recently three case reports of successful treatment of HIT with hirulog were published.[5] Other successfully completed compassionate-use cases at our hospital strongly support the use of thrombin inhibitors in HIT and HITTS. In particular, Novastan appears to be clinically effective in rescuing patients with HITTS from almost sure amputation or death. Treatment of thrombosis with Novastan provides adequate anticoagulation to resolve the clot, and the HIT antibody titer is simultaneously reduced (Fig. 2). Clinical trials are in progress. Recombinant hirudin was also successfully used in patients suffering from HIT.[12,28] Hirulog and argatroban offer an additional

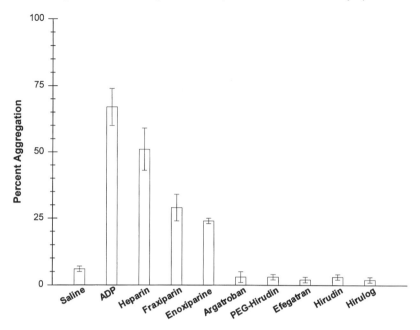

FIGURE 1.   HIT platelet aggregation assay results comparing thrombin inhibitors with unfractionated heparin and adenosine diphosphate (ADP—positive control). These results consist of data from 5 normal donor platelet-rich plasmas and 10 sera from known HIT-positive patients. Results, shown as mean ± SEM, demonstrate that thrombin inhibitors do not potentiate platelet aggregation in the presence of HIT-positive serum.

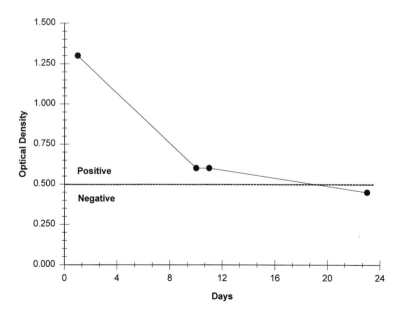

FIGURE 2.   Antibody to heparin–platelet factor 4 complex as determined by the HPIA ELISA kit (Diagnostica Stago) in an HIT-positive patient receiving Novastan for the treatment of deep venous thrombosis. The antibody titer decreased during treatment.

advantage in that the level of anticoagulation can be monitored with standard testing of activated partial thromboplastin time (APTT).

Recent clinical trials of antithrombin agents in angioplasty or as adjunct agents to thrombolytic therapy have revealed adverse effects of bleeding, rebound phenomenon, and perturbation of the regulatory role of activated protein C and thrombin.[32] These effects may be due to nonoptimized dosage, drug interactions, or individual predisposing factors in the tested population. For proper development, additional studies are warranted. Several other developmental issues related to the use of thrombin inhibitors also remain unresolved, including nonavailability of the antagonists, potential generation of neutralizing antibodies after prolonged use, and valid therapeutic monitoring. Although thrombin inhibitors appear to be highly beneficial agents, these issues need to be addressed prior to full-scale clinical acceptance.

Laboratory Validation

The platelet aggregation assay for HIT has been clinically performed for decades and is the clinically accepted method throughout the world. Other assay systems either do not lend themselves to all laboratories (e.g., radioactivity handling) or have not been universally accepted. Clinical laboratorians who know the platelet aggregation assay are fully aware of its limitations and have, therefore, instituted specific protocols to maintain sensitivity and specificity to reduce false-negative and false-positive results. Until another practical assay that is validated as clinically relevant becomes available, the aggregation assay is likely to remain.

Platelet Factor 4–Heparin Antibody

Based on the mechanism of HIT as an immune-mediated process involving antibodies to the heparin–PF4 complex, an enzyme-linked immunosorbent assay (ELISA) has been developed. In a previous publication the validity of the assay measuring antiheparin–PF4 antibody has been questioned.[10] In our institution the currently available commercial assay, HPIA ELISA Kit (Diagnostica Stago, Gennevilliers, France), that detects this antibody proved to be unreliable in providing clinically relevant diagnostic information because of both false-positive and false-negative results. In a study of patients from the Prophylaxis Against Restenosis Angioplasty Trial (PARAT) at Loyola, 80 patients underwent coronary angioplasty with heparin.[25] After the procedure, 40 patients received 80 mg/day of a low-molecular-weight (LMW) heparin (Certoparin, Sandoz, Germany) subcutaneously for 3 months and 40 patients received placebo. At baseline and 2 weeks, both the placebo and the treated groups exhibited a high titer of antiheparin–PF4 antibody (Fig. 3). None of these patients showed signs of clinical thrombocytopenia or a positive HIT aggregation test. The increase in antiheparin–PF4 antibody titer, with a delayed onset, may have been due to the initial heparinization.

In another investigation three groups of patients (n = 20–30/group) were treated therapeutically with 20 U/kg/hr of unfractionated heparin, 15 anti-Xa U/kg/hr of LMW heparin intravenously, or 4000 anti-Xa units of LMW heparin subcutaneously twice daily for up to 16 days. Platelet counts and the antiheparin–PF4 antibody titer were measured at baseline and at 4, 8, 12, and 16 days. Beginning on day 4, the heparin-treated group showed an increase in the antiheparin–PF4 antibody titer (Fig. 4). A progressive increase at days 8 and 12 was noted in all groups; however, the heparin group remained significantly higher than either LMW heparin group at all times. On day 16, the antibody titer leveled off at 3–4-fold higher than baseline levels in all groups. Both the intravenously and subcutaneously LMW heparin-treated groups showed a delayed onset in the increase of antiheparin–PF4 antibody titer (on day 4 there was no significant difference from baseline). The heparin-treated group showed a trend toward the generation of a higher antibody titer. Both the intravenously and subcutaneously treated LMW heparin groups showed a similar progression in the antibody titer increase, but both LMW heparin groups were

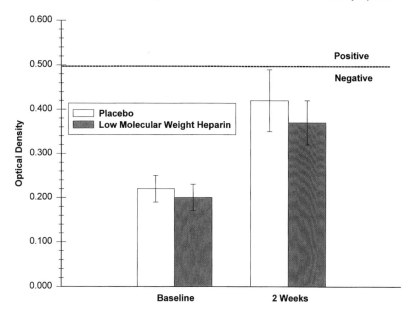

FIGURE 3.   Antibody to heparin–platelet factor 4 complex as determined by the HPIA ELISA kit (Diagnostica Stago) in patients undergoing percutaneous transluminal coronary angioplasty (n = 40/group) and treated with heparin for the procedure and either low-molecular-weight heparin (Certoparin, Sandoz, 80 mg/day subcutaneously) or subcutaneous placebo for 2 weeks after the procedure. The antibody titer increased and was no different for low-molecular-weight heparin or placebo treatment. No patient was clinically diagnosed with heparin-induced thrombocytopenia.

lower than the heparin-treated group. No patient in any of the three groups developed clinical thrombocytopenia during treatment.

These studies demonstrate that the heparin–PF4 antibody can be detected during heparin or LMW heparin therapy. Although this titer may bear no relevance to clinical HIT, such data suggest that LMW heparin may not be the drug of choice as a heparin substitute in patients with HIT. This observation also points to the fact that a reliable method is not yet available for the laboratory diagnosis of HIT. Clearly IgG antibodies (as used in the assay method) are not the only type of antibody in HIT.[30] Effects of the HIT antibodies on blood and vascular cells have not been defined at this time, although such interactions are known to exist.[34] Furthermore, the complex pathophysiology of HIT may involve additional platelet-specific processes, potentially including the generation of proaggregatory substances, such as platelet-activating factor (e.g., from the mast cell on stimulation), interleukins, leukotrienes, thomboxane, platelet-derived phospholipid, and leukocyte interaction. Thus, the sole activation through the IgG Fc receptor, as currently theorized, may not be valid, and a clinically relevant laboratory assay has yet to be developed.

Flow Cytometry

Flow cytometry is an accepted tool in research and clinical laboratories for various applications. The most common application is the immunophenotyping of cell surface antigens of leukocytes for the classification and/or monitoring of various leukocyte diseases, such as HIV infection and leukemia, or for typing and cross-matching leukocytes for organ transplantation.[4] In addition, flow cytometry has enabled the investigation of DNA from solid human tumors in efforts to determine the diagnosis and prognosis of patients suffering from carcinoma.[20] More recently, monoclonal antibodies to platelet receptors have been

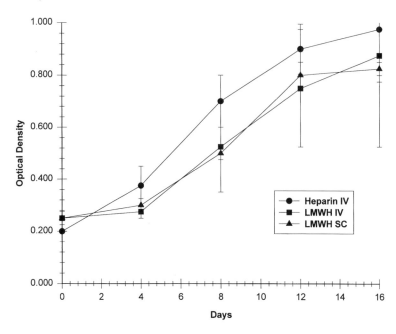

FIGURE 4.   Antibody to heparin–platelet factor 4 complex as determined by the HPIA ELISA kit (Diagnostica Stago) in patients treated for established thrombosis. Patients (n = 20–30/group) were given intravenous heparin (20 U/kg/hr), intravenous low-molecular-weight heparin (15 anti-Xa U/kg/hr), or subcutaneous low-molecular-weight heparin (4000 × 2 = 8000 anti-Xa U/day) for 16 days. The antibody titer increased in all groups after 4 days of treatment. No patient was clinically diagnosed with heparin-induced thrombocytopenia.

developed that allow direct measurement of platelet activation and aggregation.[14,22,24] Two frequently used platelet monoclonal antibodies are directed toward glycoprotein (GP) IIIa (CD-61) and P-selectin (CD-62) (Becton-Dickenson, San Jose CA).

Previous studies from our laboratory using flow cytometry to analyze platelet function have shown that the use of whole blood rather than platelet-rich plasma or washed platelets is advantageous for many reasons.[14] Whole blood eliminates centrifugation steps that may be time-consuming and produce higher levels of autoaggregation and activation of platelets. Autoaggregation occurs without any known stimulus and can be characterized by the expression of surface receptors not normally observed on resting platelets and/or platelet aggregation. In addition to platelet cellular responses, whole blood flow cytometry allows the study of the binding of platelets to leukocytes and the formation of platelet microparticles. Platelet–platelet or platelet–leukocyte aggregation is determined by an increase in cell size as detected by an increase in forward angle light scatter in a predetermined gated area for a particular range of cell size. The GP IIIa (CD-61) antibody is used to identify platelets in whole blood. P-selectin expression, a measure of platelet activation, is determined by an increase in fluorescence from the bound antibody. With the binding of platelets to leukocytes, platelet microparticle formation, and platelet aggregation, a comprehensive analysis of platelets can be performed in one test. The simultaneous analysis of the three platelet-related populations in relation to platelet activation (P-selectin expression) and the interrelationships among them may provide greater insight into platelet physiology. We have applied this technique to the study of HIT.[36,38]

In our flow cytometric HIT experiments, analysis of platelet activation was performed by measuring P-selectin expression separately in the three different platelet-related

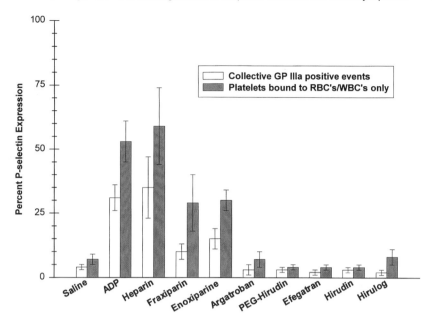

FIGURE 5.   Percent P-selectin expression in different anticoagulant systems using normal whole blood (n = 10) and HIT-positive serum (n = 15) as measured by flow cytometry. Results, shown as mean ± SEM, show that low-molecular-weight heparins are strongly reactive, whereas thrombin inhibitors show no platelet activation in comparison with heparins, and that more activity is observed consistently in the platelet-leukocyte region than in the platelet-platelet region.

populations. In the region of platelets bound to erythrocytes and leukocytes, we observed a 20–50% higher P-selectin expression than the collective mean of all platelet (GP IIIa)-positive events in the three regions. The region containing only whole platelets demonstrated equivalent P-selectin expression to the mean activation level, whereas the microparticle region exhibited only 0–4% P-selectin expression. This finding suggests that the platelet–leukocyte interaction may be a more reactive process than the platelet–platelet interaction.

Figure 5 compares the P-selectin expression of the collective mean of all GP IIIa-positive events vs. the P-selectin expression of only the platelets bound to erythrocytes or leukocytes. The assay system was composed of whole blood that was collected in the indicated agent (e.g., heparin, hirudin [no citrate]), HIT patient serum, and monoclonal antibodies (CD-61, CD-62). The heparin samples and ADP (citrate)-positive control exhibited similar results (35 ± 10%, 31 ± 4% P-selectin expression, respectively) as measured by the collective mean of all GP IIIa-positive events. But the platelets bound to erythrocytes or leukocytes demonstrated higher levels of P-selectin expression: 59 ± 12% for the heparin system and 53 ± 4% for the ADP (citrate)-positive control.

Figure 5 also compares thrombin inhibitors with heparin as an anticoagulant agent. Blood from normal donors collected in different thrombin inhibitors (in place of heparin), supplemented with HIT-positive patient serum, revealed a significantly lower level of platelet activation for the thrombin inhibitors, such that no platelet activation was observed in the system strongly positive with heparin (p < 0.05). On the other hand, blood collected in LMW heparins, Fraxiparin and Enoxiparine, exhibited more P-selectin expression than the thrombin inhibitors (p < 0.05). Although the LMW heparin activation was less than the heparin response, it was significantly higher than the saline control.

TABLE 4.   Effect of ReoPro on Heparin-induced Aggregation

ReoPro (µg/ml)	% Aggregation
0	81 ± 7
0.62	14 ± 6
1.25	10 ± 4
2.5	7 ± 3
5.0	5 ± 3
10.0	5 ± 2

Results represent the mean ± 1 standard deviation (n = 8) in the HIT platelet aggregation assay. Unfractionated heparin from Sanofi/Choay (Paris) was used in these studies.

Ex vivo and in vitro assays for testing HIT require further clinical validation, and results should be cautiously assessed. Regardless of any laboratory result, clinical observations are of foremost importance in diagnosing HIT. No diagnostic assay currently provides a high enough sensitivity and specificity for clinical accuracy. However, the preliminary data from the flow cytometry technique are promising.

Glycoprotein IIb/IIIa Antagonists and Antithrombin Agents

Numerous GPIIb/IIIa inhibitors are under development as antithrombotic drugs for both cardiovascular and cerebrovascular indications. These drugs are potent antiplatelet agents and thus may be useful for the inhibition of platelet activation in HIT. Two GPIIb/IIIa inhibitors, ReoPro (Centocor; Malvern, PA) and YM 337 (Yamanouchi; Tokyo, Japan), were evaluated using the in vitro assay for heparin-induced platelet activation, which is based on platelet aggregation in the presence of heparin and HIT patient serum.

At concentrations greater than 1.25 µg/ml, ReoPro showed complete inhibition of heparin-induced aggregation (Table 4). Figure 6 shows the results of the inhibitory effects of another GPIIb/IIIa antibody, YM 337. This agent produced complete inhibition

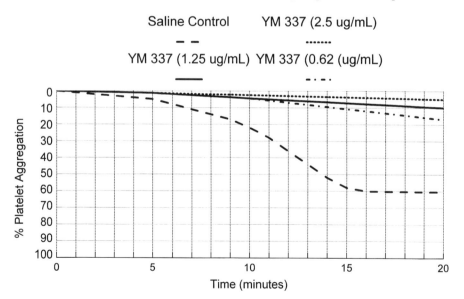

FIGURE 6.   Platelet aggregation showing that the addition of GPIIb/IIIa antibody, YM 337, to platelet-rich plasma, HIT-positive serum, and heparin inhibited the platelet aggregation response. Inhibition of platelet aggregation induced by heparin and HIT serums was complete.

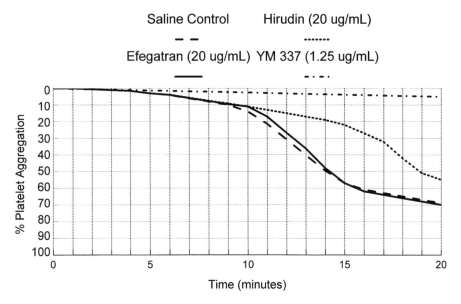

FIGURE 7.   Platelet aggregation tracing showing that the thrombin inhibitors, hirudin and efega-tran, at high concentrations up to 20 mg/ml, were unable to inhibit the platelet aggregation response induced by heparin and HIT-positive patient serum (saline), whereas the GPIIb/IIIa inhibitor, YM 337, was able to prevent the platelet aggregation response.

of heparin-induced platelet aggregation at a concentration of 0.62 µg/ml. These data suggest that GPIIb/IIIa inhibitors may be useful for the pharmacologic control of HIT. Platelet activation induced by heparin in patients with HIT may be suppressed by administering GPIIb/IIIa antagonists. However, additional studies are needed.

Figure 7 shows a comparison of YM 337 with hirudin and efegatran, two thrombin inhibitor peptides currently under clinical investigations, in the platelet aggregation assay with HIT-positive serum and heparin. In contrast to the thrombin inhibitors, YM 337 strongly inhibited the heparin-mediated activation of platelets. At a high concentration of 20 µg/ml, efegatran was ineffective, and hirudin produced only partial inhibition of heparin-induced platelet activation.

These results suggest that GPIIb/IIIa-targeting antibodies are strong inhibitors of heparin-induced platelet activation but that thrombin inhibitors cannot produce an equivalent effect. Thus, GPIIb/IIIa inhibitors may be useful to treat established HIT by stopping the stimulus for thrombocytopenia and thrombosis. Thrombin inhibitors may be useful for anticoagulation needed in patients with HIT but do not eliminate the heparin-induced platelet activation stimulus for thrombosis. The question of whether heparin can be administered simultaneously with GPIIb/IIIa inhibitors remains to be clinically resolved.

Clinical Use

The decision to treat patients with HIT prophylactically with direct thrombin inhibitors can be guided by the division of patients into three groups.

1. The first group consists of patients who are given heparin for documented clinical thrombosis, such as DVT, pulmonary embolism, unstable angina, myocardial infarction, and peripheral arterial thrombosis, and then develop HIT antibodies. Such patients have a clear indication for anticoagulation and should be treated with thrombin inhibitors until adequate laboratory evidence of anticoagulation can be documented with administration of warfarin. For treatment of patients with HITTS, a direct thrombin inhibitor is begun and

TABLE 5.   Treatment of Heparin-induced Thrombocytopenia and Thrombosis
with Thrombin Inhibitors

1. Plasmapheresis
2. Immunglobulin therapy if positive HIT antibody after 3 treatments
3. Titrate thrombin inhibitor to therapeutic dose
4. Initiate warfarin treatment after 48 hours
5. Terminate thrombin inhibitor when warfarin levels are therapeutic
6. Add aspirin treatment after thrombocytopenia resolves and thrombin inhibitor is discontinued
7. Thrombolytic therapy infusion for limb- or life-threatening thrombosis

titrated to therapeutic levels using the APTT as a guideline (Table 5). Warfarin is initiated after the thrombin inhibitor has been administered for 48 hours. Warfarin is initiated in small doses, and the thrombin inhibitor is continued until therapeutic levels of warfarin are documented. Caution in laboratory monitoring is needed, because the thrombin inhibitors can interfere in most clot-based assays.[37] It is important to recognize that patients who are treated with plasmapheresis have mechanical depletion of clotting factors. Therefore, during plasmapheresis only small doses of thrombin inhibitors and warfarin are administered, because factor-depleted patients are highly sensitive to anticoagulant drugs. Aspirin is usually started only after thrombocytopenia has resolved to a level of at least 100,000/µl platelets.

2. The second group consists of patients with HIT who have no documented thrombus but require long-term anticoagulation for prophylaxis. Examples include patients with mechanical prosthetic valves, atrial fibrillation and underlying hypercoagulable states. The ideal management strategy for such patients is to initiate oral anticoagulation while maintaining therapeutic levels of anticoagulation with an intravenous thrombin inhibitor. Once the international normalized ratio (INR) for warfarin is stable within the therapeutic range, the intravenous thrombin inhibitor is tapered and finally discontinued.

3. The third group of patients with HIT who present a management dilemma have no documented thrombus and no coincident condition that requires chronic anticoagulation. The literature reported to date suggests that patients with documented HIT antibody carry a 35% probability of developing a clinically significant thrombotic event during hospitalization.[39] Warkentin's observation with screening venography—that nearly all patients with HIT had at least subclinical venous thrombosis[40]—suggests that the probability of thrombosis in patients with HIT may be even higher. In addition, our group has observed an average of approximately two thrombotic events in every patient with HIT. Finally, numerous reports suggest that patients who develop HIT thrombosis have a mortality rate of 25–30%.[39] The high probability of developing thrombosis in patients with HIT, combined with the high mortality rate once thrombosis develops, has led to our bias for prophylactic treatment even in patients with no other indication for anticoagulation. Our current approach is initiation of a thrombin inhibitor while warfarin is titrated to therapeutic levels of anticoagulation. The thrombin inhibitors are initiated with low levels of anticoagulation until the thrombocytopenia resolves. Once platelet counts exceed 100,000/µl, full anticoagulation is achieved. Low-dose aspirin is added to the regimen once warfarin is therapeutic and the thrombin inhibitor is discontinued. This regimen is continued until the HIT antibody is no longer detected by laboratory testing.

Perhaps the greatest obstacle to overcome in the management of patients with HIT antibody is treatment of those who require coronary revascularization or cardiac valve surgery. Such patients require anticoagulation for successful percutaneous coronary interventions, coronary bypass surgery, or cardiac valve surgery. Historically, procedural anticoagulation has been achieved with a brief exposure to heparin, Orgaran (ORG 10172), or ancrod. All of these options have serious drawbacks. Reexposure to heparin carries the obvious risk of reactivating the HIT antibody and creating a prothrombotic state. Orgaran may cross-react with the HIT antibody, dosing guidelines are not well defined, and intraoperative laboratory monitoring of the level of anticoagulation is difficult because special laboratory facilities are required. Orgaran is therefore associated with significant postoperative bleeding, and no antidote is available for reversal.

The procedural applications of ancrod are equally cumbersome. Ancrod requires a loading period to establish therapeutic levels of anticoagulation. Laboratory monitoring requires the measurement of fibrinogen levels, which cannot be rapidly processed. The postoperative duration of anticoagulation is prolonged and creates a problem with postoperative hemostasis. No antidote is available to reverse the anticoagulant properties of ancrod.

Recent clinical observations with LMW heparins confirm their efficacy in the treatment of DVT and pulmonary embolism. The LMW heparins appear to be associated with a lower frequency of HIT antibody induction. However, in vitro cross-reactivity of LMW heparin and HIT antibody has been seen.[38] The low sensitivity of in vitro HIT antibody testing suggests that even patients who have negative in vitro results with LMW heparin probably carry significant risk for exacerbation of the clinical expression of HIT antibody. Intraoperative laboratory monitoring of levels of anticoagulation with LMW heparin is an additional problem.[35]

Applications of thrombin inhibitors in these areas are currently under investigation. The preliminary clinical findings suggest that the thrombin inhibitors will provide proper anticoagulation for clinical procedures without aggravating the HIT response.

Anticoagulation with the older alternatives to heparin is typically associated with significantly increased bleeding, particularly in the postoperative setting. The management of patients with HIT is difficult enough, and the drugs used for anticoagulation are not without efficacy and safety problems. It is hoped that the newly developed synthetic agents based on thrombin inhibition may prove to be clinically acceptable for anticoagulation in HIT with or without thrombosis. Several thrombin inhibitors, which are in clinical trial, produce anticoagulation without activating platelets. They are chemically and immunologically inert in the HIT reaction, as shown in the classical platelet aggregation system and by the ELISA and flow cytometry analysis of platelet activation and aggregation. Because the mechanism of action and the pharmacokinetics of thrombin inhibitors are clearly defined and the drug levels can be easily controlled and monitored, they may prove to be the anticoagulant drug of choice for patients with HIT.

REFERENCES

1. Abhyankar V, Kouides P, Phatak P: Heparin-induced thrombocytopenia is a cause of thromboembolism following coronary by-pass surgery. Blood 86(Suppl 1):846a, 1995.
2. Amiral J, Bridey F, Dreyfus M, et al: Platelet factor 4 complexed to heparin is the target for antibodies generated in heparin-induced thrombocytopenia. Thromb Haemost 68:95–96, 1992.
3. Bajusz S, Széll E, Bagdy D, et al: Highly active and selective anticoagulants D-Phe-Pro-Arg-H, a free tripeptide aldehyde prone to spontaneous inactivation, and its stable N-methyl derivative, D-MePhe-Pro-Arg-H. J Med Chem 33:1729–1735, 1990.
4. Byers, CD: Clinical applications of flow cytometry. Clin Lab Sci 6:174–176, 1993.
5. Chamberlin JR, Lewis B, Leya F, et al: Successful treatment of heparin-associated thrombocytopenia and thrombosis using hirulog. Can J Cardiol 11:511–514, 1995.
6. Chong BH, Pitney WR, Castaldi PA: Heparin-induced thrombocytopenia: Association of thrombotic complications with heparin-dependent IgG antibody that induces thromboxane synthesis and platelet aggregation. Lancet 2:1246, 1982.
7. Chong BH, Pilgrim RL, Cooley MA, Chesterman CN: Increased expression of platelet IgG Fc receptors in immune heparin-induced thrombocytopenia. Blood 81:988–993, 1993.
8. Cohen JI, Cooper MR, Greenberg CS: Streptokinase therapy of pulmonary emboli with heparin-associated thrombocytopenia. Arch Intern Med 135:1725–1726, 1985.
9. Fiessinger JN, Aiach M, Roncato M, et al: Critical ischemia during heparin-induced thrombocytopenia. Treatment by intra-arterial streptokinase. Thromb Res 33:235–238, 1984.
10. Greinacher A, Potzsch B, Amiral J, et al: Heparin-associated thrombocytopenia: Isolation of the antibody and characterization of a multimolecular PF4-heparin complex as the major antigen. Thromb Haemost l71: 247–251, 1994.

11. Greinacher A, Alban S, Dummel V, et al: Characterization of the structural requirements for a carbohydrate based anticoagulant with a reduced risk of inducing the immunological type of heparin-associated thrombocytopenia. Thromb Haemost 74:886–892, 1995.

12. Greinacher A, Völpel H, Pötzsch B: Recombinant hirudin in the treatment of patients with heparin-associated thrombocytopenia type II (HAT). Ann Hematol 72(Suppl 1):A92, 1996.

13. Horne MK, Alkins BR: Platelet binding of IgG from patients with heparin-induced thrombocytopenia. Blood 86(Suppl 1):550a, 1995.

14. Koza MJ, Jato J, Shankey TV, et al: Optimization of experimental conditions for the study of platelet activation using flow cytometry. Blood 82((Suppl 1):607a, 1993.

15. Lefkovits J, Topol EJ: Direct thrombin inhibitors in cardiovascular medicine. Circulation 90:1522–1536, 1994.

16. Lewis BE, Rao RC, Robinson JA, et al: Early plasmapheresis reduces mortality in patients with heparin-induced thrombosis. Blood 86(Suppl 1):919a, 1995.

17. Maraganore JM, Bourdon P, Jablonski J, et al: Design and characterization of hirulogs: A novel class of bivalent peptide inhibitors of thrombin. Biochemistry 29:7095–7101, 1990.

18. Markwardt F, Fink G, Kaiser B, et al: Pharmacological survey of recombinant hirudin. Pharmazie 43:202–207, 1988.

19. Matsuo T, Kario K, Kodama K, Okamoto S: Clinical applications of the synthetic thrombin inhibitor, argatroban (MD-805). Semin Thromb Hemost 18:155–160, 1992.

20. Merkel DE, McGuire WL: Ploidy, proliferative activity, and prognosis-DNA flow cytometry of solid tumors. Cancer 65:1194-–205, 1990.

21. Messmore HL, Nand S, Godwin J: Heparin-induced thrombocytopenia and platelet activation in cardiovascular surgery. In: Pifarré R, (ed): Anticoagulation, Hemostasis, and Blood Preservation in Cardiovascular Surgery. Philadelphia, Hanley & Belfus, 1993, pp 185–199.

22. Metzelaar MJ, Sixma JJ, Nieuwenhuis HK: Detection of platelet activation using activation specific monoclonal antibodies. Blood Cells 16:85–96, 1990.

23. Nand S, Robinson J: Plasmapheresis in the management of heparin associated thrombocytopenia with thrombosis. Am J Hematol 28:204–206, 1988.

24. Pifarré R, Walenga JM, Koza MJ: Studies on platelet activation in native blood by multiparametric flow cytometry. Thromb Haemost 73:1001, 1995.

25. Raible MD, Wolf H, Leya F, et al: Post- PTCA generation of hep-PF4 antibodies is associated with previous exposure to unfractionated heparin. Studies with the chronic administration of LMWH. Blood 86(Suppl 1):551a, 1995.

26. Raible M, Walenga JM, Lewis BE, Pifarré R: Plasmapheresis successfully removes heparin-platelet factor 4 antibodies from patients with heparin-induced thrombocytopenia. Blood 86(Suppl 1):906a, 1995.

27. Rao RC, Lewis BE, Johnson SA: Thrombolytic experience for treatment of thrombosis in patients with postoperative heparin-induced thrombocytopenia. Blood 86(Suppl 1):551a, 1995.

28. Schiele F, Vulleneout A, Kramarz P, et al: Use of recombinant hirudin as antithrombotic treatment in patients with heparin induced thrombocytopenia. Am J Hematol 50:20–25, 1995.

29. Suh JS, Aster RH, Visentin GP: Affinity-purified antibodies from patients with heparin-induced thrombocytopenia (HITP) recognize multiple sites on heparin: PF4 complexes and react with platelets and endothelial cells. Blood 86(Suppl 1):444a, 1995.

30. Suh JS, Malik MI, Aster RH, Visentin GP: Characterization of the humoral immune response in heparin-induced thrombocytopenia/thrombosis (HITP). Blood 86(Suppl 1):444a, 1995.

31. Teger-Nilsson A, Eriksson U, Gustafsson D, et al: Phase I studies on Inogatran, a new selective thrombin inhibitor. J Am Col Cardiol 117A–118A, 1995.

32. Theroux P, Lidon R: Anticoagulants and their use in acute ischemic syndromes. In Topol EJ (ed): Textbook of Interventional Cardiology. Philadelphia, W.B. Saunders, 1994.

33. Topol EJ, Bonan R, Jewitt D, et al: Use of a direct antithrombin, hirulog, in place of heparin during coronary angioplasty. Circulation 87:1622–1629, 1993.

34. Visentin GP, Ford SE, Scott JP, Aster RH: Antibodies from patients with heparin-induced thrombocytopenia/thrombosis are specific for platelet factor 4 complexed with heparin or bound to endothelial cells. J Clin Invest 93:81–88, 1994.

35. Walenga JM, Koza M, Park S, et al: Can heparin be replaced by LMW heparin in cardiopulmonary bypass surgery? Thromb Haemost 69:935, 1993.

36. Walenga JM, Koza MJ, Shankey TV, et al: Heparin induced thrombocytopenic potential of unfractionated heparin and low molecular weight heparins as measured by a flow cytometeric method. Blood 82(Suppl 1):612a, 1993.

37. Walenga JM, Koza MJ, Khenkina Y, et al: Coagulation assessment and laboratory monitoring of patients given the thrombin inhibitor Novastan. Blood 86(Suppl 1):891a, 1995.

38. Walenga JM, Koza MJ, Lewis BE, Pifarré R: Relative heparin induced thrombocytopenic potential of low molecular weight heparins and new antithrombotic agents. Clin Appl Thromb Hemost 2(Suppl 1):S21–S27, 1996.

39. Wallis DE, Lewis BE, Pifarré R, Scanlon PJ: Active surveillance for heparin-induced thrombocytopenia on thromboembolism. Presented at the American College of Chest Physicians, October 30–November 3, 1994.

40. Warkentin TE, Levine MN, Hirsh J, et al: Heparin-induced thrombocytopenia in patients treated with low-molecular-weight heparin or unfractionated heparin. N Engl J Med 332:1330–1335, 1995.

CHAPTER 21

A Survey of New Antithrombin Agents: Potential Use in Open Heart Surgery

DEMETRA D. CALLAS, Ph.D.
JAWED FAREED, Ph.D.

Thrombin is known to play a key role in the development of various thrombotic conditions, such as stroke, myocardial infarction, pulmonary embolism, and hypercoagulable states. Therefore, it is the primary biochemical and pharmacologic target for developing newer antithrombotic drugs. The hypothesis underlying this approach is that inhibition of thrombin at blood and vascular sites is sufficient for the control of thrombogenesis and cellular activation processes.

Venous insufficiency, blood plasma-related disorders, fibrinolytic deficit, and an imbalance of regulatory proteins result in activation of the hemostatic process. Postsurgical trauma, inflammation, and sepsis also activate the hemostatic process, leading to venous thrombosis. The primary process in venous thrombosis is generation of thrombin. During cardiovascular bypass surgery, in addition to plasmatic activation, several cellular sites are also activated. Thus, drugs targeting coagulation protease activation are useful in the treatment of venous disorders.[72-82]

Thrombin has a distinct mode of proteolytic action; it possesses three important exosites, adjacent to its catalytic site, that serve to align protein substrates and inhibitors optimally. The human thrombin molecule is composed of two chains, A (36 residues) and B (259 residues), linked by a single disulfide bridge. The function of the A chain remains unknown, although it may be implicated in conformational stability of the protein. From crystallographic[27] and computer-generated models[20,21,83-90,95] of the thrombin molecule, the structure and nature of the molecule have been characterized. The B chain of thrombin assumes a round conformation with a substrate groove resembling a deep narrow canyon. The catalytic site of thrombin, composed of the catalytic triad His-57, Asp-102, and Ser-195, lies in the center of the global mass in the groove. The interior of the groove is composed of apolar residues and lined on the exterior with charged groups.[83-90] The region above the catalytic site is also highly hydrophobic. The region of the groove next to the catalytic site is notably hydrophobic and forms the apolar binding site of thrombin.[17,204,205] On the opposite site of the catalytic site across from the apolar binding site is the anion-binding exosite I, which is composed of a long peptide segment rich in arginines and lysines.[83-90] This cluster of positively charged residues is involved in fibrinogen recognition and hirudin complexation.[83–90] Alpha thrombin possesses an anion-binding exosite II, which seems to play a synergistic role with the anion binding exosite I in the binding of heparin.[51,52] This second anion-binding exosite is located above the catalytic groove.

A unique mechanism regulates the generation of thrombin from prothrombin. Thrombin is generated from prothrombin by the double proteolytic activity of factor Xa in the prothrombinase complex. The activated thrombin then activates factors V and VIII to create a burst of coagulant activity.[168] These steps are the targets of the natural antithrombins (antithrombin and heparin cofactor II). Thrombin downregulates its own activity by binding to thrombomodulin, which results in loss of thrombin's ability to convert fibrinogen to fibrin. Furthermore, thrombomodulin-bound thrombin activates protein C, which degrades factors V and VIII with protein S as a cofactor, thus blocking the generation of thrombin.[69,70] This mechanism is an important regulatory step in the control of microvascular thrombotic events that may be involved in ischemic and thrombotic disorders.

In addition to proteolytic activities, thrombin exhibits several nonenzymatic or hormonal activities. Thrombin activates platelets and other factors to promote hemostasis. In vitro, the addition of thrombin to platelets causes phosphatidyl inositol hydrolysis, eicosanoid formation, protein phosphorylation, increase in cytosolic free calcium ions and change in their shape, granule secretion, and fibrinogen receptor expression. Thrombin also suppresses synthesis of cyclic adenosine monophosphate (cAMP) and acts on endothelial cells (stimulation of prostaglandin I_2 [PGI_2] formation, proliferation, angiogenesis, neovascularization), fibroblasts (production of cAMP, proliferation, chemotaxis), and vascular smooth muscle cells, all of which may be implicated in platelet activation. For example, PGI_2 inhibits platelet activation by stimulating cAMP synthesis. Other hormonal activities of thrombin include monocyte[13] and neutrophil chemotaxis and aggregation,[23] mitogenesis in certain macrophage-like cells,[13] albumin transport across endothelial cell monolayers,[150] and inhibition of neurite outgrowth.[108,113]

Thrombin activates various cellular receptors. It interacts with a specific high-affinity receptor on platelets to cleave the amino terminus, thus exposing a tethered ligand that activates the receptor.[227a] This receptor is linked to an inhibitory G protein, and its activation results in inhibition of adenylate cyclase and a decrease in cAMP.[197,198] The same receptor also regulates the sodium/hydrogen ion exchange in platelets during stimulation with thrombin. This receptor is thought to be linked through another G protein to phospholipase A_2, which may be the main source of arachidonate production.[125,201,202] Thrombin also interacts with a lower-affinity receptor on the platelets, but this receptor is thought to be linked through a G protein to phospholipase C and protein kinase C.[164] Activation of this receptor may be the source of the thrombin-induced elevations in cytoplasmic levels of calcium ions.

Cultured fibroblasts also have a high-affinity thrombin receptor, activation of which leads to an increase in cAMP[44–46]; it is identical to the high-affinity receptor found on platelets. The same thrombin receptor is also expressed by endothelial cells, smooth muscle cells, and lymphocytes.[28] Thrombomodulin is the thrombin-specific receptor found on endothelial cells.[2] This receptor recognizes the fibrinogen recognition site on thrombin, which is independent of its catalytic site.[117] The endothelial cells appear to have over 1 million low-affinity receptors with a K_d of about 30 nM.[16,119] Some of the biologic activation processes involve thrombin. Through inhibition of these events, cellular contribution to thrombotic activation can be controlled.

HEPARIN AS AN ANTITHROMBIN AGENT

Heparin, the traditional anticoagulant used clinically, inhibits thrombin through potentiation of antithrombin and heparin cofactor II (HC-II). Furthermore, heparin exhibits polypharmacologic behavior and targets several plasmatic and vascular sites.[123, 147] On the other hand, thrombin inhibitors represent chemically pure homogeneous agents. In addition to the antithrombin- and HC-I-mediated inhibition of thrombin, heparin produces its over-all antithrombotic effects through various mechanisms, whereas thrombin inhibitors are believed to act only through inhibition of thrombin. Thus, whereas heparin is capable of inhibiting other coagulation factors via antithrombin and HC-II, antithrombin agents an-tagonize the final stages of coagulation. In addition, heparin interacts ionically with the vascular lining to mediate a series of antithrombotic and profibrinolytic effects, such as release of tissue-type plasminogen activator (tPA), tissue factor pathway inhibitor (TFPI), and antithrombotic glycosaminoglycans from the endothelial lining.[225,226] Heparin also can inhibit platelet functions, whereas antithrombin agents inhibit only thrombin-induced aggregation.

On the other hand, most of the antithrombin agents are smaller in size and therefore can inhibit clot-bound thrombin, which may be important in clot stabilization and its sub-sequent lysis.[18,96,97] The main reason for clinical interest in antithrombin agents as a poten-tial replacement for heparin is the fact that heparin has certain limitations, which include wide subject-to-subject variability, poor response, and allergic manifestations. One of the most serious adverse effects is heparin-induced thrombocytopenia (HIT), a deleterious immune reaction in which the patient's platelets aggregate in response to heparin to form white clots. Both heparin and the higher-molecular-weight thrombin inhibitors (hirudin) exhibit immunogenicity.[61] The exact clinical implications of the antihirudin antibodies are not clear at this time. Another reason for evaluating alternative antithrombotic agents is the limited subcutaneous bioavailability of heparin. A major problem for all direct thrombin inhibitors is their pharmacologic neutralization. Although heparin is readily neutralizable by protamine, there is no currently available pharmacologic antagonist for any of the direct thrombin inhibitors.

DEVELOPMENT OF NONHEPARIN ANTITHROMBIN AGENTS

Table 1 lists the potential uses for thrombin inhibitors in cardiovascular surgery and interventional cardiologic indications. There is a strong need for an alternate anticoagulant for use in patients who cannot be treated with heparin. In particular, patients who develop HIT are in a desperate situation; without an anticoagulant, they may develop a life-threat-ening condition. Heparin itself is a polypharmacologic agent. It can produce several phar-macologic actions in addition to its anticoagulant effect. Furthermore, heparin can also activate the endogenous processes, resulting in activation of the fibrinolytic system and in-hibition or activation of platelets. A single-target drug such as hirudin may be more suit-able for cardiovascular indications.

The major reason for the use of anticoagulants during cardiovascular surgery is to keep the blood in fluid state and to mention the steady flow of blood through the extracorporeal circuit. In addition, platelet activation is also controlled to minimize the formation of platelet thrombi on the surface of the circuit. An ideal anticoagulant is therefore expected to control both the plasmatic and platelet/cellular activation processes. Antithrombin agents

TABLE 1.   Potential Uses of Thrombin Inhibitors in Cardiovascular Surgery and Interventional Cardiologic Procedures

Use	Rationale	Advantage
Coronary angiography	Anticoagulation, inhibition of thrombin	Direct inhibition of coagulation
Cardiac catheterization	Anticoagulation	No activation of platelets
Open heart surgery	Anticoagulation	Predictable anticoagulation
Cardiac transplantation	Anticoagulation, antiinflammatory action	No additional effects
Coronary angioplasty	Patency, inhibition of abrupt closure	No additional effects
Stenting	Anticoagulation, antithrombotic and anti-stenotic actions	Direct anticoagulation, no additional effects

are capable of inhibiting thrombin and thrombin-mediated activation of cells. Some of the other actions of antithrombin agents may also influence the vascular responses. Thus, preclinical studies are needed to determine such effects.

Interventional and surgical cardiovascular procedures are risky, and an associated thrombotic process may lead to serious events, such as myocardial infarction and stroke. Thus optimal anticoagulation in all of these procedures is mandatory. Because thrombin inhibitors are relatively fast-acting, they can be used with a controlled-delivery mode and may not require neutralizing agents such as protamine. Endogenous proteases also may contribute to the individual anticoagulant responses, which in turn contribute to the large variations in the clinical responses among patients treated with heparin. This may not be the case with antithrombin agents.

Thus, thrombin inhibitors may be quite useful in both interventional cardiologic and cardiovascular surgical procedures. Newer clinical trials to demonstrate their usefulness in these indications are therefore needed. At present, only limited data are available about the application of thrombin inhibitors in the cardiovascular surgical indications.

The development of substrate-related synthetic inhibitors of thrombin began with the discovery of the specificity of thrombin for hydrolysis of arginyl bonds. A broad spectrum of interests underlies work related to thrombin inhibitors, including identification of reactive groups in the active site, demonstration of similarities and differences between binding areas of related enzymes, selective inhibition of one protease in the presence of another, and in vivo anticoagulation. Physical methods such as nuclear magnetic resonance (NMR) and x-ray crystallography for topography of the thrombin active site have contributed substantially to these developments. Direct inhibitors of thrombin can be classified according to source and structure into endogenous analogs of natural substrates, and recombinant and synthetic inhibitors. Some of these are directed against the catalytic site of thrombin, whereas others bind to the exosites of thrombin. In addition, some are reversible inhibitors, whereas others are irreversible. The relative size of these inhibitors differs with the sites that are targeted. Figure 1 depicts a representative schematic of currently available thrombin inhibitors. The di- and tripeptide antithrombin agents directed against the catalytic site of thrombin are the smallest inhibitors with molecular weights of around 500 Da. Larger peptidomimetics have also been developed with molecular weights of 1,000–2,000 Da. Hirudin and its analogs interact with two sites on thrombin and are thus larger molecules with molecular weights of around 7,000 Da. Hirudin fragments coupled to tripeptides, such as hirulog, are smaller agents with a molecular weight of about 2,500 Da. All direct thrombin inhibitors are relatively small compared with heparin, which is a heterogeneous drug composed of glycosaminoglycan chains ranging from 2,000–30,000 Da.

The most direct method of controlling the actions mediated by thrombin is direct inhibition of thrombin itself. The thrombin inhibitors described below are designed or selected for this direct approach. Understanding the structure-activity relationship of thrombin is important, because inhibitors of different epitopes of the thrombin molecule result in differential modulation of thrombin's spectrum of activity.

INHIBITORS OF PLASMA ORIGIN

The natural inhibitors of thrombin belong to a class of serpins called antithrombins. The most important are antithrombin and HC-II, which recognizes the anion binding site as well as the catalytic site of thrombin.[118] Antithrombin, also referred to as antithrombin III, is a globular glycoprotein with a molecular weight of 58,000 Da; at a circulating plasma level of 2.6 μM, it directly inactivates thrombin, as well as factor Xa. Antithrombin inactivates heparin-bound thrombin faster than free thrombin.[106,170,186] Additional targets of antithrombin include factors IXa, XIa, and XIIa; kallikrein; and plasmin. The activity of antithrombin is catalyzed by the presence of heparin, which acts as a cofactor by binding to antithrombin to form a noncovalent ternary complex. Additional actions of antithrombin

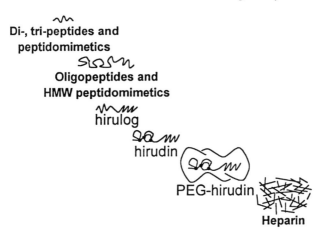

FIGURE 1. Schematic representation of antithrombin agents.

include inhibition of factors IXa, Xa, XIa, and XIIa; kallikrein; and plasmin. HC-II, a glycoprotein with a molecular weight of about 66,000 Da, is present in plasma at concentrations approximately half the concentrations of antithrombin. HC-II and antithrombin have a similar mechanism of action in that both are catalyzed in the presence of heparin.[25] The physiologic roles of antithrombin and HC-II differ in that HC-II is a specific inhibitor of thrombin without reacting with other serine proteases; in contrast to antithrombin, it can slowly inactivate chymotrypsin-like proteases.[51,52,182]

Both HC-II and antithrombin are relatively weaker inhibitors of thrombin and require heparin and related glycosaminoglycans for their antithrombin activities. Antithrombin is primarily used for the treatment of hypercoagulable state and sepsis. Its use in cardiovascular surgical procedure is rather limited. However, it can be used as an adjunct agent.

In addition to the above thrombin inhibitors, thrombin forms complexes and is inhibited by two other proteins secreted from platelets upon activation: platelet protease nexin and thrombospondin.[55] Platelet protease nexin is secreted from activated platelets and inactivates thrombin by forming a 77,000-molecular weight complex through thrombin's anion binding exosite.[55] Thrombospondin is a 420,000-molecular weight glycoprotein secreted by activated platelets; it binds to many cells and proteins[143] and is incorporated into polymerizing fibrin[11] and extracellular matrix.[121] The nexin-thrombin complex is further complexed with thrombospondin via a disulfide bond.[55]

SYNTHETIC INHIBITORS

Before the development of peptide-based inhibitors of thrombin, several nonpeptidic inhibitors were described.[98] Synthetic cationic compounds were used to decipher the spatial relationship of the specificity site of thrombin and to establish an optimal structure for hydrophobic binding and ionic interactions with the negatively charged aspartate moiety at the bottom of the pocket.[98] Of the benzene analogs, those with an amidino side chain rather than an aminomethyl or a guanidino side chain exhibited a stronger K_i.[98] This finding led to incorporation of benzamidine as a building block in more complex thrombin inhibitors. Ring systems other than benzene had an even tighter fit because of improved hydrophobic interaction with the pocket.[98] Introduction of a pyruvic acid group in the para position to the amidino side chain of benzamidine increased inhibitory potency. The augmented inhibition extended to plasmin, trypsin, and enterokinase.[98]

An alternative building block for these molecules was arginine and its modified forms. The D-configuration of arginine had little activity, whereas chemical modifications on the guanidino part or the α-amino part of L-arginine decreased the antithrombin activity.[220]

The following compounds were molecularly designed by attaching a side chain to a starter compound (usually benzamidine). The side chains were aliphatic, aromatic, or aryl aliphatic. Only the agents resulting from the link-up of two benzamidine groupings were active,[98] more so than benzamidine alone; they led to the study of factors affecting potency (length, nature and bulkiness of central chain, presence of various substituents, position of amidino groups). Diamidines proved effective, and it was shown that the second amidino group is essential for full potency, especially for inhibition of kallikrein.[98]

Based on the work done with arginine as a building block, C-terminal modifications of L-arginine were synthesized and studied. Ester compounds were easily hydrolyzed by thrombin and other trypsin-like enzymes; nonhydrolyzable tertiary amides that were found to combine only with thrombin were emphasized.[129,176,220] Modifications of the N-terminal of L-arginine were also studied.[129,176] Dansyl group incorporation as well as other bulky aromatic substituents increased the antithrombin activity of arginine.

An alternative building block used to develop small inhibitors for the catalytic site of thrombin is amidinopiperidine. Modifications of this molecule yielded competitive inhibitors of thrombin with Ki values of 20–50 nM.[116] Further modifications of the central building block have led to the development of napsagatran (Ro 46-6240) as a reversible thrombin inhibitor with a Ki of 0.27nM. This compound has been found to be an effective antithrombotic agent in various animal models.[47,96,97]

The compounds synthesized with L-arginine as the building block and incorporating both C- and N-terminal optimal modifications were found to be highly toxic because of inhibition of butyl cholinesterase.[115] The introduction of a COOH group on the carboxy terminal resulted in decreased affinity for butyl cholinesterase (and therefore less toxicity), and after further modifications an isomer named argatroban (MD805, MCI9038, or argipidine) was generated as a selective inhibitor of thrombin (Ki = 0.039 μM).[115] This compound also has a sizeable affinity for trypsin (Ki = 5.0 μM).[115] It has been characterized pharmacologically and has a plasma half-life of 40 minutes in humans.[213,214] Argatroban is also effective in preventing thrombus formation in various animal models at low concentrations (> 1 μM).[110,111,115,126,159,160] This compound is being tested clinically for several indications.[136,161–163,177, 234]

Inogatran (pINN) is a new low-molecular-weight compound that competitively inhibits thrombin with a Ki of 15 nM.[217,218] Preclinical and phase I studies have been completed in numerous investigations.[63–67,109] Inogatran was found to be selective for thrombin compared with other serine proteases. It was also found to have more effective antithrombotic effects than hirudin and hirulog in an in vivo rat model of arterial thrombosis. No interaction with fibrinolytic processes was noted when inogatran was studied in rat and dog models of thrombolysis. The half-life of inogatran is about 1 hour.[217,218] This compound also has a substantial oral bioavailability that is species- and gender-specific.[63–67,109]

The nonpeptidic thrombin inhibitors exhibit relatively shorter biologic half-lives and therefore may be useful for short-term anticoagulation during interventional cardiovascular or surgical procedures. Furthermore, the anticoagulant effects of these agents are rather specific for thrombin and can be controlled rather easily.

PEPTIDE INHIBITORS

With the elucidation of the primary structure of procoagulant proteins and the identification of the proteolytic activation cleavage sites, specific chromogenic substrates for serine proteases were developed by synthesis of peptides that mimic the amino acid sequence adjacent to the substrate's cleavage site and have a para nitro-aniline (pNA) group attached to the carboxy terminus.[12] A comprehensive study reported the effects of many peptide inhibitors belonging to various classes of serine proteases using clotting and novel amidolytic systems.[72–82]

Aldehyde Derivatives

In 1975 a series of tripeptide aldehydes containing arginine were developed as the first reversible peptide thrombin inhibitors. The prototype compound to be synthesized was D-Phe-Pro-Arg-H (GYKI 14166),[7–10] which was a selective and potent inhibitor of thrombin but highly unstable in neutral aqueous solution, where it cyclized and was inactivated.[7–10] To prevent cyclization, a derivative was synthesized with a protective amino terminal t-butyloxycarbonyl (Boc) group: Boc-D-Phe-Pro-Arg-H (GYKI 14451).[7–10] This compound was more stable than its parent compound but was not as specific for thrombin because it inhibited plasmin as well. To achieve compounds that are both stable and specific for thrombin, a series of N-alkyl derivatives were synthesized (a basic amino terminus promotes thrombin specificity). From this series the methyl derivative D-MePhe-Pro-Arg-H (GYKI 14766)[7–10] was found to be as potent and selective for reversible inhibition of thrombin as the prototype aldehyde. The Ki for the aldehyde derivatives is around 0.1 μM. The aldehydes D-Phe-Pro-Arg-H and D-MePhe-Pro-Arg-H have been studied pharmacologically. From toxicity studies in mice and rabbits, the LD_{50} for both compounds was about 40–45 mg/kg. Both agents were devoid of hemorrhagic effects as determined by a rabbit-ear bleeding model. The unprotected aldehyde, however, produced a blood pressure-lowering effect (40% decease) when injected intravenously, which may have been due to contaminants. When these aldehydes were administered to rabbits and dogs orally, they produced persistent anticoagulant effects, although the bioavailability may have been low. Similar results indicated a high bioavailability when the compounds were administered subcutaneously. The biologic half-life of both aldehydes after intravenous administration to primates was estimated to be 90–180 minutes. The anticoagulant activities of the compounds were evident in the global clotting tests and were independent of antithrombin.[3–10] Both agents inhibited thrombin-induced platelet aggregation in a concentration-dependent manner, but the platelet count was not reduced after systemic administration. All three of the tripeptide aldehydes had antithrombotic activities as tested in various models of thrombosis (rats, rabbits, baboons). The free aldehyde and the methylated derivative were effective antithrombotics after intravenous, subcutaneous, oral and postoperative administration, whereas the Boc derivative was active only after intravenous administration.

An analog of the D-MePhe-Pro-Arg-H aldehyde, D-1-Piq-Pro-Arg-H (LY303496), is under development as an orally effective thrombin inhibitor. This compound has been shown to be an effective antithrombotic agent in rat models of deep venous thrombosis[231] and arterial thrombosis.[138]

Like the peptidomimetic antithrombin agents, aldehyde derivatives also exhibit a relatively shorter biologic half-life and can be administered in controlled-delivery mode. Some of these peptide inhibitors are also able to inhibit several other serine proteases, such as plasmin and plasminogen activator. These effects may produce several additional physiologic effects.

Chloromethyl Ketone Derivatives

Peptides of arginine chloromethyl ketones correspond to the primary structure of physiologic substrates of target proteases.[127,128] Chloromethyl ketones inactivate serine proteases by the formation of an intermediate, reversible, substrate-like complex with the protease followed by irreversible alkylation of the active site histidine. Peptides of arginine chloromethyl ketone are more effective than lysine analogs, because thrombin hydrolyzes only specific arginine bonds in its substrates. Testing of these cleavage site analogs revealed that the tripeptide chloromethyl ketone analogs of factor XIII cleavage site (Val-Pro-Arg-CH_2Cl) and the prothrombin cleavage site (Ile-Pro-Arg-CH_2Cl and

Val-Ile-Pro-Arg-CH$_2$Cl) are the most potent thrombin inhibitors; the tetrapeptide is the optimal as well as the most specific thrombin inhibitor. These inhibitors also inactivate plasmin, kallikrein, and urokinase—but slowly and to a limited extent. Binding at secondary sites contributes to the compounds' selectivity for trypsin-like proteases. The most effective irreversible inhibitor of thrombin synthesized from this class of substrates is D-Phe-Pro-ArgCH$_2$Cl (PPACK or FPRCH$_2$Cl).[127,128] This compound exhibits high specificity for thrombin as opposed to other serine proteases. Thus, D-Phe-Pro-ArgCH$_2$Cl has been used in biochemical studies of thrombin and hemostasis as well as in pharmacologic studies. The toxicity of this tripeptide chloromethyl ketone is species-dependent. For example, although mice show no toxic effects after intravenous infusions of up to 50 mg/kg, in rabbits nearly all platelets agglutinate, even though clotting is prevented. The biologic half-life of this agent, as measured after intravenous administration to rabbits, is about 3 minutes; it is also absorbed in an active form subcutaneously. The anticoagulant effects of the ketone are detectable in a concentration-dependent manner with thrombin time and activated partial thromboplastin time as well as with the thromboelastogram (TEG) whole blood clotting test. However, such effects are lost after incubation with plasma, suggesting inactivation of the compound by plasma components. In various animal models (rats, dogs, and rabbits) D-Phe-Pro-ArgCH$_2$Cl has proved to be an effective antithrombotic after both intravenous and subcutaneous administration.

The chloromethyl ketone derivatives are rather toxic and, therefore, are not suitable for clinical use. They have been used for the collection of blood samples and instrument use.

Nitrile Derivatives

Tripeptide derivatives with α-nitrile groups have been synthesized as competitive inhibitors of thrombin. The peptide derivative D-Phe-Pro-Arg-CN is a strong competitive inhibitor of thrombin with a Ki = 0.7 μM. This agent has been studied pharmacologically in mice, rats, and rabbits. The LD$_{50}$ is 30–40 mg/kg intravenously in mice. Intravenous infusion of the agent to rats has serious blood pressure-lowering effects (70–80% reduction). This effect may be related to the generation of nitric oxide. The bleeding effects are minimal,[209] an indication that primary hemostasis is not affected. The biologic half-life after intravenous injection in rabbits is around 12 minutes; it is also effective after subcutaneous administration. The biliary route accounts for about 30% of excretion of the total amount administered. This tripeptide nitrile exhibits anticoagulant effects in a concentration-dependent manner as detected by the global clotting tests and the TEG whole blood clotting assay. It is also an effective antithrombotic in various rat models of thrombosis.

Boronic Acid Derivatives

The search for selective and potent inhibitors of thrombin has led to the development of three more classes of reversible tripeptide inhibitors: (1) trifluoromethyl ketones (e.g., D-Phe-Pro-Arg-CF$_3$,[169] with a Ki in the nM range) (2) α-aminophosphonic acid tripeptide derivatives with Ki values in the nM range, and (3) α-aminoboronic acid derivatives. The boronic acid derivatives were initially developed as inhibitors of elastase and chymotrypsin. To develop a compound specific for thrombin, the arginine in the sequence D-Phe-Pro-Arg has been replaced with its boronic acid derivative. This led to the synthesis of Ac-(D)-Phe-Pro-boroArg (Ki = 41 pM), Boc-(D)-Phe-Pro-boroArg (Ki = 3.6 pM), and H-(D)-Phe-Pro-boroArg (Ki < 1 pM).[127,128] The boroarginine derivatives are a recent development, and their pharmacologies are not complete. Ac-(D)-Phe-Pro-boroArg appears to have a biologic half-life of around 15 minutes after intravenous administration to rabbits, and it is an effective anticoagulant after subcutaneous administration. The anticoagulant effects are dose-dependent and detectable with the global clotting tests after administration to rats, rabbits, and baboons. The agent also exhibits antithrombotic effects as demonstrated by two thrombosis models. H-(D)-Phe-Pro-boroArg also exhibits anti-thrombotic effects in a baboon model of thrombosis. Compared with the adelhyde analog (D)-Phe-Pro-Arg-H, the boronic acid derivative achieves the same effect at a dose 20 times lower.

In attempting to develop a more specific, orally bioavailable thrombin inhibitor, the above boronic acid derivatives have been modified to yield the compound Ac-D-Phe-N-cyclopentylGly-boroArg (S18326).[224] Although this compound is more specific than Ac-D-Phe-Pro-boroArg and does not interfere in vitro with fibrinolysis, it possesses sizable inhibitory activities against other fibrinolytic enzymes.[224] However, S18326 has potent antithrombotic activities in rat models of arterial and venous thrombosis and is bioavailable orally.[224]

The above boronic acid derivatives lack specificity for thrombin. In an attempt to overcome this drawback, the C terminal of the tripeptides has been extended.[127,128] However, the resulting compounds still lack specificity for thrombin. Tapparelli et al.[215,216] replaced the boroArg in the third position (corresponding to the S1 pocket site of thrombin) with a neutral boron-containing moiety. The compound Z-D-Phe-Pro-boromethoxypropyl-Gly-pinendiol has a lower Ki for thrombin (8.9 nM) than its predecessors, but the specificity for thrombin is improved.[215,216] However, this compound is a weak anticoagulant in the global clotting tests and does not inhibit thrombin-induced platelet aggregation in vitro or in vivo.

Another series of boronic acid derivatives has been developed as specific inhibitors of thrombin: Z-D-Phe-Pro-boroMpgOPin (TRI50), Z-D-Phe-Pro-boroMpgOPinacol (TR1506), and Z-D-Phe-Pro-boroPgIOPin (TRI11).[68] The most promising antithrombin agent appears to be the pinacol ester derivative, TRI50b, with a Ki of 7 nM. This compound is also an effective antithrombotic in various animal models of arterial and venous thrombosis after intravenous and intraduodenal administration.[99,103] Although these anticoagulants are relatively potent, some produce potent effects on blood cells and vasculature. In addition, they are also capable of inhibiting several other serine proteases, which may result in nonspecific effects.

Other Peptide Analogs

Substituting amidinoPhe for Arg in the D-Phe-Pro-Arg prototype sequence led to the development of a series of compounds with inhibitory activities for various enzymes. The compound N-α-(2-napthylsulfonylGly)-4amidinoPhe piperidine (NAPAP) was found to be the most optimal thrombin inhibitor with a Ki of 6 nM.[210] NAPAP was an effective antithrombotic in a series of animal models.[124] However, in addition to adverse side effects (hypotension and respiratory depression), NAPAP has an even shorter half-life than most thrombin inhibitors (< 10 min vs. > 20 min[124]); thus clinical development has been abandoned.

Another direct thrombin inhibitor currently under development is CVS-1123 [(CH$_3$CH$_2$CH$_2$)$_2$-CH-CO-Asp(OCH$_3$)-Pro-Arg-CHO)].[227] This compound has an oral bioavailability of > 30% when administered to cynomolgous monkeys and is an effective antithrombotic in a dog model of coronary artery thrombosis.[53] Peptide analogs may be useful in producing oral antithrombotic effects and warrant faster development.

RECOMBINANT INHIBITORS

Aptamers

Aptamers are oligonucleotides (double- or single-stranded DNA or single-stranded RNA) that act directly on proteins to inhibit disease processes. Thirty-two such aptamers have been recently isolated as inhibitors of thrombin with binding affinities in the range of 20-200 nM.[26] One of the most potent aptamers interacts with thrombin's anion-binding exosite, competing with substrates that interact with that specific site, such as fibrinogen and platelet thrombin receptors.[148,180] This aptamer has been shown recently to reduce arterial platelet thrombus formation in an animal model as well as to inhibit clot bound thrombin in an in vitro system.[145] Recently, a second pool of aptamers, with a different sequence composition from the first class and modified bases, has shown promising anticoagulant activities.[142] Another recent development is the isolation of two RNAs that bind thrombin with high affinity (K_d in the nM range). These oligonucleotides have been shown to inhibit fibrinogen clotting in an in vitro test.[135] Because of their effects on blood and vascular sites, the aptamers may be useful as adjunct drugs with other anticoagulants for cardiovascular indications.

Hirudin and Its Variants

Hirudin is the most potent family of natural thrombin inhibitors, found in the saliva of the leech *Hirudo medicinalis.* It is a single polypeptide chain of 64–66 amino acid residues, stabilized in a characteristic conformation by three disulfide bridges in the N-terminal.[183] The Tyr moiety in position 63 is sulfated and important in imparting inhibitory potency against thrombin.[225,226] The mode of interaction of hirudin with thrombin has been elucidated from x-ray studies of the crystallized thrombin-hirudin complex.[107,192] The amino terminus of this polypeptide interacts with the apolar binding site of thrombin,[228] whereas the carboxy terminus, which is highly acidic, interacts with the anion-binding exosite for fibrinogen recognition.[49,50] Thus, by binding to these two sites on thrombin, hirudin masks the catalytic site, rendering thrombin inactive. Because hirudin recognizes two different exosites on thrombin rather than its catalytic site, it is a highly specific inhibitor of thrombin.

Several isotypes of hirudin exist, all with similar thrombin inhibitory potencies. These variants, named HV-1,[57–59] HV-2,[112] and HV-3,[57–59] were produced by recombinant technology;[57–59,112,193] the expression systems include *Eschericia coli, Bacillus subtilis,* and *Saccharomyces cerevisiae.* The recombinant forms differ from the natural forms in that the Tyr residue in position 63 is not sulphated. Although this lack of sulfation reduces the antithrombin activity of hirudin, the reduction is negligible, because the formation of the thrombin-hirudin complex is almost irreversible.[225,226] The recombinant hirudins are also named desulfatohirudins or desirudins because of the lack of sulfation at position 63. The hybrid recombinant hirudin CX-397 has been synthesized from the N-terminal fragment of HV-1 and the C-terminal fragment of HV-3.[133] This hybridization results in a molecule that has an improved inhibitory potency for thrombin over the natural hirudins. Point mutations to develop variant forms of hirudin have been used.[193]

Binding of recombinant hirudin to dextran has been reported in an attempt to prolong its biologic half-life.[153–156] More recently, polyethylene glycol (PEG) has been coupled with recombinant hirudin to develop longer-lasting agents.[137,235] This modification results in a molecular weight increase from 7,000 to 17,000 Da, which prevents extravasation and retards renal elimination, substantially increasing the biologic half-life.[31,190] Furthermore, the PEG-hirudin metabolites differ from those of hirudin, suggesting different renal metabolism.[141] Hirudin is capable of inhibiting clot-bound thrombin compared with heparin.[96,97] PEG-hirudin has also been shown to be effective in a rabbit model of disseminated intravascular coagulation (DIC).[235] Another application of PEG-hirudin is stent-coating;[206] expansion of this usage to reduce the thrombogenicity of other biomaterials, such as catheters, vascular prostheses, and oxygenators, is under consideration.

In addition to PEG, albumin also has been linked to the carboxy terminus of hirudin to prolong its half-life without impairing its antithrombin activity.[212] The albumin-hirudin product has not been tested in vivo.

Extensive pharmacologic studies have been completed with recombinant hirudin, which repeatedly has been shown to be effective in rat, rabbit, and pig models of venous and arterial thrombosis.[225,226] The effects are always dose-dependent at μmol/kg doses, even after subcutaneous injection. Of interest, the pharmacokinetics of desirudin reveal that it is distributed in extracellular compartments and that renal metabolism and excretion are important components of the overall excretion profile.[225,226] Recombinant hirudin may be of value in both arterial and venous thrombosis and warrants clinical development.

INHIBITORS OF THROMBIN NOT DIRECTED AGAINST ITS CATALYTIC SITE

Based on the structure of the carboxy terminus of hirudin, which interacts with the anion-binding exosite of thrombin, a series of synthetic peptides cyclized via disulfide linkages were synthesized as inhibitors of thrombin.[134] These inhibitors block the anion-binding exosite of thrombin, thus preventing fibrinogen cleavage and subsequent fibrin clot formation; optimal N terminal substitution of these peptides can lead to inhibition of fibrin formation.[178,179]

A 22- and a 27-amino acid peptide have been synthesized, modelled after the sequence of HC-II that interacts with thrombin's anion-binding exosite, which prevents proteolytic cleavage of fibrinogen. The IC_{50} values for these two peptides in inhibiting thrombin are 38 and 28 μM, respectively. Neither peptide, however, interferes with thrombin's catalytic site.[118]

The same group that studied HC-II analogs[118] compared them with a fibrinogen (18 residues) and a thrombomodulin (19 residues) cleavage site analog and with a peptide corresponding to the 12 terminal amino acids of hirudin. The IC_{50} values for these compounds are 130, 140, and 1.3 μM, respectively.

A fibrinogen analog has also been synthesized as a thrombin inhibitor.[22] This 24-amino acid peptide is modelled after the sequence of fibrinogen downstream of the thrombin cleavage site (different from the one studied by Glen et al. above). It is able to prevent fibrinogen clotting with a Ki of around 190 μM.[22] This peptide does not block the thrombin catalytic site.

A new thrombin inhibitor, triabin, is a protein with a molecular weight of 17,000 Da, isolated and cloned from the saliva of the assassin bug, *Triatoma pallidipanis*.[173] Triabin inhibits thrombin by binding to its anion-binding exosite but does not interfere with its catalytic site. A recent report[102] shows that triabin is potent in inhibiting thrombin-mediated platelet aggregation and smooth muscle contraction. Although these inhibitors are useful in understanding the mechanism of the antithrombin actions of hirudin-related antithrombotic drugs, their clinical value is questionable.

CHIMERIC THROMBIN INHIBITORS

Coupling of peptides that mimic the carboxy terminal of hirudin to peptides that are specific for inhibition of the catalytic site of thrombin (D-Phe-Pro-Arg) has led to the development of a series of chimeric molecules termed hirulogs. The amino terminus consists of the catalytic site-directed peptides, whereas the carboxy terminus consists of the 12 terminal residues of hirudin. The two moieties are linked by a bridge of glycine residues of variable length.[56,151,152] Thus, hirulogs inhibit thrombin by binding to both its catalytic site and its anion-binding exosite, thus conferring specificity for thrombin. Hirulog-1 has been developed aggressively for several cardiovascular indications.[42,43,219,221,222] However, its superiority over heparin has not been established.

The recently reported synthetic thrombin inhibitor, CVS#995,[227] is composed of 19 amino acids. Recognition sequences for the catalytic and primary exosite binding domains of thrombin have been linked by a transition state analog.[227] The Ki value for thrombin is in the pM range for this slow and tight-binding thrombin inhibitor. Compared with hirulog-1, CVS#995 is claimed to be superior at inhibiting platelet aggregation and venous thrombosis in a rat model.[19,227]

In another chimeric molecule, the 12 terminal residues of hirudin are coupled to the tripeptide Arg-Gly-Asp.[51,52] This tripeptide is a sequence found in thrombin and the adhesive proteins, fibrinogen, fibronectin, vitronectin, and von Willebrand factor; it is recognized by the platelet surface receptor GPIIb/IIIa, which mediates platelet cell adhesion and aggregation.[184,185,191] The chimeric molecule inhibits platelet adhesion to surfaces as well as inactivates thrombin. The implications of this type of structuring are that thrombin inactivation can be targeted to specific cells trapped in thrombi. Based on this hybrid molecule and the crystal structure of the hirudin-thrombin complex, a new class of recombinant hirudin variants has been developed, called hirudisins.[132] These recombinant hirudins have residues 32–35 replaced by the sequence Arg-Gly-Asp-Ser or Lys-Gly-Asp-Ser to yield molecules with characteristics similar to those of the Arg-Gly-Asp-C-terminal of hirudin chimera.

In a novel approach to target a thrombin inhibitor to the surface of a clot, hirudin was covalently linked to a fibrin-specific monoclonal antibody.[27] This chimeric agent was shown to be more effective than hirudin alone in preventing platelet deposition and clot formation in vitro and in a baboon model of arteriovenous shunt. The development of chimeric thrombin inhibitors not only results in functional enhancement but also may lead to agents with multiple targets at plasmatic and cellular sites.

THROMBIN-DIRECTED ANTIBODIES

Acquired antithrombin autoantibodies are rare and have been poorly characterized. In one reported case,[200] the patient had mild bleeding symptoms and markedly prolonged clotting times and eventually died of cerebral hemorrhage. The antibody was found to be an immuoglobulin that recognized at least in part the apolar binding site of thrombin, adjacent to the catalytic site. Another patient developed antibodies against thrombin and factor Xa after exposure to topical treatment with bovine thrombin.[236] Polyclonal antibodies against thrombin have been raised by using the human α-thrombin B chain.[172] These antibodies were found to inhibit the functions of thrombin that require involvement of its anion-binding site, such as activation of protein C when bound to thrombomodulin, cleavage of fibrinogen, and binding to hirudin. On the other hand, the catalytic site of thrombin was not inhibited; thus the enzyme retained its activity to activate protein C and interact with small chromophores (directed against thrombin's catalytic site). These antibodies are useful tools in capturing complexes of thrombin[139,140] as well as in studying requirements of thrombin sites in other interactions.[49,50,172] Unlike the use of GpIIb/IIIa antibodies for their antiplatelet effects, the use of the antithrombin antibodies is rather questionable in the management of thrombotic disorders.

CLINICAL APPLICATIONS OF THROMBIN INHIBITORS

Since their introduction, most of the clinical indications for the new anticoagulants have been in interventional cardiovascular procedures.[114] Initial focus has been on the prevention of abrupt closure during coronary angioplasty.[221,222] These agents also have been tested for the prevention of both early and late reocclusion after percutaneous transluminal coronary angioplasty (PTCA).[211] In addition, some of the thrombin inhibitors have been used for treatment of unstable angina.[221,222] More recently, others have been tested for their efficacy in stenting.[32,206,223] Although several reports have been published about experimental use of these agents in cardiovascular surgery in animal models, only isolated reports in human studies are available.[60,189] Concerns over the use of these agents have been expressed.[60]

Thrombin inhibitors are attractive to both clinicians and surgeons as substitute anticoagulants, particularly in heparin-compromised patients. Several trials are currently in progress in patients with HIT who require anticoagulation to test the efficacy of new antithrombin agents.[48,60]

Interest in the use of these agents in the prevention and treatment of deep venous thrombosis is growing.[30] Eriksson[63–69] reported the successful use of recombinant hirudin in the prophylaxis of postorthopedic surgery. He compared unfractionated heparin (5000 IU subcutaneously 3 times/day) with hirudin (15 mg subcutaneously 2 times/day) and found hirudin to be superior. Several other trials of different antithrombin agents are currently underway. The cost of recombinant drugs is rather high. Therefore, objective pharmaco-economic analyses that compare cost with standards of care may be a major consideration in the clinical acceptance of recombinant hirudin.

Antithrombin

The major application of antithrombin is in disorders associated with antithrombin deficiency, acquired or hereditary. Antithrombin replacement therapy in patients with hereditary antithrombin deficiency is in phase I and phase II clinical studies. Supplementation of antithrombin before and after various surgical procedures, with or without other treatments, has proved effective.[166] The combination of antithrombin and heparin is effective in prophylaxis of venous thrombosis after total hip and total knee replacement surgery.[94] The role of antithrombin replacement in prophylaxis of thrombotic episodes during pregnancy remains controversial.[178,179] A study by Demers et al.[54] suggests that replacement of antithrombin in people who are deficient should be a mode of prophylaxis only during periods of high risk for thrombotic phenomena. In addition, antithrombin has been evaluated in clinical trials in patients with septic shock and DIC.[24,93,149] The outcomes of these trials proved that antithrombin is effective in early attenuation and correction of DIC, but the mortality rate is not affected. The role of antithrombin as an anticoagulant is rather questionable. Thus, antithrombin itself may not be developed for the same indications as other agents.

Argatroban

Although argatroban has been studied in wide range of animal models and has been approved for treatment of peripheral arterial occlusive disease in Japan for some years, only recently have European and American groups begun to evaluate its clinical usefulness.

In an initial study in the U.S., argatroban was evaluated in patients with unstable angina.[104] Although myocardial ischemia did not occur during infusion of argatroban, some patients had recurrent angina within 6 hours after discontinuing the infusion. However, the outcomes may be improved by changing the infusion protocol. Recurrent angina was correlated with an increase in the thrombin-antithrombin complex and was described as a rebound phenomenon. This observation was explained by either the premature cessation of argatroban infusion, which resulted in inhibition of thrombin but was not enough to inhibit generation of thrombin,[104] or by heparin withdrawal before infusion of argatroban, which results in recurrent angina.[230] Furthermore, heparin alone promotes antithrombin clearance, so that antithrombin levels may have been artificially low before infusion of argatroban.[230]

Argatroban is currently under evaluation as an adjunct to thrombolytic agents and aspirin in two phase II trials in North and South America. The Argatroban in Myocardial Infarction (AMI) study at the Montreal Heart Institute uses two doses of argatroban in conjunction with streptokinase and aspirin in patients with acute myocardial infarction. The Myocardial Infarction with Novastan and tPA (MINT) study at Massachusetts General Hospital compares two doses of argatroban with heparin in patients diagnosed with acute myocardial infarction and receiving tPA and aspirin. Argatroban is also under evaluation in phase II trials at Loyola University Medical Center and the University of Calgary in patients with HIT. The University of Calgary study compares argatroban with ancrod (a defibrinating enzyme). Results of both studies are expected to be available in early 1997.

Argatroban is also proposed as an anticoagulant for cardiovascular bypass surgery. Several other indications for argatroban in various medical and surgical indications are currently under exploration.

Efegatran

The tripeptide aldehyde D-MePhe-Pro-Arg-H is currently marketed under the generic name efegatran sulfate by Eli Lily. Although efegatran has been examined in various animal models and has been studied experimentally for several years with promising results, only in the last two years has it been considered for clinical usage. Five clinical studies have been performed with efegatran in normal male volunteers to assess safety and pharmacokinetics/pharmacodynamics. Of interest, some participants experienced short-lived headaches, postural dizziness, and vasovagal episodes when moving from a lying to a sitting position after intravenous infusion of efegatran. It is currently under study in a phase II trial in patients with acute myocardial infarction (the Prevention of Reocclusion by Inhibition of thrombin during Myocardial Events [PRIME] study). The PRIME trial is comparing adjunct usage of tPA and aspirin with efegatran at different doses vs. adjunct usage of tPA and aspirin with heparin. Results are expected in 1996.

Inogatran

Although inogatran is a new competitive thrombin inhibitor and limited information about its pharmacology is available, phase I studies are already completed.[217,218] Results indicate that inogatran is an effective anticoagulant with a biologic half-life of about 1 hour, which is longer than the other thrombin inhibitors currently under clinical evaluation. Inogatran appears to have no metabolites and is excreted evenly in urine and faeces. However, it prolongs the capillary bleeding time in some healthy human subjects. Currently, inogatran is evaluated in a phase II trial in patients with unstable angina.

Napsagatran

Like inogatran, napsagatran is a newly developed reversible thrombin inhibitor. It is currently under evaluation in phase II clinical trials for prevention of postoperative thrombosis and treatment of established venous thrombosis.

Hirudin

The antithrombotic and anticoagulant effects of recombinant hirudin have been well established in experimental animal models. Hirudin also has been studied in various clinical trials for a range of indications. The Thrombolysis in Myocardial Infarction (TIMI 5) Trial compared hirudin with heparin in patients with acute myocardial infarction who were treated with tPA and aspirin.[42,43] Despite an improvement in clinical endpoints with hirudin compared with heparin, hirudin had no dose-dependent effect on outcomes. The TIMI 6 Trial compared hirudin with heparin in patients with acute myocardial infarction who received streptokinase and aspirin[144] and found a trend for improved outcome with the higher dose of hirudin compared with the lower dose of hirudin and heparin. However, the subsequent larger phase III Hirudin for Improvement of Thrombolysis (HIT III) trial, which compared hirudin with heparin in patients with acute myocardial infarction who were treated with tPA and aspirin,[171] was stopped prematurely because of excessive intracranial bleeding in the hirudin-treated group. The Global Use of Strategies to Open Occluded Arteries (GUSTO) II trial also was stopped prematurely because of excessive intracerebral bleeding.[237,238] Hirudin was again compared with heparin in patients with acute coronary syndromes (unstable angina or myocardial infarction). The incidence of hemorrhagic strokes increased in patients receiving concomitant thrombolytic therapy. Another interesting finding is that hirudin, regardless of dose, is less effective in inhibiting thrombin generation than heparin.[237,238] The Thrombolysis and Thrombin Inhibition in Myocardial

Infarction (TIMI) 9A trial, designed to compare heparin and hirudin as adjuncts to thrombolytic therapy, was also prematurely stopped because of increased incidence of hemorrhagic strokes in patients receiving either heparin or hirudin.[1] Both the GUSTO II and TIMI 9A trials were reinitiated with lower doses of hirudin and heparin under the acronyms GUSTO IIb and TIMI 9B.[225,226] In Gusto IIb, over 12,000 patients from 373 hospitals in 13 countries were included to compare intravenous recombinant hirudin and heparin. At the 45th Annual Scientific Session of the American College of Cardiology Meeting in Orlando, FL, Topol described the study as validating the direct thrombin hypothesis of acute myocardial infarction. However, this conclusion is poorly supported by the results; the differences between the hirudin- and heparin-treated groups are small and not sustained at 30 days. Furthermore, even at the adjusted dose, which produced no difference in the incidence of stroke in the two treatment groups, the hirudin-treated group showed increased hemorrhagic strokes in one of the non-ST elevation subgroups.

The HIT-SK trial, designed to compare hirudin and heparin as adjunct treatments to streptokinase in patients with acute myocardial infarction,[167] was recently completed. The results showed no clear dose-response relationship, and major bleeding events were increased.

Hirudin has also been evaluated for use in coronary angioplasty in a phase III trial, Hirudin in a European Restenosis Prevention Trial Versus Heparin in Treatment of PTCA Patients (HELVETICA).[199] Compared with heparin-treated patients, the hirudin-treated group showed an improvement in clinical outcomes (fewer myocardial infarctions, bypass surgeries and ischemic events) in the early stages of treatment, but at 7-month follow-up there was no difference in the rate of restenosis between the two groups.

In patients with unstable angina, hirudin has been compared with heparin and found to decrease the rate of subsequent myocardial infarction (OASIS, Organization to Assess Strategies for Ischemic Syndromes).[92] However, there was no dose-response relationship in the hirudin-treated group. Another problem is an increase in ischemic events after hirudin or heparin is stopped. A recent study of coagulation markers in patients with unstable angina who were treated with heparin or hirudin in conjunction with aspirin showed that although coagulation was suppressed during treatment, it was reactivated when treatment was stopped.[92] Therefore, treatment should be continued for longer time periods (> 72 hours).

Hirudin has been compared with heparin in patients undergoing elective total hip replacement in small phase II trials.[62–67] In a recent report a fixed dose of 15 or 20 mg of hirudin administered preoperatively and subcutaneously twice daily for at least 9 days, was shown to be superior to heparin and to provide prophylaxis against thromboembolic complications in patients undergoing total hip replacement surgery. However, such a study should have compared hirudin with the standard treatment, which is currently low-molecular-weight heparin administered subcutaneously twice daily. Thus, there is a need for additional clinical trials of hirudin for this indication.

A recent report describes the use of hirudin in 10 patients with severe venous thromboembolism.[30,194,195] It was concluded that thrombin generation was only partial and that the dose of hirudin should be increased in subsequent studies and compared with heparin or low-molecular-weight heparin.

Novel and successful applications of hirudin have been reported in two patients who developed HIT. One patient successfully underwent cardiopulmonary bypass surgery by using hirudin instead of heparin for anticoagulation.[187,188] The second patient with HIT successfully underwent cardiopulmonary bypass surgery with an aortic valve replacement after being anticoagulated with hirudin instead of heparin.[189] Since these two isolated reports, an additional 11 patients with HIT have been treated successfully with hirudin during cardiopulmonary bypass surgery.[187,188] Hirudin was administered as an initial bolus of 0.25 mg/kg, and the heart-lung machine was primed with a bolus of 0.2 mg/kg.

Additional hirudin boli were administered to keep the plasma levels above 2.0 µg/ml, as monitored by APTT and ecarin clotting time. This regimen was found to be optimal. No intraoperative bleeding complications occurred in any of the 11 patients, and the hirudin plasma concentrations fell below 1.25 µg/kg in 30 min, making reversal of the anticoagulant effects unnecessary. Concerns about replacement of heparin with hirudin during cardiopulmonary bypass surgery include the absence of an antidote to hirudin and the questionable ability of hirudin to suppress thrombin generation.[60] Another novel application of hirudin was in a patient with diabetic nephropathy and HIT.[74] The continual usage of hirudin in conjunction with hirudin-impermeable dialyzers proved to be safe and efficacious.

Although hirudin has been regarded as a weakly immunogenic agent, a recent study reports the detection of IgG anti-hirudin antibodies in 38 of 82 patients with HIT who were treated successfully for more than 6 days with hirudin.[61,105] Although no allergic reactions were induced in any of the patients, the effects of the antibodies on the pharmacologic responses of hirudin are not clear.

The recombinant hirudin CX-397, a chimeric molecule between HV-1 and HV-3, has been compared with heparin in two groups of 5 patients receiving aspirin before coronary angiography.[91] CX-397 is shown to be a strong anticoagulant that warrants further investigations in patients undergoing coronary angioplasty.

The interactions of PEG-hirudin with aspirin were studied recently in 9 healthy human volunteers.[29] PEG-hirudin in combination with aspirin may be associated with a higher risk of bleeding. The additive bleeding effects were not correlated with any of the platelet function tests or with any of the coagulation parameters. To avoid bleeding complications, it was suggested that the PEG-hirudin dose should be decreased or that aspirin should be given after PEG-hirudin treatment was completed.

Phase I clinical studies of PEG-hirudin have shown that it is a safe thrombin inhibitor in healthy human volunteers after intravenous or subcutaneous injection.[71] Because of its prolonged half-life compared with hirudin, PEG-hirudin appeared to be a promising agent for prophylactic development as a once-daily subcutaneous injection. The relatively rapid clearance of PEG-hirudin from the central compartment after intravenous injection also indicates that it may be suitable for low-dose continuous infusions.

Hirulog

The biochemistry of hirulog peptides has been characterized extensively. Hirulog peptides are specific thrombin inhibitors, and in in vitro clotting studies they appear to be potent anticoagulants.[151,152,175,232] Hirulog has been compared with heparin as an adjunct to streptokinase and aspirin in patients with acute myocardial infarction.[146] Based on the favorable findings for hirulog, a larger trial is now underway for the same indication.[229]

A large phase III trial, the Hirulog Angioplasty Study, compared hirulog with heparin in patients undergoing coronary angioplasty for unstable angina or ongoing ischemia after myocardial infarction.[207,208] Hirulog was found to be superior in high-risk patients undergoing angioplasty after myocardial infarction, although there was no overall difference in the rate of primary outcome events (mortality, myocardial infarction, emergency bypass). The same study also revealed that hirulog does not prevent restenosis after coronary angioplasty,[33] although the thrombin rebound effect is more suppressed with hirulog than with heparin.[207,208]

In the TIMI 7 trial, the effects of hirulog were examined in patients with unstable angina who were receiving aspirin. Although death and myocardial infarction were reduced at the higher doses of hirulog, no heparin controls were included in the study.

Hirulog also has been evaluated in prophylaxis of venous thrombosis in high-risk patients undergoing major orthopedic surgery. The highest hirulog dose proved to be as effective as other forms of prophylaxis, including low-molecular-weight heparin.[101] Because

TABLE 2. Classification of Thrombin Inhibitors Based on Serine Protease Inhibitory Spectrum

Monospecific	Hirudin, hirulog, argatroban, heparin cofactor II, aptamers
Narrow spectrum	Napsagatran, inogatran, antithrombin
Broad spectrum	Ac-(D)Phe-Pro-boroARG-OH, peptide arginals

of its relatively smaller molecular weight, hirulog may have cost advantages over hirudin in terms of shorter half-life, less immunogenicity, and increased accessibility to clots and clot-bound thrombin.

CONCLUSION

The development of thrombin inhibitors has added a new dimension to the management of thrombotic and vascular disorders. Although the major clinical indications include interventional cardiovascular procedures and DVT prophylaxis, little is known about their use for surgical and therapeutic anticoagulation. Many of the newer thrombin inhibitors, such as hirulog and hirudin, may be developed as anticoagulants and substituted for heparin. Synthetic tripeptides with a broader serine protease inhibitory spectrum offer unique tools to control thrombogenesis at different levels and may prove to be more useful in chronic indications, including prophylaxis. The usefulness of various thrombin inhibitors for a given medical or surgical indication can be proved only in properly designed clinical trials. A classification of thrombin inhibitors can thus be generated on the basis of their serine protease activities (Table 2). Hirudin, hirulog, and their analogs; argatroban; HC-II; and aptamers are monospecific agents that interact solely with thrombin. On the other hand, agents such as Ac-(D)Phe-Pro-boroArg-OH interact with almost every serine protease involved in systems other than coagulation, including the fibrinolytic system. Agents with limited serine protease inhibitory activities but not restricted to thrombin are included in the narrow spectrum class of thrombin inhibitors. Examples are napsagatran, inogatran, and antithrombin; in addition to their antithrombin activities, they also exhibit weaker inhibition of other coagulation factors.

In coming years, newer antithrombin agents with varying degrees of specificity for thrombin and other serine proteases will be introduced. In addition to the inhibition of serine proteases, these agents also produce effects on blood and vascular cellular targets, including receptor sites. Furthermore, they also may have direct interactions with plasmatic proteins and cellular sites. Such interactions may influence their pharmacologic profile and clinical outcome. The endogenous transformation of these agents also may play an important role, and observed clinical effects can be strongly influenced by this process. Thus, the factors resulting in endogenous transformations and interactions may have to be taken into account in the optimal development of antithrombin agents. Therefore, another classification of thrombin inhibitors can be proposed on the basis of the spectrum of their pharmacologic actions (Table 3). Antithrombin agents can be grouped into three major categories:

1. Hirudin, hirulog, and their analogs clearly have only plasmatic actions, solely targeting the generated thrombin and its regulatory functions.

2. Agents such as heparin and aptamers mediate diverse pharmacologic actions, including vascular, anti-inflammatory, antiplatelet, and antiproliferative effects.

TABLE 3. Classification of Thrombin Inhibitors Based on Pharamacologic Actions

Agents with plasmatic actions only	Hirudin, hirulog
Agents with dual mechanism of action (plasmatic and vascular)	Peptides, peptidomimetics
Agents with additional regulatory effects (antiproliferative, platelet interactions, antiinflammatory)	Heparin, aptamers

3. Agents such as tripeptide and peptidomimetic thrombin inhibitors possess vascular effects in addition to their plasmatic actions, placing them in a category between the two described above.

Thrombin inhibitors represent suitable alternatives in patients who are not treatable with heparin. In such conditions as HIT, thrombin inhibitors may be especially useful. Although no antagonist is currently available for neutralization of these agents, it is likely that controlled delivery, along with some approaches to neutralization, will be available soon.

Because of their defined chemical nature, thrombin inhibitors can be coupled with other pharmacologic entities to develop hybrid multiple effects. Thus, a bifunctional hybrid to target desired activation sites can be developed. Many of these agents can also be conjugated with inert linker or carrier molecules to obtain desired biologic half-life and site specificity. This potential introduces the concept of designer antithrombin agents. Biotechnology, organic synthesis, and knowledge of natural products may lead to many molecularly developed antithrombin agents.

Thrombin inhibitors also can be used as adjunct anticoagulants with such drugs as the thrombolytic agents, GpIIb/IIIa inhibitors, aspirin, and ticlopidine. In addition, the new anticoagulants can be used for the coating of biomaterials and stent implantation. Additional studies are needed to investigate drug interactions.

In addition to systemic administration, the newer thrombin inhibitors can also be developed for oral, nonparenteral, and on-site delivery. Furthermore, they can be incorporated with biomaterials and formulated for depot delivery. Iontophoresis, phonophoresis, and other delivery modalities can be used for mobilize these agents. Thrombin inhibitors, therefore, provide a wide spectrum of newer anticoagulant and antithrombotic drugs that can be developed for multiple indications to control thrombosis and related pathophysiologic events. However, it must be understood that these agents are not heparin; each product represents a distinct drug entity and must be developed as a new drug for a given indication. Thus, safety and efficacy must be evaluated individually.

REFERENCES

1. Antmann EM, for the TIMI 9A Investigators: Hirudin in acute myocardial infarction: Safety report from the thrombolysis and thrombin inhibition in myocardial infarction (TIMI) 9A trial. Circulation 90:1624–1630, 1994.
2. Awbrey BJ, Hoak JC, Owen WG: Binding of human thrombin to cultured human endothelial cells. J Biol Chem 254:4092–4095, 1979.
3. Bagdy D, Barabás E, Bajusz S, et al: Comparative studies in vitro and ex vivo on the anticoagulant effects of a reversible and an irreversible tripeptide inhibitor of thrombin. Thromb Res 67:221–231, 1992.
4. Bagdy D, Barabás E, Bajusz S, Széll E: In vitro inhibition of blood coagulation by tripeptide aldehydes— a retrospective screening study focused on the stable D-MePhe-Pro-Arg-H•H_2SO_4. Thromb Haemost 67:325–330, 1992.
5. Bagdy, D, Barabás E, Szabó G, et al: In vivo anticoagulant and antiplatelet effect of D-Phe-Pro-Arg-H and D-MePhe-Pro-Arg-H. Thromb Haemost 67:357–365, 1992.
6. Bagdy D, Szabó G, Barabás E, Bajusz S: Inhibition by D-MePhe-Pro-Arg-H (GYKI-14766) of thrombus growth in experimental models of thrombosis. Thromb Haemost 68:125–129, 1992.
7. Bajusz S, Barabás E, Széll E, Bagdy D: Peptide aldehyde inhibitors of the fibrinogen-thrombin reaction. In Meienhofer J (ed): Peptides-Chemistry, Structure and Biology. Ann Arbor, MI, Ann Arbor Science, 1975, pp 603–608.
8. Bajusz S, Barabás E, Tolnay P, et al: Inhibition of thrombin and trypsin by tripeptide aldehydes. Int J Peptide Protein Res 12:217–221, 1978.
9. Bajusz S, Széll E, Bagdy D, et al: US Patent No. 4.703.036, 1987.
10. Bajusz S: The story of D-MePhe-Pro-Arg-H, the likely anticoagulant and antithrombotic of the future. Biokémia 14:127–134, 1990.
11. Bale MD, Mosher DF: Thrombospondin is a substrate for blood coagulation factor XIIIa. Biochemistry 25:5667–5673, 1986.
12. Bang NU, Mattler LE: Thrombin sensitivity and specificity of three chromogenic peptide substrates. In Lundblad RL, Fenton JW, Mann KG (eds): Chemistry and Biology of Thrombin. Ann Arbor, MI, Ann Arbor Science, 1977, pp 305–310.

13. Bar-Shavit R, Kahn A, Wilner GD, Fenton JW II: Monocyte chemotaxis: Stimulation by specific exosite region in thrombin. Science 220:728–731, 1983.

14. Barabás E, Bagdy D, Bajusz S, Széll E: Studies on the questionable antifibrinolytic effect of some synthetic thrombin inhibitors of the tripeptide type. Thromb Haemost 65:1291, 1991.

15. Barabás E, Széll E, Bajusz S: Screening for fibrinolysis inhibitory effect of synthetic thrombin inhibitors. Blood Coagul Fibrinol 4:243–248, 1993.

16. Bauer PI, Machovich R, Aranyi P, et al: Mechanism of thrombin binding to endothelial cells. Blood 61:368–372, 1983.

17. Berliner LJ, Shen YYL: Physical evidence for an apolar binding site near the catalytic center of human α-thrombin. Biochemistry 16:4622–4626, 1977.

18. Berry CN, Girardot C, Lecoffre C, Lunven C: Effects of the synthetic thrombin inhibitor argatroban on fibrin- or clot-incorporated thrombin: comparison with heparin and recombinant hirudin. Thromb Haemost 72:381–386, 1994.

19. Biemond BJ, Friederich PW, Levi M, et al: Sustained antithrombotic effects of novel, specific inhibitors of thrombin and factor Xa in experimental thrombosis. Thromb Haemost 73:1311, 1995.

20. Bing DH, Andrews JM, Cory M: Affinity labelling of thrombin and other serine proteases with an extended reagent. In Lundblad RL, Fenton JW, Mann KG (eds): Chemistry and Biology of Thrombin. Ann Arbor, MI, Ann Arbor Science, 1977, pp 159–178.

21. Bing DH, Laura R, Robinson DJ, et al: A computer generated three-dimensional model of the B chain of bovine a-thrombin. Ann NY Acad Sci 370:496–510, 1981.

22. Binnie CG, Lord ST: A synthetic analog of fibrinogen alpha 27-50 is an inhibitor of thrombin. Thromb Haemost 65:165–168, 1991.

23. Bizios R, Lai L, Fenton JW II, Malik AB: Thrombin-induced chemotaxis and aggregation of neutrophils. J Cel Physiol 128:485–490, 1986.

24. Blauhut B, Kramar H, Vinazzer H, et al: Substitution of antithrombin III in shock and DIC: A randomized study. Thromb Res 39:81–89, 1985.

25. Blinder MA, Marasa JC, Reynolds CH, et al: Heparin cofactor II. cDNA sequence, chromosome localization, restriction fragment length polymorphism, and expression in Escherichia coli. Biochemistry 27:752–759, 1988.

26. Bock LC, Griffin LC, Latham JA, et al: Selection of single-stranded DNA molecules that bind and inhibit human thrombin. Nature 355:564–566, 1992.

27. Bode C, Mehwald P, Peter K, et al: Enhanced antithrombotic potency of fibrin-targeted recombinant hirudin in a non-human primate model [abstract]. Ann Hematol I:A52, 1996.

28. Brass LF: Issues in the development of thrombin receptor antagonists. Thromb Haemost 74:499–505, 1995.

29. Breddin HK, Radziwon P, Eschenfelder V, et al: PEG-hirudin and acetylasalicylic acid show a strong interaction on bleeding time [abstract]. Ann Haematol I:A53, 1996.

30. Bridey F, Dreyfus M, Parent F, et al: Recombinant hirudin (HBW 023). Biological data of ten patients with severe venous thromboembolism. Am J Hematol 49:69–72, 1995.

31. Bucha E, Kossemehl A, Nowak G: Animal experimental studies on the pharmacokinetics of PEG-hirudin [abstract]. Ann Hematol I:A55, 1996.

32. Buchwald AB, Sandrock D, Unterberg C, et al: Platelet and fibrin deposition on coronary stents in mini-pigs: effect of hirudin versus heparin. J Am Coll Cardiol 21:249–254, 1993.

33. Burchenal JEB, Marks DS, Schweiger MJ, et al: Hirulog does not prevent restenosis after coronary angio-plasty [abstract]. Circulation 92:2913, 1995.

34. Callas D, Bacher P, Iqbal O, et al: Fibrinolytic compromise by simultaneous administration of site-directed inhibitors of thrombin. Thromb Res 74:193–205, 1994.

35. Callas D, Fareed J: Comparative pharacology of site directed antithrombin agents. Implication in drug development. Thromb Haemost 74:473–481, 1995.

36. Callas D, Iqbal O, Fareed J: Comparison of the anticoagulant activities of thrombin inhibitors as assessed by thrombelastographic analysis. Semin Thromb Hemost 21:76–79, 1995.

37. Callas DD, Bacher P, Fareed J: Studies on the thrombogenic effects of recombinant tissue factor: in vivo versus ex vivo findings. Semin Thromb Hemost 21: 166–176, 1995.

38. Callas DD, Fareed J: Direct inhibition of protein Ca by site directed thrombin inhibitors: Implications in anticoagulant and thrombolytic therapy. Thromb Res 78:457–460, 1995.

39. Callas DD, Hoppensteadt D, Fareed J: Comparative studies on the anticoagulant and protease generation inhibitory actions of newly developed site-directed thrombin inhbitory drugs: Efegatran, argatroban, hirulog, and hirudin. Semin Thromb Hemost 21:177–183, 1995.

40. Callas DD, Hoppensteadt D, Iqbal O, Fareed J: Ecarin clotting time (ECT) is a reliable method for the monitoring of hirudins, argatroban, efegatran and related drugs in therapeutic and cardiovascular indications [abstract]. Ann Hematol I: A58, 1996.

41. Callas DD, Iqbal O, Hopensteadt D, Fareed J: Fibrinolytic compromise by synthetic and recombinant thrombin inhibitors. Implications in the management of thrombotic disorders. Clin Appl Thromb Hemost 1:114–124, 1995.

42. Cannon CP, Braunwald E: Hirudin: initial results in acute myocardial infarction, unstable angina and angioplasty. J Am Coll Cardio 25(Suppl 7):30S–37S, 1995.

43. Cannon CP, Maraganore JM, Loscalzo J: Anticoagulant effects of hirulog, a novel thrombin inhibitor, in patients with coronary artery disease. Am J Cardiol 71:778–782, 1993.

44. Carney DH, Glenn KC, Cunningham DD: Conditions which affect initiation of animal cell division by trypsin and thrombin. J Cell Physiol 95:13–33, 1978.

45. Carney DH, Redin W, McCroskey L: Role of high-affinity thrombin receptors in postclotting cellular effects of thrombin. Semin Thromb Hemost 18:91–103, 1992.

46. Carney DH, Stiernberg J, Fenton JW II: Initiation of proliferative events by α-thrombin requires both receptor binding and enzymatic activity. J Cell Biochem 26:181–195, 1984.

47. Carteaux JP, Gast A, Tschopp TB, Roux S: Activated clotting time as an appropriate test to compare heparin and direct thrombin inhibitors such as hirudin or Ro 46-6240 in experimental arterial thrombosis. Circulation 91:1568–1574, 1995.

48. Chamberlin JR, Lewis B, Leya F, et al: Successful treatment of heparin-associated thrombocytopenia and thrombosis using hirulog. Can J Cardiol 11:511–514, 1995.

49. Chang AC, Detwiler TC: The reaction of thrombin with platelet-derived nexin requires a secondary recognition site in addition to the catalytic site. Biochem Biophys Res Commun 177:1198–1204, 1991.

50. Chang JY, Ngai PK, Rink H, et al: The structural elements of hirudin which bind to the fibrinogen recognition site of thrombin are exclusively located within its acidic C-terminal tail. FEBS Lett 261:287–290, 1990.

51. Church FC, Noyes CM, Griffith MJ: Inhibition of chymotrypsin by heparin cofactor II. Proc Natl Acad Sci USA 82:6431–6434, 1985.

52. Church FC, Phillips JE, Woods JL: Chimeric Antithrombin Peptide. J. Biol Chem 266:11975–11979, 1991.

53. Cousins GR, Friedrichs GS, Sudo Y, et al: Orally efective CVS-1123 prevents coronary artery thrombosis in the conscious canine [abstract]. Circulation 92:1442, 1995.

54. Demers C, Ginsberg JS, Hirsh J, et al; Thrombosis in antithrombin-III-deficient persons. Report of a large kindred and literature review. Ann Intern Med 116:754–761, 1992.

55. Detwiler TC, Chang AC, Speziale MV, et al: Complexes of thrombin with proteins secreted by activated platelets. Semin Thromb Hemost 18:60–66, 1992.

56. DiMaio J, Gibbs B, Munn D, et al: Bifunctional thrombin inhibitors based on the sequence of hirudin 45-65. J Biol Chem 265:21698–21703, 1990.

57. Dodt J, Kohler S, Schmitz T, Wilhelm B: Distinct binding sites of ala48-hirudin1-47 and Ala48-hirudin48-65 on alpha thrombin. J Biol Chem 265:713–718, 1990.

58. Dodt J, Machleidt W, Seemüller U, et al: Isolation and characterization of hirudin isoinhibitors and sequence analysis of hirudin PA. Biol Chem Hoppe-Seyler 367:803–811, 1986.

59. Dodt J, Müller HP, Seemüller U, Chang JY: The complete amino acid sequence of hirudin, a thrombin specific inhibitor. FEBS Lett 165:180–184, 1984.

60. Edmunds LH: HIT, HITT, and desulfatorhirudin: Look before you leap. J Thorac Cardiovascu Surg 110:1–3, 1995.

61. Eichler P, Greinacher A; Anti-hirudin antibodies induced by recombinant hirudin in the treatment of patients with heparin-induced thrombocytopenia (HIT) [abstract]. Ann Hematol I:A4, 1996.

62. Ekman S, Baur M, Eriksson BI, et al: An effective and safe prophylaxis of thromboembolic complications in patients undergoing a primary total hip replacement with recombinant hirudin, TMRevasc, CIBA [abstract], Ann Hematol I:A55, 1996.

63. Eriksson Bi, Ekman S, Kälebo P, et al: Prevention of deep-vein thrombosis after total hip replacement: Direct thrombin inhibition with recombinant hirudin, CGP 39393. Lancet 347:635–639, 1996.

64. Eriksson BI, Kälebo P, Ekman S, et al: The most effective and safe prophylaxis of thromboembolic complications in patients undergoing total hip replacement with recombinant hirudin, TMRevasc, (CGP 39393), Ciba [abstract]. Circulation 92:3294, 1995.

65. Eriksson BI, Kälebo P, Ekman S, et al: Direct thrombin inhibition with rec-hirudin CGP 39393 as prophylaxis of thromboembolic complications after total hip replacement. Thromb Haemost 72:227–231, 1994.

66. Eriksson BI, Lindbratt S, Toerholm C, et al: Recombinant hirudin, CGP 39393 15 mg (TMRevasc-Ciba), is the most effective and safe prophylaxis of thromboembolic comlications in patients undergoing total hip replacement. Thromb Haemost 73:1093, 1995.

67. Eriksson UG, Renberg L, Vedin C, Strimfors M: Pharmacokinetics of inogatran, a new low molecular weight thrombin inhibitor, in rats and dogs. Thromb Haemost. 73(6):1318, 1995.

68. Esmail AF, Dupe RJ, Goddard M, et al: Antithrombotic and anticoagulant properties of novel peptide boronic acid thrombin inhibitors: Comparison with heparin and hirudin. Thromb Haemost 73:1318, 1995.

69. Esmon CT: The regulation of natural anticoagulant pathways. Science 235:1348–1352, 1987.

70. Esmon NL, DeBault LE, Esmon CT: Proteolytic formation and properties of γ-caroxyglutamic acid-domainless protein C. J Biol Chem 258:5548–5553, 1983.

71. Esslinger HHU, Haas S, Lassmann A, et al: Phase I results on PEG-hirudin (LU 57291), a safe and effective anticoagulant with prolonged activity [abstract]. Thromb Haemost 73:1452, 1995.

72. Fareed J, Callas DD: Pharmacological aspects of thrombin inhibitors: A developmental perspective. Vessels 1:15–24, 1995.
73. Fareed J, Hoppensteadt D, Calabria R, et al: Studies on the anticoagulant and antiprotease actions of a synthetic tripeptide (D-MePhe-Pro-Arg-H), recombinant hirudin and heparin. Implications in the development of newer antithrombotic drugs. Thromb Haemost 65:1288, 1991.
74. Fareed J, Hoppensteadt D, Walenga JM, Bick RL: Current trends in the development of anticoagulant and antithrombotic drugs. Med Clin North Am 78:713–731, 1994.
75. Fareed J, Kindel G, Kumar A: Modulation of smooth muscle responses by serine proteases and related enzymes. Semin Thromb Hemost 12:265–276, 1986.
76. Fareed J, Messmore HL, Kindel G, Balis JU: Inhibition of serine proteases by low molecular weight peptides and their derivatives. Ann NY Acad Sci 370:765–784., 1981.
77. Fareed J, Pifarre R, Leya F, et al: Platelet factor 4 and antithrombin-III are not the sole determinants of heparinization responses. Circulation 90:968, 1994.
78. Fareed J, Walenga JM, Hoppensteadt D, et al: neutralization of recombinant hirudin: some practical considerations. Semin Thromb Hemost 17:137–144, 1991.
79. Fareed J, Walenga JM, Hoppensteadt DA, et al: Pharmacologic profiling of defibrotide in experimental models. Semin Thromb Hemost 14:27–37, 1988.
80. Fareed J, Walenga JM, Iyer L, et al: An objective perspective on recombinant hirudin: A new anticoagulant and antithrombotic agent. Blood Coagul Fibrinol 2(1):135–147, 1991.
81. Fareed J, Walenga JM, Kumar A, Rock A: A modified stasis thrombosis model to study the antithrombotic actions of heparin and its fractions. Semin Thromb Hemost 11:155–175, 1985.
82. Fareed J, Walenga JM, Leya F, Bacher P, et al: Some objective considerations for the use of heparins and recombinant hirudin in percutaneous transluminal coronary angioplasty. Semin Thromb Hemost 17:455–470, 1991.
83. Fenton II JW, Fasco MJ, Stackrow AB, et al: Human thrombins. Production, evaluation, and properties of α-thrombin. J Biol Chem 252:3587–3598, 1977.
84. Fenton II JW: Structural regions and bioregulatory functions of thrombin. In Boynton AL, Leffert HL (eds): Cell Proliferation: Recent Advances. New York, Academic Press, 1986.
85. Fenton JW II, Bing DH: Thrombin active-site regions. Semin Thromb Hemost 12:200–208, 1986.
86. Fenton JW II, Landis BH, Walz DA, et al: Human thrombins. In Lundblad RL, Fenton II JW, Mann KG (eds): Chemistry and Biology of Thrombin. Ann Arbor, MI, Ann Arbor Science, 1977, pp 43–70.
87. Fenton JW II, Olson TA, Zabinski MP, et al: Anion-binding exosite of human α-thrombin and fibin(ogen) recognition. Biochemistry 27:7106–7112, 1988.
88. Fenton JW II: Regulation of thrombin generation and functions. Semin Thromb Hemost 14:234–240, 1988.
89. Fenton JW II: Thrombin bioregulatory functions. Adv Clin Enzymol 6:186–193, 1988.
90. Fenton JW II: Thrombin. Ann NY Acad Sci 485:5–15, 1986.
91. French P, Finet G, Ovize M, et al: Sustained antithrombotic effects of CX-397, a new recombinant hirudin after intravenous bolus in patients undergoing coronary angiography. Circulation 92(8):2324, 1995.
92. Flather M, for the Organization to Assess Strategies for Ischaemic Syndromes (OASIS) Pilot Study Investigators: Recombinant hirudin in the treatment of patients with unstable angina pectoris: Preliminary results of the OASIS pilot study [abstract]. Ann Hematol I: A92, 1996.
93. Fourrier F, Huart JJ, Runge I, et al: Results of a double-blind, placebo-controlled trial of antithrombin III concentrates in septic shock with DIC. In Müller-Berghaus G, Madlener K, Blombäck M, et al (eds): DIC: Pathogenesis, Diagnosis and Therapy of Disseminated Intravascular Fibrin Formation. Amsterdam, Excerpta Medica, 1993, pp 221–226.
94. Francis CW, Pellegrini VD Jr, Harris CM, et al: Prophylaxis of venous thrombosis following total hip and total knee replacement using antithrombin III and heparin. Semin Hematol 28:39–45, 1991.
95. Furie B, Bing DH, Feldman RJ, et al: Computer-generated modes of blood coagulation factor Xa, IXa, and thrombin based upon structural homology with other serine proteases. J Biol Chem 257:3875–3882, 1982.
96. Gast A, Tschopp TB, Baumgartner HR: Thrombin plays a key role in late platelet thrombus growth and/or stability. Effect of a specific thrombin inhibitor on thrombogenesis induced by aortic subendothelium exposed to flowing rabbit blood. Arterioscler Thromb Vasc Biol 14:1466–1474, 1994.
97. Gast A, Tscopp TB, Schmid G, Hilpert K, Ackermann J: Inhibition of clot-bound and free (fluid phase thrombin) by a novel synthetic thrombin inhibitor (Ro 46-6240), recombinant hirudin and heparin in human plasma. Blood Coagul Fibrinol 5:879–887, 1994.
98. Geratz JD, Tidwell RR: The development of competitive reversible thrombin inhibitors. In Lundblad RL, Fenton JW, Mann KG (eds): Chemistry and Biology of Thrombin, Ann Arbor, MI, Ann Arbor Science, 1977, pp 179–196.
99. Gerrard DJ, Dupe R, Esmail A, et al: Prevention of thrombosis in a pig coronary model, comparison of the efficacy of a specific thrombin inhibitor TRI50b with aspirin. Thromb Haemost 73:1307, 1995.
100. Gilboa N, Villannueva GB, Fenton JW II: Inhibition of fibrinolytic enzymes by thrombin inhibitors. Enzyme 40:144–148, 1988.

101. Ginsberg JS, Nurmohamed MT, Gent M, et al: Use of hirulog in the prevention of venous thrombosis after major hip or knee surgery. Circulation 90:2385–2389, 1994.
102. Glusa E, Daum J, Noeske-Jungblut C: Inhibition of thrombin-mediated cellular effects by triabin [abstract]. Ann Hematol I:A53, 1996.
103. Goddard M, Esmail AF, Dupe RJ, et al: Pharmacokinetics and bioavailability of a novel direct thrombin inhibitor in rats following intravenous and intraduodenal administration. Thromb Haemost 73:1308, 1995.
104. Gold HK, Torres FW, Garabedian HD, et al: Evidence for rebound coagulation phenomenon after cessation of a 4-hour infusion of a specific thrombin inhibitor in patients with unstable angina pectoris. J Am Coll Cardiol 21:1039–1047, 1993.
105. Greinacher A, Völpel H, Pötzsch B: Recombinant hirudin in the treatment of patients with heparin-associated thrombocytopenia type II (HAT) [abstract]. Ann Hematol I:A92, 1996.
106. Griffith MJ: Kinetics of the heparin-enhanced antithrombin III/thrombin reaction. Evidence for a template model for the mechanism of action of heparin. J Biol Chem 257:7360–7365, 1982.
107. Grutter MG, Priestle JP, Rahuel J, et al: Crystal structure of the thrombin-hirudin complex: a novel mode of serine protease inhibition. EMBO J 9:2361–2365, 1990.
108. Gurwitz D, Cunningham DD: Thrombin modulates and reverses neuroblastoma neurite outgrowth. Proc Natl Acad Sci USA 85:3440–3444, 1988.
109. Gustafsson D, Elg M, Lenfors S, et al: Effects of inogatran, a new low molecular weight thrombin inhibitor, on rat models of thrombosis. Thromb Haemost 73:1319, 1995.
110. Hara T, Iwamoto M, Ishihara M, Tomikawa M: Preventive effect of argatroban on ellagic acid-induced cerebral thromboembolism in rats. Haemostasis 24:351–357, 1994.
111. Hara T, Yokoyama A, Ishihara H, et al: DX-9065a, a new synthetic, potent anticoagulant and selective inhibitor for factor Xa. Thromb Haemost 71:314–319, 1994.
112. Harvey RP, Degryse E, Stefani L, et al: Cloning and expression of cDNA coding for the anticoagulant hirudin from the bloodsucking leech, *Hirudo medicinalis*. Proc Natl Acad Sci USA 83:1084–1088, 1986.
113. Hawkins RL, Seeds NW: Effect of proteases and their inhibitors on neurite outgrowth from neonatal mouse sensory ganglia in culture. Brain Res 398:63–70, 1986.
114. Herrmann JP, Serruys PW: Thrombin and antithrombotic therapy in interventional cardiology. Tex Heart Inst J 21:138–147, 1994.
115. Hijikata-Okunomiya A, Okamoto S: A strategy for a rational aproach to designing synthetic selective inhibitors. Semin Thromb Hemost 18:135–149, 1992.
116. Hilpert K, Ackermann J, Banner DW, et al: Design and synthesis of potent and highly selective thrombin inhibitors. J Med Chem 37:3889–3901, 1994.
117. Hofsteenge J, Taguchi H, Stone SR: Effect of thrombomodulin on the kinetics of the interaction of thrombin with substrate and inhibitors. Biochem J 237:243–251, 1986.
118. Hortin GL, Tollefsen DM, Benutto BM: Antithrombin activity of a peptide corresponding to residues 54–75 of heparin cofactor II. J Biol Chem 264:13979–13982.
119. Isaacs JD, Savion N, Gospodarociz D, et al: Covalent binding of thrombin to specific sites on corneal endothelial cells. J Am Chem Soc 20(2):398–403, 1981.
120. Jackson JV, Wilson HC, Growe VG, et al: Reversible tripeptide thrombin inhibitors as adjunctive agents to coronary thrombolysis: a comparison with heparin in a canine model of coronary artery thrombosis. J Cardiovasc Pharmacol 21:587–594, 1993.
121. Jaffe EA, Leung LLK, Nachman RL, et al: Cultured human fibroblasts synthesize and secrete thrombospondin and incorporate it into the extracellular matrix. Proc Natl Acad Sci USA 80:998–1002, 1983.
122. Jang IK, Gold HK, Leinbach RC, Fallon JT, Collen D: In vivo thrombin inhibition enhances and sustains arterial recanalization with recombinant tissue-type plasminogen activator. Cir Res 67:1552–1561, 1990.
123. Jeske W, Hoppensteadt D, Fareed J, Bermes E: Measurement of functional and immunologic levels of tissue factor pathway inhibitor. Some methodologic considerations. Blood Coagul Fibrinol 6:S73–S80, 1995.
124. Kaiser B, Hauptmann J, Weiss A, Markwardt F: Pharmacological characterisation of a new highly effective synthetic thrombin inhibitor. Biomed Biochim Acta 44:1201–1210, 1985.
125. Kajiyama Y, Murayama T, Nomura Y: Pertussis toxin-sensitive GTP-binding proteins may regulate phospholipase A2 in response to thrombin in rabbit platelets. Arch Biochem Biophys 274:200–208, 1989.
126. Kawai H, Umemura K, Nakashima M: Effects of argatroban on microthrombin formation and brain damage in the rat middle cerebral artery thrombosis model. Jpn J Pharacol 69:143–148, 1995.
127. Kettner C, Mersinger L, Knabb R: The selective inhibition of thrombin by peptides of boroarginine. J Biol Chem 265:18289–18297, 1990.
128. Kettner C, Shaw E: The selective inactivation of thrombin by peptides of chloromethyl ketone. In Lundblad RL, Fenton JW, Mann KG (eds): Chemistry and Biology of Thrombin. Ann Arbor, MI, Ann Arbor Science, 1977, pp 129–144.
129. Kikumoto R, Tamao Y, Ohkubo K, et al: Thrombin inhibitors. 2. Amide derivatives of Nα-substituted L-arginine. J Med Chem 23:830–836, 1980.
130. Klement P, Borm A, Hirsh J, et al: The effect of thrombin inhibitors on tissue plasminogen activator induced thrombolysis in a rat model. Thromb Haemost 68:64–68, 1992.

131. Klement P, Hirsh J, Maraganore J, Weitz J: The effect of thrombin inhibitors on tissue plasminogen activator-induced thrombolysis in a rat model. Thromb Haemost 65:735, 1991.
132. Knapp A, Degenhardt T, Dodt J: Hirudisins: hirudin-derived thrombin inhibitors with disintegrin activity. J Biol Chem 267:24230–24234, 1992.
133. Komatsu Y, Misaawa S, Sukesada A, Ohba Y, Hayashi H: CX-397, a novel recombinant hirudin analog having a hybrid sequence of hirudin variants-1 and 3. Biochem Biophys Res Commun 196:773–779, 1993.
134. Krstenansky JL, Owen TJ, Yates MT, Mao SJ: Design, synthesis and antithrombin activity for conformationally restricted analogs of peptide anticoagulants based on the C-terminal region of the leech peptide, hirudin. Biochim Biophys Acta 957:53–59, 1988.
135. Kubik MF, Stephens AW, Schneider D, et al: High-affinity RNA ligands to human α-thrombin. Nucl Acids Res 22:2619–2626, 1994.
136. Kumon K, Tanaka K, Nakajima N, et al: Anticoagulation with a synthetic thrombin inhibitor after cardiovascular surgery and for treatment of disseminated intravascular coagulation. Crit Care Med 12:1039–1043, 1984.
137. Kurfurst MM: Detection and molecular weight determination of polyethylene glycol-modified hirudin by staining after sodium dodecyl sulfate-polyacrylamide gel electrophoresis. Ann Biochem 200:244–248, 1992.
138. Kurz KD, Smith T, Shuman RT, Wilson A: Oral thrombin inhibitors (TIS) LY303496 and efegatran: a comparison in the rat [abstract]. Blood 86 (Suppl 1):919.
139. Lackman M, Geczy CL: Radioimmunoassay for the detection of active-site specific thrombin inhibitors in biological fluids. II: Heparin affects the binding of hirudin to α-thrombin. Thromb Res 63:609–616, 1991.
140. Lackman M, Hoad R, Kakakios A, Geczy CL: Radioimmunoassay for the detection of active-site specific thrombin inhibitors in biological fluids. I. Assay characteristics and quantitation of recombinant hirudin. Thromb Res 63:595–607, 1991.
141. Lange U, Lehr A, Nowak G: Biologically active metabolites of recombinant and PEG-hirudin in rat urine—isolation and biochemical characterization [abstract]. Ann Hematol I:A58, 1996.
142. Latham JA, Johnson R, Toole JJ: The application of a modified nucleotide in aptamer selection: novel thrombin aptamers contining 5-(1-pentynyl)-2'-deoxyuridine. Nucleic Acids Res 22:2817–2822, 1994.
143. Lawler J: The structural and functional properties of thrombospondin. Blood 67:1197–1209, 1986.
144. Lee LV, for the TIMI-6 Investigators. Initial experience with hirudin and streptokinase in acute myocardial infarction: results of the Thrombolysis in Myocardial Infarction (TIMI) 6 trial. Am J Cardiol 75:7–13, 1995.
145. Li WX, Kaplan AV, Grant GW, et al: A novel nucleotide-based thrombin inhibitor inhibits clot-bound thrombin and reduces arterial platelet thrombus formation. Blood 83:677–682.
146. Lidon RM, Théroux P, Bonan R, et al. A pilot early angiographic patency study using a direct thrombin inhibitor as adjunctive therapy to stretptokinase in acute myocardial infarction. Circulation 89:1567–1572, 1994.
147. Lindahl AK, Abilgaard U, Larsen ML, et al: extrinsic pathway inhibitor (EPI) and the post-heparin anticoagulant effect in tissue thromboplastin-induced coagulation. Thromb Res 64:155–168, 1991.
148. Macaya RF, Schultze P, Smith FW, et al: Thrombin-binding DNA aptamer forms a unimolecular quadruplex structure in solution. Proc Natl Acad Sci USA 90:3745–3749, 1993.
149. Maki M, Terao T, Ikehouse T, et al: Clinical evaluation of antithrombin III concentrate (BI 6.013) for disseminated intravascular coagulation in obstetrics: well controlled multicenter trial. Gynecol Obstet Invest 23:230–240, 1987.
150. Malik AB, Lo SK, Bizios R: Thrombin-induced alterations in endothelial permeability. Ann NY Acad Sci 485:293–309, 1986.
151. Maraganore JM, Bourdon P, Jablonski J, et al: Design and characterization of hirulogs: A novel class of bivalent peptide inhibitors of thrombin. Biochemistry 29:7095–7101, 1990.
152. Maraganore JM, Bourdon P, Jablonski J, et al: Design and characterization of hirulogs: A novel class of bivalent peptide inhibitors of thrombin. Biochemistry 29:7095–7101, 1990.
153. Markwardt F, Nowak G, Hoffmann J: Comparative studies on thrombin inhibitors in experimental microthrombosis. Thromb Haemost 49:235–237, 1983.
154. Markwardt F, Nowak G, Stürzebecher J: Clinical pharmacology of recombinant hirudin. Haemostasis 21(suppl 1): 133–136, 1991.
155. Markwardt F, Sturzebecher J: Inhibitors of trypsin and trypsin-like enzymes with a physiological role. In Sandler M, Smith HJ (eds): Design of Enzyme Inhibitors as Drugs. Oxford University Press, 1989, pp 619–649.
156. Markwardt F: Development of hirudin as an antithrombotic agent. Semin Thromb Hemost 15:269–282, 1989.
157. Martin U, Fischer SS, Sponer G: Influence of heparin and systemic lysis on coronary blood flow after reperfusion induced by the novel recombinant plasminogen activator B < 06.022 in a canine model of coronary thrombosis. J Am Coll Cardiol 22:914–920, 1993.
158. Martin U, Spooner G, Strein K: Hirudin and sulotroban improve coronary blood flow after reperfusion induced by the novel recombinant plasminogen activator BM 06.22 in a canine model of coronary artery thrombosis. Int J Hematol 56:143–153, 1992.

159. Maruyama I, Salem HH, Majerus PW: Coagulation factor Va binds to human umbilical vein endothelial cells and accelerates protein C activation. J Clin Invest 74:224–230, 1984.
160. Maruyama I: Synthetic anticoagulant. Jpn J Clin Hematol 31:776–781, 1990.
161. Matsuo T, Kario K, Chikahira Y, et al: Treatment of heparin-induced thrombocytopenia by use of argatroban, a synthetic thrombin inhibitor. Br J Haematol 82:627–629, 1992.
162. Matsuo T, Kario K, Kodama K, Okamoto S. Clinical applications of the synthetic thrombin inhibitor, argatroban (MD-805). Semin Thromb Hemost 18:155–160, 1992.
163. Matsuo T, Kario K, Sakamoto S, et al: Hereditary heparin cofactor II deficiency and coronary artery disease. Thromb Res 65:495, 1992.
164. McGowan EB, Detwiler TC: Modified platelet response to thrombin. Evidence of two types of receptors or coupling mechanisms. J Biol Chem 261:739–746, 1986.
165. Mellott MJ, Connolly TM, York SJ, Bush LR: Prevention of reocclusion by MCI-9038, a thrombin inhibitor, following t-PA-induced thrombolysis in a canine model of femoral arterial thrombosis. Thromb Haemost 64:526–534, 1990.
166. Menache D. Replacement therapy in patients with hereditary antithrombin III deficiency. Semin Hematol 28:31–38, 1991.
167. Molhoek GP, Laarman GJ, Lok DJA, et al: Effects of recombinant hirudin on early, complete and sustained coronary patency in patients with acute myocardial infarction treated with streptokinase (final results on the HIT-SK study) [abstract]. Ann Hematol I:A91, 1996.
168. Mosesson MW, Church WR, DiOrio JP, et al: Structural model of factor V and Va based on scanning transmission electron microscope images and mass analysis. J Biol Chem 265:8863–8868, 1990.
169. Neises B, Tarnus C: Thrombin inhibition by the tripeptide trifuloromethyl ketone D-Phe-Pro-Arg-CF$_3$ (MDL 73756). Thromb Haemost 65:1290, 1991.
170. Nesheim ME: A simple rate law that describes the kinetics of heparin-catalyzed reaction between antithrombin III and thrombin. J Biol Chem 258:14708–14717, 1983.
171. Neuhaus KL, von Essen R, Tebbe U, et al: Safety observations from the pilot phase of the randomized r-hirudin for improvement of thrombolysis (HIT-III) study: A study of the Arbeitsgemeinschaft Leitender Kardiologischer Krankenhausartze (ALKK). Circulation 90:1638–1642, 1994.
172. Noe G, Hofsteenge J, Rovelli G, Stone SR: The use of sequence-specific antibodies to identify a secondary binding site in thrombin. J Biol Chem 263:11729–11735, 1988.
173. Noeske-Jungblut C, Haendler B, Donner P, et al: Triabin, a highly potent exosite inhibitor of thrombin. J Biol Chem 270:28269–28634, 1995.
174. Nowak G, Bucha E, Brauns I, Butti A: The use of r-hirudin as anticoagulant in regular haemodialysis in an HAT-II patient over a long period [abstract], Ann Hematol I: A56, 1996.
175. Ofosu FA, Fenton JW II, Maraganore J, et al: Inhibition of the amplification reactions of blood coagulation by site-specific inhibitors of α-thrombin. Biochem J 283 (Pt 3):893–897, 1992.
176. Okamoto S, Kinjo K, Hijikata A, et al: Thrombin inhibitors. 1. Ester derivatives of Nα-(Arylsulfonyl)-arginine. J Med Chem 23:827–830, 1980.
177. Oshiro T, Kanbayashi J, Kosaki G: Antithrombotic therapy of patient with peripheral arterial reconstruction-clinical study on MD805. Blood Vessel 14:216–218, 1983.
178. Owen J: Antithrombin III replacement therapy in pregnancy. Semin Hematol 28:46–52, 1991.
179. Owen TJ, Krstenansky JL, Yates MT, Mao SJ: N-terminal requirements of small peptide anticoagulants based on hirudin54–65. J Med Chem 31:1009–1011, 1988.
180. Paborsky LR, McCurdy SN, Griffin LC, et al: The single-stranded DNA aptamer binding-site of human thrombin. J Biol Chem 268:20808, 1993.
181. Parent F, Bridey F, Dreyfus M, et al: Treatment of severe venous thromboembolism with intravenous Hirudin (HBW 023): an open pilot study. Thromb Haemost 70:386–388, 1993.
182. Parker KA, Tollefsen DM: The protease specificity of heparin cofactor II. Inhibition of thrombin generated during coagulation. J Biol Chem 260:3501–3505, 1985.
183. Petersen TE, Roberts HR, Sottrup-Jensen L, Magnusson S: Primary structure of hirudin, a thrombin-specific inhibitor. In Peters H(ed): Peptides of the Biological Fluids. Oxford, Pergamon, 1976, pp 145–149.
184. Phillips DR, Charo IF, Parise LV, Fitzgerald LA: The platelet membrane glycoprotein IIb-IIIa complex. Blood 71:831–843, 1988.
185. Plow EF, Ginsberg MH: Cellular adhesion: GPIIb-IIIa as a prototypic adhesion receptor. Prog Hemost Thromb 9:117–156, 1989.
186. Pomerantz MW, Owen WG: A catalytic role of heparin. Evidence for a ternary complex of heparin cofactor thrombin and heparin. Biochim Biophys Acta 535:66–77, 1978.
187. Pötzsch B, Greinacher A, Riess FC, et al: Recombinant hirudin as anticoagulant in cardiac surgery: experiences with eleven patients [abstract]. Ann Hematol I: A4, 1996.
188. Pötzsch B, Iversen S, Riess FC, et al: Recombinant hirudin as an anticoagulant in open-heart surgery: A case report. Ann Hematol 68:A53, 1994.
189. Riess FC, Löwer C, Seelig C, et al: Recombinant hirudin as a new anticoagulant during cardiac operations instead of heparin: successful for aortic valve replacement in man. J Thorac Cardiovasc Surg 110:265–267, 1995.

190. Rübsamen K, Eschenfelder V: Effect of recombinant hirudin (LU 52369) on reocclusion rates after thrombolysis in rabbits. Haemostasis 21(Suppl 1): 93–98, 1991.
191. Ruoslahti E, Pierschbacher MD: New perspectives in cell adhesion. RGD and integrins. Science 238:491–497, 1987.
192. Rydel TJ, Ramachandran KG, Tulinsky A, et al: The structure of a complex of recombinant hirudin and human α-thrombin. Science 249:277–280, 1990.
193. Scharf M, Engels J, Tripier D: Primary structures of new "iso-hirudins". FEBS Lett 255:105–110, 1989.
194. Schiele F, Eriksson H, Wallmark A, et al, on behalf of the International Multicentre Hirudin Study Group. A multicentre dose-ranging study of subcutaneous recombinant hirudin in the treatment of deep vein thrombosis [abstract]. Circulation 92:2325.
195. Schiele F, Vuillemenot A, Kramarz P, et al: Use of recombinant hirudin as antithrombotic treatment in patients with heparin-induced thrombocytopenia. Am J Hematol 50:20-25, 1995.
196. Schneider J: Heparin and the thrombin inhibitor argatroban enhance fibrinolysis by infused or bolus-injected saruplase (r-scu-PA) in rabbit femoral artery thrombosis. Thromb Res 64:677–689, 1991.
197. Seiler SM, Goldenberg HJ, Michel IM, et al: Multiple pathways of thrombin-induced platelet activation differentiated by desensitization and a thrombin exosite inhibitor. Biochem Biophys Res Commun 181:636–643, 1991.
198. Seiler SM, Peluso M, Michel IM, et al: Inhibition of thrombin and SFLLR-peptide stimulation of platelet aggregation, phospholipase A2 and Na+/H+ exchange by a thrombin receptor antagonist. Biochem Pharmacol 49:519–528, 1995.
199. Serruys PW, Herrman JP, Simon R, et al, for the HELVETICA Investigators. A comparison of hirudin with heparin in the prevention of restenosis after coronary angioplasty. N Engl J Med 333:757–763, 1995.
200. Sie P, Bezeaud A, Dupouy D, Archipoff G, et al: An acquired antithrombin autoantibody directed toward the catalytic center of the enzyme. J Clin Invest 88:290–296, 1991.
201. Siess W, Weber PC, Lapetina EG: Activation of phospholipase C is dissociated from arachidonate metabolism during platelet shape change induced by thrombin or platelet-activating factor. J Biol Chem 259: 8286–8292, 1984.
202. Silk ST, Clejan S, Witkom K: Evidence of GTP-binding protein regulation of phospholipase A2 activity in isolated human platelet membranes. J Biol Chem 264:21466–21469, 1989.
203. Sitko GR, Ramjit DR, Stabilito II, et al: Conjunctive enhancement of enzymatic thrombolysis and prevention of thrombotic reocclusion with the selective factor Xa inhibitor, tick anticoagulant peptide. Circulation 85:805–815, 1992.
204. Sonder SA, Fenton II JW: Proflavin binding within the fibrinopeptide groove adjacent to the catalytic site of human α-thrombin. Biochemistry 23:1818–1823, 1984.
205. Sonder SA, Fenton II JW: Thrombin specificity with tripeptide chromogenic substrates: comparison of human and bovine thrombins with and without fibrinogen clotting activities. Clin Chem 32:934–937, 1986.
206. Stemberger A, Schmidmaier E, Beilharz C, et al: Rendering stents blood compatible through degradable coatings with incorporated anticoagulants [abstract]. Ann Hematol I: A30, 1996.
207. Strony J, Ahmed WH, Meckel CR, et al, on behalf of the Hirulog Angioplasty Study Investigators: Clinical evidence for thrombin rebound after stopping heparin but not hirulog [abstract]. Circulation 92:2915, 1995.
208. Strony J, Bittl JA, Deutsch E, et al: Hirulog vs. heparin during percutaneous transluminal coronary angioplasty in patients with post-infarction angina: results of the myocardial infarction arm of the Hirulog Angioplasty Trial [abstract]. J Am Coll Cardiol 25:357A, 1995.
209. Stüber W, Kosina H, Heimburger N: Synthesis of a tripeptide with a C-terminal nitrile moiety and the inhibition of proteinases. Int J Pept Protein Res 31:63–70, 1988.
210. Stürzebecher J, Markwardt F, Voigt B, et al: Cyclic amides of Nα-arylsulfonylaminoacylated 4-amidinophaenylalanine-tight binding inhibitors of thrombin. Thromb Res 29:635–642, 1983.
211. Suzuki S, Sakamoto S, Adachi K, et al: Effect of argatroban on thrombus formation during acute coronary occlusion after balloon angioplasty. Thromb Res 77:369–373, 1995.
212. Syed S, Sheffield WP: Maintenance of tight-binding inhibition of hirudin fused to albumin via its corboxy- but not amino-terminus [abstract]. Blood 86(Suppl 1):358a, 1995.
213. Tamao Y, Yamamoto T, Hirata T, et al: Effect of argipidine (MD-805) on blood coagulation. Jpn Pharmacol Ther 14:869–874, 1986.
214. Tamao Y, Yamamoto T, Kimuoto R, et al: Effect of a selective thrombin inhibitor MCI-9038 on fibrinolysis in vitro and in vivo. Thromb Haemost 56:28–34, 1986.
215. Tapparelli C, Metternich R, Ehrhardt C, Cook NS: Synthetic low-molecular weight thrombin inhibitors: molecular design and pharmacological profile. Trends Pharmacol Sci 14:366–376, 1993.
216. Tapparelli C, Metternich R, Ehrhardt C, et al: In vitro and in vivo characterization of a neutral boron-containing thrombin inhibitor. J Biol Chem 268:4734–4741, 1993.
217. Teger-Nilsson AC, Eriksson U, Gustafsson D, et al: Phase I studies on inogatran, a new selective thrombin inhibitor [abstract]. J Am Coll Cardiol 117A, 1995.
218. Teger-Nilsson AC, Gyzander E, Andersson S, et al: In vitro properties of inogatran, a new selective low molecular weight inhibitor of thrombin [abstract]. Thromb Haemost 73:1325, 1995.

219. Théroux P, Lidon R: Anticoagulants and their use in acute ischemic syndromes. In Topol EJ (ed): Textbook of Interventional Cardiology. Philadelphia, W.B. Saunders, 1994, pp 23–45.
220. Tonomura S, Kikumoto R, Tamao Y, et al: A novel series of synthetic thrombin inhibitors. II. Relationships between structure of modified OM-inhibitors and thrombin inhibitory effect. Kobe J Med Sci 26:1–9, 1980.
221. Topol EJ, Bonan R, Jewitt D, et al: Use of a direct antithrombin, hirulog, in place of heparin during coronary angioplasty. Circulation 87:1622–1629, 1993.
222. Topol EJ: Novel antithrombotic approaches to coronary artery disease. Am J Cardiol 75:27B–33B, 1995.
223. van Beusekom HM, Serruys PW, van der Giessen WJ: Coronary stent coatings. Coron Artery Dis 5:590–596, 1994.
224. Verbeuren TJ, Rupin A, Simonet S, et al: Anti-thrombotic properties of S 18326, a new potent orally active tripeptide boronic acid thrombin inhibitor. Thromb Haemost 73:1310, 1995.
225. Verstraete M, Zoldhelyi P: Novel antithrombotic drugs in development. Drugs 49:856–884, 1995.
226. Verstraete M: Desirudin. Review of Its Pharmacology and Prospective Clinical Uses. Norwich, GB, Royal Society of Medicine Press, 1995.
227. Vlasuk GP, Demsey EM, Oldeschulte GL, et al: Evaluation of a novel small protein inhibitor of blood coagulation factor Xa (rNAP-5) in animal models of thrombosis [abstract]. Circulation 92:3287, 1995.
227a. Vu et al. 1991.
228. Wallace A, Dennis S, Hofsteenge J, Stone SR: Contribution of the N-terminal region of hirudin to its interaction with thrombin. Biochemistry 28:10079–10084, 1989.
229. Weitz JI, Califf RM, Ginsberg JS, et al: New antithrombotics. Chest 108:471S–485S, 1995.
230. Willerson JT, Cascells W: Thrombin inhibitors in unstable angina: rebound or continuation of angina after argatroban withdrawal? J Am Coll Cardiol 21:1048–1051, 1993.
231. Wilson A, Smith T, Shuman RT, Kurz KD: Antithrombotic efficacy of an oral thrombin inhibitor (TI) in a conscious rat model of deep venous thrombosis (DVT) with and without aspirin (ASA) [abstract]. Blood 86(Suppl 1):91a, 1995.
232. Witting JI, Bourdon P, Brezniak DV, et al: Thrombin-specific inhibition by and slow cleavage of hirulog-1. Biochem J 283(Pt 3):737–743, 1992.
233. Yasuda T, Gold HK, Yaoita H, et al: Comparative effects of aspirin, a synthetic thrombin inhibitor and a monoclonal antiplatelet glycoprotein IIb/IIIa antibody on coronary artery reperfusion, reocclusion and bleeding with recombinant tissue-type plasminogen activator in a canine preparation. J Am Coll Cardiol 16:714–722, 1990.
234. Yonekawa Y, Handa H, Okamoto S, et al: Treatment of cerebral infarction in the acute stage with synthetic antithrombin MD805: Clinical study among multiple institutions. Nippon Geka Hokan 55:711–726, 1986.
235. Zawilska K, Zozulinska M, Turowiecka Z, et al: The effect of a long-acting recombinant hirudin (PEG-hirudin) on experimental disseminated intravascular coagulation (DIC) in rabbits. Thromb Res 69:315–320, 1993.
236. Zehnder JL, Leung LL: Develoment of antibodies to thrombin and factor V with recurrent bleeding in a patient exposed to topical bovine thrombin. Blood 76:2011–2016, 1990.
237. Zoldhelyi P, Bichler J, Owen WG, et al: Persistent thrombin generation in humans during specific thrombin inhibition with hirudin. Circulation 90:2671–2678, 1994.
238. Zoldhelyi P, Janssens S, Lefèvre G, et al, for the GUSTO-2A Investigators. Effects of heparin and hirudin (CGP 39393) on thrombin generation during thrombolysis for acute myocardial infarction [abstract]. Circulation 92:3555, 1995.

CHAPTER 22

Comparative Pharmacology of Heparin and Newer Antithrombin Drugs

DEMETRA D. CALLAS, Ph.D.
JAWED FAREED, Ph.D.

Because thrombin plays a key role in the development of various thrombotic conditions (e.g., stroke, myocardial infarction, pulmonary embolism, hypercoagulable states), it is the primary biochemical and pharmacologic target for developing newer antithrombotic drugs. One of the hypotheses underlying this approach is that sole inhibition of thrombin at blood and vascular sites is sufficient for the control of thrombogenesis and cellular activation processes. This central question is addressed by determining the relative inhibitory effects of four agents in the control of thrombogenesis: recombinant (r) hirudin, a monospecific inhibitor of thrombin; the synthetic tripeptide antithrombin agent, D-MePhe-Pro-Arg-H (efegatran sulfate); the peptidomimetic thrombin inhibitor, argatroban; and unfractionated heparin.

The newer agents are in various phases of clinical development. However, a comparative account of their biochemical and pharmacologic actions has not been available until now. Several studies indicate that they differ not only from heparin but also from each other in terms of mechanisms of action and pharmacologic properties. Because each of the thrombin inhibitors exhibits a specific structural and biochemical profile, this comparative study provides valuable information about their structure-activity relationships. Furthermore, a direct comparison with heparin provides additional insight into the role of endogenous macromolecular ligands and receptors in the mediation of the pharmacologic actions of the newly developed synthetic and recombinant agents.

Except for heparin, the agents included in this study are homogeneous, structurally characterized peptides or peptidomimetics, with pharmacologic actions that can be expressed in terms of molarity in relation to their interactions with endogenous enzymes, ligands, and other sites. Thus, their anticoagulant and antiprotease actions can be quantified and compared in defined terms. A direct comparison of these data with heparin also provides new information about mechanisms for mediation of their actions. This chapter presents an integrated account of the pharmacologic properties of several thrombin inhibitors that not only differ in structural characteristics but also exhibit varying degrees of specificity toward thrombin. The experimental approaches are designed to test the hypothesis that inhibition of thrombin may not be the sole determinant of their endogenous antithrombotic and hemorrhagic actions. It is likely that several other endogenous factors are responsible for their pharmacologic effects at both plasmatic and cellular sites.

Heparin is used as a reference anticoagulant. However, unlike the antithrombin agents studied, heparin produces its actions through potentiation of antithrombin and heparin cofactor II (HC-II). Furthermore, heparin exhibits polypharmacologic behavior and targets several plasmatic and vascular sites.[1,2] On the other hand, the synthetic and recombinant thrombin inhibitors represent chemically pure homogeneous agents.

In addition to the antithrombin-mediated inhibition of thrombin, heparin produces its overall antithrombotic effects through various mechanisms, whereas thrombin inhibitors are believed to act only through inhibition of thrombin. Thus, whereas heparin is capable of inhibiting other coagulation factors via antithrombin and HC-II, antithrombin agents antagonize the final stages of coagulation. In addition, heparin interacts ionically with the vascular lining to mediate a series of antithrombotic and profibrinolytic effects, such as release of tissue-type plasminogen activator (tPA), tissue factor pathway inhibitor (TFPI), and antithrombotic glycosaminoglycans from the endothelial lining.[3] Heparin also inhibits platelet functions, whereas antithrombin agents inhibit only thrombin-induced aggregation. On the other hand, most of the antithrombin agents are smaller in size and therefore capable of inhibiting clot-bound thrombin, which may be important in clot stabilization and its subsequent lysis.[4–6]

The main reason for clinical interest in antithrombin agents as a potential replacement for heparin is the fact that heparin has certain limitations, which include wide subject-to-subject variability, poor response, and allergic manifestations. One of the most serious adverse effects is heparin-induced thrombocytopenia (HIT), a deleterious immune reaction in which platelets aggregate in response to heparin to form white clots. Both heparin and the higher-molecular-weight thrombin inhibitors (e.g, hirudin) exhibit immunogenicity.[7] The clinical implications of the antihirudin antibodies are not clear at this time. Another reason for evaluating alternative antithrombotic agents is the limited subcutaneous bioavailability of heparin. Heparin has a subcutaneous bioavailability of 20–30%, whereas the thrombin inhibitors have a subcutaneous bioavailability of 80–100%. The oral bioavailability of the thrombin inhibitors ranges from 5–30%, whereas heparin has limited absorption (< 5%) by this route. Another major problem that needs to be addressed for all direct thrombin inhibitors is pharmacologic neutralization. Whereas heparin is readily neutralizable by protamine, no pharmacologic antagonist is currently available for any of the direct thrombin inhibitors.

Thrombin inhibitors have significant structural variations. Recombinant hirudin is a protein analog of natural hirudin with absolute specificity for thrombin. The tripeptide arginals, such as efegatran, are low-molecular-weight peptide derivatives with strong antithrombin potency. However, they also exhibit varying degrees of inhibitory actions toward other serine proteases. The peptidomimetic agent argatroban is a relatively weaker inhibitor of thrombin with a high degree of specificity.

Although the antiprotease spectrum of these agents has been extensively investigated,[8] little is known about their interactions with the cellular components of blood and vasculature. It is generally perceived that their antithrombin actions correlate directly with their in vivo pharmacologic effects. Theoretically, this hypothesis appears logical, although experimental validation is not available. The data reported in this chapter compare the different antithrombin agents in defined biochemical systems mimicking thrombogenic processes, and valid pharmacologic models are used to investigate their relative antithrombotic and bleeding actions. This research provides an integrated account of the biochemical and pharmacologic actions of antithrombin agents that may be useful in predicting their relative therapeutic index.

Despite extensive trials of the new thrombin inhibitors for appropriately chosen clinical indications, supportive studies of their biochemical and pharmacologic influences have been rather limited. As a result, problems with both safety and efficacy have been obvious during the newer clinical trials. The comparative studies reported in this chapter address the following key questions:

1. Is the sole inhibition of thrombin sufficient to control thrombogenesis in various thrombotic states?
2. Are thrombin inhibitors similar to heparin in their pharmacologic action?
3. Are there any differences among the currently available thrombin inhibitors?
4. Do thrombin inhibitors manifest non–thrombin-mediated pharmacologic actions?

MATERIALS AND METHODS

The tripeptide aldehyde D-MePhe-Pro-Arg-H•H_2SO_4 (GYKI 14766) was synthesized and obtained from the Institute for Drug Research (Budapest) in dried powder form and kept in refrigerated desiccators. The procedures for its synthesis and its chemical characterization have been described elsewhere.[9,10] The compound is currently marketed under the generic name efegatran sulfate by Eli Lily (Indiana). Argatroban, (2R,4R)-4-methyl-1-(N^2-((3 methyl-1,2,3,4-tetrahydro-8-quinolinyl)sulfonyl]-L-arginyl)]-2-piperidine carboxylic acid, consists of a mixture of the diastereoisomers 21-(R)- and 21-(S)-around the 2- and 4- positions of the piperidine ring in a ratio of approximately 65:35. The method for its synthesis was described by Okamoto and Hijikata.[11] Argatroban was obtained from Texas Biotechnology Corporation (Houston) in a 0.5-mg/ml solution. Light-resistant vials containing 10 mg of argatroban in 20-ml sterile isotonic solution were kept at room temperature. Recombinant hirudin variant 1 (rHV-1) was obtained from Knoll AG (Ludwigshafen, Germany) in lyophilized form in vials containing 20 mg/17,000 ATU/mg (batch no. 00300AL). It was produced in *Escherichia coli* as a single 65-amino acid polypeptide chain. The purity was > 95% with 0.5% moisture; the additives were succinate and sodium chloride. The molecular weight of rHV-1 is 6,963 Da. Unfractionated porcine mucosal heparin (PMH, lot no. RB 21055) was obtained from Sanofi-Choay Institut (Paris) in a white powder form as a sodium salt. The molecular weight for this compound is 10,700 Da. Its specific activity was found to be 160 U/mg. Aprotinin, a broad-spectrum serine protease inhibitor, was obtained in powder form from Pentapharm AG (Basel), 6,120 KIU mg. This Kunitz-type inhibitor consists of a single 58-amino acid polypeptide chain with a molecular weight of 6,512 Da. It is extracted from bovine lungs.[12]

Thrombin Titration Assay

An amidolytic method was used to determine the direct antithrombin actions of various thrombin inhibitors.[13] This assay as developed by Iyer and Fareed[14] for determination of the specific activity of r-hirudin and as a tool for quality assurance and determination of batch-to-batch variation. Because an antithrombin unit (ATU) is defined as the amount of thrombin inhibitor that inhibits 1 NIH unit of thrombin, the assay was developed so that the final concentration of thrombin in the system was 1 NIH unit/ml. Therefore, the amount of thrombin inhibitor that produces 100% inhibition of thrombin activity is designated as the potency of a thrombin inhibitor in ATU/mg. Alpha-thrombin (lot α375, specific activity 3,369 U/mg, protein concentration 0.68 mg/ml) was obtained from John Fenton II, M.D., New York State Department of Health (Albany). The amidolytic activity of thrombin was detected with the chromogenic substrate Spectrozyme TH (American Diagnostica, Greenwich, CT). Cleavage of this substrate by thrombin results in release of the yellow chromophore pNA.

Residual thrombin activity after incubation with a thrombin inhibitor was expressed as a percentage of the saline control by dividing the two respective rates of change in absorbance. The final concentration of the thrombin inhibitor was plotted against the residual thrombin activity.

The order of the regression analysis was the lowest that yielded regression coefficients > 0.99. The thrombin inhibitor concentration that produced 50% residual thrombin activity was the concentration that inhibited 0.5 NIH U/ml thrombin; therefore, the ATU of the thrombin inhibitor was twice that concentration. From these values, the relative antithrombin activity of each agent was calculated in terms of ATU/mg or ATU/nmole. Each concentration-response curve was repeated in triplicate on separate runs.

Thrombin Time in a Fibrinogen-based System

The fibrinogen-based thrombin time (TT) is a biochemically defined functional method for measuring the antithrombin effects of thrombin inhibitors, using human fibrinogen as the substrate. To perform the TT assay, a known amount of preformed human thrombin is added to the fibrinogen sample (containing varying amounts of a thrombin inhibitor), and the time required for clot formation measures the rate at which the fibrin is formed. TT measurements were carried out using a solution of human fibrinogen (IMCO, Stockholm, > 97% clottable fibrinogen) at 100 mg/dl; the solution was made in Owren's Veronal Buffer (Baxter Dade, Miami). Each of the thrombin inhibitors was diluted at various concentrations in the buffered fibrinogen solution. Fibrindex brand of human thrombin (lyophilized, 50 U/ampule, Ortho Diagnostic Systems, Raritan, NJ) at a concentration of 10 NIH U/ml in 0.025 M calcium chloride or sterile saline solution was used to initiate fibrinogen conversion to fibrin. In this procedure 100 μl of 10 U/ml human thrombin prewarmed at 37° C were added to 200 μl of fibrinogen prewarmed at 37° C for 3 minutes, and the clotting time was measured. Each concentration-response curve was repeated in triplicate on separate days.

Antithrombin and Anti-Xa Assays

The antithrombin and anti-Xa assays measure the concentration of thrombin inhibitor, assessing the inhibitory effect against the amidolytic activity of thrombin (Fibrindex) or factor Xa (0.65 ng/ml, Enzyme Research, South Bend, IN), as quantitated by a chromogenic substrate for thrombin (Spectrozyme TH) or factor Xa (Spectrozyme FXa, American Diagnostica, Greenwich, CT). These methods were initially described by Walenga et al.[15] After in vitro supplementation of normal human plasma with thrombin inhibitors at various concentrations and incubation with thrombin or factor Xa, the residual thrombin or factor Xa was detected amidolytically by the addition of the factor-specific chromogenic substrate. The thrombin and factor Xa inhibition by each agent at each concentration was calculated by the following formula:

% thrombin or factor Xa inhibition by agent = $[1 - \text{agent } \Delta A_{405}/\text{saline } \Delta A_{405}] \times 100$

The agent concentration vs. percent of inhibition graphs provided the basis for the calculation of the inhibitory concentration of 50% (IC_{50}) for each agent. Because the molecular weight of each agent is known, all data were converted to molar concentrations. Each concentration-response curve was repeated in triplicate on separate days.

Inhibitory Effects of Thrombin Inhibitors on Specific Serine Proteases

The following assays were designed to examine the inhibitory effects of thrombin inhibitors on other serine proteases, as measured by their amidolytic activity in purified systems.[16] The assays were conducted with a fast kinetic centrifugal analyzer (ACL 300 plus). Generally, each thrombin inhibitor was diluted in sterile saline solution at various concentrations. Ten microliters of the thrombin inhibitor were incubated with 100 μl of a known amount of the specific enzyme for 1 minute. At the end of the incubation period, 40 μl of chromogenic substrate specific for the enzyme were added, and the optical density was measured over a period of 999 seconds. The serine protease inhibition by each thrombin inhibitor at each concentration was calculated by the following formula:

% protease inhibition = $[1 - \text{inhibitor } \Delta A_{405}/\text{saline } \Delta A_{405}] \times 100$

The thrombin inhibitor concentration vs. percent of inhibition graphs provided the basis for the calculation of the inhibitory concentration of 50% (IC_{50}) for each agent. Because heparin has no direct serpin activities and its actions are mediated primarily through potentiation of antithrombin, the stock solution of heparin was made as 10 mg/ml in 1 U/ml of antithrombin (Kabi Vitrum, Stockholm). In addition to the thrombin inhibitors, aprotinin was also tested as a positive control for evaluation of the thrombolytic enzymes. Because the molecular weight of each agent is known, all data were converted to molar concentrations.

Inhibition of Chymotrypsin.   Chymotrypsin (Zolyse) from ox pancreas, 750 U.S.P. units/vial, was obtained from Ben Venue Laboratories (Bedford, OH). Chymotrypsin was used at a final assay concentration of 6.67 U/ml. The chromogenic substrate used to detect the activity of chymotrypsin was S-2586 (Kabi Diagnostica, Kabi Vitrum, Stockholm) at a final assay concentration of 0.27 mM.

Inhibition of Trypsin.   Porcine pancreatic trypsin (type II, crude; trypsin activity = 1740 BAEE units/mg; chymotrypsin activity = 1150 ATEE units/mg) was obtained from Sigma Chemical Company, St. Louis. Trypsin was used at a final assay concentration of 66.67 µg/ml. The chromogenic substrate used to detect the activity of trypsin was S-2423 (Kabi Diagnostica, Kabi Vitrum, Stockholm) at a final assay concentration of 0.27 mM.

Inhibition of Activated Protein C.   Activated protein C (APC) was obtained from the American Red Cross (Holland Laboratories, Rockville, MD) in lyophilized form, 5 mg/vial. The final assay concentration of APC was 62.5 µg/ml. S-2288 (Kabi Diagnostica, Kabi Vitrum, Stockholm) was the chromogenic substrate used to detect the activity of APC at a final assay concentration of 0.27 mM.

Inhibition of Glandular Kallikrein.   Pancreatic kallikrein (4.7 units/mg solid, 4.8 units/mg protein) was obtained from Sigma Chemical Company, St. Louis. Kallikrein was used at a final assay concentration of 0.67 mg/ml. The chromogenic substrate used to detect the activity of kallikrein was S-2303 (Kabi Diagnostica, Kabi Vitrum, Stockholm) at a final assay concentration of 0.27 mM.

Inhibition of Tissue Plasminogen Activator.   Tissue plasminogen activator (tPA) was obtained from Genentech, South San Francisco, CA (Activase, Alteplase, recombinant, 50 mg or 29 million IU/vial). The final assay concentration of tPA was 0.67 mg/ml. Spectrozyme TH was the chromogenic substrate used to detect tPA activity at a final assay concentration of 0.27 mM.

Inhibition of Urokinase.   A low-molecular-weight form of urokinase (Abbokinase, 250,000 IU/vial), acquired from human kidney cells by tissue culture, was obtained from Abbott Laboratories, North Chicago, IL. The final assay concentration of urokinase was 6,667 U/ml. The chromogenic substrate used to detect urokinase activity was S-2444 (Kabi Diagnostica, Kabi Vitrum, Stockholm) at a final assay concentration of 0.27 mM.

Inhibition of Plasmin.   Plasmin (6 nKat/vial) was obtained from Diagnostica Stago, Asnieres-sur-Seine, France. Plasmin was used at a final assay concentration of 1.2 nKat/ml. The chromogenic substrate used to detect the activity of plasmin was S-2251 (Kabi Diagnostica, Kabi Vitrum, Stockholm) at a final assay concentration of 0.27 mM.

Inhibition of Extrinsic and Intrinsic Activation Systems in Fibrinogen-deficient Human Plasma by Thrombin Inhibitors

Plasmatic methods developed by Kaiser et al.[17] were used to determine the inhibitory effects of various thrombin inhibitors on generation of thrombin and factor Xa after extrinsic activation of the coagulation cascade. Coagulation was initiated extrinsically or intrinsically, and the generated thrombin and factor Xa were measured amidolytically. The materials used were chromogenic substrate specific for thrombin (Spectrozyme TH), chromogenic substrate specific for factor Xa (Spectrozyme FXa), fibrinogen-deficient plasma (fibrinogen < 15 mg/dl, George King Biomedical, Overland Park, KS), extrinsic activator (lyophilized acetone-dehydrated, rabbit brain Thromboplastin C, Dade, Miami), and intrinsic activator (Actin, Dade, Miami). The instrument used was a fast kinetic centrifugal analyzer (ACL 300 plus). The procedure for the assays was as follows: each thrombin inhibitor at a specific concentration was incubated with fibrinogen-deficient plasma for 300 seconds, after which the chromogenic substrate (for either thrombin or factor Xa), mixed with either extrinsic or intrinsic activator, was added, and the optical density was measured for 999 seconds.

The inhibition of extrinsic or intrinsic thrombin and factor Xa generation by each thrombin inhibitor at each concentration was calculated by the following formula:

% thrombin or factor Xa generation inhibition = $[1 - \text{agent } \Delta A_{405}/\text{saline } \Delta A_{405}] \times 100$

The thrombin inhibitor concentration vs. percent of inhibition graphs provided the basis for the calculation of the IC_{50} for each thrombin inhibitor. Because the molecular weight of each agent is known, all data were converted to molar concentrations.

Anticoagulant Effects of Thrombin Inhibitors in Normal Human Pooled Plasma

Amidolytic methods based on intrinsic and extrinsic activation of plasma provide information about the effects of agents on the generation of thrombin and factor Xa, using the amidolytic activities of these factors. To study the functional inhibitory effects on clot formation or the anticoagulant effects of thrombin inhibitors and which pathways are inhibited most effectively, each agent was added in vitro to normal human pooled plasma (NHP) and tested in the global clotting tests described below. The tests were performed on a fibrometer (Becton, Dickinson and Company, Cockeysville, MD) according to the specifications by each of the manufacturers. NHP was obtained from the Loyola Blood Bank.

Prothrombin Time.   Prothrombin time (PT) was assessed by the method originally described by Quick et al.[18] Thromboplastin, added to a known amount of plasma, activates factor VII to factor VIIa, thus activating the extrinsic pathway of coagulation. After 100 μl of plasma were incubated for 3 minutes at 37° C, 200 μl of Thromboplastin C, prewarmed at 37° C, were added, and clotting time was measured.

Activated Partial Thromboplastin Time.   Activated partial thromboplastin time (APTT) is based on the method originally described by Proctor and Rapaport.[19] This method measures the intrinsic coagulation factors (factors VIII, IX, XI, and XII), the factors common to extrinsic and intrinsic systems (factors V and X and prothrombin), and the conversion of fibrinogen to fibrin. The time to clot formation after citrated plasma has been activated by a platelet substitute (a rabbit brain phospholipid with micronized silica as activator) and calcium ions is measured. APTT was measured using the reagent from Organon Teknika Corporation (Durham, NC). After 100 μl of plasma were incubated for 5 minutes with 100 μl of APTT reagent (platelet substitute), 100 μl of 0.025 M calcium chloride, prewarmed at 37° C, were added, and clotting time was measured.

Thrombin Time.   Thrombin time (TT) is based on the method described by Bonsnes and Sweeney.[20] In the determination of citrated plasma TT, a known amount of preformed human thrombin is added to plasma, and the time required for clot formation measures the rate at which fibrin is formed. TT was measured using Fibrinidex human thrombin at a concentration of 10 NIH U/ml in 0.025 M calcium chloride. After 100 μl of human thrombin, prewarmed at 37° C, were added to 200 μl of plasma, prewarmed at 37° C for 3 minutes, clotting time was measured.

Ecarin Clotting Time.   Ecarin clotting time (ECT) is a new plasma-based clotting method, originally described by Nowak and Bucha.[21] Ecarin is an enzyme purified from the venom of the *Echis carinatus* snake. Ecarin activates prothrombin to meizothrombin and other intermediates rather than to fully functional thrombin. However, meizothrombin also has procoagulant activities, although it is weaker than thrombin. The ECT assay was carried out with a fast kinetic centrifugal analyzer (ACL 300 plus).[16] After 100 μl of citrated plasma were incubated for 2 minutes at 37° C, 100 μl of ecarin (Knoll AG, Ludwigshafen, Germany) were added, and time to clotting was measured.

Heptest.   The Heptest assay, originally developed by Yin et al.,[22] measures the ability of an agent to inhibit exogenous factor Xa. Heptest clotting time is measured using the Heptest reagents (Haemachem, St. Louis): bovine factor Xa and Recalmix (calcium chloride and brain cephalin in a bovine plasma fraction). After 100 μl of plasma were incubated with 100 μl of bovine factor Xa reagent for 2 minutes at 37° C, 100 μl of Recalmix were added, and clotting time was measured. At the final stage of this assay, thrombin is generated and results in the formation of a detectable clot.

Anticoagulant Effects of Thrombin Inhibitors in Native Human Whole Blood

The following thrombin inhibitors were studied in whole blood assays: D-MePhe-Pro-Arg-H, argatroban, hirudin, and heparin. Whole blood was collected from normal healthy human volunteers via venipuncture. The first 3 ml of blood drawn were discarded.

Activated Clotting Time.   Activated clotting time (ACT), which measures whole blood clotting time, was originally described by Hattersley in 1966.[23] In determining the ACT of freshly drawn blood samples, special prefilled glass tubes containing celite (an intrinsic system activator) were used. The ACT was measured with a Hemochron coagulation timing instrument (International Technidyne Corporation, Edison, NJ). The procedure for determining the ACT was carried out as specified by the manufacturer. In brief, 2 ml of freshly drawn whole blood were added to a glass tube prefilled with celite (International Technidyne Corporation, Edison, NJ), the tube was inserted immediately into the Hemochron coagulation timing instrument, and the timer was started.

Thrombelastographic Analysis.   The Thrombelastograph Coagulation Analyzer (Haemoscope Corporation, Skokie, IL) automatically records the viscoelastic changes in a sample of whole blood as the sample clots, retracts, and/or lyses. The resulting profile is a measure of the kinetics of clot formation and dissolution and of clot quality. Thrombelastographic measurements were made on freshly drawn whole blood samples, preincubated at 37° C in a glass tube for 3 minutes using a Hellige thrombelastograph (Haemoscope Corporation, Skokie, IL). The thrombelastograms (TEGs) generated in this manner were analyzed using the standard procedure described by Fiedel and Ku.[24] The length from the beginning of the recording until the point at which the graph reaches a 2-mm divergence was recorded as the r value.

Rabbit Model of Venous Stasis-Thrombosis

A modified Wessler stasis-thrombosis model[25] was used for determination of the in vivo antithrombotic effects of D-MePhe-Pro-Arg-H, hirudin, and heparin. The underlying principle of this model is that clot formation in the jugular segments of the rabbit in response to a thrombogenic trigger can be prevented by administration of antithrombotic agents before administration of the thrombogenic trigger. Recombinant tissue factor (rTF; 1.38 μM in 2.57 mM of phospholipid, biosynthesized and reconstituted as described by Bach et al.[26] and provided by Yale Nemerson, M.D., Mount Sinai School of Medicine, New York) was used as the trigger for clot formation in the jugular segments.

White male New Zealand rabbits weighing 2.5–3.5 kg were obtained from LSR Industries (Union Grove, WI) and housed individually. The animals were kept on standard rabbit chow diet and had free access to water. Ketamine hydrochloride at an intramuscular dose of 50 mg/kg, in combination with xylazine at an intramuscular dose of 25 mg/kg, was used to anesthetize each rabbit. Both jugular veins were carefully isolated. The left marginal ear vein was cannulated for intravenous administration of the thrombogenic and antithrombotic agents or saline. After 5 minutes of the saline or thrombin inhibitor injection, rTF was injected through the cannulated marginal ear vein as the thrombogenic challenge.

Twenty seconds after intravenous administration of rTF, the jugular segments were tied. Ten minutes after injection of rTF, the right segment was dissected in a petri dish and the contained thrombi were graded. Twenty minutes after the administration of rTF, the same procedure was repeated on the left segment. The grading system for the thrombi was a scale from 0 to +4, as established by Fareed et al. in 1985. The animal was euthanized with an intravenous injection of 0.5 ml of sodium pentobarbital and phenytoin sodium solution (Beuthanasia-D, Steris Laboratories, Phoenix, AZ).

To determine the dose-dependent antithrombotic effects of the thrombin inhibitors after intravenous administration in the rabbit stasis-thrombosis model, each thrombin inhibitor was injected through the marginal ear vein of the left ear, 5 minutes before injecting rTF at 0.68 pmol/kg. Each thrombin inhibitor was injected at various doses to obtain a dose-response curve. Groups of 6 rabbits were tested at each dose. Blood samples were collected at baseline and 5 minutes after injection of the antithrombin agent.

Rat Model of Laser-induced Arterial Thrombosis

The rat model of laser-induced thrombosis was selected to study the antithrombotic effects of the thrombin inhibitors in the arterial system, as described in detail by Weichert et al.[27] Male Wistar rats weighing 300–350 gm (LSR Industries, Union Grove, WI) were anesthetized with sodium pentobarbital, 100 mg/kg, administered intraperitoneally (Butler Company, Colombus, OH). An intestinal loop was exposed through a hypogastric incision and continuously irrigated with sterile saline solution, spread on a stage mounted on a microscope table (Nikon, inverted microscope, Diaphot-TMD, Nippon Kogaku K.K., Tokyo). Vascular lesions were induced with an argon laser system (INNOVA 70-2 Argon Laser, Coherent, Inc., Santa Clara, CA). The laser beam was directed through the optical path of the microscope on small mesenteric arterioles (inside diameter of 10–15 μm) of the fat-free portion of the mesentery. The laser beam pathway was controlled by means of a camera shutter (Uniblitz VS1452Z0) and driver (Uniblitz T132, Vincent Associates, Rochester, NY). The effective constant energy was 50 mW, as measured with a power meter on the microscope stage (model 200/10W, Coherent, Inc., Santa Clara, CA). The exposure time of the laser lesions was 150 msec. The time interval between laser shots was 1 minute. Results were evaluated by direct microscopic observation of occlusive changes in the blood vessel. The number of laser injuries required to induce a thrombus that was of a length equal to 1.5 × inside diameter of the vessel or that produced complete occlusion was the endpoint. The rat was sacrificed at the end of the experiment by intravenous injection of sodium pentobarbital (Beuthanasia, 0.5 ml/kg).

Each thrombin inhibitor was diluted in sterile saline to various concentrations so that the agent concentration corresponded to the dose (e.g., 1 mg/ml of thrombin inhibitor for dosing at 1 mg/kg). Thus, the volume injected in the rat was always 1 ml/kg animal weight. After the rat was prepared and placed on the microscope stage and a suitable vessel was located, each thrombin inhibitor was injected intravenously through one of the rat tail veins at various concentrations. Each thrombin inhibitor was allowed to circulate for 5 minutes before initiation of the laser-induced vascular lesion. Groups of 6 rats were tested at each dose for each thrombin inhibitor.

Rabbit Ear Bleeding Model

To study the hemorrhagic effects of thrombin inhibitors, a rabbit model of ear blood loss, as described by Cade et al.,[28] was used. White male New Zealand rabbits weighing 2.5–3.5 kg were obtained from LSR Industries. The animals were kept on standard rabbit chow diet and had free access to water. Ketamine at an intramuscular dose of 50 mg/kg, was injected in combination with xylazine at an intramuscular dose of 25 mg/kg to induce anesthesia. The marginal ear vein was cannulated for intravenous administration of antithrombin agents at various doses. After a constant circulation time, the right ear was immersed in a 950-ml, 37° C saline bath for a few seconds. Then five uniform, full-thickness incisions were made in the ear in areas free of major vascularization, and the ear was returned to the saline bath for 10 minutes. The saline was collected, and the red blood cells were counted using a hemacytometer (Brightline, Improved Neubauer, Hausser Scientific; 0.100 mm deep). The same procedure was repeated on the other ear 15 minutes after the procedure was initiated on the first ear. At the end of the experiment, hemostasis was ensured, and the animal was returned to its cage.

Each thrombin inhibitor was diluted in sterile saline (Baxter Healthcare Corporation, Deerfield, IL) to concentrations corresponding to 10-fold the dose to be used so that the volume of the injected agent remained constant at 0.1 ml/kg (intravenous or subcutaneous) animal weight for every rabbit. To determine the dose-dependent hemorrhagic effects of the thrombin inhibitors after intravenous administration, each thrombin inhibitor was injected through the marginal ear vein of the left ear, 5 minutes before making the incision in the right ear, as described above. The incisions in the left ear were made 20 minutes after intravenous injection of the antithrombotic agent. Each thrombin inhibitor was injected at various doses to obtain a dose-response curve. Groups of 6 rabbits were tested at each dose, and groups of 6 rabbits were used for each treatment.

Statistical Analysis

The experimental data derived from the in vitro assays were compiled as mean ± SD (standard deviation of the sample). The data derived from the in vivo studies were compiled as mean ± SEM (standard error of the mean). The sample mean was the average of the measurements within each group. The SEM was reported along with the mean to provide an indication of the precision of estimation of the population mean and to facilitate comparison among means of different groups. The data in the figures are presented as mean ± SD or mean ± SEM, depending on whether they were derived from in vitro or in vivo procedures. All figures were drawn using SigmaPlot software. The error bars were not shown if they were smaller than the size of the symbols in the figure.

The statistical tests performed on the data included one-way analysis of variance (ANOVA), followed by Neuman-Keuls multiple comparison test when the one-way ANOVA revealed a significant difference. These statistical tests were used to evaluate the results from all studies except the clot scores from the stasis-thrombosis model. The Kruskal-Wallis test was used to examine the differences among clot scores obtained in the rabbit stasis-thrombosis model.

RESULTS

The comparative biochemical profile of heparin and representative thrombin inhibitors included studies of potency evaluation, inhibitory profile using purified serine proteases, and effects on generation of protease in both coagulation- and fibrinolytic-based systems. The global anticoagulant effects of each inhibitor are reported in terms of its ability to prolong the clotting profile of normal human plasma. The ecarin clotting time (ECT) is used to determine relative anticoagulant potency. Whole blood studies using normal human whole blood assays in the TEG and ACT analyses are also included. All results are reported in statistically defined molar values.

The inhibition of thrombin activity can be explored in vitro by using the amidolytic and clotting activities of thrombin, chromogenic substrates that yield color when cleaved by thrombin, and fibrinogen that is converted to fibrin when digested by thrombin. The studies were designed to explore the relative in vitro inhibition of the formed thrombin by various agents, amidolytically with the thrombin titration assay and functionally with thrombin time in the fibrinogen-based assay. In addition, inhibition of the plasma-based antithrombin assay and thrombin generation was explored in the fibrinogen-deficient plasma assays. The effect of the thrombin inhibitors on other serine proteases, such as factor Xa, chymotrypsin,

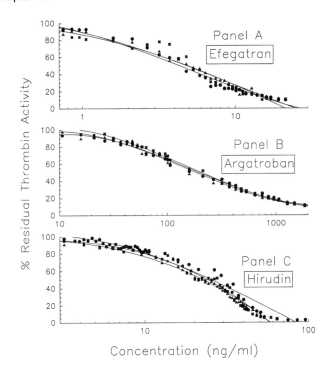

FIGURE 1.   Concentration-dependent inhibition of the amidolytic activity of thrombin by antithrombin agents. *A,* Results produced by D-MePhe-Pro-Arg-H. *B,* Results produced by argatroban. *C,* Results produced by hirudin. Each agent was tested in triplicate.

trypsin, activated protein C, tissue-type plasminogen activator, urokinase, and plasmin, was studied in assays based on the amidolytic activity of the enzymes. The effects of the antithrombin agents on generation of some of these enzymes were also examined in the thrombin and factor Xa generation assays.

The thrombin titration assay, an amidolytic method, was used to compare the direct antithrombin activity of thrombin inhibitors.[13] The results of the studies of inhibition of the amidolytic activity of thrombin by specific thrombin inhibitors are depicted in Figure 1. The concentration of each antithrombin agent that resulted in 50% inhibition of thrombin was the agent concentration that inhibited 0.5 thrombin units, since a total of 1 thrombin unit/L was present in the assay. Therefore, based on this value, the amount of thrombin units inhibited by 1 mg or 1 nmol of each thrombin inhibitor was calculated. The specific activities in terms of ATU potencies for each thrombin inhibitor, based on the results depicted in Figure 1, are reported in Table 1. On a gravimetric basis, the most potent thrombin inhibitor appeared to be the aldehyde D-MePhe-Pro-Arg-H with

TABLE 1.   Specific Activities of Thrombin Inhibitors as Assessed by Amidolytic Assay*

	ATU/mg	**ATU/nmol**
D-MePhe-Pro-Arg-H	102,422 ± 6,342	52,747 ± 3,266
Argatroban	2,774 ± 138	1,476 ± 73
Hirudin	22,382 ± 1,929	155,849 ± 13,432

* Each value represents the mean ± 1 SD of three separate determinations. On the ATU/mg and ATU/nmol bases, all values were significantly different from each other (p < 0.05; ANOVA followed by Student-Newman-Keuls test).

FIGURE 2. Concentration-dependent prolongation of fibrinogen-based thrombin time (TT) by various agents. *A*, Effects produced by thrombin inhibitors in the fibrinogen-based TT system in which thrombin was reconstituted in saline. *B*, Effects produced by antithrombin agents in the fibrinogen-based TT system in which thrombin was reconstituted in calcium chloride. (•) D-MePhe-Pro-Arg-H, (▲) argatroban, (♦) hirudin, (■) heparin. Each point represents mean ± 1 SD of three individual determinations.

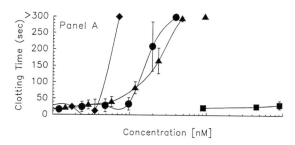

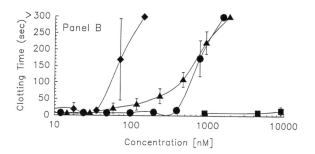

a specific activity of about 102,400 ATU/mg. Hirudin exhibited weaker activity (22,400 ATU/mg), and argatroban appeared to be the weakest thrombin inhibitor (2,800 ATU/mg).

The order of potency for each thrombin inhibitor on a molar basis was found to be different from the order of potency on a gravimetric basis. On a molar basis, hirudin was found to be the strongest thrombin inhibitor (155,800 ATU/nmol), followed by D-MePhe-Pro-Arg-H (about 52,700 ATU/nmol). Argatroban was again the weakest thrombin inhibitor (1,500 ATU/nmol).

A buffered fibrinogen-based clotting assay was developed to evaluate the comparative antithrombin effects of individual inhibitors on the clotting function of thrombin in an isolated test system. Human thrombin was added to a human fibrinogen solution to mediate clotting, with no feedback and amplification processes involved (unlike a plasmatic medium, in which other factors are present). The results of these studies are depicted in Figure 2. To evaluate the comparative effects of thrombin inhibitors, an index was devised whereby the concentration of thrombin inhibitor required to prolong the fibrinogen clotting time to 100 seconds (CT_{100}) was calculated (Table 2). The order of potencies for

TABLE 2. Antithrombin Potencies of Thrombin Inhibitors as Determined in Fibrinogen Clotting Systems*

	Prolongation of Clotting Time to 100 Seconds (nM)	
	10 U TT	10 Ca²⁺ TT
D-MePhe-Pro-Arg-H	134 ± 10	592 ± 12
Argatroban	140 ± 24	422 ± 128
Hirudin	47± 3	56 ± 3
Heparin	> 9,090	> 9,090

* Each value represents the mean ± 1 SD of three separate determinations. In the 10 U TT assay, none of the values were statistically different from each other. In the 10 U Ca²⁺ TT assay, all values were significantly different from each other except for the following pair: D-MePhe-Pro-Arg-H vs. argatroban ($p < 0.05$; ANOVA followed by Student-Newman-Keuls test).

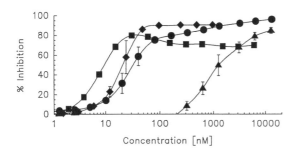

FIGURE 3. Concentration-dependent inhibition of the amidolytic activity of thrombin by various agents in the NHP-based system. (•) D-MePhe-Pro-Arg-H, (▲) argatroban, (♦) hirudin, (■) heparin. Each point represents mean ± 1 SD of three individual determinations.

each inhibitor was similar in both assays: hirudin was consistently found to be the strongest anticoagulant with a CT_{100} of 47 and 56 nM in the saline and calcium chloride tests, respectively.

Heparin had no effects at concentrations as high as 9 μM. In the saline/thrombin system, D-MePhe-Pro-Arg-H (CT_{100} of 134 nM) was more potent than argatroban (CT_{100} of 140 nM), whereas in the calcium chloride thrombin assay argatroban (CT_{100} of 422 nM) was more potent than D-MePhe-Pro-Arg-H (CT_{100} of 592 nM). With the exception of heparin, all thrombin inhibitors were capable of prolonging the clotting time to > 300 seconds at nM concentrations. Hirudin appeared to have an all-or-none anticoagulant effect, whereas the other thrombin inhibitors exhibited a more graded concentration-anticoagulant response relationship.

As in the thrombin titration assay, the evaluation of the antithrombin potential of thrombin inhibitors in plasma is based on the ability of antithrombin agents to inhibit the amidolytic activity of thrombin, as detected by the release of pNA from a specific chromogenic substrate. The thrombin inhibitors are diluted in plasma rather than buffer to mimic the matrix of circulating plasma. Thus, this assay represents a more physiologic condition for observing the effects of plasmatic factors on the antithrombin agents.

The results of the antithrombin activities of various agents after in vitro supplementation in normal human pooled plasma (NHP) are depicted in Figure 3. With the exception of heparin, all other thrombin inhibitors exhibited a sigmoidal concentration-response curve that eventually reached 100% thrombin inhibition. After calculating the IC_{50} for each thrombin inhibitor (Table 3), it was apparent that although heparin did not completely inhibit the amidolytic activity of thrombin, it seemed to be the strongest inhibitor (IC_{50} of 9.6 nM). Hirudin followed closely with an IC_{50} of 32 nM. The weakest inhibitor was found to be argatroban (IC_{50} of 1,250 nM). Whereas most thrombin inhibitors reached maximal thrombin inhibition in the nM range, argatroban produced its effects only in the μM range. This assay is based on the ability of thrombin inhibitors to suppress the amidolytic activity of factor Xa, as detected by a specific chromogenic substrate. As

TABLE 3.   Antithrombin Potencies of Thrombin Inhibitors as Determined in Amidolytic Systems in Normal Pooled Human Plasma and NRP*

	IC_{50} (nM) in Normal Pooled Human Plasma
D-MePhe-Pro-Arg-H	32.2 ± 7
Argatroban	1,250 ± 140
Hirudin	21 ± 2
Heparin	9.6 ± 0.5

* Each value represents the mean ± 1 SD of three separate determinations. In the NHP-based antithrombin amidolytic assay, only the value produced by argatroban was significantly different from all others (p < 0.05, ANOVA followed by Student-Newman-Keuls test).

FIGURE 4. Concentration-dependent inhibition of the amidolytic activity of factor Xa by thrombin inhibitors in the NHP-based system. (•) D-MePhe-Pro-Arg-H, (▲) argatroban, (♦) hirudin, (■) heparin. The broken line denotes that results may be due to a precipitation effect mediated by heparin. Each point represents mean ± 1 SD of three individual determinations.

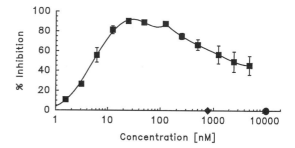

in the antithrombin assay, the thrombin inhibitors were diluted in plasma to demonstrate any matrix effects.

The results of the anti-Xa activities of thrombin inhibitors after in vitro supplementation in NHP are depicted in Figure 4. With the exception of heparin, none of the thrombin inhibitors exhibited anti-factor Xa activity. After calculating the IC_{50} for heparin (Table 4), it was apparent that although heparin failed to achieve complete inhibition of the amidolytic activity of factor Xa, it was a potent inhibitor with an IC_{50} value in the nM range (5.4 nM). Of interest, a gradual decrease in the inhibitory activity of heparin against factor Xa was noted at concentrations > 100 nM.

To evaluate the antiprotease spectrum of thrombin inhibitors, amidolytic assays with enzyme-specific synthetic substrates were used.[8] Only one enzyme was present in purified form, thus ensuring that inhibition of amidolytic activity was due to inhibition of the particular enzyme. Because heparin has no direct antiprotease activities and its mechanism of action is mediated primarily through antithrombin, stock solutions of heparin were made with antithrombin and then further diluted in saline before studying the effects of heparin on each of the serine proteases. In addition to the thrombin inhibitors, aprotinin was also included as a broad-spectrum serine protease inhibitor and positive control.

Figure 5 depicts the inhibitory activities of various agents against the amidolytic activity of chymotrypsin. None of the thrombin inhibitors were capable of inhibiting amidolytic activity at high concentrations: D-MePhe-Pro-Arg-H > 26 µM, argatroban > 25 µM, hirudin > 1.9 µM, and heparin > 1.2 µM. However, aprotinin produced a concentration-dependent inhibition of chymotrypsin with an IC_{50} of 0.8 µM (Table 5).

Figure 6 depicts the results from the trypsin inhibitory studies for various agents. Argatroban, hirudin, and heparin had relatively weaker inhibitory activities against the amidolytic activity of trypsin at concentrations > 125, 1.9, and 1.2 µM, respectively. D-MePhe-Pro-Arg-H demonstrated a concentration-dependent inhibition of trypsin. According to the IC_{50} values for each thrombin inhibitor (see Table 5), the most potent thrombin inhibitor was D-MePhe-Pro-Arg-H (IC_{50} of 0.18 µM). The antifibrinolytic agent aprotinin, used as the positive control, also exhibited a concentration-dependent anti-trypsin effect (IC_{50} of 0.39 µM).

TABLE 4. Anti-factor Xa Potencies of Thrombin Inhibitors as Determined in Amidolytic Systems in Normal Human Pooled Plasma and NRP*

	IC_{50} (nM) in Normal Human Pooled Plasma
D-MePhe-Pro-Arg-H	> 10,500
Argatroban	> 10,000
Hirudin	> 800
Heparin	5.4 ± 0.2

* Each value represents the mean ± 1 SD of three separate determinations.

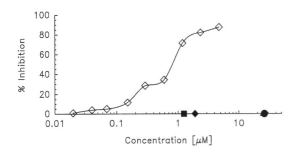

FIGURE 5. Concentration-dependent inhibition of the amidolytic activity of chymotrypsin by various agents. (•) D-MePhe-Pro-Arg-H, (▲) argatroban, (◆) hirudin, (■) heparin, (◇) aprotinin.

The inhibitory effects of thrombin inhibitors against the amidolytic activity of APC are depicted in Figure 7. Heparin, hirudin, and argatroban exhibited no inhibitory actions at high concentrations (> 9, > 10, and $> 100 \mu M$, respectively); D-MePhe-Pro-Arg-H, with an IC_{50} value of $8.4 \mu M$ (see Table 5) was clearly the most potent inhibitor. Aprotinin was slightly weaker than D-MePhe-Pro-Arg-H but also inhibited APC in a concentration-dependent manner (IC_{50} of $16.6 \mu M$). Both agents completely inhibited APC amidolytic activity at concentrations around $100 \mu M$.

Representative data about the inhibition of glandular kallikrein by various thrombin inhibitors are depicted in Figure 8. Only heparin exhibited a concentration-dependent inhibitory effect against the amidolytic action of glandular kallikrein. Compared with aprotinin (IC_{50} of $0.32 \mu M$), heparin was found to be a relatively weaker inhibitor. Furthermore, heparin was not capable of completely inhibiting kallikrein at concentrations higher than $60 \mu M$ (see Table 5 for IC_{50} values).

The amidolytic activity of tPA was inhibited by D-MePhe-Pro-Arg-H (Fig. 9). Argatroban, hirudin, heparin, and aprotinin did not affect the amidolytic activity of tPA at higher concentrations up to 60, 10, 62, and $5 \mu M$, respectively. D-MePhe-Pro-Arg-H exhibited a concentration-dependent inhibition of tPA (for estimated IC_{50} values, see Table 5).

Figure 10 depicts the inhibitory activities of various agents on the amidolytic action of urokinase. D-MePhe-Pro-Arg-H, argatroban, hirudin, heparin, and aprotinin failed to inhibit the amidolytic activity of urokinase at high concentrations (> 60, > 10, > 62, and $> 5 \mu M$, respectively).

With the exception of hirudin, the amidolytic activity of plasmin was inhibited by all thrombin inhibitors as well as aprotinin (Fig. 11). Argatroban exhibited the weakest

TABLE 5. Inhibition of Serine Proteases by Thrombin Inhibitors as Determined in Biochemically Defined Amidolytic Systems*

	IC_{50} (μM)						
	Chymo-trypsin	Trypsin	APC	Glandular Kallikrein	tPA	Urokinase	Plasmin
D-MePhe-Pro-Arg-H	> 26	0.18 ± 0.02	8.4 ± 0.8	> 65	52.7 ± 2.9	> 65	1.58 ± 0.10
Argatroban	> 25	> 125	> 115	> 115	> 115	> 115	> 115
Hirudin	> 1.9	> 1.9	> 9.6	> 9.6	> 9.6	> 9.6	> 9.6
Heparin	> 1.2	> 1.2	> 62	> 62	> 62	> 62	> 62
Aprotinin	0.8	0.39 ± 0.09	16.6 ± 0.2	0.322 ± 0.015	> 5	> 5	0.057 ± 0.005

APC = activated protein C; tPA = tissue-type plasminogen activator.

* Each value represents the mean ± 1 SD of three separate determinations. In the trypsin assay, aprotinin was significantly different from D-MePhe-Pro-Arg-H. In the APC assay, D-MePhe-Pro-Arg-H and argatroban were significantly different from each other. In the plasmin assay, the values produced by D-MePhe-Pro-Arg-H and aprotinin were significantly different from each other ($p < 0.05$, ANOVA followed by Student-Newman-Keuls test).

FIGURE 6. Concentration-dependent inhibition of the amidolytic activity of trypsin by thrombin inhibitors. (•) D-MePhe-Pro-Arg-H, (▲) argatroban, (♦) hirudin, (■) heparin, (◇) aprotinin. Each point represents mean ± 1 SD of three individual determinations.

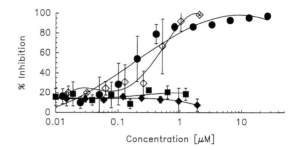

FIGURE 7. Concentration-dependent inhibition of the amidolytic activity of APC by various agents. (•) D-MePhe-Pro-Arg-H, (▲) argatroban, (♦) hirudin, (■) heparin, (◇) aprotinin. Each point represents mean ± 1 SD of three individual determinations.

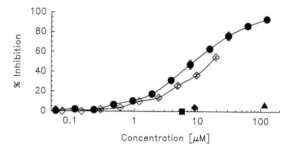

FIGURE 8. Concentration-dependent inhibition of the amidolytic activity of kallikrein by thrombin inhibitors. (•) D-MePhe-Pro-Arg-H, (▲) argatroban, (♦) hirudin, (■) heparin, (◇) aprotinin. Each point represents mean ± 1 SD of three individual determinations.

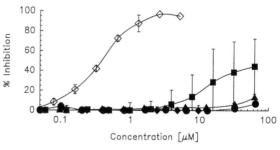

FIGURE 9. Concentration-dependent inhibition of the amidolytic activity of tissue-type plasminogen activator by antithrombin agents. (•) D-MePhe-Pro-Arg-H, (▲) argatroban, (♦) hirudin, (■) heparin, (◇) aprotinin. Each point represents mean ± 1 SD of three individual determinations.

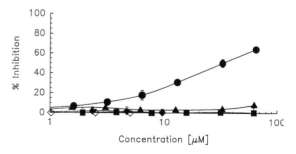

FIGURE 10. Concentration-dependent inhibition of the amidolytic activity of urokinase by various agents. (•) D-MePhe-Pro-Arg-H, (▲) argatroban, (♦) hirudin, (■) heparin, (◇) aprotinin. Each point represents mean ± 1 SD of three individual determinations.

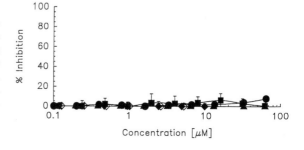

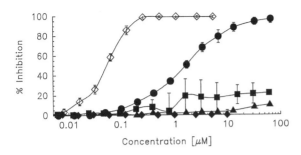

FIGURE 11. Concentration-dependent inhibition of the amidolytic activity of plasmin by thrombin inhibitors. (•) D-MePhe-Pro-Arg-H, (▲) argatroban, (♦) hirudin, (■) heparin, (◇) aprotinin. Each point represents mean ± 1 SD of three individual determinations.

inhibitory activity; even the highest concentration (115 µM) did not achieve 50% inhibition of plasmin. Of interest, heparin exhibited an inhibitory activity against plasmin at concentrations > 10 µM that was not concentration-dependent and plateaued around 20% inhibition. All tripeptide thrombin inhibitors and aprotinin exhibited concentration-dependent antiplasmin activity, and all were capable of maximal plasmin inhibition at µM concentrations. After calculating the IC_{50} value for each inhibitor (see Table 5), the most potent plasmin inhibitor was aprotinin (IC_{50} of 0.057 µM), followed by D-MePhe-Pro-Arg-H (IC_{50} of 1.58 µM).

Although the antithrombin and anti-Xa assays provided data about the direct inhibitory activities of thrombin inhibitors against thrombin and factor Xa, their effects on protease generation were not addressed. The coagulation cascade is a complex enzyme network with feedback mechanisms and amplification loops. Thus, it is conceivable that even if a thrombin inhibitor is effective in directly inhibiting thrombin or factor Xa, it may not inhibit the generation of various proteases and thrombin. Therefore, inhibitory effects on the generation of thrombin and factor Xa were studied in fibrinogen-deficient plasma, in which specific activators of the extrinsic and intrinsic assay systems were used. Clot formation was avoided to minimize clotting interference.

Figure 12A depicts data about the inhibition of thrombin generation after extrinsic activation by various thrombin inhibitors. All agents produced a concentration-dependent inhibition of thrombin. Although hirudin was the most efficacious inhibitor (IC_{50} of 0.02 µM), the maximal inhibitory activity plateaued around 80%. D-MePhe-Pro-Arg-H completely inhibited the generation of thrombin at higher concentrations. According to the IC_{50} values for each thrombin inhibitor (Table 6), after hirudin the most potent inhibitor was heparin (IC_{50} of 0.2 µM), followed by D-MePhe-Pro-Arg-H (IC_{50} of 5.1 µM). Argatroban was found to be the weakest inhibitor.

Figure 12B depicts the results of the inhibition of factor Xa after extrinsic activation by various agents. All inhibitors produced a concentration-dependent inhibition of factor Xa. Hirudin appeared to be a weak inhibitor of extrinsic factor Xa generation; only about 20% of factor Xa generation was maximally inhibited at a concentration as high as 5 µM. D-MePhe-Pro-Arg-H completely inhibited the generation of factor Xa. According to IC_{50} values for each antithrombin agent (see Table 6), the most potent inhibitor was heparin (IC_{50} of 0.045 µM), followed by D-MePhe-Pro-Arg-H (IC_{50} of 13 µM). Argatroban was the weakest inhibitor (IC_{50} > 62 µM).

Extrinsic activation and intrinsic activation of the coagulation cascade trigger different sequences of clotting factors. Therefore, the proportions of active factors generated, as well as the speed at which they are generated, are different. To study the effects of thrombin inhibitors on the coagulation cascade after intrinsic activation, their effects on the generation of thrombin and factor Xa were studied. Human plasma was activated intrinsically, and the amount of thrombin and factor Xa generated was detected with specific chromogenic substrates. As with the extrinsic assays, fibrinogen-deficient human plasma was used.

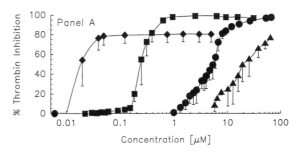

FIGURE 12. Concentration-dependent inhibition of the extrinsic activation of coagulation by antithrombin agents in the fibrinogen-deficient system. *A,* Effects mediated by various agents in the extrinsic thrombin generation system. *B,* Effects mediated by agents in the extrinsic factor Xa generation system. (•) D-MePhe-Pro-Arg-H, (▲) argatroban, (♦) hirudin, (■) heparin. Each point represents mean ± 1 SD of three individual determinations.

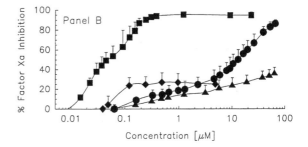

Figure 13A depicts the concentration-dependent inhibition of thrombin generation after intrinsic activation by various thrombin inhibitors. Although heparin was found to be the most potent inhibitor (IC_{50} of 0.032 μM), followed closely by hirudin (IC_{50} of 0.04 μM), the maximal inhibitory activity of both agents plateaued around 80%. D-MePhe-Pro-Arg-H appeared to be weaker than heparin and hirudin but completely inhibited the generation of thrombin at higher concentrations. According to the IC_{50} values for each thrombin inhibitor (see Table 6), after hirudin and heparin the most potent inhibitor was D-MePhe-Pro-Arg-H (IC_{50} of 1.4 μM). Argatroban was found to be the weakest inhibitor (IC_{50} of 6.5 μM) and appeared to plateau around 65%.

Figure 13B presents the concentration-dependent inhibition of factor Xa generation after intrinsic activation by various agents. All agents completely inhibited factor Xa generation at higher concentrations. The order of potency was as follows: heparin (IC_{50} of 0.006 μM), hirudin (IC_{50} of 0.018 μM), D-MePhe-Pro-Arg-H (IC_{50} of 0.07 μM), and argatroban (IC_{50} of 0.17 μM).

TABLE 6.   Inhibition of Generation of Thrombin and Factor Xa by Thrombin Inhibitors as Determined in Fibrinogen-deficient Amidolytic Systems*

	Extrinsic Generation, IC_{50} (μM)		Intrinsic Generation, IC_{50} (μM)	
	Thrombin	Factor Xa	Thrombin	Factor Xa
D-MePhe-Pro-Arg-H	5.1 ± 0.5	13 ± 1.5	1.4 ± 0.4	0.106 ± 0.005
Argatroban	19 ± 3	> 60	6.5 ± 0.6	0.17 ± 0.03
Hirudin	0.02 ± 0.01	> 5	0.04 ± 0.005	0.018 ± 0.002
Heparin	0.2 ± 0.1	0.045 ± 0.01	0.032 ± 0.004	0.006 ± 0.002

* Each value represents the mean ± 1 SD of three separate determinations. In the extrinsic activation of thrombin assay, all values were significantly different from each other except for the following pair: hirudin vs. heparin. In the extrinsic activation of factor Xa, the value produced by D-MePhe-Pro-Arg-H was significantly different compared with heparin. In the intrinsic thrombin generation assay, all values produced by thrombin inhibitors were significantly different from each other, with the exception of the following pair: hirudin vs. heparin. In the extrinsic factor Xa generation assay, all values were significantly different from each other ($p < 0.05$, ANOVA followed by Student-Newman-Keuls test).

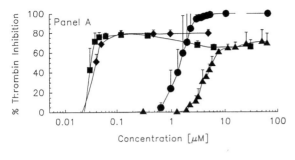

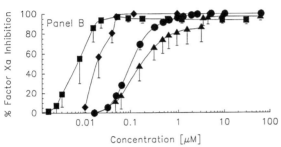

FIGURE 13. Concentration-dependent inhibition of the intrinsic activation of coagulation by antithrombin agents in the fibrinogen-deficient system. *A,* Effects mediated by various agents in the intrinsic thrombin generation system. *B,* Effects mediated by agents in the intrinsic factor Xa generation system. (•) D-MePhe-Pro-Arg-H, (▲) argatroban, (♦) hirudin, (■) heparin. Each point represents mean ± 1 SD of three individual determinations.

All of the results described previously, with the exception of the TT in the human fibrinogen-based test, were based on the inhibition of the amidolytic activity of thrombin, factor Xa, and other serine proteases. Furthermore, the TT in the fibrinogen-based test was a defined assay in which no other clotting factors except thrombin and fibrinogen were present. Therefore, the in vitro anticoagulant effects of thrombin inhibitors, based on the inhibition of thrombin clotting activity, were studied in global clotting tests, in which all clotting factors were present in normal human plasma. Each assay was based on the activation of coagulation in a distinct manner, thus providing specific data about the inhibitory actions of antithrombin agents at various sites. To compare the relative anticoagulant effects of thrombin inhibitors in these assays, the concentration of each inhibitor that resulted in prolongation of the clotting time to 100 seconds (CT_{100}) was calculated (Table 7).

TABLE 7. Comparative Anticoagulant Effects of Thrombin Inhibitors
in Normal Human Pooled Plasma*

	Concentrations that Prolong Clotting Time to 100 sec in μM				
	PT	APTT	TT	ECT	Heptest
D-MePhe-Pro-Arg-H	33 ± 1	8.2 ± 0.2	2.7 ± 0.3	0.22 ± 0.05	11.2 ± 0.4
Argatroban	28 ± 1	6.90 ± 0.20	8.9 ± 0.2	0.21 ± 0.01	3.65 ± 0.10
Hirudin	2.3 ± 0.5	1.44 ± 0.05	0.009 ± 0.006	0.065 ± 0.015	1.3 ± 0.05
Heparin	> 0.9	0.22 ± 0.03	0.155 ± 0.005	> 10.0	0.30 ± 0.05

PT = prothrombin time, APTT = activated partial thromboplastin time, TT = thrombin time, ECT = ecarin clotting time.

* Each value represents the mean ± 1 SD of three separate determinations. In the PT assay, values produced by all thrombin inhibitors (except heparin) were significantly different from each other. In the APTT assay, values produced by all thrombin inhibitors were significantly different from each other. In the 10 U Ca2+ TT assay, values produced by all thrombin inhibitors were significantly different from each other, with the exception of hirudin vs. heparin. In the ECT assay, values produced by all thrombin inhibitors (except heparin) were significantly different from each other, with the exception of D-MePhe-Pro-Arg-H vs. argatroban. In the Heptest assay, values produced by all thrombin inhibitors were significantly different from each other ($p < 0.05$, ANOVA followed by Student-Newman-Keuls test).

FIGURE 14. Comparative anticoagulant effects of antithrombin agents after supplementation in normal human pooled plasma, as studied in prothrombin time (PT). (•) D-MePhe-Pro-Arg-H, (▲) argatroban, (♦) hirudin, (■) heparin. Each point represents mean ± 1 SD of three individual determinations.

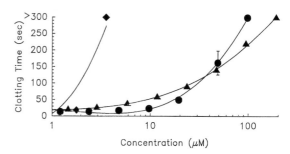

In the PT assay, thromboplastin was added to NHP to activate the coagulation cascade extrinsically (starting with factor VII), leading to thrombin generation and clot formation. The inhibitory activities of thrombin inhibitors were concentration-dependent (Fig. 14). Heparin had no effect at high concentrations (> 0.9 μM). In comparing the concentrations of each thrombin inhibitor that resulted in prolongation of the clotting time to 100 seconds (see Table 7), it was found that the most potent inhibitor of PT was hirudin (CT_{100} of 2.3 μM). Hirudin appeared to have all-or-none effects on PT. The effects of hirudin were followed by argatroban (CT_{100} of 28 μM) and D-MePhe-Pro-Arg-H (CT_{100} of 33 μM). Although argatroban produced a clotting time prolongation to 100 seconds at a lower concentration than D-MePhe-Pro-Arg-H, the latter prolonged PT to over 300 seconds at lower concentrations than argatroban (97 μM vs. 188 μM, respectively).

In the APTT assay, a contact activator was added to NHP to activate the coagulation cascade intrinsically (starting with factor XII), leading to thrombin generation and clot formation. The inhibitory activities of various thrombin inhibitors were concentration-dependent (Fig. 15). In comparing the concentrations of each thrombin inhibitor that resulted in prolongation of the clotting time to 100 seconds (see Table 7), it was found that the most potent inhibitor of APTT was heparin (CT_{100} of 0.22 μM), followed by hirudin (CT_{100} of 1.44 μM), argatroban (CT_{100} of 6.9 μM), and D-MePhe-Pro-Arg-H (CT_{100} of 8.2 μM). The inhibitory profiles of the last four thrombin inhibitors were superimposable.

In the TT assay, thrombin was added to NHP to convert the existing fibrinogen to fibrin clots. Furthermore, the added thrombin activated the coagulation cascade at multiple points (extrinsically via factors VII and V, intrinsically via factor XI, and common pathway via factor VIII), leading to additional thrombin generation and clot formation. Inhibitory activities were concentration-dependent (Fig. 16). The concentrations of each thrombin inhibitor that resulted in prolongation of the clotting time to 100 seconds are given in Table 7. The most potent inhibitor of the TT was hirudin (CT_{100} of 0.009 μM), followed by heparin (CT_{100} of 0.155 μM), D-MePhe-Pro-Arg-H (CT_{100} of 1.7 μM), and lastly argatroban (CT_{100} of 8.9 μM).

FIGURE 15. Comparative anticoagulant effects of various agents after supplementation in normal human pooled plasma, as studied in activated partial thromboplastin time (APTT). (•) D-MePhe-Pro-Arg-H, (▲) argatroban, (♦) hirudin, (■) heparin. Each point represents mean ± 1 SD of three individual determinations.

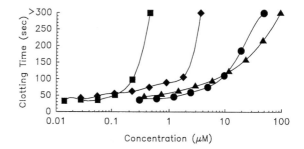

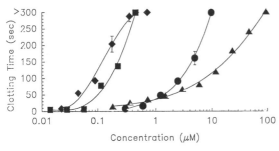

FIGURE 16. Comparative anticoagulant effects of thrombin inhibitors after supplementation in normal human pooled plasma, as studied in thrombin time (TT). (●) D-MePhe-Pro-Arg-H, (▲) argatroban, (◆) hirudin, (■) heparin. Each point represents mean ± 1 SD of three individual determinations.

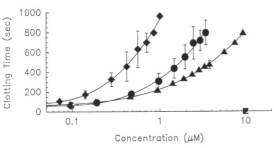

FIGURE 17. Comparative anticoagulant effects of antithrombin agents after supplementation in normal human pooled plasma, as studied in ecarin clotting time (ECT). (●) D-MePhe-Pro-Arg-H, (▲) argatroban, (◆) hirudin, (■) heparin. Each point represents mean ± 1 SD of three individual determinations.

In the ECT assay, ecarin was added to NHP to activate the existing prothrombin to meizothrombin and other intermediates with clotting activity, which led to conversion of fibrinogen to fibrin clots.[16] This test was different from the TT, in which exogenous thrombin was added to NHP. Figure 17 depicts the inhibitory activities of thrombin inhibitors. With the exception of heparin, the inhibitory activities were concentration-dependent. Table 7 shows the concentration of each thrombin inhibitor that resulted in prolongation of the clotting time to 100 seconds. The most potent inhibitor of the ECT was hirudin (CT$_{100}$ of 0.065 μM), followed by D-MePhe-Pro-Arg-H (CT$_{100}$ of 0.21 μM) and lastly by argatroban (CT$_{100}$ of 0.22 μM). Heparin had no effect at high concentrations (> 0.91 μM).

In the Heptest assay, factor Xa added to NHP activated the common pathway, which led to thrombin formation and subsequent conversion of fibrinogen to fibrin clots. The inhibitory activities of antithrombin agents were concentration-dependent (Fig. 18). In comparing the concentrations of each thrombin inhibitor that resulted in prolongation of the clotting time to 100 seconds (see Table 7), heparin was found to be the most potent inhibitor of the Heptest (CT$_{100}$ of 0.3 μM), followed by hirudin (CT$_{100}$ of 1.3 μM), argatroban (CT$_{100}$ of 3.7 μM), and D-MePhe-Pro-Arg-H (CT$_{100}$ of 11.2 μM).

The coagulation process in vivo takes place in whole blood; thus, in addition to the coagulation factors present in plasma, the rest of the blood components, such as platelets and white cells, may also play a role in the clotting process. To investigate the anticoagulant

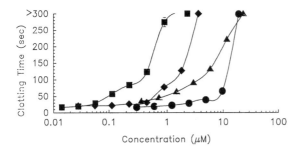

FIGURE 18. Comparative anticoagulant effects of various agents after supplementation in normal human pooled plasma, as studied in the Heptest. (●) D-MePhe-Pro-Arg-H, (▲) argatroban, (◆) hirudin, (■) heparin. Each point represents mean ± 1 SD of three individual determinations.

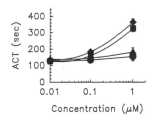

FIGURE 19. Comparative anticoagulant effects of thrombin inhibitors after supplementation in normal human whole blood, as detected in the activated clotting time (ACT) assay. (•) D-MePhe-Pro-Arg-H, (▲) argatroban, (♦) hirudin, (■) heparin. Each point represents mean ± 1 SD of three individual determinations.

activities of thrombin inhibitors in normal human whole blood, the ACT and TEG were used to compare D-MePhe-Pro-Arg-H, argatroban, hirudin, and heparin. Freshly drawn blood samples were supplemented in vitro with various concentrations of thrombin inhibitors.

The results of the concentration-dependent anticoagulant activities of thrombin inhibitors in whole blood, as studied in the ACT, are depicted in Figure 19. Hirudin and heparin produced a similar concentration-dependent pattern, with prolongation of ACT to 300–370 seconds at concentrations of 1 μM. D-MePhe-Pro-Arg-H and argatroban had weak anticoagulant activities even at the highest concentration, producing a prolongation of ACT to 150–180 seconds at 1 μM concentrations.

The results of the concentration-dependent anticoagulant activities of thrombin inhibitors in whole blood, as studied in the TEG, are depicted in Figure 20. D-MePhe-Pro-Arg-H, hirudin, and heparin produced a similar concentration-dependent pattern of prolongation of the r value of the TEG (38–47 mm) at equimolar concentrations (0.1 μM). Argatroban had weak anticoagulant activities even at the highest concentration, producing a prolongation of the TEG r value to 31 mm at 1 μM.

Injection of all four thrombin inhibitors produced dose-dependent antithrombotic effects after 10- and 20-minute stasis times in a dose range of 0.001–2 μmol/kg (Fig. 21). The strongest antithrombotic agent appeared to be heparin at doses in the nmol/kg range after both 10- and 20-minute stasis times, with ED_{50} of 0.008 and 0.009 μmol/kg, respectively. The effects of heparin were followed closely by those of hirudin (ED_{50} of 0.003 and 0.11 μmol/kg, respectively). After 20-minute stasis time, the antithrombotic effects of heparin and hirudin were superimposable at doses > 0.01 μmol/kg. D-MePhe-Pro-Arg-H was the weakest antithrombotic agent after both 10- and 20-minute stasis times, with ED_{50} of 0.242 and 1.60 μmol/kg, respectively. The estimated ED_{50} from each thrombin inhibitor dose-response curve is reported in Table 8.

The results of the studies of the antithrombotic effects of heparin, hirudin, and D-MePhe-Pro-Arg-H in the rat model of laser-induced arterial thrombosis are depicted in Figure 22. In control rats (injected with saline) 3 laser shots were needed to reach an endpoint. All thrombin inhibitors produced dose-dependent antithrombotic effects. In comparing the dose of each agent required to extend the endpoint to 6 laser shots (Table 9), heparin was the most potent antithrombotic agent (0.08 μmol/kg), followed by hirudin (0.28 μmol/kg). Consistent with the rabbit jugular vein stasis-thrombosis model, D-MePhe-Pro-Arg-H had the weakest effects in the rat laser-induced thrombosis model

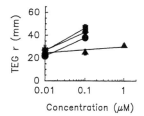

FIGURE 20. Comparative anticoagulant effects of thrombin inhibitors after supplementation in normal human whole blood, as studied in the thrombelastogram (TEG) assay. (•) D-MePhe-Pro-Arg-H, (▲) argatroban, (♦) hirudin, (■) heparin. Each point represents mean ± 1 SD of three individual determinations.

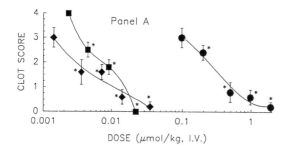

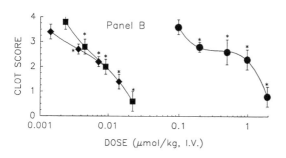

FIGURE 21. Comparative dose-dependent antithrombotic effects of various agents, as studied in the rabbit model of jugular vein stasis-thrombosis. Each thrombin inhibitor was injected intravenously and circulated for 5 minutes before initiation of the stasis procedure. *A*, Clot scores obtained after 10 minutes of stasis. *B*, Clot scores obtained after 20 minutes of stasis. (•) D-MePhe-Pro-Arg-H, (♦) hirudin, (■) heparin. Each point represents mean ± SEM (n = 6). * Denotes statistical significance (p < 0.05) compared with control (3.2 ± 0.2 after 10 minutes of stasis in *A*, 3.6 ± 0.3 after 20 minutes of stasis in *B*), as analyzed with the Kruskal-Wallis test.

(2 µmol/kg). The ceiling for heparin and hirudin appeared to be around 8 laser exposures. However, D-MePhe-Pro-ARg-H produced dose-dependent antithrombotic effects to a dose of 3.4 µmol/kg; with higher doses, the antithrombotic effects were weaker. In rats that received D-MePhe-Pro-Arg-H at doses > 3.4 µmol/kg, it was visually observed that the blood flow was reduced within 3–10 minutes after injection of the thrombin inhibitor.

To compare hemorrhagic potential, D-MePhe-Pro-Arg-H, hirudin, and heparin were studied in a rabbit model of ear bleeding,[28] and an index was devised whereby the dose of the antithrombin agent that produced bleeding of $2 \cdot 10^9$ RBC/L was estimated as the BD_2. The dose-dependent hemorrhagic effects of thrombin inhibitors after intravenous injection, as assessed in the rabbit ear bleeding model, are depicted in Figure 23. The hemorrhagic procedure was initiated 5 minutes and 20 minutes after intravenous injection of the thrombin inhibitor. Except for heparin, the other thrombin inhibitors resulted in dose-dependent hemorrhagic effects. The agent with the strongest hemorrhagic effects was hirudin, 5 and 10 minutes after intravenous injection, with BD_2 of 0.11 and 0.30 µmol/kg, respectively. The effects of hirudin were followed by D-MePhe-Pro-Arg-H (BD_2 pf 2.82 and > 4.85 µmol/kg, 5 and 20 minutes after injection). Heparin exhibited minimal hemorrhagic effects, as seen both 5 and 20 minutes after intravenous injection (BD_2 of > 0.45 µmol/kg in both cases). The dose of each thrombin inhibitor that resulted in bleeding of $2 \cdot 10^9$ RBC/L, 5 and 20 minutes after intravenous injection, is reported in Table 10.

TABLE 8.   Comparative Antithrombotic Potencies of Thrombin Inhibitors after Intravenous Injection as Determined in the Rabbit Model of Jugular Vein Stasis-Thrombosis*

| | Dose of Each Agent that Results in a Clot Score of + 2 in µmol/kg | |
	10 Min Stasis Time	20 Min Stasis Time
D-MePhe-Pro-Arg-H	0.242	1.60
Hirudin	0.003	0.011
Heparin	0.008	0.009

* Each value represents a single determination from the respective dose-response curve depicted in Figure 21.

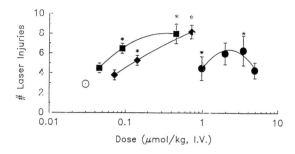

FIGURE 22. Comparative dose-dependent antithrombotic effects of various agents, as studied in the rat model of laser-induced thrombosis. Each thrombin inhibitor was injected through the rat tail vein and circulated for 5 minutes before initiation of the laser injury procedure. (•) D-MePhe-Pro-Arg-H, (♦) hirudin, (■) heparin. Each point represents mean ± SEM (n = 6). * Denotes statistical significance ($p < 0.05$) compared with control (0.100 ± 0.060), as analyzed with ANOVA followed by the Student-Newman-Keuls test.

DISCUSSION

The general order of potency of the antithrombotic effects of thrombin inhibitors in the rabbit stasis-thrombosis model was hirudin > heparin > D-MePhe-Pro-Arg-H. This order correlated well in a number of in vitro assays. Specifically, the antithrombotic effects of hirudin and D-MePhe-Pro-Arg-H correlated with their published K_i values, amidolytic thrombin potency evaluations, and fibrinogen-based clotting assay results. The antithrombotic effects of all thrombin inhibitors in the rabbit model correlated with their respective results in extrinsic and and intrinsic thrombin generation from fibrinogen-deficient plasma as well as with in vitro PT and TT clotting assays.

The order of potency of the antithrombin agents in the rat laser model correlated with only one of the in vitro assay profiles—the APTT. This observation supports the hypothesis that platelet activation and clot formation may not be due to intrinsic activation of coagulation.

The overall order of potency of the bleeding effects of antithrombin agents, as observed in the rabbit model of ear blood loss, was hirudin > D-MePhe-Pro-Arg-H > heparin. The order of the three first agents followed the same trend as their K_i values, results of the amidolytic thrombin potency evaluation studies, fibrinogen-based clotting tests, PT assay, and ECT test. However, when the antithrombotic effects of heparin are also considered, none of the in vitro assays correlate with the hemorrhagic results, indicating the necessity of in vivo evaluation of the hemorrhagic effects of antithrombin agents.

The above observations point to the usefulness of standardization of various thrombin inhibitors. Care should be taken to compare various agents in the same system and with agents such as heparin, which are not direct thrombin inhibitors; standardization is not possible in the same manner as with direct antithrombin agents. Furthermore, it may be that some in vitro assays are not suitable for comparison of agents with different mechanisms

TABLE 9. Comparative Antithrombotic Potencies of Thrombin Inhibitors, as Determined in the Rat Model of Laser-induced Thrombosis in Isolated Mesenterial Arterioles

	Dose of Each Agent that Results in Increase of Laser Shots to 6 in μmol/kg
D-MePhe-Pro-Arg-H	2.0
Hirudin	0.28
Heparin	0.08

* Each value represents a single determination from the respective dose-response curves depicted in Figure 22. Saline, as the control, required 2.9 ± 0.1 laser shots for occlusive thrombus formation.

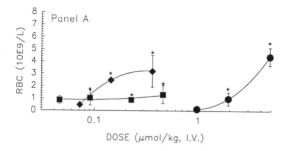

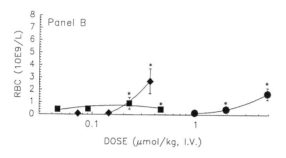

FIGURE 23. Comparative dose-dependent hemorrhagic effects of thrombin inhibitors, as studied in the rabbit ear bleeding model. *A,* Each agent was injected intravenously and allowed to circulate for 5 minutes before initiation of the incision procedure. *B,* Each agent was injected intravenously and circulated for 20 minutes before initiation of the incision procedure. (•) D-MePhe-Pro-Arg-H, (◆) hirudin, (■) heparin. Each point represents mean ± SEM (n = 6). * Denotes statistical significance (p < 0.05) compared with control (0.100 ± 0.060), as analyzed with ANOVA followed by the Student-Newman-Keuls test.

of thrombin inhibition, as is the case with argatroban and its effects on the amidolytic assays. For the same reason, although the amidolytic protease generation assays provide useful information about the mechanisms of action of thrombin inhibitors and their relative efficacies and potencies, argatroban cannot be compared with the other agents in a manner that can be related to its effects in clot-based assays or to its in vivo antithrombotic effects. Therefore, apart from the Ki comparison of agents for thrombin, clot-based assays may be more applicable in comparing thrombin inhibitors.

In terms of therapeutic monitoring of an individual thrombin inhibitor, the ECT assay may be useful because its range of sensitivity is wider than that of any other assay. Furthermore, the ECT is not affected by the presence of indirect thrombin inhibitors, which makes it ideal for monitoring thrombin inhibitors in situations in which additional antithrombotic agents may have been used. However, the suitability of the ECT for comparison of various anticoagulants and extrapolation of relative in vitro effects to relative in vivo antithrombotic effects is unclear.

The relative potency of the thrombin inhibitors included in this study is usually expressed in terms of Ki or IC_{50} values that are measured in defined in vitro systems, in which thrombin titration is used. Whether the assigned inhibitory constants translate into pharmacologic effects is not known. This study represents the first comprehensive comparison of

TABLE 10.   Comparative Hemorrhagic Potencies of Thrombin Inhibitors after Intravenous Injection, as Determined in the Rabbit Model of Ear Bleeding*

| | Dose of Each Agent that Resulted in Bleeding of $2 \cdot 10^9$ RBC/L in μmol/kg | |
	5 min after IV injection	20 min after IV injection
D-MePhe-Pro-Arg-H	2.82	> 4.85
Hirudin	0.11	0.30
Heparin	> 0.45	> 0.45

* Each value represents a single determination from the respective dose-response curves depicted in Figure 23. Saline produced bleeding of 0.100 ± 0.070 10^9 RBC/L.

the biochemical and pharmacologic actions of heparin and antithrombin agents. Although an agent may show strong antithrombin potency, because of its complex pharmacodynamics and other endogenous interactions its behavior may not be predictable simply by assigning an antithrombin potency. For example, hirudin exhibited the strongest antithrombin potency, but in the laser model of arterial thrombosis it was relatively weaker than the other thrombin inhibitors. This observation clearly suggests that factors in addition to thrombin inhibition contribute to the pharmacologic actions of antithrombin agents.

Heparin is a complex polypharmacologic agent with multiple plasmatic and vascular sites of action. Although its overall anticoagulant activity is usually standardized in anticoagulant units (USP assays), the potency designation of antithrombin agents may not be directly comparable to that assigned to heparin and related drugs. Thus, an APTT elevation to 3 or 4 times the baseline level by a thrombin inhibitor may or may not be relevant to the overall anticoagulant/antithrombotic response observed with heparin. This investigation has provided clear evidence for this hypothesis. At equivalent levels of APTT, the relative antithrombotic actions of these agents are not the same. Furthermore, thrombin inhibitors at equivalent prolongation of clotting tests exert different degrees of antithrombotic and/or hemorrhagic effects. These studies, therefore, provide evidence that bioequivalence is not predictable by any currently available test.

One of the most significant questions about the relative importance of thrombin in the mediation of thrombogenesis and its inhibition as the main target for controlling thrombotic events has been objectively addressed in this chapter. Experimental evidence indicates that the sole inhibition of thrombin is not the primary determinant of the antithrombotic actions of antithrombin agents and heparin. In the case of thrombin inhibitors, additional plasmatic and nonplasmatic processes also contribute to the control of thrombogenesis. It is obvious that the antithrombin-mediated inhibition of thrombin is only one of the multiple mechanisms for the pharmacologic action of heparin.

Another significant observation relates to the fact that antithrombin agents are considered inhibitors that target only thrombin. However, their effects on other serine proteases and modified forms of thrombin are not taken into account. Many of the thrombin inhibitors, such as D-MePhe-Pro-Arg-H and Ac-(D)Phe-Pro-boroArg-OH, significantly inhibit nonthrombin serine proteases, and this inhibition may have a complex outcome. In addition, most thrombin inhibitors inhibit thrombomodulin-bound thrombin, which can have significant implications in the management of thrombotic and cardiovascular disorders. This comparative study has provided additional insight into the potential clinical implications of the nonspecificity of these agents.

Results of these studies emphasize the importance of pharmacologic profiling for new antithrombin agents, because the direct antithrombin effects and other plasmatic or vascular actions can be evaluated only in valid pharmacologic studies. Some of the recent adjustments in clinical trials and adverse events due to compromise of both safety and efficacy resulted largely from incomplete preclinical pharmacologic information.

CONCLUSION

Direct thrombin inhibitors are potent anticoagulant agents that may be useful as alternate anticoagulants for cardiovascular surgical procedures in patients in whom heparin may not be used as an optimal anticoagulant. Furthermore, these agents primarily inhibit thrombin to produce their anticoagulant effects and therefore do not possess the adverse side effects associated with heparin. However, they have their own pharmacologic and toxicologic profile, which is distinct from heparin. Thus, they must be developed in valid pharmacologic studies to establish their therapeutic and safety profile. The developmental programs at the preclinical and clinical levels should not be based totally on the approaches taken for heparin. Additional studies are needed to validate their clinical use as anticoagulants in cardiovascular surgery.

REFERENCES

1. Lindahl AK, Abilgaard U, Larsen ML, et al: Extrinsic pathway inhibitor (EPI) and the post-heparin anticoagulant effect in tissue thromboplastin-induced coagulation. Thromb Res 64:155–168, 1991.
2. Jeske W, Hoppensteadt D, Fareed J, Bermes E: Measurement of functional and immunologic levels of tissue factor pathway inhibitor: Some methodologic considerations. Blood Coagul Fibrinol 6:S73–S80, 1995.
3. Verstraete M, Zoldhelyi P: Novel antithrombotic drugs in development. Drugs 49:856–884, 1995.
4. Gast A, Tschopp TB, Schmid G, et al: Inhibition of clot-bound and free (fluid phase thrombin) by a novel synthetic thrombin inhibitor (Ro 46-6240), recombinant hirudin and heparin in human plasma. Blood Coagul Fibrinol 5:879–887, 1994.
5. Gast A, Tschopp TB, Baumgartner HR: Thrombin plays a key role in late platelet thrombus growth and/or stability. Effect of a specific thrombin inhibitor on thrombogenesis induced by aortic subendothelium exposed to flowing rabbit blood. Arterioscler Thromb Vasc Biol 14:1466–1474, 1994.
6. Berry CN, Girardot C, Lecoffre C, Lunven C: Effects of the synthetic thrombin inhibitor argatroban on fibrin- or clot-incorporated thrombin: Comparison with heparin and recombinant hirudin. Thromb Haemost 72:381–386, 1994.
7. Eichler P, Greinacher A: Anti-hirudin antibodies induced by recombinant hirudin in the treatment of patients with heparin-induced thrombocytopenia (HIT) [abstract]. Ann Hematol 1:A4, 1996.
8. Callas DD, Hoppensteadt D, Malinowska K, Fareed J: Comparative studies on the anticoagulant and protease generation inhibitory actions of newly developed site-directed thrombin inhibitory drugs: Efegatran, argatroban, hirulog and hirudin. Semin Thromb Hemost 21:177–183, 1995.
9. Bajusz S, Barabás E, Tolnay P, et al: Inhibition of thrombin and trypsin by tripeptide aldehydes. In J Peptide Protein Res 12:217–221, 1978.
10. Bajusz S, Széll E, Bagdy D, et al: Highly active and selective anticoagulants: D-Phe-Pro-Arg-H, a free tripeptide aldehyde prone to spontaneous inactivation, and its stable N-methyl derivative, D-MePhe-Pro-Arg-H. J Med Chem 33:1729–1735, 1990.
11. Okamoto S, Kinjo K, Hijikata A, et al: Thrombin inhibitors. I: Ester derivatives of Nα-(Arylsulfonyl)-L-arginine. J Med Chem 23:827–830, 1980.
12. Fritz H, Wunderer G: Biochemistry and applications of aprotinin, the kallikrein inhibitor from bovine organs. Drug Res 33:479–494, 1993.
13. Callas DD, Fareed J: Comparative studies on the antithrombin potency of various thrombin inhibitors, as determined by using an amidolytic method. Thromb Res 83:97–102, 1996.
14. Iyer L, Fareed J: Determination of specific activity of recombinant hirudin using a thrombin titration method. Thromb Res 78:259–263, 1994.
15. Walenga JM, Fareed J, Messmore HL: Newer avenues in the monitoring of antithrombotic therapy: The role of automation. Semin Thromb Hemost 9:346–354, 1983.
16. Callas DD, Fareed J: Comparative anticoagulant effects of various thrombin inhibitors as determined in the ecarin clotting time method. Thromb Res 83:463–468, 1996.
17. Kaiser B, Fareed J, Hoppensteadt D, et al: Influence of recombinant hirudin and unfractionated heparin on thrombin and factor Xa generation in extrinsic and intrinsic activated systems. Thromb Res 65:157–164, 1992.
18. Quick AJ, Stanley-Brown M, Bancroft FW: A study of the coagulation defect in hemophilia and in jaundice. Am J Med Sci 190:501, 1935.
19. Proctor RR, Rapaport SI: The partial thromboplastin time with kaolin—a simple screening test for first stage plasma clotting factor deficiencies. Am J Clin Pathol 36:212, 1961.
20. Bonsnes RW, Sweeney WJ III: A rapid, simple semiquantitative test for fibrinogen employing thrombin. Am J Obstet 70:334–340, 1995.
21. Nowak G, Bucha E: A new method for the therapeutic monitoring of hirudin. Thromb Haemost 69:1306, 1993.
22. Yin ET, Giudice LC, Wessler S: Inhibition of activated factor X-induced platelet aggregation: The role of heparin and the plasma inhibitor to activate factor X. J Lab Clin Med 82:390–398, 1973.
23. Hattersley PG: Heparin anticoagulation. In Koepke JA (ed): Laboratory Hematology. New York, Churchill Livingstone, 1984, pp 789–818.
24. Fiedel BA, Ku CS: Further studies on the modulation of blood coagulation by human serum amyloid P component and its acute phase homologue C-reactive protein. Thromb Haemost 55:406–409, 1986.
25. Fareed J, Walenga JM, Kumur A, Rock A: A modified stasis thrombosis model to study the antithrombotic actions of heparin and its fractions. Semin Thromb Hemost 11:155–175, 1985.
26. Bach R, Gentry R, Nemerson Y: Factor VII binding to tissue factor in reconstituted phospholipid vesicles induction of cooperativity by phosphatidylserine. Biochemistry 25:4007–4020, 1986.
27. Weichert W, Breddin HK, Staubesand J: Application of a laser-induced endothelial injury model in the screening of antithrombotic drugs. Semin Thromb Hemost 14(Suppl):106–114, 1988.
28. Cade JF, Buchanan MR, Boneu B, et al: A comparison of the antithrombotic and hemorrhagic effects of low molecular weight heparin fractions: The influence on the method of preparation. Thromb Res 35:613–625, 1984.

New Antithrombin Agents: Potential for Coating Biomaterials Used in Cardiopulmonary Bypass

A. STEMBERGER, Ph.D.
G. SCHMIDMAIER
C. FÖRSTER
E. ALT, M.D.
J. KOHN, Ph.D.
A. CALATZIS

Numerous biomaterials made of plastic or metal have been developed to substitute or improve different functions of the body. Examples include catheters, vascular prostheses, heart valves, and stents. Plastic materials in oxygenators or dialysis systems have intensive contact with blood in extracorporeal circulation during heart and vascular surgery or dialysis. The fact that these artificial surfaces set off a sequence of reactions after contact with blood has been a largely unsolved problem (Fig. 1).[3,6,9,27]

Adhesive proteins, especially fibrinogen, are adsorbed on foreign surfaces and lead to activation of plasmatic coagulation and complement as well as to adhesion and aggregation of platelets.[7,16,18,21,22,31] Monocytes and neutrophils also are involved in these mechanisms. Such complex reactions depend on the type of plastic materials.[24]

Through activation of the complement system, dialysis membranes can produce symptoms suggestive of adult respiratory distress syndrome (ARDS), although they show only slight thrombogenicity.[30] During extracorporeal circulation, the mechanisms initiated on the surfaces of oxygenators can initiate the feared "whole body inflammatory response."[9,17]

After contact with blood, plastic materials adsorb fibrinogen and other adhesive proteins. These proteins initiate adhesion and aggregation of platelets. The exposed thrombocytic lipid membranes trigger plasmatic coagulation and thus promote clot formation.[34]

Even during optimal anticoagulation with heparin, the deposition of blood clots, which may lead to thrombotic or embolic complications, has been observed. A special problem exists, even with optimal anticoagulation through coumarin derivatives, when artificial materials are implanted for life-long use (e.g., vascular prostheses, heart valves, stents).[2,31]

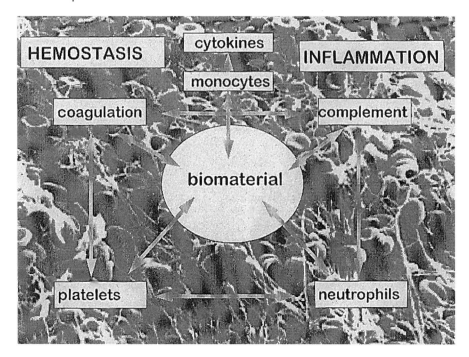

FIGURE 1.   Interaction of plasmatic and cellular components of the blood with biomaterials.

Current attempts to improve the biocompatibility of artificial surfaces often focus on chemical modifications of traditional plastics.[1,4,8,26] Additional strategies for improvement of surface characteristics include fixation of anticoagulant drugs, such as heparin or phosphatidylcholin analogs.[5,10,19,20,23,32,33] Coatings with incorporated antiplatelet agents and antibiotics, fixated by various chemical procedures, are designed to promote blood compatibility and infection resistance.[14,15,25,28]

During the past years our group has investigated the blood compatibility of traditional biomaterials and has pursued new concepts for the development of antithrombotic surfaces. An attempt was made to imitate the body's natural strategies for antithrombogenicity in the vascular endothelium.

In the body the formation of blood clots and their deposition in the vascular system are prevented by various mechanisms. Involved are inhibitors of plasmatic coagulation, such as antithrombin III (AT III), heparin cofactor II, tissue factor pathway inhibitor (TFPI), and the activated protein C system. Prostacyclin, activators of protein C, and plasminogen activators are released from the intact endothelial cells. Furthermore, the endothelial cells secrete glycosaminoglycans, which have an effect similar to that of heparin. The outer lipid membranes of endothelial cells and resting thrombocytes and intact erythrocytes are rich in phosphatidylcholin, which also possesses antithrombotic activity.[34]

Imitation of these mechanisms guided our working group to the following approach to surface modification: clinically proved devices made of plastics or metals were coated with resorbable drug carriers with incorporated anticoagulants.

COATING TECHNOLOGY AND METHODS OF STUDY

Biomaterials are coated by means of solvent casting with a solution of resorbable drug carriers in volatile organic solvents. Carbon fiber netting or thrombelastographic cuvettes made of steel are used as model substances for thrombogenic surfaces. The thrombogenicity of coated vs. uncoated hollow fibers from oxygenators (Akzo Nobel Faser AG, Wuppertal) was also studied.

As a first step, 400 mg of a drug carrier such as R 203 (d.l. lacitide, Boehringer, Ingelheim) or poly (DTO) carbonates (provided by Ertel and Kohn[11,12]) were dissolved in 6 ml of methylene chloride. Then the biomaterials were dipped in this solution and allowed to dry. For some examinations anticoagulant drugs were added. At present, 5% PEG hirudin (Knoll AG, Ludwigshafen) and/or 1% iloprost (Schering, Berlin) is added in relation to the weight of the drug carrier.

Using nonanticoagulated human blood from healthy volunteers, thrombelastography of uncoated vs. coated cups was performed with established techniques. In addition, nonanticoagulated blood from healthy volunteers was brought into contact with the coated and uncoated materials in the so-called human stasis model, which consists of commercially available, sterile, disposable faucets. The three-way faucets were inserted into one another and connected by polyvinyl chloride (PVC) tubes that contained the materials to be tested. The hollow fibers of the oxygenators were inserted directly. A large-lumen, indwelling catheter was placed into the cubital vein.

At this point control samples were taken from the catheter. The removal system with the incorporated biomaterials was then screwed onto the catheter and fixed to the arm of the volunteer with adhesive tape. The arm was at rest and lay on a cushioned work area. The three-way faucets were opened, one after the other, and with slight suction pressure the 10-ml syringes (to which a 1-ml citra solution was added previously) were filled with blood. The zero value was then determined. After 5 or 10 minutes, more blood was taken in the same manner. Then the indwelling catheter was removed, along with the complete device, and the biomaterials were taken out immediately, photographed, and put into the fixation solution for scanning electronmicroscopic (SEM) preparation.

After the biomaterials had made contact with the human blood of healthy volunteers, the markers of activated coagulation were analyzed with commercially available test kits (TAT and F_{1-2}, Behringwerke, Marburg).

RESULTS

The thrombelastogram (TEG) is a proven test procedure for determination of global coagulation in routine clinical practice. Coagulation in the TEG is initiated through contact of the sample with the coated or uncoated stainless steel surface. The TEG amplitude is a measure of the magnitude of the mechanical coupling between the pin and the cup through the clot. This mechanical coupling requires attachment of the clot to the surfaces of the pin and cup. An irregular decline of amplitude during measurement indicates disruption of this attachment. TEG is as an easy-to-use procedure for thrombogenicity testing within the context of coating technology.

Our analysis showed delayed onset of coagulation with the coated vs. uncoated cups and an irregular decline of amplitude during measurement (Fig. 2). This finding indicates that drug carriers with an aliphatic polyester composition, such as polyactides, can delay the onset of coagulation, even when anticoagulant drugs are not added. The decline of amplitude during measurement indicates disturbed deposition of adhesive proteins onto the coated surfaces.

Test kits for detection of the markers of activated coagulation, such as thrombin–antithrombin (TAT) complexes or prothrombin fragments (F_{1-2}), are suitable only for the human system and not applicable in animal models. Thus the human stasis model was developed to bring biomaterials into contact with human blood under standardized conditions. Blood is taken from the cubital vein, and the PVC tubes are filled with the incorporated biomaterials (Fig. 3). In addition, biomaterials such as vascular prostheses or hollow fibers from oxygenators can be directly inserted. Thrombogenicity of the artificial

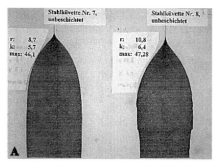
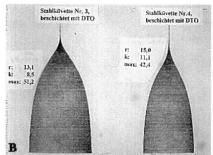
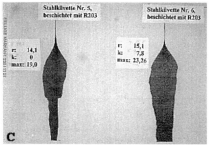

FIGURE 2. Thrombelastogram (TEG) of steel cuvettes following contact with blood. *A*, Uncoated cuvettes. *B*, Cuvettes coated with DTO. *C*, Cuvettes coated with R203.

surfaces can then be tested according to mode of coating and evaluated later with macroscopic and SEM analyses.

Uncoated carbon fibers were covered with a thick blood clot after 5 minutes of contact with blood. No coagulation plugs could be seen by macroscopic evaluation of the surface of coated carbon fibers (Fig. 4). The materials were not rinsed with an isotonic saline solution after contact with blood but instead were placed into a glutaraldehyde solution for fixation for SEM evaluation.

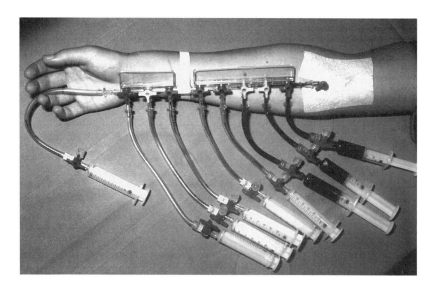

FIGURE 3. Human stasis model, with commercially available, disposable components. Blood is withdrawn by filling the PVC tubes with the incorporated or interconnected biomaterials.

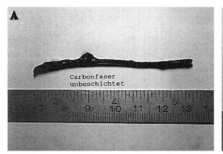
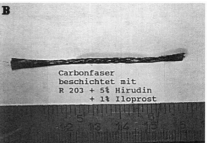

FIGURE 4. Macroscopic picture of carbon fibers following contact with blood. *A,* Uncoated carbon fibers. *B,* Coated carbon fibers (R203, 5% hirudin, 1% iloprost).

SEM pictures of the carbon fiber surfaces showed that activation of coagulation is inhibited by the R203 coating with incorporated hirudin and iloprost (Fig. 5). The formation of thrombi after blood contact with the untreated carbon fibers can be corroborated through biochemical methods because of the high levels of TAT complexes and F_{1-2}. After blood contact with the coated carbon fibers, levels of both markers were tremendously reduced (Fig. 6).

SEM pictures of the uncoated hollow fibers of the oxygenators after blood contact show the same picture: coagulation activation and deposition of a clot consisting of fibrin strands with aggregated platelets and incorporated erythrocytes (Fig. 7). The fibers coated with R203, hirudin, and iloprost showed no coagulation activation and no deposition of thrombotic materials. The coated hollow fibers remained penetrable (Fig. 8). After contact of the untreated hollow fibers with blood, high levels of the TAT complexes and split products of prothrombin during thrombin formation (F_{1-2}) were detected. In contrast, markers of activated coagulation were at much lower levels after contact of coated hollow fibers with blood (Fig. 9).

Oxygenators with hollow fibers can be coated without alteration in structure; the porous structure necessary for oxygen exchange remains intact.

DISCUSSION

The above results indicate that the coating technology developed by our group can reduce thrombogenicity of clinically established biomaterials, such as catheters, oxygenators, and vascular prostheses. All substances used for coating, including the drug carrier and incorporated anticoagulants, are currently used in humans, either systemically or

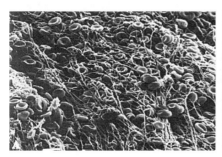
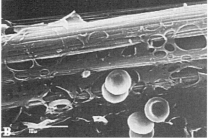

FIGURE 5. Scanning electronmicroscopic picture of uncoated and coated carbon fibers after contact with blood. *A,* Uncoated carbon fibers. *B,* Coated carbon fibers (R203, 5% hirudin, 1% iloprost).

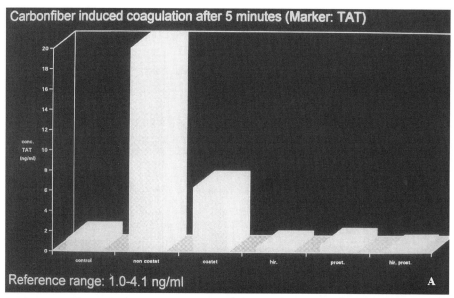

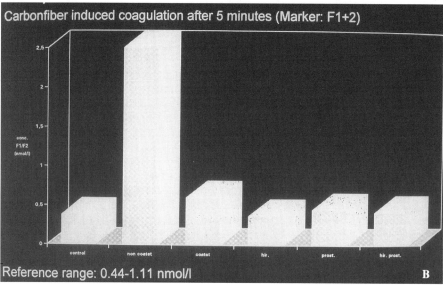

FIGURE 6. Levels of thrombin–antithrombin (TAT) and F_{1-2} in uncoated and coated carbon fibers (R203, 5% hirudin, 1% iloprost) after contact with blood. *A*, TAT levels of uncoated and coated carbon fibers. *B*, F_{1-2} levels of uncoated and coated carbon fibers.

locally, in much higher concentrations. Polymers made of lactic acid or glycolic acid and their combined polymerisates have been used in all areas of medicine—as resorbable suture material and as resorbable screws and plates for bone fixation.[29] In addition, drug carriers with aliphatic polymers are used in the formulation of slow-release systems. The biocompatibility of these polymers has been proved in numerous studies.[13]

The polylactic acid used as a carrier substance is permanently degraded and thus inhibits the adhesion of proteins and cellular components of the blood. Combinations of

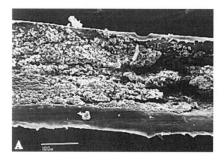
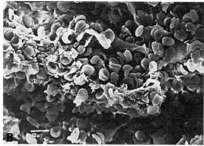

FIGURE 7.   Scanning electronmicroscopic picture of uncoated oxygenator fibers after contact with blood. *A,* Magnified × 240. *B,* Magnified × 1200.

these carriers with hirudin, a potent antithrombin agent, and iloprost, an inhibitor of thrombocyte aggregation, prevent the formation of blood clots after contact of nonanticoagulated blood with coated surfaces. Because of their low dosage and significant persistence in the coating, side effects, such as those described after systemic application, are not expected.

The drug carrier should have anticoagulant characteristics that supplement the effects of incorporated anticoagulant drugs and antiplatelet agents. This approach imitates the body's natural strategy of antithrombogenicity in the vascular endothelium.

At present, synthetic thrombin inhibitors are being tested with good results. In addition, an aseptic coating technology is under development. Medium- and long-term results of coated catheters and vascular prostheses are presently being evaluated in extensive animal experiments.

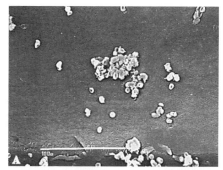
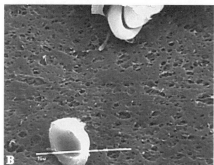

FIGURE 8.   Scanning electronmicroscopic picture of coated oxygenator fibers (R203, 5% hirudin, 1% iloprost) after contact with blood. *A,* Magnified × 600. *B,* Magnified × 6000.

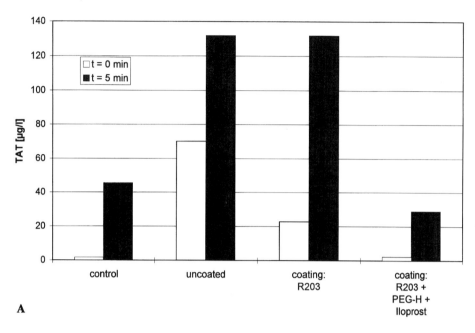

A

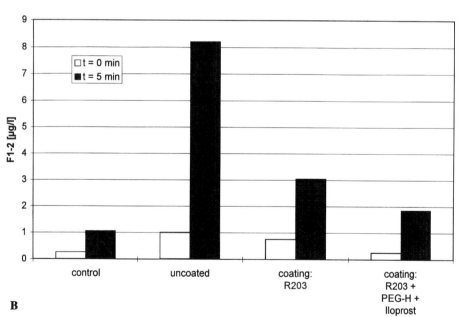

B

FIGURE 9. Levels of thrombin–antithrombin (TAT) complex and F_{1-2} in uncoated and coated oxygenator fibers (R203, 5% hirudin, 1% iloprost) after contact with blood. *A,* TAT levels of uncoated and coated oxygenator fibers. *B,* F_{1-2} levels of uncoated and coated oxygenator fibers.

REFERENCES

1. Bakker D, Van Blitterswijk CA, Daems WT, Grote JJ: Biocompatibility of six elastomers in vitro. J Biomed Mater Res 22: 423–439, 1988.
2. Bick RL: Physiology and pathology of hemostasis during cardiac surgery. In Pifarre R (ed): Anticoagulation, Hemostasis, and Blood Preservation in Cardiovascular Surgery. Philadelphia, Hanley & Belfus, 1993, pp 23–55.
3. Bick RL:Physiology and pathophysiology of hemostasis during cardiac surgery. In Pifarre R (ed): Blood Conservation with Aprotinin. Philadelphia, Hanley & Belfus, 1995, pp 1–44.
4. Bolz A, Schaldach M: Haemocompatibility optimisation of implants by hybrid structuring. Med Biol Eng Comput 31:123–133, 1993.
5. Borowiec J, Thelin S, Bagge L, et al: Heparin-coated cardiopulmonary bypass circuits and 25% reduction of heparin dose in coronary artery surgery—a clinical study. Upsala J Med Sci 97:55–66, 1992.
6. Breillatt J, Hsu L-C: Antithrombotic biomaterials for cardiovascular surgery. In Pifarre R (ed): Anticoagulation, Hemostasis, and Blood Preservation in Cardiovascular Surgery. Philadelphia, Hanley & Belfus, 1993, pp 353–362.
7. Chenoweth DE: Complement activation produced by biomaterials. Trans Am Soc Artif Intern Organs 226–232, 1986.
8. Courtney JM, Irvine L, Jones C, et al: Biomaterials in medicine—a bioengineering perspective. Int J Artif Organs 16:164–171, 1993.
9. Edmunds LH: Cardiopulmonary bypass and blood. In Pifarre R (ed): Blood Conservation with Aprotinin. Philadelphia, Hanley & Belfus, 1995, pp 45–66.
10. Elgue G, Blombäck M, Olsson P, Riesenfeld J: On the mechanism of coagulation inhibition on surfaces with end point immobilized heparin. Thromb Haemost 70:289–293, 1993.
11. Ertl SI, Kohn J, Zimmermann MC, Parsons JR: Evaluation of poly(DTH carbonate), a tyrosine-derived degradable polymer, for orthopedic applications. J Biomed Mater Res 29:1–12, 1995.
12. Ertl SI, Kohn J: Evaluation of a series of tyrosin-derived polycarbonates for biomaterial applications. J Biomed Mater Res 28:919–930, 1994.
13. Furr BJA, Hutchinson FG: A biodegradable delivery system for peptides: preclinical experience with the gonadotrophin-releasing hormone agonist Zoladex R. J Control Release 21:117–128, 1994.
14. Goeau-Brissonniere O, Leport C, Bacourt F, et al: Prevention of vascular graft infection by rifampin bonding to a gelatin-sealed dacron graft. Ann Vasc Surg 5:408–412, 1991.
15. Hall JD, Rittgers SE, Schmidt SP: Effect of the controlled local acetylsalicylic acid release on in vitro platelet adhesion to vascular grafts. J Biomater Appl 8:361–384, 1994.
16. Hayashi K, Fukumura H, Yamamoto N: In vivo thrombus formation induced by complement activation on polymer surfaces. J Biomed Mater Res 24:1385–1395, 1990.
17. Jayabalan M: Biological interactions: Causes for risks and failures of biomaterials and devices. J Biomater Appl 8:64–71, 1993.
18. Janatova J, Bernshaw NJ: A novel approach to test blood-biomaterials compatibility. Presented at the 21th Annual Meeting of the Society for Biomaterials, San Francisco, March 18–22, 1995.
19. Jozefonvicz J, Mauzac M, Aubert N, Jozefowicz M: Antithrombogenic activity of polysaccharide resins. In Williams DF (ed): Biocompatibility of Tissue Analogs, vol II. Boca Rotan, FL, CRC Press, 1985, pp 133–152.
20. Kodama K, Pasche B, Olsson P, et al: Antithrombin III binding to surface immobilized heparin and its relation to F Xa inhibition. Thromb Haemost 58:1064–1067, 1987.
21. McGriffin DC, Kirklin JK: Complement and the damaging effects of cardiopulmonary bypass. In Pifarre R (ed): Blood conservation with aprotinin. Philadelphia, Hanley & Belfus, 1995, pp 67–82.
22. Oliver WC, Nuttall GA: Platelet function and cardiopulmonary bypass. In Pifarre R (ed): Blood Conservation with Aprotinin. Philadelphia, Hanley & Belfus, 1995, pp 83–101.
23. Olsson P, Larm O: Biologically active heparin coating in medical devices. Int J Artif Organs 14:453–456, 1991.
24. Preissner KT, Müller-Berghaus G: Molekulare Wechselwirkungen zwischen Komplement-, Gerinnungs- und Fibrinolysesytem. Hämostaseologie 6:67–81, 1986.
25. San Roman J, Escudero MC, Gallardo A, et al: Application of new coatings for vascular grafts based on polyacrylic systems with antiaggregating activity. Biomaterials 15:759–765, 1994.
26. Spilezewski KL, Anderson JM, Schaap RN, Solomon DD: In vivo biocompatibility of catheter. Biomaterials 9:253–256, 1988.
27. Sundaram S, Courtney JM, Taggart DP, et al: Biocompatibility of cardiopulmonary bypass: Influence on blood compatibility of device type, mode of blood flow and duration of application. Int J Artif Organs 17:118–128, 1993.
28. Szycher M, Lee SJ: Cardiovascular devices for the 1990s. J Biomater Appl 8:31–63, 1993.
29. Törmälä P, Vasenius J, Vainionpää S, et al: Ultra-high-strength absorbable self-reinforced polyglycolide (SR-PGA) composite rods for internal fixation of bone fractures: In vitro and in vivo study. J Biomed Mater Res 25:1–22, 1991.

30. Vogt W: Anaphylatoxins: Possible roles in disease. Complement 3:177–189, 1986.
31. Webb AR, Mythen MG, Jacobson D, Mackie IJ: Maintaining blood flow in the extracorporeal circuit: Haemostasis and anticoagulation. Intens Care Med 21:84–93, 1995.
32. Yianni JP: Making PVC more biocompatible. Med Dev Technol Sept:20–29, 1995.
33. Yianni JP: Biocompatible surfaces based upon biomembrane mimicry. In Quinn PJ, Cherry RJ (eds): Structural and dynamic properties of lipids and membranes. London, Portland Press, 1992, pp 187–216.
34. Zwaal RFA, Hemker HC: Blood cell membranes and haemostasis. Haemostasis 11:12–39, 1982.

CHAPTER 24

Tissue Factor Pathway Inhibitor as an Anticoagulant and Antithrombotic Agent

DEBRA A. HOPPENSTEADT, M.S., M.T. (ASCP)
JAWED FAREED, PH.D.

Activation of the coagulation system proceeds through a series of reactions in which the zymogens of serine enzymes are sequentially activated by proteolytic cleavage. Initially the coagulation cascade was separated into two pathways, the extrinsic and intrinsic systems, which converge at the activation of factor Xa with the subsequent generation of thrombin.

More recently, tissue factor (TF) has been designated as the main activator of coagulation. Exposed TF from the cell surface of TF liberated from damaged cells binds factor FVIIa. The TF–FVIIa complex activates factors X and IX. Loeb was the first to identify a constituent of tissue factor that, when mixed with serum, led to the inhibition of coagulation.[18] In 1957, Hjort showed that adsorbed serum inhibited the factor VIIa–TF complex.[15] Control of this activation process was not understood until 1985, when Sanders and colleagues demonstrated that an inhibitor in plasma was capable of interacting with factor Xa before inhibiting the FVIIa–TF complex.[25] This inhibitor was identified as tissue factor pathway inhibitor (TFPI). In 1988, Wun and colleagues cloned and characterized TFPI.[32]

Plasma contains an inhibitor of the FVIIa–TF complex, previously referred to as lipoprotein-associated coagulation inhibitor (LACI) or extrinsic pathway inhibitor (EPI). TFPI is a kunitz-type serine protease inhibitor (Fig. 1). TFPI consists of a 28-residue signal peptide followed by the full-length TFPI molecule.[22] It consists of 276 amino acid residues (32kd) with 18 cysteine and 3 N-linked glycosylation sites.[22] The TFPI molecule has an acidic terminal followed by 3 tandem kunitz-type domains and a basic carboxy terminal region.[8,32]

TFPI is produced by endothelial cells and renal cells as well as umbilical vein endothelial cells and carcinoma cells. The presence of three kunitz-type domains is consistent with its inhibitory properties for both FVIIa–TF and factor Xa.[7] Kunitz-type inhibitors are present in both animal and plant kingdoms. They characteristically produce slow, tight-binding, competitive, and reversible inhibition.[3,11,20] Drugs such as heparin release TFPI from the vascular sites. Thus, during cardiovascular bypass surgery TFPI is released in sizable amounts and is responsible for the overall anticoagulant responses observed during heparinization.

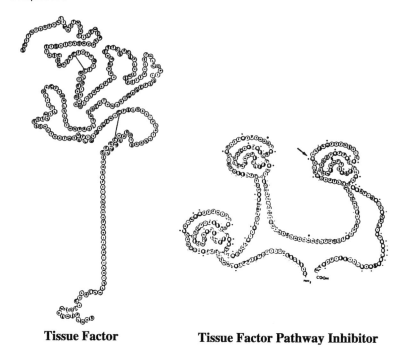

Tissue Factor   **Tissue Factor Pathway Inhibitor**

FIGURE 1.   Comparative molecular structure of tissue factor (TF) and tissue factor pathway inhibitor (TFPI). TF is a transmembrane protein. TFPI is composed of three Kunitz-type domains.

MECHANISM OF ACTION

TFPI inhibits the extrinsic pathway of coagulation by inhibiting the FVIIa–TF complex and by directly inhibiting factor Xa (Fig.2). The factor Xa interaction with TFPI has a stoichiometry of 1:1, and TFPI binds at or near the serine active site of the factor Xa.[12] TFPI also inhibits trypsin but does not effectively alter leukocyte elastase, thrombin, activated protein C, tissue-type plasminogen activator (tPA), or kallikrein. Plasmin and chymotrypsin are inhibited only slightly by TFPI.[10]

The kunitz-1 domain of TFPI is the site of FVIIa binding. This mechanism requires cell surface tissue factor. The kunitz-2 domain is responsible for the binding and inhibition of factor Xa.[13] The carboxy terminal with residues 253–276 is required for optimal inhibition of factor Xa.[30] Broze et al. have shown in vitro that heparin accelerates the reaction between TFPI and FXa.

Cleavage of TFPI by human leukocyte elastase at the Thr 87–Thr 88 bond between the kunitz-1 and kunitz-2 domains also reduces the ability of TFPI to inhibit factor Xa and releases active factor Xa already bound in the TFPI quaternary complex.[14] The release of elastase may trigger the extrinsic system activation in the presence of tissue factor and phospholipids as a result of factor Xa release. This may result in feedback activation of FVII in the absence of functional TFPI. These mechanisms suggest another link between the coagulation and inflammatory systems.

Two mechanisms for the formation of the quaternary complex Xa–TFPI–FVIIa–TF have been proposed (Fig. 3). This quaternary complex can form from the initial binding of FXa to TFPI with the subsequent binding of the factor Xa–TFPI complex to FVIIa–TF. Another proposal is that TFPI binds to the preformed FXa–FVIIa–TF complex.[7] The formation of a quaternary complex explains the need for FXa to inhibit the FVIIa–TF complex as well as the need for active factor Xa, because inactivated FX will

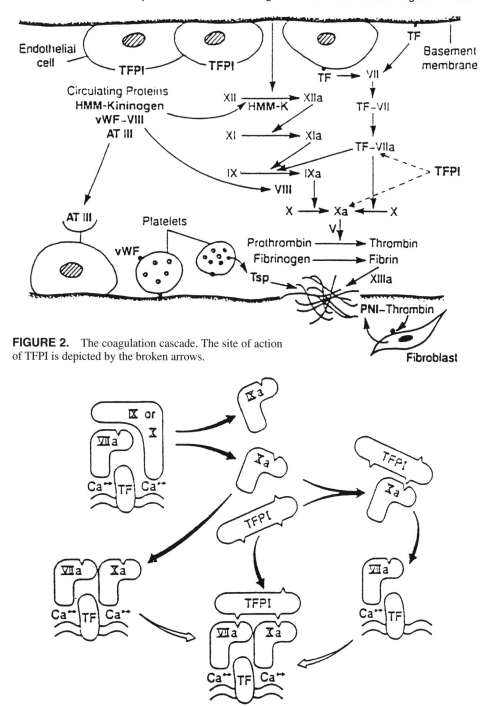

FIGURE 2. The coagulation cascade. The site of action of TFPI is depicted by the broken arrows.

FIGURE 3. Proposed mechanism of the inhibition of FVIIa–TF complex by TFPI. (From Broze JB et al: The lipoprotein-associated coagulation inhibitor that inhibits factor VII-tissue factor complex also inhibits factor X: Insight into possible mechanisms of action. Semin Hematol 29(3):159–169, 1992, with permission.)

not bind to TFPI. High concentrations of TFPI have been shown to inhibit FVIIa–TF activity directly.[24]

The physiologic role of the kunitz-3 domain is not known. However, alteration of the active site residues of the kunitz-3 domain has no effect on FXa or FVIIa–TF inhibition by TFPI.[9]

ENDOGENOUS DISTRIBUTION OF TISSUE FACTOR PATHWAY INHIBITOR

Approximately 80% of TFPI circulates bound to the lipoproteins in plasma: low-density > high-density > very-low-density lipoproteins.[16,22,28] In plasma TFPI is present in multiple molecular weight forms. The predominant forms are found at 34 kd and 40 kd.

The major form of TFPI is the 34-kd form, which is associated with low-density lipoprotein. The 40-kd form is associated with high-density lipoprotein. Very low-density lipoprotein contains both 34- and 40-kd forms.[7] The exact mechanism of the association of lipoproteins to TFPI is not known. The total amount of TFPI in plasma is influenced by the amount of lipoproteins.

Approximately 3–8% of total body TFPI is carried by alpha granules of the platelet. TFPI is released by platelets on their stimulation by thrombin or the calcium ionophore, A23187.[17,21] Therefore, TFPI may be of importance in primary hemostasis, in which platelets are the first line of defense.[7] TFPI is released as a stable soluble protein from the platelet and is not associated with the platelet membrane or shed vesicles.[21]

Another source of TFPI is heparin-releasable TFPI. Plasma levels increase 3- to 5-fold after the infusion of heparin.[23,26] Ex vivo addition of heparin does not change the plasma TFPI level. Therefore, the release of TFPI must come from some intra- or extracellular stores. Cell cultures have shown that TFPI is released from endothelial cells; it is presumed to be intima-bound to other glycosaminoglycans on the endothelial cell surface.[3] Novotny has shown that heparin-releasable TFPI is structurally different from lipoprotein-associated TFPI.[21]

TFPI is synthesized in culture by several different cells from various tissues, including liver, endothelium, monocyte, cell line U937, lung, bladder, and kidney.[1,4,10,27,29,31,32] It is suspected that endothelial cells are responsible for the plasma TFPI levels because of their amount, size, and location.[5]

TFPI circulates in the plasma in many different forms: truncated, full-length, carboxylated, and bound to lipoproteins. The physiologic significance of the different forms of TFPI in disease states and after heparinization is not known. The large increase in plasma TFPI after heparin administration suggests that plasma TFPI is only a fraction of the total TFPI that can be mobilized from several tissue sites that synthesize TFPI. Other pathologic states, such as cancer and heart disease, may cause release of TFPI from these other tissue sites.[7]

RELEASE OF TISSUE FACTOR PATHWAY INHIBITOR BY HEPARIN

TFPI levels increase 2–3 minutes after a single intravenous injection of heparin.[26] The level of TFPI depends on the dosage of heparin. After a bolus of 5000–10000 units, the TFPI activity increases approximately 3-fold.[17,26] After a bolus injection of heparin the TFPI level declines proportionally to the decrease in heparin concentration.[3] After subsequent injections of heparin, the TFPI level increases to approximately the same level as the initial rise.[3] The release of TFPI by heparin shows that the releasable fraction, which is probably intima-bound to glycosaminoglycans, is definitely larger than the circulating TFPI levels.

RESULTS OF HUMAN PLASMA STUDIES

Normal human plasma from 10 healthy donors was pooled, and heparin, recombinant TFPI, and antithrombin III (AT III) were supplemented into the pooled plasma at final concentration ranges of 10–0 µg/ml (heparin and recombinant TFPI) and 10–0 U/ml (AT III).

TEST: PT

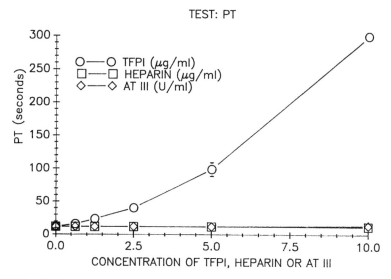

FIGURE 4.   In vitro comparison of TFPI, AT III, and heparin in normal human plasma. TFPI, heparin, and AT III were supplemented in NHP and the prothrombin time (PT) was measured. All results represent a mean of 3 individual determinations.

The effects of TFPI, AT III, and heparin were assay-dependent. TFPI showed the strongest effect in the Xa-based assays, whereas heparin and AT III demonstrated stronger anti-IIa effects.

- The results of the prothrombin time (PT) in the pooled plasma are shown in Figure 4. TFPI caused a dose-dependent elevation in PT between concentrations of 2.5–10 µg/ml. As much as 10 µg/ml of heparin and 10 U/ml of AT III caused no increase in PT.
- The activated partial thromboplastin time (APTT) was measured in the same manner (Fig. 5). Heparin demonstrated a dose-dependent anticoagulant effect. However, TFPI showed only a slight elevation. AT III had no effect on the APTT at concentrations as high as 10 U/ml.
- The results of the thrombin time (TT), using thrombin at a concentration of 5 U/ml, are shown in Figure 6. Both heparin and AT III elevated the thrombin time in a dose-dependent fashion, with heparin being more potent than AT III. TFPI had no effect on the thrombin-based assay.
- An anti-Xa amidolytic assay was also used to compare the anticoagulant effects of recombinant TFPI, heparin, and AT III (Fig. 7). A dose-dependent effect was observed with all three agents. Recombinant TFPI inhibited factor Xa to a greater extent than heparin and AT III. AT III was capable of weakly inhibiting Xa. At a concentration of 10 U/ml, AT III was capable of inhibiting only 50% of the anti-Xa effects.

Heparin, recombinant TFPI, and AT III were also tested in AT III-depleted plasma (Figs. 8–11). Recombinant TFPI and AT III showed identical results in AT III-depleted plasma and normal human pooled plasma in all assays. However, heparin lost activity in the APTT, TT, and anti-Xa assays. As in the normal plasma system, TFPI was the only agent to demonstrate an anticoagulant effect in the PT assay (Fig. 8). In the APTT assay all three agents showed very weak effects (Fig. 9). TFPI and heparin showed weak effects with a concentration of 10 µg/ml, prolonging the clotting time to only 70 seconds. Figure 10 shows the results of the 5U thrombin time. A marked decrease in thrombin clotting

TEST: APTT

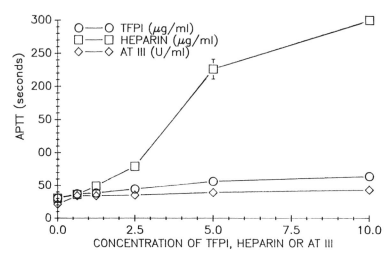

FIGURE 5. In vitro comparison of TFPI, AT III, and heparin in normal human plasma. TFPI, heparin, and AT III were supplemented in NHP and the activated partial thromboplastin time (APTT) was measured. All results represent a mean of 3 individual determinations.

time was noted in the heparin-supplemented, AT III-depleted plasma. No effect was seen in the AT III- or the TFPI-supplemented, AT III-depleted system compared with the normal plasma system.

In the chromogenic assay (Fig.11), the heparinized plasma lost all of its inhibitory function of factor Xa in the absence of AT III. The effect of TFPI and AT III remained the

TEST: THROMBIN TIME 5 U

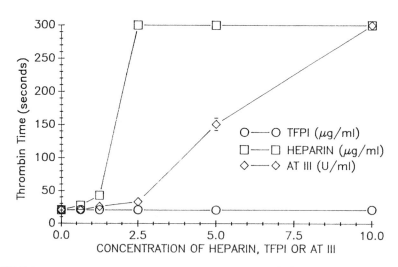

FIGURE 6. In vitro comparison of TFPI, AT III, and heparin in normal human plasma. TFPI, heparin, and AT III were supplemented in NHP and the 5U thrombin time (TT5U) was measured. All results represent a mean of 3 individual determinations.

TEST: ANTI FACTOR Xa

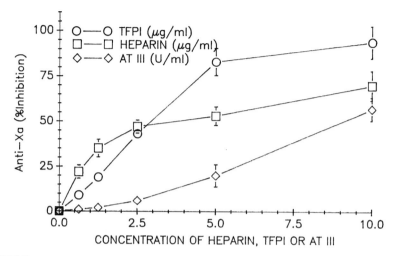

FIGURE 7.   In vitro comparison of TFPI, AT III, and heparin in normal human plasma. TFPI, heparin, and AT III were supplemented in NHP and the amidolytic anti-Xa activity was measured. All results represent a mean of 3 individual determinations.

same as in the normal plasma system. A dose-dependent increase was observed for AT III in both anti-Xa assays. Only anti-Xa showed a dose-dependent response in the TFPI-supplemented plasma, as expected.

In the AT III-depleted plasma system the results obtained with TFPI and AT III were the same as the results in the normal plasma system. However, in the heparinized AT III-depleted plasma, approximately 50–75% of the activity was lost. Heparin requires AT III

TEST: PT

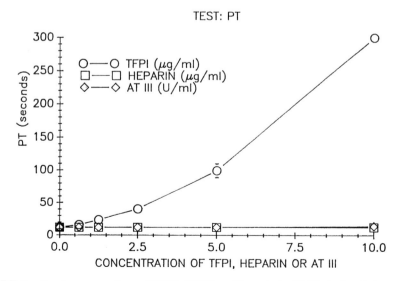

FIGURE 8.   In vitro comparison of TFPI, AT III, and heparin in AT III-depleted plasma. TFPI, heparin, and AT III were supplemented in AT III-depleted plasma and the prothrombin time (PT) was measured. All results represent a mean of 3 individual determinations.

TEST: APTT

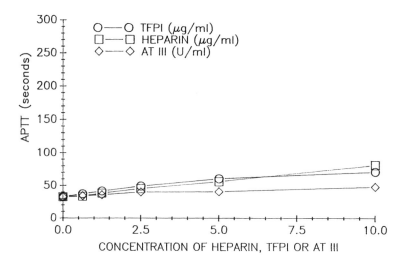

FIGURE 9.   In vitro comparison of TFPI, AT III, and heparin in AT III-depleted plasma. TFPI, heparin, and AT III were supplemented in AT III-depleted plasma and the activated partial thromboplastin time (APTT) was measured. All results represent a mean of 3 individual determinations.

as a cofactor. In the presence of heparin, the thrombin-antithrombin interaction is increased 10,000-fold and the heparin-Xa interaction is increased 4,000-fold. In the absence of AT III, the inhibition of these serine proteases occurred at a much slower rate.

Finally, the effects of the three agents were studied in TFPI-depleted plasma. Figures 12–15 show the results of the PT, APTT, 5U TT, and anti-Xa assays. The results

TEST: THROMBIN TIME 5U

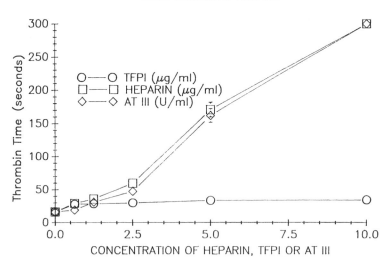

FIGURE 10.   In vitro comparison of TFPI, AT III, and heparin in AT III-depleted plasma. TFPI, heparin, and AT III were supplemented in AT III-depleted plasma and the 5U thrombin time (TT5U) was measured. All results represent a mean of 3 individual determinations.

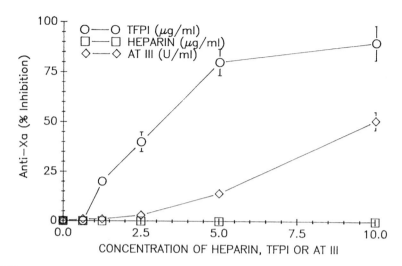

FIGURE 11. In vitro comparison of TFPI, AT III, and heparin in AT III-depleted plasma. TFPI, heparin, and AT III were supplemented in AT III-depleted plasma and the amidolytic anti-Xa activity was measured. All results represent a mean of 3 individual determinations.

of heparin, AT III, and TFPI supplementation in TFPI-depleted plasma were identical to the results in normal plasma. TFPI requires no cofactors in plasma to exert its anticoagulant effects. Furthermore, TFPI is not a cofactor for AT III or heparin.

Administration of heparin results in a 3–5-fold increase in TFPI. TFPI is mobilized from the endothelium after heparin administration. TFPI released from the endothelium results in an increase in anticoagulant effect in the plasma. In the in vitro system, in which

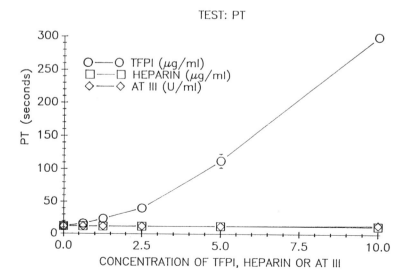

FIGURE 12. In vitro comparison of TFPI, AT III, and heparin in TFPI-depleted plasma. TFPI, heparin, and AT III were supplemented in TFPI-depleted plasma and the prothrombin time (PT) was measured. All results represent a mean of 3 individual determinations.

TEST: APTT

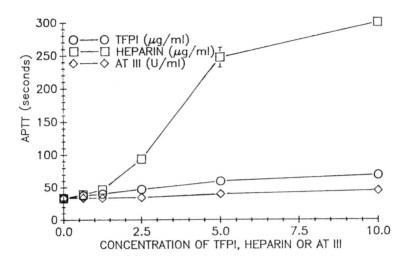

FIGURE 13. In vitro comparison of TFPI, AT III, and heparin in TFPI-depleted plasma. TFPI, heparin, and AT III were supplemented in TFPI-depleted plasma and the activated partial thromboplastin time (APTT) was measured. All results represent a mean of 3 individual determinations.

TFPI levels are low, (approximately 60 ng/ml), the contribution of TFPI to the heparin effect is difficult to quantitate. Thus, in TFPI-depleted plasma, the anticoagulant effect of heparin was the same as in normal human plasma. The synergistic effect of TFPI and heparin can be observed in vivo only in the presence of intact endothelium with large vascular stores of releasable TFPI.

TEST: THROMBIN TIME 5 U

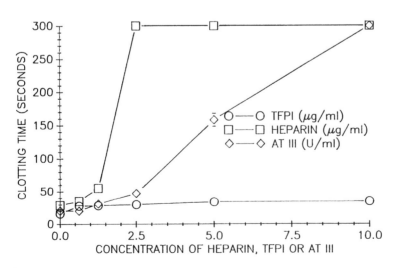

FIGURE 14. In vitro comparison of TFPI, AT III, and heparin in TFPI-depleted plasma. TFPI, heparin, and AT III were supplemented in TFPI-depleted plasma and the 5U thrombin time (TT5U) was measured. All results represent a mean of 3 individual determinations.

TEST: ANTI FACTOR Xa

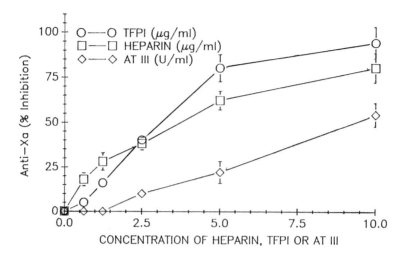

FIGURE 15. In vitro comparison of TFPI, AT III, and heparin in TFPI-depleted plasma. TFPI, heparin, and AT III were supplemented in TFPI-depleted plasma and the amidolytic anti-Xa activity was measured. All results represent a mean of 3 individual determinations.

In addition to the anticoagulant effects of TFPI, the in vivo antithrombotic effects of recombinant TFPI were also studied. A rabbit model of jugular vein stasis-thrombosis was used to test the antithrombotic effects. This model uses stasis, combined with FEIBA (Immuno AG, Austria), a prothrombin complex concentrate, as a thrombogenic challenge. Recombinant TFPI showed a dose-dependent antithrombotic response in the rabbit stasis-thrombosis model (Fig. 16). With an intravenous dose of 100 µg/kg, the mean clot score

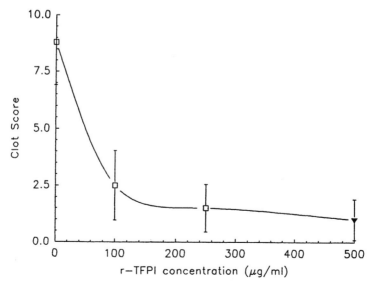

FIGURE 16. Antithrombotic actions of intravenously injected recombinant-TFPI in a rabbit model of stasis-thrombosis. All results represent a mean of 5 individual determinations ± 1 standard deviation.

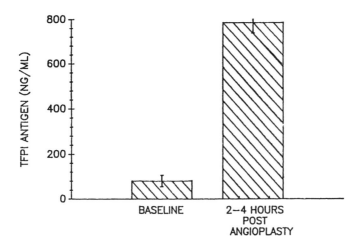

FIGURE 17.   TFPI antigen levels in patients undergoing PTCA. Patients were given a 10,000–20,000 U intravenous bolus of heparin before the PTCA procedure. Blood samples were drawn before and 2-4 hours after angioplasty. All results represent a mean of 30 individual determinations ± 1 standard deviation.

after a 10-minute stasis time was 2.5 compared with the control clot score of 8.8 (p < 0.001). Approximately 72% of clot formation was inhibited by recombinant TFPI at this dosage. With an intravenous dose of 250 μg/kg, 83% was inhibited, and with an intravenous dose of 500 μg/kg, inhibition of clot formation was complete. No bleeding effects were observed at a dosage 10 times higher than that required to obtain an antithrombotic effect.

In addition to AT III, TFPI has been shown to be an important contributor to the anticoagulant and antithrombotic action of heparin. TFPI binds factor Xa and inactivates the TF–FVIIa complex. Heparin redistributes and releases the intravascular stores of TFPI by binding to the endothelium. During interventional cardiologic procedures, such as percutaneous transluminal coronary angioplasty (PTCA) and cardiopulmonary bypass surgery, in which large preoperative dosages of heparin are administered, the TFPI antigen was quantitated. The effects on the TFPI antigen levels after heparinization in angioplasty are shown in Figure 17. After the administration of an intravenous bolus of 10,000–20,000 U of heparin, the TFPI levels increased 8–10-fold over the baseline value (p < 0.001). Approximately 2–4 hours after angioplasty the TFPI antigen levels remained elevated, indicating that large quantities of heparin-releasable TFPI were displaced from the endogenous stores. Similar results were obtained in bypass patients (Fig. 18). TFPI antigen levels were elevated 8–10-fold from baseline 30 minutes after injection of a bolus of heparin (20,000–25,000 U). These levels remained elevated throughout bypass surgery.

DISCUSSION

Exactly 50 years ago, Biggs and coworkers postulated the concept of a TF-dependent pathway or extrinsic cascade.[6] Ratanoff and coworkers independently postulated the concept of an intrinsic pathway of coagulation. Their work led to the classic concept of the coagulation cascade. Although the coagulation cascade remains an important process, the role of Morawitz's thrombokinase has been proved to exceed the original conception.[19] The extrinsic pathway of coagulation was initially thought to be a single biochemical reaction in which a vitamin K-dependent factor, namely FVII, interacted with TF in the presence of calcium to activate factor X. However, the role of TF involves the activation not only of proteases but also of several cells. Monocytes, macrophages, fibroblasts,

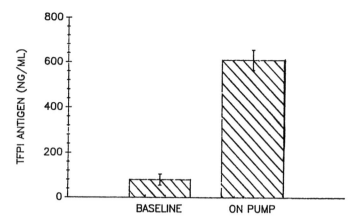

FIGURE 18. TFPI antigen levels in patients undergoing cardiopulmonary bypass surgery. Patients were administered 10,000–20,000 U intravenous bolus of heparin, 30 minutes after bypass was initiated. Blood samples were drawn before and 30 minutes on pump. All results represent a mean of 30 individual determinations ± 1 standard deviation.

and endothelium are known to possess TF receptors that, through signal transduction reaction of cellular mechanisms, regulate processes leading to thrombogenesis. Thus, TF is known to be a key player in the mediation of thrombogenesis.

The pioneering work of Broze and Wun led to the isolation and characterization of a specific inhibitor of TF, namely TFPI.[10,32] This inhibitor was later expressed in *Escherichia coli* (the recombinant equivalent of plasma TFPI), which prompted extensive biochemical and pharmacologic studies of the potential role of TFPI as one of the endogenous regulators of the actions of TF. In addition, TFPI possesses several other properties, including inhibition of factor Xa, platelet activation, and regulation of cells. Of greater interest, heparin and related drugs are known to mobilize TFPI from endogenous sites to augment their own antithrombotic effects. TFPI alone produces antithrombotic effects without circulating heparin. The availability of TFPI variants has therefore greatly facilitated our understanding of the role of TFPI as a mediator of the antithrombotic actions of pharmacologic agents.

With the availability of recombinant forms, the role of TFPI in the control of TF-mediated activation of proteases and platelets, as well as its role as an anticoagulant and antithrombotic agent, has been elucidated. AT III conventionally has been known to be the key mediator of the actions of heparin. Without AT III heparin is nonfunctional. Although heparin requires AT III as a cofactor, TFPI requires no cofactors. A parallel comparison of AT III, heparin, and TFPI demonstrates that on a molar basis TFPI is a more potent inhibitor of factor Xa than heparin and AT III. In contrast to heparin, TFPI does not inhibit thrombin.

Because of its multiple effects on the coagulation cascade and platelet function, TFPI was also tested for its antithrombotic actions in a model in which a complex mixture of activated FVII and FX was used as a thrombogenic agent. In the intravenous studies TFPI produced a dose-dependent antithrombotic effect with an apparent ED_{50} of 70 µg/kg. Thus, at an initial circulating concentration of 1.4 µg/ml (30 nM), TFPI produced a potent antithrombotic action. The pharmacokinetics of its antithrombotic action were not addressed. The initial pharmacodynamic analysis revealed complex interactions and a large volume of distribution. Thus, valid investigations to understand the mechanism involved in the compartmentalization of TFPI are warranted.

All antithrombotic drugs exhibit hemorrhagic effects at 5–10 times the dose of the antithrombotic actions. A rabbit model of ear blood loss was used to assess the hemorrhagic actions of TFPI. TFPI produced no significant bleeding effects at intravenous doses up to 1 mg/kg. This dose represents a 12-fold increase in the ED_{50} in which antithrombotic actions were noted. In contrast, a similar dose of heparin causes bleeding.

Interventional cardiologic procedures, such as PTCA and cardiopulmonary bypass surgery, require large doses of heparin, which often reach circulating concentrations of 5 U/ml. Such procedures provide a unique opportunity to determine the release of TFPI by large doses of heparin. The enzyme-linked immunosorbent assay (ELISA) demonstrated up to a 10-fold increase in levels of TFPI antigen after heparinization. Some patients were found to resist heparinization, and a parallel deficit in TFPI release was evident. Intravenous administration of large amounts of heparin at doses used for cardiovascular procedures may be enough to mobilize all of the vascular and other pools of TFPI. Heparin remains the most useful anticoagulant for cardiovascular procedures. In both PTCA and bypass surgery, massive amounts of TF are generated. Heparin mobilizes TFPI, which can effectively neutralize its effects, whereas hirudin and related antithrombin agents do not mobilize TFPI. These agents have been proposed as alternate anticoagulants to heparin for cardiovascular indications. A direct comparison of the two anticoagulant drugs will provide crucial information about the potential role of TF in the mediation of thrombogenesis and its modulation by TFPI. Data obtained in this group of patients prove unequivocally the endogenous release of TFPI by heparin. The multiple pharmacologic actions of TFPI remain to be elucidated.

DEVELOPMENTAL POTENTIAL

TFPI is currently produced by recombinant technology for pharmaceutical purposes. Both the *E. coli* and CHO cell lines have been used for expression of TFPI. The antithrombotic actions of TFPI have been extensively profiled in various animal models. A recent study reported the effects of TFPI on the effects of myocardial infarction in an animal model.[5] TFPI also has been shown to reduce reperfusion injury in similar animal models. Thus TFPI alone can be used as an anticoagulant for various surgical procedures. The circulating concentration of TFPI is enough to control the tissue factor activation of the coagulation system. However, at levels below 100 ng/ml TFPI produces no anticoagulant effects. In much the same way, physiologic levels of tPA may produce endogenous fibrinolysis but are insufficient to produce systemic lysis. Through recombinant technology both proteins can be produced in adequate amounts for clinical use. TFPI can be produced in different variant forms, with adjusted endogenous half-lives, thus providing a unique nonheparin, protein-derived anticoagulant that can be developed for several cardiovascular indications.

REFERENCES

1. Abildgaard U, Sandset PM, Andersson TR, et al: The inhibitor of FVIIa in plasma measured with a sensitive chromogenic substrate assay. Comparison with antithrombin, protein C, heparin cofactor II in a clinical material. Flia Haematol (Leipz) 115:274–277, 1988.
2. Abildgaard U, Sandset PM, Lindahl AK: Tissue factor pathway inhibitor. In Poller L (ed): Recent Advances in Blood Coagulation, 6th ed. Edinburgh, Churchill Livingstone, 1993, pp 105–124.
3. Antonini E, Ascenzi P, Menegatti E, Guarneri M: Multiple intermediates in the reaction of bovine β-trypsin with bovine pancreatic trypsin inhibitor (Kunitz). Biopolymers 22:363–375, 1983.
4. Bajaj MS, Kuppuswamy MN, Saito H, et al: Cultured normal human hepatocytes do not synthesize lipoprotein-associated coagulation inhibitor: Evidence that endothelium is the principle site of its synthesis. Proc Natl Acad Sci USA 87:8869–8873, 1990.
5. Basim K, Ferguson EW, Yu CD, et al: The effect of TFPI on myocardial infarction size. J Am Col Cardiol 81A:902–931, 1996.
6. Biggs R, Nossel HL: Tissue extract and the contact reaction in blood coagulation. Thromb Diath Haemorrh 6:1–14, 1961.
7. Broze G: The role of tissue factor pathway inhibitor in a revised coagulation cascade. Semin Hematol 29(3):159–169, 1992.
8. Broze G, Girard TJ, Novotny WF: Regulation of coagulation by a multivalent kunitz-type inhibitor. Biochemistry 29:7539–7546, 1990.

9. Broze GJ, Likert K, Higuchi D: Inhibition of factor VIIa/tissue factor by antithrombin III and tissue factor pathway inhibitor. Blood 82:1679–1681, 1993.
10. Broze GJ, Miletich JP: Isolation of the tissue factor inhibitor produced by HepG2 hepatoma cells. Proc Natl Acad Sci USA 84:1886–1890, 1987.
11. Broze GJ Jr, Warren LA, Girard JJ, et al: Isolation of the lipoprotein-associated coagulation inhibitor produced by HepG2 (human hepatoma) cells using bovine factor Xa affinity chromatography. Thromb Res 48:253–259, 1987.
12. Broze GJ, Warren LA, Novonty WF, et al: The lipoprotein-associated coagulation inhibitor that inhibits factor VII-tissue factor complex also inhibits factor X: Insight into possible mechanisms of action. Blood 71:335–343, 1988.
13. Girard TJ, Warren LA, Novonty WF: Functional significance of the kunitz-type inhibitor domains of lipoprotein associated coagulation inhibitor. Nature 338:518–520, 1989.
14. Higuchi DA, Wun TC, Likert KM: The effect of leukocyte elastase on tissue factor pathway inhibitor. Blood 79:1712–1719, 1992.
15. Hjort PF: Intermediate reactions in the coagulation of blood with thromboplastin. Scand J Clin Lab Invest 9(Suppl 27):1–173, 1957.
16. Hubbard AR, Jennings CA: Inhibition of the tissue factor-factor VII complex: Involvement of factor Xa and lipoproteins. Thromb Res 46:527–537, 1987.
17. Lindahl AK, Abildgaard U, Staalesen R: The anticoagulant effect in heparinized blood and plasma resulting from interactions with extrinsic pathway inhibitor. Thromb Res 64:155–168, 1991.
18. Loeb L, Fleischer MS, Tuttle L: The interaction between blood serum and tissue extract in the coagulation of blood. I: The combined action of serum and tissue extract on fluoride, hirudin and peptone plasma; the effect of heating on the serum. J Biol Chem 51:461–483, 1922.
19. Morawitz P: The Chemistry of Blood Coagulation. (Translated by Hartmann RC, Guenther PF). Charles C Thomas, Springfield, MA, 1958, p 194.
20. Morrison SA, Jesty J: Tissue factor-dependent activation of tritium-labeled factor IX and factor X in human plasma. Blood 63:1338–13347, 1982.
21. Novotny WF, Girard TJ, Miletich JP, et al: Platelets secrete a coagulation inhibitor functionally and antigenically similar to the lipoprotein-associated coagulation inhibitor. Blood 71:2020–2025, 1988.
22. Novotny WF, Girard TJ, Miletich JP, Broze GJ: Purification and characterization of lipoprotein-associated coagulation inhibitor from human plasma. J Biol Chem 264:18832–18837, 1989.
23. Novotny WF, Palmier M, Wun TC, et al: Purification and properties of heparin-releasable lipoprotein-associated coagulation inhibitor. Blood 78:394–400, 1991.
24. Pederson AH, Nordfang O, Norris F, et al: Recombinant human tissue factor pathway inhibitor. J Biol Chem 265:16786–16793, 1990.
25. Sanders NL, Bajaj SP, Zivelin A, et al: Inhibition of tissue factor/factor VII activity requires factor Xa and an additional plasma component. Blood 66:204–212, 1985.
26. Sandset PM, Abildgaard, Larsen ML: Heparin induces the release of extrinsic coagulation pathway inhibitor (EPI). Thromb Res 47:803–813, 1988.
27. Warn-Cramer BJ, Almus FE, Rapaport SI: Studies of the factor Xa dependent inhibitor of factor VIIa/tissue factor (extrinsic pathway inhibitor) from cell supernates of cultured human umbilical vein endothelial cells. Thromb Haemost 61:101–105, 1989.
28. Warn-Cramer BJ, Maki SL, Zivelin A, et al: Partial purification and characterization of extrinsic pathway inhibitor (the factor Xa-dependent plasma inhibitor of factor VIIa/tissue factor). Thromb Res 48:11–22, 1987.
29. Warr TA, Rao VM, Rapaport S: Human plasma extrinsic inhibitor activity: Plasma levels in disseminated intravascular coagulation and hepatocellular disease. Blood 74:994–998, 1989.
30. Wenzel HR, Tschesche H: Chemical mutation by amino acid exchange in the reactive site of a proteinase inhibitor and alteration of its inhibitor specificity. Angew Chem Int Ed 20:295–296, 1981.
31. Wun TC, Kretzmer KK, Girard TJ, et al: Cloning and characterization of a cDNA coding for the lipoprotein-associated coagulation inhibitor shows that consists of three tandem kunitz-type inhibitory domains. J Biol Chem 263:6001–6004, 1988.
32. Wun TC, Huang MD, Kretzmer KK, et al: Immunoaffinity purification and characterization of lipoprotein-associated coagulation inhibitor from HepG2 hepatoma, chang and SK hepatoma cells. J Biol Chem 265:16096–16101, 1990.

CHAPTER 25

Synthetic and Biotechnology-derived Heparin Homologs and Analogs as Potential Antithrombotic Agents

WALTER P. JESKE, Ph.D.
JEANINE M. WALENGA, Ph.D.
JAWED FAREED, Ph.D.

McLean isolated the first heparin 80 years ago. Despite its acceptance into clinical practice, the intricacies of heparin's mechanism of action still remain unclear. Unfractionated heparin is used clinically in the treatment of unstable angina and myocardial infarction and for the prevention of deep vein thrombosis (DVT). Low-molecular-weight (LMW) heparins are currently the agents of choice for the prevention of DVT in Europe, and they are quickly gaining acceptance in the United States. Other heparin-related drugs, including even lower LMW heparins and the pentasaccharide representing the minimal antithrombin (AT) III-binding sequence of heparin, are being developed for clinical use. Concerns with using heparin and heparin-like anticoagulants include hemorrhage and heparin-induced thrombocytopenia. Consequently, the pharmaceutical industry has been interested in newer and more effective antithrombotic drugs. This chapter discusses the pharmacology of synthetic and biotechnology-derived homologs and analogs of heparin.

Analogs and homologs of heparin can be divided into three categories, as listed in Table 1. The synthetic analogs of heparin include the AT III binding pentasaccharides, sulfated lactobionic acid derivatives, and cyclic polysulfones. The semi-synthetic, biotechnology derived analogs include K5 derived heparin polysaccharides and pentosan polysulfate. Chemically modified heparins include such agents as O-desulfated heparins and supersulfated heparins.

SYNTHETIC ANALOGS OF HEPARIN

Synthetic analogs of heparin offer several advantages over unfractionated heparin. Perhaps the most important is that they are pure substances. Whereas unfractionated and LMW heparins are mixtures of glycosaminoglycan chains of different size and contain microheterogeneity in the sulfation and carboxylation of the molecular backbones, the structures of the synthetic agents are fully known. Another advantage of the synthetic analogs is the absence of contaminating materials. Heparins are produced from natural

TABLE 1.   Analogs and Modifications of Heparin

Synthetic analogs of heparin
  Pentasaccharide
  Bis-lactobionic acid derivatives
  Polysulfonates
Semisynthetic analogs of heparin
  Pentosan polysulfate
  K5-derived analogs
  Heparan sulfate and dermatan sulfate
    Marine products
    Fish-skin derived products
Chemically and physically modified heparins
  Astenose
  Supersulfated heparins
  Desulfated heparins

sources that have the potential of viral contamination, such as bovine spongiform encephalopathy or hoof and mouth disease. Other glycosaminoglycans, such as dermatan sulfate or heparan sulfate, or nucleic acid residues can also be present in heparin preparations. Finally, because they are produced synthetically, these analogs provide a framework for structure-activity studies. Side groups and various functional groups can be readily modified to provide molecules that may exhibit a targeted mechanism of action.

Pentasaccharide

Heparin is an antithrombotic and anticoagulant agent because it interacts with the plasma serum protease inhibitor antithrombin III (AT III) and thereby markedly potentiates the inhibition of serine proteases of the coagulation cascade, particularly thrombin and factor Xa. By measuring the AT III affinity of a series of heparin fragments, it was determined that the minimal AT III binding sequence resides in an irregular region of heparin and is a pentasaccharide in size.[10,44,58] This pentasaccharide, which is present in approximately 25–30% of heparin chains, contains a unique 3-O sulfate group. The importance of this sulfate group to both in vitro anticoagulant and in vivo antithrombotic activities has been demonstrated.[74] After its discovery, this pentasaccharide was chemically synthesized.[53] Higher yields of the methyl α-glycoside derivative of the pentasaccharide have been achieved; its chemical structure is depicted in Figure 1. This derivative exhibits the same biologic properties as the native agent.

Studies have shown that the pentasaccharide has no measurable activity in the assays for prothrombin time or activated partial thromboplastin time (APTT). In addition, pentasaccharide is known to be ineffective in both coagulant and amidolytic antithrombin assays.[73] It does, however, exhibit a high antifactor Xa potency.[11] Pentasaccharide has been

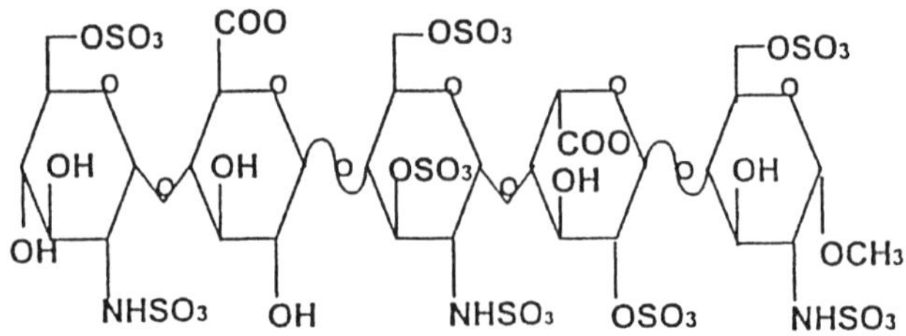

FIGURE 1.   The chemical structure of a methyl α-glycoside derivative of the high-affinity binding pentasaccharide of heparin. The pentasaccharide contains the unique 3-O sulfate group required for high-affinity binding to antithrombin III. The molecular weight of this agent is 1728 Da.

shown to inhibit thrombin generation in normal human plasma in a concentration-dependent manner.[45] Thrombin generation was more potently inhibited after extrinsic pathway activation than after intrinsic pathway activation. This weaker inhibition of the intrinsic pathway is likely due to the pentasaccharide's inability to inhibit formation of factors V and VIII.[51] It has been shown both in vitro and in vivo that thrombin generation is not completely inhibited by pentasaccharide. At doses of pentasaccharide that completely prevented thrombus formation in a modified Wessler model, thrombin generation was inhibited by only 60%.[75] Clots contained predominantly red cells and fibrin but few platelets. The thrombi formed in the arteriovenous shunt model contain red cells, fibrin strands, and a large amount of platelets. Pentasaccharide was able to inhibit thrombus formation in both models. In a rat thrombosis model, Hobbelen showed that pentasaccharide inhibited thrombosis caused by various triggers in a dose-dependent manner.[24] In addition, this study has shown that pentasaccharide causes a smaller increase in blood loss than heparin at antithrombotically active doses. Impaired thrombin generation rather than anti-Xa activity was observed to correlate with prevention of stasis-induced thrombus formation.[69]

The antithrombotic effect of pentasaccharide has also been tested in baboons using a modified arteriovenous shunt in which both arterial-type and venous-type thrombi can form.[8] Although both types of thrombi were inhibited by pentasaccharide, higher doses were needed to achieve a comparable level of inhibition on the arterial side. The pentasaccharide was also observed to have no effect on platelet function as measured by the template bleeding time. The pentasaccharide has been observed to reduce thrombus formation after an electrical stimulation injury in rabbit carotid arteries and to enhance clot lysis induced by tissue plasminogen activator.

A series of structural analogs of the native pentasaccharide sequence has been synthesized.[48] These analogs contain an additional 3-O sulfate group on glucosamine residue H. In addition, some of the analogs also contained a 3-O or 4-O sulfate group on glucosamine residue D. All of the analogs with additional 3-O sulfate groups exhibited a higher anti-Xa potency than the native pentasaccharide (1230 anti-Xa U/mg vs. 700 anti-Xa U/mg). The higher specific activity is thought to be due to a tighter two-site binding to AT III. As expected, all of the analogs were active in a rat model of stasis thrombosis. The duration of the antithrombotic effect was 4–5 times longer for the highly sulfated pentasaccharides than for the natural pentasaccharide. The half-life of the anti-Xa activity of the modified analogs was approximately twice that of the natural pentasaccharide. Conversion of the N-sulfate groups on the parent pentasaccharide to O-sulfates has been shown to increase AT III affinity twofold, whereas O-methylation was observed to lead to an eightfold increase in AT III affinity.[23]

Bis-Lactobionic Acid Derivatives

Sulfated bis-aldonic acid amides are a new class of synthetic LMW polyanions that possess antithrombotic activity. These agents are synthesized by conversion of aldonic acids to their corresponding cyclic ester, or lactone. Two such lactone molecules are linked via amide bonds with an alkylene diamine. The intermediate is then fully sulfated with a pyridine-SO_3 complex, resulting in a homogeneous product.[36] Lactobionic, D-gluconic, L-mannonic, D-galactonic, milibionic, and maltobionic acids have been used as starting materials and were linked by alkylene diamine bridges ranging from 2–12 units in length. The compound that has shown the best anticoagulant and antithrombotic profile consists of two lactobionic acid moieties linked by a trimethylene diamine.[37,38] This compound is known as aprosulate (Fig. 2). A unique feature of aprosulate is its high degree of sulfation: every hydroxyl group on both disaccharides contains an O-linked sulfate group. The molecular weights of these compounds are lower than those of the LMW heparins (6000 Da); the molecular weight of aprosulate is 2388 Da.

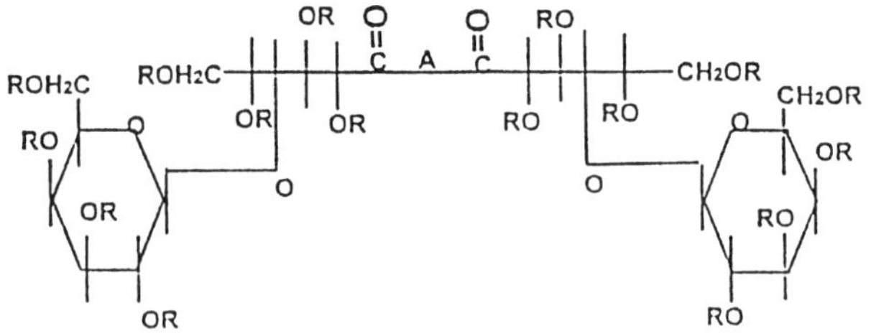

$$A = NH\text{-}(CH_2)_3\text{-}NH$$
$$R = \text{-}SO_3Na$$

FIGURE 2.   The chemical structure of aprosulate, which is characterized by two fully sulfated disaccharides linked via amide bonds by a propylene chain. The molecular weight of aprosulate is 2388 Da.

The anticoagulant properties of several aldonic acid amides have been reported.[32,56,66] These agents exhibited anticoagulant activity in the APTT and Heptest assays, indicating that they inhibit the intrinsic coagulation pathway enzymes. This activity was low compared with heparin. Activity in a chromogenic anti-factor Xa assay was reported to be 200 times less than that of heparin.[56]

Fareed et al. examined the pharmacodynamics of aprosulate in Rhesus monkeys (*Macaca mulatta*) after both intravenous and subcutaneous injection.[14] The APTT, 5U thrombin time, and Heptest were prolonged by aprosulate in a dose-dependent manner. The amidolytic activity of thrombin was inhibited only up to 30 minutes after injection. Based on these data, the biologic half-life of aprosulate was estimated to be 45 minutes.

In vitro, ex vivo, and in vivo neutralizations of aprosulate have been examined with protamine sulfate. In in vitro samples, complete neutralization in the Heptest and thrombin time assays was observed with a 2–4-fold gravimetric excess of protamine. Despite this high level of protamine, the APTT values remained elevated.[27] Aprosulate's effects on the amidolytic anti-IIa and anti-Xa assays were completely neutralized by equigravimetric amounts of protamine. Protamine effectively neutralized aprosulate when an intravenous injection of aprosulate was followed by an equigravimetric intravenous injection of protamine, as measured using the Heptest or thrombin time.[27,35] In addition, protamine neutralizes the antithrombotic activity of aprosulate in a dose-dependent manner, as measured in a rat jugular vein-clamping model of thrombosis. A 2.5-fold gravimetric excess of protamine was required to neutralize the antithrombotic activity completely. The anticoagulant activity of aprosulate was not affected by high concentrations of the native heparin inhibitor, platelet factor 4.[37]

The mechanism of action of aprosulate has been examined in several studies. Aprosulate was observed to inhibit approximately 50% of thrombin activity in the presence of plasma at 5–20 µg/ml. If purified AT III was substituted for the plasma, aprosulate was completely ineffective at inhibiting thrombin. Heparin, in contrast, is more potent in the presence of purified AT III. To examine further aprosulate's interaction with AT III, the APTT was measured with and without the presence of rabbit anti-AT III antibodies. Addition of the antibodies did not affect the prolongation of the APTT by aprosulate, whereas heparin's ability to prolong the APTT was almost completely neutralized in the presence of the antibodies.[37] Aprosulate is able to inhibit thrombin in a dose-dependent manner when incubated with purified heparin cofactor II.[25,32] Ofosu et al. demonstrated that aprosulate was able to inhibit intrinsic prothrombin activation by a mechanism similar to that of dermatan sulfate, via heparin cofactor II. Even at high concentrations, aprosulate is unable to prevent the activation of tissue factor-dependent factor X and factor V.[51] The lag time for intrinsic prothrombin activation is, however, increased by aprosulate. Although several bis-aldonic acid amides have been shown to release tissue plasminogen activator in an isolated pig ear perfusion model, aprosulate does not.[37] It is also a potent stimulator of the release of tissue factor pathway inhibitor (TFPI).

Aprosulate is an effective antithrombotic agent in vivo, as shown in several animal models. In the Harbauer model[21] of venous thrombosis in rabbits, 1 mg/kg of aprosulate, administered intravenously, almost completely prevents thrombosis. The same effect was observed 2 hours after subcutaneous administration of the same dose. A significant inhibition of thrombus formation was seen at least 6 hours after subcutaneous administration. This effect is stronger than that seen with an equigravimetric dose of heparin.[54] In a rat jugular vein-clamping model,[55] 1 mg/kg of aprosulate is observed to be an effective antithrombotic agent.[56] With increasing doses, an increased number of clampings is required to elicit thrombus formation. Aprosulate is less potent than heparin in preventing thrombosis in this model. Aprosulate has been shown to be effective in an arteriovenous shunt model of thrombosis.[65] Antithrombotically effective doses of aprosulate are not associated with significant bleeding risks.

Polysulfonates

GL-522-Y-1 (Genelabs, Redwood City, CA) is a synthetic sulfonated calix[8]arene that exhibits weak antithrombotic properties. This compound does not have a saccharidic backbone like heparin, yet maintains a degree of antithrombotic activity. It does not derive its polyanionic character from sulfate groups but rather from sulfonate groups (Fig. 3). Unlike heparin, GL-522-Y-1 exhibits anticoagulant activity in global clotting assays only at very high concentrations. In addition, negligible activity is observed in chromogenic antithrombin and anti-factor Xa assays at these concentrations.[30] GL-522-Y-1 exhibits no affinity to antithrombin III and only a weak affinity for heparin cofactor II; however, it inhibits factor Xa and thrombin generation, as measured in amidolytic, fibrinogen-deficient plasma systems. GL-522-Y-1 is a protease generation inhibitor following both intrinsic and extrinsic pathway activation. This inhibition is more potent than that of either pentasaccharide or aprosulate and is observed at lower concentrations than those required to activate heparin cofactor II. The mechanism by which GL-522-Y-1 achieves this inhibition is not known.

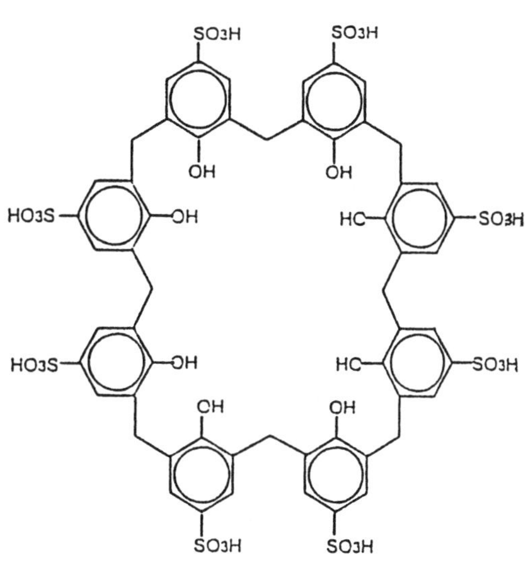

FIGURE 3. The chemical structure of GL-522-Y-1. This agent is not saccharidic but is a cyclic polymer of phenol residues alternately separated by methyl groups. The anionic charge is derived from sulfonate groups rather than sulfate groups as in heparin. The molecular weight of GL-522-Y-1 is 1488 Da.

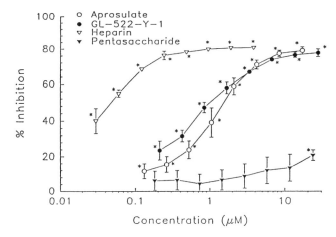

FIGURE 4.   Effect of aprosulate, GL-522-Y-1, pentasaccharide, and heparin on the heparin co-factor II-mediated inhibition of thrombin. Thrombin inhibition was measured using a plasma-free amidolytic assay.

GL-522-Y-1 has been shown to be effective as an antithrombotic agent in the rabbit model of stasis thrombosis.[31] It is effective after both intravenous and subcutaneous administration.[42] GL-522-Y-1 is also effective in a laser injury model of thrombosis after intravenous and oral administration.[18] The antithrombotic activity after oral administration has a duration of 6 hours. Administration of GL-522-Y-1 to primates (*Macaca fascicularis*) results in an increase in plasma levels of functional TFPI.[32]

Comparisons of Pentasaccharide, Aprosulate, GL-522-Y-1, and Heparin

Comparison of the above described synthetic agents on a chemical basis reveals that their molecular weights are about one-third to one-half that of a typical LMW heparin. Moreover, based on their structural differences, they have varying charge densities. Figure 4 shows the potencies of these analogs in comparison with heparin in a purified biochemical system in which the heparin cofactor II-mediated inhibition of thrombin is measured. Heparin is by far the most potent of these agents in inhibiting thrombin via heparin cofactor II. Aprosulate and GL-522-Y-1 exhibit approximately tenfold lower potency than heparin in inhibiting thrombin, whereas pentasaccharide does not inhibit thrombin via heparin cofactor II. If, in a similar system, AT III is substituted for heparin cofactor II, heparin is clearly the only agent capable of inhibiting thrombin via AT III (Fig. 5). None of the synthetic analogs are able to inhibit thrombin by this mechanism. In contrast, pentasaccharide and heparin are approximately equipotent in their ability to inhibit the amidolytic activity of factor Xa. Neither aprosulate nor GL-522-Y-1 significantly inhibits factor Xa.

These agents have also been tested for their antithrombotic activity in an in vivo rabbit model of stasis thrombosis (Fig. 6). An activated prothrombin complex concentrate is injected intravenously as a thrombogenic challenge before ligation of the jugular segments. After 10 minutes the jugular segments are removed from the animal, and the clot is removed from the vessel segment and graded. Each of these agents, despite their varying mechanisms of action, inhibit clot formation in a dose-dependent manner. Because of its ability to inhibit both thrombin (via interactions with AT III and heparin cofactor II) and factor Xa (via AT III), heparin was the most potent of these agents. Pentasaccharide also exhibited a potent antithrombotic effect. Both agents were more potent than the agents that do not mediate their actions via AT III. Notably, the two agents that inhibit thrombin via

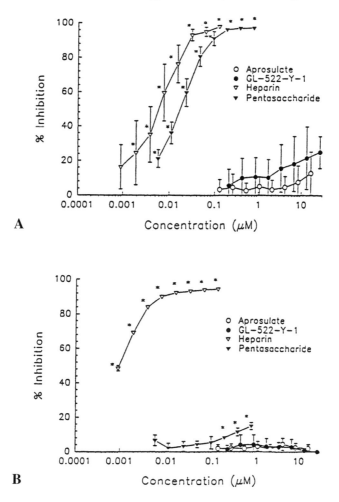

FIGURE 5.   Effect of aprosulate, GL-522-Y-1, pentasaccharide, and heparin on the antithrombin III-mediated inhibition of *(A)* factor Xa and *(B)* thrombin. Inhibition was determined using plasma free amidolytic assays.

heparin cofactor II, aprosulate and GL-522-Y-1, showed a sevenfold difference in their in vivo potency, which was not observed in the in vitro assay of thrombin inhibition via heparin cofactor II.

The hemorrhagic effect of the synthetic analogs was assessed with a rabbit model of ear bleeding. Two of the compounds tested, heparin and GL-522-Y-1, increased the amount of blood loss from the rabbit ear in a dose-dependent manner (Fig. 7). Neither aprosulate nor pentasaccharide increased the amount of blood loss. The doses of heparin that caused an increase in bleeding were approximately tenfold higher than the doses that produced effective antithrombotic activity in the rabbit model of stasis thrombosis. GL-522-Y-1 exhibited a stronger bleeding effect than heparin at doses comparable to those that were effective at inhibiting clot formation in the rabbit model of stasis-thrombosis.

Tissue factor pathway inhibitor is a tri-Kunitz inhibitor of the coagulation cascade that is primarily bound to the vascular endothelium. The positive amino acids that are clustered on the carboxy terminus of this molecule are thought to form a heparin-binding

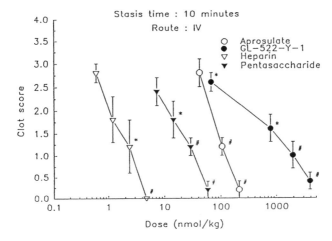

FIGURE 6. Comparison of the antithrombotic actions of synthetic heparin analogs in a rabbit model of stasis-thrombosis using an activated prothrombin complex concentrate as the thrombogenic stimulus. Stasis was induced 5 minutes after intravenous administration of each heparin analog. Clot scores were determined 10 minutes after the induction of stasis. Results represent the mean ± SEM (n = 5/group). Saline treatment resulted in a clot score of 2.9 ± 0.1 in control rabbits.

domain.[43] The mechanism of action of TFPI occurs in two steps.[19] In the first step, factor Xa binds to the second Kunitz domain of TFPI. In the second step, the factor VIIa–tissue factor complex binds to the first Kunitz domain of the factor Xa–TFPI complex, thereby inhibiting the extrinsic pathway of coagulation at two points.

According to reports in the literature, heparin and heparinlike compounds displace TFPI from the vascular endothelium and increase the plasma concentrations of TFPI.[3,76] The effect of GL-522-Y-1 on plasma levels of TFPI was examined with an antigenic method after administration of GL-522-Y-1 to monkeys. After an intravenous bolus of GL-522-Y-1, there was a rapid increase in plasma TFPI levels of 2–2.5-fold compared with normal human plasma (Fig. 8). The TFPI levels gradually decreased to baseline as the drug was eliminated. When pentasaccharide was administered to monkeys, no change in

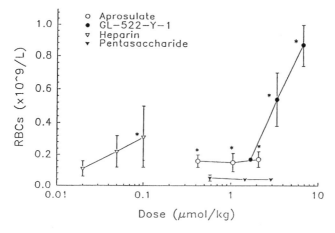

FIGURE 7. Comparison of the hemorrhagic effects of synthetic heparin analogs in a rabbit model of ear bleeding after intravenous administration. Results represent the mean ± SEM (n = 5/group).

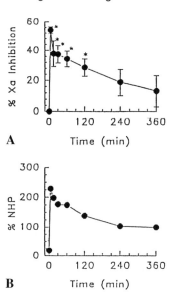

FIGURE 8. Release of tissue factor pathway inhibitor (TFPI) in monkeys after intravenous administration of 10 mg/kg GL-522-Y-1. TFPI levels were measured using *(A)* an amidolytic functional assay (n = 3) and *(B)* an immunologic assay (n = 1).

the plasma levels of TFPI antigen was observed despite a dose-dependent increase in the Heptest clotting time.

Heparin-induced thrombocytopenia (HIT) is thought to be mediated through the formation of a heparin–PF4 complex that results in the production of antiplatelet antibodies.[2] The FcRII receptor on platelets is also thought to be involved in the pathophysiology of HIT. Other studies have shown that the antibody is not heparin-specific. In 1995, Greinacher et al.[20] showed that the high level of sulfation rather than AT III-binding capacity, is the determining factor in whether an agent will produce HIT. Figure 9 compares the synthetic analogs with heparin in a screening assay for HIT. Platelet-rich plasma from normal human volunteers is incubated with varying concentrations of these agents, and serum obtained from known HIT-positive patients. Both heparin (as expected) and the highly sulfated aprosulate increased the amount of platelet aggregation in a concentration-dependent manner. Neither GL-522-Y-1 nor pentasaccharide induced significant aggregation.

These data indicate that the pharmacologic actions of heparin and its analogs are mediated by their interactions at several sites, including the plasmatic serine protease inhibitors AT III and heparin cofactor II and the release of TFPI from the vascular endothelium. The

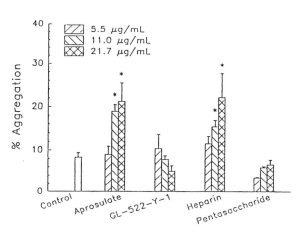

FIGURE 9. Effect of synthetic heparin analogs in a heparin-induced thrombocytopenia screening test. Aggregation in platelet-rich plasma from a normal donor is induced by the test agent and serum from a patient with heparin-induced thrombocytopenia.

plasmatic anticoagulant actions are primarily mediated via AT III, although at higher doses heparin cofactor II and TFPI release appear to contribute to their pharmacologic actions.

No toxic effects have been observed in the clinical development of pentasaccharide. By allometry, it has been estimated that the half-life of pentasaccharide in humans is approximately 14 hours.[22] The first clinical study of pentasaccharide in humans confirmed its long duration of action after subcutaneous administration.[7] Half-lives of 13.1–13.9 hours were observed in healthy volunteers. The peak plasma concentrations were linearly related to dose, and plasma clearance was threefold higher than that of typical LMW heparins. Pentasaccharide has been reported to be well tolerated, with no prolongation of the bleeding time, APTT, or PT. Van Amsterdam has shown that unbound pentasaccharide is cleared rapidly from the plasma but that AT III-bound pentasaccharide is cleared much like endogenous AT III.[71]

After subcutaneous administration of pentasaccharide to normal volunteers, thrombin generation was observed to be inhibited for as long as 18 hours.[46] TFPI release was not observed with subcutaneously administered pentasaccharide doses as high as 12,000 anti-Xa units. This study concluded that thrombin generation by pentasaccharide is mediated exclusively through selective AT III-mediated inhibition of factor Xa. Pentasaccharide, which is under joint development by Sanofi and Organon, is currently being tested in a phase-II hip replacement study. Because of its low ability to induce HIT, it appears to have a strong potential for use in these patients.

In contrast, both aprosulate and GL-522-Y-1 appear to promote an increase in liver enzyme concentration and inflammation of the liver and kidneys. Thus their development has been limited. Aprosulate has been administered to humans in two phase I clinical trials. In the first trial, ascending doses from 0.25–2.0 mg/kg were administered to healthy individuals on alternate days. Both APTT and the Heptest were elevated in a dose-dependent manner. No effect was observed on the thrombin time, and there was no indication of a thrombocytopenic response.[52] In the second trial, three doses of aprosulate were studied in a repeated administration protocol for 1 week. An increase in plasma levels of TFPI antigen was observed after each administration of aprosulate. The levels of TFPI antigen were observed to correlate with the plasma levels of aprosulate.[33] GL-522-Y-1 remains in preclinical development with no current trials underway.

SEMISYNTHETIC HEPARIN ANALOGS

Semisynthetic heparin analogs are either highly sulfated or somewhat desulfated in comparison with heparin; they exhibit multiple effects, much like the heparin analogs. They can enhance fibrinolysis, inhibit smooth muscle cell proliferation, and display other actions that are similar to heparin, including antilipemic, antiviral or antiarthritic effects.

Pentosan Polysulfate

Another potential antithrombotic agent is pentosan polysulfate, a fully sulfated linear polymer of 1-4 linked ß-xylopyranose units derived from the beech tree. This hypersulfated agent is a highly potent stimulator of TFPI release both in clinical and experimental settings and also modulates the fibrinolytic system, probably through its release of tissue-type plasminogen activator (tPA). Like unfractionated heparin, pentosan polysulfate has multiple pharmacologic actions. It has been widely used as an antilipemic agent,[4] selectively inhibits HIV-1 replication,[5] and has antitumor effects in animals.[77]

Unlike heparin, pentosan polysulfate prevents coagulation by two mechanisms, both independently of AT III.[17,60] First, it prevents thrombin generation through its ability to inhibit the thrombin-dependent activation of factor V, thereby inhibiting the formation of the prothrombinase complex. Second, it promotes the inhibition of preformed thrombin via HC-II.[61] Pentosan polysulfate has been shown to have low anticoagulant potency in vitro.[60,64] The potency of pentosan polysulfate has been reported as 12 anti-IIa U/mg and 8 anti-Xa U/mg.

Despite its low anticoagulant activity, a number of investigators have demonstrated the antithrombotic efficacy of pentosan polysulfate. In a rabbit model of stasis thrombosis, it was shown to inhibit factor Xa, thrombin and thromboplastin-induced thrombogenesis to varying degrees. Thromboplastin-induced thrombosis was most potently inhibited.[72] Similarly, in rats pentosan polysulfate was observed to increase the number of laser injuries required to induce thrombogenesis in a dose-dependent manner, although at much higher doses than were required for heparin or LMW heparin.[40]

The major side effects of pentosan polysulfate are reported to be similar to those of heparin. A recent report indicates that pentosan polysulfate induces thrombocytopenia and thrombosis in patients receiving repeated administrations.[67] Positive cross-reactivity with heparin and LMW heparin was observed in a large number of HIT cases studied in vitro.

K5-Derived Agents

Casu et al.[9] have prepared heparinlike compounds by modification of the *Escherichia coli* capsular polysaccharide, K5. The *E. coli* K5 polysaccharide has the same chemical structure as the heparin precursor N-acetyl heparosan, which can be converted through a series of epimerizations, sulfations, and acetylations to an agent that is structurally similar to an LMW heparin. To make a heparinlike substance, this precursor is first deacetylated with hydrazine[29] and then N-sulfated. The resultant sulfamino heparosan undergoes C5 epimerization to produce iduronic acid moieties,[41] and finally O-sulfation produces a substance resembling mammalian heparin. Nuclear magnetic resonance (NMR) analysis of the resultant polysaccharides indicates strong signals characteristic of N-sulfated groups, glucosamine, and glucuronic acid residues.[29] These modified polysaccharides also contain the 3-O sulfate group on glucosamine, which is required for high-affinity heparin binding to AT III. These agents produce similar in vitro anticoagulant and in vivo antithrombotic effects as LMW heparin.[15]

Potential advantages of the K5-derived analogs of heparin include freedom from viral contaminants. Because these agents are produced through a series of controlled chemical modifications, the degree of sulfation and other molecular characteristics can be readily modified and controlled.

Figure 10 compares the anticoagulant activity of a K5-derived material with that of a commercially available LMW heparin, Fraxiparin, after supplementation to normal human plasma using the Heptest. Both agents exhibit a similar concentration-dependent prolongation of the clotting time. Figure 11 depicts the dose-response curves for the antithrombotic activity of SR 80486A and Fraxiparin in the rabbit model of stasis thrombosis. Over the dose range of 0–100 μg/kg administered intravenously, the antithrombotic activity of SR 80486A was observed to be equivalent to that of Fraxiparin. At a dose of 100 μg/kg, both agents completely inhibited clot formation.

Comparison of the hemorrhagic effects of the K5-derived material and two LMW heparins showed the typical small increase in bleeding with LMW heparins but a smaller increase in bleeding after SR 80486A administration (Fig. 12).

Heparan Sulfate and Dermatan Sulfate

Several other glycosaminoglycans have been studied as potential antithrombotic agents. These agents typically have been derived from bovine and porcine sources; more recently, however, marine products and fish skin have been used. Examples include dermatan sulfate, a galactosaminoglycan, and heparan sulfate, which contains a backbone similar to heparin. Heparan sulfate generally contains more than 20% N-acetylated glucosamine and nearly equal amounts of N- and O-sulfation. In contrast, the ratio of O- to N-sulfation in heparin is almost 4 to 1. Like heparin, heparan sulfate primarily inhibits proteases via activation of AT III and has been shown to catalyze the formation of thrombin–antithrombin

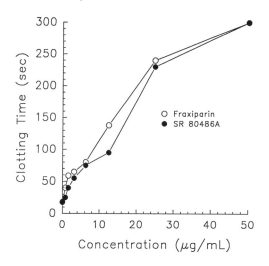

FIGURE 10. Comparative anticoagulant actions of SR 80486A and Fraxiparin as measured by the Heptest. Each agent was supplemented to normal human plasma over a concentration range of 0–50 µg/ml.

complexes. Because it does not completely inhibit prothrombin activation, it is much less effective than heparin. The antithrombotic dosage of heparan sulfate has been shown to be approximately 500–600 µg/kg compared with 60–70 µg/kg of heparin.

Dermatan sulfate is a glycosaminoglycan polymer of iduronic acid and N-acetylated galactosamine. Because of a difference in the molecular backbone, dermatan sulfate is unable to interact with AT III[50] but rather complexes with heparin cofactor II to mediate thrombin inhibition.[70] The anticoagulant potency of dermatan sulfate is less than that of heparan sulfate.[68] Anticoagulant activity, as measured by the APTT and thrombin time, is nearly undetectable.[63] Dermatan sulfate inhibits thrombin as it is formed rather than prevents its generation. Inhibition of thrombin generation by dermatan sulfate is much less than for an equigravimetric amount of heparin.[47] At a dosage of 150 µg/kg, dermatan sulfate

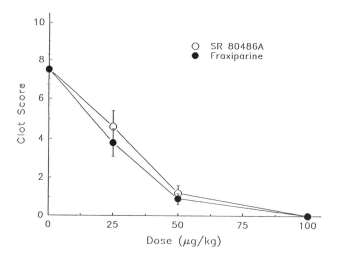

FIGURE 11. Comparison of the antithrombotic actions of SR 80486A and Fraxiparin in a jugular vein stasis-thrombosis model using an activated prothrombin complex concentrate as the thrombogenic stimulus. Stasis was induced 5 minutes after intravenous administration of heparin. Clot scores were determined 10 minutes after the induction of stasis. Results represent the mean ± SEM (n = 5/group). Saline treatment resulted in a clot score of 7.5 ± 0.3 in control rabbits.

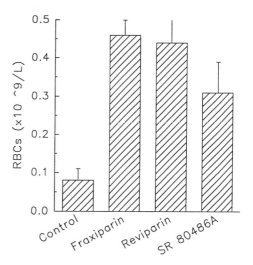

FIGURE 12. Comparison of the hemorrhagic effects induced by low-molecular-weight heparins and SR 80486A after intravenous administration. Results represent the mean ± SEM (n = 5/group),

caused a 28% inhibition of thrombin generation compared with an 83% inhibition by heparin. Although dermatan octasaccharides bind heparin cofactor II, 12–14 residues are required for thrombin inhibition. Dermatan sulfate chains with a higher charge density appear to bind to heparin cofactor II better than those with a lower charge.

Dermatan sulfate is active in vivo as an antithrombotic agent in the rabbit model of stasis thrombosis but to a lesser extent than heparin.[47] Although both agents inhibited thrombus formation to the same extent at an equigravimetric dosage of 150 μg/kg after 10 minutes of stasis, dermatan sulfate was ineffective at inhibiting thrombus formation after 20 minutes stasis time at a dose 8 times higher than that of heparin. The advantage of dermatan sulfate over heparin as an antithrombotic agent is a lower risk of bleeding complications.[13,16] Dermatan sulfate does not significantly increase bleeding, compared with a saline control, at doses that are antithrombotically effective.

The decreased bleeding seen with dermatan sulfate is thought to result from its minor effects on platelets. Sie et al. have shown that whereas thrombin-induced platelet aggregation is inhibited by dermatan sulfate in the presence of heparin cofactor II, arachidonic acid, ADP and collagen induced aggregations were not affected.[63] In addition, dermatan sulfate has a smaller effect than heparin on heparin-induced thrombocytopenic, serum-induced platelet aggregation.[26]

Dermatan sulfate is currently under limited development in Italy. It requires a relatively higher dosage to achieve its pharmacologic effects and is also somewhat costly to produce. LMW derivatives are currently being developed. Heparan sulfate has been used only in experimental settings to date. ORG 10172, a mixture of chondroitin sulfate, heparan sulfate, and dermatan sulfate, is in limited clinical use for prophylaxis against venous thrombosis. Although it appears to have a lower bleeding risk, its extremely long half-life precludes its use in certain situations.

CHEMICALLY MODIFIED HEPARINS

Astenose

Astenose is produced by a periodate oxidation of heparin, followed by a borohydride reduction that leads to a cleavage in the AT III-binding region of heparin, thereby attenuating a large portion of its anticoagulant activity. Astenose retains the ability to inhibit thrombin via HCII activation (Fig. 13).

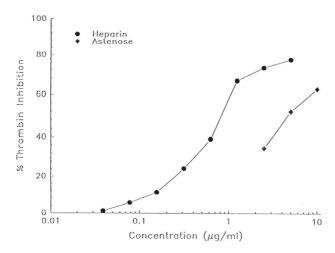

FIGURE 13. Comparison of the heparin cofactor II-mediated inhibition of thrombin by heparin and Astenose. Thrombin inhibition was measured with a plasma free amidolytic assay.

Several studies with Astenose have been reported,[1] including platelet activation and adhesion studies showing that Astenose is fourfold more potent than heparin in the inhibition of von Willebrand factor. Astenose is a potent inhibitor of bFGF-stimulated proliferation and also inhibits proliferation of rat and human smooth muscle cells. Consequently, a possible use of Astenose is in the prevention of restenosis. An investigational new drug (IND) application was filed for Astenose early in 1994, but it was subsequently withdrawn because of the drug's remaining anticoagulant and bleeding tendencies.

Hypersulfated Heparins

The anticoagulant and antithrombotic actions of heparins containing higher than normal degrees of sulfation have been examined in several studies. In a laser model of thrombosis, a supersulfated LMW heparin was observed to require a tenfold lower dose than native heparin or LMW heparin to achieve a comparable antithrombotic effect.[40] In another study, oversulfation of LMW heparin reduced the ex vivo anticoagulant activity relative to LMW heparin that has not been oversulfated. Addition of sulfate groups, however, did not affect the antithrombotic activity in a rat model of venous stasis thrombosis and did not significantly increase the bleeding time.[49] The release of lipoprotein lipase by the supersulfated LMW heparin was twice that of heparin. In a pure biochemical system, the inhibition of thrombin via heparin cofactor II by supersulfated LMW heparin was approximately 100-fold stronger than for LMW weight heparin.

Hypersulfated heparins and LMW heparins are being developed by several companies, including Iketon and Recordati in Italy and Sanofi/Choay in France. Phase I studies have been completed with the Iketon compound, whereas the other two compounds remain in the preclinical stages.

Hypersulfated LMW heparins exhibit several distinct characteristics compared with standard LMW heparin. First, inhibition of thrombin is greatly enhanced (Fig. 14). The heparin cofactor II-mediated inhibition of thrombin by LMW heparin occurs at much higher concentrations than required for hypersulfated LMW heparin. A second interesting feature of hypersulfated LMW heparins is their apparent oral bioavailability in animal models of thrombosis. The hypersulfated LMW heparin was given at doses ranging from 2.5–10 mg/kg via a nasogastric tube to rabbits that ingested nothing by mouth

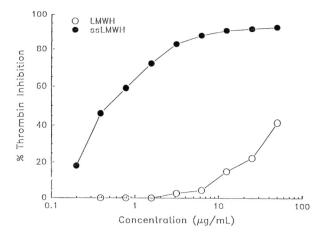

FIGURE 14.   Comparison of the heparin cofactor II-mediated inhibition of thrombin by a standard low-molecular-weight heparin (LMWH) and a supersulfated (ss) LMWH.

overnight. The administration of hypersulfated LMW heparin resulted in a dose-dependent decrease in the clot score in a standard rabbit model of jugular vein stasis thrombosis (Fig. 15).

The hypersulfated heparins have also been compared in a rat model of restenosis (Fig. 16). The carotid arteries were injured by balloon angioplasty in the presence of 1 mg/kg of intravenous Enoxaparin, a typical LMW heparin, or a hypersulfated heparin administered at a dose of 2.5 mg/kg subcutaneously for 2 weeks. Both the hypersulfated heparin and LMW heparin decreased the amount of growth of the neointima compared with controls.

Desulfated Heparins

The anticoagulant and antithrombotic effects of desulfated heparins have also been examined. A partially N-desulfated heparin had no measurable anticoagulant or antiprotease

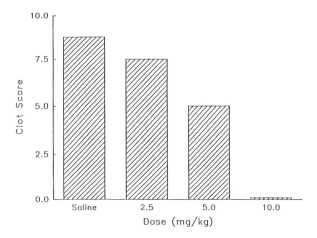

FIGURE 15.   Antithrombotic activity of a supersulfated low-molecular-weight heparin after oral administration as measured using a rabbit model of stasis-thrombosis. Clot scores were measured 2 hours after administration of the agent (n = 3/dose).

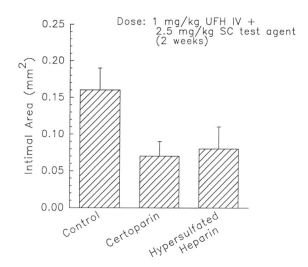

FIGURE 16. Effect of low-molecular-weight heparin, Certoparin, and a hypersulfated heparin in a rat model of carotid restenosis. After balloon damage of the carotid artery, rats were treated with a bolus of 1 mg/kg of unfractionated heparin and 2.5 mg/kg/day subcutaneously of either Certoparin or hypersulfated heparin for 2 weeks. Intimal area was measured after 2 weeks of treatment.

activity but impaired thrombogenesis in vivo in a dose-dependent manner.[59] A completely N-desulfated heparin derivative lacked both in vitro and in vivo activity.[28] Other investigators have shown that N-desulfated heparins have minimal anticoagulant activity.[6,12] The weak anticoagulant activity is attributable to the lack of interaction with AT III.[12] N-desulfated heparin has been shown to be cleared approximately sixfold faster than native heparin.[6] Rajtar demonstrated that N-desulfated heparins were less effective at inhibiting platelet function than native heparin.[57]

Gamma-irradiated Heparins

Because fractionation of heparin has proved to be an inefficient means to obtain LMW heparins, other methods utilizing nitrous acid, alkaline solutions, or heparin-degrading enzymes have been developed. Although these methods are effective in producing therapeutically useful agents, they can induce structural alterations in the molecule that may affect bioactivity. LMW heparins have now been produced by exposing heparin to gamma irradiation. This process has been shown to cleave heparin chains without loss of sulfation. In addition, the duration of irradiation is correlated with mean molecular size. Depolymerized material with a molecular weight of approximately 5 kDa has been shown to have a similar anticoagulant and antithrombotic profile to commercially available LMW heparins.[34] Heparins depolymerized by this method and exhibiting higher or lower molecular weights may be optimized for additional clinical indications.

CONCLUSIONS

Several issues drive the search for alternative antithrombotic agents. First is the need to find effective antithrombotic agents that do not promote bleeding. Second is the need to develop agents that are suitable for use in settings in which heparin therapy is not optimal, such as HIT and restenosis. Third is the recent concern over the use of bovine-derived glycosaminoglycans, which may be contaminated with such viral entities as BSE. This concern will have a profound effect on public acceptance of such products and has further reinforced the development of alternate sources for sulfated glycosaminoglycan-based analogs with antithrombotic activity. Finally, because of the widespread use of porcine raw material to make LMW heparins, the supplies of such material may become depleted. By the year 2000, almost all of the porcine raw material could be used for the production of LMW heparins; hence the need to develop agents that are obtained through alternate means.

Recent research in the development of synthetic and biotechnology-derived heparin analogs has produced several newer drugs with defined pharmacologic actions. Both AT III-dependent and AT III-independent mechanisms appear to mediate the actions of these agents. Current research on synthetic analogs of heparin may be extended to obtain anticoagulant drugs that mimic heparin's actions. Pentasaccharide behaves as a true analog of heparin and can be molecularly manipulated to exhibit additional properties of heparin through alteration of charge density and saccharidic chain extension. The therapeutic index of each of these agents can be adjusted through structural alterations. These agents also represent important tools for the study of the mechanism of action of heparin and related drugs, whether or not they turn out to be efficient drugs on their own. The analogs of heparin produce their effects through multiple mechanisms of action, including modulation of both plasmatic and cellular systems. They can be obtained in desirable amounts and do not depend on the supply of raw materials of animal origin. Based on some of the preclinical data and potential costs of developing these agents, it appears that the AT III-binding oligosaccharides (e.g., pentasaccharide) and K5-derived analogs of heparin may hold a high developmental potential. In contrast, agents such as highly sulfated heparins and some of the other hypersulfated agents may have a somewhat smaller developmental potential because of their tendency to produce thrombocytopenia.

REFERENCES

1. Ackerman NR: Astenose®: A non-anticoagulating heparin—its utility in restenosis and thrombosis. In Advances in Anticoagulant, Antithrombotic and Thrombolytic Drugs. Boston, 1993.
2. Amiral J, Bridley F, Wolf M, et al: Antibodies to macromolecular platelet factor factor 4-heparin complexes in heparin-induced thrombocytopenia: A study of 44 cases. Thromb Haemost 73:21–28, 1995.
3. Ariens RAS, Faioni EM, Mannucci PM: Repeated release of the tissue factor pathway inhibitor. Thromb Haemost 72:327–328, 1984.
4. Baba M, Nakajima M, Schols D, et al: Pentosan polysulfate, a sulfated oligosaccharide, is a potent and selective anti-HIV agent in vitro. Antiviral Res 9:335–943, 1988.
5. Barrowcliffe TW, Gray E, Merton RE, et al: Anticoagulant activities of pentosan polysulfate (Hemoclar) due to release of hepatic triglyceride lipase (HTGL). Thromb Haemost 56:202–206, 1986.
6. Bjornsson TD, Schneider DE, Hecht AR: Effects of N-deacetlyation and N-desulfation of heparin on its anticoagulant activity and in vivo disposition. J Pharmacol Exp Ther 245:80–88, 1988.
7. Boneu B, Necciari J, Cariou R, et al: Pharmacokinetics and tolerance of the natural pentasaccharide (SR90107/OGR31540) with high affinity to antithrombin III in man. Thromb Haemost 74:1468–1473, 1995.
8. Cadroy Y, Hanson SR, Harker LA: Antithrombotic effects of synthetic pentasaccharide with high affinity for plasma antithrombin III in non-human primates. Thromb Haemost 70:631–635, 1993.
9. Casu B, Grazioli G, Razi N, et al: Heparin-like compounds prepared by chemical modification of capsular polysaccharide from E. coli K5. Carbo Res 263:271–284, 1994.
10. Choay J, Lormeau JC, Petitou M, et al: Anti-Xa active heparin oligosaccharides. Thromb Res 18:573–578, 1980.
11. Choay J, Petitou M, Lormeau JC, et al: Structure-activity relationship in heparin: a synthetic pentasaccharide with high affinity for antithrombin III and eliciting high anti-factor Xa activity. Biochem Biophys Acta 116:492–499, 1983.
12. Danishefsky I, Ahrens M, Klein S: Effect of heparin modification on its activity in enhancing the inhibition of thrombin by antithrombin III. Biochim Biophys Acta 498:215–222, 1977.
13. Desnoyers P, Bara L, Samama M: Dermatan sulfate and the prevention of experimental venous thrombosis. Pathol Biol 37:759–767, 1989.
14. Fareed J, Coker S, Iqbal O, et al: Pharmacodynamics of a sulfated lactobionic acid amide antithrombotic agent (aprosulate) in primates. Semin Thromb Hemost 17(Suppl 2):147–152, 1991.
15. Fareed J, Jeske W, Hoppensteadt D, et al: Biochemical and pharmacologic equivalence of a semi-synthetic GAG (SR 80486A) and fraxiparine. Thromb Haemost 73:1318, 1995.
16. Fernandez F, Niguyen P, Van Ryn J, et al: Hemorrhagic doses of heparin and other glycosaminoglycans induce a platelet defect. Thromb Res 43:491–495, 1986.

17. Fischer AM, Barrowcliffe TW, Thomas DP: A comparison of pentosan polysulfate (SP54) and heparin. I: Mechanism of action on blood coagulation. Thromb Haemost 47:104–108, 1982.

18. Giedrojc J, Radziwon P, Chen J, Breddin HK: On the effects of GL-522(Y-1), a polysulfonate, on laser-induced thrombus formation and on platelet induced thrombin generation [abstract]. Thromb Haemost 69:673, 1993.

19. Girard TJ, Warren LA, Novotny WF, et al: Functional significance of the Kunitz-type inhibitory domains of lipoprotein-associated coagulation inhibitor. Nature 338:518–520, 1989.

20. Greinacher A, Alban S, Dummel V, et al: Characterization of the structural requirements for a carbohydrate based anticoagulant with a reduced risk of inducing the immunological type of heparin-associated thrombocytopenia. Thromb Haemost 74:886–892, 1995.

21. Harbauer G, Hiller W, Hellstein P: In Koslowski L (ed): Chirurgisches Forum 84 fur Experementelle und Klinische Forschung. Springer Verlag, Berlin, 1984, pp 69–72.

22. Herault JP, Barzu T, Bernat A, et al: Pharmacokinetics of three synthetic AT-III binding pentasaccharides in various animal species—extrapolation to humans. Thromb Haemost 73:1321, 1995.

23. Herault JP, Barzu T, Crepon B, et al: Biochemical and pharmacological properties of O-sulfated, O-methylated analogues of the natural pentasaccharide. Thromb Haemost 73:1321, 1995.

24. Hobbelen PMJ, van Dinther TG, Vogel GMT, et al: Pharmacological profile of the chemically synthesized antithrombin III binding fragment of heparin (pentasaccharide) in rats. Thromb Haemost 63:265–270, 1990.

25. Hoppensteadt D, Ahsan A, Walenga JM, Fareed J: Activation of heparin cofactor II by sulfated lactobionic acid. Blood 72:298, 1988.

26. Hoppensteadt D, Walenga JM, Fareed J: Effect of dermatan sulfate and heparan sulfate on platelet activity compared to heparin. Semin Thromb Hemost 17:60–64, 1991.

27. Hoppensteadt D, Walenga JM, Fareed J: Protamine sulfate neutralization of lactobionic acid amides. Semin Thromb Hemost 17(Suppl 2):153–157, 1991.

28. Inoue Y, Nagasawa K: Selective N-desulfation of heparin with dimethyl sulfoxide containing water or methanol. Carbohydr Res 46:87–95, 1976.

29. Jann K, Jann B, Casu B, et al: Anticoagulants and processes for preparing such. Patent WO 92/17507, 1992.

30. Jeske W, Lojewski B, Fareed J: Biochemical and pharmacologic studies on a novel polysulfonated oral antithrombotic agent (GL-522-Y-1) [abstract]. Blood 80(Suppl 1):322a , 1992..

31. Jeske W, Nelson S, Lee T, et al: Tissue factor pathway inhibitor (TFPI) release induced by a novel sulfonic acid polyphenol (GL-522) following IV administration to cynomologous monkeys. FASEB J 7:A210, 1993.

32. Jeske W, Fareed J: Antithrombin III and heparin cofactor II mediated anticoagulant and antiprotease actions of heparin and its synthetic analogues. Semin Thromb Hemost 19(Suppl 1):241–247, 1993.

33. Jeske W, Hoppensteadt D, Klauser R, et al: Effect of repeated aprosulate and enoxaparin administration on tissue factor pathway inhibitor antigen levels. Blood Coag Fibrinol 6:119–124, 1994.

34. Jeske W, Iqbal O, Gonnella S, et al: Pharmacologic profile of a low molecular weight heparin depolymerized by gamma irradiation. Semin Thromb Hemost 21:201–211, 1995.

35. Kijowski R, Hoppensteadt D, Jeske W, Fareed J: Protamine sulfate neutralization of the anticoagulant activity of Aprosulate, a synthetic sulfated lactobionic acid amide. Thromb Res 73:349–359, 1994.

36. Klauser RJ, Meinetsberger E, Raake W: Biochemical studies on sulfated lactobionic acid amides. Semin Thromb Hemost 17(Suppl 1):118–125, 1991.

37. Klauser RJ, Raake W, Meinetsberger E, Zeiller P: Antithrombotic and anticoagulant properties of synthetic polyanions: Sulfated bis-aldonic acid amides. J Pharmacol Exp Ther 259:8–14, 1991.

38. Klauser RJ: Interaction of the sulfated lactobionic acid amide LW 10082 with thrombin and in endogenous inhibitors. Thromb Res 62:557–565, 1991.

39. Klocking HP, Hoffmann A, Fareed J: Influence of hypersulfated lactobionic acid amides on tissue plasminogen activator release. Semin Thromb Hemost 17:379–384, 1991.

40. Krupinski K, Breddin HK, Casu B: Anticoagulant and antithrombotic effects of chemically modified heparins and pentosanpolysulfate. Haemostasis 20:81–92, 1990.

41. Kusche M, Hannesson HH, Lindahl U: Biosynthesis of heparin. Use of Escherichia coli K5 capsular polysaccharide as a model substrate in enzymatic polymer-modification reactions. Biochem J 275:151–158, 1991.

42. Lee TC, Jeske W, Chen J, et al: Anticoagulant and antithrombotic profile of a series of novel polysulfonates. Thromb Haemost 69:894, 1993.

43. Lindahl AK, Sandset PM, Abildgaard U: The present status of tissue factor pathway inhibitor. Blood Coag Fibrinol 3:439–449, 1992.

44. Lindahl U, Backstrom G, Hook M, et al: Structure of the antithrombin-binding site of heparin. Proc Natl Acad Sci USA 76:3198–3202, 1979.

45. Lormeau JC, Herault JP: Comparative inhibition of extrinsic and intrinsic thrombin generation by standard heparin, a low molecular weight heparin, and a synthetic AT-III binding pentasaccharide. Thromb Haemost 69:152–156, 1993.

46. Lormeau JC, Herault JP: The effect of the synthetic pentasaccharide SR90107/ORG31540 on thrombin generation ex vivo is uniquely due to ATIII-mediated neutralization of factor Xa. Thromb Haemost 74:1474–1477, 1995.

47. Merton RE, Thomas DP: Experimental studies on the relative efficacy of dermatan sulphate and heparin as antithrombotic agents. Thromb Haemost 58:839–842, 1987.

48. Meuleman DG, Hobbelen PM, van Dinther TG, et al: Anti-factor Xa activity and antithrombotic activity in rats of structural analogues of the minimum antithrombin III binding sequence: Discovery of compounds with a longer duration of action than the natural pentasaccharide. Semin Thromb Hemost 17(Suppl 1): 112–117, 1991.

49. Naggi A, Torri G, Casu B, et al: "Supersulfated" heparin fragments, a new type of low-molecular weight heparin. Physico-chemical and pharmacological properties. Biochem Pharmacol 36:1895–1900, 1987.

50. Ofosu FA, Fernandez F, Gauthia D, Buchanan M: Heparin cofactor II and other endogenous factors in the mediation of the antithrombotic and anticoagulant effects of heparin and dermatan sulfate. Semin Thromb Hemost 11:1333–1337, 1985.

51. Ofosu F: Modulation of the enzymatic activity of a-thrombin by polyanions: Consequence of intrinsic activation of FV and FVIII. Haemostasis 21:240–247, 1991.

52. Papoulias UE, Wyld PJ, Haas S, et al: Phase I-study with aprosulate, a new synthetic anticoagulant. Thromb Res 72:99–108, 1993

53. Petitou M, Duchaussoy P, Lederman I, et al: Synthesis of heparin fragments: A chemical synthesis of the pentasaccharide O-(2-deoxy-2-sulfamido-6-O-sulfo-D-glucopyranosyl)-(1-4)-O-(ß-D-glucopyranosyluronic acid)-(1-4)-O-(2-deoxy-2-sulfamido-3,6-di-O-sulfo-D-glucopyranosyl)-(1-4)-O-(2-O-sulfo-L-idopyranosyluronic acid)-)1-4)-2-deoxy-2-sulfamido-6-O-sulfo-D-glucopyranose decasodium salt. A heparin fragment having high affinity for antithrombin III. Carbohyr Res 147:221–236, 1986.

54. Raake W, Klauser RJ, Elling H, Meinetsberger E: Anticoagulant and antithrombotic properties of synthetic sulfated bis-lactobionic acid amides. Thromb Res 56:719–730, 1989.

55. Raake W, Elling H: Rat jugular vein hemostasis—a new model for testing antithrombotic agents. Thromb Res 53:73–77, 1989.

56. Raake W, Klauser RJ, Meinetsberger E, et al: Pharmacologic profile of the antithrombotic and bleeding actions of sulfated lactobionic acid amides. Semin Thromb Hemost 19(Suppl 1):129–135, 1991.

57. Rajtar G, Marchim E, deGaetano G, Cerletti C: Effects of glycosaminoglycans on platelet and leukocyte function: Role of N-sulfation. Biochem Pharmacol 46:958–960, 1993.

58. Rosenberg RD, Lam L: Correlation between structure and function of heparin. Proc Natl Acad Sci USA 76:1218–1222, 1979.

59. Sache E, Maillard M, Malazzi P, Bertrand H: Partially N-desulfated heparin: some physico-chemical and biological properties. Thromb Res 55:247–258, 1989.

60. Scully MF, Weerasinge KM, Ellis V, et al: Anticoagulant and antiheparin activities of a pentosan polysulfate. Thromb Res 31:87–97, 1983.

61. Scully MF, Kakkar VV: Identification of heparin cofactor II as the principle plasma cofactor for pentosan polysulfate (SP54). Thromb Res 36:187–194, 1984.

62. Sie P, Dupouy D, Dol F, Boneu B: Determination of plasma dermatan sulfate at relevent pharmacological concentrations. Semin Thromb Hemost 17(Suppl 2):181–185, 1991.

63. Sie P, Fernandez F, Caranobe C, et al: Inhibition of thrombin induced platelet aggregation and serotonin release by antithrombin III and heparin cofactor II in the presence of heparin, dermatan sulfate and pentosan polysulfate. Thromb Res 35:231–236, 1982.

64. Soria C, Soria J, Ryckewaert JJ, et al: Anticoagulant activities of a pentosan polysulfate: comparison with standard heparin and a low molecular weight heparin. Thromb Res 19:455–463, 1980.

65. Sugidachi A, Asai F, Koike H: In vivo pharmacology of aprosulate, a new synthetic polyanion with anticoagulant activity. Thromb Res 69:71–80, 1993.

66. Sugidachi A, Asai F, Koike H: Anticoagulant and antiprotease activities of aprosulate sodium, a new synthetic polyanion, in human plasma and purified systems. Blood Coag Fibrinol 5:773–779, 1994.

67. Tardy-Poncet B, Tardy B, Grelac F, et al: Pentosan polysulfate-induced thrombocytopenia and thrombosis. Am J Hematol 45:252–257, 1994.

68. Teien A, Abildgaard U, Hook M: The anticoagulant effect of heparan sulfate and dermatan sulfate. Thromb Res 8:859–867, 1976.

69. Thomas DP, Merton RE, Gray E, Barrowcliffe TW: The relative antithrombotic effectiveness of heparin, a low molecular weight heparin, and a pentasaccharide fragment in an animal model. Thromb Haemost 61:204–207, 1989.

70. Tollefsen DM, Pestka CA, Monafo WJ: Activation of heparin cofactor II by dermatan sulfate. J Biol Chem 258:6713–6716, 1983.

71. van Amsterdam RG, Vogel GMT, Visser A, et al: Plasma disappearance of synthetic pentasaccharides derived from heparin explained by antithrombin III binding. Thromb Haemost 69:893, 1993.

72. Van Ryn-McKenna J, Gray E, Weber E, et al: Effects of sulfated polysaccharides on inhibition of thrombus formation initiated by different stimuli. Thromb Hemost 61:7–9, 1989.

73. Walenga JM, Fareed J: Preliminary biochemical and pharmacologic studies on a chemically synthesized pentasaccharide. Semin Thromb Hemost 11:89–99, 1985.
74. Walenga JM, Bara L, Petitou M, et al: Importance of a 3-O-sulfate group in heparin pentasaccharide for anti-thrombotic activity. Thromb Res 52:553–563, 1988..
75. Walenga JM, Bara L, Petitou M, et al: The inhibition of the generation of thrombin and the antithrombotic effect of a pentasaccharide with sole anti-factor Xa activity. Thromb Res 51:23–33, 1988.
76. Warn-Cramer BJ, Maki SL, Rapaport SI: Heparin-releasable and platelet pools of tissue factor pathway inhibitor on rabbits. Thromb Haemost 69:221–226, 1993.
77. Wellstein A, Zugmaier G, Califano JA, et al: Tumor growth dependent on Kaposi's sarcoma-derived fibroblast growth factor inhibited by pentosan polysulfate. J Natl Cancer Inst 83:716–720, 1991.

CHAPTER 26

Ancrod as a Practical Alternative to Heparin

C. WILLIAM COLE, M.D., FRCSC, FACS

Effective anticoagulation is required for most operations that involve vascular anastomoses and for the nonoperative management of vascular complications such as thromboembolism. In the majority of cases heparin is the drug of choice because it is effective and can be initiated and reversed almost instantaneously. In certain situations, however, heparin is inappropriate or contraindicated. Examples include heparin-associated thrombocytopenia and thrombosis, in which the inciting thrombotic agent is heparin itself, and antithrombin III deficiency, in which heparin is not effective. In these and other conditions, ancrod has been shown to be a highly effective alternative to heparin. This chapter discusses the use of ancrod as an effective anticoagulant and antithrombotic agent with an expanding role in clinical practice.

HISTORICAL BACKGROUND

Dr. Alistair Reid, a tropical medicine specialist, observed that the venom of the Malayan pit viper (*Agkistrodon rhodostoma*) caused hypofibrinogenemia. This clinical observation was pursued in the laboratory and eventually led to the purification of the active principle, ancrod, and to its use in clinical medicine as an antithrombotic agent. It has been available in many parts of the world since the 1960s and has been tested in a number of clinical situations.[20] Clinical trials in which ancrod was compared with heparin have consistently shown that ancrod is as effective as heparin as an anticoagulant and antithrombotic agent and has fewer bleeding complications.[2] However, ancrod requires more time to become effective and is more costly. Besides, apart from bleeding, complications that require complete avoidance of heparin are rare. Consequently, it is usually only when heparin cannot be used that alternatives are sought. The alternatives that may be used depend on availability; ancrod is not generally available in the United States at the time of this writing, but an application for approval is now under review by the Food and Drug Administration.

WHAT IS ANCROD? HOW DOES IT WORK?

Ancrod is a purified enzyme derived from the venom of the Malayan pit viper. Fibrinogen is the substrate for both ancrod and thrombin (Fig. 1). Thrombin cleaves both the A- and B-fibrinopeptides from fibrinogen, but ancrod affects only the A-fibrinopeptide. This results in polymerization of partially effective fibrin/fibrinogen into an unstable configuration that is susceptible to rapid degradation by plasmin.[24] In addition, ancrod does

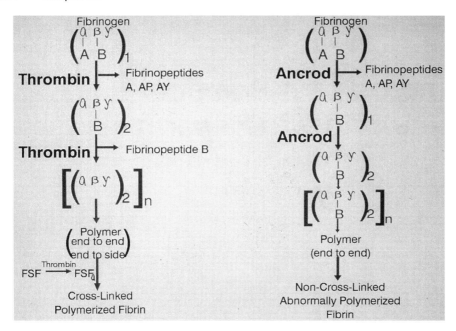

FIGURE 1. Fibrinogen is the principal substrate for both ancrod and thrombin. Thrombin cleaves both the A- and B-fibrinopeptides and also activates factor XIII, which stabilizes the normal clot. Ancrod cleaves only the A-fibrinopeptide, resulting in a partially generated fibrin/fibrinogen polymer that is unstable and susceptible to digestion by plasmin. Ancrod does not activate factor XIII. A constant infusion of ancrod results in depletion of the circulating fibrinogen. When fibrinogen is in the range of 0.2–0.5 gm/L, the patient is effectively anticoagulated.

not activate factor XIII, another feature that distinguishes the ancrod-formed thrombus from normal clot.

Ancrod has other actions at the level of the endothelial cell. Prostacyclin (PGI_2) production by endothelial cells is augmented by ancrod[4] and tissue plasminogen activator (tPA) is increased, probably because ancrod binds the inhibitor of tPA.[27] Ancrod is *not* a fibrinolytic agent and has no direct effect on plasminogen, nor does it affect normally formed thrombus. This probably accounts for the low frequency of bleeding complications.

Ancrod has an indirect action on platelet aggregation. The principal intermediary between aggregating platelets is fibrinogen, which binds to the IIb-IIIa receptor on the platelet surface[27] (Fig. 2). Experimentally, elimination of fibrinogen has been shown to inhibit platelet aggregability.[3]

In heparin-associated thrombocytopenia and thrombosis, in which platelet aggregation is driven by an immunologic response to heparin,[11] platelet aggregation can be effectively inhibited by depleting the available fibrinogen. In this situation complete discontinuation of heparin is essential, and depleting fibrinogen with ancrod appears to provide optimal therapy.[8]

FIBRINOGEN AS A RISK FACTOR FOR VASCULAR DISEASE

The importance of fibrinogen as a risk factor for chronic vascular disease has been well documented, but its role in promoting acute changes is often not appreciated. Figure 3 illustrates the potential mechanisms for fibrinogen to act on the vessel wall.

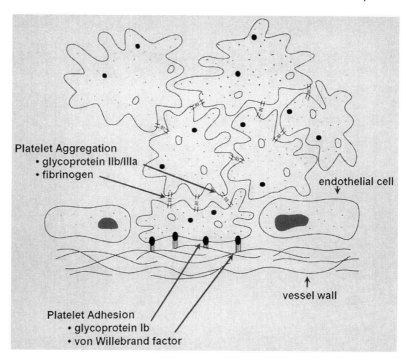

FIGURE 2.   One of the principal mechanisms that bind platelets together is fibrinogen. Platelet aggregation can be inhibited by depletion of fibrinogen.

Acute Changes

One of the normal acute phase reactions to injury, including surgery, is an increase in circulating fibrinogen. This may be of some survival advantage in the trauma victim, for example, in whom hemostasis is the primary concern, but in controlled situations such as operative intervention, an elevation in circulating fibrinogen may not be advantageous once hemostasis has been achieved. Early after injury, elevation in circulating fibrinogen contributes to hypercoagulability and increased blood viscosity. In marginally perfused tissue beds, these two features may contribute to microvascular stasis and thrombosis and eventually tissue ischemia. Taken together, increased fibrinogen concentration has a number of effects that may, in the aggregate, contribute to intravascular thrombosis, ischemia, and organ failure.

Prolonged immobilization is a common requirement in severely injured patients, especially those with long bone and pelvic fractures. Venous stasis and thromboembolic complications torment the clinical course of a large proportion of these patients,[15] and although the risk attributable to elevated fibrinogen has not been precisely determined, some data suggest that a clinical benefit may derive from depleting it with ancrod.[9]

Chronic Changes

Chronic elevation in fibrinogen concentration is a risk factor for a number of vessel wall changes. Figure 3 also illustrates some of the possible mechanisms by which fibrinogen may contribute to atherosclerosis. As endothelial injury occurs, from cigarette smoking, for example, an increased concentration of fibrinogen pushes the balance between thrombosis and thrombolysis toward the former. Fibrin binds low-density lipoproteins, and fibrin degradation products stimulate smooth muscle cell proliferation and recruit

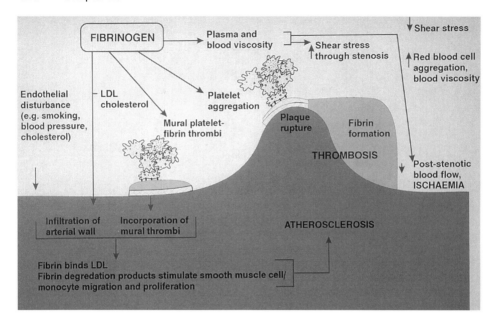

FIGURE 3.   Increased circulating fibrinogen concentration may contribute to (1) increased blood viscosity and slower blood flow; (2) platelet aggregation, macro- and microvascular stasis, and thrombosis, causing ischemia of marginal tissue beds; (3) incorporation of LDL-cholesterol in the arterial wall; and (4) promotion of inflammatory cell migration into the arterial wall.

monocytes into the arterial wall. Chronic elevation of circulating fibrinogen may accelerate the changes associated with aging.

Several large population studies illustrate the effect of a chronically elevated fibrinogen concentration in terms of the risk for ischemic heart disease and stroke (Fig. 4). The results of the Prospective Cardiovascular Munster (PROCAM) study illustrate the point.[16] Plasma fibrinogen was found to be an independent risk indicator for coronary heart disease. Over 6-year follow-up, individuals with high low-density lipoprotein (LDL) cholesterol and high plasma fibrinogen concentrations had a 6.1-fold increase in coronary risk. And contrary to what might have been expected, individuals with low plasma fibrinogen had a low incidence of coronary events even when LDL was high. Higher levels of plasma fibrinogen markedly increase the predictive power of high LDL cholesterol. Clinical trials for fibrinogen-lowering agents have been suggested,[25] and one of the obvious choices for such a trial is ancrod.

CLINICAL USE OF ANCROD

Heparin-induced Thrombocytopenia and Thrombosis

The principal use of ancrod today is as a substitute for heparin in patients with heparin-induced thrombocytopenia and thrombosis (HITT; see chapter 7). A fundamental rule in these patients is that all heparin must be immediately discontinued, but when anticoagulation is still required, the clinician will find that the alternatives to heparin are few and most of them have similar risks or are not as effective as heparin. Low-molecular-weight heparin has been reported to have a cross-reactivity with unfractionated heparin antibody. This phenomenon is more evident with the heparinoid ORG 10172; cross-reactivity with the heparin-directed antibody occurs in as many as 18% of cases.[5] Whenever possible, patients who are receiving prophylactic heparin may be converted to warfarin, provided the enteral route of drug administration is available. In others, however, full systemic

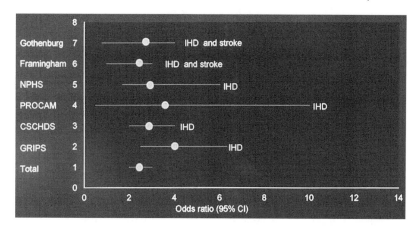

FIGURE 4. Studies of chronically elevated concentrations of fibrinogen. Gothenburg = 70-year-old people in Gothenburg, Sweden[26]; Framingham = The Framingham Study[18]; NHPS = Northwick Park Heart Study[19]; CSCHDS = Caerphilly and Speedwell Collaborative Heart Disease Studies[29]; GRIPS = Gottingen Rise Incidence and Prevalence Study.[10]

anticoagulation is required to perform vascular procedures. In all of these situations the best alternative is ancrod.

Ancrod has been used to perform peripheral vascular reconstructions[7] as well as coronary artery bypass grafts[28,30] and angioplasty.[23] The complication rate, especially bleeding complications, is at least no worse than with heparin—and several reports suggest that it is less. Table 1 summarizes the recent literature on the clinical use of ancrod.

Dose and Method of Use

Ancrod should be administered intravenously in most cases. Rapid infusion occasionally may be necessary because of the critical nature of the problem,[11] but it is important to

TABLE 1.   Clinical Use of Ancrod

Author and Year	Description
Becker, 1988[1]	Case reports—glomerulonephritis
Bell, 1988[2]	Review of clinical trials in acute stroke, DVT prophylaxis
Cole, 1988[6]	Case series, 7 patients—HITT, HIT, antithrombin III deficiency
Cole, 1989[8]	Case series, 9 patients—HIT and HITT
Cole, 1991[7]	Randomized trial, 28 patients—heparin vs. ancrod in distal bypass grafts
Cole, 1994[9]	Case series, 30 patients—DVT prophylaxis in multiple trauma
Demers, 1991[11]	Case series, 11 patients—HIT
Dion, 1989[12]	Case report—HIT, HITT, right ventricular thrombus
Doskum, 1984[13]	Case report—systemic lupus erythematosus
Hossmann, 1983[17]	Randomized, single-blind study, 30 patients with acute stroke
O-Yurvati, 1994[21]	Case report, HIT with Greenfield filter in right atrium
Pollak, 1990[22]	Case series—acute stroke
Pothoulakis, 1995[23]	Case report—HIT
Teasdale, 1989[28]	Case report—HITT and surgery to repair ventricular septal defect
Zulys, 1989[30]	Case series—20 patients having coronary artery bypass surgery

DVT = deep venous thrombosis; HIT = heparin-induced thrombocytopenia; HITT = heparin-induced thrombocytopenia and thrombosis.

remember *not* to administer ancrod as a bolus. It must be given no faster than the native fibrinolytic system can remove the ancrod-formed fibrin. In our experience, an infusion of 70 units in normal saline over 6–12 hours results in a fibrinogen concentration of 0.2–0.5 gm/L in most patients. Fibrinogen can then be maintained at that level with an infusion of 70 units in normal saline over 24 hours. The infusion rate may be titrated, depending on the urgency of the situation, but unless faced with a compelling reason, we have found that depleting fibrinogen over 12 hours seems to be the most satisfactory course.

Monitoring Ancrod

When the concentration of fibrinogen is very low, it is difficult to measure accurately, yet it is extremely important to know whether fibrinogen has been completely eliminated or is simply present in concentrations too low to measure by standard laboratory methods. Blood will not clot if fibrinogen is totally absent, but only 10–15% of the normal amount is required for hemostasis.[14] Experience with patients and experimental animal models shows that a concentration of fibrinogen in the range of 0.2–0.6 g/L can support ongoing hemostasis but effectively prevents spontaneous clotting or thrombosis. The prothrombin time (PT) is a valuable indicator of the fibrinogen concentration, because it will remain normal or within 1 or 2 seconds of normal until fibrinogen is reduced to zero. When fibrinogen has been reduced to 0.2–0.6 g/L or when the laboratory report indicates that the level of fibrinogen is below the concentration that can be measured, we monitor the PT. If the PT is prolonged more than 1 or 2 seconds, we consider the concentration of fibrinogen to be reduced to zero and stop the ancrod infusion until the fibrinogen is restored to a measurable quantity or until the PT is normal.

Bleeding

Bleeding is always a concern when patients are anticoagulated. However, ancrod appears to be associated with a lower risk of bleeding than heparin.[20] If bleeding does occur, it may be because the concentration of fibrinogen has been reduced to zero, in which case temporarily stopping the infusion may be sufficient treatment. If the response to discontinuation of the infusion of ancrod is too slow for timely correction, fibrinogen can be administered in the form of cryoprecipitate.

An antidote to ancrod is available. It is a purified globulin prepared from the sera of goats hyperimmunized with venom. We have not used it and are not aware that it has ever been used; there are no reports in the published literature. In our experience and that of others,[11] bleeding is an uncommon event if fibrinogen is not completely reduced to zero. In any case, fibrinogen can be restored quickly with cryoprecipitate and the risk associated with goat serum can be avoided.

CONCLUSION

Ancrod is a purified enzyme that acts on fibrinogen and causes the formation of an unstable fibrin/fibrinogen polymer that is rapidly digested by plasmin. A constant infusion results in steady depletion of the circulating fibrinogen. Reduction of circulating fibrinogen to very low levels (0.2–0.6 g/L) effectively anticoagulates the patient. This can usually be achieved in 6–12 hours and more quickly if the situation demands. This method of providing anticoagulation has been shown to be safe and effective for the conduct of major vascular reconstructions, including coronary artery as well as peripheral vascular bypass grafts. Ancrod is usually indicated when heparin is contraindicated (e.g., HITT) or ineffective (e.g., antithrombin III deficiency).

REFERENCES

1. Becker GJ: Ancrod in glomerulonephritis. Quart J Med 69: 849–850, 1988.
2. Bell WRJ: Clinical trials with ancrod. In Pirkle H, Markland FSJ (eds): Hemostasis and Animal Venoms. New York, Marcel Dekker, 1988, p. 541–551.

3. Chang, MC, Huang TF: The antiplatelet activity of ancrod on administration to rabbits. J Lab Clin Med 125: 508–516, 1995.
4. Chang MC, Wang CY, Huang TF: Ancrod-formed fibrin stimulates prostacycline production of human umbilical vein endothelial cells via de novo synthesis of cyclooxygenase. Biochem Biophys Res Commun 203: 1920–1926, 1994.
5. Chong BH, Ismail F, Cade J , et al: Heparin induced thrombocytopenia: studies with a new low molecular weight heparanoid, ORG 10172. Blood 73:1592–1596, 1989.
6. Cole CW, Bormanis J: Ancrod: A practical alternative to heparin. J Vasc Surg 8: 59–63, 1988.
7. Cole CW, Bormanis J, Luna GK, et al: Ancrod versus heparin for anticoagulation during vascular surgical procedures. J Vasc Surg 17: 288–293, 1993.
8. Cole CW, Fournier LM, Bormanis J: Heparin-associated thrombocytopenia and thrombosis: Optimal therapy with ancrod. Can J Surg 33: 207–210, 1990.
9. Cole CW, Shea B, Bormanis J: Ancrod as prophylaxis or treatment for thromboembolism in patients with multiple trauma. Can J Surg 38: 249–254, 1995.
10. Cremer P, Nagel D, Labrot B, et al: Lipoprotein Lp(a) as predictor of myocardial infarction in comparison to fibrinogen, LDL cholesterol and other risk factors: Results from the prospective Gottingen Risk Incidence and Prevalence Study (GRIPS). Eur J Clin Invest 24: 444–453, 1994.
11. Demers C, Ginsberg, JS, Brill-Edwards P, et al: Rapid anticoagulation using ancrod for heparin-induced thrombocytopenia. Blood 78: 2194–2197, 1991.
12. Dion D, Dumesnil JG, LeBlanc P: In situ right ventricular thrombus secondary to heparin induced thrombocytopenia. Can J Cardiol 5: 308–310, 1989.
13. Dosekun AK, Pollak VE, Blas-Greenwalt P, et al: Ancrod in systemic lupus erythematosus with thrombosis. Arch Intern Med 144:37–42, 1984.
14. Furukawa, K, Isimaru S: Use of thrombin-like snake venom enzymes in the treatment of vascular occlusive disease. In Stocker KT (ed): Medical Use of Snake Venom Proteins. Boca Raton, FL, CRC Press, 1990, pp 161–173.
15. Geerts WK, Code, KI, Jay RM, et al: A prospective study of venous thromboembolism after major trauma. N Engl J Med 331:1601–1606, 1994.
16. Heinrich, J, Balleisen L, Schulte H, et al: Fibrinogen and factor VII in the prediction of coronary risk. Results from the PROCAM study in healthy men. Arterioscler Thromb 14:54-59, 1994.
17. Hossmann V, Heiss W, Bewermeyer H, Wiedemann G: Controlled trial of ancrod in ischemic stroke. Arch Neurol 40:803–808, 1983.
18. Kannel WB, Wolf PA, Castelli WP, D'Agostino RB: Fibrinogen and risk of cardiovasclar disease. The Framingham Study. JAMA 258:1183–1186, 1987.
19. Kelleher CC: Plasma fibrinogen and factor VII as risk factors for cardiovascular disease. Eur J Epidemiol 1:79–82, 1992.
20. Latallo ZS: Report of the Task Force on Clinical Use of Snake Venom Enzymes. Thromb Haemost 39: 768–774, 1978.
21. O-Yurvati AH, Laub GW, Southgate TJ, McGrath LB: Heparinless cardiopulmonary bypass with ancrod [review]. Ann Thorac Surg 57: 1656–1658, 1994.
22. Pollak VE, Glas-Greenwalt P, Olinger CP, et al: Ancrod causes rapid thrombolysis in patients with acute stroke. Am J Med Sci 299: 319–325, 1990.
23. Pothoulakis AJ, Neerukonda SK, Ansel G, Jantz RD: Ancrod for coronary angioplasty. Tex Heart Inst J 22:342–346, 1995.
24. Prentice CR, Hampton KK, Grant PJ, et al: The fibrinolytic response to ancrod therapy: characterization of fibrinogen and fibrin degradation products. Br J Haematol 83: 276–281, 1993.
25. Resch KL, Ernst E, Matrai A, Paulsen HF: Fibrinogen and viscosity as risk factors for subsequent cardiovascular events in stroke survivors. Ann Intern Med 117:371–375, 1992.
26. Rosengren AL, Wilhelmsen L, Welin A, et al: Social influences and cardiovascular risk factors as determinants of plasma fibrinogen concentration in a general population sample of middle aged men. BMJ 300: 634–638, 1990.
27. Soszka T, Kirschbaum NE, Stewart GJ, Budzynski AZ: Direct effect of fibrinogen clotting enzymes on plasminogen activator secretion from human endothelial cells. Thromb Haemost 54:164–169, 1985.
28. Teasdale SJ, Zulys VJ, Mycyk T, et al: Ancrod anticoagulation for cardiopulmonary bypass in heparin-induced thrombocytopenia and thrombosis. Ann Thorac Surg 48:712–713, 1989.
29. Yarnell JW, Baker IA, Sweetnam PM, et al: Fibrinogen, viscosity, and white blood cell count are major risk factors for ischemic heart diseases. The Caerphilly and Speedwell collaborative heart disease studies. Circulation 83:836–844, 1991.
30. Zulys VJ, Teasdale SJ, Michel ER, et al: Ancrod (Arvin) as an alternative to heparin anticoagulation for cardiopulmonary bypass. Anesthesiology 71: 870–877, 1989.

CHAPTER 27

A Survey of Anti-Xa-Based Drugs: Potential Use in Cardiovascular Indications

BRIGITTE KAISER, M.D.

Thromboembolic processes play an important role in the pathogenetic mechanisms of various cardiovascular disorders. Although the balanced activity of the clotting system is necessary to prevent blood loss after injury, the activation of coagulation within the blood vessels can lead to unfavorable, often fatal effects, such as myocardial infarction, stroke, pulmonary embolism, deep vein thrombosis, and disseminated intravascular coagulation.

After initiation of coagulation via the extrinsic or intrinsic pathway, a cascadelike activation of inactive zymogens into active enzymes leads to the generation of thrombin and finally to fibrin formation. The serine protease thrombin is the central bioregulatory enzyme in the coagulation system; it possesses procoagulant as well as anticoagulant properties and causes various cellular effects via the reaction with its specific receptors. In the coagulation cascade, thrombin catalyzes the conversion of fibrinogen to clottable fibrin and activates factor XIII to cross-link soluble fibrin and form the final clot. It activates platelets, converts cofactors V and VIII to their active forms, and also acts as an anticoagulant via the protein C pathway.

In addition to thrombin, factor Xa is also a central and crucial enzyme in the coagulation cascade at the stage of the conversion of extrinsic and intrinsic pathways. Factor X is synthesized in the liver as a vitamin K-dependent protein and secreted into the blood stream as an inactive precursor. It circulates in plasma as a two-polypeptide chain glycoprotein with a molecular weight of 58,000 Da. Factor X is converted to factor Xa by both the factor VIIa–tissue factor complex (extrinsic pathway) and the factor IXa–factor VIIIa–calcium–phospholipid complex (intrinsic pathway). Activated platelets, endothelial cells at sites of vascular injury, vascular smooth muscle cells, and fibroblasts are capable of supporting the activation of factor X to Xa via the extrinsic or intrinsic pathway.[2] After activation, factor Xa in the presence of calcium associates stoichiometrically with factor Va on phospholipid surfaces to form the prothrombinase complex (Fig. 1). The required membrane surfaces are provided after vascular cell damage and activation of platelets. In addition to the exposition of negatively charged phospholipids on the platelet surface on which the prothrombinase complex can be formed, stimulated platelets and platelet-derived microvesicles also express some membrane-bound factor Xa activity.[20] After its formation, the prothrombinase complex converts prothrombin to α-thrombin by splitting off the F1+2 prothrombin fragment.

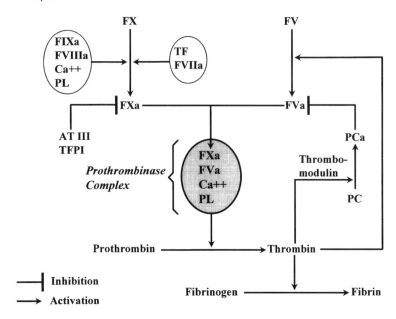

FIGURE 1.   Formation of the prothrombinase complex as a key event in the coagulation process.

In contrast to thrombin, which acts on several important protein substrates, factor Xa exerts its action mainly on the substrate prothrombin. The catalytic capacity of factor Xa alone is extremely low and is insufficient to generate thrombin and produce a fibrin–platelet clot at the site of vascular injury.[33,35,37] On formation of the prothrombinase complex, however, the catalytic efficiency of thrombin synthesis by factor Xa is enhanced more than 300,000-fold, leading to sufficient coagulation by cleavage of prothrombin.

The activity of clotting enzymes, including factor Xa, is controlled by several endogenous inhibitors. Antithrombin III (AT III) is a potent inhibitor of the blood coagulation system that inactivates factor Xa as well as thrombin and other serine proteases. However, factor Xa that is bound to factor Va on the membrane surface does not seem to be susceptible to AT III-mediated inhibition.[33,34] After activation by the thrombin–thrombomodulin complex (PCa) in the presence of the cofactor protein S, protein C inactivates factors Va and VIIIa. After cleavage by PCa, the factor Va molecule is incompetent in binding factor Xa and prothrombin. The inhibition of the extrinsic coagulation pathway is mediated by tissue factor pathway inhibitor (TFPI). In a first step, TFPI binds and inhibits factor Xa; in a second step, the TFPI–factor Xa complex forms a quaternary complex with TF–factor VIIa, thus interrupting the clotting process.

As a result, thrombosis causes many cardiovascular and other diseases, and there is a great need for effective antithrombotic prophylaxis and therapy. Inhibition and modulation of the effect of clotting enzymes is one way to control coagulation and thrombosis. Development of synthetic low-molecular-weight thrombin inhibitors and the natural anticoagulant hirudin has been rapid.[3,4,15,19,21,24,25,36] An effective and specific thrombin inhibitor, however, neutralizes both the procoagulant actions of the enzyme (fibrin formation) and its anticoagulant effects (activation of the protein C pathway). On the other hand, the important role of factor Xa in the coagulation cascade and the amplification of its procoagulant action by prothrombinase complex formation (a key event in the coagulation process) makes factor Xa a promising target for the development of highly effective and specific inhibitors for clinical use as anticoagulants and antithrombotics.

TABLE 1.   Strategies for Inhibition of Coagulation at the Stage of Factor Xa

---

• Direct inactivation of factor Xa
  Naturally occurring factor Xa inhibitors
    Antistasin (ATS) (from *Haementeria officinalis*)
    Tick anticoagulant peptide (TAP) (From *Ornithodorus moubata*)
    FXaI/yagin (from *Hirudo medicinalis*)
  Synthetic, low-molecular-weight factor Xa inhibitors
    DX-9065a
    SEL 2711

• Potentiation of inactivation of factor Xa by endogenous inhibitors
  Synthetic pentasaccharides

• Inhibition of activity of prothrombinase complex
  Inactive forms of factor Xa

DEVELOPMENT OF FACTOR Xa INHIBITORS

In recent years, knowledge of the causes and mechanisms of thromboembolic disorders has increased rapidly, and several new concepts for antithrombotic therapy have been developed. Development of factor Xa inhibitors, however, has not been as rapid as development of synthetic or naturally occurring thrombin inhibitors. Only a few systematic studies of factor Xa inhibitors comprehensively characterized their in vitro inhibition of various coagulation enzymes and their in vivo antithrombotic effectiveness.[26] Because of the dramatic increase in the catalytic activity of factor Xa after assembly of the prothrombinase complex, an effective factor Xa inhibitor must have an extremely high affinity for the enzyme. Synthetic, directly acting factor Xa inhibitors developed and studied in the past had only less selectivity over thrombin; furthermore, because of their modest potency, no final conclusions about the anticoagulant and antithrombotic potential of the inhibition of factor Xa could be drawn.[18,52] During the past few years potent factor Xa inhibitors have been isolated from natural sources or chemically synthesized (Table 1).[46] The naturally occurring factor Xa inhibitors are now available as recombinant polypeptides.

Various highly effective and selective polypeptide inhibitors of factor Xa were isolated from blood-sucking animals and characterized biochemically as well as pharmacologically (Table 2). Antistasin (ATS), which was isolated from the salivary glands of the

TABLE 2.   Characteristics of Various Inhibitors of Factor Xa

	Antistasin	Tick Anticoagulant Peptide	FXaI/Yagin	DX-9065a	SEL 2711
Origin	*Haementeria officinalis* (recombinant)	*Ornithodorus moubata* (recombinant)	*Hirudo medicinalis* (recombinant)	Synthetic	Synthetic
Chemical structure	Polypeptide (119 amino acids)	Polypeptide (60 amino acids)	Polypeptide (85 amino acids)	(Amidinoaryl) propanoic acid derivative	Pentapeptide
Molecular weight	15 kDa	6.9 kDa	14.4 kDa	—	760 Da
Ki factor Xa [nmol/L]	0.3–0.6	0.18 (free FXa) 0.006 (FXa complex)	10 (free FXa) 0.12 (FXa complex for FXaI) 0.05 (FXa complex for yagin)	41	3
Selectivity for factor Xa	High	High	High (except for trypsin)	High	High
Orally active	No	No	No	Yes	Yes
References	7, 40, 41, 54	22, 23, 30, 55, 57	45	12,27,28,39	49

Mexican leech (*Haementeria officinalis*), is a selective inhibitor of factor Xa that reacts with the active site of the enzyme, forming a stable complex.[40,41,54] Tick anticoagulant peptide (TAP) was originally isolated from the tick *Ornithodorus moubata*.[57] TAP is a reversible, slow-acting, tight-binding inhibitor of factor Xa. A first low-affinity binding of TAP to a site distinct from the catalytic site is followed by formation of a stable enzyme–inhibitor complex.[22,23] The affinity of TAP for factor Xa in the prothrombinase complex is greater than that for the free enzyme.[30,55] Another factor Xa inhibitor, FXaI, was isolated from the saliva of the medicinal leech (*Hirudo medicinalis*). Yagin is a novel recombinant factor Xa inhibitor from *H. medicinalis*.[45] Both FXaI and yagin are slow-acting, tight-binding, and (except for trypsin) selective inhibitors of factor Xa with a highly similar inhibition pattern. Both FXaI and yagin are more effective in inhibiting factor Xa in the prothrombinase complex than the free factor Xa in solution.[45]

A novel synthetic factor Xa inhibitor is DX-9065a (also called APAP).[62] It is a non-peptide, low-molecular-weight compound that has been described as a potent inhibitor of factor Xa with constant potency in the nanomolar range. It is also highly selective for factor Xa and absorbed orally.[12,27,28,39] Another synthetic active-site factor Xa inhibitor is SEL 2711,[49] a pentapeptide that is available orally and inhibits factor Xa in a reversible, competitive manner.

In addition to direct inhibition of the catalytic activity of the enzyme, factor Xa can also be inactivated by potentiation or acceleration of its inhibition by AT III. Synthetic pentasaccharide, which represents the AT III-binding region of heparin, catalyzes the AT III-mediated inactivation of factor Xa but not of thrombin.[31,42] Another possibility is inhibition of the activity of the prothrombinase complex by inactive forms of factor Xa,[1,50] which do not have catalytic activity but are still capable of associating into prothrombinase complexes. Competitive inhibition of plasma factor Xa needed for assembly of the prothrombinase complex by inactive forms reduces thrombin generation and thus controls thrombotic processes.[50]

ANTICOAGULANT ACTION OF FACTOR Xa INHIBITORS

In the past, because of the lack of highly potent and selective factor Xa inhibitors, no final conclusion about the anticoagulant effectiveness of factor Xa inhibition could be drawn. In general, the anticoagulant action of prothrombinase inhibitors is studied with routine coagulation assays such as thrombin time (TT), activated partial thromboplastin time (APTT), and prothrombin time (PT). Based on the amplification mechanisms in the coagulation cascade and the outstanding effectiveness of the prothrombinase complex, interference with the coagulation process at the level of factor Xa can be expected to lead to effective anticoagulation.

For anticoagulant and antithrombotic actions besides the direct inactivation of coagulation enzymes, the inhibition of their generation is of great interest. The inactivation of factor Xa by specific inhibitors has no effect on the activity of preformed thrombin. Because of their mechanism of action, however, factor Xa inhibitors may prevent the further generation of thrombin and thus inhibit thrombin-mediated feedback reactions that enhance thrombin production through autoamplification.

According to in vitro as well as in vivo studies with global clotting assays, neither naturally occurring nor synthetic factor Xa inhibitors show an effect on TT, whereas APTT and PT are prolonged in a concentration- or dose-dependent manner. The factor Xa inhibitors DX-9065a and SEL 2711 demonstrated anticoagulant activities in ex vivo blood samples after intravenous, subcutaneous, and oral administration, proving their oral bioavailability.[12,14,49] For unknown reasons, some factor Xa inhibitors, such as ATS and DX-9065a, showed clear differences in their anticoagulant actions in different species.[13,17,41] Studies of the anticoagulant effects of ATS and TAP revealed differences in potency both in vitro[6] and in vivo.[47,56] In measurements of ex vivo clotting times, at nearly

TABLE 3. Effective Concentrations of Hirudin and Antistasin for Doubling the Clotting Time in Human Plasma in Three Coagulation Assays

	Concentration for Doubling Clotting Time (μmol/L)				
Inhibitor	**TT**	**PT**	**APTT**	**Ki of FIIa (nmol/L)**	**Ki of FXa (nmol/L)**
Antistasin	> 100	0.036	0.16	—	0.3
Hirudin	0.011	0.78	0.10	0.00048	> 5

TT = thrombin time, PT = prothrombin time, APTT = activated partial thromboplastin time.
From Hauptmann J, Kaiser B: Anticoagulant potential of synthetic and recombinant inhibitors of factor Xa and thrombin in vitro. Blood Coag Fibrinol 4:577–582, 1993, with permission.

equal antithrombotic efficiency TAP was less potent than ATS in prolonging APTT.[47,56] These results may reflect kinetic differences in the rate of factor Xa inactivation, but they also demonstrate that the antithrombotic efficacy of a given anticoagulant cannot be predicted by APTT values alone.

In an in vitro study comparing the thrombin inhibitor hirudin with the factor Xa inhibitor ATS, the PT assay was found to be most sensitive to the anticoagulant effect of the factor Xa inhibitor (Table 3). The APTT assay seems to be more dependent on the antithrombin potential of an inhibitor.[16] Furthermore, a combination of hirudin with various amounts of ATS showed that as little as 1% ATS in the combination nearly doubled its anticoagulant potency in the PT assay compared with hirudin alone; 10% ATS increased the potency 5-fold, and 33% led to a 10-fold increase (Fig. 2).[16]

ANTITHROMBOTIC EFFECTS OF FACTOR Xa INHIBITORS

The formation of venous or arterial thrombi in different regions of the vascular system is a complex process that results mainly from changes in blood flow, in the vessel wall, or in blood constituents. In experimental studies intravascular thrombosis in venous

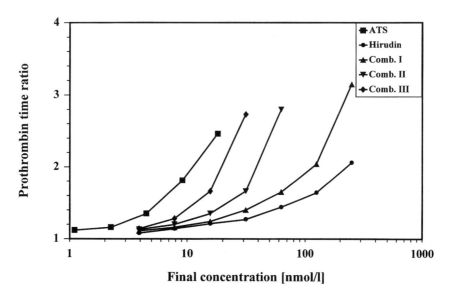

FIGURE 2. Anticoagulant potency of antistasin and hirudin alone or in various combinations in the prothrombin time assay. Combination I: 1% antistasin + 99% hirudin; combination II: 10% antistasin + 90% hirudin; combination III: 33% antistasin + 67% hirudin. (From Hauptmann J, Kaiser B: Anticoagulant and antithrombotic action of the factor Xa inhibitor antistasin (ATS). Thromb Res 71:169–174, 1993, with permission.)

or arterial vessels can be induced by activation of the coagulation system with activated clotting factors; mechanical or chemical damage of the vessel wall; alterations in blood flow; or contact of the blood with artificial surfaces.

Thrombin-induced platelet reactions and fibrin formation are major factors in the development of intravascular thrombosis. Therefore, substances that inhibit the generation of thrombin are expected to prevent the formation of thrombi or their progression, both under experimental conditions and in clinical situations. The antithrombotic principle for factor Xa inhibitors is based on their interference with the thrombotic process at a relatively early stage of coagulation activation—the action of the prothrombinase complex. Because active prothrombinase complexes may persist at the site of vascular injury and contribute to perpetuation of thrombotic processes, inactivation of factor Xa in plasma and especially of factor Xa bound in the complex may prevent both further formation of prothrombinase complexes and production of thrombin.

The antithrombotic efficacy of factor Xa inhibitors has been studied in various models of experimental thrombosis in animals, in which the underlying pathophysiologic mechanisms of arterial and venous thrombosis or of disseminated intravascular coagulation corresponded largely to those in humans. Experimental studies with ATS, TAP, yagin, DX-9065a, and SEL 2711 indicate that inhibitors of factor Xa have considerable potential as antithrombotic agents (Table 4). Because of the inactivation of factor Xa, formation of thrombi in the jugular vein of rats or rabbits initiated by thromboplastin or activated human serum was reduced or completely prevented in a dose-dependent manner (Fig. 3).[17,49,56,59] In various models of arterial thrombosis, factor Xa inhibitors were shown to prevent platelet and fibrin deposition as well as thrombus formation in arteriovenous shunts;[10,14,47–49,59,62] to accelerate reperfusion during thrombolysis; and to prevent acute reocclusion.[29,37,38,51] Interesting results were obtained in a rabbit model of restenosis after balloon angioplasty of atherosclerotic femoral arteries.[44] A brief infusion of ATS or TAP significantly reduced restenosis of the vessels 28 days after angioplasty and led to less luminal narrowing by plaque formation.

Several studies compared the antithrombotic effectiveness of factor Xa inhibitors and heparin or hirudin. In a model of mild disseminated intravascular coagulation, the effect of ATS was comparable to that of standard heparin when equally effective anticoagulant doses were given.[5] Nearly equal antithrombotic actions of heparin and factor Xa inhibitors were also seen in venous thrombosis,[9,56] coronary arterial thrombosis,[32] and vascular graft thrombosis.[48,49] In femoral or coronary artery thrombosis treated by lysis with recombinant tissue-type plasminogen activator, ATS and TAP were even more effective than heparin or hirudin in shortening the time until reperfusion and in preventing reocclusion and restenosis.[37,44,51] Thus, under experimental conditions, the inhibition of thrombin generation with specific inhibition of factor Xa is at least as effective in preventing thrombosis as the direct inactivation of thrombin by selective thrombin inhibitors.

TABLE 4. Studies of Directly Acting Factor Xa Inhibitors Showing Antithrombotic Effectiveness in Experimental Models of Thrombosis

- Rat and rabbit models of venous thrombosis: antistasin,[17,56] tick anticoagulant peptide,[9,56] yagin,[59] and SEL 1711.[49]
- Rat and baboon models of arteriovenous shunt thrombosis: antistasin,[47] tick anticoagulant peptide,[48] yagin,[10,59] DX-9065a,[14,62] and SEL 2711.[49]
- Canine model of coronary artery thrombosis: tick anticoagulant peptide.[32]
- Rabbit and canine model of arterial thrombolysis and acute reocclusion after rt-PA: antistasin,[37] tick anticoagulant peptide,[38,51] and yagin.[29]
- Rabbit model of restenosis after balloon angioplasty: antistasin[44] and tick anticoagulant peptide.[44]
- Mice and rat model of acute disseminated intravascular coagulation: yagin[59] and DX-9065a.[14,53,60,61]
- Monkey model of hemodialysis: DX-9065a.[11]

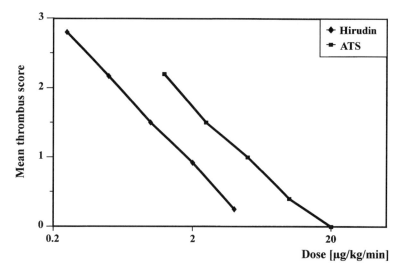

FIGURE 3.   Prevention of stasis-induced venous thrombosis in the jugular vein of rats by intravenous injection of antistasin or hirudin. (From Hauptmann J, Kaiser B: Anticoagulant and antithrombotic action of the factor Xa inhibitor antistasin (ATS). Thromb Res 71:169–174, 1993, with permission.)

POTENTIAL USE OF FACTOR Xa INHIBITORS FOR CLINICAL INDICATIONS

The principal criteria for clinical application of factor Xa inhibitors are effectiveness and safety. Preclinical studies with factor Xa inhibitors showed that interaction with the coagulation system at the level of factor Xa and/or prothrombinase complex formation by highly specific and selective inhibitors is an effective approach for an anticoagulant and antithrombotic therapy (Table 5). In various models of experimental thrombosis in animals, factor Xa inhibitors were found to be antithrombotically effective. Experimental findings indicate that these agents are potentially useful in a number of different therapeutic areas, especially for thrombotic disorders (Table 6).

Because of the interruption of the blood coagulation process at a relatively early step in the coagulation cascade and in accordance with experimental in vivo studies, inhibition of factor Xa by highly effective agents may be useful to prevent and treat venous thromboembolism.

The binding of thrombin to fibrin is thought to be an important mechanism by which thrombi exhibit procoagulant activity that leads to recurrent thrombosis after thrombolysis and to propagation of thrombi.[58] Newer results, however, indicate that the procoagulant activity of residual thrombi during or after fibrinolysis does not depend primarily on

TABLE 5.   Hemostatic Characteristics of Specific Factor Xa Inhibitors

Anticoagulant action in global clotting assays	Most effective in prothrombin time and activated partial thromboplastin time
Usefulness for whole blood anticoagulation	Not known
Inhibition of preexisting thrombin	No
Inhibition of thrombin generation	Yes
Inhibition of clot-bound factor Xa	Yes
Antithrombotic effectiveness in experimental models of thrombosis	Yes
Therapeutic usefulness in thrombotic disorders	Prophylaxis and therapy of venous and arterial thrombosis

TABLE 6.   Possible Clinical Indications for Factor Xa Inhibitors

- Perioperative thrombosis prophylaxis (e.g., in orthopedic surgery [hip replacement])
- Adjunction administration in thrombolytic therapy
- Prevention of restenosis after angioplasty or thrombolysis
- Administration of orally effective agents in patients requiring long-term anticoagulation
- Administration of orally effective agents in patients with unstable angina or coronary ischemia

preexisting, clot-bound thrombin but rather on de novo activation of prothrombin mediated by factors Xa and Va.[8,43] Both thrombin and factor Xa bound to clot seem to be protected from inhibition by AT III. Therefore, the clot-associated factor Xa activity is resistant to inhibition by AT III-dependent inhibitors such as pentasaccharide, but it is inhibited by specific factor Xa inhibitors such as TAP.[8] Because factor Xa appears to be an important determinant of the procoagulant activity of whole-blood clots and arterial thrombi, inhibitors of factor Xa may be highly effective in interrupting the progression of thrombotic processes and preventing rethrombosis and restenosis after thrombolytic therapy. In addition, the therapeutic effect may be enhanced by a combination of factor Xa inhibitors with directly acting, potent thrombin inhibitors.[43]

The most important safety factor of antithrombotic therapy is related to bleeding complications, which often limit the therapeutic range of inhibitors of coagulation enzymes. At antithrombotically effective doses factor Xa inhibitors, unlike unfractionated heparin, did not affect bleeding time or blood loss.[10,14,37,38,47,48,53,59,61] Factor Xa inhibitors such as DX-9065a are not expected to impair hemostatic mechanisms because they do not affect platelet aggregation.[12] Furthermore, as competitive inhibitors they do not suppress the formation of thrombin completely. Small amounts of thrombin are able to initiate primary hemostasis (i.e., to form the hemostatic plug at a site of vascular injury), but they cannot catalyze the conversion of fibrinogen to fibrin in sufficient quantities. Because of their effective blockade of the coagulation process without compromise of the hemostatic functions of platelets, factor Xa inhibitors can be used as adjunctive drugs in thrombolysis as well as in combination with antiplatelet agents without increasing the risk of hemorrhagic side effects.

In addition to their anticoagulant and antithrombotic profile and possible hemorrhagic side effects, other pharmacologic properties of factor Xa inhibitors have to be taken into consideration to assess their therapeutic usefulness. Pharmacokinetic behavior includes the time course of antithrombotic action, bioavailability and effectiveness after different routes of administration, biologic half-life, and metabolism and excretion. Because of their polypeptide nature, compounds such as ATS or TAP have to be administered parenterally and thus are more limited in their therapeutic use than substances that are absorbed after oral administration, such as DX-9065a. Orally available factor Xa inhibitors are especially appropriate for patients who require long-term anticoagulation, provided that their biologic half-life is long enough to reach effective plasma concentrations over a sufficient period.

Other pharmacodynamic actions of factor Xa inhibitors also need to be investigated, such as effects on the cardiovascular and respiratory systems as well as antigenicity, which is especially important for inhibitors with a polypeptide structure.[5] The induction of an immunologic response by foreign proteins limits either duration of application or possibly even their initial use. The inhibition of factor Xa appears to be a promising antithrombotic treatment in patients with thromboembolic disorders, but further clinical evaluations are required to make a final statement about their usefulness in various diseases.

SUMMARY

The inhibition of factor Xa by highly effective and selective inhibitors leads to control of both intrinsic and extrinsic pathways of the coagulation cascade. The resulting decrease or even prevention of thrombin generation, as well as thrombin-mediated feedback mechanisms and platelet reactions, is an effective approach to prevent thrombus formation in venous and arterial vessels, even after events that lead to rethrombosis and restenosis.

Unlike heparin, directly acting factor Xa inhibitors demonstrate anticoagulant and antithrombotic activity independently of AT III or any other endogenous inhibitor. Furthermore, they were shown to have a greater efficacy and safety profile, especially with regard to bleeding complications, because they do not compromise hemostatic functions of platelets. Inhibition of thrombin generation by direct inactivation of factor Xa may be an effective way for suppressing thrombosis without impairing hemostasis.

Factor Xa inhibitors may become useful antithrombotic agents with favorable benefit-to-risk properties. They may provide therapeutic benefit in a wide range of clinical indications. However, these agents are still in the phase of preclinical investigations. Clinical studies must clarify whether factor Xa inhibitors have antithrombotic effects in humans and whether they have real advantages over established drugs for use in cardiovascular indications.

REFERENCES

1. Benedict CR, Ryan J, Todd J, et al: Active site-blocked factor Xa prevents thrombus formation in the coronary vasculature in parallel with inhibition of extravascular coagulation in a canine thrombosis model. Blood 81:2059–2066, 1993.
2. Brinkmann HM, Mertens K, Holthuis J, et al: The activation of human blood coagulation factor Xa on the surface of endothelial cells: A comparison with various vascular cells, platelets and monocytes. Br J Haematol 87:332–342, 1994.
3. Bush LR: Argatroban, a selective, potent thrombin inhibitor. Cardiovasc Drug Rev 9:247–263, 1991.
4. Callas D, Fareed J: Comparative pharmacology of site directed antithrombin agents. Implications in drug development. Thromb Haemost 74:473–481, 1995.
5. Dunwiddie CT, Nutt EM, Vlasuk GP, et al: Anticoagulant efficacy and immunogenicity of the selective factor Xa inhibitor antistasin following subcutaneous administration in the rhesus monkey. Thromb Haemost 67:371–376, 1992.
6. Dunwiddie CT, Smith DE, Nutt EM, Vlasuk GP: Anticoagulant effects of the selective factor Xa inhibitors tick anticoagulant peptide and antistasin in the APTT assay are determined by the relative rate of prothrombinase inhibition. Thromb Res 64:787–794, 1991.
7. Dunwiddie CT, Thornberry NA, Bull HG, et al: Antistasin, a leech-derived inhibitor of factor Xa. Kinetic analysis of enzyme inhibition and identification of the reactive site. J Biol Chem 264:16694–16699, 1989.
8. Eisenberg PR, Siegel JE, Abendschein DR, Miletich JP: Importance of factor Xa in determining the procoagulant activity of whole-blood clots. J Clin Invest 91:1877–1833, 1993.
9. Fioravanti C, Burkholder D, Francis B, et al: Antithrombotic activity of recombinant tick anticoagulant peptide and heparin in a rabbit model of venous thrombosis. Thromb Res 71: 317–324, 1993.
10. Hanson SR, Harker LA, Levanon A, et al: Inhibition of factor Xa in baboon thrombosis models. Thromb Haemost 73: 1311, 1995.
11. Hara T, Morishima Y, Kunitada S: Selective factor Xa inhibitor, DX-9065a, suppressed hypercoagulable state during haemodialysis in cynomorgus monkeys. Thromb Haemost 73:1311, 1995.
12. Hara T, Yokoyama A, Ishihara H, et al: DX-9065a, a new synthetic, potent anticoagulant and selective inhibitor for factor Xa. Thromb Haemost 71:314–319, 1994.
13. Hara T, Yokoyama A, Morishima Y, Kunitada S: Species differences in anticoagulant and anti-Xa activity of DX-9065a, a highly selctive factor Xa inhibitor. Thromb Res 80: 99–104, 1995.
14. Hara T, Yokoyama A, Tanabe K, et al: DX-9065a, an orally active, specific inhibitor of factor Xa, inhibits thrombosis without affecting bleeding time in rats. Thromb Haemost 74:635–639, 1995.
15. Harker LA: Strategies for inhibiting the effects of thrombin. Blood Coag Fibrinol 5:S47–S58, 1994.
16. Hauptmann J, Kaiser B: Anticoagulant potential of synthetic and recombinant inhibitors of factor Xa and thrombin in vitro. Blood Coag Fibrinol 4:577–582, 1993.
17. Hauptmann J, Kaiser B: Anticoagulant and antithrombotic action of the factor Xa inhibitor antistasin (ATS). Thromb Res 71:169–174, 1993.
18. Hauptmann J, Kaiser B, Nowak G, et al: Comparison of the anticoagulant and antithrombotic effects of synthetic thrombin and factor Xa inhibitors. Thromb Haemost 63:220–223, 1990.
19. Hauptmann J, Markwardt F: Pharmacologic aspects of the development of selective synthetic thrombin inhibitors as anticoagulants. Semin Thromb Hemost 18:200–217, 1992.

20. Holme PA, Brosstad F, Solum NO: Platelet-derived microvesicles and activated platelets express factor Xa activity. Blood Coag Fibrinol 6:302–310, 1995.
21. Johnson PH: Hirudin—clinical potential of a thrombin inhibitor. Annu Rev Med 45:165–177, 1994.
22. Jordan SP, Mao SS, Lewis SD, Shafer JA: Reaction pathway for inhibition of blood coagulation factor Xa by tick anticoagulant peptide. Biochemistry 31:5374–5380, 1992.
23. Jordan SP, Waxman L, Smith DE, Vlasuk GP: Tick anticoagulant peptide: Kinetic analysis of the recombinant inhibitor with blood coagulation factor Xa. Biochemistry 29:11095–11100, 1990.
24. Kaiser B: Anticoagulant and antithrombotic actions of recombinant hirudin. Semin Thromb Hemost 2:130–136, 1991.
25. Kaiser B, Hauptmann J: Pharmacology of synthetic thrombin inhibitors of the tripeptide type. Cardiovasc Drug Rev 10:71–87, 1992.
26. Kaiser, B, Hauptmann, J. Factor Xa inhibitors as novel antithrombotic agents: Facts and perspectives. Cardiovasc Drug Rev 12:225–236, 1994.
27. Katakura S, Nagakara T, Hara T, Iwamoto M: A novel factor Xa inhibitor: Structure-activity relationships and selectivity between factor Xa and thrombin. Biochem Biophys Res Commun 197:965–972, 1993.
28. Katakura S, Nagakara T, Hara T, et al: Molecular model of an interaction between factor Xa and DX-9065a, a novel factor Xa inhibitor: Contribution of the acetimidoylpyrrolidine moiety of the inhibitor to potency and selectivity for serine proteases. Eur J Med Chem 30:387–394, 1995.
29. Kornowsky R, Eldor A, Werber M, et al: Enhancement of rTPA thrombolysis with a selective factor Xa inhibitor derived from the leech: Comparison to heparin and hirudin in a rabbit thrombosis model. Thromb Haemost 73:1317, 1995.
30. Krishnaswamy S, Vlasuk GP, Bergum PW: Assembly of the prothrombinase complex enhances the inhibition of bovine factor Xa by tick anticoagulant peptide. Biochemistry 33:7897–7907, 1994.
31. Lormeau JC, Herault JP: The effect of the synthetic pentasaccharide SR 90107/ORG 31540 on thrombin generation ex vivo is uniquely due to ATIII-mediated neutralization of factor Xa. Thromb Haemost 74:1474–1477, 1995.
32. Lynch JJ, Sitko GR, Lehman ED, Vlasuk GP: Primary prevention of coronary arterial thrombosis with the factor Xa inhibitor rTAP in a canine electrolytic injury model. Thromb Haemost 74:640–645, 1995.
33. Mann KG: The assembly of blood clotting complexes on membranes. Trends Biochem Sci 12:229–233, 1987.
34. Mann KG, Nesheim ME, Church WR, et al: Surface-dependent reactions of the vitamin K-dependent enzyme complexes. Blood 76:1–16, 1990.
35. Mann KG, Kalafatis M: The coagulation explosion. Cerebrovasc Dis 5:93–97, 1995.
36. Markwardt F: Prospective clinical use of hirudin as an anticoagulant. Biomed Prog 2:19–23, 1990.
37. Mellott MJ, Holahan MA, Lynch JJ, et al: Acceleration of recombinant tissue-type plasminogen activator-induced reperfusion and prevention of reocclusion by recombinant antistasin, a selective factor Xa inhibitor, in a canine model of femoral arterial thrombosis. Circ Res 70:1152–1160, 1992.
38. Mellott MJ, Stranieri MT, Sitko GR, et al: Enhancement of recombinant tissue plasminogen activator-induced reperfusion by recombinant tick anticoagulant peptide, a selective factor Xa inhibitor, in a canine model of femoral arterial thrombolysis. Fibrinolysis 7:195–202, 1993.
39. Nagahara T, Katakura S, Yokoyama Y, et al: Design, synthesis and biological activities of orally active coagulation factor Xa inhibitors. Eur J Med Chem 30(Suppl):140s–143s, 1995.
40. Nutt E, Gasic T, Rodkey J, et al: The amino acid sequence of antistasin. J Biol Chem 263:10162–10167, 1988.
41. Nutt EM, Jain D, Lenny AB, et al: Purification and characterization of recombinant antistasin: a leech-derived inhibitor of coagulation factor Xa. Arch Biochem Biophys 285:37 44, 1991.
42. Olson ST, Björk I, Sheffer R, et al: Role of antithrombin-binding pentasaccharide in heparin acceleration of antithrombin-proteinase reactions. J Biol Chem 267:12528–12538, 1992.
43. Prager NA, Abendschein DR, McKenzie CR, Eisenberg PR: Role of thrombin compared with factor Xa in the procoagulant activity of whole blood clots. Circulation 92:962–967, 1995.
44. Ragosta M, Gimple LW, Gertz SD, et al: Specific factor Xa inhibition reduces restenosis after balloon angioplasty of atherosclerotic femoral arteries in rabbits. Circulation 89:1262–1271, 1994.
45. Rigbi M, Jackson CM, Atamna H, et al: FXa inhibitor from the saliva of the leech Hirudo medicinalis. Thromb Haemost 73:1306, 1995
46. Ripka W, Brunck T, Stanssens P, et al: Strategies in the design of inhibitors of serine proteases of the coagulation cascade—factor Xa. Eur J Med Chem 30(Suppl):88s–100s, 1995.
47. Schaffer LW, Davidson JT, Vlasuk GP, et al: Selective factor Xa inhibition by recombinant antistasin prevents vascular graft thrombosis in baboons. Arterioscler Thromb 12:879–885, 1992.
48. Schaffer, LW, Davidson JT, Vlasuk GP, Siegl PKS: Antithrombotic efficacy of recombinant tick anticoagulant peptide. A potent inhibitor of coagulation factor Xa in a primate model of arterial thrombosis. Circulation 84:1741–1748, 1991.
49. Seligman B, Stringer SK, Ostrem JA, et al: SEL 2711: A specific, orally available, active-site inhibitor of factor Xa discovered using synthetic combinatorial chemistry. In Speaker Presentations at the Sixth IBC International Symposium: Advances in Anticoagulants and Antithrombotics. Washington, DC, 1995.

50. Sinha U, Hollenbach S, Wolf DL: Macromolecular complex assembly of prothrombinase is a central process of thrombosis. Ann N Y Acad Sci 714:32–40, 1994.

51. Sitko GR, Ramjit DR, Stabilito II, et al: Conjunctive enhancement of enzymatic thrombolysis and prevention of thrombotic reocclusion with the selective factor Xa inhibitor tick anticoagulant peptide. Comparison to hirudin and heparin in a canine model of acute coronary artery thrombosis. Circulation 85:805–815, 1992.

52. Stürzebecher J, Stürzebecher U, Vieweg H, et la: Synthetic inhibitors of bovine factor Xa and thrombin. Comparison of their anticoagulant efficiency. Thromb Res 54:245–252, 1989.

53. Tanabe K, Honda Y, Kunitada S: An orally active, specific inhibitor of factor Xa does not facilitate haemorrhage at the effective doses in rat thrombosis model. Thromb Haemost 73:1312, 1995.

54. Tuszynski GP, Gasic TB, Gasic GJ: Isolation and characterization of antistasin. An inhibitor of metastasis and coagulation. J Biol Chem 262:9718–9723, 1987.

55. Vlasuk GP: Structural and functional characterization of tick anticoagulant peptide (TAP): A potent and selective inhibitor of blood coagulation factor Xa. Thromb Haemost 70:212–216, 1993.

56. Vlasuk GP, Ramjit D, Dunwiddie CT, et al: Comparison of the in vivo anticoagulant properties of standard heparin and the highly selective factor Xa inhibitors antistasin and tick anticoagulant peptide (TAP) in a rabbit model of venous thrombosis. Thromb Haemost 65:257–262, 1991.

57. Waxman L, Smith DE, Arcuri KE, Vlasuk GP: Tick anticoagulant peptide (TAP) is a novel inhibitor of blood coagulation factor Xa. Science 248:593–596, 1990.

58. Weitz JI, Hudoba M, Massel D, et al: Clot-bound thrombin is protected from inhibition by heparin-antithrombin III but is susceptible to inactivation by antithrombin III-independent inhibitors. J Clin Invest 86:385–391, 1990.

59. Werber MM, Zeelon E, Levanon A, et al: Yagin, a leech-derived FXa inhibitor, expressed in and recovered from E. coli: Antithrombotic potency in vitro and in vivo. Thromb Haemost 73:1312, 1995.

60. Yamazaki M, Asakura H, Aoshima K, et al: Effects of DX-9065a, an orally active, newly synthesized and specific inhibitor of factor Xa, against experimental disseminated intravascular coagulation in rats. Thromb Haemost 72:393–396, 1994.

61. Yamazaki M, Asakura H, Saito M, et al: Effects of DX-9065a, an orally active, newly synthesized and specific inhibitor of factor Xa against experimental disseminated intravascular coagulation in rats. Thromb Haemost 73:1312, 1995.

62. Yokoyama T, Kelly AB, Marzec UM, et al: Antithrombotic effects of orally active synthetic antagonists of activated factor X in nonhuman primates. Circulation 92:485–491, 1995.

CHAPTER 28

Aspirin and Antiplatelet Drugs: Effects during Cardiopulmonary Bypass

HANS KLAUS BREDDIN, M.D.

PLATELET FUNCTION DURING CARDIOPULMONARY BYPASS

During extracorporeal circulation platelets are activated by the nonendothelial artificial surfaces of the oxygenator, tubings, roller pumps, and other materials. The activated platelets undergo shape change, aggregation, and release, depending on the intensity of activation or the strength of the agonists. Activated platelets stick to the artificial surfaces and form aggregates that may block microcirculatory vessels. This process leads to a drop in platelet count, which may be attenuated if thrombin is formed either during or at the end of extracorporeal circulation.

Platelets have receptors for agonist molecules such as adenosine diphosphate (ADP), collagen, or proteases (e.g., thrombin). Platelets as adhesive cells also bind to many subendothelial and plasma molecules. Activation is associated with changes in the cytoskeleton and outside-in signalling. The originally disk-shaped plaletets swell, and membrane glycoproteins such as GPIIb/IIIa and GpIb, along with other activation proteins, are released. Low-affinity platelet glycoprotein receptors for adhesive molecules on the platelet membrane, such as GP IIb/IIIa, are activated, leading to high affinity for substances such as fibrin and to subsequent aggregation. GPIIb/IIIa changes its confirmation during this activation process, so that it can bind fibrinogen, von Willebrand factor (VWF), or fibronectin.[12] Fibrinogen bound to GPIIb/IIIa also binds to resting platelets, thereby leading to their activation. Platelet adhesion and aggregation at high shear stress are mediated by GPIb and GP IIb/IIIa. Other activation antigens include P-selectin (CD62). This and other molecules can be detected by the combination of monoclonal antibodies and immunohistologic staining or by flow cytometry. The GPIb–V-IX complex is involved in platelet interactions with exposed subendothelium and with VWF. GPIb is the VWF receptor.

Loss of platelets and impaired platelet function contribute to the impaired hemostasis and bleeding complications after cardiac surgery. However, to what extent platelet dysfunction is responsible for intra- and postoperative bleeding is still under debate because no generally accepted tests are available.

The combined use of aspirin and heparin significantly increases the bleeding time.[3] Platelet function in open heart surgery has recently been studied with different methods. Platelet function tests, however, have limitations, because they depend on sampling techniques; no global platelet function test is available. In addition to platelet count and aggregation in response to different inducing agents, general targets of investigation with flow cytometry include platelet adhesion or retention, release of platelet factor 4, platelet spreading, and platelet activation.

Stern et al. studied 51 patients undergoing CPB with a system that measures viscoelastic properties of recalcified whole blood (Sonoclot Analyzer). Despite a significant decrease in clot retraction in patients taking nonsteroidal antiinflammatory drugs, the test results did not predict postoperative bleeding.[51] Dorman et al. studied 60 patients before coronary artery bypass surgery with the thrombelastogram, bleeding time, and different coagulation tests. Only the bleeding time, platelet count, and prothrombin time had a significant predictive value.[18]

Using an in vitro bleeding time method (Thrombostat 4000), Tabuchi et al. studied patients undergoing cardiac surgery. They found that platelet function was impaired shortly after the start of CPB and partly recovered at its conclusion. During CPB aspirin-treated platelets were more severely affected than non–aspirin-treated platelets. The degree of platelet dysfunction at the end of the operation correlated significantly with blood loss from the chest drain.[52] Ratnatunga et al., using the same test system, studied 205 patients before cardiac surgery and concluded that the bleeding risk could not be predicted preoperatively, probably because of the platelet abnormalities that occur later during CPB.[41]

The extent of anticoagulation clearly affects the amount of platelet loss during extracorporeal circulation.[8,62] Platelet retention is reduced in hemolytic blood. Hemodilution preserves platelets. Excessive use of protamine bears the risk of thrombin formation and may lead to dramatic changes in platelet count and platelet function. Menys et al. studied micro- and macroaggregation in hirudinized whole blood and platelet-rich plasma (PRP) from patients who had undergone CPB.[37] In aspirin-treated patients collagen-induced micro-and macroaggregation were markedly impaired. Irani et al.[27] concluded that preoperative and intraoperative whole blood lumiaggregometry may not predict postoperative blood loss in patients receiving PRP intraoperatively during CPB surgery. On the other hand, prolongation of bleeding time does not predict peri- and postoperative bleeding in CPB surgery.[16]

Platelet volume can be measured easily using electric conductivity methods. Boldt et al.[8] found a significant correlation between changes in mean platelet volume and changes in aggregation variables (ADP or collagen as inducers) and concluded that increased platelet volume indicates abnormalities in platelet function in the postbypass period. As reported by George et al.,[23] thrombin-induced platelet activation leads to a decrease in platelet surface concentration of GpIb and GpIIb with no increase in glycoprotein membrane protein 140 or thrombospondin.

Several authors have proposed the use of platelet function inhibitors to preserve platelet function during CPB, with the intention of reducing postoperative bleeding. Uthoff et al.[59] treated dogs during CPB with the GPIIb/IIIa inhibitor Integrelin or with placebo. Six hours after CPB platelet number and function were better preserved in the integrelin group, which also had less postoperative blood loss in comparison with placebo. Utley[60] suggested the postoperative use of aspirin and platelet transfusions in patients with heparin-induced thrombocytopenia. Teoh et al. described the reduction of blood loss during CPB by using membrane oxygenators and preoperative oral treatment with dipyridamole.[54,55]

In summary, platelets are activated and reduced in number during CPB. As a result, they are also functionally impaired. This impairment probably contributes significantly to intra- and postoperative bleeding. All platelet function inhibitors to some extent increase the risk of bleeding. Whether short-acting platelet inhibitors can preserve platelets during CPB, with a resulting improvement of hemostatic function, is an interesting hypothesis.

MODE OF ACTION OF ANTIPLATELET DRUGS

Aspirin, dipyridamole, ticlopidine, and prostacyclin impair platelet activation.

Aspirin

Aspirin has antithrombotic effects by inhibiting platelet function. It mildly prolongs the bleeding time. Aspirin inhibits thromboxane A_2 formation by inhibiting cyclooxygenase in platelets and vascular synthesis of PGI_2. Cyclooygenase exists in two isoforms, COX-1 and COX-2.[38] Acetylsalicylic acid (ASA) at low antithrombotic doses inhibits COX-1; it also inhibits the enzymatic function of cyclooxygenase after acetylation of the aminoacid Tyr 385 and binds to Ser 530, thereby preventing arachidonic acid from reaching the enzyme.[32] After single doses of aspirin above 100 mg, thromboxane synthesis in platelets is almost totally suppressed. Aspirin mildly prolongs the bleeding time and has an inhibitory effect on thrombin generation,[9,29] which is not seen with ticlopidine.

Aspirin Resistance

Response to aspirin varies in healthy volunteers and patients, who may be hypo- or hyperresponders. Aspirin resistance has been described not only in single patients but also under certain clinical conditions. Authorities debate whether higher doses of ASA are needed in cerebrovascular disease than in coronary disease and whether some diabetics are more resistant.[4,38] The COX-2 gene is probably expressed in atherosclerotic vessels leading to a hundredfold expression of prostaglandin synthesis in the vessel wall.[44] Under these conditions a retrograde transfer of precursors from the vessel wall to adhering platelets may increase their thromboxane synthesis. This mechanism may explain the generally increased thromboxane synthesis in cardiovascular diseases.[20]

High doses of aspirin (500 mg) inhibit thrombin formation in whole blood.[29] Lower doses (300 mg/day) inhibit thrombin formation in PRP with a marked intraindividual variation.[9] How such mechanisms are correlated with the inhibition of thromboxane synthesis in platelets and to what extent they may explain aspirin resistance in a clinical setting need further evaluation.

Ticlopidine and Clopidogrel

The thienopyridines ticlopidine and clopidogrel are inactive in vitro. Their in vivo inhibiting effect on platelet aggregation is probably due to the formation of an active metabolite in the liver. Both drugs inhibit ADP-induced aggregation. This effect is retarded and reaches its peak after 4–5 days of treatment. It is probably caused by the antagonization of a G-protein receptor for ADP on the platelet membrane. The binding of fibrinogen to the GP IIb/IIIa complex triggered by ADP is dramatically inhibited. This inhibition is not due to direct modification of the glycoprotein complex. Clopidogrel is about 6 times as active as ticlopidine in inhibiting ADP-induced platelet aggregation in humans. Both ticlopidine and clopidogrel mildly prolong the bleeding time. Aspirin and ticlopidine inhibit only amplification pathways of platelet activation.

Both aspirin and ticlopidine have a long-lasting effect because they irreversibly inhibit circulating platelets in contrast to dipyridamole and prostacyclin and its analogs. As new platelets enter the circulation, platelet inhibition is gradually reduced. The risk of bleeding is reduced about 3 or 4 days after the last intake. The maximal aggregation-inhibiting effect of the standard dose of ticlopidine (250 mg/twice daily) is reached after 5 days of oral administration. The sensitivity to aspirin and ticlopidine has a marked individual variation in terms of the time required to inhibit aggregation and intensity of inhibition as well as effects on platelet activation and bleeding time.

Combination of Aspirin and Ticlopidine

Recently many cardiologists have advocated the combined use of aspirin and ticlopidine in patients receiving Palmaz-Schatz stents. In an early interaction study[56] in healthy volunteers, ticlopidine potentiated the effect of aspirin on collagen-induced aggregation and led to an additive prolongation of bleeding time. This finding was recently confirmed.[15]

Dipyridamole

Dipyridamole stimulates platelet membrane adenylate-cyclase. It inhibits phosphodi-esterase, thus preventing the degradation of cyclic adenosine monophosphate (cAMP) to adenosine monophosphate. In addition, it decreases adenosine uptake and degradation and increases plasma levels of adenosine.[7] The platelet-inhibiting effects of dipyridamole are relatively shortlasting. After single oral doses of 75 mg the antiaggregating effect lasts for about 3 hours. The short duration of platelet inhibition may be mainly responsible for the lack of increased bleeding in patients receiving dipyridamole during CPB. Whether treatment before cardiac surgery with a newly developed, long-acting dipyridamole preparation is similarly well tolerated remains to be established.

Prostacyclin and Other Prostaglandins

Prostacyclin and its analogs increase the intracellular level of cAMP probably by platelet receptor-mediated activation of adenyl cyclase. In vascular smooth muscles this process leads to vasodilation. At higher doses in vitro and in animal models, iloprost dramatically decreases platelet response to all antagonists. However, such effects have not been measured ex vivo with the agents and doses currently in clinical use. It is likely that the blood levels necessary for marked impairment of platelet function are not reached with the clinically used doses of prostaglandins. After intravenous infusion of these drugs is discontinued, blood levels decrease within minutes, and no platelet-inhibiting effect is present.

Platelet Membrane Glycoprotein Inhibitors

Platelet membrane GPIIb/IIIa inhibitors, such as Abciximab, Tirofiban, Integrelin, and MK 852, block platelet fibrinogen receptors and have much stronger effects than aspirin and ticlopidine. After intravenous infusion of the presently available drugs is discontinued, however, platelet function partially normalizes within a relatively short time (1 or 2 days). Available data are limited.

The heterodimer GP IIb/IIIa complex is a member of the integrin family of receptors, which mediates platelet aggregation and adhesion to collagen. Expression of the GP IIb/IIIa complex and its binding to fibrinogen is the final common pathway for all platelet agonists. The amino acid sequence Arg-Gly-Asp (RGD) or RGDS of fibrinogen, VWF, and fibronectin bind to the activated GP IIb/IIIa receptor. The first drug to be effectively used in clinical trials was the chimeric monoclonal 7E3 Fab (Abciximab), which was created via genetic recombination. This new hybrid molecule consists of mouse-derived variable antibody regions linked to the constant region derived from human immunoglobulin. Abciximab has been successfully used in large trials in high-risk patients undergoing percutaneous transluminal coronary angioplasty (EPIC, EPILOG) and in patients with unstable angina (CAPTURE). The EPIC trial, however, reported a 2–3-fold increase in intraprocedural bleeding complications in treated patients than in patients receiving placebo.[2] The reduction of heparin apparently reduced excessive bleeding in the EPILOG and CAPTURE trials.

In addition to different snake venom polypeptides that prevent binding of adhesive protein to GP IIb/IIIa, a series of highly potent synthetic peptides containing RGD (e.g., Integrelin[57]) or similar sequences has been developed, along with nonpeptide inhibitors of GP IIb/IIIa.[61] If the receptor inhibition exceeds 80%, these agents also inhibit platelet-induced thrombin formation and platelet adhesion.

BLEEDING RISK WITH ANTIPLATELET AGENTS

Aspirin in Cardiac Surgery

Approximately 5% of patients undergoing coronary artery bypass grafting (CABG) are believed to require reoperation to control hemorrhage or to relieve pericardial tamponade caused by hemorrhage. Many patients with ischemic heart disease who wait for cardiac surgery take aspirin.

Bashein et al. carried out a case-control study of patients who underwent CABG-only operations. Ninety analyzable cases with reoperation for bleeding before discharge were matched with 180 controls. The proportions of patients who received aspirin within 7 days before surgery were 34.4% (reoperative patients) and 22.2% (controls) with an estimated odds ratio for reoperation after aspirin ingestion of 1.82 (95% confidence interval: 1.23–3.32). The differences in preoperative template (simplate) bleeding time were statistically significant but said to be clinically unimportant in reoperative patients and controls (5.5 ± 2.2 vs. 4.9 ± 1.1, mean ± SD, respectively).[6]

The assessment of the extent of post-CPB bleeding shows wide variations. Judgment of the effects of aspirin is no exception. In multicenter studies the involvement of several surgeons and different CPB techniques is probably responsible for variation in bleeding volumes. Many authors strongly advise against the preoperative use of aspirin, especially because early postoperative administration seems to provide the same protective effect for CABG patency,[22,25,47,52] whereas others[40,42] claim that the increase in bleeding risk related to aspirin is marginal and clinically irrelevant. However, in one of the studies patients had taken aspirin for only two days before cardiac surgery.

Most but not all studies suggest that patients taking aspirin before CPB have excessive and prolonged mediastinal bleeding and are at higher risk for reoperations.[43,53] Increased bleeding complications were reported with preoperative aspirin treatment compared with aspirin started 6 hours postoperatively.[29] Patients received 325 mg aspirin or placebo on the night before surgery. After surgery all patients received 325 mg/day of aspirin, with the first dose administered through a nasogastric tube 6 hours postoperatively. The reoperation rate for bleeding was 6.3% in the group receiving preoperative aspirin compared with 2.4% in the placebo group. More transfusions were also required (median = 900 vs. 725 ml). Median chest-tube drainage within the first 6 hours was slightly increased (500 vs. 448 ml).

Menys et al. reported that ASA reduces macroaggregation and collagen-induced microaggregation in patients undergoing CPB.[37] This effect was suggested by the results of an earlier trial, conducted by the same investigators, in which preoperative aspirin was compared with placebo throughout the study period. Patients receiving aspirin showed an increase in mediastinal bleeding, transfusions, and reoperation rate (4–9%).

The clinical trials devoted to the effects of aspirin on CABG provide an objective assessment of aspirin-related bleeding risk but only under the particular circumstances of each study and with postoperative continuation of aspirin. They are not relevant to the management of the relatively large number of patients who receive only preoperative aspirin. Taggart et al. studied 202 patients, of whom 102 received preoperative aspirin (44 at 75 mg/day, 28 at 150 mg/day and 29 at 300 mg/ day). The mean blood loss in the aspirin-treated patients was significantly higher than in the controls. Aspirin treatment did not prolong the postoperative hospital stay.[53]

Torosian et al.[58] studied 100 consecutive patients operated by the same surgeon. The only surgical procedure was CABG, and the surgical technique remained constant throughout the 5-month study period. Thirteen patients received preoperative aspirin, with administration terminated 2–7 days before surgery. For the second to fourth hours, hourly chest-tube drainage was significantly increased in these patients compared with 64 patients who received no treatment impairing hemostasis (< 100 ml/hr). Mean mediastinal loss was about 900 ml vs. about 400 ml, and mean chest tube duration was 35 ± 6 vs. 20 ± 1 hours (mean ± SEM) in the aspirin-treated group and control group, respectively. Only 3 patients, including one who received aspirin, returned to the operating room for reexploration related to excessive postoperative bleeding. Each had a surgically correctable lesion.

Ferraris et al. carried out a small nonblinded study of 34 patients scheduled for urgent or elective CABG. Patients were randomized to receive either 1 aspirin tablet (325 mg) or no aspirin the day before operation.[19] Sixteen aspirin-treated patients were compared with 18 controls. Aspirin-treated patients showed an increase in chest-tube drainage 12 hours after surgery (1513 ± 977 vs. 916 ± 482 ml, respectively) and a statistically significant increase in transfusion requirements (packed red blood cells, platelets, fresh-frozen plasma). Six patients in the aspirin-treated group had postoperative bleeding that required intervention in the form of hemostatic drugs such as 1-deamino-8-D-arginine vasopressin (DDAVP), epsilon-amino-caproic acid (EACA), or reoperation (2 patients). A subset of patients seemed to be highly sensitive to aspirin.

In some studies,[35,53,64] preoperative anticoagulant therapy was compared with preoperative treatment with aspirin and dipyridamole. The rate of perioperative complications was higher in the anticoagulant group. Bleeding complications did not differ significantly between the groups. The authors conclude that there is no advantage to preoperative oral anticoagulation.

The overall evidence is quite conclusive: bleeding risk is increased by preoperative administration of aspirin. Therefore, most authors recommend that preoperative aspirin should be avoided whenever possible. Although fewer data are available, the same holds true for ticlopidine. In addition, the Third North American Consensus Conference stated that aspirin started 6 hours after CABG at 325 mg/day is safer than aspirin of the same dose started before operation and results in a similar rate of occlusion. If postoperative bleeding prevents the administration of aspirin at 6 hours after surgery, initiation of therapy as soon as possible thereafter is advised.

What is the appropriate treatment of patients with inadvertent aspirin use for whom surgery cannot be deferred? Patients vary in their response to aspirin in terms of bleeding time and to ticlopidine in terms of bleeding time and platelet aggregation. If one also takes into account the at least rough relationship between prolongation of bleeding time and type and degree of inherited platelet or VWF defect, bleeding time may help to identify patients on antiplatelet therapy who are at highest risk of bleeding.

However, the clinical value of the bleeding time is as controversial as the methods of measurement, although the Ivy technique with a horizontal incision is by far the most studied. Moreover, despite progress in standardization with availability of automatic devices, the observer's skill remains of crucial importance. The predictive value of bleeding time for surgical bleeding risk is not yet established, and even with the new GPIIb/IIIa inhibitor Abciximab no predictive value of the bleeding time and bleeding episodes can be shown. However, other factors that are correctable should be considered, including surgical technique. The quality of intraoperative hemostasis, hematocrit (threshold for prolongation of the bleeding time due to low hematocrit is about 30%!), and use of other drugs, such as nitrates or betalactam antibiotics, that impair hemostasis are important. If, despite these precautionary measures, serious bleeding occurs intraoperatively, platelet transfusions should be quickly effective.

Ticlopidine in Cardiac Surgery

A few small prospective studies were designed to improve CABG patency with preoperative treatment with ticlopidine. Ticlopidine was administered 3–5 days before surgery. It is likely that the maximal antiplatelet effect was not yet reached at the time of operation. A trend for increased bleeding was noticed, but the rate of reoperation was not significantly higher. No increase in bleeding risk was reported, but graft patency was significantly increased.[32] The authors conclude that postoperative ticlopidine may be a safe alternative for aspirin in allergic patients, at least in terms of perioperative bleeding.

Combined Use of Aspirin and Ticlopidine in Stenting

Recent reports by cardiologists[5,13,21,46] have led to a wide acceptance of the combination of ASA and ticlopidine in patients receiving coronary stents. These studies indicate that the combined use of ticlopidine and aspirin after stenting reduces the bleeding incidence in comparison with use of vitamin K antagonists and that the reocclution rate after stenting is markedly less than that seen with oral anticoagulation. Thebauldt et al.[56] reported in 1977 that aspirin does not increase the effect of ticlopidine on ADP-induced aggregation, although ticlopidine increases the effect of aspirin on collagen-induced aggregation. Aspirin and ticlopidine prolonged the bleeding time slightly in comparison with aspirin alone. The combination of high-dose aspirin with ticlopidine led to a marked prolongation of the bleeding time in all volunteers except one. It is not yet clear whether the combined use of aspirin and ticlopidine improves the patency rate after coronary stenting or whether the changes in technology and stent material are responsible for these effects. Beyond doubt, however, patients taking both drugs will come to emergency CABG more frequently in the future because combined use is increasing. In a small study, Hall et al. observed no difference in rates of rethrombosis and patency between stented patients taking aspirin and stented patients taking ticlopidine plus aspirin.[26]

Prostacyclin and Iloprost

A double-blind study compared 25 patients receiving iloprost (TK 36374) and 25 patients without iloprost, all of whom underwent coronary surgery.[49] The results showed preservation of platelets and fewer platelets sequestered in the extracorporeal circuit in the iloprost-treated group. There was no difference in postbypass bleeding, but significant hypotension was reported in patients receiving iloprost.[49]

A chemically synthetized prostacyclin, known as epoprostenol, has been studied in 4 controlled trials with doses up to 15 ng/kg/min. With a higher dose some platelet preservation was reported as well as a trend toward decreased blood loss and blood transfusion. These results illustrate the paradox that preservation of platelets from consumption and from alterations due to CPB by intraoperative administration of an antiplatelet agent may in fact improve postoperative hemostasis.

Iloprost, a chemically stable analog of prostacyclin, was infused into 11 patients with heparin-induced thrombocytopenia and thrombosis who required cardiac or vascular surgery and thus were reexposed to unfractionated heparin. The maximal dose for each patient, which varied from 10–48 ng/kg/min, was reportedly sufficient to prevent further platelet activation in vivo in the presence of heparin. No perioperative complications occured. Iloprost was also studied by Massonet et al. in a double-blind, randomized, placebo-controlled pilot study involving 30 patients undergoing CABG with a mean CPB duration of 90 minutes.[36] Iloprost was infused in incremental doses up to 12 ng/kg/min. The infusion was begun before CPB and stopped at the time of protamine injection. No significant difference in postbypass bleeding was observed between the iloprost-treated and placebo groups. Iloprost appeared to preserve platelet function. Two patients in the iloprost group experienced severe hypotension, and the infusion had to be stopped prematurely. Some data suggest that both prostacyclin and iloprost can potentiate the effects of unfractionated heparin on coagulation tests.

GP-IIb/IIIa Inhibitors

A higher bleeding tendency must be expected if emergency operations are performed during or shortly after stopping the infusion of the GPIIb/IIIa inhibitor, Fabiximab.

Use of Desmopressin in Patients Taking Aspirin during CPB

Among the treatments for bleeding in patients undergoing CPB, especially those on aspirin, DDAVP and aprotinin have been proposed in addition to platelet transfusion. Desmopressin acetate increases the plasma levels of VWF in most patients, and aprotinin, a strong plasmin inhibitor, inhibits fibrinolysis. Several randomized, double-blind studies have shown no benefit, in general, from desmopressin infusions in patients undergoing

CPB.[31,43,49] However, most investigators found that desmopressin had favorable effects on the bleeding tendency of patients who were taking aspirin during CPB,[17,25,28,48] despite a few studies[30,45] that demonstrated no benefit. In a metaanalysis of 17 double-blind, placebo-controlled studies of the effect of desmopressin on reducing blood loss in cardiac surgery, Cattaneo et al.[11] concluded that desmopressin significantly reduced postoperative blood loss by 9% but had no statistically significant effect on transfusion requirements. Two studies in the metaanalysis demonstrated a beneficial effect of desmopressin on reducing either excessive blood loss[25] or postoperative blood transfusion[17] in patients on aspirin therapy.

The studies published so far make clear that routine administration of desmopressin to aspirin-taking patients undergoing CPB is not to be recommended. However, aspirin-treated patients who bleed excessively after operation may benefit from desmopressin infusions.

HEPARIN-INDUCED THROMBOCYTOPENIA AND ANTIPLATELET THERAPY

Walks et al. reviewed data from 3438 patients, of whom 46 had heparin-dependent antiplatelet antibodies.[62] Five patients known to have the antibodies before open heart surgery were pretreated with platelet-inhibiting drugs before reexposure to heparin. No thromboembolic events occured in this group. In 41 patients antibodies were diagnosed after surgery. Bleeding complications occurred in 21 and thromboembolic complications in 13 patients. The hospital mortality rate was 37%. Successful treatment with aspirin and dipyridamole before heparin reexposure in patients with HIT was also described.[34]

Addonizio et al. reported successful treatment of three patients with HIT by continuous intravenous infusion of iloprost until protamine neutralization of heparin during CPB.[1] Similar results were obtained by Corbeau et al.[14]

In the above studies the diagnosis of HIT was based mainly on the presence of positive in vitro antibody or aggregation tests. Later findings have led to strong doubts about the specificity for HIT of all presently available tests. Many patients taking heparin apparently develop antibodies against heparin without developing the clinical syndrome of HITT II. The diagnosis of HITT II, therefore, is still based only on clinical symptoms (thrombocytopenia and thrombotic complications with heparin). Hopefully more specific tests will soon be available.

REFERENCES

1. Addonizio VP, Fisher CA, Kappa JR, Ellison N: Prevention of heparin induced thrombocytopenia during open heart surgery with iloprost (ZK36374). Surgery 102:796–807, 1987.
2. Aguirre FV, Topol EJ, Ferguson JJ, et al: Bleeding complications with the chimeric antibody to platelet glycoprotein IIb/IIIa integrin in patients undergoing percutaneous coronary intervention. Circulation 91:2882–2890, 1995.
3. Bang CJ, Talstad BR, Berstad A: Interaction between heparin and acetylsalicylic acid on gastric mucosal and skin bleeding in humans. Scand J Gastroenterol 27:489–492, 1992.
4. Barnett HJM, Kaste M, Meldrum H, Eliasziw M: Aspirin dose in stroke prevention. Beautiful hypotheses slain by ugly facts. Stroke 27:588–592, 1996.
5. Barragan P, Sainsous J, Silvestri M, et al: Ticlopidine and subcutaneous heparin as an alternative regimen following coronary stenting. Cathet Cardiovasc Diagn 32:133–138, 1994.
6. Bashein G, Nessly ML, Rice AL, et al: Preoperative aspirin therapy and reoperation for bleeding after coronary artery bypass surgery. Arch Intern Med 151:89–93, 1991.
7. Best LC, McGuire MB, Jones PBB, et al: Mode of action of dipyridamole on human platelets. Thromb Res 16:367–379, 1979.
8. Boldt J, Schindler E, Welters I, et al: The effect of the anticoagulation regimen on endothelial related coagulation in cardiac surgery patients. Anaesthesia 50:954–960, 1995.
9. Breddin HK, Lindemann R: Aspirin inhibits Platelet induced thrombin generation [in preparation].
10. Brown MR, Swygert TH, Whitten CW, Hebeler R: Desmopressin acetate following cardiopulmonary bypass: Evaluation of coagulation parameters. J Cardiothorac Anesth 3:762–729, 1989.
11. Cattaneo M, Harris AS, Stromberg U, Mannucci PM: Effects of desmopressin on reducing blood loss in cardiac surgery—a metaanalysis of double blind, placebo controlled trials. Thromb Haemost 74:1064–1070, 1995.
12. Clemetson KJ: Platelet activation: Signal transduction via membrane receptors. Thromb Haemost 74:111–116, 1995.

13. Colombo A, Hall P, Nakamura S, et al: Intracoronary stenting without anticoagulation accomplished with intravascular ultrasound guidance. Circulation 91:1677–1688, 1995.
14. Corbeau JJ, Jacob JP, Moreau X, et al: Iloprost (Ilomedine registered) et circulation extracorporelle avec heparinisation conventionelle chez un patient ayant une thrombopenie a l'heparine. Ann Fr Anesth Reanim 12:55–59, 1993.
15. De Caterina R, Sicari R, Bernini W, et al: Benefit/risk profile of combined antiplatelet therapy with ticlopidine and aspirin. Thromb Haemost 65:504–510, 1991.
16. De-Caterina R, Lanza M, Manca G, et al: Bleeding time and bleeding: An analysis of the relationship of the bleeding time with parameters of surgical bleeding. Blood 84:3363–3370, 1994.
17. Dilthey G, Dietrich W, Spannagl M, Richter J.A: Influence of desmopressin acetate on homologous blood requirements in cardiac surgical patients pretreated with aspirin. J Cardiothoracic Vasc Anesth 7:425–430, 1993.
18. Dorman BH, Spinale FG, Baily MK, et al: Identification of patients at risk for excessive blood loss during coronary artery bypass surgery: Thrombelastograph versus coagulation screen. Anesth Analg 76:694–700, 1993.
19. Ferraris VA, Ferraris SP, Lough FC, Berry WR: Preoperative aspirin ingestion increases operative blood loss after coronary artery bypass grafting. Ann Thorac Surg 59:1036–1037, 1995.
20. FitzGerald GA, Healy C, Daugherty J: Thromboxane A_2 biosynthesis in human disease. Fed Proc 46:154–158, 1987.
21. Garcia-Cantu E, Spaulding C, Corcos T, et al: Stent implantation in acute myocardial infarction. Am J Cardiol 77:454–454, 1996.
22. Gavaghan TP, Gebski V, Baron DW: Immediate postoperative aspirin improves vein graft patency early and late after coronary artery bypüass graft surgery. A placebo-controlled, randomized study. Circulation 83:1526–1533, 1991.
23. George JN, Pickett EB, Saucerman S: Platelet surface glycoproteins. Studies on resting and activated platelets and platelet membrane microparticles in normal subjects, and observations in patients during adult resiratory distress syndrome and cardiac surgery. J Clin Invest 78:340–348, 1986.
24. Goldman S, Copeland J, Moritz T, et al: Starting aspirin therapy after operation: Effects on early graft patency. Circulation 84:520–526, 1991.
25. Gratz, I, Koehler J, Olsen D, et al: The effect of desmopressin acetate on postoperative hemorrhage in patients receiving aspirin therapy before coronary artery bypass operations. J Thorac Cardiovasc Surg 104:1417–1422, 1992.
26. Hall P, Nakamura S, Maiello L, et al: A randomized comparison of combined ticlopidine and aspirin therapy versus aspirin therapy alone after successful intravascular ultrasound guided stent implantation. Circulation 93:215–222, 1996.
27. Irani MS, Izzat NN, Jones JW: Platelet function, coagulation tests and cardiopulmonary bypass: Lack of correlation between preoperative and intraoperative whole blood lumiaggregometry and perioperative blood loss in patients receiving autologous platelet rich plasma. Blood Coag Fibrinol 6:428–432,1995.
28. Kam PCA: Use of desmopressin in controlling aspirin induced coagulopathy after cardiac surgery. Heart Lung J Crit Care 23:333–336, 1994.
29. Kessels H, Beguin S, Nandree H, Hemker HC: Measurement of thrombin generation in whole blood—the effect of heparin and aspirin. Thromb Haemost 72:78–83,1994.
30. Lazenby WD, Russo I, Zadeh BJ, et al: Treatment with desmopressin acetate in routine coronary artery bypass surgery to improve postoperative haemostasis. Circulation 82:IV-413–IV-419, 1990.
31. Hackmann T, Gascoyne RD, Naiman SC, et al: A Trial of desmopressin (1-desamino-8-arginine vasopressin) to reduce blood loss in uncomplicated cardiac surgery. N Engl J Med 321:1437–1443, 1989.
32. Limet R, David JI, Magotteaux P, et al: Prevention of aortocoronary bypass graft occlusions. Beneficial effect of ticlopidine on early and late patency rates of venous coronary bypass grafts. A double blind study. J Thorac Cardiovasc Surg. 94:773–783, 1987.
33. Loll PJ, Picot D, Garavito M: The structural basis of aspirin activity inferred from the crystal structure of inactivated prostaglandin H2 synthase. Nature Struct Biol 2:637–643, 1995.
34. Makhoul RG, McCann RL, Austin EH: Management of patients with heparin-associated thrombocytopenia and thrombosis requiring cardiac surgery. Ann Thorac Surg 43:617–621, 1987.
35. Malouf JF, Alam S, Gharzeddine W, Stefadouros MA: The role of anticoagulation in the development of pericardial effusion and late tamponade after cardiac surgery. Eur Heart J 14:1451–1457, 1993.
36. Massonet-Castel S, Farge D, Tournay D: Utilisation d'une prostacycline de synthese en circulation extracorporelle. Presse Med 21:113–118, 1992.
37. Menys VC, Belcher PR, Noble MIM, et al: Macroaggregation of platelets in plasma, as distinct from microaggregation in whole blood (and plasma), as determined using optical aggregometry and platelet counting, respectively, is specifically impaired following cardiopulmonary bypass in man. Thromb Haemost 72:511–518, 1994.
38. Mori TA, Vandongen T, Douglas AJ, Mcculloch RK, Burke V: Differential effect of aspirin on platelet aggregation in IDDM. Diabetes 41:261–266, 1992.

39. Otto JC, Smith WL: Prostaglandin endoperoxide synthases 1 and 2. J Lipid Med 12:139–156, 1995.
40. Rajah SM, Salter MCP, Donaldson DR, et al: Acetylsalicylic acid and dipyridamoile improve the early patency of aorta-coronary bypass grafts. J Thorac Cardiovasc Surg 90:373–377, 1985.
41. Ratnatunga CP, Rees GM, Kovacs IB: Preoperative hemostatic activity and excessive bleeding after cardiopulmonary bypass. Ann Thorac Surg 52:250–257, 1991.
42. Rawitscher RE, Jones JW, McCoy TA, Lindsley DA: A prospective study on aspirin's effect on red blood cell loss in cardiac surgery. J Cardiovasc Surg 32:1–7,1991.
43. Reich DL, Patel GC, Vela Cantos F, et al: Aspirin does not increase homologous blood requirements in elective coronary bypass surgery. Anesth Analg 78:4–8, 1994.
44. Rimarachin JA, Jacobson JA, Szabo P, et al: Regulation of cyclooxygenase-2 expression in aortic smooth muscle cells. Arterioscler Thromb 46:154–158, 1994.
45. Salmenpera M, Kuitunen A, Hynynen M, Heinonen J: Hemodynamic responses to desmopressin acetate after CABG: A double blind trial. J Cardiothoracic Vasc Anesth 5:146–149, 1991.
46. Serruys PW, Emanuelsson H, van der Giessen W, et al: Heparin coated Palmaz-Schatz stents in human coronary arteries: Early outcome of the Benestent II pilot study. Circulation 93:412–422, 1996.
47. Sethi GK, Copeland JG, Goldman S, et al: Implications of preoperative administration of aspirin in patients undergoing coronary bypass grafting. J Am Coll Cardiol 15:15–20, 1990.
48. Sheridan DP, Card RT, Pinilla JC, et al: Use of desmopressin acetate to reduce blood transfusion requirements during cardiac surgery in patients with acetylsalicylic-acid induced platelet dysfunction. Can J Surg 37:33–36, 1994.
49. Spyt TJ, Wheatley DJ, Walker ID, et al: Placebo-controlled study of Iloprost (ZK 36374) in cardiopulmonary bypass surgery. Perfusion 3:179–186, 1988.
50. Spyt TJ, Weerasena NA, Bain WH, Lowe GDO: The effects of desmopressin acetate (DDAVP) on haemostasis and blood loss in routine coronary artery bypass surgery: A randomized double blind trial. Perfusion 5(Suppl):57–61, 1990.
51. Stern MP, DeVos-Doyle K, Viguera MG, Lajos TZ: Evaluation of post cardiopulmonary bypass Sonoclot signatures in patients taking nonsteroidal anti-inflammatory drugs. J Cardiothoracic Anesth 3:730–733, 1989.
52. Tabuchi N,Tigchelaar I, Van Oeveen W: Shear-induced pathway of platelet function in cardiac surgery. Semin Thromb Hemost 21(Suppl 2):66–70, 1995.
53. Taggart DP, Siddiqwi A, Wheatly DJ: Low dose preoperative aspirin therapy, postoperative blood loss, and transfusion requirements. Ann Thorac Surg 50:425–428, 1990.
54. Teoh KH, Christakis GT, WeiselL RD, et al: Dipyridamole preserved platelets and reduced blood loss after cardiopulmonary bypass. J Thorac Cardiovasc Surg 96:332–341, 1988.
55. Teoh KH, Christakis, Weisel RD: Blood conservation with membrane axygenators and dipyridamole. Ann Thorac Surg 44:40–47, 1987.
56. Thebault, JJ, Blatrix CE, Blanchard JF, Panak EA: The interactions of ticlopidine and aspirin in normal subjects. J Int Med Res 5:405–411, 1977.
57. Tcheng JE, Harrington RA, Kottke-Marchant K, et al: Multicenter, randomized, double blind, placebo-controlled trial of the platelet integrin glycoprotein IIb/IIIa blocker Integrelin in elective coronary intervention. Circulation 91:2151–2157, 1995.
58. Torosian M, Michelson EL, Morganroth J, MacVaugh H: Aspirin and coumadin related bleeding after coronary bypass graft surgery. Ann Intern Med 89:325–328, 1978.
59. Uthoff K, Zehr KJ, Geerling R, et al: Inhibition of platelet adhesion during cardiopulmonary bypass reduces postoperative bleeding. Circulation 90(Suppl II):II269–II274, 1994.
60. Utley JR: Pathophysiology of cardiopulmonary bypass: Current issues. J Card Surg 5:177–189, 1990.
61. Verstraete M, Zoldhelyi P: Novel antithrombotic drugs in development. Drugs 49:856–884, 1995.
62. Walks JT, Curtis JJ, Silver D, Boley TM: Heparin-induced thrombocytopenia in patients who undergo open heart surgery. Surgery 108:686–693, 1990.
63. Woodmann RC, Harker CA: Bleeding complications associated with cardiopulmonary bypass. Blood 76:1680–1697, 1990.
64. Yli-Mayry S, Huikuri HV, Korlonen UR, et al: Efficacy and safety of anticoagulant therapy started preoperatively in preventing coronary vein graft occlusion. Eur Heart J 13:1259–1264, 1992.

CHAPTER 29

Hemostatic Restoration during Cardiopulmonary Bypass

FRIEDRICH SCHUMANN, Ph.D.

If blood is considered an organ, the response of this organ to the stress introduced by cardiopulmonary bypass (CPB) with extracorporeal circulation has little to do with physiologic hemostasis as a response to isolated vessel or tissue trauma. Evolution has not had enough time to equip modern humans with the biologic mechanisms that could counteract the complications associated with high-tech medicine and intensive care. The pattern by which the body reacts to major trauma and aggressive surgery still follows the atavistic principle of seeking rescue in fight or flight or being sacrificed with no opportunity to propagate the genome.

Strange and complex mechanisms affect patients undergoing open heart surgery and their blood organ, the biologic sense of which is hard to understand. First are the still incompletely elucidated consequences of foreign surface contact of circulating blood with the oygenator, tubes, and filters of the heart-lung machine, resulting in a so-called "total body inflammatory response." Second is an acquired platelet function defect that leads to prolonged oozing and leakage at the capillary level. Third is the so-called postoperative fibrinolytic shut-down phenomenon, which exposes the patient to an increased risk of thrombosis when the level of plasminogen-activator inhibitor (PAI-1) starts to rise.[78, 83]

Physiologic hemostasis probably does not require the intrinsic pathway of coagulation, starting with factor XII, because the activation process is dominated by the extrinsic pathway, which starts with the release of tissue factor and activation of factor VII. However, in extracorporeal circulation, in which all circulating blood comes into rapid and extensive contact with nonendothelial surfaces, the situation is different, and the intrinsic pathway of blood coagulation no longer plays an insignificant role. The quality of anticoagulation in patients undergoing heart surgery is assessed by measuring the prolonged response time of heparinized blood to the procoagulatory stimulus of an active surface material such as celite or kaolin, which is the conventional method of determining the activated clotting time (ACT). This assessment demonstrates the pathophysiologic relevance of foreign surface contact. Otherwise the conventional ACT would not be the right instrument.

This chapter does not aim to plunge into the depths of the biochemical mechanisms caused by contact phase activation or to discuss the relative contribution of both enzymes, plasmin and thrombin, to the evolving platelet function defect during extracorporeal circulation. Moreover, the pros and cons of the classic heparin anticoagulation regimen in comparison with new, alternative anticoagulants and antithrombotic agents are extensively discussed elsewhere in this book. Rather, this chapter concentrates on one of the main aspects of heart surgery during and early after the operation. The patients bleed, and they bleed to an extent that still requires donor blood transfusion in about 50% of all patients,[81] independent of the hemorrhagic risk category and the general acceptance of low intra- and postoperative hemoglobin levels. In recent years there has been much discussion of the optimization of transfusion strategies and adequate "transfusion trigger" as well as of the desirability and feasibility of autologous blood transfusion. Yet the most effective correction of blood loss would be to avoid it from the beginning rather than to replace lost volume and red cells by one or the other sophisticated technique.

This chapter is restricted to restoration of adequate hemostasis by prophylactic pharmacologic intervention and does not deal with nonpharmacologic means of blood saving. Because of the widespread consensus that desmopressin, dipyridamole, prostacyclin, and other earlier drugs did not fulfill their promises,[32] the following overview is further limited to aprotinin and the lysine analog, tranexamic acid. Much of the information about tranexamic acid also may be valid for epsilon-aminocaproic acid (EACA), although in most countries EACA has become obsolete and been replaced by tranexamic acid. Among the newer, still experimental drugs, nafamstat mesilate[90] has undergone limited clinical investigation in open heart surgery[88,114]; however, the quality of this investigation and the resulting information are not comparable with those available for aprotinin or tranexamic acid and do not justify a similar discussion. Nafamstat mesilate may become the subject of future review articles, when its development has made further progress.

Many articles address the detrimental changes imposed on the blood by CPB with extracorporeal circulation, related to its functional capacity to maintain fluidity for oxygen and nutrient transport and to repair vascular leaks with a seal of fibrin and platelets.[5,29,43,73,123] Open heart surgery is not possible without heparin or an alternative anticoagulant of at least comparable efficacy and safety. The search for a nonthrombogenic artificial surface has not brought the ultimate solution, despite much improvement in biocompatibility. As Edmunds observed, "The endothelial cell is the only known non-thrombogenic surface; no other cell or surface is non-thrombogenic."[29] Hence the need for anticoagulation. Long-term results with heparin-coated devices in patients subjected to extracorporeal membrane oxygenation[120] are not representative of routine cardiac surgery with median sternotomy and the resulting major bone and tissue trauma. Although one can use a heparinized system, it is preferable to give some systemic heparin, because clotting problems may occur not only in the system but also in the patient.[96] The desired effect of heparin is to reduce the coagulatory function of blood, whereas the undesired effect of heparin and heparin–protamine complex is to increase contact phase and complement activation[29,85]; both effects, however, are pathophysiologic mechanisms that will affect hemostasis as long as heparin cannot be safely replaced by other drugs in the practice of cardiac surgery.

Apart from the negative effects of hemodilution, hypothermia, and heparinization, hemostasis is impaired by two important mechanisms during and early after CPB. Plasmin is generated by plasminogen activators—not only by the endothelium-derived tissue-type plasminogen activator (tPA) but also by plasma-derived urokinase as a direct consequence of contact phase activation via activated Hageman factor and kallikrein.[59,60,110] Studies consistently show an excessive formation of specific fibrin degradation products, D-dimers, which indicate ongoing fibrinolysis during and early after open heart surgery. This excess is the result of plasmin activity in vivo, since administration to the patient of the proteinase inhibitor aprotinin, which is a good plasmin inhibitor in vitro, predictably diminishes the increase in D-dimer levels.[10,27,47,78]

Hyperfibrinolysis was seen as the cause of catastrophic hemorrhage during open heart surgery—a major problem in the early days of extracorporeal circulation when the equipment was more primitive and less biocompatible than today. This rationale was behind the first investigational use of aprotinin as an effective antifibrinolytic agent to combat hyperfibrinolytic hemorrhage in cardiac surgery.[82,115] It is not precisely known why alpha$_2$-antiplasmin, the natural specific serpin that normally keeps plasmin under tight control, does not work efficiently enough in CPB with extracorporeal circulation. Apparently, not only relations of summary concentrations and enzyme kinetics are important, but also the volatility of the enzyme-inhibitor reaction partners in their microenvironments.

Thrombelastography (TEG) has shown a correlation between blood loss and TEG findings indicating a hypocoagulable state.[61] The hypocoagulability observed in TEG is due to the second mechanism responsible for impaired hemostasis in patients undergoing open heart surgery—loss of adhesive platelet function. Platelets assemble on their surface not only most of the coagulation proteins but also the proteins necessary for the generation of plasmin (i.e., plasminogen and plasminogen activators).[93] Whether platelet activation in the setting of CPB starts with trace amounts of plasmin or thrombin via the platelet-specific thrombin receptor may eventually become a minor question. Some evidence, however, suggests that plasmin diminishes the availability of the platelet membrane glycoprotein receptors GPIb and GPIIb/IIIa,[17,40,79,80,122] leaving them less functional for the formation of a hemostatic plug. After the end of extracorporeal circulation platelet counts have usually dropped to a low that cannot be explained by hemodilution alone. A part of the platelet population has responded to the stimuli provided by the surgical wound, foreign surface contact, and changes in shear forces and has disappeared from the circulating blood. The remaining platelet population is less responsive to a stimulus such as collagen.[67,87,99,109] This platelet dysfunction is responsible for the observed oozing and prolongation of skin bleeding time after surgery. The hemostatic problem is aggravated when platelet cyclooxygenase has been inhibited by aspirin pretreatment.

This admittedly rather condensed description of a highly complex pathophysiology highlights the role of two key enzymes: plasmin and kallikrein (Fig. 1). The role of

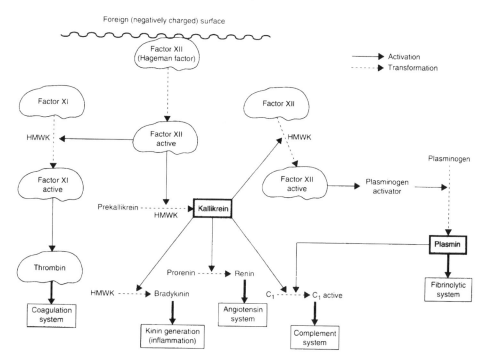

FIGURE 1. The role of kallikrein and plasmin as mediators in the coagulation, fibrinolytic, kinin, complement, and angiotensin systems after activation by foreign surface contact of the blood. (From Davis R, Whittington R: Aprotinin: A review of its pharmacology and therapeutic efficacy in reducing blood loss associated with cardiac surgery. Drugs 49:954–983, 1995, with permission.)

kallikrein gains more weight when more emphasis is placed on the trigger function of contact phase activation and the intrinsic activation pathway of the plasmatic enzyme cascade.[23,24,121] A concept of active pharmacologic intervention to counteract the mainly proteolytic activation mechanisms during CPB has been termed "blood anesthesia" by Edmunds[43]; it is partly met by treatment with the proteinase inhibitor, aprotinin.

APROTININ

Aprotinin, also known as the bovine pancreatic trypsin inhibitor (BPTI), is a member of the Kunitz family of naturally occurring serine proteinase inhibitors. It was independently discovered by Frey, Kraut, and Werle as a kallikrein inhibitor[62] in 1930 and by Kunitz and Northrop as a trypsin inhibitor[64] in 1936. It consists of a single polypeptide chain of 58 amino acids with 3 cystin disulfide bridges that give the molecule an unusual compactness and physical stability. Aqueous solutions of aprotinin are stable at room temperature, without loss of activity, within a broad pH range. As molecular models have demonstrated for the enzyme-inhibitor complex (e.g., aprotinin and porcine pancreatic kallikrein), the reactive inhibitor domain fits almost perfectly into the pocket of the enzyme where the contact region for the normal enzyme substrate is located.[37] The inhibitor acts as a pseudo-substrate that prevents further proteolytic activity while it remains tightly bound to the enzyme. Although in the literature aprotinin has occasionally been referred to as a "polyvalent" proteinase inhibitor, the list of enzymes inhibited at clinically relevant concentrations is limited. It includes trypsin; the kallikreins from organs, tissue, and plasma; and the fibrinolytic enzyme plasmin.

Aprotinin forms 1:1 complexes with the inhibited enzymes. For practical considerations, the equilibrium between the complex and the single reaction partners is shifted almost completely to the side of the complex. This enzyme–inhibitor complex has a short biologic half-life, like most of the complexes between enzymes and their natural inhibitors, the serpins. Although the inhibitory mechanism has correctly been described by biochemists as reversible, for considerations of clinical application it may be more appropriate to speak of "pseudo-irreversible" inhibition, according to Bieth.[9] An objective criterion for the quality of reversible enzyme inhibition by a peptide inhibitor is the Ki value. The lower the Ki value (in M), the more potent the inhibitor for a specific enzyme. For the reaction between plasmin and aprotinin the Ki is about 1×10^{-10}, whereas for human plasma kallikrein the Ki is about 1×10^{-8}. Under clinical conditions aprotinin in the conventional dosage is at first a potent plasmin inhibitor; however, at plasma concentrations that are still efficacious in respect to its antifibrinolytic action, inhibition of plasma kallikrein may become insufficient. It is necessary to recall this different enzyme specificity in discussing the rationale for an "optimal" dosage scheme in the sense of "blood anesthesia."[43]

For historical reasons, quantities and concentrations of aprotinin usually are indicated in kallikrein inactivator units (KIU): 1×10^6 KIU is equivalent to 0.14 gm of aprotinin; 46.5×10^3 KIU are equivalent to 1 μmol; and a solution of 46.5 KIU or 6.5 μg of aprotinin per ml represents a micromolar concentration. Aprotinin has to be administered by intravenous infusion; as a protein, it is not absorbed systemically after oral administration. Therapeutic doses result in plasma concentrations of 1–8 μM. After single dose administration of 1 and 2 million KIU of aprotinin, the maximal plasma concentration (C_{max}) is about 20–30 and 60 mg/L, equivalent to about 140–210 and 430 KIU/ml, respectively.[74,104] Plasma concentrations of aprotinin decrease biphasically, with distribution and elimination half-lives of 0.32–0.50 hours and 5.25–8.28 hours for the two phases, respectively.[56,104]

The clinically relevant half-life (i.e., after the early rapid distribution into the extravascular spaces) rather than the terminal half-life is about 1.5 hours.[56] Amidolytic assays of plasmin and kallikrein activity in nonhuman primate plasma with increasing aprotinin concentrations have shown that 100% plasmin inhibition is achieved with 4 μM of aprotinin, whereas a concentration of about 15 μM results in only about 90% kallikrein inhibition.[30] To sustain effective antiprotease concentrations for more than 2 hours, it would thus appear necessary to administer aprotinin in repeated bolus doses or by constant infusion.

Clinical Efficacy of Aprotinin in Open Heart Surgery

Although earlier clinical reports and even prospective clinical studies had shown a reduction of blood loss by aprotinin during open heart surgery,[2,44,52,82,84,98,115] a new interest in the hemostatic action of aprotinin suddenly arose in 1987 when blood loss and transfusion data were published from clinical trials in which aprotinin had been administered in a novel high-dose scheme. The first trial, conducted by Royston and Bidstrup at Hammersmith Hospital in London, had originally been planned with the objective of studying the effect of aprotinin on complement activation during CPB. The so-called Hammersmith regimen of aprotinin had no effect on the levels of complement factors C3a and C4a, but the mean thoracic drainage volume and the amount of transfused blood was significantly reduced by about 50%.[117] The second trial, performed in 22 patients with either repeat cardiac valve replacement or repeat coronary artery bypass graft (CABG) operations, showed a drastic hemostatic improvement, resulting in a reduction of the mean transfusion requirement from 3.7 units in the control group to 0.5 units in the aprotinin-treated group.[101]

The Hammersmith regimen, consisting of a bolus dose of 2 million KIU given at the start of the operation, followed by a constant infusion of 500,000 KIU/hr until the end of the operation, plus an additional dose of 2 million KIU in the priming solution for the oxygenator of the heart-lung machine, has since been successfully investigated in a series of independent clinical studies, all parallel, randomized, placebo-controlled, and double-blinded, with similar protocols but in various surgical and cardiotechnical environments. The results are summarized in Table 1.

Obviously there are large differences between the placebo groups of the various studies, which may reflect different techniques as well as different patient characteristics. There is no global standard for "normal" blood loss or transfusion patterns in open heart surgery, and many different factors other than those routinely checked and sometimes taken into account by stratification in a randomized clinical trial may influence these variables. This observation constitutes a caveat to data pooling and metaanalyses of efficacy data. On the other hand, it is comforting to see the consistency of the statistically significant and clinically relevant reductions in blood loss or transfusion requirements.

Aprotinin has been shown to be equally effective in primary and repeat open heart surgery. Because of the known increased bleeding tendency in repeat cases, the blood-saving potential of aprotinin is higher in patients with repeat cardiac surgery. Aprotinin has also been studied specifically in patients pretreated with aspirin, which is a well-known risk factor for increased perioperative hemorrhage, and the differences in blood loss and transfusion requirements between placebo and treatment groups were of the same degree as observed in trials with patients not pretreated or weaned from aspirin before surgery.[6,89] In the subset of aspirin-pretreated patients from two major clinical studies with repeat CABG,[16,75] the effect of high-dose aprotinin on the transfusion of blood and blood products was most pronounced (Table 2). High-dose aprotinin diminished the transfusion-associated risk for transmission of infectious diseases—or any other transfusion risk —by > 75%, as the mean number of units of donor blood or blood products transfused in the treatment group was only 23% of the number transfused in the placebo group.

Because the Hammersmith regimen was developed empirically and was not the result of formal dose-finding studies, it frequently has been challenged. Lower-dose regimens have been proposed, and some have been evaluated in controlled clinical trials. Most common are the so-called "half-Hammersmith" and "pump-prime-only" schemes. The first regimen uses a loading dose of 1 million KIU, followed by a constant infusion of

TABLE 1. Summary of Double-blind Trials Comparing Aprotinin Treatment in the Full Hammersmith Regimen with Placebo

Author	Type of Surgery	Percentage of Patients Receiving Donor Blood		Mean Transfusion Requirements (Units)		Mean Total Blood Loss (ml)	
		Aprotinin	Placebo	Aprotinin	Placebo	Aprotinin	Placebo
Bidstrup,[7] 1989	Primary CABG (n = 80)	20	95	0.3	2.0	309	573
Bidstrup,[8] 1993	Primary CABG (n = 96)	20	49	NA		390	620
Bidstrup,[6] 1995	Primary CABG* (n = 60)	23	57	NA		195	504
Murkin,[89] 1994	Primary CABG* or valves (n = 55)	57	87	1.6	4.3	720	1485
Dietrich,[27] 1990	Primary CABG (n = 20)	37	75	1.7	3.2	739	1442
Harder,[45] 1991	Primary CABG (n = 80)	32	57[†]	NA		559	911
Neuhof,[107] 1990 [data on file]	Primary CABG (n = 78)	22	66	1.5	2.4	338	447
Fraedrich,[34] 1989	Primary CABG (n = 80)	42	68	1.8	2.8	652	1204
Fraedrich,[106] 1990 [data on file]	Primary CABG (n = 60)	25	52	NA		536	871
Dementjeva,[20,21] 1995	Primary CABG (n = 100)	22	56[†]	NA		392	690
Swart,[113] 1994	Primary CABG or valves (n = 100)	68	86	1.8	2.8	506	783
Casas,[14] 1995	Primary CABG or valves (n = 99)	26	56	0.7	1.8	195	489
Lemmer,[71] 1994	Primary CABG (n = 151)	38	52	1.1	2.2	855	1503
Lemmer,[71] 1994	Repeat CABG (n = 65)	30	72	0.4	3.3	1255	1979
Cosgrove,[16] 1992	Repeat CABG (n = 115)	46	79	NA		720	1121
Minami,[86] 1993	Repeat CABG (n = 49)	28	52	NA		441	772
Levy,[75] 1995	Repeat CABG (n = 145)	54	75	1.6	3.4	900	1700

NA = not available; CABG = coronary artery bypass graft.
* Exclusively in aspirin-treated patients.
† Postoperative blood transfusion only.

250,000 KIU/hr until the end of surgery, plus an additional dose of 1 million KIU in the oxygenator prime. With the pump-prime-only regimen, the administration of aprotinin is restricted to 2 million KIU given via the extracorporeal circulation at the start of CPB. In a large multicenter study with patients undergoing repeat CABG,[75] the high dose was marginally better than the half dose for all patients; however, it was significantly better for repeat patients pretreated with aspirin (see Table 2). The pump-prime-only dosage was clearly inferior to full and half Hammersmith regimens (Table 3).

TABLE 2. Transfusion Requirements in Aspirin-pretreated Patients Undergoing Repeat CABG: Comparison of Full and Half Hammersmith Regimens of Aprotinin with Placebo*

	Aprotinin High Dose (n = 53)	Aprotinin Half Dose (n = 46)	Placebo (n = 51)	p = High vs. Placebo High vs. Half Dose
Required donor blood (%)	45	54	86	0.000 0.384
Mean units of donor blood	1.3	2.2	3.4	0.004 0.044
Required donor blood or blood products (%)	45	63	90	0.000 0.095
Mean units of donor blood or blood products	2.1	5.2	9.1	0.000 0.010

* Data on file, Bayer AG.

In patients undergoing primary elective CABG, the three dose regimens have also been studied in a parallel, double-blind, placebo-controlled multicenter study. The efficacy data in terms of blood loss and transfusion requirement were almost identical for all three active treatment groups in comparison with the placebo group.[69] Aprotinin significantly reduced the amount of transfused donor blood and blood products by more than 50% (Table 4). This recent study strongly supports the concept that there is room for improvement of hemostasis by pharmacologic means even in primary elective CABG.

The study thus confirmed that in primary CABG a lower dose than the full Hammersmith dosage regimen is effective. In addition, improved hemostasis in the aprotinin-treated groups was reflected not only in diminished transfusion needs but also in a significantly reduced rate of early reoperations due to bleeding. In the combined aprotinin-treated groups, 6 of 526 patients valid for safety (1.1%) underwent reoperation for bleeding, whereas in the placebo group 13 of 178 (7.3%) such patients demonstrated either diffuse bleeding or a surgically correctable source of blood loss and had to be reopened. The probability that a significant difference had occurred by chance was low ($p < 0.0001$) because of the large number of patients in the study. Reducing the incidence of resternotomy for bleeding is of great clinical relevance, because resternotomy has been identified as a marker for increased morbidity and mortality in cardiac surgery.[116]

TABLE 3. Transfusion Requirements in Repeat Coronary Artery Bypass Grafting: Comparison of Full Hammersmith, Half Hammersmith, and Pump-Prime-Only Regimens of Aprotinin with Placebo

	Aprotinin High Dose (n = 61)	Aprotinin Half Dose (n = 59)	Aprotinin Pump Prime Only (n = 68)	Placebo (n = 65)	p = High vs. Placebo Pump Prime Only vs. Placebo
Required donor blood (%)	54	46	72	75	0.007 0.663
Mean units of donor blood	1.6	1.6	2.5	3.4	0.001 0.293
Required donor blood or blood products (%)	54	53	74	85	< 0.001 0.125
Mean units of donor blood or blood products	2.2	3.4	5.1	10.3	< 0.001 0.001

From Levy JH, Pifarre R, Schaff IV, et al: A multicenter, double-blind, placebo-controlled trial of aprotinin for reducing blood loss and the requirement for donor-blood transfusions in patients undergoing repeat coronary artery bypass grafting. Circulation 92:2236–2244, 1995.

TABLE 4.   Transfusion Requirements in Primary Elective Coronary Artery Bypass Grafting: Comparison of Full Hammersmith, Half Hammersmith, and Pump-Prime-Only Regimens of Aprotinin with Placebo

	Aprotinin High Dose (n = 61)	Aprotinin Half Dose (n = 59)	Aprotinin Pump Prime Only (n = 68)	Placebo (n = 65)	p = High vs. Placebo Pump Prime Only vs. Placebo
Required donor blood (%)	33	35	33	52	< 0.05
					< 0.05
Units of donor blood (mean)	0.8	0.9	0.9	1.8	< 0.001
					< 0.001
Required donor blood or blood products (%)	34	37	35	55	< 0.001
					< 0.001
Units of donor blood or blood products (mean)	1.5	1.6	1.7	4.1	0.001
					0.001

From Lemmer JH, Dilling EW, Moton JR, et al: Aprotinin for primary coronary artery bypass surgery: A multicenter, randomized, double-blind, placebo-controlled trial of three dose regimens. Ann Thorac Surg 1996 [in press].

Tolerability and Clinical Safety of Aprotinin

Aprotinin in general has remarkably few side effects and is well tolerated, even in the highest doses applied in cardiovascular surgery.[19,119] For good reasons, the safety assessment of drugs administered to patients undergoing heart surgery or other complex procedures with subsequent intensive care should be based on carefully collected treatment-emergent event data from prospective, randomized, parallel, placebo-controlled trials. The trials should be sufficiently sized so that a reasonable statistical chance is provided for the detection of drug-related adverse events. With a certain level of suspicion, but without a control group that is treated under more or less identical circumstances, a multitude of adverse events that are not uncommon in certain types of patients may be associated erroneously with the drug treatment. Historical control groups are of limited value, because treatment conditions, technical and operational as well as comedication, change over time. In multicenter studies it is necessary to balance the proportion of patients treated with the drug under investigation or with placebo or a reference drug for each participating center at any time during the study. The double-blind requirement is essential, because investigator bias necessarily leads to over- or underreporting of adverse events.

Although these methodical requirements constitute a heavy burden on drug development, demanding also considerable investment of finances and resources, the reward is harvested when the review process by health authorities comes to a positive conclusion about a favorable risk-to-benefit ratio for the drug in its proposed indication. In the United States, aprotinin (Trasylol) has been licensed by the Food and Drug Administration to reduce perioperative blood loss and the need for blood transfusions in repeat and high-risk primary CABG, including primary CABG in patients treated with aspirin.

One study of repeat CABG operations at the Cleveland Clinic[16] found a trend for a higher incidence of myocardial infarction in the aprotinin-treated groups. This finding led to a second study[75] with larger numbers of patients, multicentric design, improved anticoagulation regimen based on a heparin-protamine titration assay rather than on the celite-activated ACT, and standardized evaluation of all relevant data for the diagnosis of myocardial infarction by an outside blinded expert. Table 5 shows the results of this search for signs and symptoms of myocardial infarctions in the second large aprotinin study of repeat CABG operations.

When the same methods for the assessment of perioperative signs of myocardial infarction were applied to patients from an even larger study of primary CABG,[69] a weak trend for a higher incidence compared with placebo was detected, but only in the

TABLE 5. Incidence of Myocardial Infarction in Repeat Coronary Artery Bypass Grafting: Comparison of Full Hammersmith, Half Hammersmith, and Pump-Prime-Only Regimens of Aprotinin with Placebo

	Aprotinin High Dose (n = 68)	Aprotinin Half Dose (n = 68)	Aprotinin Pump Prime Only (n= 70)	Placebo (n = 67
Definite MI by ECG data (%)	12	15	9	12
Definite or probable MI, all data (%)	29	30	24	29
Definite, probable, or possible MI, all data (%)	32	32	24	31
Definitely no MI, all data (%)	68	68	76	69

n = Patients valid for safety.
MI = myocardial infarction, ECG = electrocardiography.
From Levy JH, Pifarre R, Schaff IV, et al: A multicenter, double-blind, placebo-controlled trial of aprotinin for reducing blood loss and the requirement for donor-blood transfusions in patients undergoing repeat coronary artery bypass grafting. Circulation 92:2236–2244, 1995.

treatment group with the lowest dose of aprotinin (2 million KIU pump prime only). This result—at first glance paradoxical—leads to interesting speculation about the importance of the inhibition of plasma kallikrein as well as plasmin, which requires a higher concentration of aprotinin in the blood. Pure antifibrinolytic activity may be not as good as antifibrinolytic activity plus interference with the early intrinsic coagulation pathway by high-dose aprotinin when thrombin is inhibited by heparin. Aprotinin itself is not an anticoagulant; it does not inhibit thrombin. Thus the risk-to-benefit ratio is less favorable for the pump-prime-only regimen than for the full and half Hammersmith regimens.

The question of whether intraoperative aprotinin therapy may affect the rate of early graft occlusion in patients after CABG operations has been addressed in several placebo-controlled, double-blind studies.[8,55,66,71] None of these studies found a significant increase in the rate of early postoperative graft closure. Conflicting reports, such as the recently published restrospective evaluation of an uncontrolled series from one center of a multi-center study with a different study objective,[118] carry little weight in view of the appropriate methodology outlined above.

Aprotinin is stored and metabolized by the proximal tubular cell of the kidney. This physiologic mechanism of mammals recycles small-sized proteins and their amino acids, which pass the glomerular filter into the urine. The renal uptake of aprotinin, which has been investigated in detail,[54] is a typical example of the renal handling of small proteins[4,33] The results of specific measurements of marker proteins for tubular function indicate reversible microproteinuria due to a transient, isolated defect of tubular protein absorption after high-dose aprotinin.[35] The question of whether this finding has any bearing on the clinical status of patients undergoing open heart surgery can now be answered from a sufficiently large number of patients for whom data related to creatinine and adverse renal events have been collected during placebo-controlled, double-bind studies.[72,75] There were no significant differences between the aprotinin-treated groups and the placebo group in the number of patients showing peak increases of postoperative serum creatinine levels ≥ 0.5 mg/dl or > 2.0 mg/dl. A slight increase in serum creatinine levels below a delta of 0.5 mg/dl, however, has been observed and seems to be reproducible. In the large multicenter study of patients undergoing repeat CABG[75] 19 of 215 aprotinin-treated patients (8.8%) and 6 of 72 placebo-treated patients (8.3%) were documented by the attending clinician as suffering from renal failure, acute renal failure, or abnormal renal function in the postoperative period. Limited clinical experience suggests that aprotinin can also be administered to patients with renal failure undergoing open heart surgery.[70,102] In view of these results from well-controlled clinical trials and in high-risk patients, warnings and cautionary comments based solely on laboratory assessment[31] appear to be of limited concern.

Negative experience with aprotinin in an uncontrolled series of patients undergoing reconstruction of the thoracic aorta in total circulatory arrest with deep hypothermia[112] has led to a warning statement in the manufacturer's product brochure. However, this experience has not been confirmed by others, who recently reported positive results with aprotinin in operations on the intrathoracic aorta and concluded that aprotinin may be safely and effectively used in patients undergoing deep hypothermia and circulatory arrest.[41,92]

The safety of aprotinin for use in infants and children has been shown in several placebo-controlled, double-blind studies of pediatric cardiac surgery. However, the pooled database from controlled clinical trials is not as extensive for children as for adults. Moreover, the efficacy of aprotinin in pediatric cardiac surgery has not been shown with the same consistency as in adult cardiac surgery. Of the few prospective, parallel, randomized, placebo-controlled, double-blind studies that have been reported so far, only the studies by Dietrich et al.[26] and Herynkopf et al.[48] have shown a clinically relevant benefit, whereas the study by Boldt et al.[12] failed to show significant differences in blood loss and homologous blood requirement. A recently published prospective, open, randomized study of low-dose aprotinin in only 25 acyanotic children (11 aprotinin, 14 controls)[108] demonstrated no significant benefit from low-dose aprotinin treatment. The problem with any study in infants and children is the large variation in body weight. The larger the variation in body weight, the smaller the chances that the study produces mean values and standard deviations that lead to a statistically significant difference of hemostatic target variables between treatment groups. Adequate doses of aprotinin are important; some evidence supports the concept that small children may need a higher dose per kg body weight than adults to achieve the same effectiveness.[25] The use of aprotinin in pediatric cardiac surgery is still a matter of intense discussion; it appears to have strong-minded proponents.[25,53,95]

As a nonhuman protein, aprotinin may cause anaphylactic reactions in sensitized individuals. Signs and symptoms vary in intensity and duration, ranging from flushing, urticaria, isolated drop in blood pressure, tachycardia or bradycardia, and airway obstruction to severe hypotension and anaphylactic shock that, in rare cases, is fatal. Hypersensitivity reactions are very rare in patients with no prior exposure to aprotinin. The incidence after repeat exposure may reach 5%, as found by retrospective analysis of several small series of patients with documented aprotinin treatment at their first and second operations.[42,105] When the time interval between first and second treatment was more than 3 months, the incidence appeared to decrease.[28] Prophylactic administration of H_1 and H_2 antagonists appeared to reduce substantially the severity and incidence of hypersensitivity reactions.[65]

TRANEXAMIC ACID

Tranexamic acid is *trans*-aminomethylcyclohexanoic acid (AMCHA), a synthetic lysine analog similar to EACA. Both compounds have been known as synthetic antifibrinolytic agents since the fundamental work of Okamoto in the fifties and early sixties.[91] Because the distance between the two functional groups in the AMCHA molecule is fixed by a cyclic structure, the potency of tranexamic acid in comparison with EACA is increased by a factor of 6–10, depending on the test system. In addition, the pharmacokinetic properties of tranexamic acid offer advantages over EACA. Therefore, in most countries EACA preparations have been replaced by AMCHA preparations.Good review articles about the clinical pharmacology and clinical application of theses substances are available.[3,119]

The mechanism of action of tranexamic acid is different from that of aprotinin. The lysine analogs do not inactivate the enzyme plasmin in a direct manner.[1,77] They primarily occupy the lysine-binding site of the plasminogen molecule, producing a conformational change in the molecule that makes plasminogen even more susceptible to the attack of plasminogen activators in vitro. However, blockade of the lysine-binding site by tranexamic acid is biologically much more important, because curtailment of plasminogen attachment to the fibrin strands via the lysine binding site thus results in a fibrin polymer with greater resistance to natural fibrinolysis. Plasminogen activators, when released, find less substrate that can be converted into plasmin on their target surface. This is probably true not only for fibrin as a target surface but also for platelet and other cell membranes.[3,63,103] In a series of ex vivo clot lysis assays, Longstaff recently showed that the pattern of fibrinolysis is differently influenced by tranexamic acid and aprotinin. He suggested that aprotinin may be an even more effective inhibitor of fibrinolysis in vivo than the two physiological inhibitors, α_2-antiplasmin and α_2-macroglobulin.[77]

The usual dose of tranexamic acid in its various applications as an antifibrinolytic agent is an intravenous injection of 10–15 mg/kg body weight 2 –3 times/day or an oral dose of 1–1.5 gm up to 4 times/day.[119]

Clinical Efficacy of Tranexamic Acid in Open Heart Surgery

A fresh interest in the use of antifibrinolytic drugs to prevent or treat the hemostatic deficiency associated with CPB was generated by the remarkable effects of aprotinin and the ensuing reports from the group at the Hammersmith Hospital in London.[7,101,117] Although investigational use of the lysine analog EACA in open heart surgery was documented much earlier,[38,39] antifibrinolytics had been generally regarded as problematic drugs with a rather restricted indication because of a perceived risk of microthrombosis and disseminated intravascular coagulation (DIC).

Later studies performed in open heart surgery with EACA or tranexamic acid have been expertly reviewed by others.[36,46] A well-controlled study with EACA in 40 patients undergoing primary CABG[18] showed that a total dose of 30 gm significantly decreased the postoperative cumulative blood loss. Five patients in the placebo group received donor blood or blood components versus 1 patient in the treatment group. However, the majority of studies with lysine analogs investigated the effect of tranexamic acid, either in the conventional dose of about 1.5 gm or—more recently—in an increased dose of 10 gm administered before the start of CPB. Tables 6 and 7 summarize the available clinical efficacy data for tranexamic acid in open heart surgery.

Study design and assessment of relevant target variables have varied greatly in clinical trials of tranexamic acid. Lemmer[68] rightfully pointed to the lack of uniformity and completeness in reporting the results of blood conservation interventions. Despite these shortcomings, however, there can be no doubt that the 10-gm dosage scheme of tranexamic acid is efficacious.[58]

Numerous small studies have attempted to compare the clinical effectiveness of tranexamic acid and aprotinin. Most do not meet the standards of valid methodology for clinical research. Conclusions based on the absence of a statistically significant difference may be erroneous if the sample size is small and the study lacks sufficient statistical power to detect a difference. This is true for both efficacy variables and safety data. For example, a Canadian study[97] compared randomized treatment of 13 patients with 10 gm of tranexamic acid, 16 patients with the full Hammersmith dosage of aprotinin, and 7 control patients. The difference in the mean red cell transfusion requirements of 2.6 units in the tranexamic acid-treated group versus 1.5 units in the aprotinin-treated group was not significant ($p > 0.05$), but the authors concluded that aprotinin and tranexamic acid were equal in controlling blood loss in CPB.[97]

Tolerability and Clinical Safety of Tranexamic Acid

The few known side effects of tranexamic acid occur rarely and are described as nausea, vomiting, diarrhea, and orthostatic dysregulation.[119] Because of experimental

TABLE 6.   Summary of Studies Comparing Treatment with Tranexamic Acid (About 1.5 gm) vs. Placebo or No Treatment Controls

Author	Type of Surgery (AMCHA/Control)	% of Patients Receiving Donor Blood		Mean Transfusion Requirements (Units)		Mean Total Blood Loss	
		AMCHA	Control	AMCHA	Control	AMCHA	Control
Horrow,[51] 1995	CABG or valves[1] (n = 21/27)	29	29	NA		365 gm	552 gm
Horrow,[50] 1991	CABG or valves[2] (n = 37/34)	32	36	NA		328 gm	462 gm
Horrow,[49] 1990	CABG or valves[3] (n = 18/20)	NA		1.1	0.9	496 ml	750 ml
DePeppo,[22] 1995	CABG or valves[4] (n = 15/15)	7	20	0.07	0.4	534 ml	724 ml
Speekenbrink,[111] 1995	Primary CABG[5] (n = 15/15)	NA		2.9	3.1	352 ml	674 ml
Blauhut,[11] 1994	Primary CABG[6] (n = 15/14)	47	60	0.8	1.6	403 ml	453 ml
Corbeau,[15] 1995	Primary CABG[7] (n = 41/20)	37	60	0.8	1.7	1015 ml	1416 ml

AMCHA = tranexamic acid, NA = data not available from referenced publication, CABG = coronary artery bypass grafting.
1. Placebo-controlled, double-blind, part of 6-armed dose comparison protocol; dosage 10 mg/kg loading plus 1 mg/kg/hr constant infusion for 12 hr; transfusion requirement until day 5 postoperativley; blood loss measured in gm for 12 hr.
2. Placebo-controlled, double-blind, part of comparative study with desmopressin; dosage 10 mg/kg loading plus 1 mg/kg/hr constant infusion for 12 hr; blood loss measured in gm for 12 hr postoperatively (p < 0.001).
3. Placebo-controlled, double-blind; dosage 10 mg/kg loading plus 1 mg/kg/hr constant infusion for 10 hr; blood loss measured for 12 hr postoperatively (p = 0.006); mean volume of transfused packed red blood cells = 275 vs. 227 ml.
4. Placebo-controlled, double-blind, part of comparative study with aprotinin and EACA; dosage 10 mg/kg loading plus 1 mg/kg/hr constant infusion for 10 hr; 24 hr postoperative blood loss; differences in blood loss and transfusion data not significant.
5. Randomized prospective clinical trial, part of comparative study with aprotinin and dipyridamole vs. untreated controls; dosage 10 mg/kg loading plus 1 mg/kg/hr up to a total dose of 1000 mg; blood loss measured for 6 hr postoperatively (p = 0.019).
6. Randomized prospective controlled trial, part of a comparative study with aprotinin vs. untreated controls; dosage 10 mg/kg loading plus 1 mg/kg/hr constant infusion for 10 hr; no significant difference in 24-hr postoperative blood loss and blood transfusion.
7. Randomized prospective controlled trial, part of a comparative study with aprotinin vs. untreated controls; dosage 30 mg/kg in 2 fractions during surgery; total postoperative blood loss (p < 0.05); blood transfusion over 48 hr postoperatively.

findings from chronic administration of high doses, tranexamic acid is contraindicated in patients with visual impairment. However, no retinal changes were found in patients receiving tranexamic acid clinically over periods ranging from several weeks to 6 years.[119] Because of the observation of lysis-resistant extravascular blood clots in the renal pelvis or bladder in the presence of lysine analogs, tranexamic acid is also contraindicated for massive bleeding from the upper urinary tract, especially in hemophiliac patients.[13]

Few hard data support the repeated concerns about a potential increase in the rate of thromboembolic events as a consequence of therapeutic or prophylactic use of antifibrinolytic drugs. Retrospective epidemiologic assessment of tranexamic acid treatment in noncardiac patients who appear to be predisposed to thrombotic complications provided no evidence of a thrombogenic effect.[76] Whereas the safety data of large well-controlled clinical trials with aprotinin in cardiac surgery have been published,[71,72,75] safety data from prospective, placebo-controlled, double-blind studies with lysine analogs in open heart surgery are lacking or, at best, anecdotal. Most of the information on which the discussion

TABLE 7. Summary of Studies Comparing Treatment with Tranexamic Acid (10 gm) vs. Placebo or No Treatment Controls

Author	Type of Surgery (AMCHA/Control)	% of Patients Receiving Donor Blood		Mean Transfusion Requirement (Units)		Mean Total Blood Loss (ml)	
		AMCHA	Control	AMCHA	Control	AMCHA	Control
Katsaros,[58] 1996	CABG or valves* (n = 104/106)	11	25	0.2	0.5	474	906
Karski,[57] 1995	CABG or valves† (n = 49/48)	40	40	0.8	0.8	640	980
Rousou,[100] 1995	Primary CABG‡ (n = 206/209)	NA		0.7	1.3	804	1114

AMCHA = tranexamic acid, NA = data not available from referenced publication, CABG = coronary artery bypass grafting.

* Placebo-controlled, double-blind; 86% primary CABG; dose, 10 gm; blood loss measured for 24 hr postoperatively (p < 0.001); significant difference in blood transfusion data (p < 0.05).

† Placebo-controlled, double blind; 70% CABG, 18% reoperations; dose 10 gm (20-gm group not shown); difference in 24 hr postoperative blood loss (p = 0.0001); precise transfusion data not given.

‡ Sequential design, no-treatment control group first; dose, 10 gm; difference in total postoperative blood loss (p < 0.001); difference in total blood product use (p < 0.005).

of potential thrombotic risk is founded either was based on theoretical considerations or resulted from casuistic clinical reports and retrospective evaluation of clinical data.[94] The recent study of Katsaros et al.[58] states that 10 gm of tranexamic acid showed no increased incidence of postoperative myocardial infarction, cerebrovascular accident, pulmonary embolism, or thrombosis-related morbidity or mortality. Given the difference in the mechanism of action between aprotinin and the lysine analogs, which favors the formation of more lysis-resistant clots under high-dosage treatment with tranexamic acid or EACA, the apparent absence of thromboembolic reactions with these compounds is, after all, surprising. Perhaps the advent of aprotinin for open heart surgery has started a new chapter in the book of therapeutics that ultimately will lead to a revised opinion of the risk-to-benefit ratio of the lysine analogs. However, one should not dismiss too early the requirement of a sufficiently large database for any judgment of clinical safety—and that, at present, appears to be available only for aprotinin.

REFERENCES

1. Alston TA, Baggio RF: Aminocaproic acid enhances inactivation of plasmin by aprotinin [abstract]. Anesth Analg 80(Suppl):SCA129, 1995.
2. Ambrus JL, Schimert G, Lajos TZ, et al: Effect of antifibrinolytic agents and estrogens on blood loss and blood coagulation factors during open heart surgery. J Med 2:65–81, 1971.
3. Åstedt B: Clinical pharmacology of tranexamic acid. Scand J Gastroenterol 22(Suppl 137):22–25, 1987.
4. Bianchi C, Donadio C, Tramonti G, et al: Renal handling of cationic and anionic small proteins: Experiments in intact rats. Contr Nephrol 68:37–44, 1988.
5. Bick RL: Physiology and pathophysiology of hemostasis during cardiac surgery. In Pifarré R (ed): Blood Conservation with Aprotinin. Philadelphia, Hanley & Belfus, 1995, pp 1–44.
6. Bidstrup BP: Pretreatment with aprotinin and aspirin. In Pifarré R (ed.): Blood Conservation with Aprotinin. Philadelphia, Hanley & Belfus, 1995, pp 287–291.
7. Bidstrup BP, Royston D, Sapsford RN, Taylor KM: Reduction in blood loss and blood use after cardiopulmonary bypass with high dose aprotinin (Trasylol). J Thorac Cardiovasc Surg 97:364–372, 1989.
8. Bidstrup BP, Underwood SR, Sapsford RN: Effect of aprotinin (Trasylol) on aorta-coronary bypass graft patency. J Thorac Cardiovasc Surg 105:147–153, 1993.
9. Bieth JG: In-vivo significance of kinetic constants of protein proteinase inhibitors. Biochem Med 32:387–397, 1984.
10. Blauhut B, Gross C, Necek S, et al: Effects of high-dose aprotinin on blood loss, platelet function, fibrinolysis, complement, and renal function after cardiopulmonary bypass. J Thorac Cardiovasc Surg 101:958–967, 1991.
11. Blauhut B, Harringer W, Bettelheim P, et al: Comparison of the effects of aprotinin and tranexamic acid on blood loss and related variables after cardiopulmonary bypass. J Thorac Cardiovasc Surg 108:1083–1091, 1994.

12. Boldt J, Knothe C, Zickmann B, et al: Comparison of two aprotinin dosage regimens in pediatric patients having cardiac operations. J Thorac Cardiovasc Surg 105:705–711, 1993.
13. Bundesverband der Pharmazeutischen Industrie (eds): Rote Liste 1996 [German Drug Inventory]. Aulendorf/Württ., ECV Editio Cantor, 1996.
14. Casas JI, Zuazu-Jausoro I, Mateo J, et al: Aprotinin versus desmopressin for patients undergoing operations with cardiopulmonary bypass. J Thorac Cardiovasc Surg 110:1107–1117, 1995.
15. Corbeau JJ, Monrigal JP, Jacob JP, et al: Comparaison des effets de l'aprotinine et de l'acide tranexamique sur le saignement en chirurgie cardiaque [Comparative effects of aprotinin and tranexamic acid on blood loss in cardiac surgery]. Ann Fr Anesth Réanim 14:154–161, 1995.
16. Cosgrove DM III, Heric B, Lytle BW, et al: Aprotinin therapy for reoperative myocardial revascularization: a placebo-controlled study. Ann Thorac Surg 54:1031–1038, 1992.
17. Cramer EM, Lu H, Caen JP, et al: Differential redistribution of platelet glycoproteins Ib and IIb-IIIa after plasmin stimulation. Blood 77:694–699, 1991.
18. Daily PO, Lamphere JA, Dembitsky WP, et al: Effect of prophylactic epsilon-aminocaproic acid on blood loss and transfusion requirements in patients undergoing first-time coronary artery bypass grafting. J Thorac Cardiovasc Surg 108:99–108, 1994.
19. Davis R, Whittington R: Aprotinin. A review of its pharmacology and therapeutic efficacy in reducing blood loss associated with cardiac surgery. Drugs 49:954–983, 1995.
20. Dementieva II, Dzemeshkevich SL, Charnaya MA, Shabalkin BV: The use of high doses of aprotinin to decrease blood loss in aortocoronary bypass surgery. J Cardiovasc Surg 35(Suppl 1):185–186, 1994.
21. Dementjeva II, Charnaya MA, Dzemeshkevich SL, et al: Effects of high aprotinin doses on the intra- and postoperative blood loss in cardiopulmonary bypass surgery. Anesteziol Reanim 2:91–93, 1995.
22. DePeppo AP, Pierri MD, Scafuri A, et al: Intraoperative antifibrinolysis and blood-saving techniques in cardiac surgery. Tex Heart Inst J 22:231–236, 1995.
23. Dietrich W: Reducing thrombin formation during cardiopulmonary bypass: Is there a benefit of the additional anticoagulant action of aprotinin? J Cardiovasc Pharmacol 27(Suppl I):S50–S57, 1996.
24. Dietrich W, Dilthey G, Spannagl M, et al: Influence of high-dose aprotinin on anticoagulation, heparin requirement, and celite- and kaolin-activated clotting time in heparin-pretreated patients undergoing open-heart surgery. Anesthesiology 83:679–689, 1995.
25. Dietrich W, Mössinger H: The use of aprotinin in pediatric cardiopulmonary bypass. In Pifarré R (ed): Blood Conservation with Aprotinin. Philadelphia, Hanley & Belfus, 1995, pp 275–286.
26. Dietrich W, Mössinger H, Spannagl M, et al: Hemostatic activation during cardiopulmonary bypass with different aprotinin dosages in pediatric patients having cardiac operations. J Thorac Cardiovasc Surg 105:712–720, 1993.
27. Dietrich W, Spannagl M, Jochum M, et al: Influence of high-dose aprotinin treatment on blood loss and coagulation patterns in patients undergoing myocardial revascularization. Anesthesiology 73:1119–1126, 1990.
28. Dietrich W, Späth P, Ebell A, Richter JA: Incidence of anaphylactic reactions to aprotinin—analysis of 248 reexposures to aprotinin [abstract]. Anesthesiology 83(Suppl):A104, 1995.
29. Edmunds LH: Cardiopulmonary bypass and blood. In Pifarré R (ed): Blood Conservation with Aprotinin. Philadelphia, Hanley & Belfus, 1995, pp 45–66.
30. Fareed J, Hoppensteadt D, Koza MJ, et al: Pharmacokinetics of aprotinin and its relevance to antifibrinolytic and other biological effects. In Pifarré R (ed): Blood Conservation with Aprotinin. Philadelphia, Hanley & Belfus, 1995, pp 131–149.
31. Feindt PR, Walcher S, Volkmer I, et al: Effects of high-dose aprotinin on renal function in aortocoronary bypass grafting. Ann Thorac Surg 60:1076–1080, 1995.
32. Ferraris VA, Ferraris SP: Limiting excessive postoperative blood transfusion after cardiac procedures. Tex Heart Inst J 22:216–230, 1995.
33. Foulkes EC: Tubular reabsorption of low molecular weight proteins. Physiologist 25:56–59, 1982.
34. Fraedrich G, Engler H, Kanz L, Schlosser V: High dose aprotinin regimen in open heart surgery—A prospective randomised double blind trial. Circulation 80(Suppl2):II158, 1989.
35. Fraedrich G, Neukamm K, Schneider T, et al: Safety and risk/benefit assessment of aprotinin in primary CABG. In Friedel N, Hetzer R, Royston D (eds): Blood Use in Cardiac Surgery. Darmstadt, Steinkopff Verlag, 1991, pp 221–231.
36. Fremes SE, Wong BI, Lee E, et al Metaanalysis of prophylactic drug treatment in the prevention of postoperative bleeding. Ann Thorac Surg 58:1580–1588, 1994.
37. Fritz H, Wunderer G: Biochemistry and applications of aprotinin, the kallikrein inhibitor from bovine organs. Arzneim Forsch/Drug Res 33:479–494, 1983.
38. Gans H, Krivit W: Problems in hemostasis during open heart surgery. III: Epsilon-aminocaproic acid as an inhibitor of plaminogen activator activity. Ann Surg 155:268–276, 1962.
39. Gans H, Subramanian V, John S, et al: Theoretical and practical (clinical) considerations concerning proteolytic enzymes and their inhibitors with particular reference to changes in the plasminogen-plasmin system observed during assisted circulation in man. Ann N Y Acad Sci 146:721–736, 1968.

40. George JN, Shattil SJ: The clinical importance of acquired abnormalities of platelet function. N Engl J Med 324:27–39, 1991.
41. Goldstein DJ, DeRosa CM, Mongero LB, et al: Safety and efficacy of aprotinin under conditions of deep hypothermia and circulatory arrest. J Thorac Cardiovasc Surg 110:1615–1622, 1995.
42. Goldstein DJ, Oz MC, Smith CR, et al: Safety of repeat aprotinin administration for LVAD recipients undergoing cardiac transplantation. Ann Thorac Surg 61:692–695, 1996.
43. Gorman JH, Edmunds LH: Blood anesthesia for cardiopulmonary bypass. J Card Surg 10:270–279, 1995.
44. Hannekum A, Reuter HD, Dalichau H, et al: Anlage und zusammenfassendes Ergebnis einer klinischen Doppelblindstudie bei Operationen am offenen Herzen. Einfluß von Aprotinin auf Thrombozytenzahl und - funktion. In Dudziak R, Kirchhoff PG, Reuter HD, Schumann F (eds.): Proteolyse und Proteinaseninhibition in der Herz- und Gefäßchirurgie. Stuttgart, Schattauer, 1985, pp 221–233.
45. Harder MP, Eijsman L, Roozendaal KJ, et al: Aprotinin reduces intraoperative and postoperative blood loss in membrane oxygenator cardiopulmonary bypass. Ann Thorac Surg 51:936–941, 1991.
46. Hardy JF, Bélisle S: Natural and synthetic antifibrinolytics in adult cardiac surgery: efficacy, effectiveness and efficiency. Can J Anaesth 41:1104–1112, 1994.
47. Havel M, Teufelsbauer H, Knöbl P, et al: Effect of intraoperative aprotinin administration on postoperative bleeding in patients undergoing cardiopulmonary bypass operation. J Thorac Cardiovasc Surg 101:968–972, 1991.
48. Herynkopf F, Lucchese F, Pereira E, et al: Aprotinin in children undergoing correction of congenital heart defects. A double-blind pilot study. J Thorac Cardiovasc Surg 103:517–521, 1994.
49. Horrow JC, Hlavacek J, Strong MD, et al: Prophylactic tranexamic acid decreases bleeding after cardiac operations. J Thorac Cardiovasc Surg 99:70–74, 1990.
50. Horrow JC, van Riper DF, Strong MD, et al: Hemostatic effects of tranexamic acid and desmopressin during cardiac surgery. Circulation 84:2063–2070, 1991.
51. Horrow JC, van Riper DF, Strong MD, et al: The dose-response relationship of tranexamic acid. Anesthesiology 82:383–392, 1995.
52. Huth C, Hoffmeister HE: Einsatz von Proteinaseninhibitoren während der extrakorporalen Zirkulation - Wirkungsverbesserung durch Optimierung der Dosis in einer klinischen Studie. In Dudziak R, Kirchhoff PG, Reuter HD, Schumann F (eds): Proteolyse und Proteinaseninhibition in der Herz- und Gefäßchirurgie. Stuttgart , Schattauer, 1985, pp 243–250.
53. Jonas RA: Advances in surgical care of infants and children with congenital heart disease. Curr Opini Pediatr 7:572–579, 1995.
54. Just M: In vivo interaction of the Kunitz protease inhibitor and of insulin with subcellular structures from rat renal cortex. Naunyn-Schmiedeberg's Arch Pharmacol 287:85–95, 1975.
55. Kalangos A, Tayyareci G, Pretre R, et al: Influence of aprotinin on early graft thrombosis in patients undergoing myocardial revascularization. Eur J Cardio-thorac Surg 8:651–656, 1994.
56. Kaller H, Patzschke K, Wegner LA, Horster FA: Pharmacokinetic observations following intravenous administration of radioactive labelled aprotinin in volunteers. Eur J Drug Metab Pharmacokin 3:79–85, 1978.
57. Karski JM, Teasdale SJ, Norman P, et al: Prevention of bleeding after cardiopulmonary bypass with high-dose tranexamic acid. J Thorac Cardiovasc Surg 110:835–842, 1995.
58. Katsaros D, Petricevic M, Snow NJ, et al: Tranexamic acid reduces postbypass blood use: A double-blinded, prospective, randomized study of 210 patients. Ann Thorac Surg 61:1131–1135, 1996.
59. Kluft C: Pathomechanisms of defective hemostasis during and after extracorporeal circulation: Contact phase activation. In Friedel N, Hetzer R, Royston D (eds): Blood Use in Cardiac Surgery. Darmstadt, Steinkopff Verlag, 1991, pp 10–15.
60. Kluft C, Dooijewaard G, Emeis JJ: Role of the contact system in fibrinolysis. Semin Thromb Hemost 13:50–68, 1987.
61. Koza MJ, Walenga JM, Khenkina YN, et al: Thrombelastographic analysis of patients receiving aprotinin with comparison to platelet aggregation and other assays. Semin Thromb Haemost 21(Suppl 4):80–85, 1995.
62. Kraut H, Frey EK, Werle E: Über die Inaktivierung des Kallikreins. Hoppe-Seyler's Zeitschrift für physiol Chemie 192:1–21, 1930.
63. Krishnamurti C, Vukelja SJ, Alving BM: Inhibitory effects of lysine analogues on t-PA induced whole blood clot lysis. Thromb Res 73:419–430, 1994.
64. Kunitz M, Northrop JH: Isolation from beef pancreas of crystalline trypsinogen, trypsin, a trypsin inhibitor, and an inhibitor-trypsin compound. J Gen Physiol 19:991–1007, 1936.
65. Lamparter-Schummert B, Mugaragu I, Hetzer R, Adt M: Aprotinin re-exposure in patients undergoing repeat cardiac surgery: Effect of prophylaxis with H1- and H2-receptor antagonists [abstract]. Br J Anaesth 74(Suppl):3, 1995.
66. Lass M, Welz A, Kochs M, et al: Aprotinin in elective primary bypass surgery. Graft patency and clinical efficacy. Eur J Cardiothorac Surg 9:206–210, 1995.
67. Lavee J, Savion N, Smolinsky A, et al: Platelet protection by aprotinin in cardiopulmonary bypass: Electron microscopic study. Ann Thorac Surg 53:477–481, 1992.

68. Lemmer JH: Reporting the results of blood conservation studies: The need for uniform and comprehensive methods. Ann Thorac Surg 58:1305–1306, 1994.

69. Lemmer JH, Dilling EW, Morton JR, et al: Aprotinin for primary coronary artery bypass surgery: A multi-center, randomized, double-blind, placebo-controlled trial of three dose regimens. Ann Thorac Surg 1996 [in press].

70. Lemmer JH, Metzdorff MT, Krause AH, et al.: Aprotinin use in patients with dialysis-dependent renal failure undergoing cardiac operations. J Thorac Cardiovasc Surg 112:192–194, 1996.

71. Lemmer JH, Stanford W, Bonney SL, et al: Aprotinin for coronary bypass operations: Efficacy, safety, and influence on early saphenous vein graft patency. J Thorac Cardiovasc Surg 107:543–553, 1994.

72. Lemmer JH, Stanford W, Bonney SL, et al: Aprotinin for coronary artery bypass grafting: Effect on post-operative renal function. Ann Thorac Surg 59:132–136, 1995.

73. Leonard EF, Turitto VT, Vroman L (eds): Blood in contact with natural and artificial surfaces. Ann N Y Acad Sci 516:1–688, 1987.

74. Levy JH, Bailey JM, Salmenperae M: Pharmacokinetics of aprotinin in preoperative cardiac surgical patients. Anesthesiology 80:1013–1018, 1994.

75. Levy JH, Pifarré R, Schaff HV, et al: A multicenter, double-blind, placebo-controlled trial of aprotinin for reducing blood loss and the requirement for donor-blood transfusion in patients undergoing repeat coronary artery bypass grafting. Circulation 92:2236–2244, 1995.

76. Lindoff C, Rybo G, Åstedt B: Treatment with tranexamic acid during pregnancy, and the risk of thrombo-embolic complications. Thromb Haemost 70:238–240, 1993.

77. Longstaff C: Studies on the mechanisms of action of aprotinin and tranexamic acid as plasmin inhibitors and antifibrinolytic agents. Blood Coagul Fibrinol 5:537–542, 1994.

78. Lu H, du Buit C, Soria J, et al: Postoperative hemostasis and fibrinolysis in patients undergoing cardiopulmonary bypass with or without aprotinin therapy. Thromb Haemost 72:438–443, 1994.

79. Lu H, Soria C, Cramer EM, et al: Temperature dependence of plasmin-induced activation or inhibition of human platelets. Blood 77:996–1005, 1991.

80. Lu H, Soria C, Li H, Soria J, et al: Role of active center and lysine binding sites of plasmin in plasmin-induced platelet activation and disaggregation. Thromb Haemost 65:67–72, 1991.

81. Magovern JA, Sakert T, Benckart DH, et al: A model for predicting transfusion after coronary artery bypass grafting. Ann Thorac Surg 61:27–32, 1996.

82. Mammen EF: Natural protease inhibitors in extracorporeal circulation. Ann N Y Acad Sci 146:754–762, 1968.

83. Manucci L, Gerometta PS, Mussoni L, et al: One month follow-up of haemostatic variables in patients undergoing aortocoronary bypass surgery. Effect of aprotinin. Thromb Haemost 73:356–361, 1995.

84. Masiak M: Trasylol as an inhibitor of fibrinolysis in ECC. In Fritz H, Dietze G, Fidler F, Haberland GL (eds): Recent Progress on Kinins. Basel, Birkhäuser, 1982, pp 690–699.

85. McGiffin DC, Kirklin JK: Complement and the damaging effects of cardiopulmonary bypass. In Pifarré R (ed): Blood Conservation with Aprotinin. Philadelphia, Hanley & Belfus, 1995, pp 67–82.

86. Minami K, Notohamiprodjo G, Buschler H, et al: Alpha-2-plasmin inhibitor –plasmin complex and postoperative blood loss: Double-blind study with aprotinin in reoperation for myocardial revascularization. J Thorac Cardiovasc Surg 106:934–936, 1993.

87. Mohr R, Goor DA, Lusky A, Lavee J: Aprotinin prevents cardiopulmonary bypass-induced platelet dysfunction. A scanning electron microscope study. Circulation 86:II405 –II409, 1992.

88. Murase M, Usui A, Tomita Y, et al: Nafamostat mesilate reduces blood loss during open heart surgery. Circulation 88:432–436, 1993.

89. Murkin JM, Lux J, Shannon NA, et al: Aprotinin significantly decreases bleeding and transfusion requirements in patients receiving aspirin and undergoing cardiac operations. J Thorac Cardiovasc Surg 107: 554–561, 1994.

90. Okajima K, Uchiba M, Murakami K: Nafamostat Mesilate. Cardiovasc Drug Rev13:51–65, 1995.

91. Okamoto S, Oshiba S, Mihara H, Okamoto U: Synthetic inhibitors of fibrinolysis: in vitro and in vivo mode of action. Ann N Y Acad Sci 146:414–429, 1968.

92. Okita Y, Takamoto S, Ando M, Morota T, Kawashima Y: Is usage of aprotinin safe with deep hypothermic circulatory arrest in aortic surgery? Investigations on blood coagulation [abstract]. Circulation 92(Suppl): 1457, 1995.

93. Ouimet H, Loscalzo J: Reciprocating autocatalytic interactions between platelets and the activation system. Thromb Res 70:355–364, 1993.

94. Ovrum E, Holen EA, Abdelnoor M, et al: Tranexamic acid (cyclocapron) is not necessary to reduce blood loss after coronary bypass operations. J Thorac Cardiovasc Surg 105:78--83, 1993.

95. Penkoske PA, Entwistle LM, Marchak BE, et al: Aprotinin in children undergoing repair of congenital heart defects. Ann Thorac Surg 60:S529–S532, 1995.

96. Pennington DG, Hahn CJ (moderators): Discussion of ECMO for cardiac support. Ann Thorac Surg 61:340–341, 1996.

97. Podlosky L, Clarke G, Boshkov L, et al: Platelet glycoproteins (GPs), fibrinolysis and blood loss in reoperative cardiac patients on tranexamic acid or aprotinin [abstract]. Transfusion 34(Suppl): S120, 1994.

98. Popov-Cenic S, Murday H, Kirchhoff PG, et al: Anlage und zusammenfassendes Ergebnis einer klinischen Doppelblindstudie bei aorto-koronaren Bypass-Operationen. In Dudziak R, Kirchhoff PG, Reuter HD, Schumann F (eds): Proteolyse und Proteinaseninhibition in der Herz- und Gefäßchirurgie. Stuttgart, Schattauer, 1985, pp 171–186.

99. Primack C, Walenga JM, Koza MJ, et al: Aprotinin modulation of platelet activation in patients undergoing cardiopulmonary bypass operations. Ann Thorac Surg 61:1188–1193, 1996.

100. Rousou JA, Engelman RM, Flack JE, et al: Tranexamic acid significantly reduces blood loss associated with coronary revascularization. Ann Thorac Surg 59:671–675, 1995.

101. Royston D, Bidstrup BP, Taylor KM, Sapsford RN: Effect of aprotinin on need for blood transfusion after repeat open-heart surgery. Lancet ii:1289–1291, 1987.

102. Royston D, Bidstrup BP, Taylor KM, et al: Reduction of bleeding after open heart surgery with aprotinin (Trasylol): Beneficial effects in patients taking aspirin and in those with renal failure. In Birnbaum DE, Hoffmeister HE (ed.): Blood Saving in Open Heart Surgery. Stuttgart, Schattauer, 1990, pp 66–75.

103. Rubens F, Wells P: Tranexamic acid use during coronary artery bypass grafting [letter]. Ann Thorac Surg 61:774–775, 1996.

104. Schall R, Müller FO, Hundt HKL, et al: Pharmacokinetic profile of high doses of aprotinin in patients undergoing primary elective hysterectomy. A meta-analysis of two clinical trials. Drug Invest 7:200–208, 1994.

105. Schulze K, Graeter T, Schaps D, Hausen B: Severe anaphylactic shock due to repeated application of aprotinin in patients following intrathoracic aortic replacement. Eur J Cardio-thorac Surg 7:495–496, 1993.

106. Schumann F: Report on a clinical double-blind study, comparing postoperative renal function in patients treated with Trasylol or placebo during aorto-coronary bypass operation (Investigator: G. Fraedrich). Bayer Pharma Report No PH-21343, 1992.

107. Schumann F, Dirksen MSC: Report on a clinical double-blind study with Trasylol (aprotinin) in open heart surgery (Investigator: H. Neuhof). Bayer Pharma Report No R-5124, 1990.

108. Seghaye MC, Duchateau J, Grabitz RG, et al: Influence of low-dose aprotinin on the inflammatory reaction due to cardiopulmonary bypass in children. Ann Thorac Surg 61:1205–1211, 1996.

109. Shinfeld A, Zippel D, Lavee J, et al: Aprotinin improves hemostasis after cardiopulmonary bypass better than single-donor platelet concentrate. Ann Thorac Surg 59:872–876, 1995.

110. Spannagl M, Dooijewaard G, Dietrich W, Kluft C: Protection of single-chain urokinase-type plasminogen activator (scu-PA) in aprotinin treated cardiac surgical patients undergoing cardiopulmonary bypass. Thromb Haemost 73:825–828, 1995.

111. Speekenbrink RGH, Vonk ABA, Wildevuur CRH, Eijsman L: Hemostatic efficacy of dipyridamole, tranexamic acid, and aprotinin in coronary bypass grafting. Ann Thorac Surg 59:438–442, 1995.

112. Sundt TM, Kouchoukos NT, Saffitz JE, et al: Renal dysfunction and intravascular coagulation with aprotinin and hypothermic circulatory arrest. Ann Thorac Surg 55:1418–1424, 1993.

113. Swart MJ, Gordon PC, Hayse-Gregson PB, et al: High-dose aprotinin in cardiac surgery—A prospective, randomized study. Anaesth Intens Care 22:529–533, 1994.

114. Tanaka K, Kondo C, Sato T, et al: Nafamostat mesilate (FUT-175) improves hemostatic function after cardiopulmonary bypass by its effect on both platelets and coagulofibrinolytic system [abstract]. Thromb Haemost 69:1073, 1993.

115. Tice DA, Reed GE, Clauss RH, Worth MH: Hemorrhage due to fibrinolysis occurring with open-heart operations. J Thorac Cardiovasc Surg 46:673–679, 1963.

116. Unsworth-White MJ, Herriot A, Valencia O, Poloniecki J, et al: Resternotomy for bleeding after cardiac operation: a marker for increased morbidity and mortality. Ann Thorac Surg 59:664–667, 1995.

117. van Oeveren W, Jansen NJ, Bidstrup BP, et al: Effects of aprotinin on hemostatic mechanism during cardiopulmonary bypass. Ann Thorac Surg 44:640–645, 1987.

118. van der Meer J, L.Hillege H, Ascoop CAPL, et al: Aprotinin in aortocoronary bypass surgery: increased risk of vein-graft occlusion and myocardial infarction? Supportive evidence from a retrospective study. Thromb Haemost 75:1–3, 1996.

119. Verstraete M: Clinical application of inhibitors of fibrinolysis. Drugs 29:236–261, 1985.

120. von Segesser LK: Heparin-bonded surfaces in extracorporeal membrane oxygenation for cardiac support. Ann Thorac Surg 61:330–335, 1996.

121. Wachtfogel YT, Kucich U, Hack CE, et al: Aprotinin inhibits the contact, neutrophil, and platelet activation systems during simulated extracorporeal perfusion. J Thorac Cardiovasc Surg 106:1–10, 1993.

122. Wenger RK, Lukasiewicz H, Mikuta BS, et al: Loss of platelet fibrinogen receptors during clinical cardiopulmonary bypass. J Thorac Cardiovasc Surg 97:235–239, 1989.

123. Woodman RC, Harker LA: Bleeding complications associated with cardiopulmonary bypass. Blood 76:1680–1697, 1990.

CHAPTER 30

New Anticoagulants for Adjunct Use in Angiography

OMER IQBAL, M.D.

With the significant increase in the number of effective and less invasive procedures, interventional radiologists are faced with a growing challenge of pre-, peri-, and postinterventional patient care involving the use and monitoring of sophisticated anticoagulant therapy for prevention and management of thromboembolic complications. Homeostasis may be defined as a physiologic homeostasis, resulting from a dynamic equilibrium between coagulation and fibrinolysis. An intact endothelium serves as a unique hemostatic tool in the regulation of coagulation by synthesizing procoagulant substances, such as thromboxane, von Willebrand factor, phospholipids, platelet-activating factor, tissue factor, interleukin-1, and plasminogen activator inhibitor type I, and anticoagulant substances, such as tissue factor pathway inhibitor (TFPI), tissue-type plasminogen activator (tPA), prostacyclin, protein C, protein S, thrombomodulin, heparan sulfate, and urokinase.[71] The use of catheters, the different catheter techniques and materials, and the interaction of various contrast media with blood components and endothelium disturb the delicate hemostatic balance and create an optimal environment for a procoagulant state that necessitates use of an anticoagulant.

HEPARIN: AN OVERVIEW

The mechanism of action, side effects, and complications of heparin, a conventionally used anticoagulant, are essential to mention before the newer anticoagulants are discussed. Heparin was a chance discovery made by medical student Jay McLean in 1916.[56] Howell and Holt introduced the term heparin,[41] purified the material,[42] and published a detailed report about its chemical and physiologic actions.[43] It was first used clinically in 1937 by Crafoord, a Swedish surgeon who anticoagulated patients suffering from postoperative pulmonary emboli.[16] A little over half a century has passed since the initial clinical trials of heparin. The National Institutes of Health Consensus Conference in 1986 concluded that heparin was the drug of choice for the prophylaxis of postoperative thrombosis. Heparin retained this status despite its drawbacks and undesired side effects, such as hemorrhage, short duration of action requiring frequent administration, heparin-induced thrombocytopenia (HIT), heparin-induced thrombosis or white clot syndrome, alopecia, osteoporosis, and lipolysis. HIT is diagnosed when the platelet count decreases by 50% from the pretreatment level or has dropped below 100,000/μl with no apparent cause other than heparin therapy and has persisted for 2 days or more.[2] The immediate step after a diagnosis of HIT is suspected is to stop heparin therapy and to draw blood for in vitro testing, preferably after 4–6 hours, when as a rule heparin is not available in the circulation.

471

Heparin-induced thrombosis and its thromboembolic sequelae can be devastating for the patient, with a mortality rate of about 30%. About 25% of the cases of thrombosis are seen in the veins and 75% in the arteries; amputation is required in 20% or more.[47] Continuation of heparin therapy after the diagnosis of HIT is made can be dangerous, resulting in even more thromboembolic complications.

Heparin and warfarin sodium have become the most commonly used anticoagulant drugs for the parenteral anticoagulation and long-term oral treatment of thrombotic disorders. Native heparin is a mixture of mucopolysaccharide chains of variable lengths, ranging from 5,000–30,000 Da. Heparin becomes effective in the presence of the plasma protein, antithrombin III (AT III), with which it forms a complex. Heparin augments the activity of AT III and neutralizes coagulation factors X, II, XII, XI, and IX. Embolus due to catheter clot formation can be avoided by the routine use of heparinized saline for catheter flushing. In patients with HIT and white clot syndrome, however, heparinized saline cannot be used; other anticoagulant drugs must be found as alternatives.

Heparin is not always effective. In some conditions, excessive doses are required to achieve therapeutic effects—a phenomenon referred to as heparin resistance. Because heparin acts by potentiating the effect of AT III, resistance can be seen in patients with AT III deficiency. Such a deficiency is found in up to 10% of patients under 45 years of age with venous thromboembolism. Low levels of antithrombin (40–60% of normal concentration) may be seen in severe infections, cancer, liver failure, and hereditary thrombophilia; during the first 3 days of heparin treatment; and in patients undergoing cardiopulmonary bypass (CPB). One can monitor heparin levels and anticoagulant effects by activated partial thromboplastin time (APTT), Heptest, factor Xa inactivation (clotting assays and chromogenic substrate assays), and activated clotting time (ACT). In normal plasma, the specific assays may detect 0.01–0.02 U/ml of heparin. Higher levels of heparin achieved during angiography can be measured (≈ 5.0 U/ml) by ACT.

Heparin overdosage should be treated immediately by administration of protamine sulfate. The anticoagulant effect of heparin is reversed by slow injection of 1 mg of protamine sulfate per 100 U of circulating heparin. When 5,000 U of heparin are administered with an estimated half-life of 90 minutes, at the end of the procedure the circulating heparin is about 2,500 U. Reversal is achieved by injecting 1 mg of protamine per 100 U of heparin to a total of 25 mg. Protamine should be injected slowly to avoid hypotension, bradycardia, or flushing. The dose of protamine sulfate should be optimal. Insufficient reversal may lead to excessive blood loss, and protamine overdosage results in many side effects, including platelet inhibition and prolongation of APTT.[70] Other problems with administration of protamine are systemic hypotension, pulmonary hypertension,[14,21] and anaphylaxis as a result of consumption of complement.[9,67]

Heparin rebound denotes the reemergence of heparin activity after protamine sulfate neutralization. Heparin rebound is a well-reported cause of excessive blood loss after CPB.[20] Kesteven defined heparin rebound as reappearance of heparin 2 hours after complete neutralization as determined by prolongation of APTT.[49] Heparin rebound was observed in 29% of cases and occurred in patients with the highest circulating load of heparin before reversal. Patients in whom rebound was observed had a significantly lower ratio of total administered protamine sulfate to total circulating load of heparin. The ratio was less than 1.6 in all cases.

ANGIOGRAPHY: AN OVERVIEW

About two decades before the discovery of heparin and within a few months of Roentgen's discovery of x-rays in 1895, the first report of the arteriogram was published. The arteriogram was obtained by injecting a radiopaque paste into the brachial artery of a cadaver. In vivo angiography was first performed in the 1920s and improved with the availability of safer intravascular contrast media in the 1930s. The development of percutaneous techniques of injection in the 1940s and 1950s led to percutaneous arteriography as a routine radiologic procedure. Swick first developed the water-soluble radiopaque contrast media.[72,73] The ionic contrast media are basically tri-iodinated derivatives of benzoic acid and are formulated as salts with cations of sodium or meglumine. Typical reactions to contrast media include nausea and vomiting,[5] scattered-to-extensive urticaria, hypotension, bronchospastic reaction, anaphylactoid reaction, vagal reaction, cardiac arrest, and convulsions. Transformation of the ionizing carboxyl group at the number-one position of the benzene ring to a nondissociating amide group results in a nonionic contrast medium (NICM). In 1969 Almén introduced metrizamide (Amipaque, Winthron-Breon, New York), the first commercial NICM, classified as low-osmolality contrast media (LOCM).[1] Newer LOCMs have since been introduced, such as Iohexol (Omnipaque, Winthrop Pharmaceuticals), Iopamidol (Isovue, E.R. Squibb & Sons), and Ioversol (Opitray, Mallinckrodt), which are classified as NICMs, and Ioxaglate (Hexabrix, Guerbet, Aulnay-sous-Bois, France), which is classified as ionic.

The NICMs cause fewer side effects than ionic contrast media. However, several clinical and experimental investigators have reported potential thrombogenic risks. Robertson reported blood clot formation in angiographic syringes containing NICM.[62] Kopko and coworkers indicated that thrombin can be generated in mixtures of blood and NICM.[52] Grollman reported thrombotic complications during coronary angiography.[38] Gasparetti reported the association of NICM with thrombus formation in percutaneous transluminal coronary angioplasty (PTCA).[32] Grines observed the effects of ionic and nonionic contrast media in a canine model of thrombosis caused by acute arterial injury.[37] Hwang and coworkers demonstrated the risks of thromboembolism during diagnostic and interventional cardiac procedures with NICM.[45] Esplugas reported the risk of thrombosis during coronary angioplasty with low-osmolality contrast media.[19] Rasuli reported blood clot formation in angiographic syringes containing NICM,[61] and Mamon reported the lack of inhibition of thrombin generation by NICM.[53] However, the clot formation that may occur when blood is mixed directly with NICM during angiographic procedures has not been observed by all clinicians. Jacobson and Rosenquist raised an important point about the medical, economic, and legal issues pertaining to the appropriate use of contrast media and stated that the NICM-LOCM should be reserved for high-risk patients.[46] Thus, some clinicians are concerned about the safety of NICMs in interventional radiologic diagnosis. A pragmatic approach to the study and understanding of these agents will elicit basic findings about their anticoagulant or procoagulant nature.

Anticoagulation-related Concerns

The high-osmolarity ionic contrast media have a potent anticoagulant effect that may be potentiated by the synergistic effect of heparin. Hemorrhagic complications can be prevented when the two drugs need to be combined, as in extracorporeal circulation immediately after diagnostic computed tomography (CT) or angiography for a ruptured thoracic aorta. The bleeding complications with the combination of ionic contrast media and heparin can be minimized by postprocedure protamine neutralization of heparin or by use of NICM and heparin. However, the use of heparin involves the potential risk of developing HIT or white clot syndrome. Furthermore, some patients may resist heparinization because of endogenous AT III deficiency or platelet factor 3 release and, therefore, require an alternative anticoagulant.

A NEW FAMILY OF ANTICOAGULANT DRUGS

During the past decade, various new heparin analogs, antiplatelet agents, endothelial and viscosity modulators, and biotechnology-based proteins have emerged as alternatives to the conventional heparin and warfarin regimens. Longer duration of action, higher bioavailability, improved safety and efficacy, and simplified modes of administration characterize some of these new compounds, which may be used as logical coadjuncts for

TABLE 1.   New Antithrombotic Drugs

Heparin-related drugs	**Biotechnology-based proteins** (cont'd.)
Low-molecular-weight heparins	Antithrombin III
Medium-molecular-weight heparins	Antithrombin III–heparin complexes
High-molecular-weight heparins	Recombinant heparin cofactor II
Chemically modified heparins	Glycoprotein-targeting proteins and peptides
Dermatans	Protease-specific inhibitors
Heparans	Recombinant tissue factor pathway inhibitor
Semisynthetic heparin derivatives (Suleparoide)	**Peptides and related antithrombotic peptides**
Chemically synthesized antithrombotic oligo-	Hirulogs
saccharides	D-Me-Phe-Pro-Arg-derived antithrombotic drugs
Sulfated dextrans	Argatroban
Synthetic hypersulfated compounds	Inogatran
Polyanionic agents	Borohydride derivatives
Marine polysaccharides	**Synthetic inhibitors of thrombin**
Antiplatelet drugs	Peptide inhibitors
Ticlopidine and related antiplatelet drugs	Heterocyclic conjugates
Platelet and related phosphodiesterase inhibitors	Nucleic acid derivatives
Prostanoid modulators (Iloprost)	Others
Eicosanoids and related drugs	**Recombinant inhibitors of thrombin**
ω-3 Fatty acids and fish oil-related products	Hirudin and related proteins
Antibodies targeting membrane glycoproteins	Site-specific proteins
Peptides and proteins modulating platelet function	Others
Endothelial-lining modulators	**Polytherapy**
Nucleic acid derivatives (defibrotide)	Heparin and antiplatelet drugs
Sulfomucopolysaccharide mixtures	Coumadin and antiplatelet drugs
1-Deamino-8-D-arginine vasopressin (DDAVP)	Thrombolytic agents and heparin
and related peptides	Thrombolytic agents and antiplatlet drugs
Growth factor-related peptides	Recombinant drugs and conjugates
Protein digests	Thrombolytic agents and hirudin
Vitamins	Hirudin and glycoprotein-targeting antibodies
Viscosity modulators	Thrombolytic agents and hirudin, other thrombin
Synthetic and natural polymers	inhibitors
Pentoxifylline	**Newer drug delivery systems and formulations**
Venoms (defibrinating agents)	Oral agents
Polyelectrolytes	Ointments
Biotechnology-based proteins	Transdermal agents
Tissue-type plasminogen activator and mutants	Pulmonary agents
Hirudin, mutants, and fragments	Sustained-release formulations
Activated protein C	Target-specific antithrombotic drugs (antibody-
Thrombomodulin	directed)
Thrombomodulin–thrombin complexes	Catheters and devices capable of targeted drug delivery

angiography, angioplasty, atherectomy, intravascular laser and ultrasonic procedures, and thrombolysis. Significant advances in biotechnology and separation techniques have resulted in development of newer antithrombotic drugs (Table 1).[22–29]

The large number of new antithrombotic drugs acting on the vascular endothelium, platelets, viscosity, and various steps of the coagulation cascade represents a major challenge to the practicing radiologist, who must become familiar with the pharmacologic and physiologic actions of the new agents as they begin to be used in the angiographic suite. Recently, the Food and Drug Administration granted approval for a low-molecular-weight heparin (LMWH), enoxaparin, for postsurgical prophylaxis of thromboembolism in patients undergoing hip replacement surgery. This agent is claimed to exhibit higher safety and efficacy profiles than heparin and may be used during angiographic procedures. Recombinant hirudin and hirulog are highly potent anticoagulants that can be readily used as substitutes for heparin. However, they are currently undergoing clinical trials. It is expected that several of the newer agents will become available for anticoagulation in the future and may be of value to interventional radiologists.

TABLE 2.   Comparison of Unfractionated Heparin and Low-Molecular-Weight Heparin

Unfractionated Heparin	Low-Molecular-Weight Heparin
Similar manufacturing methods	Different manufacturing methods
Molecular weight 12–60 kd	Molecular weight 3–7 kd
Standardization by United States Pharmacopeia method	No uniform methods for standardization
Products can be interchanged for prophylactic and therapeutic indications	Products cannot be interchanged for any indication
Product equivalence in both in vitro and in vivo settings	Product inequivalence in both in vitro and in vivo settings

Low-Molecular-Weight Heparin

For nearly 50 years, unfractionated heparin (UFH) remained unchallenged by other anticoagulants. To recognize that native heparin is not always the optimal means of anticoagulation is the first step toward the use of heparin derivatives, which have greater safety and improved efficacy.

Thus, the development of LMWHs has started a new era in management of thrombotic disorders. These agents are now considered to be the gold standard for the prophylaxis of deep vein thrombosis. LMWHs provide an attractive option for anticoagulation because of their safety profile, especially in interventional radiology. Because of their lesser anticoagulant yet improved antithrombotic efficacy, they may prove to be valuable alternatives to heparin. LMWHs are manufactured by chemical or enzymatic depolymerization of the benzylic esters of UFH and exhibit different biochemical and pharmacologic properties.

Because of their lower molecular weight and charge density characteristics, LMWHs are almost completely absorbed when given subcutaneously. In contrast, heparin is only partially absorbed. Table 2 compares UFH and LMWH. The advantages of LMWHs are listed in Table 3. The relative significance of the use of heparin, LMWH, and hirudin in angiography is summarized in Table 4.

LMWHs may be used as a heparin substitute in patients with HIT and heparin-induced platelet aggregation (HIPA). They produce the following effects:

1. Less bleeding
2. Lower incidence of HIT and HIPA
3. Longer duration of action
4. Fewer synergistic actions with ionic contrast media

The potential uses of LMWHs in interventional radiology include the following:

1. Substitute anticoagulant during angiography
2. Prophylaxis for contrast media-induced phlebothrombosis

TABLE 3.   Advantages of Low-Molecular-Weight Heparins

• Stronger antithrombotic effect on a lower anticoagulant level than heparin

• Higher safety index due to lesser anticoagulant action

• Higher bioavailability

• Subcutaneous administration

• Sustained anticoagulant and antithrombotic actions

• Use in patients with congenital antithrombin III (AT III) deficiency because LMWHs produce their actions via non-AT III pathways

• Less platelet interaction than heparin; hence smaller incidence of thrombocytopenia and platelet activation

• Less neutralization by endogenous antiheparin agents such as platelet factor 4 and histidine-rich glycoproteins

• Monitoring may not be necessary in prophylaxis

TABLE 4. Heparin vs. Low-Molecular-Weight Heparin and Hirudin in Angiography

	Heparin	LMWH	Hirudin
Anticoagulation during PTCA	++++	++	++++
Drug interaction during PTCA	+	±	±
Platelet activation control	+	+	–
Tissue factor release inhibition	–	–	–
Inhibition of formed thrombin	++	+	++
Inhibition of vascular spasm	+	+	–
Growth factor released	+	++	–

LMWH = low-molecular-weight heparin, PTCA = percutaneous transluminal coronary angioplasty.
From Fareed J, Walenga JM, Leya I, et al: Some objective considerations for the use of heparins and recombinant hirudin in percutaneous transluminal coronary angioplasty. Semin Thromb Hemost 17:455–469, 1991.

3. Prophylaxis in patients at high risk for the following:
   Hyperviscosity syndrome
   Hemoconcentration
   Sickle-cell disease
   Paraproteinemias
   Thrombophilia with hemostatic deficit (protein C, protein S, AT III)
   Antiphospholipid syndrome
   Pregnancy-associated thrombosis (LMWHs do not cross placenta)
4. Prophylaxis against postoperative angiography-related thromboembolism
5. Postprocedure discharge prophylaxis
6. Prophylaxis against restenosis after angiography, atherectomy (laser, ultrasound)

Hirudin and Hirulog

The recognition of thrombin as the main mediator of thrombogenesis has led to the development of recombinant and synthetic drugs that mainly target this enzyme. Medicinal leeches have been known to secrete a potent anticoagulant, hirudin. Through biotechnology, this 65-amino acid-containing protein is now commercially produced. Currently, several versions of r-hirudin are in clinical trials for various anticoagulation indications. Hirulog (Biogen, Cambridge, MA), a synthetic analog of hirudin, has been extensively tested in angioplasty and other interventional procedures. These two anticoagulants may have substantial advantages compared with conventional heparin. Unlike heparins, hirudin and Hirulog require no endogenous cofactors such as AT III. Thus they produce their anticoagulant effect with no mediator, and hemodilution does not affect their potency. Because both agents can be mixed with contrast media and exhibit no incompatible behavior, they may be the anticoagulants of choice for interventional radiologists.

Hirudin, the anticoagulant agent derived from leeches (*Hirudo medicinalis*)[54] and now available by recombinant DNA technology, has been shown to be more effective than heparin in preventing thrombosis.[44,55] Hirudin binds strongly and specifically to thrombin. After binding with hirudin, thrombin loses its effects on platelets, particularly thrombin-induced platelet aggregation. Thrombin acts as an agonist for a number of cellular activators, such as those producing stimulation of endothelial and smooth muscle cells and proliferation of fibroblasts.[8,7,69] Thrombin also plays an essential role in recurrent stenosis after PTCA. Recombinant hirudin and synthetic hirudin are currently being evaluated.[44,55,65,78]

The advantages of hirudin over heparin include the following:
- Recombinant hirudin is 3–5 times more potent than heparin in its anticoagulant actions.
- For acute anticoagulation, hirudin does not produce side effects such as heparin-induced thrombocytopenia or thrombosis.

- Hirudin does not require protamine for neutralization.
- Because its anticoagulant actions last for a short time, hirudin can be given by controlled delivery systems.
- Recombinant hirudin is not known to induce activation of fibrinolysis during surgery, unlike heparin; hence, no bleeding complications are seen.

Hirulog, a 20-amino acid, hirudin-based synthetic peptide and selective thrombin inhibitor, has emerged as as new antithrombotic drug that, unlike heparin, can effectively inhibit clot-bound thrombin and escape neutralization by activated platelets. It may be used as a surgical anticoagulant because of its anticoagulant actions. In a recent clinical trial, Topol et al. concluded that for the first time it is possible to perform coronary angioplasty with an anticoagulant other than heparin in patients pretreated with aspirin. They also observed that Hirulog was associated with a rapid-onset, dose-dependent anticoagulant effect.[77] In another clinical trial, Canon et al. concluded that Hirulog provided a predictable level of anticoagulation and appeared to have a potent yet well-tolerated anticoagulant profile in patients with coronary artery disease.[6]

The advantages of Hirulog over heparin include the following:
- Its shorter half-life requires adjustment of dose by controlled delivery system.
- No endogenous modulator, such as AT III, is needed for anticoagulant action.
- Hirulog can inactivate clot-bound thrombin; hence, proteolytic activation of platelets and cleavage of fibrinogen are prevented.
- Hirulog is not neutralized by components of platelet release reaction, such as PF4 and heparinase.

Table 5 compares heparin and recombinant hirudin for use in coronary angiography.

Hirudin and Hirulog represent a unique approach to anticoagulation that is much easier to manage during interventional radiologic procedures. Because of their homogeneous chemical nature as simple proteins, these agents do not exhibit incompatibility with contrast media. Both agents are direct thrombin inhibitors and require no endogenous plasmatic cofactors. Hemodilution and separation from blood do not alter their anticoagulant properties. More importantly, both agents are 3–5 times more potent as anticoagulants than heparin. Because of their shorter half-life, protamine neutralization is not required. Neither agent produces HIT or white clot syndrome. Both agents can be all-purpose anticoagulants during angioplasty. Because of their direct thrombin action, they do not activate fibrinolysis and compromise hemostasis.

The development of dry reagent technology (TAS Analyzer, Cardiovascular Diagnostics, Raleigh, NC), based on the principle of motion of paramagnetic iron oxide particles (PIOP), offers a rapid point of care monitoring of anticoagulant drugs. Clotting tests such as prothrombin time (PT), APTT, and the Heparin Management Test (HMT), can be performed with this technology. Supplementation of the dry reagent formulation with ecarin has resulted in the development of ecarin test cards for monitoring of antithrombin agents.

TABLE 5. Heparin vs. Recombinant Hirudin for Anticoagulation During Coronary Angioplasty

Heparin	Recombinant Hirudin
1–5 U/ml, depending on procedure	10–30 µg, depending on procedure
Generally administered via intravenous bolus	Administered via intravenous bolus or continuous infusion
Requires protamine neutralization	May not require neutralization
Adverse effects include thrombocytopenia, thrombosis, and allergic reactions	No similar effects
Bleeding complications (spinal anesthesia)	May not have bleeding complications if dose is carefully titrated
Hemodilution alters degree of anticoagulation	Hemodilution alters degree of anticoagulation

THERAPEUTIC FIBRINOLYSIS

Hemostasis is a delicate balance between coagulation and fibrinolysis. Fibrinolysis involves fragmentation of fibrin into fibrin split products. Urokinase or tissue-type plasminogen activator (tPA) activates the circulating or thrombus-entrapped plasminogen into plasmin. This step can be inhibited by plasminogen activator inhibitor (PAI-1). Plasmin acts by degrading fibrinogen into fibrinogen degradation products and fibrin into fibrin split products. Plasmin is inhibited by α_2-macroglobulin, α_2-antiplasmin, and AT III. The presence of fibrin split products in the plasma is evidence that fibrinolysis is taking place.

Therapeutic fibrinolysis involves administration of various thrombolytic agents, such as streptokinase, urokinase, and tPA. Indications include (1) occlusion of venous vessels (e.g., superior mesenteric, pulmonary, coronary, and peripheral arteries); (2) thrombosed arterial grafts; (3) deep vein thrombosis with massive pulmonary embolism, and (4) occluded heart valves. The recommended dosages are as follows:

Urokinase: 20,000–100,000 U/hr or 10,000 U/min

Streptokinase: 5,000–30,000 U/hr or 3000 U every 2 minutes

tPA: 0.02–0.05 mg/kg/hr

Thrombolytic therapy should be followed by heparin, because it results in the depletion of plasminogen, which leads to thrombosis. Low-dose heparin during thrombolytic therapy prevents pericatheter thrombosis.[18]

Complications of therapeutic fibrinolysis include local hemorrhage at the catheter insertion site, retroperitoneal or cerebral hemorrhage, distal embolization, and pericatheter thrombosis and secondary embolization. Gofette at al. have shown severe complications in 18–50% of cases using streptokinase and 5–16% using urokinase.[34]

Absolute contraindications include active bleeding, cerebral tumor, cerebrovascular accident, and uncontrolled coagulopathy. Relative contraindications include recent history of bleeding, recent surgery, postpartum status, major trauma, gastric ulcer, ulcerative colitis, arterial hypertension, cardiac thrombi, bacterial endocarditis, and hepatic or renal insufficiency.

Thrombolysis is reversed by stopping the thrombolytic infusion; use of epsilon amino caproic acid (EACA), aprotinin, fresh frozen plasma, or cryoprecipitate (fibrinogen); or platelet transfusion.

Table 6 compares various thrombolytic agents in regard to cost, safety, and efficacy. Guidelines for prevention of postlytic occlusion are given in Table 7.

Fibrinogen should not be depleted in patients undergoing thrombolytic therapy. Thus, it should be monitored when large doses of thrombolytic agents are used. Patients who have large titers of plasminogen activator and antistreptolysin resist thrombolysis. Thus, these parameters should be measured. Table 8 summarizes replacement of heparin with LMWH. Table 9 lists the sources of currently available LMWHs, hirudin, and Hirulog.

The peripheral angiogram in a patient with HIT is shown in Figure 1. The peripheral angiogram showing recanalization after the use of Hirulog as an adjunct to peripheral angioplasty and thrombolytic therapy is shown in Figure 2. Table 10 lists the advantages of synthetic peptide inhibitors and Table 11 the advantages of alternative anticoagulants.

TABLE 6.   A Comparison of Various Thrombolytic Agents

Thrombolytic Agent	Cost	Safety	Efficacy
Streptokinase	+	++	++++
Urokinase	++	+++	+++
tPA	++++	++++	+++
APSAC	+++	++	++++
Prourokinase (SCU-PA)	+++	++	++

tPA = tissue-type plasminogen activator, APSAC = acylated plasminogen streptokinase activator complex, SCU-PA = single-chain urokinase-type plasminogen activator.

TABLE 7. Guidelines for Prevention of Postlytic Occlusion

1. Optimal use of thrombolytic agent
2. Objective appraisal of lytic process
3. Use of adjunct anticoagulants (hirudin and heparin)
4. Periodic reevaluation of lytic region

TABLE 8. Replacement of Heparin with Low-Molecular-Weight Heparin*

Conventional angiography
   Heparin: 5–10,000 U
   Low-molecular-weight heparin: 2–3 mg/kg

Angioplasty procedures
   Heparin: 10,000–15,000 U
   Low-molecular-weight heparin: 250–300 mg
   Hirudin: 150–200 mg
   Hirulog: dose to be determined

Average approximate amounts. Adjusted dosage for underweight and overweight patients improves safety and efficacy.

TABLE 9. Sources of New Anticoagulants

Trade Name	Manufacturer	Method of Preparation
Currently available LMWHs		
Fraxiparin, Seleparin	Sanofi, Paris	Fractionation, optimized nitrous acid depolymerization
Enoxaparin, Clexane, Lovenox	Rhone-Poulenc Rorer, Paris	Benzylation followed by alkaline hydrolysis
Fragmin	Kabi, Stockholm	Controlled nitrous acid depolymerization
Fluxum	Opocrin, Corlo, Italy	Peroxidative cleavage
Ardeparin, Normiflo	Wyeth, Philadelphia	Peroxidative cleavage
Logiparin	Novo, Copenhagen	Heparinase digestion
Innohep	Leo, Copenhagen	Heparinase digestion
Sandoparin, Certoparin	Sandoz AG, Ludwigshafen, Germany	Isoamyl nitrate digestion
Reviparin, Clivarin	Knoll AG, Ludwigshafen, Germany	Nitrous acid digestion
Boxol	Rovi, Madrid	β-Elimination or nitrous acid digestion
Miniparin	Syntex, Buenos Aires	Nitrous acid digestion
Clivarin	Knoll AG, Ludwigshafen, Germany	Controlled nitrous acid depolymerization followed by chromatographic purification
Sources of hirudin		
Hoechst (Frankfurt)		
Ciba-Geigy (Basel)		
Souces of Hirulog		
Biogen (Cambridge, MA)		

LMWHs = low-molecular-weight heparins.

TABLE 10. Advantages of Synthetic Peptide Inhibitors

• Pure material
• Usually single mechanism of action (thrombin inhibitors have been shown to be effective anticoagulants)
• No dependence on cofactor for activity expression
• Short half-life

TABLE 11. Advantages of Alternative Anticoagulants

• Reduced or no platelet interaction	• No plasma cofactors needed for action
• Specific activity	• Consistent lot-to-lot preparations
• Short half-life	• Pure material

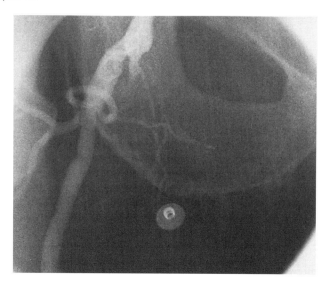

FIGURE 1. Peripheral angiogram in a patient with heparin-induced platelet aggregation and thrombosis, performed by percutaneous insertion of the catheter into the left axillary artery by the Seldinger technique, with 20 ml of Iohexol and 20 ml of Hexabrix. The right proximal superficial femoral artery was 100% obstructed with a large clot. The profunda is patent. The dye was injected proximal to the take-off of the profunda.

Table 12 summarizes the rebound phenomenon seen with the use of thrombin inhibitors; Table 13, the coupling of thrombin inhibitors with other agents for target-specific use; and Table 14, the cost consideration of thrombin inhibitors in the management of cardiovascular disorders.

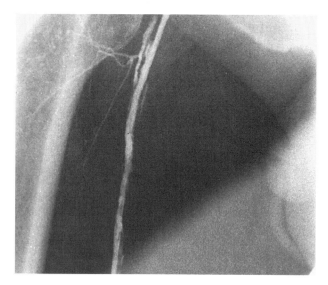

FIGURE 2. Peripheral angiogram showing recanalization of the right superficial femoral artery after thrombolytic therapy (100,000 U of urokinase) and angioplasty. Hirulog was used after angioplasty. Dye was injected distal to the take-off of the profunda, demonstrating reestablishment of flow in the superficial femoral artery.

TABLE 12.   Thrombin Inhibitors: The Rebound Phenomenon

- Increased thrombin formation after withdrawal of argatroban
- Increased symptoms of angina after withdrawal of thrombin inhibitor
- Concomitant use of aspirin may prevent rebound phenomenon

TISSUE FACTOR PATHWAY INHIBITOR

The concept of in vivo and in vitro inhibition of the procoagulant effect of tissue extracts by serum led Hjort in 1957 to show that, although serum did not inhibit either factor VII or tissue factor individually, it did inhibit the factor VII–tissue factor complex (convertin).[40] This inhibitor was later designated as extrinsic pathway inhibitor (EPI)[60] or lipoprotein-associated coagulation inhibitor (LACI).[3] Recently it has been named tissue factor pathway inhibitor (TFPI) by the ISTH subcommittee.

Biochemistry and Molecular Biology

TFPI is a protein of 276 amino acid residues with a molecular weight of 32 kd. It consists of three Kunitz-type domains, an acidic N-terminus, and a basic C-terminus. The C-terminus of TFPI is essential to its anticoagulant activity[57] and is thought to be involved in the binding of TFPI to heparin. The first Kunitz-type domain has been identified as the site of binding of the TF–FVIIa complex, and the second domain binds FXa.[33] The function of the third Kunitz domain is unknown. The circulating free TFPI amounts to approximately 5% of the plasma TFPI. About 80–90% of TFPI is bound to lipoprotein (low-density lipoprotein > high-density lipoprotein > very-low-density lipoprotein). In addition, 3–5% of the total TFPI is carried by alpha granules of the platelets. The TFPI gene has been cloned, and now TFPI is available through recombinant DNA technology.

TFPI is the feedback inhibitor of the factor VIIa–TF complex formed on the initiation of the extrinsic pathway of coagulation after vascular injury.[17] It has been postulated that initially TFPI binds and inhibits factor Xa.[64] This complex then binds and inactivates the TF–FVIIa complex, forming a quaternary TFPI–Xa–TF–VIIa inhibitory complex.[4,33,79]

Endothelial cells are considered to be the most important sites for the production of TFPI. About 50–90% of the total intravascular pool of TFPI is bound to the endothelium. The other two intravascular pools of TFPI are plasma and platelets. Less than 2.5% of the total intravascular pool of TFPI is located in platelets and released on platelet activation.

Plasma levels of TFPI can be determined by functional chromogenic-based assay, functional clot-based assay, immunologic and radioimmunoassays that quantitate TFPI antigen, and ligand and Western blot techniques.

Clinical Implications

1. Although TFPI is currently under development as a new anticoagulant agent, it will be some time before validation studies are completed for its use in surgical medicine.

2. Sequential compression devices mediate their antithrombotic action via endogenous release of TFPI.

3. Heparin and LMWH release endogenous TFPI, implying that TFPI is important to heparin's effect.

TABLE 13.   Coupled Thrombin Inhibitors for Target-specific Use

1. Coupling with glycoprotein IIb/IIIa-targeting peptides and Fab fragments
2. Coupling to fragments of antibodies against fibrin beta chain
3. Coupling with heparin pentasaccharide
4. Coupling with tissue factor pathway inhibitor
5. Polyetheylene glycol (PEG) coupling for longer-lasting effects and targeted use

TABLE 14.   Cost Considerations of Thrombin Inhibitors in the Management
of Cardiovascular Disorders

1. High cost in comparison with heparin
2. Three-day course of intravenous hirudin costs more than $1000
3. Additional monitoring for efficacy and safety also add to cost

Summary

1. Recombinant (r) TFPI is a potent anticoagulant capable of producing its effects independently of any endogenous mediators.

2. In comparison with AT III and unfractionated heparin, r-TFPI is a stronger antithrombotic agent in experimental systems. However, UFH–AT III complexes may exhibit stronger actions in other systems.

3. Unlike r-hirudin, r-TFPI does not inhibit thrombin. However, it strongly inhibits FXa, elastase, and trypsin.

4. TFPI also inhibits tissue factor-mediated activation of platelets, as measured by flow cytometry.

5. UFH and some of its analogs increase plasma levels of TFPI antigen.

6. Molecular alterations of full-length TFPI may modulate its biochemical and pharmacologic actions.

With the development of newer anticoagulant agents, it is now possible to use alternatives to heparin. The development of LMWHs through chemical or enzymatic depolymerization of heparin has signalled a new era in the anticoagulant and antithrombotic management of thrombotic disorders. LMWHs have less anticoagulant yet improved antithrombotic efficacy.

Aprosulate, a sulfated derivative of lactobionic acid, a synthetic analog of heparin, was developed by Luitpold Pharma, Munich; it is currently in phase II trials.[50] Recombinant and synthetic hirudins are currently under evaluation. These specific thrombin inhibitors are more effective than heparin in preventing thrombosis. Hirulog, a hirudin-based synthetic peptide, effectively inhibits clot-bound thrombin. Topol et al. have shown that it is now possible to perform coronary angioplasty with an anticoagulant other than heparin.[77] In an adjunctive therapy with r-tPA, hirudin was given to patients suffering from acute myocardial infarction. This approach led to early, complete, and sustained patency with a reduction in reocclusion rates. Patency rates after adjunctive therapy with streptokinase and hirudin are under investigation (38th Congress of the German Society for Research in Thrombosis and Hemostasis GTH, February 16–19, 1994, Munich). TFPI has emerged as a potential anticoagulant drug. The critical role played by the activation of the extrinsic pathway in thrombotic reocclusion after vascular injury has prompted the idea of possible use of TFPI for prevention of restenosis after angioplasty.

ANTIPLATELET DRUGS

In view of the hemostatic effects of contrast media, it is important to consider the use of antiplatelet drugs in diagnostic interventional radiology. Aspirin is an effective antiplatelet agent for both primary and secondary prevention of thrombotic events by inhibiting thromboxane A_2 (TXA_2)-dependent platelet function with low risk of bleeding.[31,35,36,59,63,80] Acute arterial occlusion as a complication of atherosclerosis, vascular injury, or hypercoagulable states warrants the use of antiplatelet drugs. Antiplatelet drugs inhibit the formation of platelet-rich thrombi on atherosclerotic plaques.[30] Aspirin is far less effective for the prevention of atherogenesis and restenosis after angioplasty or arterial surgery. The platelet glycoprotein (GP) IIb/IIIa receptor is platelet-specific, mediates platelet aggregation by all physiologic agonists, and does not abolish platelet adhesion. Endothelial damage results in exposure of adhesive glycoproteins such as von Willebrand factor (VWF) and collagen.

Platelets first adhere and, with the help of the GPIIb/IIIa receptors, form a single layer of platelets. The conformation of the GPIIb/IIIa receptors is modified after activation of the platelets, which enables its binding to fibrinogen and VWF. Further platelet recruitment results in the formation of aggregates, which, if large, can cause mechanical vascular obstruction and may also release vasospastic substances such as TXA_2 and serotonin, resulting in functional vascular occlusion. Dislodgement of platelet aggregates may result in embolization with ischemia of the microcirculation.[10] Blocking of the GPIIb/IIIa receptor by antiplatelet agents blocks platelet aggregation induced by all agonists, prevents thrombus formation, and keeps platelet adhesion intact. Various agents, such as 7E 3 monoclonal antibody,[11,12] snake venom proteins, oligopeptides, and oligopeptidomimetics, are available.[13,15] Because of antigenicity, snake venoms had limited development as therapeutic agents. The other nonpeptide GPIIb/IIIa inhibitors are RO44-9883 (Hoffman-LaRoche) and MK-383 (Merck).[13,15] Orally active agents are SC 54684 (Searle), RO43-8857 (Hoffman-LaRoche), GR 144053 (Glaxo), and DMP 728 (Dupont-Merck). Chronic GPIIb/IIIa blockade can be achieved using orally active antiplatelet agents.

Many of the GPIIB/IIIa inhibitors are undergoing clinical trials. Results of phase I and phase II studies with Integrelin, MK-383, RO44-9883, and C7E3 Fab in PTCA, unstable angina, and acute myocardial infarction are quite promising.[48,51,58,66,68,74–76]

CONCLUSIONS AND FUTURE CONSIDERATIONS

Heparin, despite its limitations, is still considered the gold standard in the effective anticoagulant management of thrombotic disorders. However, in patients who have HIT, heparin-induced thrombosis or white clot syndrome, heparin resistance, or AT III deficiency, there is a genuine need for newer anticoagulants as alternatives to heparin. LMWHs have a stronger antithrombotic effect, higher safety index, higher bioavailability, and more sustained anticoagulant and antithrombotic actions than heparin. The antithrombin drugs provide significant advantages over conventional heparin. However, the lack of an effective antagonist to these antithrombin drugs and the serious complication of intracerebral bleeding observed in various clinical trials pose a major limitation to their use. Because thrombin acts as an agonist for stimulation of endothelial and smooth muscle cells and proliferation of fibroblasts, antithrombin drugs may play an essential role in the effective management of recurrent restenosis after PTCA. Similarly, tissue factor-induced coagulation mediated by activation of the extrinsic pathway plays a key role in thrombotic reocclusion after vascular injury. Haskel et al. have shown that TFPI prevents restenosis after thrombolysis.[39]

Further understanding of the pathophysiology of restenosis will enable the development of newer or improvised pharmacologic modes of prevention of restenosis after angioplasty. Although some of the antithrombin drugs are approved for clinical use on a compassionate basis, in view of their potential to cause severe bleeding complications due to the lack of an effective antagonist, careful dose selection and titration on an individual basis are essential in patients undergoing major surgery or interventional radiologic procedure. Furthermore, the pharmacokinetics and pharmacodynamics of these agents may be quite different in patients with multiple organ failure or toxicity due to existing pathology, adjunct medications (e.g., contrast media), or their possible interactions. Animal experimental data are carefully interpreted for antithrombin dose selection because of the species differences in pharmacokinetics and pharmacodynamics of these agents as well as species differences in hemostatic parameters and responses.

The development of newer antiplatelet drugs such as GPIIb/IIIa inhibitors has initiated a new era in the effective management of arterial thrombosis and prevention of atherogenesis and restenosis after angioplasty by inhibiting platelet aggregation without abolishing platelet adhesion. The combination of unfractionated heparin and GPIIb/IIIa inhibitors may have synergistic anticoagulant effects. However, the interaction of ionic and nonionic contrast media with a combination of unfractionated heparin and GPIIb/IIIa inhibitors has shown no synergistic advantage in anticoagulant responses, as measured by HMT with dry reagent technology (Cardiovascular Diagnostics, Raleigh, NC), when these agents were supplemented ex vivo in human whole blood. Further experiments are being carried out to validate these interactions and to evaluate their clinical implications.

A bewildering array of newer anticoagulant drugs is available for interventional radiologic procedures or adjunctive use in various underlying conditions. An astute physician or interventional radiologist should be familiar with the pharmacokinetics and pharmacodynamics of these agents, drug–drug interactions, and drug combination–contrast media interactions to ensure improved safety and efficacy. The 1990s will witness many advancements in anticoagulant management of patients undergoing interventional radiologic procedures.

REFERENCES

1. Almén T: Contrast agent design: Some aspects on the synthesis of water soluble contrast agents of low osmolality. J Theor Biol 24:216–226, 1969.
2. Bell WR: Heparin associated thrombocytopenia and thrombosis. J Lab Clin Med 111:600–605, 1988.
3. Broze GJ, Girard TJ, Novotny WF: Regulation of coagulation by multivalent Kunitz type inhibitor. Biochemistry 29:7539–7546, 1990.
4. Broze GJ, Warren LA, Novotny WF, et al: The lipoprotein associated coagulation inhibitor that inhibits the factor VIIa–tissue factor complex also inhibits factor Xa: Insight into the possible mechanisms of action. Blood 71:335–343, 1988.
5. Bush WH, Swanson DP: Acute reactions to intravascular contrast media: Types, risk factors, recognition and specific treatment. Am J Radiol 157:1153–1161, 1991.
6. Canon CP, Maraganore JM, Loscalzo J, et al: Antiocoagulant effects of hirulog, a novel thrombin inhibitor in patients with coronary artery disease. Am J Cardiol 71:778–782, 1993.
7. Chesebro JH, Zoldhelyi P, Badimon L, Fuster V: Role of thrombin in arterial thrombosis: Implications for therapy. Thromb Haemost 66:1–5, 1991.
8. Chesebro JH, Fuster V: Antithrombotic therapy for acute myocardial infarction: Mechanism of prevention of deep venous, left ventricular and coronary artery thromboembolism. Circulation 74(Suppl III):1110–1111, 1986.
9. Chin RC, Samson R: Complement (C3, C4) consumption in cardiopulmonary bypass, cardioplegia and protamine administration. Ann Thorac Surg 37:229, 1984.
10. Coller BS, Anderson K, Weisman HF: New antiplatelet agents: Platelet GPIIb/IIIa antagonists. Thromb Hemost 74:302–308, 1995.
11. Coller BS, Scudder LE, Beer J, et al: Monoclonal antibodies to platelet GPIIb/IIIa as antithrombotic agents. Ann N Y Acad Sci 614:193–213, 1991.
12. Coller BS: A new murine monoclonal antibody: Reports on activation dependent change in the conformation and/or microenvironment of the platelet glycoprotein IIb/IIIa complex. J Clin Invest 76:101–108, 1985.
13. Cook NS, Kottirsch G, Zerwes HG: Platelet glycoprotein IIb/IIIa antagonists. Drugs Future 19:135–159, 1994.
14. Courin A, Streisan RL, Greineder JK, Stuckey JH: Protamine sulfate administration and the cardiovascular system. J Thorac Cardiovasc Surg 62:193, 1971.
15. Cox D, Aoki T, Seki J, et al: The pharmacology of integrins. Med Res Rev 14:195–228, 1994.
16. Crafoord C: Preliminary report on post-operative treatment with heparin as a preventive of thrombosis. Acta Chirur Scand 79:407–426, 1937.
17. Davie EW, Fujikawa E, Kiesel W: The coagulation cascade: Initiation, maintenance and regulation. Biochemistry 30:10363–10370, 1991.
18. Dondelinger RF: Use of anticoagulant and clotting agents. In Steinbrich W, Gross-Fengells W (eds): Interventional Radiology, Adjunctive Medication and Monitoring. New York, Springer Verlag, 1991, pp 102–121.
19. Esplugas E, Cequier A, Jara F, et al: Risk of thrombosis during coronary angioplasty with low osmolality contrast media. Am J Cardiol 68:1020–1024, 1991.
20. Fabian I, Aronson M: Mechanism of heparin rebound in in vitro study. Thromb Res 18:535, 1980.
21. Fadall MA, Ledbetter M, Papacostas CA, et al: Mechanism responsible for the cardiovascular depressant effect of protamine sulfate. Ann Surg 180:232, 1974.
22. Fareed J, Bacher P, Messmore HL, et al: Pharmacologic modulation of fibrinolysis by antithrombotic and cardiovascular drugs. Prog Cardiovasc Dis 6:379–398, 1992.
23. Fareed J, Callas DD, Hoppensteadt D, et al: Recent development in antithrombotic agents. Exp Opin Invest Drugs 4:389–412, 1995.
24. Fareed J, Walenga JM, Lassen M, et al: Pharmacologic profile of a low molecular weight heparin (Enoxaparin): Experimental and clinical validation of the prophylactic antithrombotic effects. Acta Chirur Scand 556(Suppl):75–90, 1990.

25. Fareed J, Walenga JM, Pifarre R, et al: Some objective considerations for the neutralization of the anticoagulant actions of recombinant hirudin. Haemostasis 21:64–72, 1991.
26. Fareed J, Walenga JM, Hoppensteadt D, et al: Study on the in vitro and in vivo activities of seven low molecular weight heparins. Haemostasis 18:3–15, 1988.
27. Fareed J, Walenga JM, Racanelli A, et al: Validity of the newly established low molecular weight heparin standard in cross-referencing low molecular weight heparins. Hemostasis 18:33–47, 1988.
28. Fareed J, Walenga JM, Pifarre R: Newer approaches to the pharmacologic management of acute myocardial infarction. Card Surg State Art Rev 6:101–111, 1992.
29. Fareed J, Walenga JM, Hoppensteadt D, et al: Chemical and biochemical heterogeneity in low molecular weight heparins: Implications for clinical use and standardization. Semin Thromb Hemost 15:440–463, 1989.
30. Fuster V, Badimon L, Badimon JJ, Chesebro JH: The pathogenesis of coronary artery disease and acute coronary syndromes (Parts 1 and 2). N Engl J Med 326:242–250, 310–318, 1992.
31. Fuster V, Dyken ML, Volkonas PS, Hennekens C: Aspirin as a therapeutic agent in cardiovascular disease. Circulation 87:659–675, 1993.
32. Gasperetti CM, Feldman MD, Burwell LR, et al: Influence of contrast media on thrombus formation during coronary angioplasty. J Am Coll Cardiol 18:433–450, 1991.
33. Girard TJ, Warren LA, Novotny WF, et al: Functional significance of the Kunitz type inhibitor domain of lipoprotein associated coagulation inhibitor. Nature 338:518–520, 1989.
34. Gofette P, Kurdziel JC, Dondelinger RF: Local arterial thrombolytic infusion: Therapeutic effects and complications. Acta Radiol 32:305–310, 1991.
35. Goodnight SH, Coull BM, McAnulty JH, Taylor LM: Antiplatelet therapy (Parts 1 and II). West J Med 158:385–392, 506–514, 1993.
36. Goodnight SH: Antiplatelet therapy in cardiovascular disease. In Hull RD, Pineo GF (eds): Disorders of Thrombosis. Philadelphia, W.B. Saunders, 1995, pp 31–43.
37. Grines CL, Diaz C, Mickelson J: Acute thrombosis in a canine model of arterial injury: Effect of ionic versus non-ionic contrast media. Circulation 80(Suppl 2):411, 1989.
38. Grollman JH, Chi C, Astone RA: Thromboembolic complications in coronary angiography associated with the use of non-ionic contrast media. Cathet Cardiovasc Diag 14:159–164, 1988.
39. Haskel EJ, Torr SR, Day KC, et al: Prevention of arterial reocclusion after thrombolysis with recombinant lipoprotein associated coagulation inhibitor. Circulation 84:821–827, 1991.
40. Hjort PF: Intermediate reactions in the coagulation of blood with thromboplastin. Scand J Clin Lab Invest 9(Suppl 27):1–173, 1957.
41. Howell WH, Holt E: The purification of heparin and its chemical and physiologic reactions. Bull Johns Hopkins Hosp 42:199–207, 1928.
42. Howell WH, Holt E: The purification of heparin and its presence in the blood. Am J Physiol 71:553–559, 1925.
43. Howell WH, Holt E: Two new factors in blood coagulation: Heparin and proantithrombin. Am J Physiol 47:328–334, 1918.
44. Hubbard T, Olivier T, Bacher P, et al: Use of recombinant hirudin to increase the patency rate of microanastomosis in a rabbit model. Blood Coag Fibrinol 2:101–103, 1991.
45. Hwang MH, Piao ZE, Murdock DK, et al: The potential risk of thrombosis during angiography using non-ionic contrast media [abstract]. J Am Coll Cardiol 11:55, 1988.
46. Jacobson PD, Rosenquist CJ: The introduction of low osmolar contrast agents in radiology: Medical, economic, legal and public policy issues. JAMA 260:1586–1592, 1988.
47. Kelton JG: Heparin induced thrombocytopenia. Hemostasis 16:173–186, 1986.
48. Keriakes D, Kleiman N, Ambrose J, et al: A dosing study in high risk PTCA of MK-383, a platelet IIb/IIIa antagonist [abstract]. Circulation 90:1–21, 1994.
49. Kesteven PJ, Pasoglu IT, Savidge GF: Significance of the whole blood activated clotting time in cardiopulmonary bypass. J Cardovasc Surg 27:85, 1986.
50. Klause RJ: Interaction of sulfated lactobionic acid amide LW 10082 with thrombin and its endogenous inhibitors. Thromb Res 62:557–656, 1991.
51. Kleiman NS, Ohman ME, Califf RM, et al: Profound inhibition of platelet aggregation with monoclonal antibody 7E3 Fab following thrombolytic therapy: Results of the TAMI 8 pilot study. J Am Coll Cardiol 22:381–389, 1993.
52. Kopko P, Smith DG, Bull BS: Thrombin generation in non-clottable mixtures of blood and non-ionic contrast agents. Radiology 174:459–461, 1990.
53. Mamon JF, Fareed J, Hoppensteadt D, Moncada R: Lack of inhibition of thrombin generation by non-ionic contrast media [brief communication]. Thromb Res 61:165–170, 1991.
54. Markwardt F, Fink J, Kaiser B, et al: Pharmacological survey of recombinant hirudin. Pharmazie 43:202–207, 1988.
55. Markwardt F: Hirudin and derivatives as anticoagulant agents. Thromb Haemost 66:141–152, 1991.
56. McLean J: The discovery of heparin. Circulation 19:75–78, 1959.

57. Nordfang B, Bjorn SE, Valentin S, et al: The C-terminus of tissue factor pathway inhibitor is essential to its anticoagulant activity. Biochemistry 30:10371–10376, 1991.
58. Ohman M, Kleiman N, Talley D, et al for the IMPACT-AMI study group: Simultaneous platelet glycoprotein IIb/IIIa integrin blockade with accelerated tissue plasminogen activator in acute myocardial infarction [abstract]. Circulation 90:I-564, 1994.
59. Patrono C: Drug therapy: Aspirin as an antiplatelet drug. N Engl J Med 330:1287–1294, 1994.
60. Rapaport SI: The extrinsic pathway inhibitor: A regulator of tissue factor dependent blood coagulation. Thromb Haemost 66:6–15, 1991.
61. Rasuli P: Blood clot formation in angiographic syringes containing non-ionic contrast media [letter]. Radiology 165:582, 1987.
62. Robertson HJ: Blood clot formation in angiographic syringes containing non-ionic contrast media [letter]. Radiology 162:621–622, 1987.
63. Roth GJ, Calverley DC: Aspirin, platelets and thrombosis: Theory and practice. Blood 83:885–898, 1994.
64. Sanders NL, Bajaj SP, Zivelin A, Rapaport SI: Inhibition of tissue factor/factor VIIa activity in plasma requires factor X and an additional plasma component. Blood 6:204–212, 1985.
65. Sarembock IJ, Gertz DS, Gimple LW, et al: Effectiveness of recombinant desulfato hirudin in reducing restenosis after balloon angioplasty of atherosclerotic femoral arteries in rabbits. Circulation 84:232–243, 1991.
66. Schulman SP, Goldschmidt-Clermont PJ, Navetta FI, et al: Integrelin in unstable angina: A double-blind randomized trial [abstract]. Circulation 88:I-608, 1993.
67. Sharath MD, Metzger WJ, Richerson HB, et al: Protamine induced fatal anaphylaxis. Prevalence of antiprotamine immunoglobulin E antibody. J Thorac Cardiovasc Surg 90:86, 1985.
68. Simoons ML, de Boer MJ, Van den Brand MJ, et al: The European Cooperative Study Group: Randomized trial of GPIIB/IIIa platelet receptor blocker in regulatory unstable angina. Circulation 89:596–603, 1994.
69. Stead NW: Therapeutic fibrinolysis. Circulation 84:905–948, 1991.
70. Stefaniszyn HJ, Novick RJ, Salerno TA: Toward a better understanding of the hemodynamic effects of protamine and heparin interaction. J Thorac Cardiovasc Surg 87:678, 1984.
71. Sutton D, Young JWR: A Concise Textbook of Clinical Imaging, 2nd ed. St. Louis, Mosby, 1995.
72. Swick M: Radiographic media in urology. The discovery of excretion urography: Historical and developmental aspects of the organically bound urographic media and their role in the varied diagnostic angiographic areas. Surg Clin North Am 58:977–994, 1978.
73. Swick M: Urographic media. Urology 4:750–757, 1974.
74. Tcheng JE, Ellis SG, Kleiman NS, et al: A multicenter, randomized, double-blind, placebo controlled trial of the platelet integrin glycoprotein IIb/IIIa blocker integrelin in elective coronary intervention. Circulation 91(8):2151–2157, 1995.
75. Theroux P, White H, David D, et al: A heparin-controlled study of MK-383 in unstable angina [abstract]. Circulation 90:I-231, 1994.
76. Theroux P, Kouz S, Knudston M, et al: A randomized double blind controlled trial with the non-peptide platelet GPIIb/IIIa antagonist RO 44-9883 in unstable angina [abstract]. Circulation 90:I-232, 1994.
77. Topol EJ, Bonan R, Jewitt D, et al: Use of a direct antithrombin, hirulog, in place of heparin during coronary angioplasty. Circulation 87:1622–1629, 1993.
78. Walenga JM, Bakhos M, Messmore HL, et al: Comparison of recombinant hirudin and heparin as an anticoagulant in a cardiopulmonary bypass model. Blood Coag Fibrinol 2:105–111, 1991.
79. Warn Cramer BJ, Rao LVM, Maki SL, Rapaport SL: Modification of extrinsic pathway inhibitor (EPI) and factor Xa that affects their ability to interact and to inhibit factor VIIa/tissue factor: Evidence for a two step model of inhibition. Thromb Haemost 60:453–456, 1988.
80. Willard JE, Lange RA, Hillis LD: Current concepts: The use of aspirin in ischemic heart disease. N Engl J Med 327:175–181, 1992.

CHAPTER 31

Orgaran Anticoagulation for Cardiopulmonary Bypass in Patients with Heparin-induced Thrombocytopenia

H. N. MAGNANI, M.B., M.Sc., Ph.D.
R. J. R. BEIJERING, M.D
J. W. TEN CATE, M.D., Ph.D.
B. H. CHONG, M.B., Ph.D.

Because of the combination of cooling, nonphysiologic flow patterns, and foreign surface activation of both the clotting cascade and platelets, cardiopulmonary bypass (CPB) surgery has complex effects on hemostasis. Technical advances and improved surgical techniques have been developed to handle such effects, but increased postoperative bleeding remains a problem.[2,13,26] Heparin is the most frequently used anticoagulant for CPB, but if heparin sensitivity develops, a safe, effective replacement must be found, often in an emergency setting. The most common type of heparin sensitivity is type II heparin-induced thrombocytopenia (HIT), which has an incidence of 1/2500 to 1/500 and high thrombotic morbidity and mortality rates.[32] If HIT develops in a patient about to undergo CPB, heparin is contraindicated. Anticoagulation is mandatory, but of the possible alternatives some may be unavailable or unsuitable, especially if cross-reactivity with the heparin-induced antibody is demonstrable. Of the present alternatives, Orgaran (ORG 10172, or danaparoid sodium; previously known as Lomoparan) has proved to be effective in a wide variety of clinical situations in routine patients and patients with HIT.[19] Patients with HIT have been treated in a compassionate use program that has grown rapidly and now includes 650 patients, of whom 572 have had HIT and a continuing need for antithrombotic and anticoagulant therapy.

The first patient in the compassionate use program to undergo CPB presented in 1985 for coronary artery bypass grafting (CABG). The dosing schedule was based on previous pharmacologic studies;[6,27] the fact that high intravenous infusions (up to 10,000 U/day) had already been used safely and successfully in patients with recent hemorrhagic stroke and either acute DVT or intracardiac thrombus;[9] and a study in dogs undergoing CPB.[14] The regimen attempted to limit the amount of Orgaran used according to a maximal intra-operative plasma anti-Xa activity of 1.5–2.0 U/ml. Despite successful surgery, the first patient developed severe postoperative bleeding but recovered without sequelae. Protamine sulphate was without obvious effect, as in earlier animal models of Orgaran-induced bleeding. No controlled study of Orgaran in patients undergoing CPB has been undertaken, but in view of the results in the first patient, over 50 more have since received Orgaran anticoagulation during CPB, generally with satisfactory results.

This chapter assesses 10 years of experience with Orgaran use for CPB in patients with HIT, draws conclusions about its risk-benefit profile, and proposes an improved dosing schedule.

COMPOSITION OF ORGARAN

Orgaran is a heterogeneous mixture of glycosaminoglycuronans: heparan sulphate (~84%), dermatan sulphate (~12%), and a small amount (up to 5 %) of chondroitin sulphate[20] isolated from animal intestinal mucosa. The final product has been shown by physicochemical analyses to be free of heparin.[12] The heparan sulphate fraction includes a small subfraction (~5%) with high affinity for AT III. This subfraction is responsible for Orgaran's anti-factor Xa activity and about half of its smaller degree of antithrombin activity. The dermatan sulphate fraction also mediates a portion of the antithrombin activity via heparin cofactor II.[31] However, fractionation shows that these two subfractions are responsible for only about one-half of the antithrombotic activity of Orgaran;[20] the other half is due to an unknown mechanism. The anti-Xa to anti-IIa ratio of Orgaran is at least 22, which clearly differentiates it from unfractionated heparin (UFH) and low-molecular-weight heparins (LMWHs), which have ratios from 1–5. Orgaran's almost single mode of action on the clotting cascade results in a more linear dose-response curve than UFH.[21] This fact, along with the lack of bleeding-inducing antiplatelet activity, indicates a potentially wider safety margin and hence improved benefit-risk ratio.

PHARMACOLOGY OF ORGARAN

Animal studies demonstrated that Orgaran not only possesses a better antithrombotic-bleeding ratio than UFH and LMWHs, but also is more potent at preventing the extension of preexisting thrombi,[5] thus confirming its improved benefit-risk ratio. Thrombus inhibition is mediated principally by prevention of fibrin formation, whereas platelet deposition is hardly affected. In humans the half-life of biologic activity depends on the clotting cascade effect under consideration.[11] The plasma anti-Xa response has been the most extensively studied and in animal models has been shown to bear a linear dose-response relationship with both antithrombotic and bleeding effects over a wide dosing range.[20] In humans, however, the anti-Xa response is probably useful only as an indicator of the amount of drug in the circulation, because the clinical dose range, based on body weight, is relatively narrow compared with the range used in animal experiments. Furthermore, as previously stated, at least half of the antithrombotic activity is not explained by Orgaran's known effects on the coagulation cascade. The half-life of anti-Xa activity in humans is 25 hours, whereas the half-life of the antithrombin effect and prothrombinase inactivation (which results in thrombin generation inhibition [TGI]) is much shorter.[11,15] Experiments suggest that TGI best reflects Orgaran's antithrombotic activity, but the assay does not lend itself to routine use. On the basis of these findings, twice-daily intravenous or subcutaneous injections of Orgaran are recommended as the most effective dosage for the present approved indication (DVT prophylaxis). The principal route of elimination is renal ; no hepatic metabolism has been demonstrated.[6,21] The half-lives of the various biologic activities are independent of the dose and route of administration, and the bioavalability approaches 100%. Orgaran has only a small linear effect on routine clotting tests (e.g., prothrombin time [PT], activated partial thromboplastin time [APTT], thrombin time [TT], and activated clotting time [ACT]), which are thus unsuitable for monitoring biologic activity or dose-setting. If dose monitoring is needed, the effect on anti-Xa activity is best measured with an amidolytic assay.[28] The Heptest, a simple clotting assay, provides results that cannot be directly correlated with the amidolytic results in all patients. The amidolytic assay must use Orgaran to generate the standard curve to avoid errors due to nonparallelism with the curves produced by using UFH or LMWH.

Preclinical development revealed no toxic or adverse effects other than those associated at high doses (at least 50 times the highest doses/kg body weight used in humans) with an exaggerated pharmacologic effect[21] (i.e., hematoma formation and anemia). Lack of toxicity was confirmed during the clinical development of Orgaran, when the only adverse experience was a low incidence of transient skin reactions at the subcutaneous injection sites. Intolerance and major bleeding with subcutaneous regimens designed for venous thromboprophylaxis in humans[23] and higher subcutaneous or intravenous doses used to treat venous[30] or arterial thrombosis[1] and acute promyelocytic leukemia[22] (a disorder particularly associated with high bleeding risk) have not been a problem. Efficacy has been demonstrated by randomized, controlled trials in a variety of clinical situations requiring DVT prophylaxis or treatment[23,29,30] and renal dialysis.[17]

METHODS

Patient Referral for Bypass Surgery and Data Collection

All patients were referred for CPB surgery by their physicians or surgeons because of a present or past history of HIT and the need for anticoagulant treatment during extracorporeal circulation. They were admitted to the program according to the requirements of a simple protocol. Orgaran was used under the following conditions: (1) other causes of platelet count reduction (of this magnitude) had been excluded; (2) the prognosis of the patient's underlying disease, if any, was at least 3 months; (3) the local Investigational Review Board approved its use for the specific patient ; and (4) the patient gave written informed consent. In some countries, a letter of intent had to be sent to the local national health authority. Orgaran was then supplied from the local company or from NV Organon in the Netherlands. Plasma anti-Xa activity levels, measured in less than 50% of the patients, were available to the surgeons only postoperatively because of the time required for the assay. Hence the anti-Xa activity levels were of no use for intraoperative dose-level evaluation.

Age, gender, weight, concomitant diseases, method of HIT diagnosis, platelet counts, plasma anti-Xa responses (if performed), perioperative details, and postoperative clinical progress (including adverse experiences) until hospital discharge were requested for all patients. Routine hematologic, biochemical, and hemostatic laboratory data were also provided by some investigators. Deaths and other adverse experiences were also reported for up to 6 weeks after stopping Orgaran treatment. Clinical and laboratory data were collected on forms provided by the company. Because this was not a formal study, investigators were not obligated to provide the requested information; some did not, or did so only in part.

Orgaran Dosing

The recommended dosing schedule in this series of patients was 8750 U by intravenous bolus after thoracotomy but before bypass hook-up and 7500 U in the priming fluid of the bypass machine. Booster intravenous injections of 1500 U Orgaran could be administered intraoperatively, if necessary (because of clot or fibrin formation), on an hourly basis. However, the surgeons were advised that the final injection, if possible, should not be given < about 1 hour before the expected end of the operation. If body weight was < 60 kg or > 90 kg, then the postthoracotomy bolus was either reduced to 5000 U or increased to 10,000 U, respectively. Some investigators modified the recommended dosing schedule—for example, in an attempt to obtain the same ACT prolongation as achieved with the usual initial bolus injection of UFH or from the mistaken assumption that Orgaran dosing is similar to that of heparin. As a result, two patients received double the recommended postthoracotomy/prebypass dose of Orgaran or had more than the recommended dose added to the priming fluid.

Assessment of Orgaran Use

The endpoints for evaluation of the clinical outcomes were defined as follows:

Adequate outcome: (1) surgery could be performed, (2) no life-threatening event was attributed by the investigator to Orgaran, and (3) HIT did not recur.

Failure: (1) surgery had to be abandoned as a result of clotting or bleeding; (2) the patient died or suffered a life-threatening event that was attributed to Orgaran; or (3) the patient developed clinical sensitivity to Orgaran.

The following events were not considered as drug failures: postoperative death (unless the investigator stated that Orgaran had been or contributed significantly to the cause), minor amounts of intraoperative clotting (which could not be overcome with booster injections of Orgaran), and excessive postoperative bleeding (unless it was considered life-threatening).

Finally, a *nonevaluable* (NE) category was used for patients with no or inadequate outcome information.

Bleeding

Bleeding was reported by the investigators in different ways but rarely as actual volumes lost. Hence a global assessment for analysis was made in relation to the number of units of replacements that were needed perioperatively. *None* indicates the usual replacement requirement (up to 7 units), whereas *mild, moderate (mod)*, and *severe* indicate increased bleeding that required 8–12, 13–20, and > 20 units, respectively, to correct the hemostatic or hematologic deficit. Replacements consisted of various proportions of packed cells, fresh frozen plasma, fresh platelets, or clotting factor concentrates, as considered necessary by the attending physician. Although the need for reoperation to explore the surgical site or to evacuate a hematoma was recorded, it was not necessarily taken as an indication of drug failure, especially if, as in some patients, the bleeding resulted from surgical error.

Monitoring of Plasma Anti-Xa Activity

Although not essential, the plasma anti-Xa activity was measured perioperatively for about one-half of patients, using the method of Teien et al.[28] as a check on the dosing schedule. However, because neither bleeding induction nor antithrombotic effects are related directly to anti-Xa activity,[21] it is not recommended for monitoring hemostasis. The results were often unreliable because of the use of either UFH or the World Health Organization LMWH standard for the calibration curve. Since both these compounds are neutralized by endogenous plasma factors, whereas Orgaran is not, the plasma anti-Xa activity induced by Orgaran was underestimated. In practice, the underestimation was not a problem, because the results were not available until after the operation was completed. Later, however, the results provided some insight into the responses of patients with body weight outside the range of 55–90 kg.

Results

Between 1985 and 1996 a total of 53 patients with HIT have undergone CPB surgery. For the 47 whose treatment outcome is known, the gender distribution was 21 women and 26 men; the mean age was 59 years (median: 66 yr; range: 16–78 yr); and the mean body weight (n = 40) was 65 kg (median: 70 kg; range: 55–92 kg).

Because of occasional modification of the recommended dosing schedule or lack of adequate information, the total Orgaran dose given to some patients throughout the bypass procedure can only be approximated; for two of the 47 patients it is unknown.

TABLE 1.   HIT Status of Patients

Clinical HIT Status	HIT Test Results		
	Positive	Negative	Not Done
Current (n = 32)*	26	2	4
Past (n = 15)	7[†]	0	8

* Circulating antibody demonstrable or expected to be present.
[†] Diagnosis or test for HIT was performed in the past; the antibody had disappeared from the circulation.

HIT Status (Table 1)

Current HIT (i.e., acute or recent HIT[19]) indicates that even if the platelet count has recovered, the specific heparin-induced antiplatelet antibody is still circulating. Past HIT means that sufficient time has elapsed since the acute episode for the specific antibody to have disappeared from the circulation; most patients had developed HIT at least 1 year previously. Of the two patients with current HIT and negative tests for the antiplatelet antibody, one was positive for thrombocytopenia on rechallenge. Furthermore, 8 patients treated with Orgaran had positive cross-reactivity tests with one or more of the low-molecular-weight heparins; thus Orgaran was the only alternative treatment available.

Comorbid Disorders

In addition to undergoing the operations indicated in Table 2, many of the patients had comorbid problems, including severe heart failure (9), cardiomyopathy (3), multiple organ failure (4), sepsis (2), and disseminated intravascular coagulation (2). One patient was a heroin addict. In addition, all patients had current or previous HIT, which was either confirmed (see Table 1) or strongly suspected for clinical reasons. Thus an alternative to heparin was necessary.

Operations Performed

Many details of the operations (e.g., duration, degree of cooling, surgical approach, and type of bypass procedure) are lacking. Most patients underwent CABG (see Table 2). Both intraoperative and postoperative blood loss volumes are unknown for most patients; hence, severity of postoperative blood loss was judged according to the remarks of the investigators and the volume of transfusions specifically given to reverse bleeding and its effects.

Orgaran Dosing

The dosing of Orgaran for patients in this series is summarized in Table 3, which shows that of the 47 patients whose outcome is known, most received an initial intravenous bolus of 8750 U immediately after thoracotomy. For most patients the extracorporeal circuit was then primed with a further 7500 U of Orgaran. One or more additional intravenous bolusses of 1500 U Orgaran/hr, as necessary, were given after it was known from the first few patients that intraoperative clotting may occur. Some patients were already being treated with Orgaran preoperatively, and several investigators introduced their own modifications in an attempt to adjust for preoperative dosing.

TABLE 2.   Types of Operation Performed

Type of Operation	Number
Coronary artery bypass graft	31
Valve replacement	10
Cardiac transplant	4
Pulmonary embolectomy	1
Proximal aortic aneurysm repair	1

TABLE 3.   Summary of Dosing Schedule Used for Bypass Surgery

Dosing Times	N	Orgaran Dose (Anti-Xa Units)		
		Mean	Mode	Range
Postthoracotomy bolus	47	8224	8750	2000–23400
Added to priming fluid	44*	6375	7500	2500–10000
Intraoperative bolus	30†	3527	2500	1250–11900
Total dose	45‡	17500	16250	10000–33400

* For 3 patients unknown.
† For 5 patients unknown. One patient received a continuous intraoperative infusion. The remaining 11 patients did not have intraoperative booster injections.
‡ Total dose not even approximately known for 2 patients.

Of the 47 patients, 30 are known to have received intraoperative booster injections, but for one the amount is not available. One patient received a continuous infusion throughout the operation, and another 5 patients possibly had boosters (if so, the amount is unknown). Thus 11 patients definitely had no intraoperative booster injections of Orgaran. The 29 patients for whom the volume is known received an average of 3527 U (range: 1250–11900 U; mode: 2500 U) given as 1 or more extra injections intraoperatively. The actual timing of these injections in relation to surgical closure is not known.

Of the 47 patients for whom data are available, 28 had the recommended dose after thoracotomy and 29 were given the correct dose in the priming fluid, but only 23 (49%) received both doses correctly, according to the dosing schedule. Thus 24 (51%) of the patients were not given Orgaran as recommended.

OUTCOME OF SURGERY

Efficacy

Of the 47 CPB procedures, 45 were considered successful or adequate at the time of wound closure; that is, the operation could be completed. The remaining two patients were considered Orgaran-resistant, and surgery had to be abandoned. Both were in the group of 18 in whom "clots" were seen either in the operative field or in the bypass circuit. One other patient developed clots toward the end of the procedure; the operation was stopped, then restarted with a further dose of Orgaran because his condition mandated immediate return to bypass. The operation was completed successfully. In the remaining 15 patients who developed clotting, booster injections of Orgaran were given intraoperatively to provide a greater antithrombotic effect. Of the 18 patients for whom intraoperative clotting was reported, 16 (88%) definitely received an intraoperative booster injection; for 1 patient, the data are uncertain. For 14 of the 18 patients who developed intraoperative clots, body weight is known; 6 received less Orgaran than recommended for weight range for the postthoracotomy plus priming fluid dose (Table 4).

Thus the relationship between clot formation and dosing shows that correct or increased dosing is more likely to avoid clot formation. However, this result is not guaranteed. Of 5 patients who received excessive Orgaran injections as a result of adjustment for

TABLE 4.   Intraoperative Clotting in Relation to Initial Dose of Orgaran

Intraoperative Hemostasis	Thoracotomy + Priming Fluid Dose		
	Correct/Increased	Reduced	Unknown
No clots seen	19	7	3
Clots seen	8	6	4

ACT or failure to adjust as recommended for body weight, two also developed intraoperative clotting. No information was provided about the duration of surgery or the actual time into surgery that the clots were seen.

The tendency to form intraoperative clots was also examined in relation to the type of HIT presentation and showed no difference in frequency between patients who still had or were expected to have circulating heparin-induced antiplatelet antibody and patients who did not.

Safety (Bleeding)

The severity of both intraoperative and postoperative blood loss was assessed by the judgment of the surgeons and anesthetists and the volumes of tranfusions (e.g., blood, platelets, fresh frozen plasma, clotting factor concentrates) given specifically to reverse bleeding or its effects. Blood loss was assumed to be unexceptional if the surgeon made no comment and a total of 7 units or less of transfusion fluids was required. For 45 patients, intraoperative bleeding was not considered to be remarkable, but for two patients it was reported to be more than expected. Postoperative bleeding was defined arbitrarily by the amount of replacement transfusions needed to correct the hemostatic defect. Of the 46 patients for whom data were supplied, postoperative bleeding was as expected in 20 (43%). In the remaining 26 patients, it was mildly, moderately, or severely increased in 6 (13%), 9 (20%), and 11 (24%) patients, respectively. Figure 1 presents the postoperative blood loss in relation to the total dose of Orgaran during the operation.

The 11 patients with severe postoperative bleeding (▲) were equally divided between those who received the correct or incorrect dosing schedule at the start of the operation—5 of 23 (22%) and 6 of 24 (25%), respectively. Figure 1 illustrates the overlap between the various postoperative bleeding intensities in relation to the total dose of Orgaran.

Two of the patients with severe postoperative bleeding were in a small subgroup of 5 patients who received inappropriately high postthoracotomy plus priming fluid doses of

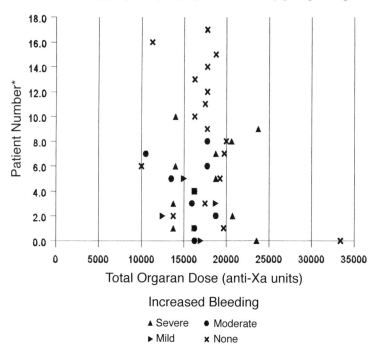

FIGURE 1.   Total dose of Orgaran and postoperative bleeding. * Each symbol represents a different patient.

Orgaran. This sub-group includes the two patients who received twice the recommended dose because of the small effect of Orgaran on ACT. One of the patients developed increased intraoperative bleeding. Both patients received several booster injections of Orgaran because clots were seen during surgery. However, information about the duration of surgery and timing of observation of clots was not provided. For the remaining three patients in this subgroup, bleeding was not reported to be unusual during the perioperative period, and no intraoperative clotting was observed.

The percentage of patients who received ≥ 2000 U (2 or more injections) of Orgaran as booster intraoperative injections and who bled severely postoperatively (8 of 21 [38%]) was little different from that of patients who received only 1500 U Orgaran (3 of 9 [33%]). Of the 11 patients definitely known not to have received booster intraoperative injections, the 6 patients for whom no information about the actual volume was given, and the one patient who received a continuous infusion, none was reported to have bled severely postoperatively (Table 5).

Five of the patients suffered bleeding due to surgical "problems," i.e., from the ends of the graft (1 patient), holes in the graft (1 patient), and retroperitoneal bleeding from the groin due to iliac artery damage during insertion of a balloon catheter (1 patient). In the two remaining patients the bleeding point was not specified. All patients had received the recommended or reduced Orgaran dosing, and all responded promptly to surgical repair. The increase in postoperative bleeding was severe in 2 patients, moderate in 2, and mild in 1.

The intensity of postoperative bleeding was also examined for any relationship to the type of HIT. The frequency of the various degrees of postoperative bleeding was about the same in patients with or without circulating specific antibody.

Three patients received Orgaran treatment postoperatively after an interval of 3–6 days. None developed bleeding during the additional Orgaran treatment despite mild or moderate increases in bleeding in the immediate postoperative period.

Measures to Arrest Postoperative Bleeding

The following drugs were given postoperatively in an attempt to reduce the bleeding: protamine sulphate (PS, 4 patients); 1-deamino-8-D-arginine vasopressin (DDAVP, 2 patients); PS and DDAVP (1 patient); epsilon-aminocaproic acid (EACA, 2 patients); and Amicar (1 patient). None of the attending physicians noted an appreciable effect on the rate of blood loss. As a result of the bleeding, 17 patients returned to the operating room, including 8 of the 11 patients with severe increases in bleeding (including 2 patients with surgical bleeding), 7 of the 9 with moderate increases (including 2 patients with surgical bleeding), and 2 of the 6 with mild increases (1 surgical bleed and 1 patient with hepatic dysfunction). None of the patients with no increase in postoperative blood loss required reoperation.

Postoperative Adverse Events

Other than increased postoperative bleeding, adverse events in the early (within 48 hr) and late (up to 6 weeks) postoperative period for the 47 patients are summarized in

TABLE 5.   Intraoperative Booster Doses of Orgaran and Severity of Postoperative Bleeding

	Unexpected Increase in Postoperative Blood Loss			
Intraoperative Booster Injections (Volume)	None*	Mild[†]	Moderate[‡]	Severe
None	6	3	2	0
1250–1500 ml	3	0	3	3
> 2000 ml	7	2	3	8

* Of the remaining 5 patients, 1 had an infusion; for 4, no information is available.

[†] For 1 patient, no information is available.

[‡] For 1 patient, no information is available.

TABLE 6. Adverse Events in the Follow-up Period

Postoperative Event*	Number†
Hemopericardium	2/0
Ischemic cerebrovascular accident	0/2
Bowel infarction	1/0
Myocardial infarction/unstable angina	0/2
Pulmonary embolus	0/1
Cardiac failure	4/0
Renal failure	0/1
Multiple organ failure	2/2
Sepsis	1/3
Disseminated intravascular coagulation	3/0
Sweet's syndrome	1/0
Atrial fibrillation	1/0

* Some patients had more than one event.
† Within 48 hours/between 2 days and 6 weeks.

Table 6. The investigators rarely reported adverse events unless they were fatal or life-threatening.

Of the 47 known outcomes at 6 weeks, 36 patients (77%) were alive. The causes and time of death in the others are summarized in Table 7. Three patients died within 48 hours after surgery: 1 from heart failure secondary to severe bleeding that required massive replacement transfusions (the patient was already in heart failure preoperatively); 1 from heart failure that proved intractable despite placement of an aortic balloon pump; and 1 from a large bowel infarct. The third patient already had multiple organ failure and had required large transfusions preoperatively. All other deaths occurred between 12 days and 6 weeks postoperatively; none of these patients had received additional Orgaran postoperatively.

Only one death, which occurred in the patient with heart failure who had suffered massive postoperative bleeding, was attributed to Orgaran.

Overall Outcome Assessment

Taking into account the result of surgery and the effect of postoperative bleeding, the eventual outcome in this group of patients with HIT who underwent CPB surgery with Orgaran anticoagulation was assessed as successful or adequate in 40 (85%) patients. In 6 (13%) patients the procedure was judged to have failed because of Orgaran resistance (2 patients); extensive intraoperative clotting, although the operation was completed

TABLE 7. Causes of Death

| Cause of Death | Time of Death | |
	< 48 hr	Late*
Heart failure	2	0
Arterial thrombosis	1	3‡
Pulmonary embolus	0	1
Multiple organ failure	0	1
Hepatic failure	0	1
Sweet's syndrome	0	1
Unknown	0	1

* Late = between 2 and 6 weeks after surgery.
† For one patient the actual day of death is unknown.

(1 patient); fatal postoperative bowel infarction (1 patient); or severe bleeding (2 patients). In 1 other patient preoperative hepatic dysfunction and disseminated intravascular coagulation led to severe postoperative bleeding that was considered "nonevaluable."

DISCUSSION

Overview

Heparin has long been the drug of choice for CPB surgery because it is effective and relatively safe (since its level can be controlled using the ACT and/or APTT). It has a fairly short half-life, and increased postoperative bleeding responds reasonably well to administration of protamine. Recent reports,[4,7] however, have shown that thrombin generation is not completely inhibited even when high doses of heparin are used, and postoperative bleeding remains a problem in such patients.[2,14] Factors contributing to the hemostatic defect include abnormal platelet function, increased fibrinolysis, and changes in clotting factors induced by the clinical disorder, bypass machine, cooling of the patient, and surgery per se.

There have also been reports[7,25] that heparin sensitivity in the form of HIT is more common than hitherto suspected, particularly in association with CPB surgery, perhaps because patients are more likely to have received heparin in the past. Although it is possible to use heparin in such patients, it is generally inadvisable because of the real risk of fatal thrombosis. Until recently, however, there has been little choice for an alternative immediate-acting anticoagulant. Organan has been useful in patients with HIT generally,[10,19] because the chances of developing cross-reactivity during treatment are small (~3%) once possible cross-reactivity is excluded before use. Organan has the added advantage of not interfering with platelet function, apart from a minor effect on thrombin-induced activation due to its weak direct antithrombin activity. It is both safe and effective, even at high intravenous doses. However, patients with HIT who require surgery using extracorporeal circuits pose additional problems, largely because of their poor clinical status, the high doses of Organan needed, and Organan's long plasma retention time coupled with the lack of an effective antidote. Thus, to date the use of Organan in CPB surgery has been limited to patients with HIT enrolled in a compassionate-use program; no other available alternative was considered to be suitable.

Organan proved to be effective for anticoagulation during CPB surgery in the above series of 47 patients with HIT and intolerance of heparin. No patient has shown evidence of cross-reactivity. Although the platelet count at the end of surgery is generally low, it has not been attributed to the use of Organan. The count has always recovered, except in the two patients who died in the early postoperative period. Nevertheless, use of Organan poses problems that need further consideration.

Clotting, Bleeding, and Dosing Schedule

The nature of the intraoperative clots remains uncertain. They may be true fibrin clots and represent insufficient anticoagulation with Organan, or they may be due to platelet activation and aggregation as a result of the bypass machine and cooling of the patient. At this early stage it is too soon for possible cross-reactivity to manifest, and there was no later evidence of continued platelet activation, despite persistence of Organan in the circulation due to its long half-life. Because Organan has only a small direct antithrombin activity, thrombin formed explosively as a result of the bypass machine may go largely unneutralized and lead to clot formation.[4] Unfortunately, however, the surgeon does not have sufficient time to consider whether the clots are composed of fibrin and must decide urgently whether to give additional bolus injections of Organan.

Because about one-third of the patients in this series developed intraoperative clots, seen either in the wound area or the bypass machine, and about 23% suffered severe postoperative bleeding, it has become necessary to reexamine the current dosing recommendations for CPB surgery. In two patients the clotting was so severe as to occasion the term *Organan resistance*, and in another patient a greatly increased dose was needed to complete the operation. The reasons are unclear, but the same phenomenon may occur with heparin.[24] Possibly it could occur if heparin-bonded circuitry were used, but no information is available. All three patients had a history of HIT and no evidence of acute thrombotic problems, and in all three the phenomenon occurred early during elective surgery. Hence it is unlikely that cross-reactivity could have developed so quickly; furthermore, in one of the patients surgery was completed without further complication using a higher dose of Orgaran.

Gender, age (using three ranges: $\leq$ 55 yr, 56–70 yr, and > 70 yr), and body weight per se (using five ranges: $\leq$ 60, 61–70, 71–80, 81–90, and > 90 kg) appeared to be related to neither clotting propensity nor degree of blood loss. In general, the platelet counts at the end of surgery had no relationship to the severity of postoperative bleeding, but the three lowest counts (22, 22, and 37×10^9/L) were seen only in patients who developed severe (2) or moderate (1) increases in blood loss.

Because severe postoperative bleeding occurred in 23% of patients and, as expected, various potential antidotes (e.g., protamine sulphate, DDAVP, EACA) had no effect, the total doses of Orgaran given for CPB surgery were examined for their relationship to bleeding exacerbation (Table 8). This table uses a cut-off level of 16,250 U of Orgaran based on the mode for the 45 patients for whom the complete dosing schedule is at least approximately known (see Table 3).

This analysis, however, revealed no differentiation of patients likely to suffer severe bleeding. The relationship was therefore reexamined (Fig. 2, Table 9), correcting the doses for the patient's body weight. The cut-off at 232 U/kg body weight represents the mode of the total Orgaran dose (16,250 U; see Table 3) divided by the median body weight (70 kg) of the patients in the series.

Figure 2 shows that all patients with severe postoperative bleeding (▲) received $\geq$ 250 U of Orgaran/kg body weight. Taking into consideration the mode of the total Orgaran dose administered in this series of patients (16,250 U) and a suitable safety margin, a dose of 232 U/kg body weight was used for the cut-off in Table 9, which includes all patients for whom body weight is known. All patients who bled severely received a total of > 232 U of Orgaran per kg body weight throughout the procedure, but administration of Orgaran beyond this level did not necessarily lead to increased bleeding. Thus other factors must be involved.

One such factor is the administration of a booster injection during surgery, especially if more than one is given. The booster injections were necessary, however, because nearly one-half of the patients developed intraoperative clotting, usually as a result of inadequate initial dosing. What is not clear from the information provided is whether a booster injection was given closer to surgical closure than the recommended 45–60 minutes. Although Orgaran may be used in extracorporeal circuits to prevent platelet activation on the extensive areas of nonbiologic surface, there is no record in this series of such use. However, heparin-bonded surfaces can reactivate HIT, leading to platelet aggregation; accordingly, they are prohibited in patients with HIT.

Other factors also may be involved in bleeding induction and exacerbation:

1. Many of the patients were severely ill and required the use of other antithrombotics before surgery, including thrombolytics (producing hypofibrinogenemia), oral anticoagulants (leading to reduced clotting factors), and aspirin (resulting in reduced platelet function).

TABLE 8.   Intensity of Blood Loss Related to Orgaran Dose

Orgaran Dose (Anti-Xa Units)	N	Unexpected Increase in Blood Loss			
		None	Mild	Moderate	Severe
$\leq$ 16,250	22	7 (32%)	4 (18%)	6 (27%)	5 (23%)
> 16,250	23	12 (52%)	2 (9%)	3 (13%)	6 (26%)

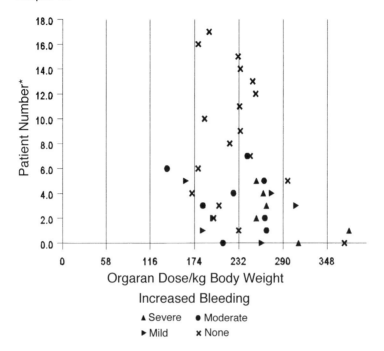

FIGURE 2.   Orgaran dose (kg body weight) and postoperative bleeding. * Each symbol represents a different patient.

2. Other disorders associated with hemostatic defects, such as disseminated intravascular coagulation, hepatic dysfunction, and sepsis, were often present and probably contributed to the global hemostatic defect.

3. Nature and extent of surgery

4. Use of the extracorporeal circuit

5. Use and degree of cooling

6. Use of cell-saver techniques may allow reinfusion of Orgaran at the end of surgery when the level should be decreasing (also a possible disadvantage of late booster injections). Two of the 3 patients known to have received cell-saver blood at the end surgery had severe postoperative bleeding, which may have been due at least partly to this procedure.[8]

7. Surgical errors

The presence of circulating HIT antibody, however, did not appear to play a role in either formation of intraoperative clots or exacerbation of postoperative bleeding.

The experience gained so far with Orgaran in CPB surgery clearly indicates that prevention of clot formation is more effective than treatment. The long half-life of Orgaran is a probable factor in the finding that booster doses during surgery contribute greatly to the severity of postoperative bleeding. Therefore, the current recommendation is to follow the initial postthoracotomy and priming fluid doses with a continuous infusion, which should be stopped 45–60 minutes before final closure. This protocol avoids intraoperative fluctuations

TABLE 9.   Degree of Blood Loss Related to Dose

Orgaran Dose (Anti-Xa U/kg BW)	N	Unexpected Increase in Blood Loss			
		None	Mild	Moderate	Severe
≤ 232	18	11 (61%)	3 (17%)	4 (22%)	0
> 232	20	7 (35%)	3 (15%)	4 (20%)	6 (30%)

in circulating levels and higher levels just before wound closure due to late intravenous booster injections. The effect of Orgaran on plasma anti-Xa activity during and after surgery was measured in less than one-half of patients. Furthermore, despite advice on the method to be used, the actual assay procedure in most centers was far from ideal, and measured levels bore little relationship to recommended levels. In addition, assay results were available only after the operation was completed and, therefore, were of no use to the surgeon.

Revised Treatment Schedule for Bypass Surgery

The treatment schedule for Orgaran has been revised not only to maintain continuous anticoagulant activity in the patient and to combat the thrombotic potential of the bypass machine, but also to reduce the potential for severe increases in postoperative bleeding. The revised schedule is as follows:

1. Intravenous bolus after thoracotomy: 125 U/kg body weight
2. Dose in priming fluid: 3 U/ml
3. Intravenous infusion: 7 U/kg/hr (started at the time of bypass hook-up and stopped 45 minutes before expected end of bypass)

For a 70-kg person undergoing an operation of about 4 hours, the total dose of Orgaran would be approximately 16,250 U or 232 U/kg—a level at which no patient so far has developed severely increased postoperative bleeding (see Fig. 2 and Table 9). This schedule is designed to eliminate the fluctuations associated with the previous regimen and to reduce the risk of both "fibrin" formation and exacerbated postoperative bleeding. Postoperative use of Orgaran for continuing prophylaxis should await establishment of adequate hemostasis and then begin without an initial intravenous bolus dose. Either the intravenous or subcutaneous route may be used, as indicated. Use of cell-saver techniques to reinfuse blood left in the bypass machine at the end of surgery is discouraged. If reinfusion is absolutely necessary, it should be delayed until hemostasis is under adequate control. Thus some possible contributory factors to bleeding exacerbation can be controlled or prevented.

CONCLUSION

Orgaran is generally a safe, well-tolerated, and effective alternative antithrombotic agent for patients with heparin sensitivity. However, because its clinical development has not taken into account all clinical settings that may involve patients with HIT, which vary from DVT prophylaxis to anticoagulation for heart transplantation, dosing recommendations should be carefully followed. As with all antithrombotics, the doses for different clinical indications vary; thrombotic risk must be balanced against the risk of bleeding.

The 47 patients in the Orgaran compassionate-use program constitute the largest series of patients with HIT undergoing bypass surgery. Results confirm the usefulness of Orgaran for this procedure, despite intraoperative clotting and severe postoperative bleeding in some patients. The data make clear that the dosing schedule is partly to blame; other important contributing factors include poor preoperative clinical status of many of the patients, inexperience with the use of Orgaran, and surgical technique. In the absence of controlled studies, the true risk-benefit potential of Orgaran for situations such as bypass surgery has not been properly evaluated. Nevertheless, the present experience shows that it can be a life-saving drug in patients requiring bypass for whom no alternative anticoagulant agent is available. It is hoped that the dosing modification described in this chapter leads to even better control of hemostasis intra- and postoperatively.

REFERENCES

1. Adams HP Jr, Woolson RF, Biller J, Clarke W: Studies of Org 10172 on patients with acute ischemic stroke. Haemostasis 22:99–103, 1992.
2. Bachmann F, McKenna R, Cole ER, Nafjafi A: The haemostatic mechanism after open-heart surgery. I: Studies on plasma coagulation factors and fibrinolysis in 512 patients after extra-corporeal circulation. J Thorac Cardiovasc Surg 70:76–85, 1975.

3. Bick RL: Physiology and pathology of hemostasis during cardiac surgery. In Pifarre R (ed): Anticoagulation, Hemostasis, and Blood Preservation in Cardiovascular Surgery. Philadelphia, Hanley & Belfus, 1993, pp 23–55.
4. Boisclair MD, Lane DA, Philipou H, et al: Thrombin production, inactivation and expression during open heart surgery measured by assays for activation fragments including a new ELISA for prothrombin fragment F_{1+2}. Thromb Haemost 70:253–258, 1993.
5. Boneu B, Buchanan MR, Cade JF, et al: Effects of heparin, its low molecular weight fractions and other glycosaminoglycans on thrombus growth in vivo. Thromb Res 40:81–89, 1985.
6. Bradbrook I, Magnani HN, Moelker HCT, et al: ORG 10172, a low molecular weight anticoagulant with a long half-life in man. Br J Clin Pharmacol 23:667–675, 1987.
7. Brister SJ, Ofosu FA, Buchanan MR: Thrombin generation during cardiac surgery: Is heparin the ideal anticoagulant? Thromb Haemost 70:259–262, 1993.
8. Bull SB, Bull MH: Cardiopulmonary bypass and the salvaged blood syndrome. In Pifarre R (ed): Anticoagulation, Hemostasis, and Blood Preservation in Cardiovascular Surgery. Philadelphia, Hanley & Belfus, 1993, pp 85–93.
9. ten Cate H, Henny ChP, Buller HR, et al: Use of heparinoid in haemorrhagic stroke patients with thromboembolic disease. Ann Neurol 15:268–270, 1984.
10. Chong BH, Magnani HN: Orgaran in heparin-induced thrombocytopenia. Haemostas 22:85–91, 1992.
11. Danhof M, de Boer A, Magnani HN, Stiekema JCJ: Pharmacokinetic considerations on Orgaran (Org 10172) therapy. Haemostasis 22:73–84, 1992.
12. van Dedem GWK: Composition of Orgaran. Thromb Haemost 69:652, 1993.
13. Gomes MMR, McGoon DC: Bleeding patterns after open-heart surgery. J Thorac Cardiovasc Surg 60:87–97, 1970.
14. Gram J, Janetzko T, Jerpersen J, Bruhn HD: Enhanced effective fibrinolysis following the neutralisation of heparin in open heart surgery increases the risk of post surgical bleeding. Thromb Haemost 63:241–245, 1990.
15. Hobbelen PMJ, Vogel GMT, Meuleman DG: Time courses of the antithrombotic effects, the bleeding effects and the interaction with factor Xa and thrombin after administration of the low molecular weight heparinoid Org 10172. Thromb Res 48:549–58, 1987.
16. Henny ChP, ten Cate H, ten Cate JW, et al: A randomised blind study comparing standard heparin and a new low molecular weight heparinoid in cardiopulmonary by-pass surgery. J Lab Clin Med 106:187–196, 1985.
17. Ireland H, Lane DA, Flynn A, et al: The anticoagulant effect of heparinoid during dialysis: An objective assessment. Thromb Haemost 55:271–275, 1986.
18. Kyritsis AP, Williams AC, Schitta HS: Cerebral venous thrombosis due to heparin-induced thrombocytopenia. Stroke 21:1503–1505, 1990.
19. Magnani HN: Heparin-induced thrombocytopenia (HIT): An overview of 230 patients treated with Orgaran (ORG 10172). Thromb Haemost 70:554–561, 1993.
20. Meuleman DG, Hobbelen PMJ, van Dedem G, Moelker HCT: A novel antithrombotic heparinoid (ORG 10172) devoid of bleeding inducing capacity. Thromb Res 27:353–363, 1982.
21. Meuleman DG: Orgaran (ORG 10172): Its pharmacological profile in experimental models. Haemostasis 22:58–64, 1992.
22. Nieuwenhuis HK, Sixma JJ: Treatment of disseminated intravascular coagulation in acute promyelocytic leukaemia with low molecular weight heparinoid ORG 10172. Cancer 58:761–764, 1986.
23. Nurmohamed MT, Fareed J, Hoppensteadt D, et al: Pharmacological and clinical studies with Lomoparan, a low molecular weight glycosaminoglycan. Semin Thromb Haemost 17:205–213, 1991.
24. Pifarre R, Istanbouli M, Sinno J: Protocol for anticoagulation during cardiopulmonary bypass. In Pifarre R (ed): Anticoagulation, Hemostasis, and Blood Preservation in Cardiovascular Surgery. Philadelphia, Hanley & Belfus, 1993, pp 57–64.
25. Prull A, Nechwatal R, Maurer W: Fulminante venöse und arterielle Thrombosen unter Heparintherapie. Dtsch Med Wschr 115:456–459, 1990.
26. Roche JK, Stengle JM: Open-heart surgery and the demand for blood. JAMA 225:1517–1521, 1973.
27. Stiekema JCJ, Wijnand HP, van Dinther ThG, et al: Safety and pharmacokinetics of the low molecular weight heparinoid ORG 10172 administered to healthy elderly volunteers. Br J Clin Pharmacol 27:39–48, 1989.
28. Teien AN, Lie M, Abildgaard U: Assay of heparin in plasma using a chromogenic substrate for activated factor X. Thromb Res 8:413–416, 1976.
29. Turpie AGG: Orgaran in the prevention of deep vein thrombosis in stroke patients. Haemostasis 22:92–98, 1992.
30. de Valk HW, Banga JD, Wester JWJ, et al: Comparing subcutaneous danaparoid with intravenous subcutaneous heparin: A randomised controlled clinical trial. Ann Intern Med 123:1–9, 1995.
31. Verhamme IMA, van Dedem GWK: Effect of the buffer composition and the presence of ORG 10172 and some glycosaminoglycans on the inhibition of alpha-thrombin by heparin cofactor II [abstract]. Thromb Haemost 58:422, 1987.
32. Warkentin TE, Kelton JG: Heparin-induced thrombocytopenia. Prog Haemost Thromb 10:1–34, 1991.

CHAPTER 32

Efficacy of Iloprost in Preventing Heparin-induced Platelet Activation during Cardiac Surgery

JEFFREY R. KAPPA, M.D.
CAROL A. FISHER, A.B.
V. PAUL ADDONIZIO, M.D.

Since McLean's initial description of heparin in 1916,[60] its use as an effective yet reversible anticoagulant has led to major advances in both cardiac and vascular surgery. In contrast to its fairly well-characterized interactions with coagulant proteins, the interaction of heparin with platelets, particularly platelets at a synthetic surface interface, remains incompletely defined. Indeed, some of these interactions can be detrimental.

A mild, transient decrease in circulating platelets was first noted in dogs and mice in 1942[25] and is now recognized as a nearly universal occurrence.[14,23,35] This mild thrombocytopenia is believed to result from platelet agglutination and is of no clinical consequence (heparin-induced thrombocytopenia [HIT] type I).[14,15,54] Type I, however, must be distinguished from a severe form of thrombocytopenia and thrombosis that can also complicate heparin therapy.[21,48,54,64,71] This syndrome, termed heparin-induced thrombocytopenia and thrombosis (HITT, type II), is believed to be immune-mediated.[19–21,37,54,71] The morbidity and mortality rates of HITT have been reported as high as 61% and 23%, respectively.[71] Thus, if the diagnosis of HITT is made, avoidance of all exposure to heparin, including heparin flush and even heparin-bonded catheters, is mandatory.[17,56] Unfortunately, in certain clinical situations, such as urgent cardiac surgery, reexposure to heparin is unavoidable. Under such circumstances, patients with HITT require alternative strategies to avoid the extreme complications of heparin administration.[31,48,54,64,71]

This chapter reviews the diagnosis, mechanism and management of heparin-induced platelet activation in patients requiring reexposure to heparin. It also summarizes our experience with iloprost, a synthetic prostacyclin analog, to prevent both heparin-induced and surface-mediated platelet activation.

CLINICAL PRESENTATION

HIT should be suspected in any patient who develops new thrombocytopenia (< 100,000/μl), who requires increasing amounts of heparin to maintain therapeutic anticoagulation, or who demonstrates extension or de novo occurrence of a thrombotic event while receiving seemingly appropriate heparin therapy. Typically, thrombocytopenia occurs 7–14 days after the initiation of heparin therapy. Intravenous and subcutaneous administration of heparin as well as heparin flush have been associated with the development of HITT.[48] In addition, prior exposure to heparin seems to accelerate its appearance, and thrombocytopenia or thrombosis may occur immediately in previously sensitized patients.[21,22,71] No age predilection and no difference in male/female prevalence have been noted.

Once a patient develops heparin-induced thrombcytopenia or thrombosis, morbidity and mortality rates are exceptionally high, particularly if heparin exposure is continued.[73] The thrombotic complications, which are frequently severe, include arterial emboli or thromboses, deep venous thromboses, myocardial infarctions, cerebrovascular accidents, mesenteric infarctions, and skin infarctions;[48,71,81] they often prolong hospitalization for more than 50 days.[71] When reexposure of heparin occurs during cardiopulmonary bypass, aortic thrombosis, extremity ischemia with necrosis, renal failure, and death are common sequelae.[31]

DIAGNOSIS OF HEPARIN-INDUCED PLATELET ACTIVATION

In our group of patients, heparin-dependent platelet aggregation was assessed by means of both platelet aggregation and C^{14}-serotonin release.[47–53,70] To assess for the presence of heparin-dependent platelet-activating factor, either bovine lung or porcine mucosa heparin (0.1–3U/ml) was added to a mixture of aspirin-free donor's platelet-rich plasma (300 µl) and patient's platelet-poor plasma (200 µl).[12,30,34] After heparin was added, at least 20% platelet aggregation within 15 minutes or 6% serotonin release within 45 minutes was considered positive. Platelets were also challenged with 5 or 10 µmol/L of adenosine diphosphate (ADP) to ensure normal platelet reactivity. Similarly, activity of the in vitro aspirin preparation and compliance with aspirin ingestion by donors was thus ensured. In addition, our lot and iloprost dilutions were tested independently to guarantee potency. Samples were also spun at 1200 rpm at 37°C, with no platelet agonist added, to assess spontaneous aggregation and/or release. If the patient's platelet count at the time of laboratory testing permitted preparation of platelet-rich plasma with > 100,000/µl, this assessment was also performed with the patient's own platelet-rich plasma.[1,62] Both aspirin and iloprost were evaluated for their ability to prevent heparin-induced platelet activation and were added to the aggregometer cuvette two minutes before the addition of heparin. Platelet aggregation and release were measured.

Figure 1 shows a representative in vitro platelet aggregation tracing in response to heparin. All patients demonstrated at least 20% platelet aggregation and/or 6% C^{14}-serotonin release in response to heparin. The lag phase between the addition of heparin and the beginning of platelet aggregation varied from < 1 minute to > 10 minutes. Some patients were evaluated with both bovine and porcine heparin and demonstrated positive responses to both. It was previously thought that patients are antigenically more reactive to the bovine form,[12,38] but this is not the case.[45]

In patients who were available for retesting, rechallenge with heparin 7–42 days after cessation of heparin therapy still resulted in a positive diagnosis, regardless of the laboratory test used. In patients whose platelet-poor plasma was no longer capable of activating normal donor platelets, their own platelet-rich plasma still demonstrated a response to heparin. Of interest, heparin-induced platelet activation persisted in the platelet-rich plasma of one patient 10 months after his last exposure to heparin.

The direct addition of aspirin (4 mmol/L) to the aggregometer cuvette before heparin exposure or use of aspirinized donor platelets reduced the extent of platelet aggregation and C^{14}-serotonin release. However, this response was quite variable and ranged from complete efficacy in preventing platelet activation to absence of measurable inhibition. Indeed, despite the addition of tenfold more aspirin to the cuvette before heparin administration, one

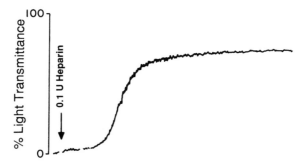

FIGURE 1.   Representative in vitro platelet aggregation in response to heparin (0.1 U/ml). Percentage of light transmittance is plotted against time. (From Kappa JR, Fisher CA, Berkowitz HB, et al: Heparin-induced platelet activation in sixteen surgical patients: Diagnosis and management. J Vasc Surg 5:101–109, 1987, with permission.)

patient still exhibited platelet activation (Fig. 2). In contrast, when iloprost (0.01 μmol/L) was added to the cuvette, both platelet aggregation and release were completely prevented in all patients tested.

Heparin-induced platelet granule release and generation of thromboxane B_2 were also assessed in patients whose own platelet count permitted preparation of platelet-rich plasma after cessation of heparin therapy. Heparin (3 U/ml, a dose that correlates with plasma levels during cardiac surgery)[77] was added to multiple samples of platelet-rich plasma in the absence and presence of either aspirin or iloprost. Studies were performed in two HITT-positive patients: an aspirin responder and an aspirin failure. For the aspirin responder, addition of either aspirin (4 mmol/L) or iloprost (0.01 μmol/L) prevented heparin-induced platelet dense, alpha, and lysosomal granule release of C^{14}-serotonin, platelet factor 4, and N-acetyl-β-glucosaminidase, respectively, each a marker to determine the strength of the activating stimulus. For the patient in whom aspirin was not an effective antiplatelet agent, heparin caused significant release of the dense, alpha, and lysosomal platelet granules (Fig. 3). Furthermore, similar results were obtained for both patients when plasma levels of thromboxane B_2, the stable end product of thromboxane A_2 (TXA_2) and a potent vasoconstrictor and proaggregatory agent, were measured (Fig. 4).

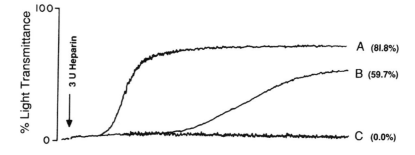

FIGURE 2.   In vitro heparin-induced platelet aggregation for one patient with no platelet inhibitors added *(A)*, with 40 mmol/L aspirin added *(B)*, and with 0.01 mmol/L iloprost added *(C)* to the aggregometer cuvette. Percentages in parentheses represent the percent C^{14}-serotonin release recorded for each aggregation curve. (From Kappa JR, Fisher CA, Berkowitz HB, et al: Heparin-induced platelet activation in sixteen surgical patients: Diagnosis and management. J Vasc Surg 5:101–109, 1987, with permission.)

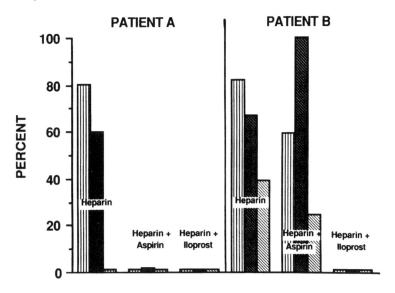

FIGURE 3.   Percent of total releasable C^{14}-serotonin (bar with vertical lines, dense granule), platelet factor 4 (black bar, alpha granule), and N-acetyl-β-glucosaminidase (bar with diagonal lines, lysosomal granule) after heparin challenge is plotted in bar form. Aspirin, iloprost, and heparin have been added to 500 μl of the patients' platelet-rich plasma to achieve a final concentration of 4 mmol/L, 0.01 μmol/L, and 3 U/ml, respectively. Patient A: aspirin responder; patient B: aspirin failure. (From Kappa JR, Fisher CA, Addonizio VP: Heparin-induced platelet activation: The role of thromboxane A_2 synthesis and the extent of platelet granule release in two patients. J Vasc Surg 9:574–579, 1989, with permission.)

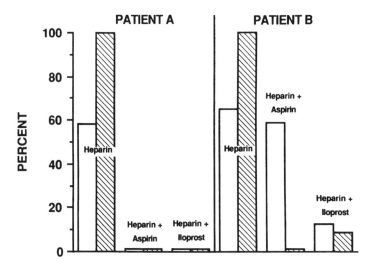

FIGURE 4.   Percent platelet aggregation (open bar) and total releasable thromboxane β_2 generation (lined bar) after heparin challenge is plotted in bar form. Otherwise, legend is identical to that of Figure 3. (From Kappa JR, Fisher CA, Addonizio VP: Heparin-induced platelet activation: The role of thromboxane A_2 synthesis and the extent of platelet granule release in two patients. J Vasc Surg 9:574–579, 1989, with permission.)

In summary, platelet activation induced by heparin appears to proceed via several biochemical pathways. In certain patients heparin can induce the release reaction, which is independent of TXA_2 synthesis. In other patients it appears to be thromboxane-dependent and can be prevented by cyclooxygenase inhibitors such as aspirin. In contrast, iloprost consistently prevented heparin-induced platelet activation in all patients evaluated in our laboratory. It is clear that patients in whom heparin behaves as a weak agonist should be protected by cyclooxygenase inhibitors such as aspirin. In contrast, patients in whom heparin behaves as a strong agonist require more effective control of platelet reactivity with a prostacyclin analog such as iloprost.

Since our assessment of iloprost as an agent for the prevention of platelet aggregation and serotonin release, many investigators have looked for diagnostic tests with improved sensitivity and specificity.[28] The platelet aggregometry test is more specific for diagnosis of heparin-induced thrombocytopenia but less sensitive.[18,33] Sensitivity can be improved by using the patient's own platelets.[1,62] The serotonin release test is more sensitive but less specific. Heparin and other large highly sulfated polysaccharides bind to platelet factor 4 to form a reactive antigen on the platelet surface.[11] IgG then binds to this complex, with activation of platelets through the platelet Fc receptors.[53] Use of an enzyme-linked immunosorbent assay (ELISA) to measure this complex now permits early and more specific diagnosis of type II HITT.[10,11]

MECHANISM OF HEPARIN-INDUCED PLATELET ACTIVATION

Although the exact mechanisms involved in the genesis of HITT and the precise pathways required for heparin-induced platelet activation remain incompletely defined, most investigators agree that HITT is an immune-mediated phenomenon.[13,20,21,37,71,78] A heparin–antibody interaction was first hypothesized by Roberts et al. as a cause for recurrent arterial emboli.[64] A factor capable of aggregating platelets in the presence of heparin was subsequently identified in the plasma of a patient with HITT.[63] Since that time, heparin-dependent platelet-aggregating factor has been isolated in the IgG and IgM fractions of patients' sera.[13,21,37,79] This factor fixes complement to platelet membranes[20,21,54,63] and requires an intact complement sequence to induce platelet activation.[21] The absorption of an immunoglobulin–heparin complex to platelet lysates in the presence of affected patients' sera has also been demonstrated.[37,43] These findings suggest that heparin acts as a hapten with an antibody directed against the heparin–platelet membrane determinant. Further studies have demonstrated that heparin and other large, highly sulfated polysaccharides bind to platelet factor 4 to form a reactive antigen on the platelet surface.[53] IgG specific to patients with HITT then binds to this complex, with activation of platelets in a complement-dependent, nonlytic fashion through the platelet Fc receptors.[21,53]

Despite significant progress in demonstrating that HITT is an immune-mediated phenomenon, the biochemical pathways of platelet activation are unknown. Using metabolic inhibitors and platelets from patients with either Glanzmann's thrombasthenia or Bernard-Soulier syndrome, Chong and Castaldi demonstrated that heparin-induced platelet activation requires metabolic energy and, thus, is not due to passive agglutination.[19,20] In addition, heparin-induced aggregation requires the membrane glycoproteins IIb/IIIa but not Ib, indicating the importance of fibrinogen in heparin-induced platelet aggregation.[19]

Further insights into the involved pathways have come from studying the effects of various platelet inhibitors on heparin-induced platelet activation. In general, depending on the strength of the stimulus, platelet activation may either require TXA_2 synthesis and release of endogenous ADP or proceed by pathways independent of TXA_2 synthesis or aggregation.[41,82,83] Thus, several investigators have demonstrated that aspirin prevents heparin-induced platelet aggregation in most patients, indicating that TXA_2 synthesis is required for platelet activation.[20,46,58] However, other investigators have found that aspirin does not prevent heparin-induced platelet activation in all patients, indicating that other metabolic pathways may be involved.[19,47–49,51] In this subset of patients, heparin causes release of lysosomal hydrolases[49] and thus appears to act as a strong platelet agonist similar to thrombin.[9,41,42] Only by elevating intracellular levels of cyclic adenosine monophosphate (AMP) with prostaglandin E_1 or the prostacyclin analog iloprost can heparin-induced platelet activation be prevented in the subset of patients in whom heparin acts as a strong agonist.[19,47,48,51] To determine whether these differing characteristics of platelet activation represent different titers or strengths of the heparin-dependent antibody or completely different antibody-platelet affinities and binding characteristics requires further investigation. The high incidence of thrombotic as opposed to hemorrhagic complications in HITT distinguishes this syndrome from other drug-induced thrombocytopenias.[39]

Heparin-dependent antibodies from patients with confirmed HITT bind to endothelial cells in culture and also fix complement to these endothelial cells even in the absence of heparin.[22] This binding damages endothelial cells and stimulates production of tissue factor. In addition, the heparin-dependent antibodies cross-react with heparan sulfate, a naturally occurring anticoagulant that binds to endothelial cells.[22] Thus, immune-mediated damage of endothelial cells may alter their surface milieu, thereby increasing the procoagulant potential of the vessel wall. In addition, sera from patients with HIT can generate platelet-derived microparticles with procoagulant activity.[80] In conjunction with activation of circulating platelets by heparin, these endothelial changes and procoagulant microparticles help to explain the high incidence of thrombotic complications.

STRATEGIES FOR MANDATORY REEXPOSURE TO HEPARIN

For some patients with confirmed HITT continued exposure or reexposure to heparin is unavoidable. Examples include patients who require cardiac or vascular surgical procedures. Indeed, the thrombotic complications associated with HITT may mandate the surgical procedure. Because reexposure to heparin can lead to intravascular activation of circulating platelets,[21,22,72] other clinical strategies are essential. Proposals have included (1) waiting for the plasma activity of the heparin-dependent platelet antibody to decline; (2) changing the form of anticoagulation; (3) controlling the effects of the coagulation cascade with defibrinating or fibrinolytic agents; and (4) preventing activation of platelets during heparin reexposure.

In patients requiring cardiac surgery, delay in the hope that the plasma activity of the heparin-dependent platelet-activating factor will decline has been proposed.[62] However, this approach is complicated by the variable length of time required for the factor to disappear[5,21] and also by the unpredictable response to even one dose of heparin.[5,47]

Because heparin is the etiologic agent in HITT, the use of other forms of anticoagulation has been evaluated. Low-molecular-weight heparins and heparinoids with fewer platelet-active properties have been used successfully in certain settings.[40,44,57–59,66,68] These fractions presumably lack the antigenic determinants of higher-molecular-weight heparins and, thus, should not cross-react. However, prevention of heparin-induced platelet activation with these agents has not been universally successful.[67] A pentasaccharide composed of the precise binding sequence that mediates heparin binding to antithrombin-III is also under investigation.[17] The use of antithrombins during cardiopulmonary bypass and other clinical situations that require anticoagulation is also under investigation and is reported elsewhere in this book. Whether these promising agents demonstrate clinical feasibility, reversibility, and lower incidence of hemorrhagic or thrombotic side effects is an area of active investigation.

Ancrod is a defibrinating agent that has also been used in patients with HITT.[24] Because it acts by depolymerizing fibrinogen, it does not prevent activation of the coagulation cascade. Predicting suitable therapeutic levels, preventing coagulation protein consumption, and reversing its anticoagulant effects remain problematic.

Because most of the complications of HITT are platelet-mediated, pharmacologic inhibition of platelet function during heparin exposure has been used with variable success.[5,46,47,51,72] Aspirin inhibits platelet activation by irreversibly acetylating cyclooxygenase, thus preventing synthesis of prostaglandin endoperoxide and TXA_2.[8,65] Since heparin-induced platelet activation does not proceed by thromboxane-dependent pathways in all patients, the success rate of aspirin is predictably variable. Janson et al. reported successful use of aspirin to permit hemodialysis in a patient with HITT.[46] However, use of aspirin in a patient requiring cardiopulmonary bypass did not prevent thrombocytopenia after heparin administration.[72] In addition, the effects of aspirin on platelet function are irreversible and often associated with excessive postoperative bleeding in patients undergoing cardiac surgery.[76]

Of the clinical agents currently available to provide antiplatelet therapy,[61] only the naturally occuring prostaglandins—prostaglandin E_1, which is produced in the seminal vesicles, and prostaglandin I_2 (prostacyclin, epoprostenal), which is synthesized by the endothelial cells—offer the dual advantages of potency and rapid reversibility. Unfortunately, their clinical utility has been limited by their vasoactive properties.[5] In addition, prostacyclin, the most potent antiplatelet agent known, has a short half-life and is chemically unstable at neutral pH. Because its therapeutic use has been limited by this inherent instability, attempts have focused on modifying the molecule to obtain an analog with greater chemical and metabolic stability and comparable physiologic activity with less pronounced vasodilation. One such effort has yielded the carbacyclin derivative, iloprost. Although the intravenous form of iloprost is no longer available in the United States, it is still available in Europe (Schering AG, Berlin, Germany).

PHARMACODYNAMIC AND PHARMACOKINETIC PROPERTIES OF ILOPROST

Iloprost differs from prostacyclin in having a triple bond at C-18 and C-19, a methyl group at C-16, and a methylene group in place of the heterocyclic oxygen atom. These modifications helped to increase the chemical stability of the analog and facilitated intravenous and oral administration.[36]

Iloprost is completely metabolized in humans through β-oxidation to the tetranor derivative and its conjugate. Excretion of the metabolites is predominantly renal with small amounts excreted through the feces. Elimination of the compound is biphasic. The initial half-life of distribution to organs and tissues is 4 minutes, and the terminal half-life, representing biotransformation and elimination, is 20–30 minutes in healthy human volunteers.[36]

Intravenous infusion of iloprost at a rate of < 2 ng/kg/min is associated with facial flushing and headache, which are the most common side effects. Increased infusion rates are associated with gastrointestinal events (nausea, vomiting, abdominal cramping, diarrhea). Other reported side effects include restlessness, sudden sweating, appearance of a red line along the infused vein, local erythema, sedation or fatigue, muscular aches, pain or numbness in the limbs, dry mouth, decreased appetite, and wheals. However, the extent to which underlying disease contributes to these adverse effects has not been established.[36] For patients with HIT who require open heart surgery and much higher doses to prevent heparin-induced platelet activation, doses in excess of 24 ng/kg/min are associated with substantial hypotension, which is well-controlled by phenylephrine or norepinephrine.[5,27] Furthermore, discontinuation of the iloprost infusion at the conclusion of cardiopulmonary bypass is associated with a rise in blood pressure.[5,27,36,47,50,51]

The proposed mechanism for the antiplatelet effect of iloprost is via the cyclic AMP system, with platelet receptor-mediated activation of adenyl cyclase. The resultant adenyl cyclase stimulation effects phospholipase activity and cytosolic calcium levels.[32,36]

ILOPROST, HEPARIN, AND SYNTHETIC SURFACES

When blood comes into contact with the synthetic surface of the extracorporeal circuit, qualitative and quantitative platelet alterations occur. Within seconds of blood contact, a layer of fibrinogen adsorbs to the synthetic surface. Soon after protein adsorption, platelets are activated; they extrude pseudopodia, adhere, aggregate, and release their granule contents. The synthetic surface acts as a soluble agonist and modulates similar, if not identical, biochemical pathways as those modulated by soluble agonists (e.g., ADP). Depending on the strength of the stimulus, the release reaction can include contents of three types of granules: dense (serotonin, ADP), alpha (platelet factor 4, β-thromboglobulin), and lysosomal (acid phosphatase, β-galactosidase, N-acetyl-β-glucosaminidase).[2,3,9] Such platelet alterations have been reduced significantly by the addition of prostaglandins E_1 and I_2 to the extracorporeal circuit.[6,7]

Because the efficacy of prostaglandins E_1 and I_2 as platelet-inhibiting agents has been well established, their equimolar potencies as antiplatelet agents were compared with iloprost.[32,69] All three prostanoids effectively inhibited both ADP- and epinephrine-induced platelet aggregation in human platelet-rich plasma in a dose-dependent manner. At equimolar doses iloprost is 100 times more potent than prostaglandin E_1 and 10 times more potent than prostaglandin I_2.[32] Use of gel-filtered platelets (platelets removed from their plasma environment through sepharose chromatography) permitted further assessment of antiplatelet action against thrombin. Iloprost was the only agent to demonstrate preferred inhibition of thrombin-induced platelet activation.[32] In vitro human whole blood studies demonstrated that platelet aggregation in response to the addition of ADP, collagen, or thrombin can be dissaggregated by iloprost.[75] Furthermore, all three prostanoids raised intracellular levels of cyclic AMP consistent with their measured pattern of platelet-induced functional inhibition.[32] In addition, increased intracellular levels of calcium have been measured.[36]

To test the hypothesis that the more potent a platelet inhibitor the greater its vasoactivity, coronary flow through a rat in-situ heart was assessed in a model of organ perfusion. With doses ≥ 6 µmol/L, coronary flow was consistently but not significantly greater in the prostacyclin-treated hearts than in the iloprost-treated hearts. With doses < 6 µmol/L, there were no observable differences.[32,74]

The efficacy of iloprost was also demonstrated in a model of extracorporeal circulation.[4] In human blood treated with 5 U/ml of heparin and recirculated for 2 hours at 37°C, iloprost (≥ 1 ng/ml) prevented platelet activation as assessed by count, functional sensitivity to ADP and epinephrine, release of platelet factor 4, and generation of thromboxane B_2. When heparin levels were reduced to 1 U/ml of whole blood, iloprost continued to demonstrate platelet inhibition.[55] This finding is consistent with the ability of iloprost to inhibit thrombin-induced platelet activation. Furthermore, use of subthreshold doses of iloprost and other classes of antiplatelet agents, such as disintegrins, also prevented surface-induced platelet alterations during simulated extracorporeal circulation.[16]

In a canine model of extracorporeal membrane oxygenation, iloprost also provided temporary control of platelet reactivity.[26] Infusion of iloprost prevented platelet adherence to the circuit and inhibited platelet aggregation. When the infusion of iloprost was discontinued, platelets demonstrate normal functional activity, although they did not adhere to the circuit. Prevention of the initial blood–synthetic surface interaction presumably permits a stereochemical configuration change in the surface-adsorbed fibrinogen molecule.[2,3] The fact that the salutary effects of iloprost outlast its presence in plasma suggests that prevention of initial platelet–synthetic interaction reduces the surface affinity for platelets, a phenomenon known as "passivation."[6]

In addition to its known antiplatelet properties, iloprost also preserved white blood cell count and prevented release of neutrophil elastase and generation of fibrinopeptide A[36,74] (the most sensitive indicator of coagulation) when human blood was recirculated through the in vitro extracorporeal circuit with only 1U/ml of heparin.[55] Of interest, this dose of heparin may represent a significant risk of thromboembolism in the clinical setting of cardiopulmonary bypass.

Iloprost also appears to possess thrombolytic properties. At least in fresh thrombi, such effects are probably mediated by an increase in fibrinolytic potential due to inhibition of the release of plasminogen activator inhibitor (PAI) from activated platelets. Indeed, it has been hypothesized that iloprost can stimulate release of tissue plasminogen activator (tPA) from blood vessel walls. A lack of consistent and significant rise in levels of tPA in the plasma suggests that an additional mechanism, perhaps inhibition of the release of tPA inhibitor from platelets, may also be involved.[74]

CLINICAL EXPERIENCE WITH ILOPROST

Use of iloprost to prevent surface-induced and heparin-induced platelet activation in patients with documented HITT who require an open heart procedure proved to be appealing for several reasons. First, iloprost is a potent antiplatelet agent with manageable vasoactive side effects. Secondly, it was efficacious in all of our in vitro studies. Finally, its use allowed for the possibility of normal platelet function with cessation of infusion because its effects are rapidly and completely reversed. A rapid return of platelet function is highly desirable for postoperative hemostasis.

Iloprost has been used in more than 70 patients with HITT who required cardiopulmonary bypass or vascular surgical procedures (personal communications, Berlex Laboratories, Wayne, NJ). The maximal infusion rate of iloprost was determined by in vitro platelet studies with titration of iloprost until heparin-induced platelet activation was completely inhibited. In all patients, iloprost effectively inhibited heparin-induced platelet activation. The results of our first 11 patients were evaluated in greatest detail.[50]

A clinical diagnosis of HITT was established in the 11 patients after thrombotic or untoward hemodynamic events associated with heparin exposure (Table 1). All studies were approved by the Institutional Review Boards of the University of Pennsylvania and Temple University, Human Research Committee of the National Inststitutes of Health, and the Veterans Administration Human Experimentation Committee Physician protocols were reviewed by the Food and Drug Administration before initiation of the clinical trial. Detailed verbal and written informed consent was obtained before sugery from each patient.

The iloprost infusion was started immediately after induction of anesthesia. Infusion rates were increased incrementally with hemodynamic monitoring until heparin-induced platelet activation was prevented in vitro (Fig. 5)—at infusion rates of 10–48 ng/kg/min. At that time, heparin was administered and the operative procedure was started. At completion of the procedure, the iloprost infusion was tapered to 6 ng/kg/min. Protamine sulfate, which forms a complex with heparin and is cleared via the reticuloendothelial system, was then administered, and the iloprost infusion was discontinued 20 minutes later. In patients undergoing cardiac operations, the mean whole blood platelet count did not change with heparin administration. Furthermore, no spontaneous platelet aggregation or platelet aggregates were observed during the period of heparin exposure. Platelet count decreased with inception of cardiopulmonary bypass and hemodilution but remained stable throughout the bypass period and well into the postoperative period (Fig. 6). Similar results were observed in patients undergoing vascular procedures. Despite preservation of platelet count, increases in plasma levels of platelet factor 4 and beta-thromboglobulin were observed after heparin administration in both patient groups (Figs. 7 and 8). Plasma levels of fibrinopeptide A decreased after heparin administration and remained essentially unchanged during the bypass and postoperative periods, indicating the absence of intravascular thrombosis (Fig. 9). Pre- and postoperative template bleeding times were 7.9 ± 1.2 and 9.6 ± 1.3 minutes, respectively (Fig. 10). At 6 and 12 hours postoperatively, chest tube drainage was 356 ± 111 and 593 ± 185 ml, respectively (Fig. 11). These findings indicate that platelet function was

TABLE 1.   Clinical Course

Pt	Age (yr)	Complications Associated with Heparin Administration	Indication for Reexposure to Heparin	Maximal Dose of Iloprost (ng/kg/min)	Perioperative Complications
1	41	Deep venous thrombosis, paradoxical emboli/CVA	Atrial septal defect, tricuspid valve replacement	10	None
2	64	Respiratory insufficiency, multiple pulmonary emboli (probable)	Aortic/mitral valve replacement	30	None
3	55	Unstable angina/myocardial infarction	CABG	30	None
4	69	Unstable angina, cardiac arrest	CABG	24	None
5	68	Cardiac ischemia	CABG	48	None
6	69	Spontaneous platelet aggregation, cardiac arrest	CABG	24	None
7	75	Unstable angina	CABG	24	Ventricular fibrillation on postoperative day 3
8	51	Thrombosis of bifemoral artery, pulmonary emboli, GI bleeding	CABG	24	None
9	72	Thrombosis of retinal artery	Aortic valve replacement	36	None
10	70	Thrombosis of femoral artery	Carotid endarterectomy	24	None
11	76	CVA, thrombosis of subclavian vein	Aortic bypass graft	36	None

Pt = patient, CABG = coronary artery bypass grafting, CVA = cerebrovascular accident, GI = gastrointestinal. (From Kappa J, Fisher C, Todd B, et al: Intraoperative management of patients with heparin-induced thrombocytopenia. Ann Thorac Surg 49:714–723, 1990, with permission.)

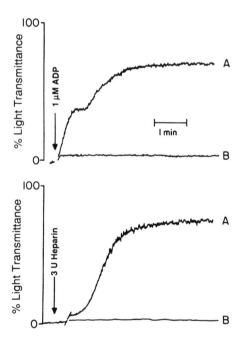

FIGURE 5.   Platelet aggregation in response to adenosine diphosphate (ADP) (upper panel) and heparin (lower panel) immediately after induction of anesthesia but before iloprost infusion *(A)* and after 20 minutes of infusing iloprost at a rate of 24 ng/kg/min *(B)*. (From Kappa JR, Horn MK III, Fisher CA, et al: Efficacy of iloprost (ZK36374) versus aspirin in preventing heparin-induced platelet activation during open cardiac surgery. J Thorac Cardiovasc Surg 94:405–413, 1987, with permission.)

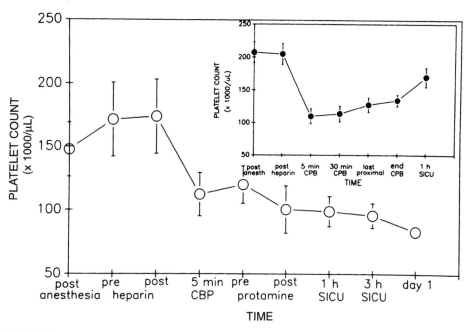

FIGURE 6. Platelet counts (mean ± standard error of the mean) are plotted against time and expressed as × 10³/μl for patients with heparin-induced thrombocytopenia/thrombosis (o—o, n = 9) and controls undergoing coronary revascularization (inset, •—•, n = 21). CPB = cardiopulmonary bypass, SICU = surgical intensive care unit. (From Kappa J, Fisher C, Todd B, et al: Intraoperative management of patients with heparin-induced thrombocytopenia. Ann Thorac Surg 49:714–723, 1990, with permission.)

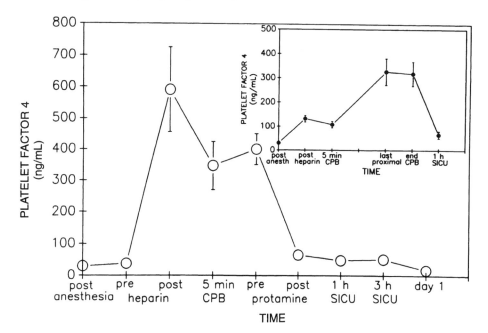

FIGURE 7. Plasma levels of platelet factor 4 (mean ± standard error of the mean) are plotted against time and expressed as ng/ml. Otherwise, legend is identical to Figure 5. (From Kappa J, Fisher C, Todd B, et al: Intraoperative management of patients with heparin-induced thrombocytopenia. Ann Thorac Surg 49:714–723, 1990, with permission.)

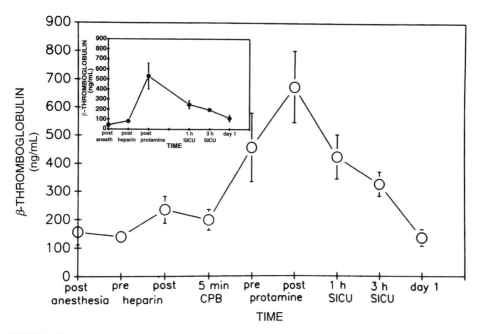

FIGURE 8. Plasma levels of β-thromboglobulin (mean ± standard error of the mean) are plotted against time and expressed as ng/ml. Otherwise, legend is identical to Figure 5. (From Kappa J, Fisher C, Todd B, et al: Intraoperative management of patients with heparin-induced thrombocytopenia. Ann Thorac Surg 49:714–723, 1990, with permission.)

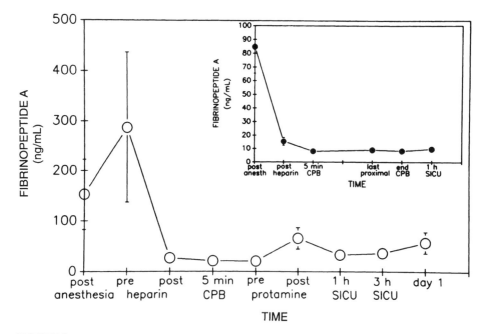

FIGURE 9. Plasma levels of fibrinopeptide A (mean ± standard error of the mean) are plotted against time and expressed as ng/ml. Otherwise, legend is identical to Figure 5. (From Kappa J, Fisher C, Todd B, et al: Intraoperative management of patients with heparin-induced thrombocytopenia. Ann Thorac Surg 49:714–723, 1990, with permission.)

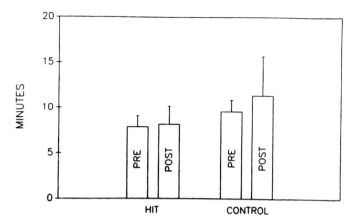

FIGURE 10.   Template bleeding time obtained immediately after anesthesia induction (PRE) and bleeding time obtained after arrival of patient in the surgical intensive care unit (POST) are plotted for patients with heparin-induced thrombocytopenia/thrombosis (HITT, n = 9) and controls (n = 21). (From Kappa J, Fisher C, Todd B, et al: Intraoperative management of patients with heparin-induced thrombocytopenia. Ann Thorac Surg 49:714–723, 1990, with permission.)

preserved and hemostasis maintained despite exposure to both heparin-induced platelet-activating factor and synthetic surface during cardiopulmonary bypass.

DISCUSSION

Iloprost is a stable analog of prostacyclin, a potent endogenous inhibitor of platelet function. Iloprost effectively prevents platelet activation by all platelet agonists evaluated in our laboratory, including thrombin. It acts by stimulating adenyl cyclase and elevating intracellular levels of cyclic AMP. In nanomolar concentrations, a level that is readily achieved clinically, iloprost prevented in vitro heparin-induced platelet aggregation and release in the sera of all patients, including those in whom heparin appears to act through thromboxane-independent pathways.

Consistent with our in vitro observations, iloprost did indeed prevent heparin-induced platelet activation in all of our patients. There was no change in circulating platelet count or

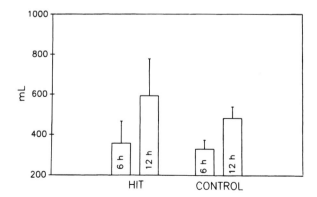

FIGURE 11.   Mean chest tube drainage amounts (mean ± standard error of the mean) at 6 and 12 hours. Otherwise, legend is identical to Figure 10. (From Kappa J, Fisher C, Todd B, et al: Intraoperative management of patients with heparin-induced thrombocytopenia. Ann Thorac Surg 49:714–723, 1990, with permission.)

formation of platelet aggregates after heparin administration. Similarly, levels of fibrino-peptide A remained low, indicating the absence of heparin-induced thrombosis. Equally important, platelet function was definitely preserved, permitting improved postoperative bleeding times and reduced blood loss. No deaths were associated with heparin or iloprost administration, even though many of the patients had severe cardiac dysfunction.

Iloprost—like its parent compound, prostacyclin—is a vasodilator. In fact, vasodilation has limited the clinical utility of prostacyclin in our experience. Fortunately, iloprost appears to be more manageable, and stable hemodynamic values were readily maintained with the aid of phenylephrine. Furthermore, no adverse side effects could be attributed to either hypotension or vasopressor administration. Thus, our experience to date has clearly demonstrated that iloprost can be administered safely even in high-risk patients.

In patients diagnosed with HITT, which is associated with extremely high morbidity and mortality rates, avoidance of reexposure to heparin is strongly recommended. For the select group of patients with HITT who require mandatory reexposure to heparin, some form of platelet inhibition is recommended. In our experience, iloprost provided this protection both safely and effectively. Because temporary inhibition of platelet function has proved so efficacious in this setting, agents with similar pharmacologic properties— i.e., those with global but rapidly and completely reversible effects against strong platelet agonists—should be a valuable addition to the management armamentarium.

REFERENCES

1. AbuRahma AF, Boland JP, Witsberger T: Diagnostic and therapeutic strategies of white clot syndrome. Am J Surg 162:175–179, 1991.
2. Addonizio VP: Platelet function in cardiopulmonary bypass and artificial organs. Hematol Oncol Clin North Am 4:145–155, 1990.
3. Addonizio VP, Colman RW: Platelets and extracorporeal circulation. Biomaterials 3:9–15, 1982.
4. Addonizio VP Jr, Fisher CA, Jenkin BK, et al: Iloprost (ZK36374), a stable analogue of prostacyclin, preserved platelets during simulated extracorporeal circulation. J Thorac Cardiovasc Surg 89:926–933, 1985.
5. Addonizio VP, Kappa JR, Fisher CA, Ellison N: Prevention of heparin-induced thrombocytopenia during open-heart surgery with ZK36374 (iloprost). Surgery 102:796–807, 1987.
6. Addonizio VP, Macarak EJ, Nicolaou KC, et al: Effects of prostacyclin and albumin on platelet loss during in-vitro simulation of extracorporeal circulation. Blood 53:1033–1042, 1979.
7. Addonizio VP, Macarak EJ, Niewiarowski S, et al: Preservation of human platelets with prostaglandin E_1 during in-vitro simulated cardiopulmonary bypass. Circ Res 44:350–357, 1979.
8. Addonizio VP, Smith JB, Guiod LR, et al: Thromboxane synthesis and platelet release during simulated extracorporeal circulation. Blood 54:371–376, 1979.
9. Addonnizio VP, Strauss JF III, Chang LF, et al: Release of lysosomal hydrolases during simulated extracorporeal circulation. J Thorac Cardiovasc Surg 84:28–34, 1982.
10. Amiral J, Bridey F, Dreyfus M, et al: Platelet factor 4 complexed to heparin is the target for antibodies generated in heparin-induced thrombocytopenia. Thromb Haemost 68:95–96, 1992.
11. Amiral J, Bridey F, Wolf M, et al: Antibodies to macromolecular platelet factor 4-heparin complexes in heparin-induced thrombocytopenia. Thromb Haemost 73:21–28, 1995.
12. Arthur CK, Isbister JP, Aspery EM: The heparin-induced thrombocytopenia syndrome (HITTS): A review. Pathology 17:82–86, 1985.
13. Babcock RB, Dumper CW, Scharfman WB: Heparin-induced immune thrombocytopenia. N Engl J Med 295:237–241, 1976.
14. Bell WR, Romasulo PA, Alving DM, Duffy TP: Thrombocytopenia occurring during the administration of heparin: A prospective study in 52 patients. Ann Intern Med 85:155–160, 1976.
15. Bell WR, Royall RM: Heparin associated thrombocytopenia: A comparison of three heparin preparations. N Eng J Med 303:902–907, 1980.
16. Bernabei A, Gikakis N, Kowalska MA, et al: Iloprost and Echistatin protect platelets during simulated extracorporeal circulation. Ann Thorac Surg 59:149–153, 1995.
17. Choay J: Biologic studies on chemically synthesized pentasaccharide and tetrasaccharide fragments. Semin Thromb Hemost 11:81–85, 1985.
18. Chong BH, Burgess J, Ismail F: The clinical usefulness of the platelet aggregation test for the diagnosis of heparin-induced thrombocytopenia. Thromb Haemost 69:344–350, 1993.
19. Chong BH, Castaldi PA: Heparin-induced-thrombocytopenia: Further studies of the effects of heparin-dependent antibodies on platelets. Br J Haematol 64:347–354, 1986.

20. Chong BH, Grace CS, Rosenberg MC: Heparin-induced-thrombocytopenia: Effect of heparin platelet antibody on platelets. Br J Haematol 49:531–540, 1981.
21. Cines DB, Kaymin P, Bina M, et al: Heparin-associated thrombocytopenia. N Engl J Med 303:788–795, 1980.
22. Cines DB, Tamaski A, Tannenbaum S: Immune endothelial cell injury in heparin-associated thrombocytopenia. N Engl J Med 316:581–589, 1987.
23. Cipolle RJ, Rodvold KA, Seifert R, Clarens R, Ramirez-Lassepas M: Heparin-associated thrombocytopenia: A prospective evaluation of 211 patients. Ther Drug Monit 5:205–211, 1983.
24. Cole CW, Bormanis J: Ancrod: a practical alternative to heparin. J Vasc Surg 8:59–63, 1988.
25. Copley AL, Robb TB: The effect of heparin on the platelet count in dogs and mice. Am J Physiol 133:248, 1941.
26. Cottrell ED, Kappa JR, Stenach N, et al: Temporary inhibition of platelet function with iloprost (ZK36374) preserves canine platelets during extracorporeal membrane oxygenation. J Thorac Cardiovasc Surg 96:535–541, 1988.
27. Ellison N, Kappa JR, Fisher CA, Addonizio VP: Extracorporeal circulation in a patient with heparin-induced thrombocytopenia. Anesthesiology 63:336–337, 1985.
28. Favaloro EJ, Barnal-Hoyos E, Exner T, Koutts J: Heparin-induced thrombocytopenia: Laboratory investigation and confirmation of diagnosis. Pathology 24:177–183, 1992.
30. Fareed J: Heparin, its fractions, fragments, and derivatives. Semin Thromb Hemost 11:1–9, 1985.
31. Feng WC, Singh AK, Bert AA, et al: Perioperative paraplegia and multiorgan failure from heparin-induced thrombocytopenia. Ann Thorac Surg 55:1555–1557, 1993.
32. Fisher CA, Kappa JR, Sinha AK, et al: Comparison of equimolar concentrations of iloprost, prostacyclin, and prostaglandin E_1 on human platelet function. J Lab Clin Med 109:184–190, 1987.
33. Frantantoni JC, Pollet R, Gralnick HR: Heparin-induced thrombocytopenia: Confirmation of diagnosis with in vitro methods. Blood 45:395–401, 1975.
34. Godal HC: Report of the International Committee on Thrombosis and Haemostasis: Thrombocytopenia and heparin. Thromb Haemost 43:222–234, 1980.
35. Gollub S, Ulin AW: Heparin-induced thrombocytopenia in man. J Lab Clin Med 59:430–435, 1962.
36. Grant SM, Goa KL: Iloprost: A review of its pharmacodynamic and pharmacokinetic properties and therapeutic potential in peripheral vascular disease, myocardial ischaemia and extracorporeal circulation procedures. Drugs 43:889–924, 1992.
37. Green D, Harris K, Reynolds N, et al: Heparin immune thrombocytopenia: Evidence for a heparin-platelet complex as the antigenic determinant. J Lab Clin Med 91:167–175, 1978.
38. Guay DRP, Richard A: Heparin-induced thrombocytopenia: Association with a platelet aggregating factor and cross-sensitivity to bovine and porcine heparin. Drug Intell Clin Pharm 18:398–401, 1984.
39. Hackett T, Kelton JG, Powers P: Drug-induced platelet destruction. Semin Thromb Hemost 8:116–137, 1982.
40. Harenburg J, Zimmerman R, Schwartz F, Kubler W: Treatment of heparin-induced thrombocytopenia with thrombosis by a new heparinoid. Lancet 1:986–987, 1983.
41. Holmsen H, Day HJ: Concepts of the blood platelet release reaction. Semin Hematol 4:3–27, 1971.
42. Holmsen H, Day HJ: The selectivity of the thrombin-induced platelet release reaction: Subcellular localization of released and retained constituents. J Lab Clin Med 75:840–855, 1970.
43. Howe SE, Lynch DM: An enzyme-linked immunosorbent assay for the evaluation of thrombocytopenia induced by heparin. J Lab Clin Med 105:554–559, 1985.
44. Huisse MG, Guillin MC, Bezeaud A, Toulemond F, Kitzis M, Andreassian B: Heparin-associated thrombocytopenia. In vitro effects of different molecular weight heparin fractions. Thromb Res 27:485–490, 1982.
45. Isenhart CE, Brandt JT: Platelet aggregation studies for the diagnosis of heparin-induced thrombocytopenia. Am J Clin Pathol 99:324–330, 1993.
46. Janson PA, Moake JL, Carpinito G: Aspirin prevents heparin-induced platelet aggregation in vivo. Br J Haematol 53:166–168, 1983.
47. Kappa JR, Cottrell ED, Berkowitz HD, et al: Carotid endarterectomy in patients with heparin-induced platelet activation: Comparative efficacy of aspirin and iloprost (ZK36374). J Vasc Surg 15:693–761, 1987.
48. Kappa JR, Fisher CA, Berkowitz HB, et al: Heparin-induced platelet activation in sixteen surgical patients: Diagnosis and management. J Vasc Surg 5:101–109, 1987.
49. Kappa JR, Fisher CA, Addonizio VP: Heparin-induced platelet activation: The role of thromboxane A_2 synthesis and the extent of platelet granule release in two patients. J Vasc Surg 9:574–579, 1989.
50. Kappa J, Fisher C, Todd B, et al: Intraoperative management of patients with heparin-induced thrombocytopenia. Ann Thorac Surg 49:714–723, 1990.
51. Kappa JR, Horn MK III, Fisher CA, et al: Efficacy of iloprost (ZK36374) versus aspirin in preventing heparin-induced platelet activation during open cardiac surgery. J Thorac Cardiovasc Surg 94:405–413, 1987.
52. Kelton JG, Sheridan D, Brian H, et al: Clinical usefulness of testing for a heparin-dependent aggregating factor in patients with suspected heparin-associated thrombocytopenia. J Lab Clin Med 103:606–612, 1984.
53. Kelton JG, Smith JW, Warkentin TE, et al: Immunoglobulin G from patients with heparin-induced thrombocytopenia binds to a complex of heparin and platelet factor 4. Blood 83:3232–3239, 1994.

54. King DJ, Kelton JG: Heparin-associated thrombocytopenia. Ann Intern Med 100:535–540,1984.
55. Korn RL, Fisher CA, Stenach N, et al : Iloprost reduces procoagulant activity in the extracorporeal circuit. J Surg Res 55:433–440, 1993.
56. Laster J, Silver D: Heparin-coated catheters and heparin-induced thrombocytopenia. J Vasc Surg 7:667–672, 1988.
57. Leroy J, Leclerc MH, Delahousse B, et al: Treatment of heparin-associated thrombocytopenia and thrombosis with low molecular weight heparin (CY216). Semin Thromb Hemost 11:326–329, 1985.
58. Makhoul RG, Greenberg CS, McCann RL: Heparin-associated thrombocytopenia and thrombosis: A serious clinical problem and potential solution. J Vasc Surg 4:522–528, 1986.
59. Messmore HL: Clinical use of heparin fractions, fragments, and heparinoids. Semin Thromb Hemost 11: 208–212, 1985.
60. McLean J: The thromboplastic action of cephalin. Am J Physiol 41:250–257, 1916.
61. Nelson JC, Lerner RG, Goldstein R, Cagen NA: Heparin-induced thrombocytopenia. Arch Intern Med 138:548–552, 1978.
62. Olinger GN, Hussey CV, Olive JA, Malik MI: Cardiopulmonary bypass for patients with previously documented heparin-induced platelet aggregation. J Thorac Cardiovasc Surg 87:673–677, 1984.
63. Rhodes GR, Dixon RH, Silver D: Heparin-induced thrombocytopenia with thrombotic and hemorrhagic manifestations. Surg Gynecol Obstet 136:409–416, 1973.
64. Roberts B, Rosato FE, Rosato EF: Heparin: A cause of arterial emboli? Surgery 55:803–808, 1964.
65. Roth GJ, Majerus PW: The mechanism of the effect of aspirin on human platelets. I. Acetylation of a particulate fraction protein. J Clin Invest 56:624–632, 1975.
66. Roussi JH, Houbouyan LL, Goguel AF: Use of low molecular weight heparin in heparin-induced thrombocytopenia with thrombotic complications. Lancet 1:1183, 1984.
67. Salem HH, Van der Weyden MD: Heparin-induced thrombocytopenia. Variable platelet-rich plasma reactivity to heparin dependent platelet aggregating factor. Pathology 15:297–299, 1983.
68. Salzman EW, Rosenberg RD, Smith MH, et al Effect of heparin fractions on platelet aggregation. J Clin Invest 65:64–73, 1980.
69. Schror K, Darius H, Matzky R, Ohlendorf R: The antiplatelet and cardiovascular actions of a new carbacyclin derivative (ZK36374) equipotent to PGI2 in vitro. Naunyn Schmiedeberg's Arch Pharmacol 316:252–255, 1981.
70. Sheridan D, Carter C, Kelton JG: A diagnostic test for heparin-induced thrombocytopenia. Blood 67:27–30, 1986.
71. Silver D, Kapsch DN, Tsoi EKM: Heparin-induced thrombocytopenia, thrombosis, and hemorrhage. Ann Surg 198:301–306, 1983.
72. Smith JP, Walls JT, Muscato MS, et al: Extracorporeal circulation in a patient with heparin-induced thrombocytopenia. Anesthesiology 62:363–365, 1985.
73. Stead RB, Schafer AI, Rosenberg RD, et al: Heterogenicity of heparin lots associated with thrombocytopenia and thromboembolism. Am J Med 77:185–188, 1985.
74. Stock G, Muller B, Krais T, Schillinger E: Iloprost, a stable analogue of PGI2: Clinical results and pathophysiological considerations. Adv Prostaglandin Thromboxane Leukotriene Res 21:583–589, 1990.
75. Sturzebecher CS, Losert W: Effects of iloprost on platelet activation in-vitro. In Gryglewski RJ, Stock G (eds): Prostacyclin and Its Stable Analogue Iloprost. Springer-Verlag, Berlin, 1987, pp 39–45.
76. Torosian M, Michelson EL, Morganroth J, McVaugh H: Aspirin and coumadin-related bleeding after coronary artery bypass graft surgery. Ann Intern Med 89:325–328, 1978.
77. Umlas J, Jaff RH, Gauvin G, Swierk P: Anticoagulant monitoring and neutralization during open heart surgery: A rapid method for measuring heparin and calculating safe reduced protamine doses. Anesth Analg 62:1095–1099, 1983.
78. Visendin GP, Ford SE, Scott JP, Aster RH: Antibodies from patients with heparin-induced thrombocytopenia/thrombosis are specific for platelet factor 4 complexed with heparin or bound to endothelial cells. J Clin Invest 93:81–88, 1994.
79. Wahl TO, Lipschitz DA, Stechschulte DJ: Thrombocytopenia associated with antiheparin antibody. JAMA 240:2560–2562, 1978.
80. Warkentin TE, Hayward CP, Boshkov LK, et al: Sera from patients with heparin-induced thrombocytopenia generate platelet-derived microparticles with procoagulant activity: an explanation for the thrombotic complications of heparin-induced thrombocytopenia. Blood 84:3691–3699, 1994.
81. Weismann RE, Tobin RW: Arterial embolism occurring during systemic heparin therapy. Arch Surg 76:219–229, 1958.
82. Weiss HJ: Platelet physiology and abnormalities of platelet function, Part I. N Engl J Med 293:531–540, 1975.
83. Weiss HJ: Platelet physiology and abnormalities of platelet function, Part II. N Engl J Med 293:580–588, 1975.

CHAPTER 33

Thrombin Participation in Cancers

JOHN W. FENTON II, Ph.D., FACB
FREDRICK A. OFOSU, Ph.D.
KATHERINE P. HENRIKSON, Ph.D.
DIANE V. BREZNIAK, M.A.
HOURIA I. HASSOUNA, M.D., Ph.D.

Thrombin has traditionally been thought of as a serine proteinase, generated from prothrombin, with central functions in thrombotic processes (e.g., platelet activation, conversion of fibrinogen into clottable fibrin), but it also participates in various physiologic and pathophysiologic processes from injury to wound healing.[1–3] In fact, thrombin seems to be a relatively recent acquisition of the pathways in hemostasis, with evolutionarily more primitive functions at the cell regulatory level.[2,3] In this regard, postthrombotic processes (e.g., thrombolysis, cell recruitment, new cell growth in repair, wound remodeling) resemble processes in cancer growth and spreading.[4] Thrombin has several activities relevant to those that are known (or envisioned) to occur in cancer (Table 1).

Because of various thrombin consumptive processes (e.g., antithrombin III [AT III], heparin cofactor II [HC II], α_2-macroglobulin [α_2M], protease nexin-1 [PN-1], cellular binding, fibrin partitioning, fluid dilution), thrombin must be continually generated to sustain its functions in thrombosis and other processes.[2] This is largely achieved by secondary thrombin generation on surfaces of activated cells in the vasculature (e.g., platelets, endothelial cells) and extravascularly, presumably through the tissue thromboplastin (TP) pathway.[3] Of note, thrombin is a potent stimulus of TP expression in many cell types, including cancer cells,[5] and in expression of tissue plasminogen (tPA) and urokinase activators (uPA) as well as plasminogen activator-1 (PA-1) (Fig. 1). Therefore, thrombin not only promotes secondary generation of more thrombin but also initiates thrombolysis with release of fibrin-entrapped thrombin.[2,3] Furthermore, thrombin activates matrix-degrading prometalloproteinase-2 (pro-MMP-2) (type IV collagenase/gelatinase),[6] which is implicated in tumor invasiveness[7] and believed to participate in wound remodeling as well as malignant spreading or metastasis (see Fig.1).

These striking similarities between processes in wound healing and cancer imply that thrombin has central functions in neoplasia (or mimics another enzyme[s] or growth factor[s] with similar functions). Thus, thrombin may be a rate-limiting factor in the growth (proliferation) and spreading (invasion) of certain cancers or may not be a requirement of other cancers. Clearly, not all cancers are alike; they may have different independent etiologies (e.g., viral, mutational, environmental stimuli).

517

TABLE 1.   Thrombin Activities Relevant to Cancer Growth and Invasion

Thrombin is a potent:
- Mitogenic substance (mitogen)
- Angiogenic substance (angiogen)[22,23]
- Chemotactic substance (chemotactin)

Thrombin also participates in:
- Edema (e.g., enhances endothelial barrier transport)
- Inflammation (e.g., substitutes for factor $\overline{\text{D}}$ in complement system, generates C3a- and C5a-like activities, induces interleukin-6 secretion,[24,25] stimulates T-cells[26])
  - Initiates thrombolysis (e.g., stimulates expression of plasminogen activators—tPA, uPA)
  - Activates matrix-degrading prometalloproteinase (pro-MMP-2)[6]

Information from references 1–3 or as cited in table.

The involvement of thrombin in certain types of cancers (e.g., small cell carcinoma) has been implicated by several lines of evidence.[4,8,9] Antithrombotic therapy with warfarin (which suppresses γ-carboxylation of essential glutamyl residues in prothrombin and other vitamin K-dependent coagulation factors) and heparin (a cofactor for AT III inhibition of thrombin and other activated cofactors) has shown benefits with such cancers. Zacharski and colleagues demonstrated the presence of thrombin in tumors of small cell sarcoma by immunologic staining with hirudin (a highly specific inhibitor of thrombin that forms a very high-affinity complex).[10] They also showed the presence of enzymatically active thrombin by immunostaining for an epitope exposed upon Bβ cleavage of fibrinogen.[11] Furthermore, the presence of fibrin deposition (e.g., fibrin cocoon) is a clear indication of thrombin. In animal models, hirudin and other thrombin inhibitors have impeded tumor genesis.[4] In one study, hirudin did not inhibit the growth of melanoma cells in tissue culture but prevented tumor formation by the same cells injected into mice.[12] Thus, thrombin may be a limiting factor for tumor invasion independent of growth, which is in accord with Figure 1.

A second major category of cancers express plasminogen activators (e.g., tPA, uPA) without the predominant indications of thrombin.[8,9] However, very low thrombin concentrations are potent stimuli of plasminogen activator expression, and γ-thrombin (which essentially lacks fibrinogen clotting activity) is second only to α-thrombin (high clotting activity) in stimulating such activity in tissue culture.[13] In addition, uPA converts α-thrombin to nonclotting forms,[14] which may account for the apparent absence of fibrin deposition, while nonclotting forms carry out cellular and other thrombin functions. Recently, a thrombin receptor (TR-1) has been cloned,[15] but knockout gene experiments[16] and other evidence[17,18] have shown that TR-1 is not the only thrombin receptor, although it behaves as the predominant receptor on various cells.[19,20] In this regard, plasmin activation of TR-1[21] may be important (see Fig. 1). As with thrombin, high local concentrations of tPA or uPA (or perhaps, plasmin) also may activate pro-MMP-2 or similar proenzyme(s) and promote invasiveness. We speculate that up-regulation of TR-1 occurs in thrombin-mediated cancer cells and that TR-1 detection on such cells should correlate with aggressiveness. In addition to the TR-1 detection per cell, the percentage of activated-to-total TR-1 may be a further indicator of a pathologic state.

Thrombin thus may be a rate-limiting factor for cancer growth and spreading. As such, individual biopsies should be (i) diagnosable by bioassays (e.g., tissue culture, invasion chambers, immunomarkers), (ii) inhibited by hirudin and/or other thrombin-directed inhibitors (e.g., argatroban, bivalirudin [hirulog]), and (iii) treatable with conventional (e.g., warfarin, heparin) or more recent antithrombotics (e.g., recombinant hirudin, argatroban, bivalirudin). Alternatively, and perhaps less expensively, quantitation of TR-1 (e.g., enzyme-linked immunosorbent assay [ELISA]) may provide a useful indication for antithrombotic intervention.

In summary, thrombin may participate in cancer growth and spreading in the apparent absence of fibrin deposition (cryptic thrombin involvement). Such cryptic involvement, moreover, should be susceptible to antithrombotic intervention.

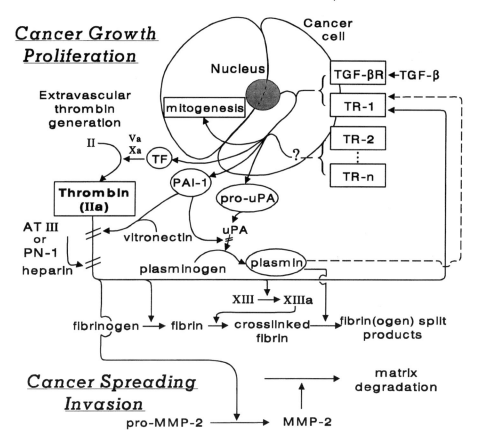

FIGURE 1. Depicted is thrombin participation in cancer growth (proliferation) and spreading (invasion). Thrombin (IIa) is generated extravascularly from prothrombin (II) by activated coagulation factor (Xa) in the presence of activated factor V (Va), activated factor VII (VIIa), and tissue factor (TF). It is inhibited by antithrombin III (AT III) or protease nexin-1 (PN-1) in the presence of heparin or plasminogen activator inhibitor (PAI-1) in the presence of vitronectin. PAI-1 also inhibits urokinase plasminogen activator (uPA) and, thus, both thrombin and plasmin pathways. Both thrombin and plasmin stimulate the known thrombin receptor (TR-1). However, thrombin can stimulate other receptors (see text). Thrombin converts fibrinogen into clottable fibrin (fibrin deposition) and stimulates cells, inducing mitogenesis and upregulating TF, PAI-1, and pro-uPA, among other cellular response proteins. Activation of pro-uPA causes plasmin generation; plasmin degrades fibrinogen and fibrin and stimulates cell responses. Thrombin activates pro-MMP-2, causing degradation of extracellular matrices and promoting cancer spreading or invasion. Thus, cancer growth (proliferation) is distinct from spreading (invasion), although the processes are envisioned to be interconnected.

REFERENCES

1. Fenton JW II: Thrombin specificity. Ann N Y Acad Sci 370:468–495, 1981.
2. Fenton JW II, Ofosu FA, Brezniak DV, Hassouna HI: Understanding thrombin and hemostasis. Hematol Oncol Clin North Am 7:1107–1119, 1993.
3. Fenton JW II: Thrombin functions and antithrombotic intervention. Thromb Haemost 74:493–498, 1995.
4. Walz DA, Fenton JW II: The role of thrombin in tumor cell metastasis. Invas Metast 14:303–308, 1995.
5. Contrino J, Hair G, Kreutzer DL, Rickles FR: In situ detection of tissue factor in vascular endothelial cells: Correlation with the malignant phenotype of human breast disease. Nature 2:209–215, 1996.
6. Galis ZS, Kranzhofer R, Fenton JW II, Libby P: Thrombin promotes activation of matrix metalloproteinase-2 produced by culture vascular smooth muscle cells. Artheroscler Thromb Vasc Biol, in revision.

7. Azzam HS, Arand G, Lippman ME, Thompson EW: Association of MMP-2 activation potential with metastatic progression in human breast cancer cell lines independent of MMP-2 production. Cancer Inst 85:1758–1764, 1993.

8. Zacharski LR, Wojtukiewicz ME, Costantini V, Ornstein DL, Memoli VA: Pathways of coagulation/fibrinolysis activation in malignancy. Semin Thromb Hemost 18:104–116, 1992.

9. Zacharski LR, Costantini V: Blood coagulation activation in cancer: Challenges for cancer treatment. Hamostaseologie 15:14–20, 1995.

10. Zacharski LR, Memoli VA, Morain WD, Schlaeppi JM, Rousseau SM: Cellular localization of enzymatically active thrombin in intact human tissues by hirudin binding. Thromb Haemost 73:793–797, 1995.

11. Zacharski LR, Memoli VA, Rousseau SM: (1987) Thrombin-specific sites of fibrinogen in small cell carcinoma of the lung [abstract]. Thromb Haemost 58:236, 1987.

12. Esumi N, Fan D, Fidler IJ: Inhibition of murine melanoma experimental metastasis by recombinant desulfatohirudin, a highly specific thrombin inhibitor. Cancer Res 51:4549–4556, 1991.

13. Levin EG, Stern DM, Nawroth PP, Marlar RA, Fenton JW II, Harker LA: Specificity of the thrombin-induced release of tissue plasminogen activator from cultured human endothelial cells. Thromb Haemost 56:115–119, 1986.

14. Bezeaud A, de Raucourt E, Miyata T, Bouton M-C, Angles-Cano E, Guillian M-C: Limited proteolysis of human α-thrombin by urokinase yields a non-clotting enzyme. Thromb Haemost 73:275 280, 1995.

15. Vu T-KH, Hung DT, Wheaton VI, Coughlin SR: Molecular cloning of a functional thrombin receptor reveals a novel proteolytic mechanism of receptor activation. Cell 64:1057–1068, 1991.

16. Connolly AJ, Ishihara H, Kahn ML, Farese JR, Coughlin SR: Role of the thrombin receptor in development and evidence for a second receptor. Nature 381:516–519, 1996.

17. Catalfamo JL, Andersen TT, Fenton JW II: Thrombin receptor activating peptides unlike thrombin are insufficient for platelet activation in most species [abstract]. Thromb Haemost 69:1195, 1993.

18. Ferraris VA, Rodriquez E, Ferraris SP, Huang M, Gupta A, Bennett JA, Andersen TT, Dunn H, Fenton FW II, Smith JB: Platelet aggregation abnormalities after cardiopulmonary bypass. Blood, 83:299–300, 1994.

19. McNamara CA, Sarembock IJ, Gimple LW, Fenton JW II, Coughlin SR, Owens GK: Thrombin stimulates smooth muscle proliferation by a proteolytic, receptor mediated mechanism. J Clin Invest 91:94–98, 1993.

20. Seiler SM, Pelusco M, Michel IM, Goldenberg H, Fenton JW II, Riexinger D, Natarajan S: Inhibition of thrombin and SFLLR-peptide stimulation of platelet aggregation, phospholipase A_2 and Na^+/H^+ exchange by a thrombin receptor antagonist. Biochem Pharmacol 49:519–528, 1995.

21. Kimura M, Andersen TT, Fenton JW II, Bahou WF, Aviv A: Plasmin-platelet interaction involves cleavage of functional thrombin receptor. Am J Physiol (Cell Physiol) 271:C54–C60, 1996.

22. Walz DA, Fenton JW II, Johnson PH: Human thrombin induces angiogenesis [abstract]. Thromb Haemost 65:1252, 1991.

23. Tsopanoglou NE, Pipili-Synetos E, Maragoudakis ME: Thrombin promotes angiogenesis by a mechanism independent of fibrin formation. Am J Physiol 264:C1302–C1307, 1993.

24. Sower LE, Froelich CJ, Carney DH, Fenton JW II, Klimpel GR: Thrombin induces IL6 production in fibroblasts and epithelial cells: Evidence for the involvement of the seven-transmembrane domain (STD)-receptor for α-thrombin. J Immunol 155:895–901, 1995.

25. Kranzhöfer R, Clinton SK, Ishii K, Coughlin SR, Fenton JW II, Libby P: Thrombin potently stimulates cytokine production in human vascular smooth muscle cells but not in mononuclear phagocytes. Circ Res 79:286–294, 1996.

26. Tordai A, Fenton JW II, Andersen TT, Gelfand EW: Functional thrombin receptors on human T lymphoblast cells. J Immunol 150:4876–4886, 1993.

CHAPTER 34

Laboratory Monitoring of New Anticoagulant and Antithrombotic Drugs

DEBRA A. HOPPENSTEADT, M.S., M.T. (ASCP)
WALTER JESKE, Ph.D.
JAWED FAREED, Ph.D.

Many recent developments in the clinical management of thrombotic and vascular disorders have been reported.[1,5,7,14] Several pharmacologic agents for the prophylactic and therapeutic management of cardiovascular disorders, such as thrombosis, acute myocardial infarction, and stroke, have been introduced. This progress is due to a better understanding of pathophysiology, including triggering events and target sites that are affected. Biotechnology and advances in separation techniques have contributed to the development of many antithrombotic, anticoagulant, and thrombolytic drugs.[2,8,13] Several new drugs, such as recombinant hirudin, hirulog, antibodies that target the glycoprotein IIb (GPIIb)–factor IIIa complex, and tissue factor pathway inhibitor, are currently undergoing clinical trials.[1,13] These new antithrombotic drugs represent a wide spectrum of natural, synthetic, and biotechnology-produced agents with marked differences in chemical composition, physicochemical properties, biochemical actions, and pharmacologic effects. The mechanism of action of the new antithrombotic agents is quite complex; therefore, monitoring is not possible with the routine clot-based assays used for heparin and oral anticoagulant drugs. Many of the new agents produce no alteration in currently measurable blood clotting parameters, but they are clinically effective therapeutic agents. Blood and vascular modulation also plays an important role in the mediation of the antithrombotic actions of newer drugs, involving red cells, white cells, platelets, endothelial cells, and proteins. Such effects are not readily measurable by any of the monitoring approaches. Polytherapy, with combinations of these agents, has also been used; it appears to be more effective in the management of cardiovascular and thrombotic disorders. Global methods to monitor the collective actions of newer drugs are not currently available.

The monitoring of the effects of newer drugs requires the development of newer methods that can measure their effects directly or indirectly, and thus assess therapeutic and adverse actions. Advances in analytical techniques have allowed monitoring of the endogenous responses that occur in a pathologic state and are modulated by the use of the newer agents.[2,3,6] As previously stated, global clotting assays are no longer sufficient

TABLE 1.   Alterations in Molecular Markers as a Result of Pathologic Events

Molecular Markers	DIC	Primary Fibrinolysis	Hyper-coagulable State	Thrombotic Stroke	Myocardial Infarction
Prothrombin fragment 1.2	↑	NC	↑	↑/NC	↑
Thrombin–antithrombin complex	↑	NC	↑	↑/NC	↑
Fibrinopeptide A	↑	NC	↑	↑/NC	↑
Tissue plasminogen acivator (tPA)	↓↑	↑	NC/↓	↓	↑
Tissue plasminogen activator inhibitor (PAI)	↓↑	NC	↑	↑	↑
Plasmin–AP complex	↑	↑	NC	NC	↑
Bβ 15-42–related peptides	↑	↑	NC	NC	↑
D-dimer	↑	↑	↑	↑	↑
Platelet factor 4	↑	NC	↑	↑	↑
β-Thromboglobulin	↑	NC	↑	↑	↑
Thromboxane β_2	↑/NC	NC	↑	↑	↑
6-keto PGF$_{1\alpha}$	NC	NC	↑	NC	NC
Endothelin	↓↑	NC	NC	↑	↑/NC
Soluble thrombomodulin	↑	NC	NC	↑	↑
Antiphospholipid antibody	↑	NC	↑/NC	↑	↑

DIC = disseminated intravascular coagulation, NC = no change.

because they measure only the effect of drugs on the clotting process. Technical advances in molecular biology and immunology have allowed the development of monoclonal and polyclonal antibody-based technology (enzyme-linked immunosorbent assays [ELISA]) to monitor the indirect effect of antithrombotic drugs, which otherwise produce no anticoagulant effects. In addition to the measurement of absolute drug concentration in plasma by high-performance liquid chromotography (HPLC), ELISA techniques have been developed to measure plasma levels of such new agents as thrombin inhibitors (hirudin) and tissue factor pathway inhibitor (TFPI, a tissue factor/Xa inhibitor).

ELISA technology also can be used to measure alterations in the coagulation, platelet, endothelium, and fibrinolytic systems that occur during pathologic events and result in the generation of specific molecular markers.[1,6] Table 1 lists alterations in these molecular markers after thrombotic stoke, hypercoagulable state, and myocardial infarction. Thus, ELISA and radioimmunoassays (RIA) can measure subclinical activation of the hemostatic system. Molecular markers are elevated in certain thrombotic and cardiovascular disorders and may be useful for the monitoring of the various effects of the new anticoagulant drugs. An increase or decrease of these markers can reflect the effects of newer drugs.

Newer clot-based methods also have been developed (Table 2). The activated clotting time (ACT) can be modified by adding thrombin or ecarin (a snake venom) to monitor the anticoagulant effects of some of the new thrombin inhibitors. These methods are being evaluated in clinical trials of many of the newer antithrombotic drugs. The ecarin clotting time is based on the activation of prothrombin to mesothrombin. This assay, which is being tested in clinical settings for the monitoring of several thrombin inhibitors, is not affected by heparin or heparin-like agents that complex with antithrombin III (AT III). Therefore, when heparin or heparin-like substances are given in combination, the thrombin inhibitor can be specifically monitored. In addition, the calcium thrombin time also can be used in place of the routinely performed thrombin time to monitor the high dosages of thrombin reagents required during cardiovascular procedures.

TABLE 2.   Newer Methods for the Monitoring of Anticoagulant Agents

• Modified activated clotting times	• Heptest clotting time
• Optimized activated partial thromboplastin time (APTT)	• Heptest-Hi
• Optimized thrombin time and calcium thrombin time	• Ecarin clotting time
• Modified bleeding time	• Point of care testing

Heptest and Heptest-Hi are two clot-based assays that are more sensitive to the agents that inhibit factor Xa and can be used for monitoring. Heptest was initially developed for the monitoring of prophylactic levels of heparin, and Heptest-Hi was developed for the monitoring of heparin levels up to 5 U/ml. This method is extremely useful in the monitoring of the low-molecular-weight heparins (LMWHs) and chemically synthesized pentasaccharide.

Synthetic substrate-based amidolytic methods are also useful for the monitoring of the new agents. These assays measure the ability of a drug to inhibit either thrombin or factor Xa by using a chromogenic substrate specific for the enzyme. Anti-Xa can be used to monitor heparin, LMWH, and factor Xa inhibitors such as TFPI. The anti-IIa assays can be used to monitor the thrombin inhibitors and the antithrombin activity of unfractionated heparin. In addition to the above tests, several newer technologies are being developed, such as point-of-care testing devices that use a card-based technology capable of performing on-site prothrombin time (PT), activated partial thromboplastin time (APTT), and several other clot-based assays in citrated whole blood or plasma.

New anticoagulant and antithrombotic agents are continually being introduced for the management of thrombotic and cardiovascular disorders.[5,8,10] As has been well documented, several adverse side effects have been observed with the use of conventional drugs such as heparin and warfarin. Because of clinical problems associated with conventional drugs, interest in the development of newer anticoagulants began to increase. By depolymerization of heparin, LMWHs were developed.[10,11] These agents have better bioavailability, requiring only 1 subcutaneous dose/day for prophylaxis of postsurgical thromboembolism. Soon after the development of LMWHs, several other heparin-related glycosaminoglycans, such as chemically synthesized heparin analogs, dermatan sulphate, and heparan sulphate, were also developed and tested for the prevention of thrombosis.[10,15] In addition to the new heparin-related drugs are the biotechnology-based agents, peptides, antithrombin agents, and several new antiplatelet drugs, including glycoprotein IIb/IIIa inhibitors, are being developed for cardiovascular indications.[8-10,12,16] The new agents represent a wide spectrum of synthetic, semisynthetic, and biotechnology-based drugs with marked variation in chemical and biochemical properties. Currently there are no valid methods for the laboratory monitoring of the newer drugs.

The endogenous actions of the newer agents are rather novel and quite distinct from heparin and oral anticoagulants.[5] Many agents produce no prolongation of the routine global clotting assays,[4] and are monospecific agents. For example, hirudin inhibits only thrombin, GPIIb/IIIa-targeting drugs inhibit GPIIb/IIIa, and receptor specific antagonists modulate only the specific receptors. Thus specific effects can be monitored with new and specific techniques.

MONITORING OF LMWHs

Monitoring of the effects of LMWHs remains controversial. The subject of conventional monitoring of LMWHs has been recently reviewed by Samama et al.[11] In contrast to a high dose of heparin, LMWHs produce no comparable effects in the ACT. However, many of the LMWHs are currently used for interventional cardiovascular procedures. Figure 1 shows the dose-response curves of heparin and LMWH in the celite ACT after supplementation in

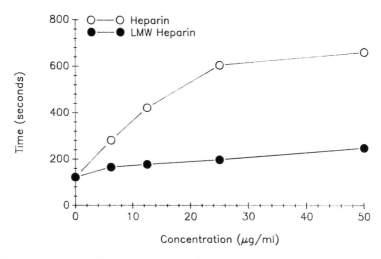

FIGURE 1.   Comparison of the antithrombotic effects of heparin and low-molecular-weight heparin (enoxaparin) in the celite activated clotting time (ACT) tests. Each agent was added to native whole blood, and celite ACT measurements were made on a Hemachron instrument.

normal human whole blood. Heparin demonstrated a strong dose-response curve in the concentration range of 50–0 µg/ml. However, LMWH only prolonged the ACT from a baseline of 122 ± 18 seconds to 248 ± 22 seconds at a concentration of 50 µg/ml. Primate studies in our laboratory demonstrated that after intravenous administration of 6 mg/kg of LMWH, the celite ACT was prolonged to only 276 ± 25 seconds. Figure 2 shows the dose-response curve obtained with heparin in primates in the celite ACT test. At 5 mg/kg of heparin, the ACT was elevated to approximately 735 seconds. These results indicate that the celite ACT is sensitive to the global clotting effects of unfractionated heparin but is not sensitive to the anticoagulant response of LMWH. Thus, when LMWHs are evaluated with the ACT test, the results should be evaluated with caution.

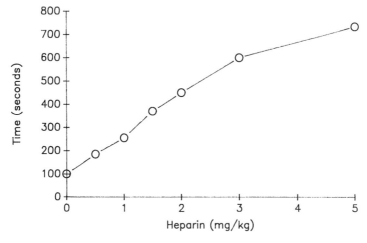

FIGURE 2.   Effect of intravenous administration of unfractionated heparin to primates. Groups of individual primates (n = 2) were given heparin, and blood samples were drawn 5 minutes later. Activated clotting time (ACT) measurements were made on the Hemachron instrument.

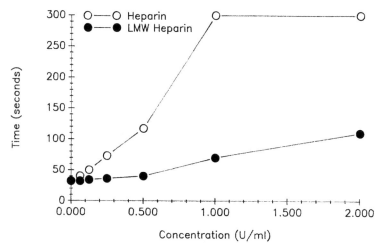

FIGURE 3.   Comparison of the anticoagulant effects of heparin and low-molecular-weight heparin (enoxaparin) in activated partial thromboplastin time (APTT) responses. Citrated plasma samples were supplemented with various amounts of each agent and APTT measurements were made.

Figures 3 and 4 compare the effects of heparin and LMWH on the APTT and thrombin time assays as performed in the citrated pool human plasma. Heparin exhibited a much stronger effect than LMWH. LMWH had a much weaker response in both APTT and thrombin time assays than heparin. Nonetheless, LMWH, given once a day, is superior to heparin for the prophylaxis of deep venous thrombosis. The results of the effects of heparin and LMWH on Heptest are shown in Figure 5. LMWH showed a strong linear response, similar to heparin, because of its inhibitory effects of factor Xa. Because each LMWH responds differently in the Heptest, however, each agent should be tested individually.[5]

The synthetic substrate-based assay for measuring the inhibition of thrombin and factor Xa also can be used to monitor the anticoagulant effects of heparin and LMWHs.

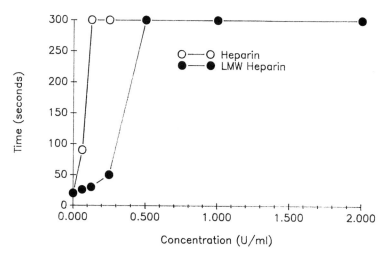

FIGURE 4.   Comparison of the anticoagulant effects of heparin and low-molecular-weight heparin in thrombin time assays. The same samples were used for this analysis as for the analyses in Figures 3 and 5.

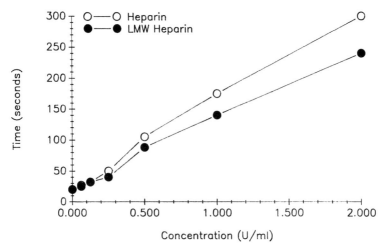

FIGURE 5. Comparison of the anticoagulant effects of heparin and a low-molecular-weight heparin in the Heptest assay. The same samples were used as in Figure 3.

The anti-Xa assay is more sensitive to the LMWHs than the anti-IIa assay and therefore can be used to monitor LMWHs.[11] Monitoring of the therapeutic dosage of LMWH is important because considerably higher amounts of heparin (up to 100 mg/once or twice daily) are used. Anti-Xa methods are quite useful for this purpose. Figure 6 shows the anti-Xa level in patients treated with Sandoz LMWH for up to 10 days. There is a progressive increase in anti-Xa levels in this group of patients. This staircasing phenomenon is important, because it may have implications for the safety and efficacy of LMWHs. The behavior of different LMWHs in terms of their anti-Xa effects can be readily assessed with the anti-Xa method. Furthermore, the efficacy of each drug in terms of its circulating level can be established. In the same study Heptest was also performed. The results are shown in Figure 7. In the Heptest study the staircasing phenomenon was not

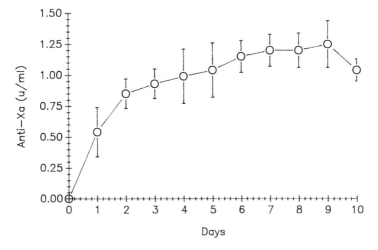

FIGURE 6. Effect of repeated administration of a subcutaneous therapeutic dose of a low-molecular-weight heparin (Certoparin) on the anti-Xa level in medical patients with established thrombosis.

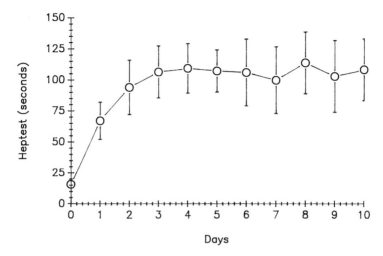

FIGURE 7.   Effect of repeated administration of a therapeutic subcutaneous dose of a low-molec-ular-weight heparin on the anti-Xa level in medical patients with established thrombosis.

observed, and a steady-state anticoagulant effect was noted after 3 days. Thus, the Heptest can be used to predict overdosing or underdosing of the drug. Because the Heptest is also an easily performed clot-based method, it is therapeutically useful for individual LMWHs.

LMWHs are now used for the treatment of established thrombosis and stroke.[5] They are administered under nursing care or a family member's care in an outpatient setting. Frequent monitoring to establish compliance may be necessary to optimize therapy. Figure 8 shows the anti-Xa level in two patient groups, one treated with 80 mg/day of Certoparin and the other with placebo. Administration of 80 mg/day of LMWH maintained anti-Xa levels of approximately 0.5 U/ml. Administration of Certoparin at 3 months showed a gradual reduction in the anti-Xa levels due to cessation of therapy. In long-term monitoring in angioplasty patients, Heptest was found to be equally effective (Fig.9). Whether high-dose long-term therapy with LMWH is needed remains to be establshed. However, it

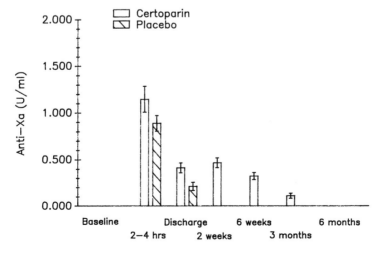

FIGURE 8.   Anti-Xa levels in patients undergoing long-term subcutaneous treatment with a low-molecular-weight heparin (Certoparin).

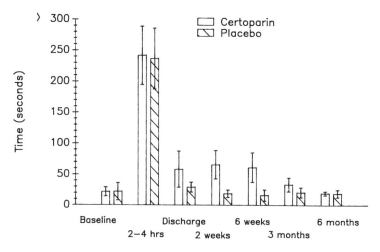

FIGURE 9.   Heptest time in patients undergoing long-term subcutaneous treatment with a low-molecular-weight heparin (Certoparin).

is clear that both Heptest and amidolytic anti-Xa assays can be used for the monitoring of LMWHs in various long-term therapeutic approaches. To prove the relevance of the results to potential bleeding or inefficacy requires well-designed clinical trials.

Heparin and LMWHs are also capable of releasing an endogenous Kunitz-type protease inhibitor, known as TFPI, from the vascular endothelium. TFPI may contribute to the mediation of the antithrombotic effect of both agents. There have been several reports of heparin mobilization of endothelium-bound TFPI. TFPI can inhibit the TF–FVIIa–FXa complex and factor Xa directly. Figure 10 shows the TFPI antigen levels in various heparinization states. The amount of TFPI released is proportional to the

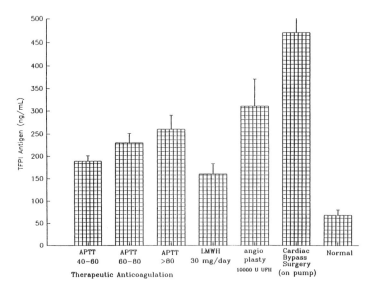

FIGURE 10.   A comparison of the tissue factor pathway inhibitor antigen level in various states of heparinization with patient groups.

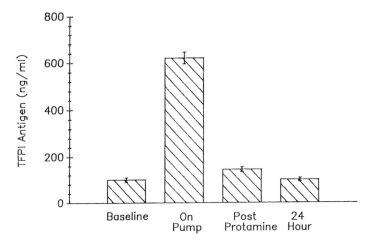

FIGURE 11.   The release of tissue factor pathway inhibitor antigen in patients undergoing cardio-vascular bypass surgery.

amount of heparinization. Both heparin and LMWH are capable of releasing TFPI, which contributes to their therapeutic and prophylactic effects. This is important during surgery, when large amounts of tissue factor (TF) are released. Figure 11 shows the release of TFPI during cardiopulmonary bypass surgery. When large dosages of heparin are used (up to 5 U/ml), a 10-fold elevation in TFPI levels has been measured. In addition, after heparin neutralization with protamine the TFPI antigen levels return to baseline, as seen in the anticoagulant assays. Therefore, TFPI appears to be an important contributor to the overall anticoagulant effect of heparin during bypass surgery. TFPI antigen levels are elevated 8–10-fold during heparinization in patients undergoing angioplasty procedures (Fig. 12). The release of TFPI is an important effect of heparin, because TFPI is a multifunctional inhibitor involved in the control of cellular, vascular, and plasma processes. Patients showing resistance to heparin may have a deficit of TFPI release. During surgical procedures, 10–20% of patients require greater amounts of heparin, perhaps because of impaired release of

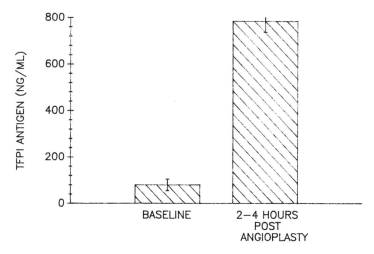

FIGURE 12.   Effect of heparin anticoagulation in patients undergoing coronary angioplasty.

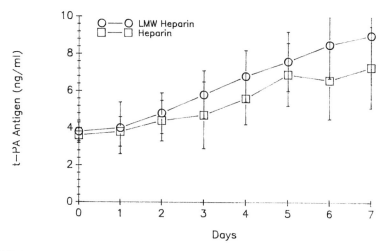

FIGURE 13. TPA antigen levels in patients treated with heparin and a low-molecular-weight heparin (Certoparin).

TFPI. Therefore, TFPI may be of major importance in the mediation of the anticoagulant actions of heparin. Once again, the clinical relevance of the circulating levels of TFPI in terms of the efficacy and safety of a given dosage of drug is not yet established.

Heparin and LMWHs also produce endothelial modulation and may release fibrinolytic activators such as tissue-type plasminogen activator (tPA), antiplatelet substances, and prostacyclin. Figure 13 shows the tPA antigen levels in patients treated with subcutaneous heparin and LMWH after general surgery. The amount of tPA increased progressively after the administration of both heparin and LMWH. TPA is produced and released from the vascular endothelium; it is known to be an activator of the fibrinolytic process and is responsible for maintaining hemostatic balance. In addition, prostacyclin is a potent vasodilator that inhibits platelet aggregation to the vascular endothelium. A stable metabolite of prostacyclin—6-keto $PGF_1\alpha$—has been measured in several clinical trials with LMWHs.

MONITORING OF ANTITHROMBIN AGENTS

Initially, the antithrombin agents were tested primarily for various cardiovascular indications. Because of safety issues, the monitoring of antithrombin agents in interventional cardiology is important; it is the only measure of total anticoagulant assurance for the cardiologist. Furthermore, bleeding complications can be relatively predictable if a proper method is used. ACT with Hemotec and Hemochron instruments has been used extensively for monitoring of heparin during cardiopulmonary bypass and percutaneous transluminal coronary angioplasty. In these indications, heparin levels of 5 U/ml are easily reached. The extent of anticoagulation is useful in establishing surgical ranges. Because the procedures have been calculated for heparin, it is logical to apply the same methods to the newly developed thrombin agents such as hirudin and argatroban. Figure 14 shows the ACT value of a group of patients undergoing angioplasty with the use of argatroban. An initial bolus of 350 µg/day followed by a 25 µg/kg/min infusion, was found to maintain the ACT > 400 seconds at the end of procedure; after termination of the infusion, ACT gradually returned to near baseline. Unlike heparinization, an infusion was necessary to maintain the level of anticoagulation. Hemotec is a different version of ACT. To compare the results of Hemotec and Hemochron ACT, parallel sampling was carried out at identical periods in the same group of patient samples. Results were somewhat increased

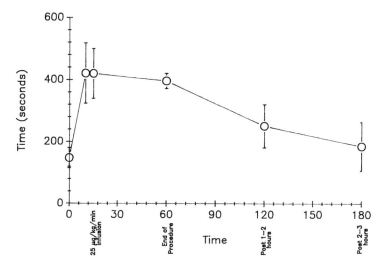

FIGURE 14.   Anticoagulant effects of argatroban as measured by Hemochron activated clotting time in patients undergoing coronary angioplasty.

in the Hemotec clotting time compared with the Hemachron clotting time (Fig.15). However, the same levels of anticoagulation were noted. Because of the emergency nature of this procedure, a point-of-care, operator-compliant technology was highly desirable. Recently, such technology has been made available, using dry chemistry methods to measure the level of heparinization. To assess its efficacy in the detection of the antithrombin anticoagulant activity, HMT brand of cards were used in conjunction with a TAS analyzer (Cardiovascular Diagnostics, Raleigh, NC). The test can be performed with one drop of blood. The results of the ACT-equivalent TAS time are shown in Figure 16. The results were nearly equivalent to those of the Hemochron ACT. Thus, this method also can be used

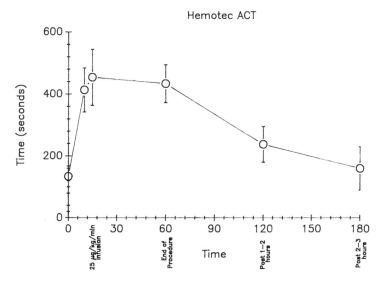

FIGURE 15.   Anticoagulant effects of argatroban as measured by Hemotec activated clotting time in patients undergoing coronary angioplasty.

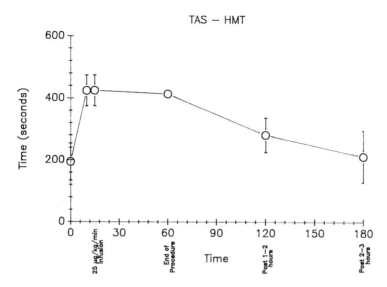

FIGURE 16.   Anticoagulant effects of argatroban as measured by a dry chemistry-based instrument using point-of-care technology.

effectively to monitor antithrombin activity. Such studies clearly demonstrate that, regardless of the type of anticoagulant, ACT maintenance in the range of 400 seconds provides adequate anticoagulation to perform interventional cardiologic procedures. Furthermore, a dry-chemistry-based, point-of-care technology can be used to assess the ACT.

Thrombin inhibitors are of natural, recombinant, and synthetic origin and represent a wide structural diversity. They can be directed against the catalytic site of thrombin or bind to the exosites of thrombin. Some are reversible, whereas others are irreversible. Argatroban, hirudin, and efegatran are now in various stages of clinical development. The dosage for each varies widely. Although the antithrombin potency of thrombin inhibitors can be adjusted, their effects on various global tests vary.

In the PT clotting assay, various thrombin inhibitors produced varying anticoagulant effects (Fig. 17). The results of the comparative anticoagulant effects of various thrombin inhibitors on APTT are shown in Figure 18. Efegatran was found to be strong, whereas hirudin was a relatively weaker inhibitor. In the Heptest assay (Fig. 19) the anticoagulant profile of each agent differed markedly. Argatroban was found to produce the strongest effects. Again, hirudin produced relatively weaker effects. These data clearly show that, although these agents produce similar effects, their relative anticoagulant effects differ markedly in different tests.

A new clot-based assay known as the ecarin clotting time was recently developed for monitoring of antithrombin agents. Ecarin is a snake venom (*Echis carnitus*) that converts prothrombin to mesothrombin, which eventually produces a clotting endpoint in citrated whole blood and plasma. Figure 20 shows the results of the ecarin clotting time obtained with several thrombin inhibitors. Each thrombin inhibitor has its own distinct anticoagulant effect. Hirulog produced the weakest effect, whereas hirudin showed the strongest effect in whole blood. Ecarin clotting time is sensitive to these antithrombin agents and can be used to monitor their effect in whole blood.

Because thrombin inhibitors can produce a strong inhibition of thrombin, several markers of thrombin generation can be used to monitor their effects. ELISA-based assays, such as prothrombin F_{1+2}, thrombin-antithrombin complex, and fibrinopeptide A can measure the effect of thrombin inhibitors at different stages of thrombotic activation. These assays also

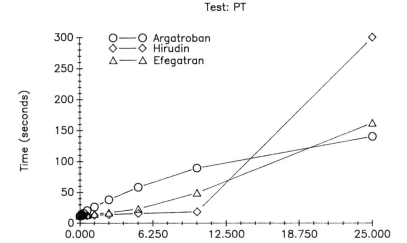

FIGURE 17.   Comparative anticoagulant effects of argatroban, hirudin, and efegatran as measured by prothrombin time.

may be helpful in monitoring the effect of other antithrombotic agents. In addition, ELISA-based assays for absolute drug concentration of hirudin and several other anti-thrombin agents, using monoclonal antibodies, have been developed. One such assay for hirudin is commercially available (Stago, Paris).

ANTIPLATELET DRUG MONITORING

Antiplatelet drugs such as aspirin have been conventionally used to manage platelet mediated disorders such as peripheral arterial disorders, stroke, and coronary artery disease.

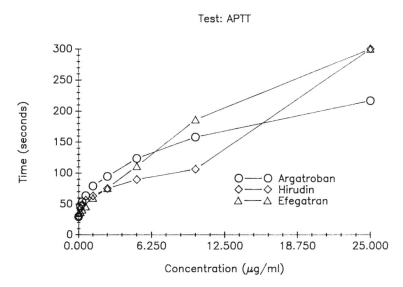

FIGURE 18.   Comparative anticoagulant effects of argatroban, hirudin, and efegatran as measured by activated partial thromboplastin time.

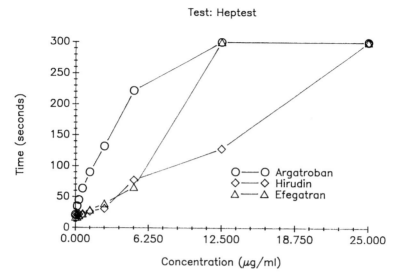

FIGURE 19.   Comparative anticoagulant effects of various thrombin inhibitors as measured by Heptest assay.

The new generation includes ticlopidine and clopidogrel, which were recently introduced for thrombotic stroke and cardiovascular indications. These drugs modify the fibrinogen binding of platelets. Although they are useful, they are capable only of inhibiting certain activation processes. Several other drugs, such as the glycoprotein IIb/IIIa antagonists, thromboxane A_2 receptor blockers, thromboxane synthase inhibitors, synthetic cyclooxygenase inhibitors, prostacyclin analogues, and serotonin receptor blockers, have been developed. Several glycoprotein IIb/IIIa monoclonal antibodies have been or are being tested for cardiovascular indication.[13,14] More specifically, these monoclonal antibodies have been tested for prevention of restenosis after percutaneous transluminal coronary angioplasty. These antibodies have no effect on the assays routinely used to monitor anticoagulant drugs. Thus

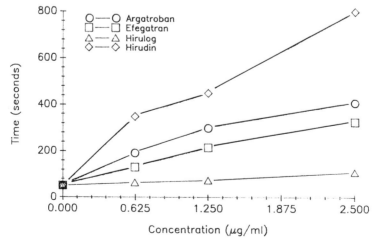

FIGURE 20.   Comparative anticoagulant effects of thrombin inhibitors as measured by ecarin clotting time.

TABLE 3. Monitoring of the Effects of Antiplatelet Drugs

Drug	Methods
Aspirin	Bleeding time/arachidonic acid-induced aggregation
Ticlopidine, Clopidogrel	Adenosine diphosphate-induced platelet aggregation
ReoPro and synthetic GPIIb/IIIa inhibitors	Thrombin receptor-activating peptide (TRAP) and adenosine diphosphate-induced glycoprotein platelet aggregation. Flow cytomety
Serotonin antagonist (Ketanserin)	Serotonin-induced platelet aggregation
P-selectin inhibitors	Flow cytometric methods

platelet aggregation is monitored with thrombin receptor-activating peptide (TRAP) and adenosine diphosphate (ADP). In addition, a newer technique has been used to measure platelet activation by using monoclonal antibodies to glycoprotein IIIa to identify platelets and P-selectin to identify activated platelets.

Antiplatelet drugs are usually monitored by using bleeding time methods or platelet aggregation techniques. Platelet counts are usually not altered by antiplatelet drugs. However, the functional characteristics of platelets, such as adhesion, aggregation, and release reactions, are usually altered. Table 3 lists various methods currently used to monitor the effect of conventional and newer antiplatelet drugs. Aspirin is usually monitored by using the aggregation methods. However, in all cases in which the antiplatelet actions of a drug are to be monitored, bleeding time provides a universal method. This method may be useful to predict overdosage of a given antiplatelet drug; however, it does not give a proper estimate of efficacy.

The effects of newer antiplatelet drugs, such as ticlopidine and clopidogrel, can be readily monitored by using simple aggregation methods such as ADP-induced aggregations. However, for the monitoring of the antiplatelet effects of newer and more specific GP IIb/IIIa inhibitors, such as ReoPro and synthetic inhibitors of GPIIb/IIIa, specific agonists such as TRAP have been found to be useful. ADP also can be used. Although the serotonin antagonists such as Ketanserin are not widely used, their antiplatelet effects can be measured by using aggregation methods with serotonin as an agonist. The newly developed P-selectin inhibitors are not yet in clinical use; however, their effects can be monitored by flow cytometric methods. Native blood can be used to monitor the antiplatelet effects of various drugs with the flow cytometric methods. Native blood is collected in plastic syringes with a platelet agonist such as ADP. The activation profile of platelets can be determined by using specific monoclonal antibodies.

Figure 21 compares the antiplatelet effects of ReoPro and a synthetic glycoprotein IIb/IIIa inhibitor in primates. TRAP was used to activate platelets. ReoPro produced a stronger inhibition of platelets and thus exhibits a much more sustained antiplatelet action. At present, no clinical trial has validated the diagnostic efficacy of this technique. Because some of these drugs (IIb/IIIa inhibitors) will be used for oral indications, their antiplatelet effects must be closely monitored for safety and efficacy. Thus, platelet aggregation techniques will be of major value in the study of GP IIb/IIIa inhibitors. Antiplatelet drugs such as GPIIb/IIIa inhibitors also inhibit the generation of platelet activation products such as thromboxane B_2, serotonin, and platelet factor 4. During active therapy, a decrease in some of these markers may be useful. At present, however, a comprehensive trial of the use of these markers is not available.

MONITORING OF ANTICOAGULANT AND ANTITHROMBOTIC DRUGS AND THEIR RELEVANCE TO INTERVENTIONAL CARDIOLOGY AND CARDIOVASCULAR SURGERY

In both interventional cardiovascular procedures and cardiovascular surgery, ACT methods (Hemotec and Hemochron) are currently used to determine the state of anticoagulation.

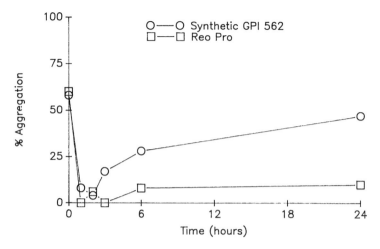

FIGURE 21.   Comparative inhibition of platelet activation by ReoPro and a synthetic GPIIb/IIIa inhibitor in primates.

The standard practice is to maintain the anticoagulant level between 300–500 seconds. Although adequate data validate this range for heparin, the extension of this range to other anticoagulant drugs, such as the antithrombins, may not be valid because of major differences in their mechanism of action. Although LMWHs are also used for various anticoagulant protocols, no satisfactory method to monitor their effect is currently available. Because of marked pharmacologic differences, these agents produce different effects on ACT and their pharmacokinetics differ significantly from heparin; thus the ACT may not be an adequate method. The GPIIb/IIIa inhibitors exert no effect on the ACT; however, they produce profound effects on the hemostatic function of platelets. At present, no valid method is available to determine the differential effects of these agents during cardiovascular procedures. Similarly, the optimal approach to monitor the effects of thrombolytic agents is to monitor various physiologic parameters. In most cases, various drugs are given in combination during cardiovascular procedures. Antiplatelet drugs, anticoagulants, and thrombolytic agents, along with various physical approaches, are used to manage cardiovascular disorders. The only monitoring consideration at present is the clotting profile of blood. Platelet function and the role of other mediators remain unmonitored. Although it is not clear that such monitoring is clinically relevant, specific evaluation may help in optimizing the use of polytherapeutic regimens. Thus, there is a need for new global tests to monitor combination anticoagulants.

At present, the ACT is the method of choice for monitoring anticoagulant effects of heparin and related drugs for both cardiologists and cardiovascular surgeons (Table 4). The use of ACT as a monitoring device also appears acceptable for other anticoagulants, such as hirudin and argatroban. At equivalent anticoagulant levels, however, heparin and antithrombin drugs produce markedly different effects on the coagulation process. Therefore, it is necessary to design valid clinical trials that determine the optimal anticoagulant range for each drug in terms of ACT values. On the other hand, the effect of many adjunct drugs, such as antiplatelet drugs, is not measurable on the ACT. Because platelets play an important role in hemostasis, it is important to monitor their functional status, particularly in postsurgical states. Thus, platelet count and a measure of platelet function should be included with the use of some of the newer drugs. The effects of newer drugs on vascular function are relatively hard to measure. However, with the availability of sensitive methods, it may be possible to determine modulatory actions on vascular function.

TABLE 4.   Laboratory Monitoring of the Anticoagulant and Antithrombotic Drugs during Interventional Cardiologic Procedures and Cardiovascular Surgery

Drugs	Laboratory Approaches
Heparin	Activated clotting time measurements
Antithrombin agents	Activated clotting times. May not reflect the same degree of anticoagulation as heparin
Low-molecular-weight heparin	No adequate method. Different anticoagulant/antithombotic ratios
GP IIb/IIIa inhibitors	Usually high dosage is used. Complete inhibition of platelets. Modified methods are needed
Thrombolytic agents	No adequate method. Only physiologic parameters
Drug combinations	None of the methods used can provide an adequate answer to the combined drug effects

With the development of sensitive assays for the molecular markers of hemostatic and vascular modulation, some data can be generated. Monitoring issues related to the use of new drugs require not only additional clinical validation of some of the newer tests, but also— and more importantly—the assessment of cost effectiveness and point of care for clinically relevant tests and instruments. Several new tests and instruments will be introduced in coming years and require clinical validation at various levels.

REFERENCES

 1. Cook NS, Kottirsch G, Zerwes HG: Platelet glycoprotein IIb/IIIa antagonists. Drugs Fut 19:135–159, 1994.
 2. EPIC Investigators: Use of a monoclonal antibody directed against the platelet glycoprotein IIb/IIIa receptor in high risk coronary angioplasty. N Engl J Med 330:956–961, 1994.
 3. Fareed J, Messmore HL, Bermes EW Jr: New perspectives in coagulation testing. Clin Chem 26:1380–1391, 1980.
 4. Fareed J: New methods in hemostatic testing. In Fareed J (ed): Perspectives in Hemostasis. New York, Pergamon Press, 1981, pp 310–348.
 5. Fareed J: Current trends in antithrombotic drug and device development. Semin Thromb Hemost 22:3–8, 1996.
 6. Fareed J, Walenga JM, Bermes EW Jr: Low molecular weight markers of hemostatic defects: Impact of automation on the quantitation of hemostatic disorders. Semin Thromb Hemost 9:354–378, 1983.
 7. Lefkovits J, Topol EJ: Direct thrombin inhibitors in cardiovascular medicine. Circulation 90:1522–1536, 1994.
 8. Markwardt F: Pharmacology of hirudin: One hundred years after the first report of the anticoagulant agent. Biophys Biochem Acta 44:1007–1013, 1985.
 9. McTavish D, Faulds D, Goa KL: Ticlopidine: An update of its pharmacology and therapeutic use in platelet-dependent disorders. Drugs 40:238–259, 1990.
10. Messmore HL: Clinical efficacy of heparin fractions: Issues and answers. CRC Clin Rev Clin Lab Sci 23:77–94, 1986.
11. Samama M: Contemporary laboratory monitoring of low molecular weight heparins. Thromb Hemost 15:119–123, 1995.
12. Teger-Nilsson A, Eriksson U, Gustafsson D, et al: Phase I studies on inogatran, a new selective thrombin inhibitor. J Am Coll Cardiol 66:117A–118A, 1995.
13. Topol EJ, Bonan R, Jewitt D, et al: Use of a direct antithrombin, hirulog, in place of heparin during coronary angioplasty. Circulation 87:1622–1629, 1993.
14. Topol EJ, Califf RM, Weisman HF, et al: Randomized trial of coronary intervention with antibody against platelet IIb/IIIa integrin for reduction of clinical restenosis: Results at six months. The EPIC Investigators. Lancet 343:881–886, 1994.
15. Walenga JM, Petitou M, Lormeau JC: Antithrombotic activity of a synthetic heparin pentasaccharide in a rabbit stasis thrombosis model using different thrombogenic challenges. Thromb Res 46:187–198, 1987.
16. Yonekawa Y, Handa H, Okamoto S, et al: Treatment of cerebral infarction in the acute stage with synthetic antithrombin MD80-clinical study among multiple institutions. Arch Jpn Chir 55:711–726, 1986.

CHAPTER 35

Monitoring of the Action of Antithrombin Agents by Ecarin Clotting Time

GÖTZ NOWAK, M.D.

For clinical anticoagulation only antithrombotics of the heparin type have been available so far. The various indications (e.g., cardiosurgery, thrombosis prophylaxis) for these agents require monitoring methods to measure blood levels. Activated partial thromboplastin time (APTT) and various modifications of activated clotting time (ACT) or prothrombin time (PT) have been used.[1] These methods, which are based on thrombin generation in the test sample, allow rapid and sufficiently accurate determination of current blood levels of heparin or heparin analogs.[37]

The same methods were used for clinical testing of hirudin, a direct-acting antithrombin.[4,7,8,13,16,23,25,36,38,40] It soon became apparent, however, that they cannot be adapted to the monitoring of blood levels of hirudin or other antithrombins. The APTT is not sensitive enough to measure clinically relevant blood levels in the therapeutic or toxic range, and individual values vary too greatly. Direct measurement using chromogenic substrates or monoclonal antibodies takes time and costs a great deal of money.[2,3,9–12,14,17,30–36,39] Moreover, they are not adaptable for universal use, especially as a bedside method.[10,15,26]

A new monitoring test, therefore, was developed for hirudin therapy—the ecarin clotting time (ECT). This test is suitable not only for hirudin but also for all other direct antithrombins.[6,19,20–22,24,28] Depending on whether optical or mechanical measurement of clotting time is used, the test can be performed in whole blood or plasma. The straightforward procedure and short measuring time allow accurate bedside diagnosis. Initial clinical studies have revealed that ECT is the method of choice to determine current blood levels of hirudin in patients subjected to extracorporeal circulation.[18] In preclinical trials, low-molecular-weight inhibitors and synthetic hirudin analogs have been measured in blood with ECT. Its low sensitivity to interference by blood constituents and the direct correlation between inhibitor concentration and clotting time in a wide range of blood levels facilitate monitoring in extracorporeal therapy.[27]

MEASURING PRINCIPLE AND BIOCHEMICAL BACKGROUND

A protease purified from the venom of *Echis carinatus* is used as the starting reagent for ECT. Ecarin and other direct prothrombin-activating proteases in venom purified from *Bothrops types, Oxyuranus scutellatus,* or *Notechis scutatus* cleave the peptide bond of the

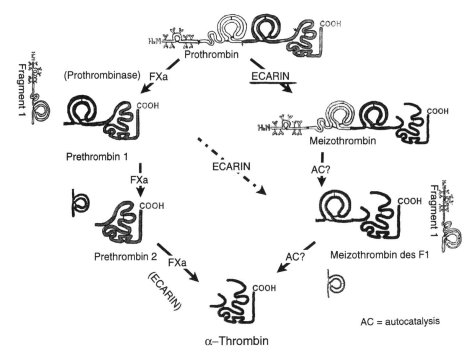

FIGURE 1.   Ecarin-induced prothrombin activation.

prothrombin molecule at ARG 320 in a highly specific manner, thereby opening the linkage between the A and B chains (Fig. 1). The resulting derivative, termed meizothrombin, already has a certain thrombin-like activity; it converts fibrinogen into fibrin and activates platelets. Its activity toward natural thrombin substrates, however, is considerably lower. Meizothrombin is activated by autocatalysis to meizothrombin-des F1 and, in a further step, to alpha-thrombin. The same general pathway underlies the usual activation of prothrombin to thrombin by the prothrombinase complex. However, the primary pathway in the induction of coagulation is "conservative" activation to alpha-thrombin via prethrombin 1 and 2, which is initiated by solid-phase activation of the high-molecular-weight prothrombinase complex using factor Xa (see Fig. 1). In determining blood concentrations of hirudin, it is important to know that hirudin also inactivates meizothrombin, with an affinity similarly high as thrombin's (K_i thrombin $\cong K_i$ meizothrombin).

This background elucidates the measuring principle of ECT. When ecarin is added to a plasma sample containing a specific amount of hirudin, it converts prothrombin into meizothrombin or meizothrombin-des F1 in a highly specific manner. Meizothrombin is then rapidly and efficiently inactivated by hirudin. Only the meizothrombin liberated after the entire amount of available hirudin has been exhausted can induce fibrinogen-to-fibrin conversion, resulting in clotting of the blood or plasma sample. The moment of clotting is recorded by a coagulometer. Hirudin, synthetic low-molecular-weight thrombin inhibitors, and direct antithrombins inhibit meizothrombin.[6] Thus, their concentrations in plasma can be measured with ECT. The reaction rate is limited by the small amount of snake venom enzyme that is added to the sample. Initially the meizothrombin inhibitors are present in excess, but subsequently they are exhausted by the constant-rate generation of meizothrombin. The addition of 0.2 EU [ecarin units] (dissolved in buffer) to an 0.2-ml sample of blood or plasma provides the optimal amount of enzymes for clinically useful ECT values.

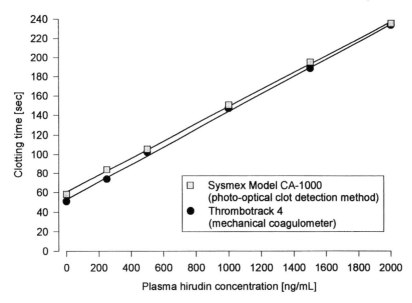

FIGURE 2. Adapting ecarin clotting time (ECT) to automatic clotting analyzers. The method has been modified to adapt to instrument-specific sample volumes. Thus, 0.1 ml of plasma was supplemented with 0.1 ml of ecarin starting reagent (stock solution: 0.9 ml of Tris buffer + 0.1 ml of ecarin [10 U/ml]). The ECTs measured on mechancial coagulometer (Thrombotrack 4) and clotting analyzer (CA-1000) provide identical standard curves.

DETERMINATION OF HIRUDIN CONTENT IN WHOLE BLOOD, PLASMA, AND URINE

ECT is equally suitable for use in whole blood or plasma. Undiluted blood or plasma, along with the selected amount of ecarin, provides a clinically useful bedside test. In general, ECT can be determined with a mechanical (Hemochrom, CL-4, or Thrombotrack) or optical coagulometer or with an automatic clotting analyzer (CA-1000 or ACL-300 plus). With the same pooled plasma sample, the hirudin standard curves established by the CL-4 and CA-1000 are nearly identical (Fig. 2). In clinical use, all possible blood levels of hirudin can be determined in a single procedure because of the wide linear range in hirudin concentration and clotting time. The standard curves in plasma and whole blood are also nearly identical (Fig. 3), and even subtherapeutic concentrations of hirudin can be determined exactly in a range up to 500 ng/ml. The linear correlation between hirudin concentration and clotting time permits measurement of therapeutic (500–2500 ng/ml) and toxic (> 2500 ng/ml) blood levels of hirudin in the same test sample without dilution. Likewise, ECT can be used to determine elimination of hirudin in urine. The determination is carried out using human pooled plasma supplemented with 0.01–0.03 ml of urine (diluted in buffer), by the method described above.[22] The hirudin content in urine can be measured with the same method (Fig. 4).

INFLUENCE OF HEPARIN ON ECARIN CLOTTING TIME

In patients subjected to an immediate change from heparin to hirudin for prophylactic or therapeutic anticoagulation, it is of great importance that heparin does not affect determination of the blood level of hirudin. Both APTT and TT are greatly influenced by heparin. Thus, neither of these methods (or any of their derivatives) can be used to determine blood levels of direct antithrombins in the presence of residual amounts of heparin or other anticoagulants of the heparin type. ECT, however, is not affected by plasma concentrations

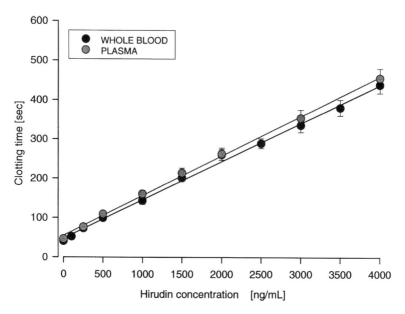

FIGURE 3. Ecarin clotting time (ECT) in whole blood and plasma. Supplementing whole blood or citrated hirudin-containing plasma from 10 healthy donors with increasing concentrations of hirudin provides near-identical ECTs.

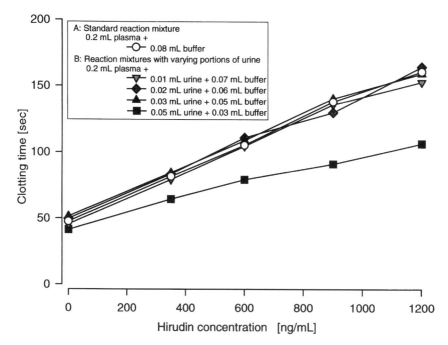

FIGURE 4. Determination of hirudin content in urine using the ecarin clotting time (ECT). The buffer of the reaction mixture is substituted by increasing amounts of urine supplemented with defined, increasing amounts of hirudin. Urine amounts up to 0.03 ml do not produce any intrinsic activity or exert any influence on ECT. In routine laboratory studies, 0.02 ml of urine should be used to measure urine hirudin concentrations.

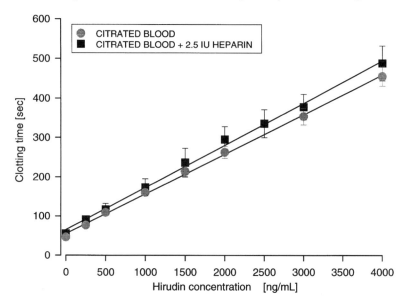

FIGURE 5.   Influence of heparin on the ecarin clotting time (ECT). Whole blood of healthy donors (n = 5) was supplemented with increasing concentrations of hirudin, both with and without addition of 2.5 U/ml of heparin. Addition of 2.5 U/ml of heparin prolonged the measured ECTs only slightly.

of heparin up to 2.5 IU/ml (Fig. 5), because heparin, when complexed with antithrombin III, does not inhibit meizothrombin generated by ecarin. Direct antithrombins such as hirudin or synthetic low-molecular-weight thrombin inhibitors, in contrast, inhibit meizothrombin directly. Therefore, the heparin–antithrombin III complex cannot exert a synergistic influence on hirudin's anticoagulant action. All fractionated and low-molecular-weight heparins behave identically, with no effect on hirudin-induced prolongation of ECT.

INFLUENCE OF COAGULATION VARIABLES

Measurement of ECT requires prothrombin and fibrinogen from blood or plasma. In patients with serious disease or acute-phase reactions, the concentration of these variables may be decreased. ECT is not significantly prolonged, however, even with a decrease in prothrombin level to residual amounts of 25% of normal (Table 1). When the fibrinogen level is decreased in steps by adding fibrinogen-deficient plasma to normal plasma, ECT is insignificantly prolonged by levels as low as 65% of normal (Table 2). This insensitivity to varying concentrations of coagulation factors results from the fact that the enzymatic action of ecarin is used to limit the reaction kinetics. Varying levels of prothrombin and fibrinogen within a wide range of blood have no significant effect on ECT.

INFLUENCE OF PHYSICAL AND CHEMICAL PARAMETERS

Reaction Temperature

The dependence of ECT on incubation temperature was studied under standardized conditions with identical concentrations of hirudin, using a mechanical multichannel coagulometer. ECT is most highly sensitive to increasing concentrations of hirudin at room temperature (22° C) (Fig. 6). The enzyme–substrate reaction runs slowly, and clotting times are prolonged accordingly. At a temperature of 45° C, the plasma sample is extremely insensitive to increasing concentrations of hirudin. Therefore, it is essential that all ECT determinations are carried out at a temperature of 37° C.

TABLE 1.   Influence of Prothrombin Concentration of Plasma on Ecarin Clotting Time

%	Plasma	Ecarin Clotting Times (sec)
100	1.0 A	44.1
90	0.9 A + 0.1 C	44.5
80	0.8 A + 0.2 C	44.2
70	0.7 A + 0.3 C	44.3
60	0.6 A + 0.4 C	45.1
50	0.5 A + 0.5 C	44.7
40	0.4 A + 0.6 C	43.8
30	0.3 A + 0.7 C	46.2
20	0.2 A + 0.8 C	47.8
10	0.1 A + 0.9 C	89.1
0	1.0 C	> 15 min

A = pooled plasma, C = $BaSO_4$-adsorbed plasma.

pH Values

Variations in pH values between 7.0 and 8.0 in human pooled plasma influence the ECT and the slope of the hirudin concentration–clotting time standard curve. The slope is steepest at pH 7.0 (Fig. 7). Acidifying the plasma increases the sensitivity of the hirudin standard curve, whereas shifting the pH to a value of 8.0 shortens the ECT compared with the standard pH of 7.5. Different pH values of plasma produce different ECTs (Fig. 8). Therefore, the ECT test has to be performed using a pH-stabilizing buffer system (e.g., Tris buffer, phosphate buffer).

Buffer Systems

Coagulometers used in laboratory diagnostics employ different, standardized buffer systems. The influence of various buffer systems on the hirudin standard curve was studied using (1) Tris or veronal acetate buffers or (2) saline. The curve rises most steeply when veronal acetate buffer is used; saline provides a substantially slower rise. These observations are important when results of different methods of determining ECT are compared. In follow-ups, it is not possible to compare directly the values obtained with different buffers. To ensure a constant measuring quality, the same measuring system, with the same buffer and physical and chemical parameters, should be used.

TABLE 2.   Influence of Fibrinogen Concentration of Plasma on Ecarin Clotting Time

%	Plasma	Ecarin Clotting Times (sec)
100	1.0 A	44.0
90	0.9 A + 0.1 B	45.2
80	0.8 A + 0.2 B	46.8
70	0.7 A + 0.3 B	47.6
60	0.6 A + 0.4 B	50.2
50	0.5 A + 0.5 B	56.8
40	0.4 A + 0.6 B	63.2
30	0.3 A + 0.7 B	87.8
20	0.2 A + 0.8 B	114.6
10	0.1 A + 0.9 B	184.6
0	1.0 B	> 15 min

A = pooled plasma, B = pooled plasma, fibrinogen-free.

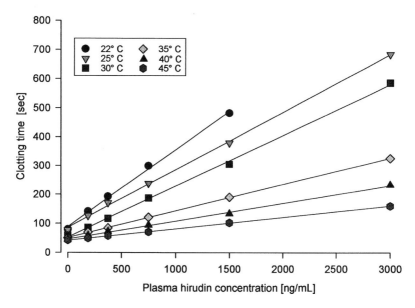

FIGURE 6.   Influence of reaction temperature on the ecarin clotting time (ECT). Citrated, pooled human plasma was supplemented with increasing concentrations of hirudin, and ECT was measured manually (wire hook) in a water bath at reaction temperatures of 22–45° C.

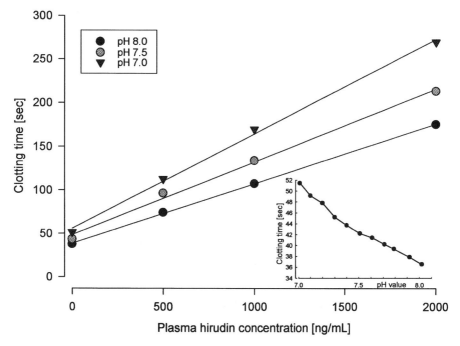

FIGURE 7.   Influence of pH value of blood and plasma on the ecarin clotting time (ECT). Citrated, pooled human plasma adjusted to pH values of 7.0–8.0 using 0.1 n HCL or 0.1 n NaOH was supplemented with increasing concentrations of hirudin, and ECT was measured. The insert shows the pH shift of ECT.

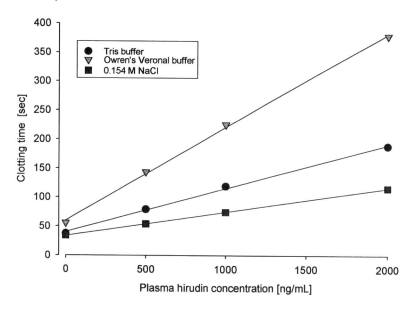

FIGURE 8.   Influence on the ecarin clotting time of the buffer used.

CLINICAL TRIALS OF ECARIN CLOTTING TIME FOR DETERMINING THE BLOOD LEVEL OF HIRUDIN

In preclinical studies of the pharmacokinetics of different hirudin variants and poly-ethylene glycol-coupled (PEG) hirudin, ECT was used routinely to determine hirudin content in blood. The consistency of standard curves established with different test mixtures and the near-identical ECT standard curves obtained for different animal species demonstrate the stability of the measuring method. Results for various laboratory animals reveal no significant differences in the hirudin standard curves (Fig. 9). In several thousand preclinical trial measurements, ECT has proved to be the method of choice for determination of the hirudin content in blood and body fluids.

The efficiency of ECT also has been demonstrated in several clinical trials of hirudin for anticoagulation in hemodialysis. Because renal insufficiency greatly affects the elimination kinetics of hirudin, dose adjustment and therapeutic monitoring of blood levels are essential for this indication. For each patient undergoing hemodialysis, the hirudin dose was adjusted by direct bedside determination of blood level. The minimal effective blood or plasma levels in extracorporeal circulation ranged between 400 and 500 ng/ml. Because hirudin was not allowed to remain beneath this level until the end of the 4- to 5-hour treatments, individual dose regimens were adjusted for each patient, depending on residual renal function. Hirudin clearance closely correlated with creatinine clearance.[5]

Patients with residual renal function undergoing hemodialysis show relatively large variations in blood level after administration of a daily dose of hirudin (Fig. 10). In contrast, the blood level curve of patients without residual excretion (nephrectomized patients) exhibits a slow rise (Fig. 11). The repeated hirudin doses for nephrectomized patients are substantially lower than those for patients with residual renal function. For comparison, other methods were used to determine blood levels of hirudin, including an enzyme-linked immunosorbent assay (ELISA) and a chromogenic substrate assay based on the ecarin-induced generation of meizothrombin. Even with these more expensive methods, comparable values of blood levels were obtained (see Figs. 10 and 11). The APTT was also measured in all patients; it was not prolonged considerably.

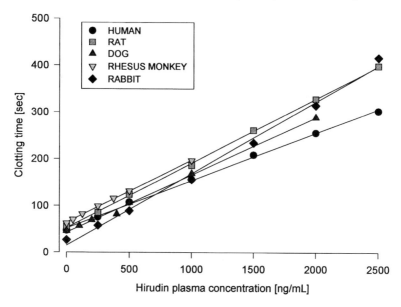

FIGURE 9.   Ecarin clotting time (ECT) in experimental preclinical research. ECT was measured in the plasma of laboratory animals, using increasing concentrations of hirudin. With the exception of rabbit plasma, the ECT curves run nearly parallel.

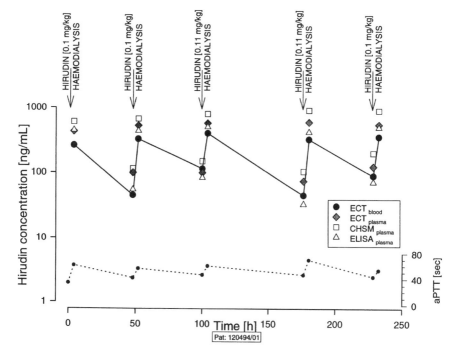

FIGURE 10.   Control of blood hirudin level in patients undergoing hemodialysis using the ecarin clotting time. Measurement of blood hirudin levels in a patient with residual renal function, anticoagulated with hirudin in 5 successive treatments. For comparison, two more hirudin determination methods were used and APTT was determined. CHSM = chromogenic substrate method.

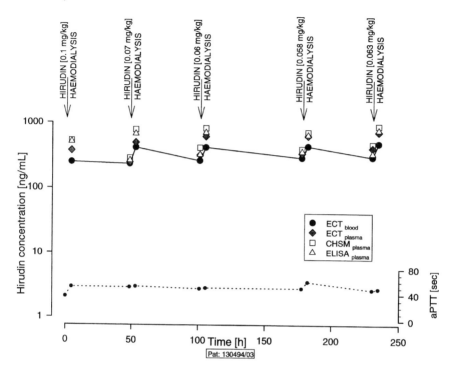

FIGURE 11.   Control of blood hirudin level in patients undergoing hemodialysis using the ecarin clotting time. Measurement of blood hirudin levels in a patient without residual renal function (nephrectomized bilaterally), anticoagulated with hirudin in 5 successive treatments. For comparison, two more hirudin determination methods were used and APTT was determined. CHSM = chromogenic substrate method.

During 6-month ambulatory hemodialysis of a patient with heparin-induced thrombocytopenia (HIT II), the dose regimen of hirudin was determined with the help of ECT. Bedside determination of blood levels allowed effective anticoagulation. Figure 12 shows the blood levels for the different doses.

In a case report, Riess et al. described the use of ECT to control blood levels in patients undergoing cardiopulmonary bypass.[27] After repeated, high doses of hirudin, the APTT was prolonged only slightly. However, ECT was highly sensitive to any deviation in hirudin level. The plasma level required for anticoagulation during bypass surgery using extracorporeal oxygenation ranged between 2 and 2.5 µg/ml.[27] Because this range often involves a relatively high risk of bleeding, short-term, continuous bedside monitoring of blood level with ECT is necessary. In patients with undisturbed renal function, the renal clearance of hirudin is high (160 ml/min). Therefore, administration of an antidote is not required.

CONCLUSIONS

The clinical use of hirudin and other antithrombin agents in patients at high risk of thromboembolic disorders requires bedside determination of current blood levels. In preclinical and clinical investigations, ECT has proved to be a rapid and precise method of determining blood levels of hirudin. Its advantages include the following:
- Ease of application
- High reproducibility
- Linearity between prolongation of clotting time and hirudin concentration over a wide range, including subtherapeutic, therapeutic, and toxic blood levels

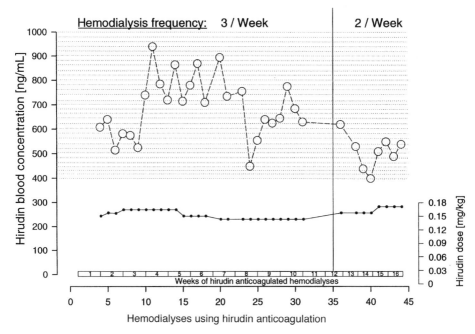

FIGURE 12.   Ecarin clotting time for drug monitoring in regular hemodialysis, anticoagulated with hirudin. Dose finding and hirudin-anticoagulated hemodialysis over several months in a patient suffering from heparin-induced thrombocytopenia (HIT II). The blood hirudin concentrations were measured at the end of each treatment. The hirudin doses are represented for comparison.

- No necessity to dilute the sample
- Possible use of whole blood
- Short time needed to obtain results
- Suitability for bedside use
- Independence of blood fibrinogen concentration in a range from 60–140% of normal
- Independence of blood prothrombin concentration (to 30% of normal)
- Possible determination of hirudin in blood containing heparin (up to 2.5 IU/ml)
- Possible determination of other direct thrombin inhibitors
- Adaptability to all available coagulation timers
- Low costs

REFERENCES

1. Bara L, Mardiguian J, et al: In vitro effect on Hep test of low molecular heparin fractions and preparations with various anti-IIa and anti-Xa activities. Thromb Res 57:585–592, 1990.
2. Berscheid G, Groetsch H ,et al: Determination of rDNA hirudin and α-human thrombin-hirudin complex in plasma samples: enzyme-linked immunosorbent assays for hirudin and complex vs. chromogenic thrombin substrate assay. Thromb Res 66:33–42, 1992.
3. Bichler H, Siebeck M, et al: Determination of thrombin-hirudin complex in plasma with an enzyme-linked immunosorbent assay. Blood Coag Fibrinol 2:129–133, 1991.
4. Breddin HK, Radziwon P, et al: Laboratory monitoring of new antithrombotic drugs [review]. Clin Lab Med 14:825–846, 1994.
5. Bucha E, Markwardt F, Nowak G: Hirudin in haemodialysis. Thromb Res 60:445–455, 1990.
6. Callas DD, Hoppensteadt D, Igbal O, Fareed J: Ecarin clotting time (ECT) is a reliable method for the monitoring of hirudins, argatroban, efegatran and related drugs in therapeutic and cardiovascular indications. Ann Hematol 72 (Suppl I):A58, 1996.
7. Dang QD, Di Cera E: A simple activity assay for thrombin and hirudin. J Protein Chem 13:367–373, 1994.

8. Eric D: Determination of the specific activity of recombinant hirudin. Thromb Res 60:433–443, 1990.
9. Griessbach U, Stuerzebecher J, et al: Assay of hirudin in plasma using a chromogenic thrombin substrate. Thromb Res 37:347–350.
10. Groetsch H, Berscheid G, et al: Interference of heparin and analogues with hirudin in the chromogenic thrombin substrate assay. Thromb Res 64:285–290, 1991.
11. Groetsch H, Damm D, et al: Comparison of two different methods for the determination of rDNA hirudin in plasma samples: HPLC vs a chromogenic thrombin substrate. Thromb Res 64:273–277, 1991.
12. Hafner G, Fickenscher K, et al: Evaluation of an automated chromogenic substrate assay for the rapid determination of hirudin in plasma. Thromb Res 77:165–173, 1995.
13. Hirsh J, Spillert CR, et al: In vitro effect of hirudin on recalcification time. J Natl Acad Med 86:627–628, 1994.
14. Iyer L, Adam M, et al: Development and validation of two enzyme-linked immunosorbent assay (ELISA) methods for recombinant hirudin. Semin Thromb 21:184–192, 1995.
15. Iyer L, Fareed J: Determination of specific activity of recombinant hirudin using a thrombin titration method. Thromb Res 78:259–263, 1995.
16. Koza MJ, Walenga JM, et al: A new approach in monitoring recombinant hirudin during cardiopulmonary bypass. Semin Thromb 19 (Suppl 1):90–96, 1993.
17. Longstaff C, Wong MY, et al: An international collaborative study to investigate standardisation of hirudin potency. Thromb Haemost 69:430–435, 1993.
18. Nowak G, Bucha E, Brauns I, Butti A: The use of r-hirudin as anticoagulant in regular haemodialysis in an HAT-II patient over a long period. Ann Hematol 72 (Suppl I):A56, 1996.
19. Nowak G, Bucha E: A new method for the therapeutical monitoring of hirudin. Naunyn-Schmiedeberg's Arch Pharmacol 346:R27, 1992.
20. Nowak G, Bucha E: A new method for the therapeutical monitoring of hirudin. Thromb Haemost 69:1306, 1993.
21. Nowak G, Bucha E: Monitoring of r-hirudin in blood with the ecarin time. Ann Hematol 66 (Suppl 1):A28, 1993.
22. Nowak G, Bucha E: Ouantitative determination of hirudin in blood and body fluids. Semin Thromb 23:197–202, 1996.
23. Nurmohamed MT, Berckmans RJ, et al: Monitoring anticoagulant therapy by activated partial thromboplastin time: hirudin assessment. An evaluation of native blood and plasma assays. Thromb Haemost 72:685–692, 1994.
24. Radziwon P, Breddin HK, Esslinger HU: Ecarin time is more suitable to monitor PEG-hirudin treatment compared to aPTT, TT, ACT or aIIa-activity. Ann Hematol 72 (Suppl I):A57, 1996.
25. Reid TJ, Alving BM: A quantitative thrombin time for determining levels of hirudin and hirulog. Thromb Haemost 70:608–616, 1993.
26. Richter M, Walsmann P, et al: A thrombin binding assay for ^{125}I-hirudin. Pharmazie 43:369–370, 1988.
27. Riess F-CH, Loewer CH, Seelig CH, et al: Recombinant hirudin as a new anticoagulant during cardiac operations instead of heparin: successful for aortic valve replacement in man. J Thorac Cardiovasc Surg 110:265–267, 1995.
28. Rübsamen K, Hornberger W, Ruf A, Bode W: The ecarin clotting time, a rapid and simple coagulation assay for monitoring hirudin and PEG-hirudin in blood. Ann Hematol 72(Suppl I):A56, 1996.
29. Rupin A, Mennecier P, et al: A screening procedure to evaluate the anticoagulant activity and the kinetic behaviour of direct thrombin inhibitors. Thromb Res 78:217–225, 1995.
30. Schlaeppi JM, Vekemans S, et al: Preparation of monoclonal antibodies to hirudin and hirudin peptides. A method for studying the hirudin-thrombin interaction. Eur J Biochem 188:463–470, 1990.
31. Schlaeppi JM: Preparation of monoclonal antibodies to the thrombin/hirudin complex. Thromb Res 62:459–470, 1991.
32. Spannagl M, Bichler H, et al: A fast photometric assay for the determination of hirudin. Haemostasis 21(Suppl 1):36–40, 1991.
33. Spannagl M, Bichler J, et al: Development of a chromogenic substrate assay for the determination of hirudin in plasma. Blood Coag Fibrinol 2:121–127, 1991.
34. Spinner S, Scheffauer F, et al: A hirudin catching ELISA for quantitating the anticoagulant in biological fluids. Thromb Res 51:617–625, 1988.
35. Spinner S, Stoffler G: Quantitative enzyme-linked immunosorbent assay (ELISA) for hirudin. J Immunol Methods 87:79–83, 1986.
36. Stuerzebecher J: Methods for determination of hirudin [review]. Semin Thromb 17:99–102, 1991.
37. Wagenvoord RJ, Hendrix HH, et al: Development of a rapid and sensitive chromogenic heparin assay for clinical use. Haemostasis 23:26–37, 1993.
38. Walenga JM, Hoppensteadt D, et al: Comparative studies on various assays for the laboratory evaluation of r-hirudin. Semin Thromb 17:103–112, 1991.
39. Walenga JM, Hoppensteadt D, et al: Laboratory assays for the evaluation of recombinant hirudin. Haemostasis 21(Suppl 1):49–63, 1991.
40. Zoldhelyi P, Webster MW, et al: Recombinant hirudin in patients with chronic, stable coronary artery disease. Safety, half-life, and effect on coagulation parameters. Circulation 88:2015–2022, 1993.

CHAPTER 36

Hemostatic Processes during Cardiovascular Bypass and Intravascular Cardiovascular Procedures

RODGER L. BICK, M.D., Ph.D., FACP
JAWED FAREED, Ph.D.

PHYSIOLOGY OF HEMOSTASIS

Hemostasis is the property of the circulation by which blood retains its fluidity within the vasculature and the ability of the system to prevent excessive blood loss upon injury. Three anatomic compartments—tissues (vasculature), blood cells (platelets), and plasma (proteins)—are involved in a series of delicately orchestrated biochemical interplays that, under normal conditions, modulate responses in a fashion compatible with maintaining the finely tuned equilibrium of hemostasis. The three specific hemostatic compartments are (1) the platelets, which must be normal in both number and function; (2) the plasma proteins, which include procoagulants, anticoagulants, and fibrinolytic proteins; and (3) the vasculature, which remains the most poorly understood component of disorders of hemostasis.

During injury, vessels constrict and generate compounds that activate platelets and plasma proteins. Platelets adhere and cohere at the site of injury, initiating a complex process that promotes further platelet aggregation, vascular constriction, and activation of coagulation components, resulting in fibrin formation. Many chemical signals designed to initiate or terminate various events serve as a system of checks and balances. Disturbances (inherited or acquired) are reflected in inappropriate responses predisposing to either thrombosis or hemorrhage—sometimes both.

To appreciate the complexity of the inter- and intracompartmental interactions, the normal hemostatic aspects of the vasculature, platelets, and plasma proteins are discussed separately. The reader is encouraged, however, to maintain a perspective of integrated function, which is the basis for efficient diagnosis of hemostatic dysfunction and the mainstay for development of targeted pharmacologic therapy.

Vascular Function

Normal vascular morphology is comprised of three discrete layers: the intima, media, and adventitia. The intima consists of a monolayer of nonthrombogenic endothelial cells and an internal elastic membrane. The media consists of smooth muscle cells; the size of

551

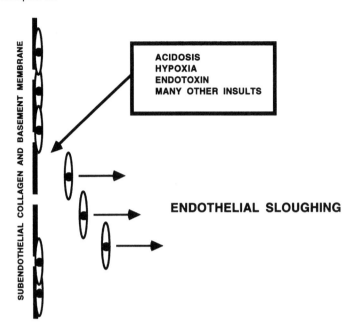

FIGURE 1. Endothelial sloughing and exposure of blood to subendothelial collagen and basement membrane.

the media varies, depending on the type (arterial/venous) and size of the vasculature. The adventitia is comprised of an external elastic lamina or membrane and supportive connective tissue.

Figure 1 illustrates the exposure of subendothelial collagen and basement membrane as a result of endothelial sloughing, which may be induced by various insults or triggers, such as acidosis, hypoxia, endotoxin, and circulating antigen–antibody complexes. Platelets are immediately recruited to fill the endothelial gap,[1–4] with the goal of forming a primary hemostatic plug that prevents blood from leaving the vascular compartment. Subsequent reparative events include migration of smooth muscle or other cells from the media through the internal elastic membrane and their differentiation into new, nonthrombogenic endothelial cells. If this is a one-time event, the reparative process is completed. Sometimes, however, formation of the primary hemostatic plug may constitute an overwhelming event that leads to a large platelet/fibrin thrombus, impedance of blood flow, and ischemic end-organ damage. This process is particularly alarming when it evolves repeatedly in the same area over a protracted period. As smooth muscle or other cells differentiate and migrate into the intima, compounds that attract macrophages are released; the macrophages, in turn, ingest cholesterol and other materials—the fundamental construct of an atherosclerotic plaque.[5–8] Figure 2 summarizes the potential consequences of vascular injury. Permeability, fragility, and vasoconstriction are properties of the vasculature. As a result of increased permeability, blood leaves the vessel and manifests as petechiae and purpura or, sometimes, large ecchymoses. Increased fragility results in rupture of the vasculature, which leads to petechiae, purpura (especially in the integument and mucous membranes), and large ecchymoses with potentially serious deep-tissue hemorrhage. Vasoconstriction is under local, neural, and humoral control. Most important is humoral control, which is effected primarily by compounds released from platelets (e.g., epinephrine, norepinephrine, adenosine diphosphate, kinins and thromboxanes). Fibrin(ogen) degradation products (FDPs) also modulate vasoconstriction.[9,10]

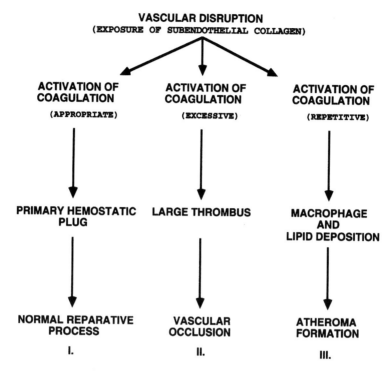

FIGURE 2.   Vascular damage and consequences of endothelial sloughing.

Endothelial cells are contractile, responding when stimulated by histamine, serotonin, kinins, or thromboxanes. The endothelial cell has been identified as a primary site of the biosynthesis of critical hemostatic proteins, including Von Willebrand factor, plasminogen activator, thrombomodulin inhibitor of active protein C, and prostaglandins.[11–15] Platelet attraction and subsequent activation occur when subendothelial basement membrane or collagen is exposed. This process also may directly activate factor XII to factor XIIa as well as factor XI to factor XIa.[16,17] Clearly, any of these processes, if left unmodulated, can lead to generalized activation of the coagulation system.[18–22]

Platelet Function

Morphologically, the platelet can be envisioned as composed of three primary zones: (1) peripheral zone, (2) sol–gel zone, and (3) organelle zone.[9] The peripheral zone is composed of an extramembranous glycocalyx, inside of which is a plasma membrane similar to other trilamellar cellular plasma membranes. Under this membrane is an open canalicular system. The sol–gel zone is composed of microtubules and microfilaments, a dense tubular system that contains primarily adenine nucleotides and calcium ions. Also in the sol-gel zone is the contractile protein, thrombosthenin, which is similar to actomyosin. The organelle zone is composed of dense bodies, alpha granules, mitochondria, and the usual array of organelles found in other cellular systems, including lysosomes and endoplasmic reticulum. Alpha granules contain and release fibrinogen and lysosomal enzymes, whereas dense bodies contain and release adenine nucleotides, serotonin, catecholamines, and platelet factor 4.[23–25]

An adequate number of platelets must be present for normal platelet function, both in vivo and in vitro. This number is usually defined as approximately 100×10^9/L. With a platelet count $< 100 \times 10^9$/L, abnormal laboratory test results are noted; for example,

TABLE 1.   Platelet Proteins

Nonspecific (Plasma) Proteins	Platelet-specific Proteins
Fibrinogen	Thrombosthenin
Factors II, V, VII, VIII, IX, X, XII, and XIII	Platelet glycoprotein
Albumin	Platelet factors 2 and 4
Plasminogen	Platelet antiplasmin
Complement components	Cathepsin A
	Beta-thromboglobulin

prolonged template bleeding times and abnormal platelet aggregation profiles. For normal function, platelets require (1) adequate energy metabolism; (2) adequate number (and contents) of storage granules, capable of releasing their contents when appropriate stimuli are presented; (3) cationic proteins, such as thrombosthenin; (4) membrane receptors responsive to appropriate stimuli; (5) divalent cations, the most important of which is calcium; and, of course, (6) adequate physical conditions, such as pH and temperature.

Table 1 summarizes the common platelet proteins. Some are not platelet-specific; many plasma proteins are found in or on the surface of platelets, including clotting factors II, V, VII, VIII, IX, X, XI, XII, and XIII.[26] Sometimes these proteins are found in a slightly different molecular form in platelets and plasma; for example, factor XIII. Platelet-specific proteins include thrombosthenin, platelet factor 4, beta-thromboglobulin, and cathepsin A. Table 2 lists the seven platelet-specific factors that have been identified and characterized. The essential ones are platelet factor 3 (platelet thromboplastin/phospholipid) and platelet factor 4 (antiheparin factor), which has become an important molecular marker of platelet reactivity.[27–29]

Compounds released from platelets include the biogenic amines (serotonin, catecholamines, and histamine); the adenine nucleotides (cyclic adenosine monophosphate [cAMP], adenosine diphosphate [ADP], and adenosine triphosphate [ATP]); various enzymes (e.g., acid hydrolases); specific ions (e.g., calcium, magnesium, and potassium); and platelet factors (e.g., platelet factors 3 and 4, beta-thromboglobulin). Additional proteins, including fibrinogen, other clotting factors, and albumin, also are released from platelets during activation.

Multiple stimuli induce platelet activation.[30,31] In addition to subendothelial collagen and basement membrane, potent inducers of a platelet release reaction include thrombin, soluble fibrin monomer, some fibrinogen degradation products (especially fragment X), endotoxin, circulating antigen–antibody complexes, gamma-globulin–coated surfaces, various viruses, ADP, catecholamines, and free fatty acids.[32–35] Many proteolytic enzymes, including trypsin, snake venoms, papain, and elastase, are used in vitro to induce platelet release. Other in vitro techniques include centrifugation, cold fracture, and addition of latex particles, carbon particles, kaolin, or celite.

When platelets are activated, they contract and form pseudopods. During contraction, the numerous intraplatelet compounds and granules are concentrated at the center of the platelet, where organelle membranes disrupt; their contents are released and subsequently transported outside the platelet via the open canalicular system. These compounds interact with neighboring platelet membrane receptors or adjacent endothelium, causing further

TABLE 2.   Platelet Factors

Platelet factor 1:	Coagulation factor V
Platelet factor 2:	Thromboplastic material
Platelet factor 3:	Platelet thromboplastin
Platelet factor 4:	Antiheparin factor
Platelet factor 5:	Fibrinogen coagulation factor
Platelet factor 6:	Antifibrinolytic factor
Platelet factor 7:	Platelet cothromboplastin

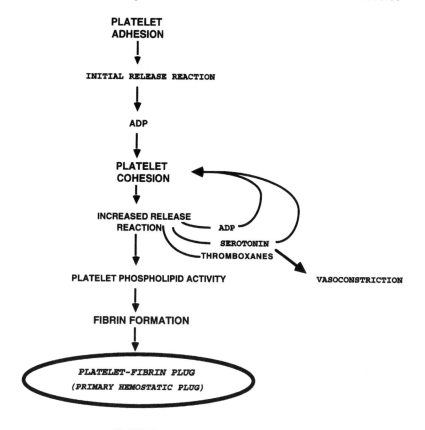

FIGURE 3.   Simplified platelet function.

platelet activation and thereby amplifying the process. Pseudopod formation enhances platelet–surface interactions (adhesion) and platelet–platelet interaction (cohesion).

Figure 3 summarizes platelet function. In the process of adhesion, a platelet adheres to something other than another platelet; for example, an artificial surface or collagen/basement membrane exposed by injury. Adhesion results in an initial release reaction that generates ADP. This process is reversible and accounts for the primary wave on an aggregation pattern (primary reversible aggregation). As the concentration of ADP increases, platelet cohesion occurs; that is, platelets stick to each other. As the process continues, released compounds (including serotonin) not only activate adjacent platelets but also induce vascular constriction. This advanced phase of activation leads to an irreversible conformational change in the platelet membrane. This change enables the activity of platelet factor 3 (platelet membrane phospholipid), which serves as a primary "surface" mediating the formation of complexes in the coagulation protein sequence. This irreversible process accounts for the secondary wave seen in a platelet aggregation pattern. In vivo, the result is the eventual formation of a platelet/fibrin thrombus or primary hemostatic plug, the function and integrity of which is facilitated by vasoconstriction.

Abbreviated intraplatelet functional biochemical sequences are outlined in Figure 4. The key modulator of intraplatelet function is cAMP,[36,37] which combines with a cAMP-dependent protein to generate kinase activity. The purpose of this activity is to phosphorylate a receptor protein, which then binds (or sequesters) calcium ions, rendering the platelet hypoaggregable and hypoadherable. Epinephrine, thrombin, collagen, and serotonin inhibit

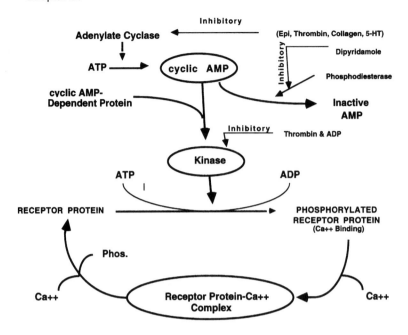

FIGURE 4.   Simplified intraplatelet biochemistry.

the enzyme adenylate cyclase, which is responsible for the conversion of ATP to cAMP. This inhibition leads to a decrease in kinase concentration and phosphorylated receptor protein and an increase in ionized (free) calcium, which renders the platelet hyperaggregable.

Balancing this biochemical sequence is the enzyme phosphodiesterase,[38,39] which is responsible for destroying cAMP. Agents such as dipyridamole, caffeine, and papaverine inhibit phosphodiesterase and thus lead to a decrease in free calcium, which makes the platelet hypofunctional. Yet another mechanism for regulating the availability of ionized calcium may relate to the activity of membrane-bound alkaline phosphatase, which is responsible for dephosphorylation of the receptor protein–Ca^{2+} complex.

Figure 5 summarizes the role of prostaglandins and their derivatives in platelet function. Phospholipids from platelets and endothelial cell membranes are converted into arachidonic acid by the enzyme, phospholipase A_2,[40] which is activated by both thrombin and collagen. Arachidonic acid is converted into prostaglandin intermediates, prostaglandin G_2 (PGG$_2$), and prostaglandin H_2 (PGH$_2$) by the enzyme cyclooxygenase. In the platelet membrane, thromboxane synthetase converts PGH$_2$ into thromboxane A_2, a potent inhibitor of adenylate cyclase and, therefore, one of the most potent aggregating agents yet described. Thromboxane A_2 also has potent vasoconstricting activity. In endothelial cells and some subendothelial muscle cells, prostacyclin synthetase converts PGH$_2$ into prostacyclin, which is a potent stimulator of adenylate cyclase and, therefore, a potent aggregation inhibitor and vasodilator.[41,42]

In this exquisitely balanced biologic system, platelets synthesize and release into the adjacent milieu a compound (thromboxane A_2) that promotes platelet function, whereas the adjacent endothelium synthesizes and releases prostacyclin, which inhibits platelet function. Therefore, the predisposition to bleeding or thrombosis may depend on the relative equilibrium between these two compounds.

Cyclooxygenase is inhibited by aspirin and sulfinpyrazone, two popular antiplatelet agents.[43] Evidence suggests that both function selectively, because their activity is directed

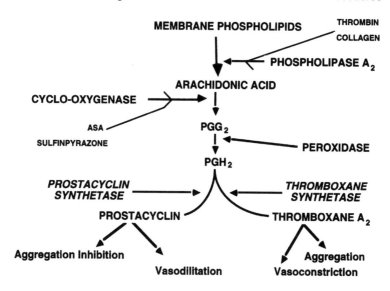

FIGURE 5.   Prostaglandins in platelet/endothelial function.

primarily toward platelets.Furthermore, in their presence endothelium continues to synthesize prostaglandins, but platelets do not. The precise mechanisms for this selectivity have not yet been elucidated.

Platelet interactions with the vasculature (adhesion), with other platelets (cohesion), and with plasma proteins occur at the platelet membrane surface and are mediated by various platelet membrane glycoproteins (PMGPs).[44] The major PMGPs and their functions, when known, are summarized in Table 3. PMGP Ia is complexed to PMGP IIa and functions to adhere platelets to subendothelial collagen, independently of von Willebrand factor.[45,46] PMGP Ib has been associated with multiple functions. It has a molecular weight of about 170,000 Da and is composed of an alpha and beta subunit, one of which fixes it to the platelet membrane. PMGP Ib is found in complex with PMGPs IX and V.[47] PMGP Ib and IX are absent from platelets in Bernard-Soulier syndrome.[48] PMGP Ib serves as a receptor for von Willebrand factor, the first step in platelet adhesion to subendothelial surfaces.[46,49] PMGP Ib is also the receptor for quinine and quinidine drug-dependent antibody, which is present in quinine and quinidine-induced thrombocytopenia.[50] PMGP Ib is also a part of the thrombin receptor complex of platelets. Although its role is not clearly defined,

TABLE 3.   Platelet Membrane Glycoproteins

GP	Function	Characteristic
Ia	von Willebrand-independent receptor for subendothelium	
Ib	von Willebrand receptor; quinidine-Ab receptor	Missing in Bernard-Soulier syndrome
Ic	No defined function	
IIa	No defined function	
IIb	von Willebrand and fibrinogen receptor; PIA-1 Ab receptor	Missing in Glanzmann's disease
IIIa	von Willebrand and fibrinogen receptor; PIA-1 Ab receptor	Missing in Glanzmann's disease
V	Thrombin receptor	Missing in Bernard-Soulier syndrome
IX		Missing in Bernard-Soulier syndrome
G	Thrombin- and collagen-induced aggregation	

GP = glycoprotein.

PMGP V is of vital importance in this mechanism of platelet activation.[51] PMGP IIb/IIIa complex is found in platelet alpha granules as well as on the membrane.[52] PMGP IIb has a molecular weight of about 125,000 Da; the molecular weight of PMGP IIIa is about 93,000 Da. Both appear to be subunits of a single glycoprotein, which depends heavily on calcium for binding of the complex.[53] PMGP IIb/IIIa is absent or markedly reduced in Glanzmann's thrombasthenia; it is the binding site for fibrinogen and serves as the apparent binding site for platelet antigen 1 antibody.[54,55] The binding of fibrinogen to PMGP IIb/IIIa is needed for optimal ADP-induced platelet aggregation. Glycoprotein G, also called thrombospondin, has a molecular weight of about 180,000 Da and is partly responsible for thrombin- and collagen-induced aggregation.[56,57] Platelet membrane glycoproteins Ic and IIa have been identified, their function in hemostasis is unknown.

Plasma Protein Function

Plasma protein function in hemostasis involves multiple interactive systems: (1) coagulation, (2) fibrino(geno)lysis, (3) complement activation, (4) kinin generation, and (5) inhibitors for these systems. Although not usually considered an integral part of hemostasis pathophysiologically, kinin generation and complement activation assume considerable importance, especially in syndromes of disseminated intravascular coagulation (DIC).[58]

Coagulation Protein System

Coagulation proteins and some synonyms are listed in Table 4. The Roman numeral system is most widely used and is preferred. The chromosome location containing genetic information for synthesis of almost all coagulation factors has been reported[59] (Table 5). The formation of a fibrin clot is best viewed as consisting of four key reactions involving the generation of proteolytic enzymes (serine proteases): (1) formation of factor IXa, (2) formation of factor Xa, (3) formation of thrombin, and (4) formation of fibrin.

Formation of Factor IXa.   The contact activation phase of coagulation begins with the generation of active Hageman factor (Factor XIIa). Surfaces (e.g., phospholipids, subendothelial collagen) and kallikrein can convert factor XII to factor XIIa, which, in turn, converts factor XI to factor XIa.[60,61] This reaction happens quickly in the presence of high-molecular-weight kininogen (a significantly prolonged activated partial thromboplastin time is noted in its absence).[62] The role of factor XIa is to convert inactive factor IX (in the presence of calcium ions) to its active form, factor IXa. Factor IXa is the enzyme responsible for the second key reaction, the generation of factor Xa. Factor XIIa converts prekallikrein into kallikrein, which enhances the generation of more factor XIIa.[63]

TABLE 4.   Coagulation Factors and Synonyms

Factor	Synonym
I	Fibrinogen
II	Prothrombin
V	AC-globulin
VII	Prothrombin conversion accelerator
VIII:C	Antihemophilic factor
IX	Christmas factor
X	Stuart-Prower factor
XI	Thromboplastin antecedent (PTA)
XII	Hageman (contact) factor
XIII	Profibrinoligase
Prekallikrein	Fletcher factor
HMW kininogen	Fitzgerald factor
Protein C	None
Protein S	None

TABLE 5.   Chromosomal Locations Containing Coagulation and Fibrinolytic Factor Information

Factor	Inheritance	Chromosome	Region
I	AD	4	q26–31
II	AD	11	p11–q12
V	AR	1	q21–25
VII	AR	13	q34
VIII:C	SLR	X	q28
von Willebrand factor	AD	12	p12–13
IX	SLR	X	q27
X	AR	13	q34
XI	AR	4	q35
XII	AR	5	q33
XIII	AD	6	p24–25
Antithrombin	AD	1	p23
Protein C	AD	2	q13–14
Protein S	AD	3	p21
Plasminogen	AD	6	q26–27
TPA	AD	8	p12
TPA-1-1	AD	7	q21–22
TPA-1-2	AD	18	q21–22
Antiplasmin	AR	18	?
Prekallikrein	AR	?	?
HMW kininogen	AR	?	?
Heparin cofactor II	AD	22	?

TPA = tissue-type plasminogen activator.
Inheritance = usual mode of inheritance. AD = autosomal dominant, AR = autosomal recessive, SLR = sex-linked recessive.

Formation of Factor Xa.   The second key reaction involves two major pathways: intrinsic and extrinsic. Intrinsic formation of factor Xa involves a five component system: (1) substrate (factor X), (2) enzyme (factor IXa), (3) determiner or cofactor (factor VIII:C), (4) surface (platelet factor 3), and (5) calcium ions.[64] The complex that is formed is mediated by calcium ions. Factor IXa cleaves a peptide from the substrate (factor X) with resultant exposure of an active serine site. Factor Xa is the product of this reaction. Factor VIII:C is modified and rendered dysfunctional in the process.

The extrinsic pathway of factor Xa formation involves the participation of thromboplastin (tissue factor), factor VII, and calcium ions. Tissue factor is a membrane-bound lipoprotein that exists in a protected state within the plasma membrane of endothelial cells. Upon injury it is released into the circulation, where it forms a complex with coagulation factor VII in the presence of calcium ions. The activity of the complex seems to depend largely on the concentration of tissue factor. However, the enzymatic activity responsible for the proteolytic activation of factor Xa resides in the factor VII molecule.[65,66] Aprotinin has been shown to inhibit the factor VIIa–tissue factor complex.[67]

Factor VII exists in plasma as a single-chain glycoprotein with close structural homology to prothrombin, factor IX, and factor X. Unlike its analogs, however, factor VII is not a zymogen in the true sense, because it has proteolytic activity—although to a limited extent. In the presence of thrombin or factor Xa and lipids and calcium ions, its proteolytic activity may be increased as much as 400-fold and is accompanied by the formation of a two polypeptide-chain molecule. With further incubation, the two-chain form of factor VII becomes inactive, and the rate of inactivation depends on the concentration of factor Xa. It has been proposed that in the activation of factor X by factor VII, the continuing generation of factor Xa results in a "pulse of factor X-converting activity that can quickly disappear."[65,66]

Formation of Thrombin.   The third key reaction is the formation of thrombin. As with the intrinsic generation of factor Xa, a five component system is involved: (1) substrate (prothrombin), (2) enzyme (factor Xa), (3) determiner/cofactor (factor V), (4) platelet factor 3, and (5) calcium ions.[68] These components form a complex on the phospholipid surface, and a new enzyme—thrombin (factor IIa)—is generated. Factor V, like factor VIII:C in the previous reaction, is modified and loses biologic activity. The role of the determiner/cofactor in both reactions is to ensure that the correct enzyme and substrate enter into complex formation. The enzymes—thrombin, factor Xa, factor IXa, factor VIIa, and others (e.g., protein C and protein S—are synthesized in liver parenchymal cells in precursor forms by a vitamin K-dependent process that involves the postribosomal attachment of calcium-binding prosthetic groups to the n-terminal region of each protein. The process involves the introduction of an extra carboxyl group on the side chain (gamma position) of several glutamic acid residues, forming gamma carboxyglutamic acid.[69] In the absence of vitamin K—for example, in a patient on vitamin K antagonist therapy[70]—a protein is synthesized, but it is dysfunctional. These abnormal vitamin K-dependent factors are called PIVKAs (proteins induced by vitamin K absence/antagonists).[71]

Formation of Fibrin.   The fourth key reaction is the formation of fibrin.[72] Figure 6 summarizes the sequence in the conversion of fibrinogen to fibrin. Thrombin specifically removes fibrinopeptide A and fibrinopeptide B from fibrinogen, a dimeric structure composed of six covalently linked polypeptide chains (two A alpha, two B beta, and two gamma chains). The removal of fibrinopeptides A and B creates a fibrin monomer.[73,74] Fibrin monomer (fibrinogen minus peptides A and B) polymerizes by aggregating end to end and side to side; these aggregates are stabilized by noncovalent bonds. The result is called "soluble fibrin" because it dissolves in 5 molar urea or 1% monochloroacetic acid. This process is called polymerization I. Thrombin, in its multiple roles as a pivotal enzyme in hemostasis,[72] also activates factor XIII to factor XIIIa. In the presence of calcium ions, factor XIIa, functioning as a transpeptidase, introduces isopeptide bonds between the epsilon amino groups of certain lysine residues and the gamma carboxyamide groups of certain glutamines in neighboring gamma and alpha chains of the fibrin polymer. This process, which renders the fibrin more elastic and less amenable to lysis,[75,76] is called polymerization II. The result is "insoluble fibrin." Figure 7 summarizes the pathways of activation for the four key reactions in coagulation.

Fibrinolytic System

Whereas fibrin deposition is viewed as a fundamental mechanism for repair of injured tissues, fibrinolysis may be viewed as its physiologic antithesis—the destruction of a fibrin clot.[77,78] Hemorrhage or thrombosis thus may depend on a delicate balance between the procoagulant system and the fibrinolytic system. Figure 8 summarizes the biology of

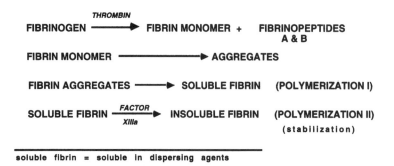

FIGURE 6.   Conversion of fibrinogen to fibrin.

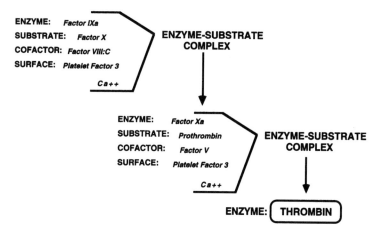

FIGURE 7.   Summary of the first two key reactions: the formation of factor Xa and thrombin.

the fibrinolytic system, which consists of a proenzyme (plasminogen) that is converted via many pathways into the active enzyme, plasmin.[79] Unlike the enzyme thrombin, which has a relatively narrow substrate specificity, the serine protease plasmin has a much broader spectrum of activity with a number of substrates. Indeed, it hydrolyzes both fibrinogen and fibrin into degradation products (FDPs) and degrades factors V, VIII, IX, and XI, adrenocorticotropic hormone (ACTH), growth hormone, insulin, components of the complement system, and many other proteins.[80–82] There are two recognized and well-characterized physiologic activation pathways of the fibrinolytic system. The primary pathway involves endothelial cell-derived plasminogen activator (TPA), which converts plasminogen to plasmin directly.[83] The second pathway, which is probably of less physiologic significance, involves factor XIIa (generated by many triggers), which converts a proactivator (prekallikrein) into an activator (kallikrein), which, in turn, converts plasminogen into plasmin.[84–86]

The fibrinolytic system is modulated by many inhibitors. Alpha-2-antiplasmin is an extraordinarily rapid inhibitor of plasmin activity.[77,87] Although present in low concentration in plasma, alpha-2-antiplasmin, with its extraordinary affinity for plasmin (resulting in an irreversible covalent complex), is the primary candidate for the major regulator of fibrinolysis in vivo. There are two known inhibitors of TPA[88,89]: plasminogen activator

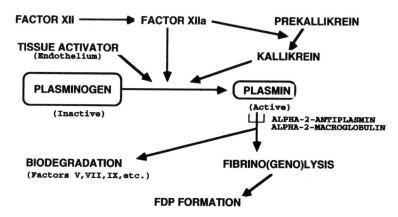

FIGURE 8.   Physiology of the fibrinolytic system.

inhibitors 1 and 2 (PAI-1 and PAI-2). PAI-1 is the primary modulator. Various cells produce this protein, including platelets, supporting the hypothesis that at sites of injury, platelet aggregation facilitates the survival of fibrin and thus the integrity of the hemostatic plug.[90] Aprotinin is a potent exogenous (pharmacologic) inhibitor of plasmin.[91]

In contrast to thrombin, which cleaves fibrinopeptides A and B from the amino terminus of fibrinogen to create fibrin monomer, plasmin begins to degrade fibrin(ogen) at the carboxy terminus of the A-alpha chain and continues to hydrolyze the matrix in various other loci, yielding soluble degradation products. Figure 9 depicts the characterized fibrin(ogen) degradation products (FDPs), which are illustrated in descending order of molecular size. Fibrinogen has a molecular weight of approximately 340,000 Da; fragment X, approximately 265,000 Da; fragment Y, approximately 155,000 Da; fragment D, approximately 95,000 Da; and fragment E, about 50,000 Da. The presence of FDPs in the circulation may seriously compromise hemostasis by interference with fibrin monomer polymerization and platelet function.[90,92,93]

Complement Activation

Although complement activation is generally not considered an integral part of the hemostatic system, its role in the pathophysiology of thrombohemorrhagic disorders is of considerable importance. It is a multimolecular, self-assembling system that constitutes the primary humoral mediator of inflammation and tissue damage.[94,95] It involves a series of sequential reactions, much like the coagulation system (Fig. 10). The primary classic activation pathway involves activation of C1 by antigen–antibody complexes, whereas the alternate (properdin) activation pathway involves direct activation of C3. The activation of C1 through C5 is called the activation phase, and the activation of C5 through C9 is called

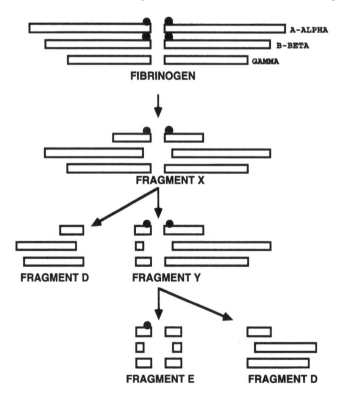

FIGURE 9. Formation of fibrinogen/fibrin degradation products.

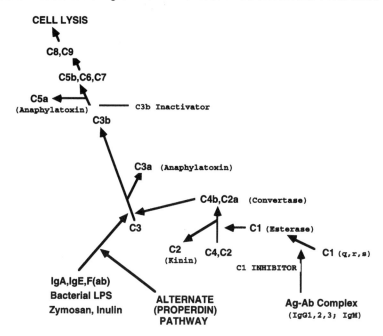

FIGURE 10. The complement system.

the attack phase, which leads to cell lysis and destruction of pathogens by phagocytes (opsonization). The attack phase includes osmotic lysis of red cells and platelets, which releases ADP and procoagulant material in the form of membrane lipoprotein, both of which accelerate the coagulation process.[96–98] Of interest, although it is difficult to assess its pathophysiologic relevance, plasmin generated either by TPA or the Hageman factor pathway can directly activate C1 or C3 independently of antigen–antibody complexes. Aprotinin can inhibit kallikrein–C1-inhibitor complexes and C1–C1-inhibitor complexes.[99] In many instances of pronounced activation of the fibrinolytic system, one may envision significant plasmin-induced activation of the complement system, which leads to serious clinical consequences.[58]

Kinin Generation

The importance of kinin generation during thrombohemorrhagic disorders has been appreciated only recently. Kinins increase vascular permeability and induce vascular dilation, leading to hypotension, shock, and potential end-organ damage—all of which are common in DIC syndromes.[58,100–102] Like complement activation, generation of kinins centers on activation of Hageman factor (factor XII). As noted earlier, factor XIIa, in addition to activating factor XI to factor XIa, converts prekallikrein (Fletcher factor) into kallikrein, which converts kininogens into kinins. In addition, factor XIIa is further digested into factor XIIa fragments by plasmin; these fragments, although void of procoagulant activity, can further activate prekallikrein to kallikrein with ensuing generation of kinins. Aprotinin is a potent inhibitor of kallikrein.[103]

Figure 11 illustrates the important interrelationships among the coagulation system, fibrinolytic system, complement system, and kinin system. Factor XII is converted to active factor XIIa by various compounds (surfaces), including collagen and phospholipids; factor XIIa converts prekallikrein to kallikrein, which, in turn, converts plasminogen to plasmin. Plasmin activates C1 and/or C3 of the complement system. In addition, plasmin-induced factor XIIa fragments convert prekallikrein to kallikrein, which, in addition to

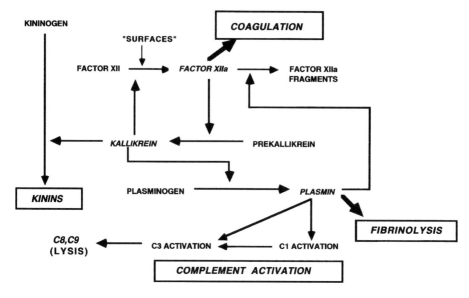

FIGURE 11.   Interactions of the systems.

generating more plasmin, convert kininogens to kinins. Although it is difficult to assess these activation pathways quantitatively, clinical observations suggest that they play important roles in the pathophysiology of DIC, often leading to catastrophic clinical consequences.[58]

Inhibitor Systems

Like other biologic processes, the blood coagulation system is governed by many inhibitory mechanisms designed to limit the extent of various biochemical reactions and possible dissemination of the coagulation process. To this extent, the regulation of coagulation is effected by a number of negative feedback loops, the involvement of specific inhibitors, and the compartmentalization of function, all of which serve to restrict clotting to a localized process. Table 6 summarizes inhibitory systems in hemostasis.[104,105] Many of these mechanisms assume major importance in pathophysiology. First is the inactivation of factors V and VIII:C by the activated protein C and protein S system.[106] This mechanism involves the interaction of the enzyme thrombin with an endothelial cell component, thrombomodulin; this interaction results in an in situ complex incapable of converting fibrinogen to fibrin but fully active in converting protein C (a proenzyme) to protein Ca (an enzyme). Protein Ca, in the presence of protein S, inactivates factors V and VIII:C by proteolysis, essentially halting further deposition of fibrin (Fig. 12). Dahlback and associates identified an "activated protein C cofactor/resistance," a molecular defect in factor V (factor V Leiden) that leads to familial thrombosis.[107] In concert

TABLE 6.   Inhibitory Systems in Hemostasis

1. Inactivation of factors V and VIII by thrombin and activated protein C and protein S system.
2. Inhibition of thrombin, factors Xa, IXa, XIa, and XIIa and kallikrein by antithrombin III.
3. Inhibition of prothrombin activation and fibrin formation by prothrombin fragments.
4. Inhibition of thrombin or factor Xa formation by suboptimal "complex" components.
5. Inhibition of thrombin activity by absorbing to fibrin.
6. Inhibition of fibrin monomer polymerization and platelet function by products of fibrino(geno)lysis (FDP).

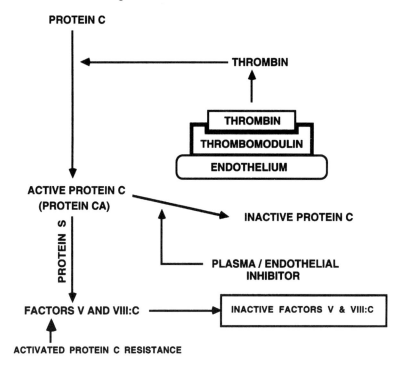

FIGURE 12.   Protein C and S system.

with procoagulant inhibitor activity is the observation that protein Ca enhances fibrinolysis, perhaps by depressing the activity of naturally occurring fibrinolytic inhibitors and/or by enhancing the activity of plasminogen activators. Aprotinin is also a potent inhibitor of activated protein C.[108] The inhibitory activity of active protein C is modulated by another endothelial cell-derived inhibitor.

Another mechanism identified as playing a primary role in modulating hemostasis is the inhibition of the serine proteases thrombin, factor Xa, factor IXa, factor XIIa, and kallikrein by antithrombin (AT). The inhibitory activity of AT is markedly enhanced by heparin.[109–113] Figure 13 illustrates the interaction of AT with serine proteases. Arginine-rich centers in AT react irreversibly with the serine center of serine proteases. In Figure 13, thrombin serves as an example. When used in therapy, heparin reacts with lysine sites in antithrombin, making the arginine-rich center more available and thereby enhancing antithrombin inhibitory activity. This ternary complex then dissociates to yield an inactive thrombin–AT complex and free heparin. The complex is cleared from the circulation. The elucidation of this mechanism has served as a fundamental rationalization for heparin/miniheparin therapy.

Although the vast majority of evidence suggests that protein C and AT are the most important modulators of coagulation, the contribution by other mechanisms listed in Table 6 is probably not trivial. For instance, the prothrombin fragments produced when thrombin is generated are known to interfere with further conversion of prothrombin and with fibrin polymerization. As fibrin is formed, it absorbs thrombin, thus decreasing its availability. In addition, FDPs may inhibit fibrin monomer polymerization and platelet function. If FDPs complex with fibrin monomer, it becomes solubilized and unavailable for polymerization. Late degradation products, especially fragments D and E, have a high affinity for platelet membranes and render platelets markedly dysfunctional. In some cases, this activity leads to significant clinical hemorrhage.[114]

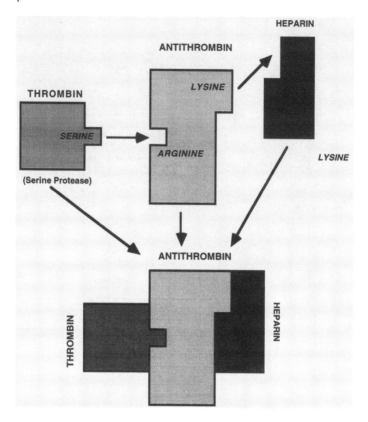

COMPLEX FORMATION

FIGURE 13.   Antithrombin inhibitory activity.

Other Interactive Components

Increasing evidence suggests that many other interactive components, including vascular proteoglycans, fibronectin, complement derivatives, neutrophils and monocytes, cytokines, and other thus far uncharacterized agents, may play important roles in modulating hemostasis.

Fibronectin is a high-molecular-weight glycoprotein that is soluble in plasma.[115] An insoluble form, found in connective tissue and basement membranes,[116] binds to collagen, fibrin, fibrinogen, and intact cells, especially fibroblasts.[116–118] It is synthesized by vascular endothelium and also found in the alpha granules of platelets.[29] Fibronectin is cleaved by thrombin and trypsin, coprecipitates with fibrin, and is covalently cross-linked to fibrin by factor XIIIa.[119–121] It is needed to support cell growth and to enhance cellular migration into a fibrin clot; it provides an extracellular matrix that eventually replaces a fibrin clot. As clot formation occurs, approximately 50% of plasma fibronectin is lost.[120] This loss is due to cross-linking of fibronectin to the alpha chain of fibrin (by factor XIIIa); fibronectin thus accounts for approximately 5% of the total protein of a fibrin clot. Fibronectin is necessary for cryoprecipitation of fibrinogen–fibrin complexes and accounts for the laboratory cryoprecipitation seen in DIC. Fibronectin is commonly decreased not only in DIC but also in postoperative states, in patients sustaining major trauma (especially burns), and in patients with solid tumor metastases.[121]

Other activities associated with fibronectin relate to the potentiation of plasminogen activators, which mediates clot lysis and matrix turnover; mediation of platelet activation by damaged tissue; opsonization of bacteria by neutrophils; attachment of bacteria to damaged tissues; and inhibition of the endothelial uptake of low-density lipoprotein. The fibronectin associated with alpha granules of platelets is released during collagen- or thrombin-induced platelet aggregation; after release, it binds to the platelet surface, further enhancing collagen-platelet adhesion and further stimulating collagen-induced platelet aggregation and release. The interaction with collagen[119] and probably other vascular proteoglycans (heparan sulfate, hyaluronic acid, and chondroitin sulfate) is mediated by cross-linking via factor XIIIa. Heparin may accelerate the binding of fibronectin to both fibrinogen and collagen; however, the binding of heparin to fibronectin does not appear to change the anticoagulant nature of the bound heparin.[121]

Vascular proteoglycans are a heterogeneous group of high-molecular-weight protein polysaccharides composed of carbohydrate polymers (glycosaminoglycans) covalently linked to a protein core.[122] The common vascular proteoglycans are hyaluronic acid, chondroitin-4-sulfate, chondroitin-6-sulfate, dermatan sulfate, keratin sulfate, heparin sulfate, heparan sulfate, and heparin.[123] Heparan sulfate is a low-sulfated D-glucuronic acid-rich polysaccharide, whereas heparin is a highly sulfated, L-iduronic acid-rich polysaccharide. The amount of each particular type of proteoglycan differs in various regions of the vasculature. Most are concentrated in the intimal layer. The concentration of dermatan and heparan sulfate correlates closely with antithrombotic activity. Selected proteoglycans inhibit collagen- and thrombin-induced platelet aggregation, accelerate AT inhibitory activity, and induce the release of platelet factor 4. Their concentrations change with the development of atherosclerotic plaques. Physiologically, vascular proteoglycans support vascular integrity, maintain the viscoelastic properties of vessels, regulate permeability of macromolecules, and regulate arterial lipid deposition. All of these properties involve modulating functions in the interaction of blood proteins with the vascular wall. Several complement derivatives, especially C3a and C5a, may play key roles in hemostasis. These components not only regulate vascular tone but also may induce a neutrophil/monocyte release of enzymes such as elastases and collagenases, which are important in the degradation of fibrinogen, fibrin, and FDPs. In addition, complement derivatives modulate release of granulocyte/monocyte procoagulant activity, may modulate platelet reactivity, and influence the neutrophil/monocyte interaction with fibronectin.[124] Granulocytes and monocytes contain procoagulant activity which may be released under pathologic conditions, such as acute leukemia.[125,126]

Conclusion

The consequences of acute insults to the hemostatic system, whether congenital or acquired, often present a considerable challenge in diagnosis and therapy. Logical and effective management depends on (1) proper identification of the hemostatic compartments involved; (2) appreciation for the considerably complex, delicately modulated interplays of various enzyme/inhibitor systems; and (3) knowledge of the mechanism by which various, apparently unrelated disease processes somtimes precipitate catastrophic events: thrombosis, embolism, and hemorrhage. The discussion of plasma proteins pays particular attention to biocybernetic principles (positive/negative feedback loops) and to the interrelationship of enzyme systems involved in coagulation, fibrinolysis, kinin generation, and complement activation, because these systems are often disrupted during cardiac surgery. A working knowledge of basic mechanisms not only provides advantages in diagnostic and therapeutic management but also serves as a firm foundation for the development of novel diagnostic and therapeutic modalities, particularly in regard to prevention, diagnosis, and management of hemorrhage associated with cardiac surgery.

PATHOLOGY OF HEMOSTASIS DURING CARDIAC SURGERY

Cardiopulmonary bypass (CPB) surgery has become routine in clinical medicine, and the severe defects in hemostasis that often accompany CPB may dramatically increase morbidity and mortality rates.

Prevention of Cardiac Surgical Bleeding

Hemorrhage associated with cardiac surgery may be devastating and life-threatening; overcautiousness in regard to prevention, diagnosis, and rapid, effective therapy is essential. Surgical hemorrhage may be minimized by uncovering hereditary, acquired, or drug-induced bleeding tendencies before CPB. A preexisting bleeding diathesis, although mild, may lead to calamitous results when coupled with the hemostatic changes induced by cardiac surgery.[127] Recently, there has been great interest in aprotinin as an agent for decreasing blood loss during cardiac surgery.[128–132]

Laboratory Screening

In general, the preoperative laboratory and hemostasis screen should be simple and incur a minimum of expense to the patient while providing adequate information; however, presurgical or precardiac bypass hemostasis screens are often insufficient.[133–135] As with an adequate history and physical examination, one must be knowledgeable in screening for defects in hemostasis when a surgical procedure is planned. When preexisting hemostatic defects are combined with the defects in hemostasis created by CPB, the resultant hemorrhage is often catastrophic. Often it can be avoided by wise screening of patients. The usually ordered SMA 12/60 biochemical screening survey, electrolytes, and complete blood and platelet count will detect the common acquired disorders often associated with a bleeding tendency, such as chronic liver disease, renal disease, and cases of hypersplenism or bone marrow failure. Most commonly, a presurgical screen consists only of prothrombin time, activated partial thromboplastin time, and platelet count. Although these simple tests detect most coagulation protein problems as well as thrombocytopenia, they provide absolutely no information about vascular or platelet function and ignore the possibility of pathologic fibrinolysis.

Most nontechnical hemorrhage associated with cardiac surgery is caused by platelet function defects; less common causes include coagulation protein or vascular defects. It is important to realize that platelet defects are a more common cause of surgical bleeding than are coagulation protein problems. Therefore, one simple procedure is added to the routine preoperative screen: the standardized template bleeding time, as described by Mielke and coworkers.[136] This test is done for all patients before a cardiac surgical procedure; it provides a reasonable screen for adequate vascular function and platelet function.[137] The template bleeding time should not be done until adequate platelet numbers ($> 100 \times 10^9$/L) are documented by count or smear evaluation. For patients undergoing CPB, thrombin time is added to the preoperative screen.[138,139] In addition, the resultant clot should be observed for 5 minutes after the test is done. A normal thrombin time ensures the absence of significant hypofibrinogenemia, dysfibrinogenemia, fibrinolysis, or FDP elevation. The use of these tests in the presurgical screen adds only minimal cost and laboratory time but provides valuable information not given by a simple prothrombin time, activated partial thromboplastin time, or platelet count. If hypothermic perfusion is to be done, cryoglobulins and cold agglutinins also should be assessed before bypass.[140–145] The preoperative surgical and bypass hemostasis screen is summarized in Table 7.[136,146–149]

Hemostasis in Cardiac Surgery

Hemorrhage during or after bypass is of more than fleeting significance, because it may lead to substantial morbidity and mortality from an elective procedure, places formidable demands on blood bank facilities, and may result in prolonged, costly hospitalizations.[139,150–153]

TABLE 7. Presurgical Hemostasis Screen (Minimal Requirements)

Complete blood count (CBC) and platelet count

Prothrombin time

Partial thromboplastin time

Template bleeding time (duplicate)

Thrombin time (cardiopulmonary bypass surgery; observe clot for 5 minutes)

Cryoglobulins and cold agglutinins (hypothermic cardiopulmonary bypass)

The actual incidence of life-threatening hemorrhage associated with CPB varies from 5–25%.[139,150–156]

Before the pathophysiology of altered hemostasis created by CPB was more clearly understood, various investigators attributed the hemorrhagic syndrome of CPB surgery to an assorted spectrum of defects. Each investigator, moreover, placed diverse degrees of importance on each defect, depending on which particular hemostatic parameters were monitored. In the past, the abnormalities most often cited to account for CPB hemorrhage included (1) inadequate heparin neutralization, (2) protamine excess, (3) heparin rebound, (4) thrombocytopenia, (5) hypofibrinogenemia, (6) primary fibrinolysis, (7) DIC, (8) isolated coagulation factor deficiencies, (9) transfusion reactions, and (10) hypocalcemia. The suggestion that all these defects may contribute to CPB hemorrhage clearly shows that despite the finding of multiple defects in hemostasis, the basic pathophysiology of altered hemostasis during CPB is bewildering to many. It is equally clear that basic mechanisms of altered hemostasis associated with CPB must be completely understood and appreciated before a useful approach to rapid diagnosis and effective therapy can be designed.

Thrombocytopenia

Early studies of hemostasis during CPB noted significant thrombocytopenia (about 50,000/cmm); many authors thought that thrombocytopenia was responsible for bypass hemorrhage. Kevy noted that thrombocytopenia was related to time on bypass and was more pronounced with perfusions lasting longer than 60 minutes.[157] A relationship between thrombocytopenia and time on bypass was also reported by Signore;[158] later studies noted similar findings.[159,160] Porter and Silver observed that in most patients undergoing CPB, the platelet count fell to one-third of the preoperative level; in addition, it was found that thrombocytopenia did not abate until several days after CPB. Earlier studies by Wright[161] and von Kaulla and Swan[162] also recognized thrombocytopenia in association with CPB, but the investigators decided that thrombocytopenia bore little, if any, relationship to actual bypass hemorrhage. Some studies finding thrombocytopenia during CPB concluded that it represented thrombocytopenia of DIC.[163–166] Bick[135,139,151,167–170] and others,[171–173] however, failed to find significant thrombocytopenia during CPB. This wide variability in experience probably represents different surgical and pumping techniques, such as flow rates, normothermic or hypothermic perfusion, specific oxygenation system used, time on bypass, and priming solution. Figure 14 shows changes in platelet number during CPB. The dotted line represents the mean platelet counts in patients with membrane oxygenation pumps, and the solid line represents patients managed with bubble oxygenation.[135,151,174] A total of 300 consecutive patients is depicted. In our experience, the type of oxygenation mechanism appears to play little, if any, role in causing clinically significant thrombocytopenia.[135,151,174] The incidence of thrombocytopenia with bubble oxygenators is slightly higher than that seen with membrane oxygenators, but the difference does not often reach clinical significance. The most commonly cited mechanisms for the development of CPB thrombocytopenia are (1) hemodilution, (2) formation of intravascular platelet thrombi, (3) platelet use in the pump or oxygenation system, and (4) peripheral utilization because of DIC. Our failure to find a correlation between CPB hematocrit and

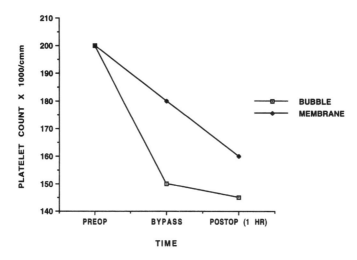

FIGURE 14.   Platelet counts during cardiopulmonary bypass: membrane vs. bubble oxygenation (300 consecutive patients).

platelet count suggests that hemodilution is not a major factor.[134,170,175] Indeed, the role, if any, of these mechanisms in producing CPB thrombocytopenia is unclear.

Platelet Function Defects

In contrast to the prolific investigations of platelet number during CPB, there has been a surprising lack of interest in assessing platelet function. Early investigators suspected that abnormalities of platelet function may occur, because faulty clot retraction was noted.[158] These results were of unclear significance, however, because other changes known to effect clot retraction, such as hypofibrinogenemia and thrombocytopenia, were also present. In an early study that assessed platelet function before but not during or after bypass,[176] abnormal preoperative platelet adhesion in glass bead columns was associated with increased postoperative bleeding. Salzman[177] studied platelet adhesion before, during, and after bypass and noted decreased adhesion to glass bead columns in patients during CPB; however, the significance of this defect was difficult to evaluate because all patients had marked thrombocytopenia, which is known to alter adhesion studies.[178–180] In addition, adhesion studies are now thought to have no particular clinical significance.[137,181,182] Salzman also observed that heparin, in doses used during CPB, did not alter platelet adhesion. He concluded that a circulating anticoagulant may be responsible for the platelet function defect, because plasma from CPB patients altered adhesion when added to normal platelets. This circulating anticoagulant probably represented FDPs.[139] Salzman's study also noted that perfusion temperature and type of priming solution did not correlate with the development of abnormal platelet function.

Platelet adhesion studies have also been performed in patients undergoing CPB without significant thrombocytopenia.[167,169,170,175] Platelet function, as measured by adhesion, decreased profoundly in all patients at the initiation of bypass; in most patients, adhesion decreased to 17% of preoperative levels. In one study, little correlation was noted between hematocrit, fibrinogen level, or FDP titer and abnormal adhesion.[169] In addition, poor correlation was noted between chest tube blood loss and abnormal platelet function, as assessed by adhesion. Although recent studies have questioned the clinical importance of platelet adhesion by the glass bead column technique,[137,181,182] this degree of abnormal platelet function would be expected to compromise hemostasis severely.

The platelet function defect is slightly more severe and tends to correct more slowly when a membrane oxygenator is used compared with a bubble oxygenator. Platelet function as assessed by template bleeding times or platelet aggregation or lumiaggregation is abnormal in patients with platelet function defects,[137,180] von Willebrand's syndrome (ristocetin aggregation only),[179] and myeloproliferative disorders.[183] Many factors, some possibly altered by CPB, may affect platelet function, including (1) pH, (2) absolute platelet count, (3) hematocrit, (4) drugs, (5) presence of FDPs, (6) type of pump prime, and (7) type of oxygenation system.[139,184–190] Although most studies poorly define the reasons for abnormal platelet function during CPB, they do suggest that several of the above mechanisms probably are not involved. The finding of platelet counts > 100,000/cmm and hematocrit values > 30% in most patients with marked platelet dysfunction 1 hour after CPB suggests that absolute platelet count and hematocrit do not account for altered platelet function. In addition, most patients have a normal or near normal pH 1 hour after bypass surgery; thus, a change in pH is unlikely to account for abnormal platelet function during bypass surgery. Heparin, at levels higher than those attained in patients undergoing CPB, has been shown not to alter platelet function.[150,177,180] Although circulating FDPs interfere with platelet function and are present in about 85% of patients undergoing CPB,[139,185,189] there is poor correlation between levels of circulating FDP and abnormal platelet function during bypass surgery.[169,175] In addition, defective platelet function is found in 100% of patients undergoing CPB; thus, circulating FDPs cannot account for altered platelet function in many instances.[134,139,151,169,175]

Other possible mechanisms of altered platelet function during CPB include platelet membrane damage by shearing force or contact with foreign material, which may result in partial release of platelet contents, platelet membrane coating with nonspecific proteins, or protein degradation products or incomplete release reaction or nonspecific platelet damage induced by flow rates. More recent studies have shown selective platelet degranulation during bypass surgery.[191] However, no studies yet reported allow conclusions to be drawn about the contribution of any of these mechanisms to altered platelet function during CPB. One preliminary study has reported platelet aggregation studies during CPB. In this series of 29 patients, only 20% developed aggregation abnormalities during CPB; however, after heparin reversal with protamine sulfate 90% of patients developed aggregation abnormalities. The authors attributed this finding to a protamine/platelet interaction and not to CPB itself.[192] We have evaluated platelets by lumiaggregation in patients undergoing CPB surgery, and in all patients platelet aggregation and platelet release were markedly altered.[150,151,193] Figures 15 and 16 depict typical mid-bypass, and post-bypass lumiaggregation patterns in patients undergoing cardiac surgery. Furthermore, in all patients assessed, the aggregation and release reaction defect occurred within 10–15 minutes of starting bypass. We also noted that in all patients levels of platelet factor 4 rise rapidly with the initiation of bypass. The aggregation defects appear to be similar with both membrane and bubble oxygenators; however, the type of priming solution (albumin vs. hydroxyethyl starch) seems to change the type of defects seen.[193]

Despite the mechanism(s) involved, studies to date clearly reveal that a significant defect in platelet function is induced in all patients undergoing CPB surgery. The magnitude of this defect certainly would be expected to have potentially serious consequences for hemostasis during and after bypass. In addition, patients who have ingested drugs known to interfere with platelet function would be expected to have more blood loss than patients not ingesting such agents. The effects of the drugs would be expected to compound the defects already induced by CPB and to potentiate the chance for hemorrhage. One small study has supplied evidence for this conclusion.[188] Although diagnosis and management of hemorrhage associated with CPB are discussed later, it should be pointed out that defects in platelet function are of major importance in post-CPB hemorrhage. In most patients with a normal platelet count, the use of platelet concentrates will promptly correct

MID-BYPASS

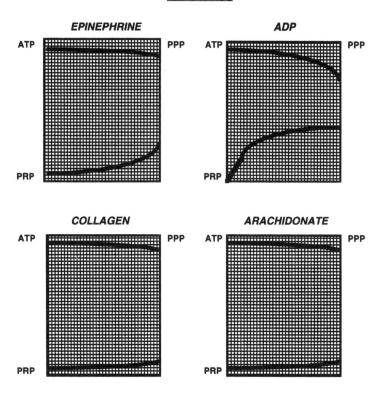

FIGURE 15. Platelet lumiaggregation patterns *during* cardiopulmonary bypass surgery. PRP = platelet-rich plasma, PPP = platelet-poor plasma, ATP = adenosine triphosphate release.

or significantly reduce most episodes of CPB or post-CPB hemorrhage. Desmopressin acetate (DDAVP) was initially thought to decrease bleeding after open heart surgery; thus, many surgeons began the empirical, and sometimes nonrational use of DDAVP during and after open heart surgery. However, more recent blinded, randomized trials have failed to show significant differences in post-CPB blood loss between DDAVP and placebo.[194–196] In addition, DDAVP releases tissue (endothelial) plasminogen activator, potentially activating the fibrinolytic system and enhancing or inducing hemorrhage; therefore, many advocates of DDAVP recommend the concomitant use of aminocaproic acid to abort possible hemorrhage.[197–200] Current evidence indicates little, if any, rationale for the empiric use of DDAVP during CPB; surgeons should be aware of the potential for enhancing hemorrhage and for increased risk of coronary artery and cerebrovascular thrombosis.

Isolated Coagulation Factor Defects
Many studies have examined and reported coagulation factor deficiencies during CPB. A wide variety of findings has been observed, like the finding of thrombocytopenia, however, they may reflect only differences in surgical or pumping techniques, such as flow rate and priming solution. Most studies have noted significant hypofibrinogenemia, which does not seem to be correlated with perfusion time.[154,159–161,169,170] We[169,170,185] and others[154,160] have found that fibrinogen levels are closely correlated with CPB fibrinolysis; however, other investigators report little correlation between hypofibrinogenemia and degree of CPB fibrinolysis.[157,201] Figure 17 depicts correlations among fibrinogen, plasminogen, circulating

POST-BYPASS

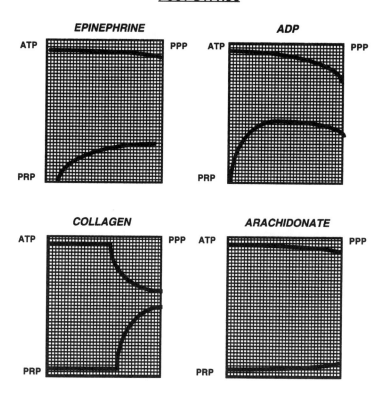

FIGURE 16.   Platelet lumiaggregation patterns *after* cardiopulmonary bypass surgery. PRP = platelet-rich plasma, PPP = platelet-poor plasma, ATP = adenosine triphosphate release.

plasmin, and FDPs during CPB. The dashed lines represent membrane-pumped patients, and the solid lines represent bubble oxygenator-pumped patients.[134,151,174] Some studies have concluded that hypofibrinogenemia is due primarily to DIC during pump surgery;[163,165,166] however, others found no evidence of hypofibrinogenemia during CPB.[202,203] It seems reasonable to conclude that hypofibrinogenemia secondary to hyperfibrinolysis may be a frequent event during CPB. Fibrinolysis occurs in about 85% of patients undergoing bypass surgery. Most studies have also noted other coagulation deficiencies in association with CPB; the deficiencies most commonly reported as playing a role in CPB hemorrhage involve factor II, factor V, and factor VIII:C.[154,157,160,161,163,166] It has been noted that some patients undergoing CPB for valvular heart disease have low levels of factor VIII:vW, high-molecular-weight monomers; levels also may increase during the CPB procedure.[195] Some conclude that such changes are secondary to DIC,[163,173] whereas others attribute them to a primary fibrinolytic syndrome and plasmin-induced degradation of coagulation proteins.[134,139,154,169,170,185] Still others found no significant decrease in most coagulation factors during bypass surgery,[157,202,203] and two authors have reported increased levels of factor VIII:C during perfusion.[202,204]

Disseminated Intravascular Coagulation

The question of DIC during bypass surgery has caused much confusion regarding altered hemostasis both during and after bypass. Many early studies of hemostasis during CPB concluded that DIC occurred.[163,165,166,205,206] However, many such studies monitored

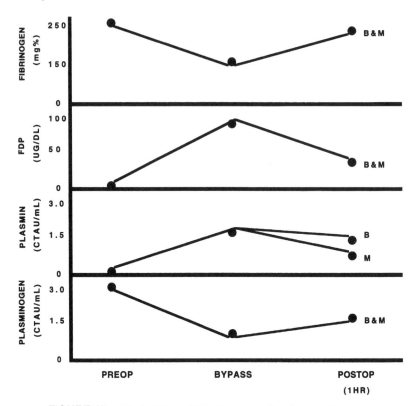

FIGURE 17. Fibrinolytic activity during cardiopulmonary bypass.

only isolated coagulation factors; the measured decreases were empirically ascribed to presumed DIC, because no other explanation was evident. Specifically, the findings of isolated deficiencies in fibrinogen, factor VIII:C,[161,165] or prothrombin complex factor[172] were often assumed, usually erroneously, to be secondary to DIC without confirmatory laboratory testing. Two more recent reports of 9 patients also concluded that DIC accounts for altered hemostasis during CPB.[173,207] The reports concluded that DIC was present after noting that several parameters of hemostasis worsened following heparin reversal with protamine. Specifically, FDP elevation, hypofibrinogenemia, and hypoplasminogenemia appeared to become accentuated after the infusion of protamine. However, our experience[134,135,139,150,169,170] and that of others[154,158,159,162,203,208] have been the opposite; in most patients, hypofibrinogenemia, hypoplasminogenemia, and FDP elevation correct rapidly and uniformly after the administration of protamine sulfate.

These findings suggest that DIC is not generally associated with CPB surgery. DIC during cardiac surgery also seems unlikely in view of massive heparinization and the absence of significant or uniform thrombocytopenia in many studies in which hemostasis appears to be markedly abnormal. Another finding that surely argues against the development of DIC during CPB is the presence of normal or near normal antithrombin (AT) levels.[134,150,154,175] Evidence suggests that decreased AT levels are a good indicator of the development of acute or chronic DIC;[209–212] only one study has shown decreased AT during CPB.[173] All of the 9 patients cited above had low levels of AT III before bypass was started; in addition, the assessment method was quite old and possibly influenced by the presence of FDPs or heparin, making interpretation of the results unclear. Furthermore, if DIC were present in patients undergoing CPB, the intravenous infusion of protamine sulfate would be expected to cause massive precipitation of soluble fibrin monomer and thus to result in extensive micro- or macrovascular occlusion. In the author's experience, only two of several thousand patients have had true DIC in association with CPB.[134,139,151] Both patients developed DIC before CPB, one from cardiac arrest and the other from septicemia. In both cases, bypass surgery was finished without incidence; however, when protamine sulfate was infused, massive vascular occlusion, including carotid and renal artery thrombosis, occurred.

Although most early and several recent studies have detected primary fibrinolysis in association with CPB, a few have concluded that DIC may occur. These conclusions probably result from the marked superficial similarities between primary fibrinolysis and DIC and the usual secondary fibrinolytic response and from the difficulty in making a clear-cut differential diagnosis between the two without sophisticated and complete coagulation studies.

Primary Fibrinolysis

Fibrinolytic activity is generally decreased or inhibited during and after most general surgical procedures.[213–216] However, most studies using a variety of laboratory tests have found increased fibrinolysis during and after CPB surgery.[134,139,151,154,169–171,185,187,193,201,208,217] Many earlier studies of hemostasis during CPB assessed fibrinolysis with euglobulin lysis time, and the finding of fibrinolysis was of unclear significance for a long time.[218,219] More recent studies of CPB hemostasis,[134,150,151,159,169,170,175] which have used more specific methods for assessing fibrinolysis (primarily synthetic substrate assays[211,220–224)] have confirmed earlier reports of a primary fibrino(geno)lytic syndrome in most patients undergoing CPB surgery (see Fig. 17). Because of early reports detecting primary fibrinolysis during CPB, the empirical use of antifibrinolytics, usually epsilon aminocaproic acid (EACA), has become commonplace. Despite attendant hazards, which include hypokalemia, hypotension, ventricular arrhythmias, local or disseminated thromboses, and DIC syndromes,[225,226] many cardiovascular surgeons have often used EACA. Controlled studies with and without antifibrinolytics have failed to show any clear-cut differences in CPB hemorrhage,[154,160,201,227,228] and Gomes and McGoon[208] and Tsuji[203] have shown a definite increase in post-CPB hemorrhage with the empirical use of antifibrinolytics. In fact, the need to use EACA to control CPB hemorrhage is extremely rare;[134,135,139,151] this agent should be used only when clear laboratory evidence of primary fibrinolysis is noted in a severely hemorrhaging CPB patient who does not respond to adequate platelet transfusions.

Several investigators finding primary fibrinolysis during CPB have concluded that it is inconsequential as a cause of postperfusion hemorrhage,[158,160] whereas others have thought that it is triggered only by specific events, such as pyrogenicity of equipment, use of rheomacrodex, or induction of anesthesia.[162,229,230] Because primary fibrinolysis occurs in most patients subjected to CPB surgery, it seems likelier that the fibrinolytic system may be activated in the oxygenation mechanism or that pump-induced accelerated flow rates may activate the plasminogen-plasmin system or alter the activity of endothelial plasminogen activator or inhibitor. Patients undergoing CPB surgery show marked activation of factor XII; about 70% of factor XII is converted to factor XIIa, possibly as a result of complement system activation.[231] The complement system is another potential activation pathway for the initiation of a primary fibrinolytic syndrome. However, the pathogenesis of fibrinolytic activation during CPB is unclear. Although many investigators have noted enhanced fibrinolysis during CPB, a few studies have found only an elevation in fibrinolytic activator activity, with no systemically circulating plasmin.[157,201,205] In addition, a few studies have found no evidence of primary fibrinolysis in association with CPB.[160,161,205,227]

Other Defects in Cardiac Surgery

Heparin rebound, which has received significant attention as a potential cause of CPB hemorrhage,[230,232–235] was observed more often in earlier studies. With the currently accepted doses of heparin and protamine, both heparin rebound and inadequate heparinization are rare.[134,139,151,164,170,173,175] Neither heparin rebound nor inadequate heparin neutralization has been documented as an actual cause of CPB hemorrhage.[134,135,151,164,165] Similarly, protamine excess has occasionally been incriminated as a cause of CPB hemorrhage; however, several studies have failed to note this phenomenon in a single patient undergoing CPB.[139,156,169,170,171,233,236] Furthermore, although protamine sulfate is a well-known in vitro anticoagulant, it is an unlikely cause of clinical hemorrhage.[237]

Several authors have reported that both coagulation defects and significant CPB hemorrhage may be associated with hypothermic perfusion;[160,162,227,230] our experience in comparing normothermic with hypothermic perfusions has led to the same conclusion.[217] Gomes and McGoon[208] and Porter and Silver[159] found no increased incidence of CPB hemorrhage with hypothermic perfusion. Many patients undergoing coronary artery bypass grafting for coronary occlusive disease have been on warfarin-type drugs. Verska and associates noted that although the prothrombin time returns to normal before CPB, patients previously receiving warfarin therapy show more hemorrhage than patients who did not receive warfarin therapy.[227] This observation also applies to general surgery patients. One study[149] noted that increased hemorrhage was associated with repeat bypass procedures; others, however, found no increased hemorrhage in association with a second procedure.[166,208] In addition, patients undergoing CPB for correction of cyanotic heart disease appear to have more severe derangements in hemostasis during perfusion and a stronger propensity to hemorrhage than patients udergoing CPB for noncyanotic heart disease.[158,208] Increased hemorrhagic risk during and after CPB surgery is associated with (1) prior use of warfarin drugs, (2) hypothermic perfusion, (3) surgery for correction of cyanotic heart disease, (4) repeat bypass procedure, (5) long perfusion/aortic cross-clamp times, and (6) preoperative ingestion of drugs interfering with platelet function.[134,135,150,151] Advancing age does not appear to be associated with increased risk of hemorrhage with CPB.[238,239]

Conclusion

Many conclusions regarding altered hemostasis and resultant hemorrhage during CPB surgery are of questionable significance; for example, overheparinization, heparin rebound, inadequate protamine neutralization, and protamine excess, although receiving at least theoretical attention as potential sources of CPB hemorrhage, have not been documented as causes of bleeding associated with bypass surgery. Similarly, thrombocytopenia, almost surely a potential source of hemorrhage, is an inconsistent finding during cardiac bypass surgery. The finding of isolated coagulation defects during CPB has added little, except confusion, to the understanding of altered hemostasis during bypass surgery; such findings probably represent isolated measurements of the results of fibrinolysis and systemically circulating plasmin.

Although some investigators claim that DIC develops during CPB, most carefully done studies have not documented this finding. The significant doses of heparin used during CPB, the absence of consistent thrombocytopenia, and the general correction of hypofibrinogenemia, hypoplasminogenemia, and the elevated levels of FDPs after heparin neutralization suggest that DIC is a rare event during cardiac surgery. DIC may be associated with cardiac surgery in the presence of another triggering event, such as sepsis, shock, massive transfusions, or frank hemolytic transfusion reaction.

Predisposing factors associated with enhanced cardiac surgery hemorrhage are listed in Table 8. Prevailing evidence suggests that most patients undergoing CPB surgery develop a primary fibrinolytic syndrome. Although the exact triggering mechanisms are unclear, the underlying cause may be activation factor XII. In any case, the resultant secondary derangements in hemostasis certainly create a potential for CPB hemorrhage. Furthermore, most patients undergoing CPB develop severe platelet dysfunction. It is unclear whether this defect results from coating of platelet surfaces by FDPs, membrane damage from the oxygenation mechanism, platelet damage from fast flow rates, or other

TABLE 8. Factors Predisposing to Hemorrhage during Cardiopulmonary Bypass

1. Long perfusion times	4. Hypothermic perfusion
2. Prior use of warfarins	5. Preoperative ingestion of antiplatelet drugs
3. Cyanotic heart disease	6. Repeat bypass procedure

unrecognized mechanisms. Whatever the triggering mechanism(s), it is quite clear that the most important alterations in hemostasis associated with CPB surgery are defective platelet function and primary fibrinolysis. These two defects, alone or in combination, certainly account for most nonsurgical and nontechnical hemorrhage in patients undergoing CPB; platelet function defects account for far more hemorrhagic episodes than primary fibrinolysis.

DIAGNOSIS OF HEMORRHAGE ASSOCIATED WITH CARDIOPULMONARY BYPASS

When bleeding occurs during or after bypass, it is extremely important to define the defect as quickly as possible; only in this manner can specific and effective therapy be delivered.[135,139,151,156,240] As mentioned earlier, many instances of CPB hemorrhage are clearly due to inadequate surgical technique, but alterations of hemostasis also may accentuate CPB hemorrhage. This discussion is limited to nontechnical causes of CPB hemorrhage. The types of hemorrhage during CPB are listed in Table 9 in descending order of probability.

The primary distinction to be made is between strictly surgical bleeding, defects in hemostasis, or a combination of the two. This distinction becomes more difficult and more important after the patient has left the operating room; a decision must be made about re-exploration and the adequacy of hemostasis for reexploration. In distinguishing between surgical and nonsurgical bleeding, many physical findings are helpful. For example, is the bleeding localized or systemic? If the patient is already in the recovery room, hematuria in association with petechiae and purpura and oozing from intravenous sites in association with increased chest tube blood loss and oozing from surgical sites (including the sternotomy wound and saphenous vein harvest site) indicate a defect in hemostasis. Increased chest tube blood loss alone, however, often signifies a technical bleeding problem. When the patient is in the operating room, the same findings hold true; the surgeon usually notes bleeding or oozing throughout the surgical field in nontechnical bleeding. Communication between the surgeon and the hematologist or internist is therefore important. Clinical suggestions of a systemic rather than a local cause of CPB hemorrhage are listed in Table 10.

When CPB hemorrhage is seen or suspected, the following laboratory tests are ordered: prothrombin time, activated partial thromboplastin time, complete blood count and platelet count, examination of a peripheral smear, levels of FDPs and D-dimer or prothrombin fragment$_{1+2}$ (PF_{1+2}), heparin assessment by synthetic substrate, thrombin time, and determination of plasminogen/plasmin levels by synthetic substrate methods.[136,150,151,156] Evaluation of the heparin level provides rapid information about the status of heparin and its potential effects on other tests of hemostasis. The resultant clot from the thrombin time

TABLE 9. Hemorrhagic Syndromes Seen with Cardiopulmonary Bypass
(in Descending Order of Frequency)

Severe platelet dysfunction
  Bypass-induced
  Drug-induced

Primary fibrinolytic syndrome

Thrombocytopenia

Hyperheparinemia or rebound??

Disseminated intravascular coagulation (exceedingly rare)

TABLE 10. Clinical Evaluation of Hemorrhage in Patients Undergoing Cardiopulmonary Bypass

Chest tube blood loss only?
or associated with
Petechiae, purpura, or ecchymoses
Hematuria
Oozing from intraarterial line sites
Oozing from intravenous sites
Oozing from venipunctures
Oozing from sternotomy wound
Oozing from saphenous graft vein site
Other systemic bleeding sites
Clots forming in chest tube?

is observed for 5 minutes for evidence of lysis, supplying rapid additional information about the presence or absence of a clinically significant primary fibrino(geno)lytic syndrome. More evidence for or against primary lysis is obtained by noting the levels of FDP and D-dimer/PF_{1+2}.[210,241–243] A peripheral blood smear and platelet count are invaluable to evaluate rapidly the potential for thrombocytopenic bleeding. Plasminogen and plasmin levels obtained by synthetic substrate technique are not time-consuming but are not used for an immediate diagnosis; however, they are invaluable in making later decisions about antifibrinolytic therapy.[136,150,151,156] If significant primary fibrinolysis is present, FDPs will be significantly elevated; levels of D-dimer/PF_{1+2} will be normal or near normal; and hypoplasminogenemia and circulating plasmin will be detected. Levels of B-beta 15–42-related peptides will be elevated but not levels of fibrinopeptide A. Excessive heparin, on the other hand, is indicated by the heparin assay; in addition, the thrombin time will be markedly prolonged. If no significant clot lysis is observed and clot is formed during measurement of the thrombin time, and if FDPs are not significantly elevated, primary fibrinolysis is unlikely. All patients undergoing CPB have a platelet function defect; when bleeding occurs, it is prudent to assume that this defect is present. Although it may not be the primary reason for hemorrhage, platelet dysfunction can be assumed to be additive to any other defect, whether due to surgical technique or altered hemostasis. Therefore, no tests of platelet function need to be done routinely, but platelets are immediately ordered for any patient who demonstrates intra- or post-bypass hemorrhage.[134,135,151] The time when hemorrhage occurs—that is, intraoperatively, after heparin neutralization, or in the recovery room—appears to bear little relationship to the cause of the primary hemostatic defect responsible for hemorrhage. Exceptions are thrombocytopenic bleeding, which usually occurs after the patient is in the recovery room, and a significant drug-induced platelet function defect, which usually manifests as significant oozing immediately after the operative procedure is started. Tests ordered for the differential diagnosis of the cause of hemorrhage during CPB surgery are listed in Table 11.

MANAGEMENT OF HEMORRHAGE ASSOCIATED WITH CARDIOPULMONARY BYPASS

When first encountering a patient with CPB hemorrhage, whether intraoperative or postoperative, it is of prime importance (1) to note the type of bleeding (systemic vs. local) (2) to order an immediate laboratory screen (as outlined earlier), and (3) to administer 6–8 units of platelet concentrates as quickly as possible. Although the use of platelet concentrates is somewhat empirical at this point, it is done for several sound reasons: (1) all patients have a significant platelet function defect, which may be the primary reason for hemorrhage and is the most common cause of a nontechnical bleed, and (2) this defect is likely to accentuate bleeding from any other cause, whether it be a surgical defect or defective hemostasis. The quick administration of platelet concentrates while waiting for

TABLE 11. Laboratory Evaluation of Bypass Hemorrhage*

Platelet count and complete blood count	D-Dimer assay
Peripheral blood smear evaluation	Heparin assay[†]
Prothrombin time	Thrombin time[‡]
Partial thromboplastin time	Plasminogen assay[†]
Fibrin(ogen) degradation products titer	Plasmin assay[†]

* To be ordered immediately.
[†] Synthetic substrate assay.
[‡] Observe for clot lysis for 5 minutes.

laboratory results stops or significantly reduces most instances of nontechnical CPB hemorrhage.[134,135,151] Recently, a fibrin glue in paste or spray form has been applied, with reasonable success, to bleeding sites in patients undergoing CPB hemorrhage; the source of the glue may be autologous or allogeneic.[244-247]

When bleeding begins immediately upon initiation of surgery, a platelet function defect, usually drug-induced, can be assumed to be present until further laboratory investigation can be done. The patient should be given 6–8 units of platelet concentrates as quickly as possible, and the surgical wound should be closed, if feasible. If a platelet function defect is responsible for the hemorrhage (no laboratory evidence of significant fibrinolysis or hyperheparinemia), 6–8 units of platelet concentrates should be repeated the evening after surgery and for 2 postoperative mornings. Thrombocytopenic CPB hemorrhage should be controlled in the same manner, although greater numbers of platelet concentrates may be needed as dictated by the initial platelet count, site and severity of hemorrhage, and response to platelet transfusions. Hyperheparinemia and heparin rebound, if thought to be a real clinical problem as documented by synthetic substrate assays, are managed by delivering 25% of the original calculated dose of protamine sulfate; this dose is repeated every 30–60 minutes until bleeding stops. Hyperheparinemia and heparin rebound are unlikely to be responsible for bleeding and should not be dwelled upon unless concrete laboratory proof of hyperheparinemia is present and evidence of primary fibrinolysis is clearly absent. The author has seen many instances of excessive heparinization resulting from mistakes in calculations and solution preparation; none of these instances was associated with significant cardiac surgical hemorrhage. Similarly, protamine excess is rarely, if ever, a clinical problem; it should not require therapy and should not be dwelled upon at the risk of ignoring other potential defects in hemostasis.

Primary fibrinolysis is common and may or may not be responsible for hemorrhage. This syndrome should not be treated empirically; antifibrinolytic therapy should be considered if the patient has failed to respond to platelet concentrates and there is documented laboratory evidence of primary fibrinolysis, as noted by the presence of hypoplasminogenemia, circulating plasmin, and elevated levels of FDPs. If appropriate testing systems are available, the absence of elevated levels of fibrinopeptide A and D-dimer and the presence of elevated levels of B-beta 15–42-related peptides offer further evidence for primary lysis. Primary fibrino(geno)lytic bleeding is generally treated with EACA, given as an initial dose of 5–10 gm by slow intravenous push, followed by 1–2 gm/hr until bleeding stops or slows to a non–life-threatening level. Because EACA may be associated with ventricular arrhythmias (tachycardia or fibrillation), hypotension, hypokalemia, localized or diffuse thrombosis, and frank DIC, it should be injected slowly and patients should be monitored carefully for cardiac status, renal output, blood pressure, and electrolytes. A newer and more potent antifibrinolytic agent now available is tranexamic acid, which is usually delivered as an intravenous dose of about 3–6 gm/24 hr.[248]

THROMBOHEMORRHAGIC COMPLICATIONS OF PROSTHETIC DEVICES, HEART TRANSPLANTATION, AND OTHER EXTRACORPOREAL CIRCUITS

Exposure of the blood to foreign surfaces is often linked with thrombosis, which provides a major clinical obstacle to the use of prosthetic devices. The use of prosthetic devices and extracorporeal circuits has become commonplace in the management of patients with cardiovascular disease and in common angiographic studies or therapeutic angioplasty.[150,249,250] The hemostatic complications that follow insertion of prosthetic devices include consumption of coagulation factors, other plasma proteins, or platelets; generation of microthrombi of little clinical consequence; and thrombosis or thromboembolism that may give rise to serious, life-threatening, or terminal vasoocclusion. Under normal circumstances, the blood remains fluid because of numerous obvious factors, including a nonthrombogenic endothelial surface; endogenous fibrinolytic activity; natural protease inhibitors such as AT III, protein C, and protein S; and dilution and dispersion of procoagulant components of the blood.[109,251,252] All of these protective mechanisms are lost, to some degree, with the use of prosthetic devices.[135,150,249]

In general, slow flow rates are associated with local thrombotic events, whereas fast flow rates are more commonly associated with a high shear force and embolization.[242] In addition, smooth prosthetic surfaces tend to favor little adhesiveness of a formed thrombus; thus, embolization is more likely to occur with a smooth than with a rough surface, which tends to favor firm fibrin clot formation and eventual neovascularization.[253] When blood is exposed to prosthetic devices or any foreign surface, including extracorporeal circuits, plasma proteins are immediately absorbed, primarily fibrinogen, albumin, alpha and beta globulins, gammaglobulin, factor VIII:C, factor XII, factor XI, and thrombin.[254,255] Factors XII and XI may simply be absorbed or may become activated. Fibrinogen, which appears to be the major plasma protein that is absorbed, promotes subsequent platelet adhesion; platelets adhere as a monolayer and then aggregate. Platelet adhesion is enhanced or induced not only by fibrinogen but also by gammaglobulin, thrombin, and subsequent activation of factors XII and XI.[256] In addition, the activation of factors XII and/or XI may induce intrinsic coagulation, with further fibrin formation generating a platelet-fibrin thrombus. As thrombotic surfaces form and embolize in the above manner, they may eventually overwhelm the ability of the reticuloendothelial system to clear them; thromboembolization with vascular occlusion and subsequent end organ infarction may result.[257]

The most common defects that may occur with prosthetic devices are as follows: (1) frank consumption of coagulation factors and platelets may result in thrombocytopenia and hemorrhage; (2) devices may cause partial platelet degranulation, with subsequent defective platelet function and hemorrhage; (3) in cases of oxygenation/dialysis membranes, fibrin-platelet deposition may render the exchange ineffective and provide a focus for thromboembolus; and (4) micro- or macrothromboemboli of platelets and/or fibrin may give rise to serious clinical vasoocclusive problems.[135,150] The use of anticoagulants, including warfarin-type drugs, heparin, and platelet suppressive agents, tends to normalize thrombotic and thromboembolic complications with prosthetic devices.[135,150] However, the problem still remains clinically significant, especially during CPB surgery, hemodialysis, angiographic studies, prosthetic heart valve placement, long-term intravenous catheterization, use of LeVeen shunts, and implantation of total artificial hearts (TAHs).[135,150]

Arterial and Venous Catheters

Intraarterial or intravenous catheters are coated with fibrin and/or platelet aggregates when used for angiographic studies, therapeutic angioplasty, long-term chemotherapy, infusions of fluids, and long-term parenteral hyperalimentation.[135,150,249,258] Thromboembolism occurs in approximately 2% of individuals catheterized for angiographic studies.[135,150,249,259] An additional complication is that an existing atherosclerotic plaque may be disrupted and embolize. The thromboembolic complications of short-term or long-term catheterization are usually minimized by the use of low dose intravenous heparin or subcutaneous low-molecular-weight (LMW) heparin. In addition to intraarterial catheters, intravenous catheters also may be associated with thrombotic events; however, they are usually associated with localized phlebitis around the introduction site. This complication may occur in as many as 20–30% of patients; only 10% of cases are diagnosed before the intravenous catheter is removed.[260] Phlebitis may be diagnosed at 60–80 hours after starting the intravenous line; it appears to occur later in diabetics and earlier in patients with intravenous catheters for peripheral hyperalimentation.[150,249,260] In addition, the incidence of local phlebitis is inordinately increased in patients who undergo intravenous therapy and have an associated infectious process.[261]

INTRAAORTIC BALLOON PUMP

Intraaortic balloon pumps (IABPs) have been in clinical use since 1968 and are commonly used for control of cardiogenic shock or low-output failure after CPB.[262–264] Common current indications also include (1) acute myocardial infarction with cardiogenic shock that remains unresponsive to immediate medical management; (2) unstable cardiac status after cardiac catheterization, coronary angiography, or coronary angioplasty; (3) impaired left ventricular function; (4) refractory low cardiac output after CPB procedures; and, occasionally, (5) arrhythmias.[262–265]

IABPs are usually constructed of polyurethane and are inserted surgically or percutaneously into the left common femoral artery.[262] The most common complications are (1) leg ischemia from diverse etiologies; (2) local or distal arterial injury or thrombosis; (3) aortic dissection; (4) destruction or activation of numerous blood elements, including red cells, platelets, and coagulation proteins; and (5) infections which are, of course, more common when the percutaneous insertion route is used.[150,266,267] Despite the high frequency of thrombus and thromboembolus formation, no uniform anticoagulation regimen is used with IABPs. Some clinicians advocate the routine use of heparin before, during, and until the point of removal of the balloons;[268] however, others use heparin only in medical patients and prefer aspirin and/or low-molecular-weight dextrans in surgical patients.[150,249,265] Other clinicians use no anticoagulants at all unless there is another underlying indication in addition to balloon assist.[269] Another approach has been to use dextran plus heparin.[264] Although it has been suggested that the routine use of anticoagulants may decrease the incidence of thrombus or thromboembolus,[157,160] no randomized studies confirm this opinion.

Several mechanisms induce thrombus, thromboembolus, and resultant end-organ infarction in patients undergoing intraaortic balloon pumping. Patients often develop thrombi adherent to the aortic intima along the path of the balloon, and emboli may easily develop.[267] Mural thrombi may detach fragments of existing thrombus, denuded endothelium, and/or platelet macroaggregates, which, in turn, may embolize downstream (during systole) or upstream (during diastole) and cause infarction of essentially any end-organ or any other site, including the upper or lower extremities, depending on the direction of embolization and size of the embolus.[267,270] After three days of balloon assist, there is marked denuding of aortic endothelium adjacent to the balloon, followed by the usual platelet hyperactivity with subsequent platelet activation and release of procoagulant and vasoactive materials. This process leads to increased platelet activation, activation of the coagulation system, and increased thrombi, emboli, thromboembolic showers, and vasoconstriction.[133] Embolization frequently affects the upper extremities, lower extremities, central nervous system, kidneys, spleen, superior mesenteric artery, or small bowel.[266,267,270,271] Embolization is noted most frequently in debilitated patients or in patients with severe cardiac failure.

Leg ischemia may develop from local thrombus formation in the aortic or iliofemoral vessels or from emboli.[265–267] Local thrombosis is especially common if the insertion is inadvertently made into the superficial femoral artery.[266] Leg ischemia due to thrombus or thromboembolus is the most frequent early complication of IABPs.[266] It has been suggested, but not proved, that the use of heparin may decrease the incidence of this serious complication.[150,153,249,266] Leg ischemia due to local thrombosis or thromboembolus may be severe enough to give rise to an anterior compartment syndrome that necessitates fasciotomy or even amputation in severe cases.[265] The incidence of leg ischemia secondary to thrombosis or thromboembolus is thought to be related to the time on balloon assist.[266] In addition, the presence of atherosclerosis in the iliofemoral system is another important predisposing factor for vasoocclusion and development of leg ischemia; the use of heparin will obviously not be preventive with this mechanism.[266] The type of balloon also may influence the incidence of thrombus or thromboembolus.[265] Even bilateral renal artery thrombi have been noted in association with IABP.[271] Limb ischemia due to thrombosis or thromboembolus associated with IABPs is common, occurring in up to 36% of patients.[150,249,264,265] Because this complication may lead to serious morbidity or even mortality, careful monitoring and use of anticoagulants, preferably heparin in nonsurgical patients, are mandatory. Evaluation of the dorsalis pedis and posterior tibial pulses, coupled with Doppler ultrasonography of the thigh vessels, should be performed every 4 hours.[265,266] Capillary filling should be assessed every 4 hours.[266] The development of leg ischemia dictates immediate removal of the balloon, if medically possible.

Hemorrhage is another potentially serious complication of IABP. Wound hemorrhage is the most common type; however, retroperitoneal hemorrhage, gastrointestinal bleeding, genitourinary bleeding, central nervous system bleeding, and frank DIC also may occur.[135,150,249,264,266] The most common cause of hemorrhage associated with IABP is thrombocytopenia;[135,264,266] the degree of thrombocytopenia is clearly related to time on the device and may be due to multiple etiologies, including consumption in an aortic mural thrombus or consumption secondary to DIC. The development of DIC also appears to be related to time on the device. Most investigators have noted DIC only in patients undergoing at least 5 days of IABP; however, DIC has also been noted with only 1 day of balloon assist.[270] There are multiple mechanisms by which DIC may develop in patients undergoing IABP. One such mechanism is simply activation of the hemostasis system by massive platelet release; another is consumption due to massive aortic intramural thrombus formation. Intravascular hemolysis may develop, especially if a patient is on the device for more than 2 days;[266] it also may trigger DIC.[272] Balloon-induced hemolytic anemia and thrombocytopenia may be so severe that support with washed packed red cells and platelet concentrates is required.[266] An additional triggering event for DIC is the high incidence of bacteremia, which is most commonly seen in patients receiving the balloon by percutaneous insertion.[266]

IABPs have become a common therapeutic modality for patients with selected indications, including cardiogenic shock and weaning from CPB in the presence of unstable hemodynamics or left ventricular dysfunction. They may be associated with severe thrombotic, thromboembolic, and hemorrhagic problems of multifaceted etiology. In general, careful monitoring of patients, judicious use of anticoagulants, and familiarity with the types of thrombotic or hemorrhagic complications are important preventive strategies.

Vascular Shunts

Surgically created arteriovenous (AV) shunts or prosthetic AV shunts are necessary for hemodialysis patients, frequently transfused patients, patients undergoing long-term parenteral hyperalimentation, patients undergoing long-term chemotherapy, and patients committed to a long-term apheresis program.[273,274] Surgically created AV shunts tend to have fewer thrombotic complications than prosthetic shunts. Although thrombosis of the shunt remains the major significant problem, infection is also of concern. Prosthetic shunts and surgically created shunts are usually declotted by the use of surgery, streptokinase, or urokinase with reasonably good success.[135,275,276] Anticoagulant therapy has not become commonplace for patients with AV shunts; however, it has been shown that dipyridamole corrects decreased platelet survival and increased platelet consumption in patients with AV shunts.[277] Aspirin alone does not decrease the incidence of shunt thrombosis. Prosthetic vascular grafts are primarily constructed of Dacron, which has sufficient porosity to allow neovascularization, thrombus organization, and nutrient blood flow. Thrombotic occlusion of prosthetic grafts is not well controlled with heparin or warfarin-type drugs; currently it is most commonly treated with platelet suppressive therapy.[135,150,249]

Peritoneovenous shunting using a LeVeen or Denver valve has become a palliative procedure for the treatment of intractable ascites associated with severe liver disease and malignancy.[278,279] A generalized hemorrhagic diathesis is frequently seen with the use of LeVeen shunts and appears to represent a straightforward DIC-type syndrome associated with accelerated destruction of fibrinogen and platelet.[58,135,249,280–284] The removal of ascitic fluid at the time of valve implantation and use of anticoagulants have been advocated to abort DIC in patients receiving LeVeen shunts.[58,135] Setting the patient upright often totally aborts or significantly blunts the DIC process; this strategy should be used as a short-term palliative measure in patients developing DIC with LeVeen shunts.[58]

Prosthetic Heart Valves

The use of prosthetic heart valves has become common and has greatly reduced morbidity and mortality in patients with valvular heart disease. However, complications such as thromboembolism, infection, hemolysis, and detachment may significantly alter morbidity and mortality rates.[285] Thromboembolism is the most common complication and can be the most serious; the most likely sites of embolism are the central nervous system, coronary arteries, retinae, and extremities.[286] Early in the history of cardiac valve placement it was discovered that warfarin can decrease but not eliminate the incidence of thromboembolic events associated with mitral and aortic valves.[287] Thromboembolism is much more common with mitral valves than aortic valves, especially if atrial fibrillation or left atrial enlargement is present.[285,287–289] Early mitral valves, which exposed blood to metal, were associated with a 50% incidence of thromboembolism; this rate was reduced to 13% with the use of warfarin.[290] Original aortic valves were associated with a 35% incidence of thromboembolism; this rate was reduced to 8% with the use of warfarin.[291] Valvular thromboemboli arise from platelets; after valve replacement platelets adhere to the foreign surface by adhesion and aggregation.[135,150,249,285,292,293] An additional impetus for platelet aggregation may also come from ADP, which is liberated during red cell hemolysis.[250] Because of this platelet consumption on valvular surfaces, many patients with prosthetic valves demonstrate decreased platelet survival and increased platelet turnover; the decreased survival appears to correlate reasonably well with the incidence of thromboemboli.[294–296] However, patients with rheumatic valve disease without prosthetic valves also demonstrate decreased platelet survival and increased platelet consumption as well as an increased incidence of thromboembolism.[297] Valvular platelet consumption has decreased progressively with new valve design, but still the problem has not been totally alleviated. Platelet deposits and thromboemboli were most pronounced with the early metal valves; the incidence decreased with second-generation cloth-bound valves, which induced neoendothelialization of the valve surface and a hopefully inert valve. Newer xenograft (porcine) valves are associated with an even greater reduction in thromboembolic complications. Despite this improvement, however, there is still a significant incidence of serious thromboembolism in patients with prosthetic aortic or mitral valves, and most are committed to long-term or life-long anticoagulation of some type.

Both dipyridamole and sulfinpyrazone normalize decreased platelet survival in patients with prosthetic valves, but aspirin alone does not have the same effect.[294,298] However, aspirin potentiates the effect of dipyridamole in normalizing platelet survival.[294]

The mechanisms are unclear, because the doses of dipyridamole and sulfinpyrazone that normalize platelet survival are lower than the doses required to alter platelet aggregation in vitro. Sulfinpyrazone also normalizes decreased platelet survival in patients with rheumatic mitral valvular disease who do not have prosthetic valves.[297] Such observations led to interest in antiplatelet drugs for the control of thromboembolism associated with prosthetic heart valves, and numerous clinical trials have proved the efficacy of several agents, including aspirin and dipyridamole.[299-303] One early trial demonstrated a reduction in incidence of thromboemboli from 14% to 1.3% with the addition of dipyridamole to a warfarin regimen.[299] Another early trial revealed that the addition of aspirin to the warfarin regimen decreased the incidence of thromboembolism by 80%.[300] The efficacy of antiplatelet agents alone remains unclear; one trial has found that aspirin plus dipyridamole alone (no warfarin) was effective,[304] but another trial found the same regimen to be ineffective.[305]

Thus, although the role of antiplatelet agents alone remains unclear, an antiplatelet agent may be considered in conjunction with warfarin in some patients with prosthetic valves. At present, there is little uniformity among anticoagulant regimens for patients with prosthetic cardiac valves. It has been suggested that the incidence of thromboembolism decreases with time and that after a given period an anticoagulant is no longer needed in selected patients.[306-308] Another recommendation is to use adequate doses of warfarin (2.5 × control time) plus aspirin or dipyridamole.[293] Yet another recommended regimen is to use warfarin in patients with mitral or double valve replacement but antiplatelet agents alone in patients with aortic valves.[289] Another author suggests a combination of antiplatelet agents alone in patients with prosthetic valves; the recommended regimen is aspirin (330 mg 3 ×/day) and dipyridamole(75 mg 3 ×/day).[295] Probably the safest recommendation is that of Frankl, who suggest that patients with aortic valves should receive adequate doses of aspirin plus dipyridamole and that patients with mitral valve replacement or double valve replacement should be treated with aspirin plus dipyridamole plus warfarin.[285]

Specific anticoagulant recommendations for patients with mechanical or bioprosthetic heart valves were offered by the American College of Chest Physicians in 1995:[309]

1. All patients with mechanical prosthetic heart valves should be anticoagulated with long-term warfarin at a dose appropriate to generate an international normalized ratio (INR) of 2.5–3.5 or higher for caged ball or caged disk valves; the addition of dipyridamole (400 mg/day) or aspirin (80–100 mg/day) may be considered an acceptable option.

2. If patients with a mechanical prosthetic heart valve suffer systemic embolization, dipyridamole (400 mg/day) or aspirin (80–100 mg/day) should be added to the above dose of warfarin.

Specific recommendations for patients with bioprosthetic heart valves are as follows:

1. All patients with bioprosthetic heart valves in the mitral position should be treated for the first 3 months with appropriate warfarin to generate an INR of 2.0–3.0; for patients with bioprosthetic valves in the aortic position who remain in normal sinus rhythm, warfarin therapy may be considered optional.

2. Patients who have a history of systemic embolization; who demonstrated a left atrial thrombus at surgery; or who have atrial fibrillation should be treated with long-term warfarin therapy to generate an INR of 2.0–3.0

3. For patients in regular sinus rhythm, long-term treatment with aspirin (325 mg/day), is optional.

4. Patients with a history of systemic embolization may be considered candidates for long-term oral anticoagulant therapy (3–12 months).

Unfortunately, these recommendations, unlike the first set (which was cosponsored by the National Heart Lung Blood Institute [NHLBI]), are sometimes based on opinion instead of level I, II, or III studies. The most recent consensus conference recommendations were not cosponsored by the NHLBI.

Transplantation of the Total Artificial Heart

Cardiac transplantation has become a routine medical procedure. However, many patients awaiting transplantation die before a human transplant becomes available or develop cardiogenic shock that remains uncontrolled by medication. Because of the number of patients awaiting transplantation, the total artificial heart (TAH) has come into use, usually as a temporizing measure. However, use of the total artificial heart has been associated with numerous complications, the most important of which is thrombus formation followed by cerebral thromboembolization. This complication, thus far, occurs in more than 50% of patients implanted with the TAH while awaiting human allogeneic heart transplant.[150,310] Most studies of both the hemodynamics and the thrombotic and thromboembolic problems with the TAH have been done in animals, with the vast majority performed in calves. Calves, however, do not have quite as high an incidence of cerebrovascular thrombosis as humans, probably because of anatomic species differences. Approximately 30–40% of calves demonstrate cerebral thromboemboli, but a higher percent develop renal emboli.[311] The mechanisms of thrombus and subsequent thromboembolic formation also have been studied primarily in the bovine species. Hartmannova implanted 8 calves and noted that 4 died of thromboembolic disease or hemorrhage.[312] The TAH was made of polymethylacrylate with polyurethane valves. The majority of thromboemboli involved the brainstem, but mesenteric thromboembolic events were also reported. The investigators noted formation of a fibrous capsule with a pseudointima in the TAH, followed by surface thrombi, primarily platelet thrombi. An additional complication was venostasis leading to a "nutmeg liver" or congestive hepatomegaly from less than ideal pump efficiency.

In studying transplanted bovine species, Vasku noted that thromboemboli arose from calcification of indigenous thrombi formed on the artificial surfaces.[313] Thus, the first event appears to be a platelet or fibrin thrombus, most commonly platelet thrombi, which later becomes calcified. The thromboemboli may be calcific, thrombotic, or a combination thereof. Vasku also noted calcification and thromboembolic events in the arteries and veins of the gastrointestinal tract as well as cerebrovascular tissue. Because thromboembolic events did not occur in the first 2–3 months of implantation of the TAH, it was concluded that temporary transplantation may be free of serious thromboembolic events if early allogeneic transplant is possible. It was believed that the development of a nidus of thrombus and subsequently the potential for thromboembolization depended on the biochemistry and physics of the TAH and was related primarily to the carbohydrate content of the coating of the biomaterial and its subsequent stretching and porosity characteristics. Vasku also noted that calcium deposits not only led to micro- and macrothrombi but also decreased driving ability of the TAH and caused mechanical damage to the driving diaphragms.

Of interest, Tolpekin and coworkers[314] implanted the TAH into 25 calves, 16 of which developed thrombi of the valves within 4–6 days, despite anticoagulation with heparin (50 U/kg) and aspirin. After 3 days of this anticoagulant regimen, the calves were changed to warfarin and pentoxifylline (Trental), and it was during this phase that the valves tended to thrombose. The investigators also noted transient thrombocytopenia during the first 24–48 hours in calves receiving a TAH. Of additional interest is that Shumakov et al. implanted 5 calves with a non-Jarvik type device that was specifically designed with an elliptical shape; vigorous anticoagulation with warfarin, aspirin, and dipyridamole (doses not specified) was instituted to keep the prothrombin time and partial thromboplastin time significantly prolonged. None of the 5 calves suffered thrombotic or thromboembolic disease.[315] The authors concluded that this was due to vigorous anticoagulation and "better hemodynamic conditions" created with an elliptical-shaped TAH.

Hughes and others studied two groups of calves receiving a TAH of the Jarvik type. In group I (n = 11) no warfarin was used, but 36% of the calves were placed on combination platelet suppressive therapy with aspirin and dipyridamole. In group II (n = 11), warfarin was used. In animals that received warfarin, the dose was adjusted to give a pro-thrombin ratio of 1.5–3.0 (15–20 seconds). It was noted that calcified thrombi developed in 9 of the 11 calves not receiving warfarin (although 36% received a combination of as-pirin and dipyridamole). However, 7 of the group II animals that were given warfarin developed calcific thrombi of the diaphragm/valvular area. The authors concluded that endogenous biomaterial surface defects led to thrombi, which then usually became calci-fied, providing a source for thromboemboli. They also concluded that the incidence could be moderately reduced with adequate warfarin.[316]

Iwaya and coworkers studied 27 calves with a TAH made of polyurethane and noted that 19% died of thrombi, primarily of the inflow or outflow of valvular tracts.[317] Thrombi of the inflow and outflow tracts led to mechanical failure, which was more commonly noted as a cause of death than thromboembolic disease. Dostal studied 7 calves with a poly-methylacrylate TAH with polyurethane valves; all animals survived for more than 100 days. Vigorous anticoagulation was provided with warfarin plus aspirin plus dipyridamole plus alpha tocopherol. Only 2 of 7 animals died of thromboembolic events, both in the central nervous system. The authors concluded that the warfarin plus combined platelet suppres-sive therapy offers adequate long-term anticoagulation for the implanted TAH.[318]

Human studies with the TAH have been far fewer than animal studies. Of the 7 pa-tients originally implanted with Jarvik-VII TAHs, over 50% developed serious throm-boembolic events to the brain.[150,311] This continues to be a problem with the Jarvik-VII device. Griffith and coinvestigators implanted 6 temporary Jarvik-VII hearts for a total of 52 patient days and noted no clinical thrombotic or thromboembolic events in any patient; when the TAHs were removed for allogeneic human heart transplantation, however, all of them had microscopic deposits of platelet and fibrin thrombi.[319] During the time of Jarvik heart implantation the patients were treated postoperatively with heparin to keep the PTT at 2.0–2.5 times control and with dipyridamole (75 mg every 8 hr). As in calf studies, the authors noted transient thrombocytopenia during the postoperative period, which then abated. Two of the 6 explanted total artificial hearts revealed large, fibrin-rich macro-thrombi; however, these thrombi did not interfere with function of the device and did not embolize. The thrombi were found primarily on the valves and valve housings. None of the 6 patients demonstrated clinical evidence of thrombotic or thromboembolic events, and the authors attributed this outcome to "good fortune," short-term use of the TAH, and vigorous anticoagulation therapy.

As stated above, the first 7 patients implanted with a Jarvik TAH suffered thrombi, emboli, or hemorrhage, most often to the central nervous system. Kolff points out that the decreased incidence of cerebral thromboemboli seen in calves vs. humans with the same Jarvik-VII type device is probably due to CNS vascular anatomic differences because the calves demonstrated a high incidence of renal thromboembolic events.[311] The same investi-gator noted that TAHs with a rough Dacron fibril intima, without quick-disconnect devices, and with tissue valves instead of mechanical valves may be the safest option yet available.

Trubel and coworkers[320] reported 3 patients implanted with a TAH while awaiting allo-geneic heart transplantation. Only 1 of the 3 died of a cerebrovascular thromboembolic event. All 3 patients were anticoagulated with intravenous heparin to keep the thrombin time at 20–30 seconds, and all three were given intravenous aspirin. None of the 3 patients had exces-sive postoperative bleeding, which is commonly seen in most patients receiving TAHs with vigorous postoperative anticoagulation. However, the investigators believed that vigorous anti-coagulation explained the absence of thromboembolic complications in 2 of the 3 patients.

Green and coworkers reported a patient implanted with a Jarvik-VII heart who de-veloped postoperative DIC.[321] The DIC was manifest by an increased level of D-dimer and fibrinopeptide A. Of interest, a 2–3-fold elevation in the level of thromboxane A_2 was also noted during treatment with heparin, warfarin, and enteric-coated aspirin. Elevation of the levels of enteric-coated aspirin was believed to be associated with alleviation of DIC;

however, as the aspirin was tapered, eventually the patient suffered a serious cerebrovascular thrombotic event followed by intracranial hemorrhage due to anticoagulant therapy. Coleman et al. reported a patient who died after sustaining a Jarvik-VII TAH for 112 days.[322] Careful examination at autopsy revealed no evidence of calcification, vegetation, or thrombus formation in the implanted device. Although small platelet thrombi were noted along the suture line in the right atrium, they did not obstruct blood flow or valve function. Microscopic thrombi, however, were found in the pumping diaphragm by scanning electron microscopy. Levinson and coworkers implanted a Jarvik-VII in a patient who was then vigorously anticoagulated with heparin; nonetheless, the patient developed a cerebrovascular thrombotic event on the seventh postoperative day. The patient recovered, however, and subsequently received an allogeneic human heart transplant.[310]

The TAH appears extremely desirable for use in suitable human candidates who are awaiting allogeneic human transplantation, particularly those who develop cardiogenic shock unresponsive to medication. However, vigorous anticoagulation, often consisting of warfarin plus heparin plus platelet suppressive therapy in various forms, has failed to alleviate an extremely high incidence of thrombotic and thromboembolic cerebral disease. In addition, vigorous anticoagulation has been associated with significant postoperative hemorrhage, which, fortunately, is often not fatal. It is hoped that major advances in biomaterials will alleviate the serious problem of thrombogenicity, which remains the rate-limiting factor in use of the TAH.

SUMMARY

This discussion has reviewed the altered hemostasis associated with CPB surgery and selected cardiovascular devices. The key to prevention of CPB hemorrhage is to obtain an adequate preoperative evaluation. An adequate history of hemorrhagic and thrombotic tendencies in both patient and family is important; in addition, a careful history of use of drugs affecting hemostasis, especially drugs known to interfere with platelet function, should be obtained. A careful physical examination, searching for clues to a real or potential bleeding diathesis, also may prevent catastrophic cases of hemorrhage. An adequate presurgical screen must be done in candidates for CPB. In addition, the usual prothrombin time, partial thromboplastin time, platelet count, standardized template bleeding time, and thrombin time should be assessed. These simple testing modalities guard against significant defects in vascular and platelet function. Most instances of nontechnical cardiovascular surgical hemorrhage are due to several well-defined defects in hemostasis that can be easily controlled if approached in a logical manner as a team effort among cardiac surgeons, pathologists, and hematologists.

REFERENCES

1. Muller-Berghaus G: Pathophysiologic and biochemical events in disseminated intravascular coagulation: dysregulation of procoagulant and anticoagulant pathways. Semin Thromb Hemost 15:58, 1989.
2. Ryan TJ: The investigation of vasculitis. In Microvascular Injury. Philadelphia, W.B. Saunders, 1976, p 333.
3. Sheppard B, French JE: Platelet adhesion in the rabbit abdominal aorta following the removal of endothelium: A scanning and transmission electron microscopic study. Proc R Soc 176:427, 1971.
4. Wessler S, Yin ET: On the mechanism of thrombosis. Prog Hematol 4:201, 1969.
5. Friedman RJ, Burns ER: Role of platelets in the proliferative response of the injured artery. Prog Hemost Thromb 4:2498, 1978.
6. Harker LA, Schwartz SM, Ross R: Endothelium and arteriosclerosis. Thromb Clin Haematol 10:283, 1981.
7. Roberts WC, Ferrans VJ: The role of thrombosis in the etiology of atherosclerosis (a positive one) and in precipitating fatal ischemic heart disease (a negative one). Semin Thromb Hemost 2:123, 1976.
8. Sinzinger H: Role of platelets in atherosclerosis. Semin Thromb Hemost 12:124, 1986.
9. Henry RL: Platelet function in hemostasis. In Murano G, Bick RL (eds): Basic Concepts of Hemostasis and Thrombosis. Boca Raton, FL, CRC Press, 1980, p 17.
10. Triplett DA: The platelet: A review. In Triplett DA (ed): Platelet Function. Chicago, ASCP Press, 1978, p 1.
11. Astrup T: Fibrinolysis: An overview. In Davidson JF, Rowan RM, Samama, MM, Desnoyers PE (eds): Progress in Chemical Fibrinolysis, vol. 3. New York, Raven Press, 1978, p 1.
12. Kwaan HC: The role of fibrinolysis in disease states. Semin Thromb Hemost 10:71, 1984.

13. Mammen EF: Inhibitor abnormalities. Semin Thromb Hemost 9:42, 1983.
14. Ruggeri ZM, Zimmerman TS: Von Willebrand factor and von Willebrand disease. Blood 70:895, 1987.
15. White GC, Shoemaker CB. Factor VIII gene and hemophilia. Blood 73:1, 1989.
16. Walsh P: The effect of collagen and kaolin on the intrinsic coagulation activity of platelets. Evidence for an alternative pathway in intrinsic coagulation not requiring factor XII. Br J Haematol 22:393, 1972.
17. Wilner GD, Nossel HL, LeRoy EL: Activation of Hageman factor by collagen. J Clin Invest 47:2608, 1968.
18. Ginbrane MA: Vascular Endothelium in Hemostasis and Thrombosis. London, Churchill Livingstone, 1986, p 250.
19. Leonard EF, Turitto VT, Vroman L: Blood in contact with natural and artifical surfaces. Ann N Y Acad Sci 516:688, 1987.
20. Ruggeri ZM, Fulcher CA, Ware J: Progress in vascular biology, hemostasis and thrombosis. Ann N Y Acad Sci 614: 311, 1991.
21. Stern DM, Nawroth PP: Vessel wall. Semin Thromb Hemost. 13:39–536, 1987.
22. Ulutin ON, et al: Modulation of endothelium and control of vascular and thrombotic disorders. Semin Thromb Hemost (Suppl) 14:114, 1988.
23. Droller MJ: Ultrastructure of the platelet release reaction in response to various aggregating agents and their inhibitors. Lab Invest 29:595, 1973.
24. Stuart MJ: Inherited defects of platelet function. Semin Hematol 12:233, 1975.
25. White JG: Identification of platelet secretion in the electron microscope. Ser Haematol 6:429, 1973.
26. Nachman RL: Platelet proteins. Semin Hematol 5:18, 1968.
27. Day NJ, Stormorken, Holmsen H: Subcellular localization of platelet factor 3 and platelet factor 4. Proceedings of the 12th Congress of the International Society of Hematology, Mexico City, 1968, p 172.
28. Packham MA, Mustard JF: Platelet reactions. Semin Hematol 8:30, 1971.
29. Thomas DP, Niewiarowski S, Ream VJ: Release of adenosine nucleotides and platelet factor 4 from platelets of man and four other species. J Lab Clin Med 75:607, 1970.
30. Born GVR, Cross MJ: The aggregation of blood platelets. J Physiol 168:178,1963.
31. Zucker MB, Peterson J: Serotonin, platelet factor 3 activity and platelet aggregating agent released by adenosine diphosphate. Blood 30:556, 1967.
32. Davis RB, Mecker WR, Bailey WL: Serotonin release after injection of *E. coli* endotoxin in the rabbit. Fed Proc 20:261, 1961.
33. Des Prez RM, Horowitz HI, Hoo EW: Effects of bacterial endotoxin on rabbit platelets. I: Platelet aggregation and release of platelet factors in vitro. J Exp Med 114:857, 1961.
34. Mueller-Eckhardt C, Luscher EF: Immune reactions of human blood platelets. I: A comparative study on the effects on platelets of heterologous antiplatelet antiserum, antigen-antibody complexes, aggregation gamma-globulin, and thrombin. Throm Diath Haemorrh 20:155, 1968.
35. Pfueller SL, Luscher F: The effects of immune complexes on blood and their relationship to complement activation. Immunochem 9:1151, 1972.
36. Haslam RJ: Interactions of the pharmacological receptors of blood platelets with adenylate cyclase. Ser Haematol 6:333, 1973.
37. Salzman EW: Cyclic AMP and platelet function. N Engl J Med 286:358, 1972.
38. Cole B, Robison GA, Hartman RC: Effects of prostaglandin E and theophylline on aggregation and cyclic AMP levels of human blood platelets. Fed Proc 29:316,1970.
39. Horlington M, Watson PA: Inhibition of 3'-5'-cyclic-AMP, phosphodiesterase by some platelet aggregation inhibitors. Biochem Pharmacol 19:955, 1970.
40. Gerrard JM, White JG: Prostaglandins and thromboxanes: "Middlemen" modulating platelet function in hemostasis and thrombosis. Prog Hemostas Thromb 4:87, 1978.
41. Gryglewski RJ, Bunting S, Moncada S, Flower RJ, Vane JR: Arterial walls are protected against deposition of platelet thrombi by a substance (prostaglandin X) which they make from prostaglandin endoperoxides. Prostaglandins 12:685, 1976.
42. Moncada S, Gryglewski R, Bunting S, Vane JR: A lipid peroxide inhibits the enzyme in blood vessel microsomes that generate from prostaglandin endoperoxides the substance (prostaglandin x) which prevents platelet aggregation. Prostaglandins 12:715, 1976.
43. Turpie AGG: Antiplatelet therapy. Thromb Clin Haematol 10:497, 1981.
44. Berndt MC, Caen JP: Platelet glycoproteins. Prog Hemost Thromb 7:111, 1984.
45. Davies GE and Palek J: Platelet protein organization: Analysis by treatment with membrane-permeable cross-linking reagents. Blood 59:502, 1982.
46. Lusher JM, et al.: Factor VIII/VWF and platelet formation and function in health and disease. Ann N Y Acad Sci 509:223, l987.
47. Berndt MC, Gregory C, Chong BH: Additional glycoprotein defects in Bernard-Soulier syndrome: Confirmation of genetic basis of parental analysis. Blood 62:800, 1983.
48. Clemetson KJ, McGregor JL, James E: Characterization of the platelet membrane glycoprotein abnormalities in Bernard-Soulier syndrome and comparison with normal by surface-labeled techniques and high-resolution two-dimensional gel electrophoresis. J Clin Invest 70:304, 1982.

49. Meyer D, Baumgartner HR: Role of von Willebrand factor in platelet adhesion to the subendothelium. Br J Haematol 54:1, 1983.
50. Kunicki TJ, Russell N, Nurden AT: Further studies of the human platelet receptor for quinine and quinidine-dependent antibodies. J Immunol 26:398, 1981.
51. Berendt MC, Phillips DR: Interaction of thrombin with platelets. Purification of the thrombin substrate. Ann N Y Acad Sci 370:87, 1981.
52. Gogstad GO, Hagen J, Korsmo R: Characterization of the proteins of isolated human platelet alpha granules, evidence for a separate alpha granule pool of the glycoproteins IIb and IIIa. Biochem Biophys Acta 670:150, 1981.
53. Fujimura K, Phillips DR: Binding of Ca++ to glycoprotein IIb from human platelet plasma membranes. Thromb Haemost 50:251, 1983.
54. McMillan R, Mason D, Tani P: Evaluation of platelet surface antigens: localization of the pla-1 alloantigen. Br J Haematol, 51:297, 1981
55. White JG: Inherited disorders of the platelet membrane and secretory granules. Human Pathol 18:123, 1987.
56. Lawler J, Hynes RO: Structural organization of the thrombospondin molecule. Semin Thromb Hemost 13:245, 1987.
57. Santoro SA: Thrombospondin and the adhesive behavior of platelets. Semin Thromb Hemost 13:290, 1987.
58. Bick, RL: Disseminated intravascular coagulation and related syndromes: A clinical review. Semin Thromb Hemost 14:299, 1988.
59. McKusick VA: Mendelian Inheritance in Man: Catalogs of Autosomal Dominant, Autosomal Recessive and X-linked Phenotypes, 9th ed. Baltimore, Johns Hopkins University Press, 1990.
60. Kaplan AP: Initiation of the intrinsic coagulation and fibrinolytic pathways of man: The role of surfaces, Hageman factor, prekallikrein, high molecular weight kininogen, and factor XI. Prog Hemost Thromb 4:127, 1978.
61. Kaplan AJ, Meier HL, Mandle R: The Hageman factor dependent pathways of coagulation, fibrinolysis, and kinin-generation. Semin Thromb Hemost 3:1,1976.
62. Griffin JH, Cochrane CG: Recent advances in the understanding of contact activation reactions. Semin Thromb Hemost 5:254, 1979.
63. Manuhalter CH: Contact phase coagulation disorders. Semin Thromb Hemost 13:130, 1987.
64. Irwin JF, Seegers WH, Andary JTJ, Fekete LF, Novoa E: Blood coagulation as a cybernetic system: Control of autoprothrombin C (Xa) formation. Thromb Res 6:431, 1975.
65. Jesty J, Maynard JR, Radcliffe RD, et al: Initiation and control of the extrinsic pathway of coagulation. In Reich E, Rifkin DB, Shaw E (eds): Proteases and Biological Control. Cold Spring Harbor, NY, Cold Spring Harbor Labs, 1975, p 171.
66. Silverberg AS, Nemerson Y, Zur M: Kinetics of the activation of bovine factor XII by components of the extrinsic pathway. J Biol Chem 252:8481, 1977.
67. Chabbat J, Porte P, Tellier M, Steinbuch M: Aprotinin is a competetive inhibitor of the factor VIIa–tissue factor complex. Thromb Res 71:205, 1993
68. Seegers WH: Prothrombin complex. Semin Thromb Hemost 7:291, 1981.
69. Stenflo J: Vitamin K, prothrombin, and gamma-carboxy-glutamic acid. N Engl J Med 296:624, 1977.
70. Denson KWE: The levels of factor II, VII, IX, and X by antibody neutralization techniques in the plasma of patients receiving phenindione therapy. Br J Haematol 20:643, 1971.
71. Mackie MJ, Douglas AS: Drug induced disorders of coagulation. In Ratnoff OD, Forbes CD (eds): Disorders of Hemostasis. Philadelphia, W.B. Saunders, 1991, p 493.
72. Walz, DA, Fenton JW, Shuman MA: Bioregulatory functions of thrombin. Ann N Y Acad Sci 485: 1–450, 1986.
73. Fenton JW, ed: Thrombin and hemostasis. Semin Thromb Hemost 19:321–424, 1993.
74. Mosesson MW, Doolittle RF: Molecular biology of fibrinogen and fibrin. Ann N Y Acad Sci 408:1–672, 1983.
75. Alami SY, Hampton JW, Race GH, Speer, RJ: Fibrin stabilizing factor (factor XIII). Am J Med 44:1, 1968.
76. Ratnoff OD: The molecular basis of hereditary clotting disorders. Prog Hemost Thromb 1:39, 1972.
77. Aoki N, Harpel PC: Inhibitors of the fibrinolytic enzyme system. Semin Thromb Hemost 10:24, 1984.
78. Wiman B, Hamsten A: The fibrinolytic enzyme system and its role in the etiology of thromboembolic disease. Semin Thromb Hemost 16:207, 1990.
79. Castellino FJ: Biochemistry of human plasminogen. Semin Thromb Hemost 10:18, 1984.
80. Aoki N: Fibrinolysis. Semin Thromb Hemost 10:107, 1984.
81. Ratnoff OD, Naff GB: The conversion of C'1s to C'1 esterase by plasmin and trypsin. J Exp Med 125:337, 1967.
82. Robbins KM: Present status of the fibrinolytic system. In Fareed J, Messmore HL, Fenton J, Brinkhous KM (eds): Perspectives in Hemostasis. New York, Pergamon Press, 1980 p 53.
83. Bachmann F, Kruithof KO: Tissue plasminogen activator: Chemical and physiological aspects. Semin Thromb Hemost 10:6, 1984.
84. Goldsmith GN, Saito H, Ratnoff OD: The activation of plasminogen by Hageman factor (factor XII) and Hageman factor fragments. J Clin Invest 21:54, 1978.

85. Kaplan AP, Austin F: The fibrinolytic pathway of human plasma. Isolation and characterization of the plasminogen proactivator. J Exp Med 135:1378, 1972.
86. Stump DC, Taylor FB, Neshein ME: Pathologic fibrinolysis as a cause of clinical bleeding. Semin Throm Hemost 16:260, 1990.
87. Schreiber AD: Plasma inhibitors of the Hageman factor dependent pathways. Semin Thromb Hemost 3:43, 1976.
88. Astedt, B, Lecander I, Ny T: The placental type plasminogen activator inhibitor: PAI-2. Fibrinolysis 1:203, 1987.
89. Loskutoff DJ, Sawdey M, Mimuro J: Type 1 plasminogen activator inhibitor. Prog Hemost Thromb 9:87, 1989.
90. Emeis JJ, Brommer EJP, Kluft C: Progress in fibrinolysis. In Poller L (ed): Recent Advances in Blood Coagulation. Edinburgh, Churchill Livingstone, 1985, p 11.
91. Yee JA, Yan L, Dominguez JC, et al: Plasminogen-dependent activation of latent transforming growth factor beta (TGF-beta) by growing cultures of osteoblast-like cells. J Cell Physiol 157:528, 1993.
92. Marder VJ: Molecular Aspects of Fibrin Formation and Dissolution. Semin Thromb Hemost 8:74, 1982.
93. Marder VJ, Shulman NR: High molecular weight derivatives of human fibrinogen produced by plasmin: Mechanism of their anticoagulant activity. J Biol Chem 244:2120, 1969.
94. Rosse WF: Complement. In Williams WJ, Beutler E, Erslev AJ, Rundles RW (eds): Hematology. New York, McGraw-Hill, 1977, p 87.
95. Ruddy S, Gigli I, Austen KF: The complement system in man. I: Activation, control, and products of the reaction sequences. N Engl J Med 278:489, 1972.
96. Gotze O: Proteases of the properdin system. In Reich E, Rifkin DB, Shaw E (eds): Proteases and Biological Control. Cold Spring Harbor, NY, Cold Spring Harbor Symposium, 1975, p 255.
97. Muller-Eberhard HJ: Complement. Annu Rev Biochem 44:667, 1975.
98. Pillomer L, Blum L, Lepow IH: The properdin system and immunity. I: Demonstration and isolation of a new serum protein, properdin, and its role in immune phenomena. Science 120:279, 1954.
99. Wachtfogel Y, Kucich U, Hack R, et al: Aprotinin inhibits the contact, neutrophil, and platelet activation systems during simulated extracorporeal circulation. J Thorac Cardiovasc Surg 106:1, 1993
100. Bennett B, Ogston D: Role of complement, coagulation, fibrinolysis, and kinins in normal haemostasis and disease. In Bloom AL, Thomas DP (eds): Haemostasis and Thrombosis. London, Churchill Livingstone, London, 1981, p 236.
101. Ryan JW, Ryan US: Biochemical and morphological aspects of the actions and metabolism of kinins. In Pisano JJ, Austen KF (eds): Chemistry and Biology of the Kallikrein-Kinin System in Health and Disease. DHEW Publ No. 76-791. Bethesda, MD, U.S. Department of Health, Education, and Welfare, 1974, p 315.
102. Van Arman CG, Bohidar HR: Role of the kallikrein-kinin system in inflammation. In Pisano JJ, Austin KF (eds): Chemistry and Biology of the Kallekrein-Kinin System in Health and Disease. Bethesda, MD, DHEW Publ No. 76-791, US Department of Health, Education and Welfare, 1974, p 471.
103. Swies J, Chopicki S, Gryglewski RJ: Kinins and thrombolysis. J Physiol Pharmacol 44:171, 1993
104. Comp PC: Hereditary disorders predisposing to thrombosis. Prog Hemostas Thromb 8:71, 1986.
105. Joist JH: Hypercoagulability: Introduction and perspective. Semin Thromb Hemost 16:151, 1990.
106. Esmon CT: Protein-C. Semin Thromb Hemost 10:109–172, 1984
107. Dalbach B, Carlsson M, Svensson PJ: Familial thrombophilia due to a previously unrecognized mechanism characterized by poor anticoagulant response to activated protein C: Prediction of a cofactor to activated protein C. Proc Nat Acad Sci, USA 90:1004, 1994.
108. Taby O, Chabbat J, Steinbuch M: Inhibition of activated Protein C by aprotinin and the use of the insolubilized inhibitor for its purification. Thromb Res 59:27, 1990
109. Bick RL: Clinical relevance of antithrombin III. Semin Thromb Hemost 8:276,1982.
110. Jaques LB, McDuffie NM: The chemical and anticoagulant nature of heparin. Semin Thromb Hemost 4:277, 1978.
111. Rosenberg RD: The effect of heparin on factor XIa and plasmin. Thromb Diath Haemorrh 33:51, 1975.
112. Rosenberg RD, Damus P: The purification and mechanism of action of human antithrombin-heparin cofactor. J Biol Chem 248:6490, 1973.
113. Seegers WH: Antithrombin III. Semin Thromb Hemost 7:263, 1981.
114. Bick RL: The clinical significance of fibrinogen degradation products. Semin Thromb Hemost 8:302, 1982.
115. Moseson MW: Cold-insoluble globulin: A circulating cell surface protein. Thromb Haemost 38:742, 1977.
116. Pearlstein E, Gold LI, Garcia-Pardo A: Fibronectin: A review of its structure and biological activity. Molec Cell Biochem 29:103, 1980.
117. Couchman JR, Austria MR, Woods A: Fibronectin-cell interactions. J Invest Dermatol 94:7, 1990.
118. Moser DF: Fibronectin. Prog Hemost Thromb 5:111, 1980.
119. Moser DF, Schad PE, Kleinman HK: Cross-linking of fibronectin to collagen by blood coagulation factor XIIIa. J Clin Invest 64:781, 1979.
120. Moseson MW, Umfleet RA: The cold-insoluble globulin of plasma. J Biol Chem 254:5728, 1970.
121. Wagner DD, Hynes RO: Domain structure of fibronectin and its relationship to function. J Biol Chem 254:6746, 1979.
122. Wight TN: Vessel proteoglycans and thrombogenesis. Prog Hemost Thromb 5:1, 1980.
123. Ofusu FA, Danishefsky I, Hirsh J: Heparin and related polysaccharides. Ann N Y Acad Sci 556:1–501, 1989.

124. Goldstein IM, Perez HD: Biologically active peptides derived from the fifth component of complement. Prog Hemost Thromb 5:41, 1980.
125. Galloway MJ, Mackie MJ, McVerry BA: Combinations of increased thrombin, plasmin, and non-specific protease activity in patients with acute leukemia. Haemost 13:322, 1983.
126. Lisiewicz J: Disseminated intravascular coagulation in acute leukemia. Semin Thromb Hemost 14:339, 1988.
127. Bick RL: Assessment of patients with hemorrhage. In Disorders of Thrombosis and Hemostasis: Clinical and Laboratory Practice. ASCP Press, 1992, p 27.
128. Taylor KM: Effect of aprotinin on blood loss and blood use after cardiopulmonary bypass. In Pifarre R (ed): Anticoagulation, Hemostasis, and Blood Conservation in Cardiovascular Surgery. Philadelphia, Hanley & Belfus, 1993 p 129.
129. Orchard MA, Goodchield CS, Prentice CR, et al: Aprotinin reduces cardiopulmonary bypass-induced blood loss and inhibits fibrinolysis without influencing platelets. Br J Haematol 85:533, 1993.
130. Schonberger JP, Bredee JJ, van Oeveren W, et al: Preoperative therapy of low-dose aspirin in internal mammary bypass operations with and without aprotinin. J Thorac Cardiovasc Surg 106:262, 1993
131. Hardy JF, Desroches J, Belisle S, et al: Low-dose aprotinin infusion is not clinically useful to reduce bleeding and transfusion of homologous blood products in high-risk cardiac surgical patients. Can J Anaesth 40:625, 1993.
132. Royston D: Controversies in the practical use of aprotinin. In Pifarre R (ed): Anticoagulation, Hemostasis, and Blood Conservation in Cardiovascular Surgery. Philadelphia, Hanley & Belfus, 1993, p 147.
133. Bick RL, Tse N: Hemostasis abnormalities associated with prosthetic devices and organ transplantation. Lab Med 23:462–486, 1992
134. Bick RL: Hemostasis Defects with Cardiac Surgery, General Surgery, and Prosthetic Devices. In Disorders of Thrombosis and Hemostasis: Clinical and Laboratory Practice. Chicago, ASCP Press, 1992, p 195.
135. Bick RL: Hemostasis defects in general surgery, cardiac surgery, transplantation, and the use of prosthetic devices. In Disorders of Hemostasis and Thrombosis: Principles of Clinical Practice. New York, Thieme, 1985, p 223.
136. Mielke CH, Kaneshiro MM, Maher LA, et al: The standardized normal Ivy bleeding time and its prolongation by aspirin. Blood 34:204, 1969.
137. Bick RL: Platelet defects. In Disorders of Hemostasis and Thrombosis: Principles of Clinical Practice. New York, Thieme, 1985, p 65.
138. Bick RL, Murano G: Primary hyperfibrino(geno)lytic syndromes. In Murano G, Bick RL (eds): Basic Concepts of Hemostasis and Thrombosis. Boca Raton, FL, CRC Press, 1980, p 181.
139. Bick RL: Syndromes associated with hyperfibrino(geno)lysis. In Disseminated Intravascular Coagulation. Boca Raton, FL, CRC Press, 1983, p 105.
140. Shahian DM, Wallach SR, Bern MM: Open heart surgery in patients with cold-reactive proteins. Surg Clin North Am 65:315, 1985.
141. Landymore R, Isom W, Barlam B: Management of patients with cold agglutinins who require open-heart surgery. Can J Surg 26:79, 1983.
142. Guena L, Kwabena KA, Addei A: Intraoperative hypothermia in a patient with cold agglutinin disease. JAMA 74:691, 1982.
143. Klein HG, Faltz LL, McIntosh CL, et al: Surgical hypothermia in a patient with a cold agglutinin. Transfusion 20:354, 1980.
144. Leach AB, Van Hasselt GL, Edwards JC: Cold agglutinins and deep hypothermia. Anaesthesia 38:140, 1983.
145. Moore RA, Geller EA, Mathews ES, et al: The effect of hypothermic cardiopulmonary bypass on patients with low-titer, non-specific cold agglutinins. Ann Thorac Surg 37:233, 1984.
146. Brecker G, Cronkite EP: Morphology and enumeration of human blood platelets. J Appl Physiol 3:365, 1950.
147. Hougie C: Fundamentals of Blood Coagulation in Clinical Medicine. McGraw-Hill, New York, p 241, 1963.
148. Proctor RR, Rapaport SI: The partial thromboplastin time with kaolin. A simple screening test for first stage plasma clotting factor deficiencies. Am J Clin Pathol 36:212, 1961.
149. Quick AJ, Stanley-Brown M, Bancroft FW: A study of the coagulation defect in hemophilia and in jaundice. Am J Med Sci 190:501, 1935.
150. Bick RL: Alterations of hemostasis associated with surgery, cardiopulmonary bypass surgery, prosthetic devices and transplantation. In Ratnoff OD, Frobes CD: Disorders of Hemostasis, 2nd ed. Philadelphia, W.B. Saunders, 1991, p 382.
151. Bick RL: Hemostasis defects associated with cardiac surgery, prosthetic devices, and other extracorporeal circuits. Semin Thromb Hemost 11:249, 1985.
152. Beall C, Yow EM, Blodwell RD, et al: Open heart surgery without blood transfusion. Arch Surg 94:567, 1967.
153. Cordell AR: Hematological complications of extracorporeal circulation. In Cordell AR, Ellison RG (eds): Complications of Intrathoracic Surgery. Boston, Little, Brown, p 27, 1979.
154. Mammen EF: Natural proteinase inhibitors in extracorporeal circulation. Ann N Y Acad Sci 146:754, 1968.
155. Koets MH, Washington BC, Wolk LW, et al: Hemostasis changes during cardiovascular bypass surgery. Semin Thromb Hemost 11:281, 1985.

156. Bick RL: Pathophysiology of Hemostasis and Thrombosis. In Sodeman's Pathologic Physiology: Mechanisms of Disease, 7th ed. Philadelphia, W.B. Saunders, 1985, p 705.

157. Kevy SV, Glickman RM, Bernhard WF, et al: The pathogenesis and control of the hemorrhagic defect in open-heart surgery. Surg Gynecol Obstet 123:313, 1966.

158. Signori EE, Penner JA, Kahn DR: Coagulation defects and bleeding in open heart surgery. Ann Thorac Surg 8:521, 1969.

159. Porter JM, Silver D: Alterations in fibrinolysis and coagulation associated with cardiopulmonary bypass. J Thorac Cardiovasc Surg 56:869, 1968.

160. Tice DA, Worth MH: Recognition and treatment of postoperative bleeding associated with open heart surgery. Ann NY Acad Sci 146:745, 1968.

161. Wright TA, Darte J, Mustard WT: Postoperative bleeding after extracorporeal circulation. Can J Surg 2:142, 1959.

162. von Kaulla KN, Swan H: Clotting deviations in man during cardiac bypass: fibrinolysis and circulating anticoagulants. J Thorac Surg 36:519, 1958.

163. Blomback M, Noren I, Senning A: Coagulation disturbances during extracorporeal circulation and the postoperative period. Acta Chir Scand 127:433, 1964.

164. Deiter RA, Neville WE, Piffare R, Jasuja M: Preoperative coagulation profiles and posthemodilution cardiopulmonary bypass hemorrhage. Am J Surg 121:689, 1971.

165. Penick GD, Averette HE, Peters RM, Brinkhous KM: The hemorrhagic syndrome complicating extracorporeal shunting of blood: An experimental study of its pathogenesis. Thromb Diath Haemorh 2:218, 1958.

166. Trimble AS, Herst R, Grady M, Crookston J: Blood loss in open heart surgery. Arch Surg 93:323, 1966.

167. Bick RL, Arbegast NR, Holtermann N, et al: Platelet function abnormalities in cardiopulmonary bypass. Circulation 50(Suppl):301, 1974.

168. Bick RL, Schmalhorst WR, Crawford L, et al: The hemorrhagic diathesis created by cardiopulmonary bypass. Am J Clin Path 63:588, 1975.

169. Bick R.L, Arbegast N R, Crawford L, et al: Hemostatic defects induced by cardiopulmonary bypass. Vasc Surg 9:228, 1975.

170. Bick RL, Schmalhorst WR, Arbegast NR: Alterations of hemostasis associated with cardiopulmonary bypass. Am J Clin Pathol 63:588, 1975.

171. Castenada AR: Must heparin be neutralized following open heart operations? J Thorac Cardiovasc Surg 52:716, 1966.

172. deVries SI, von Creveld S, Green P, et al: Studies on the coagulation of the blood in patients treated with extracorporeal circulation. Thromb Diath Haemorrh 5:426, 1961.

173. Muller N, Popov-Cenic S, Buttner W, et al: Studies of fibrinolytic and coagulation factors during open-heart surgery. II: Postoperative bleeding tendencies and changes in the coagulation system. Thromb Res 7:589, 1975.

174. Bick RL: Alterations of hemostasis during cardiopulmonary bypass: A comparison between membrane and bubble oxygenators. Am J Clin Path 73:300, 1980.

175. Bick RL, Schmalhorst SW, Arbegast NR: Alterations of hemostasis associated with cardiopulmonary bypass. Thromb Res 8:285, 1976.

176. Holswade GR, Nachman RL, Killip T: Thrombocytopathies in patients with open-heart surgery. Preoperative treatment with corticosteroids. Arch Surg 94:365, 1967.

177. Salzman W.E. Blood platelets and extracorporeaal circulation. Transfusion 3:274, 1963.

178. Bick RL, Adams T, Schmalhorst WR: Bleeding times, platelet adhesion, and aspirin. Am J Clin Pathol 65:69, 1976.

179. Bowie EJW, Owen CA, Thompson JH: Platelet adhesiveness in von Willebrand's disease. Am J Clin Pathol 52:69, 1969.

180. Bowie EJW, Owen CA: The value of measuring platelet adhesiveness in the diagnosis of bleeding diseases. Am J Clin Pathol 60:302, 1973.

181. Hirsh J: Laboratory diagnosis of thrombosis. In Coleman RW, Hirsh J, Marder VJ, Salzman EW (eds): Basic Principles and Clinical Practice. Philadelphia, J.B. Lippincott, 1982, p 789.

182. Zimmerman TS, Meyer D: Factor VIII-von Willebrand factor and the molecular basis of von Willebrand's disease. In Coleman RW, Hirsh J, Marder VJ, Salzman EW (eds): Hemostasis and Thrombosis: Basic Principles and Clinical Practice. Philadelphia, J.B. Lippincott, 1982, p 54.

183. Adams T, Schutz L, Goldberg L: Platelet function abnormalities in the myeloproliferative disorders. Scand J Haematol 13:215, 1975.

184. Mustard JF, Packham MA: Factors influencing platelet function: Adhesion, release, and aggregation. Pharmacol Rev 23:97, 1970.

185. Bick RL: The clinical significance of fibrinogen degradation products. Semin Thromb Hemost 8:302, 1982.

186. Sarin CL, Yalav E, Clement AJ, Braimbridge MV: Thrombo-embolism after Starr valve replacement. Br Heart J 33:111, 1971.

187. Hellem AJ: The advances of human blood platelets in vitro. Scand J Clin Lab Invest 51(Suppl):1, 1960.

188. Bick RL, Fekete LF: Cardiopulmonary bypass hemorrhage: Aggrevation by pre-op ingestion of antiplatelet agents. Vasc Surg 13:277, 1979.

189. Kowalski E, Kopec M, Wegrzynowicz Z: Influence of fibrinogen degradation products (FDP) on platelet aggregation, adhesiveness, and viscous metamorphosis. Thromb Diath Haemorrh 10:406, 1963.
190. Kowalski E. Fibrinogen derivatives and their biologic activities. Semin Hematol 5:45, 1968.
191. Harker LA, Malpass TW, Branson HE, et al: Mechanisms of abnormal bleeding in patients undergoing cardiopulmonary bypass: Acquired transient platelet dysfunction associated with selective alpha-granule release. Blood 56:824, 1980.
192. Stass S, Bishop C, Fosberg R, et al: Platelets as affected by cardiopulmonary bypass [abstract]. Trans Am Soc Clin Pathol 35, 1976.
193. Saunders CR, Carlisle L, Bick RL: Hydroxyethyl starch versus albumin in cardiopulmnary bypass prime solutions. Ann Thorac Surg 36:53282.
194. Salzman EW, Weinstein MJ, Weintraub RM, et al: Treatment with desmopressin acetate to reduce blood loss after cardiac surgery. N Engl J Med 314:1402, 1986.
195. Weinstein M, Ware JA, Troll J, Salzman EW: Changes in von Willebrand factor during cardiac surgery: Effect of desmopressin acetate. Blood 71:1648, 1988.
196. Rocha E, Llorens R, Paramo JA, et al: Does desmopressin acetate reduce blood loss after surgery in patients on cardiopulmonary bypass? Circulation 77:1319, 1988.
197. Mannucci PM: Desmopressin (DDAVP) for treatment of disorders of hemostasis. Prog Hemost Thromb 8:19, 1986.
198. Warrier I, Lusher JM: DDAVP: A useful alternative to blood components in moderate hemophilia A and von Willebrand's disease. J Pediatr 102:228, 1983.
199. Mariani G, Ciavarella N, Mazzucconi MG: Evaluation of the effectiveness of DDAVP in surgery and in bleeding episodes in hemophilia and von Willebrand's disease: a study of 43 patients. Clin Lab Haematol 6:229, 1984.
200. De La Fuente B, Kasper CK, Rickles FR: Response of patients with mild hemophilia A and von Willebrand's disease to treatment with desmopressin. Ann Intern Med 103:6, 1985.
201. Derman UM, Rand PW, Barker N: Fibrinolysis after cardiopulmonary bypass and its relationship to fibrinogen. J Thorac Cardiovasc Surg 51:223, 1966.
202. Bachmann F, McKenna R, Cole ER, Maiafi HJ: The hemostatic mechanisms after open-heart surgery. I: Studies on plasma coagulation factors and fibrinolysis in 512 patients after extracorporeal circulation. J Thorac Cardiovasc Surg 70:76, 1975.
203. Tsuji HK, Redington JV, Kay JH, Goesswald RK: The study of fibrinolytic and coagulation factors during open heart surgery. Ann N Y Acad Sci 146:763, 1968.
204. Woods JE, Kirklin JW, Owen CA, et al: The effects of bypass surgery on coagulation sensitive clotting factors. Mayo Clin Proc 42:725, 1967.
205. Gans H, Subramanian V, John S, et al: Theoretical and practical (clinical) considerations concerning proteolytic enzymes and their inhibitors with particular reference to changes in the plasminogen-plasmin system during assisted circulation in man. Ann N Y Acad Sci 146:721, 1968.
206. Palester-Chlebowzyk M, Strzyzewska E, Sitowski W, Olender K: Detection of the intravascular coagulation of blood clotting. II: Results of the paracoagulation test in patients undergoing open-heart surgery, with extracorporeal circulation. Pol Med J 11:59, 1972.
207. Kladetsky RG, Popov-Cenic S, Buttner W, et al: Studies of fibrinolytic and coagulation factors during open-heart surgery with ECC. Thromb Res 7:579, 1975.
208. Gomes MM, McGoon D: Bleeding patterns after open heart surgery. J Thorac Cardiovasc Surg 60:87, 1970.
209. Bick RL: Disseminated intravascular coagulation. In Disorders of Thrombosis and Hemostasis: Clinical and laboratory practice. Chicago, ASCP Press, 1992, p 137.
210. Bick RL: Disseminated intravascular coagulation and related syndromes: A clinical review. Semin Thromb Hemost 14:299,1988.
211. Bick RL: Clinical hemostasis practice: the major impact of laboratory automation. Semin Thromb Hemost 9:139, 1983.
212. Bick RL, Kovacs I, Fekete LF: A new two stage functional assay for antithrombin III (heparin cofactor): Clinical and laboratory evaluation. Thromb Res 8:745, 1976.
213. Lackner H, Javid JP: The clinical significance of the plasminogen level. Am J Clin Path 60:175, 1973.
214. Tsitouris G, Bellet S, Eilberg R, et al: Effects of major surgery on plasmin-plasminogen systems. Arch Intern Med 108:98, 1961.
215. Wuelfing D, Brandau KP: Fibrinolytic activity after surgery. Minn Med 51:1503, 1968.
216. Ygge J: Changes in blood coagulation and fibrinolysis during the postoperative period. Am J Surg 119:225, 1970.
217. Bick RL, Bishop RC, Warren M, Stemmer E: Changes in fibrinolysis and fibrinolytic enzymes during extracorporeal circulation. Trans Am Soc Hematol 109, 1971.
218. Graeff H, Beller FJK: Fibrinolytic activity in whole blood, dilute blood, and euglobulin lysis time tests. In Bang N, Beller FK, Deutsch E (eds): Thrombosis and Bleeding Disorders, Theory and Methods. New York, Academic Press, 1970, p 328.
219. Menon IS: A study of the possible correlation of euglobulin lysis time and dilute blood clot lysis time in the determination of fibrinolytic activity. Lab Pract 17:334, 1968.

220. Bick RL, Bishop RC, Shanbrom ES: Fibrinolytic activity in acute myocardial infarction. Am J Clin Pathol 57:359, 1972.
221. Bishop RC, Ekert H, Gilchrist G, et al: The preparation and evaluation of a stndardized fibrin plate for the assessment of fibrinolytic activity. Thromb Diath Haemorrh 23:202, 1970.
222. Fareed J: New methods in hemostatic testing. In Fareed J, Messmore H, Fenton J (eds): Perspectives in Hemostasis. Pergamon Press, New York, pp 310, 1981.
223. Fareed J, Messmore HL, Bermes EW: New perspectives in coagulation testing. Clin Chem 26:1380, 1980.
224. Huseby RM, Smith RE: Synthetic oligopeptide substrates: Their diagnostic application in blood coagulation, fibrinolysis, and other pathologic states. Semin Thromb Hemost 6:173, 1980.
225. Naeye RL: Thrombotic state after a hemorrhagic diathesis: A possible complication of therapy with epsilon aminocaproic acid. Blood 19:694, 1962.
226. Ratnoff OD: Epsilon aminocaproic acid: A dangerous weapon. N Engl J Med 280:1124, 1969.
227. Verska JJ, Lonser ER, Brewer LA: Predisposing factors and management of hemorrhage following open-heart surgery. J Cardiovasc Surg (Torino) 13:361, 1972.
228. Verska J: Letter to the editor. Ann Thorac Surg 13:87, 1972.
229. Brooks DH, Bahnson HT: An outbreak of hemorrhage following cardiopulmonary bypass. J Thorac Cardiovasc Surg 63:449, 1972.
230. O'Neill JA, Ende N, Collins IS, Collins HA: A quantitative determination of perfusion fibrinolysis. Surgery 60:809, 1966.
231. Bick RL, Frazier BL, Saunders CL, Arbegast NR: Alterations of hemostasis during cardiopulmonary bypass: The potential role of factor XII activation in inducing primary fibrino(geno)lysis. Blood 64:926, 1984.
232. Akkerman JW, Runne WC, Sixma JJ, Zimmerman AE: Improved survival rates in dogs after extracorporeal circulation by improved control of heparin levels. J Thorac Cardiovasc Surg 68:59, 1974.
233. Ellison N, Betty CP, Blake DR, et al: Heparin rebound: Studies in patients and volunteers. J Thorac Cardiovasc Surg 67:723, 1974.
234. Gollub S: Heparin rebound in open-heart surgery. Surg Gynecol Obstet 124:337, 1967.
235. Jaberi M, Bell WR, Benson DW: Control of heparin therapy in open-heart surgery. J Thorac Cardiovasc Surg 67:133, 1974.
236. Ellison N, Ominsky AJ, Wollman H: Is protamine a clinically important anticoagulant? A negative answer. Anesthesiology 35:621, 1971.
237. Ollendorff P. The nature of the anticoagulant effect of heparin, protamine, Polybrene, and toluidine blue. Scand J Clin Lab Invest 14:267, 1962.
238. Tsai TP, Matloff JM, Gray RJ, et al: Cardiac surgery in the octagenerian. J Thorac Surg 91:924, 1986.
239. Horneffer PJ, Gardner TJ, Manolio TA, et al: The effects of age on outcome after coronary bypass surgery. Circulation 76:v-6, 1987.
240. Soloway HB, Cornett BM, Donahoo JV, Cox SP: Differentiation of bleeding diathesis which occurs following protamine correction of heparin anticoagulation. Am J Clin Pathol 60:188, 1973.
241. Lewis JH, Wilson HJ, Brandon JM: Counterelectrophoresis test for molecules immunologically similar to fibrinogen. Am J Clin Pathol 58:400, 1972.
242. Salzman EW: The events that lead to thrombosis. Bull N Y Acad Med 48:225, 1972.
243. Bick RL, Baker WF: Diagnostic efficacy of the D-Dimer assay in DIC and related disorders. Blood 68:329, 1986.
244. Rousou JA, Engelman RM, Breyer RH: Fibrin glue: An effective hemostatic agent for nonsuturable intraoperative bleeding. Ann Thorac Surg 38:409, 1984.
245. Rousou J: Randomized clinical trial of fibrin glue sealant in patients undergoing resternotomy or reoperation after cardiac operations: A multicenter study. J Thorac Surg 97:194, 1989.
246. Garcia-Rinaldi, Simmons RP, Salcedo V, Howland C: A technique for spot application of fibrin glue during open heart operations. Ann Thorac Surg 47:59, 1989.
247. Dresdale A, Bowman FO, Malm JR, et al: Hemostatic effectiveness of fibrin glue derived from single-donor fresh frozen plasma. Ann Thorac Surg 40:385, 1985
248. Verstraete M: Clinical application if inhibitors of fibrinolysis. Drugs 29:236, 1985
249. Bick RL: Hemostasis defects associated with cardiac surgery, prosthetic devices, and other extracorporeal circuits. Semin Thromb Hemost 11:249, 1985
250. Forbes CD: Thrombosis and artificial surfaces. Clin Haematol 10:653, 1981.
251. Bick RL: Basic mechanisms of hemostasis pertaining to DIC. In Disseminated Intravascular Coagulation. Boca Raton, FL, CRC Press, 1983, p 1.
252. Esmon CT: Protein-C. Biochemistry, physiology, and clinical implications. Blood 62:1155, 1983.
253. Braunwald NS, Bonchek L: Prevention of thrombus formation on rigid prosthetic heart valves by the ingrowth of autogenous tissue. J Thorac Cardiovasc Surg 54:630, 1967.
254. Bagnall RD: Absorption of plasma proteins on hydrophobic surfaces. II: Fibrinogen and fibrinogen-containing protein mixtures. Biomed Biomater Res 12:203, 1978.
255. Hubbard D, Lucas GL: Ionic charges of glass surfaces and other materials and their possible role in the coagulation of blood. J Appl Physiol 15:265, 1960.

256. Mason RG: The interaction of blood hemostatic elements with artificial surfaces. In Spaet TH (ed): Progress in Hemostasis and Thrombosis. New York, Grune & Stratton, 1972, p 141.
257. Knieriem HJ, Chandler AB: The effect of warfarin sodium on the duration of platelet aggregation. Thromb Diath Haemorrh 18:766, 1967.
258. Lessin LS, Jensen WH, Kelser GA: Scanning electron microscopy of thrombogenesis on vascular catheter surfaces. N Engl J Med 286:139, 1972.
259. Moore CH,Wolma FJ, Brown RW, Derrick JR: Complications of cardiovascular radiology. A review of 1204 cases. Am J Surg 120:591, 1970.
260. Hershey CO, Tomford JW, McLaren CE, et al: The natural history of intravenous catheter-associated phlebitis. Arch Intern Med 144:1373, 1984.
261. Tomford JW, Hershey CO: The effect of an intravenous therapy team on peripheral venous catheter associated phlebitis. Clin Res 30:770A, 1982.
262. Bolooki H: Indications for use of IABP. In Clinical Application of Intra-Aortic Balloon Pump. Mt. Kisco, NY, Futura, 1984, p 293.
263. Okada M, Shiozawa T, Iizuka M, et al: Experimental and clinical studies on the effect of intra-aortic balloon pumping for cardiogenic shock following acute myocardial infarction. Artif Organs 3:271, 1979.
264. McEnany MT, Kay HR, Buckley MJ, et al: Clinical experience with intra-aortic balloon pump support in 728 patients. Circulation 58:124, 1978.
265. Alpert J, Bhaktan EK, Gielchinsky I, et al: Vascular complications of intra- aortic balloon pumping. Arch Surg 111:1190, 1976.
266. Balooki H: Complications of balloon pumping: Diagnosis, prevention, and treatment. In Clinical Application of Intra-Aortic Balloon Pump. Mt. Kisco, NY, Futura, 1984, p 133.
267. Isner JM, Cohen SR, Virmani R, et al: Complications of the intra-aortic ballon counterpulsation device: Clinical and morphologic observations in 45 necropsy patients. Am J Cardiol 45:260, 1980.
268. Karlson K. Discussion: Vascular complications of intra-aortic balloon pumping. Arch Surg 111:1190, 1976.
269. Curtis JJ, Barnhorst DA, Pluth JR, et al: Intra-aortic balloon assist: Initial Mayo Clinic experience and current concepts. Mayo Clin Proc 52:723, 1977.
270. Schneider MD,Kaye MP, Blatt SJ, et al: Safety of intraaortic balloon pumping: II: Physical injury to aortic endothelium due to mechanical pump action. Thromb Res 4:399, 1974.
271. Baciewicz FA, Kaplan BM, Murphy TE, Neiman HL: Bilateral renal artery thrombotic occlusion: a unique complication following removal of a transthoracic intra-aortic balloon. Ann Thor Surg 33:631, 1982.
272. Bick RL: Disseminated intravascular coagulation: Objective criteria for clinical and laboratory diagnosis and assessment of therapeutic response. Clin Appl Thromb Hemost 1:3–23, 1995
273. Bick RL, Strauss JF, Frenkel EP: Thrombosis and hemorrhage in Oncology Patients. Hematol Oncol Clin North Am 10: 875, 1996
274. Gajewski JL, Champlin RE: Vascular cccess. In Haskell CM (ed): Cancer Treatment. Philadelphia, W.B. Saunders, 1990 p 866.
275. Murano G, Bick RL: Thrombolytic therapy. In Murano G, Bick RL (eds): Basic Concepts of Hemostasis and Thrombosis. Boca Raton, FL, CRC Press, 1980, p 259.
276. Bick RL: Thrombolytic therapy. In Disorders of Hemostasis and Thrombosis. New York, Thieme, 1985 p 352.
277. Harker LA, Slichter SJ: Platelet and fibrinogen survival in man. N Engl J Med 287:999, 1972.
278. LeVeen HH, Christoudias G, Ip M, et al: Peritoneovenous shunting for ascites: Ann Surg 180:580, 1974.
279. Reinhardt GF, Stanley MM: Peritoneovenous shunting for ascites. Surg Gynecol Obstet 145:419, 1977.
280. Bick RL: Disseminated intravascular coagulation: objective laboratory diagnostic criteria and guidelines for management. Clin Lab Med 14:729, 1994.
281. Lerner RG, Nelson JC, Corines P, del Guercio LRM: Disseminated intravascular coagulation: complication of Le Veen peritoneovenous shunts. JAMA 240:2064, 1978.
282. Harmon DC, Demirjian Z, Ellman L, Fischer JE: Disseminated intravascular coagulation with the peritoneovenous shunt. Ann Intern Med 90:774, 1979.
283. Strin SF, Fulenwider JT, Ansley JD, et al: Accelerated fibrinogen and platelet destruction after peritoneovenous shunting. Arch Intern Med 141:1149, 1981.
284. Baker WF: Clinical aspects of disseminated intravascular coagulation. Semin Thromb Hemost 15:1, 1989.
285. Frankl WS: Indications for anticoagulants in cardiovascular disease. In Jepson JH, Frankl WS (eds): Hematological Complications in Cardiac Practice. Philadelphia, W.B. Saunders, p 182, 1975.
286. Kaltman AJ: Late complications of heart valve replacement. Annu Rev Med 2:343, 1971.
287. Fraser RS, Waddell J: Systemic embolization after aortic valve replacement. J Thorac Cardiovasc Surg 54:81, 1967.
288. Effler DB, Favaloro R, Groves LK: Heart valve replacement: Clinical experience. Ann Thorac Surg 1:4, 1965.
289. Mason RG, Chuang HYK, Mohammad SF, Saba HI: Thrombosis and artificial surfaces. In van de Loo J, Prentice CRM, Beller FK (eds): The Thromboembolic Disorders. Stuttgart, Schattauer Verlag, 1983, p 533.
290. Akbarian M, Austen WG, Yurchak PM, Scannel JG: Thromboembolic complications of prosthetic cardiac valves. Circulation 37:826, 1968.

291. Duvoisin GE, Brandenburg RO, McGoon DC: Factors affecting thromboembolism associated with prosthetic heart valves. Circulation 35:70, 1967.
292. Berger S, Salzman EW: Thromboembolic complications of prosthetic devices. Prog Hemost Thromb 2:273, 1974.
293. Weiss HJ: Antiplatelet drugs in clinical medicine. In Platelets: Pathophysiology and Antiplatelet Drug Therapy. New York, Alan R Liss, 1982, p 75.
294. Harker LA, Slichter SJ: Studies of platelet and fibrinogen kinetics in patients with prosthetic heart valves. N Engl J Med 283:1302, 1970.
295. Harker LA, Hirsh J, Gent M, Genton E: Critical evaluation of platelet-inhibiting drugs in thrombotic disease. Prog Hematol 9:229, 1975.
296. Weily HS, Steele PP, Davies H: Platelet survival in patients with substitute heart valves. N Engl J Med 290:534, 1974.
297. Steele PP, Weily HS, Davies H, Genton E: Platelet survival in patients with rheumatic heart disease. N Engl J Med 290:537, 1974.
298. Weily HW, Genton E: Altered platelet function in patients with prosthetic mitral valves. Effects of sulfinpyrazone therapy. Circulation 42:967, 1970.
299. Sullivan JM, Harken DE, Gorlin R: Pharmacologic control of thromboembolic complications of cardiac-valve replacement. N Engl J Med 284:1391, 1971.
300. Dale J, Myhre E, Storstein A, et al: Prevention of arterial thromboembolism with acetylsalicylic acid. Am Heart J 94:101, 1977.
301. Dale J, Myhre E, Lowe D: Bleeding during acetylsalicylic acid and anticoagulant therapy in patients with reduced platelet reactivity after aortic valve replacement. Am Heart J 99:746, 1980.
302. Altman R, Boullon F, Rouvier J, et al: Aspirin and prophylaxis of thromboembolic complications in patients with substitute heart valves. J Thorac Cardiovasc Surg 72:127, 1976.
303. Arrants JE, Hairston E: Use of persantine in preventing thromboembolism following valve replacement. Ann Surg 38:432, 1972.
304. Taguchi K, Matsumura H, Washizu T, et al: Effect of athrombogenic therapy, especially high dose therapy of dipyridamole, after prosthetic valve replacement. J Cardiovasc Surg 16:8, 1975.
305. Bjork VO, Henz A: Management of thrombo-embolism after aortic valve replacement with the Bjork-Shiley tilting disc valve. Scand J Thorac Cardiovasc Surg 9:183, 1975.
306. Sarin CL, Yalav E, Clement AJ, Braimbridge MV: Thromboembolism after Starr valve replacement. Br Heart J 33:111, 1971.
307. Gadboys HL, Litwak RS, Niemetz J, Wisch N: Role of anticoagulants in preventing embolization from prosthetic heart valves. JAMA 202:282, 1967.
308. Friedli B, Aerichide N, Grondin P, Campeau L: Thromboembolic complications of heart valve prostheses. Am Heart J 81:702, 1971.
309. Stein PD, Alpert JS, Copeland JG, et al: Antithrombotic therapy in patients with mechanical and biological prosthetic heart valves. Chest 108(Suppl) 371, 1990.
310. Levinson MM, Smith RG, Cork RC, et al: Thromboembolic complications of the Jarvik-7 total artificial heart: Case report. Artif Organs 10:236, 1986.
311. Kolff WJ: Experiences and practical considerations for the future of artificial hearts and of mankind. Artific Organs 12:89, 1988.
312. Hartmannova B, Vasku J, Dolezi S, et al: Mechanisms causing the death of 8 calves surviving with implanted artificial heart from 31 to 173 days. Sp Path 26:221, 1984.
313. Vasku J: Calcification of the driving diaphragm in a total artificial heart. Czeck Med 10:16, 1987.
314. Tolpekin VE, Ioseliani GD, Dobyshev VA, et al: Development of methods of assisted circulation with artificial heart ventricles. Artif Organs 7:112, 1983.
315. Shumakov VI, Zimin NK, Drobyshev AA, et al: Use of an ellipsoid artificial heart. Artif Organs 11:16, 1987.
316. Hughes SD, Coleman DL, Dew PA, et al: Effect of coumadin on thrombosis and mineralization in total artificial hearts Proc Trans Am Soc Artific Intern Organs 30:75, 1984.
317. Iwaya F, Hoshino S, Igari T, et al: Experimental studies in total artificial heart replacement. Jpn Circ J 48:312, 1984.
318. Dostal M, Vasku J, Cerny J, et al: Hematological and biochemical studies in calves living over 1090 days with the polymethylmethacrylate total artificial heart TNS Brno II. Int J Artif Organs 9:39, 1986.
319. Griffith BP, Hardesty RL, Kormos RL, et al: Temporary use of the Jarvik-7 total artificial heart before transplantation. N Engl J Med 316:130, 1987.
320. Trubel W, Losert U, Schima H, et al: Total artificial heard bridging: A temporary support for deteriorating heart transplantation candidates: Methods and results. Thorac Cardiovasc Surg. 35:277, 1987.
321. Green K, Liska J, Egberg N, et al: Hemostatic disturbances associated with implantation of an artificial heart. Thromb Res 48:349, 1987.
322. Coleman DL, Meuzelaar HLC, Kessler TR, et al: Retrieval and analysis of a clinical total artificial heart. J Biomed Mater Res 20:417, 1986.

CHAPTER 37

The Use of Low-Molecular-Weight Heparins in Cardiology

JEROME PREMMEREUR, M.D.

Thrombosis and embolism in cardiovascular diseases have become major causes of death in developed countries. In 1991 the National Center for Health Statistics in the United States reported 570,000 hospitalizations, with a total of 3.1 million hospital days, for the diagnosis of unstable angina pectoris. Although new therapeutic agents are under development, unfractionated heparin (UFH) is still the standard of reference in cardiology. Specific antithrombin agents, such as hirudin[1] in myocardial infarction and Hirulog during angioplasty,[2] have failed to demonstrate a better efficacy/safety ratio than UFH. In the 1980s, a new class of antithrombotics was developed in Europe, the low-molecular-weight heparin (LMWH) fractions.

The advantages of LMWHs in comparison with UFH for prevention of deep venous thrombosis (DVT) in high-risk patients is well demonstrated. For example, two meta-analyses in patients undergoing orthopedic surgery have shown that LMWHs reduce dramatically the rate of DVT (Fig. 1). Furthermore, the LMWHs, such as enoxaparin, are superior when treatment is prolonged[3] beyond a short period. In addition LMWHs are better or equivalent to UFH in the treatment of established DVT.[4] Therefore, the clinical benefit in patients with DVT may apply also to cardiovascular patients.

ADVANTAGES OVER HEPARIN

UFH and LMWH probably achieve their antithrombotic actions by catalyzing antithrombin III-mediated inhibition of several serine proteases involved in blood coagulation.[5] However, based on experience with prevention and treatment of DVT, the advantages of LMWHs in cardiology may be tremendous:

1. Better bioavailability via subcutaneous injection may be a huge advantage. The absolute bioavailability of LMWHs is usually above 90%. The first 48 hours of acute coronary syndromes (unstable angina and myocardial infarction) are crucial to patient outcomes. Dosing of UFH may be considered optimal in less than one-half of cases, based on the activated partial thromboplastin time (APTT) within 48 hours.[1]

2. Less binding with plasma proteins may offer an advantage to LMWHs in terms of pharmacodynamics and reliability of antithrombotic action, especially during the first 48 hours.[5]

3. No blood test (for assessment of APTT) is needed with LMWHs. This advantage is significant in cardiovascular emergencies and intensive care units.

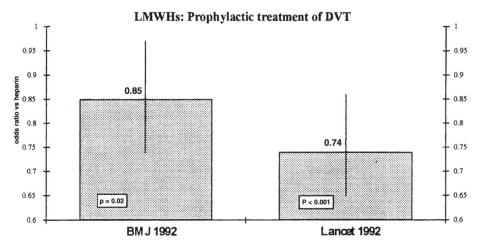

FIGURE 1.   Efficacy of low-molecular-weight heparins in prevention of deep venous thrombosis. (Data from metaanalyses by Michael T, et al. in the *Lancet* [1992] and Leizorovicz A, et al. in the *British Medical Journal* [1992]).

4. The rate of heparin-induced thrombocytopenia (HIT) was significantly less with LMWHs than with UFH[6] during prophylaxis of DVT. The rate of HIT is more important with UFH because UFH is more frequently used repeatedly in the same patient. Patients with coronary artery disease are increasingly older and have increasingly severe coronary artery disease. The mortality rate of acute coronary syndrome has decreased during the past 20 years. In 1994 the frequency of positive tests for HIT was estimated at around 4%.[7] This rate seems to be increasing. Furthermore, if only patients who develop thrombocytopenia on day 5 or later of UFH therapy are considered as the denominator (i.e., presumed to have IgG-mediated HIT), the risk of heparin-induced thrombosis may be as high as 30%.

5. LMWHs, heparan sulfate, and dermatan sulfate generally have less interaction with platelets than UFH and thus may carry lower risks of bleeding.[5] The new antiplatelet agents, such as GPIIb/IIIa inhibitors, may be used more safely in combination with LMWH than in combination with UFH without loss of efficacy. Furthermore, UFH is inhibited by platelet factor IV to a significantly greater extent than LMWHs.

6. Home treatment, already used for long-term prophylaxis of DVT[8] and treatment of established DVT,[9] may be possible in the management of cardiovascular patients. Furthermore, in high-risk patients after acute coronary syndrome or stenting, prolonged therapy with the combination of an LMWH and antiplatelet agent may be superior to classic short-term therapy with UFH and an antiplatelet agent in terms of moderating the anticoagulant activity.

7. The cardioprotective property of LMWHs has already been demonstrated to reduce reperfusion damage in animal models.[10]

POTENTIAL INDICATIONS
Although the advantages of LMWHs over UFH may be important in numerous cardiovascular settings (e.g., atrial fibrillation, stroke, bypass surgery, surgery for arterial disease of the extremities), this chapter focuses on three main indications:
1. Myocardial infarction
2. Unstable angina and non–Q-wave myocardial infarction
3. Percutaneous transluminal coronary angioplasty (PTCA) and stent

This focus was guided mainly by the annual worldwide incidence of myocardial infarction and unstable angina (3,600,000 and 2,500,000, respectively) but also by the availability of relevant data (published or in press).

Myocardial Infarction

Thrombolytic Therapy

Although the use of heparin as an adjunct to thrombolytic therapy has not been fully explored, current guidelines[11] in the United States suggest that heparin be administered with tissue plasminogen activator, whereas in patients treated with streptokinase heparin administration should be delayed until after infusion of the thrombolytic agent. The use of heparin as an adjunct to thrombolytic therapy in patients with acute myocardial infarction (AMI) is predicated on activation of the coagulation system during fibrinolysis. Both plasmin-mediated platelet activation and plasmin-mediated prothrombinase activity lead to the generation of thrombin during fibrinolytic therapy.[12]

During the TIMI 9A and GUSTO IIA trials, heparin and hirudin were compared as adjuncts to thrombolytic therapy in patients with AMI. Both trials were prematurely terminated because of an unacceptably high rate of intracerebral hemorrhage in the two treatment groups. The initial dose of both hirudin and heparin (5000 IU bolus followed by 1300 IU/hr for patients > 80 kg or 1000 IU/hour for patients < 80 kg; target APTT of 60–90 seconds) was reduced for the TIMI 9B and GUSTO IIB trials (5000 IU bolus followed by 1000 IU/hour for patients of any weight with a target APTT of 55–85 seconds). The safety results of the heparin group in TIMI 9B[1] included a major hemorrhage rate of 5.3% (vs. 4.6% for hirudin) and an intracranial hemorrhage rate of 0.9% (vs. 0.4% for hirudin). These results demonstrate that heparin has a narrow therapeutic index. LMWHs may be less heterogeneous than heparin in terms of pharmacokinetic and pharmacodynamic properties. In TIMI 9B, about 50% of heparin-treated patients had an APTT value below the target range within 48 hours, and about 18% had an APTT value above the target range within 48 hours. Therefore, if the pharmacodynamics of LMWHs is more reliable, the bleeding rate may be controlled more effectively than with heparin.

The medical need for prompt efficacy persists. High early patency is desirable because a direct correlation has been documented between the reduction in mortality achieved by thrombolytic therapy and the timeliness and completeness of reperfusion.[13] Depending on the agent prescribed, patency of the infarct-related artery is established by 90 minutes in only 60–80% of patients.[14,15] Furthermore, full anterograde perfusion (TIMI grade 3 flow) is achieved in only 30–55% of patients. The reliability of the pharmacokinetics and pharmacodynamics of LMWHs may improve the efficacy of thrombolytic therapy. Only about 40% of the heparin-treated patients had an APTT in the target range within 96 hours in the TIMI 9B study and thus could be considered well anticoagulated. In terms of reliable anticoagulation, this rate could be improved tremendously with LMWHs.

The reocclusion rate of coronary arteries opened for 90 minutes is 7–8% at hospital discharge.[16,17] Animal data indicate that the combination of an LMWH and thrombolytic agent is superior to the combination of UFH and a thrombolytic agent[18] (Fig. 2). If this advantage applies to the clinical setting, morbidity and mortality rates would be reduced.

Rescue Percutaneous Transluminal Coronary Angioplasty

LMWHs may be an interesting alternative to heparin because of their potential to reduce the reocclusion rate. The half-life of LMWHs is longer than that of UFH; the sequestration effect[19] in the endothelium may be the reason for this advantage.

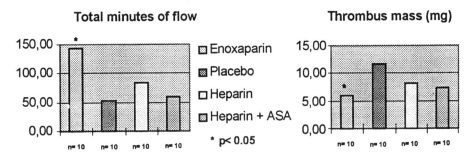

FIGURE 2.   Comparison of enoxaparin, heparin, heparin plus aspirin, and placebo for thrombolytic therapy. Recombinant tissue plasminogen activator = 100 µg/kg intravenous bolus + 20 µg/kg/min for 60 min; enoxaparin = 1 mg/kg intravenous bolus + 30 µg/kg/min for additional 1 hr; heparin = 50 U/kg intravenous bolus + 6 U/kg/min for additional 1 hr; aspirin = 5 mg/kg intravenous bolus.

Intraventricular Thrombus after Acute Myocardial Infarction

LMWHs may easily meet the need for treatment and long-term prophylaxis, especially in patients with anterior MI. The lack of flexibility in treatment with UFH or warfarin suggests a potential advantage for LMWHs.

Unstable Angina and Non–Q-wave Myocardial Infarction

The clinical course and prognosis of patients with unstable angina and acute non–Q-wave MI are similar. For this reason, and because the diagnoses frequently cannot be distinguished at presentation, most recent clinical trials include both populations. The beneficial role of either antiplatelet treatment or heparin or warfarin therapy alone in patients with unstable angina or non–Q-wave myocardial infarction has been established in randomized clinical trials.[20–27] Recently, however, three studies have demonstrated a trend toward superiority of combined antiplatelet and anticoagulation treatment over either therapy alone in such patients.[22,25,28] Pooled data from these studies show that the relative risk for infarction or death among patients with combination antithrombotic treatment compared with aspirin alone was 0.44 (95% confidence interval = 0.21–0.93).

Rationale for Use in the Acute Phase

When UFH is used as thrombolytic therapy in patients with AMI, the anticoagulant effect varies widely because of the binding of UFH molecules to several plasma proteins.[29] The amount of these proteins varies among disease states and among normal individuals. The response to UFH is therefore unpredictable and anticoagulation monitoring is needed to adjust infusions to a desired APTT. In contrast, LMWHs have minimal protein binding, excellent bioavailability,[30] and a predictable anticoagulant response. Therefore, anticoagulation monitoring is not necessary, and both inconvenience and cost are reduced.

Clinical Trials of LMWH in Acute Phase

Three studies involving patients with unstable angina or non–Q-wave myocardial infarction were recently published:

1. Gurfinkel et al.[31] randomized 211 patients with unstable angina to receive aspirin, aspirin plus UFH, or aspirin plus nadroparin. Treatment with nadroparin was associated with a significant reduction in the total number of deaths, MIs, and recurrent ischemic events compared with placebo (p = 0.003) and in episodes of recurrent ischemia compared with UFH (p = 0.002) (Fig. 3).

2. In the FRISC study,[32] patients with unstable angina or non–Q-wave MI were treated with aspirin, 75 mg/day, and then randomized in a phase III trial to either dalteparin

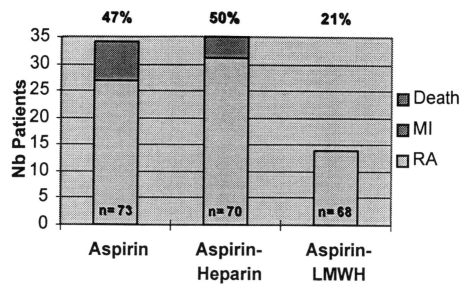

FIGURE 3. Comparison of treatment with aspirin, aspirin plus unfractionated heparin (UFH), and aspirin plus low-molecular-weight heparin (LMWH) in patients with unstable angina or non–Q-wave myocardial infraction. (Data from Gurfinkel EP, Manos EJ, Mejail RI, et al: Low molecular weight heparin versus regular heparin or aspirin in the treatment of unstable angina and silent ischemia. J Am Coll Cadiol 26:313–318, 1995).

(Fragmin), 120 IU/kg/12 hr subcutaneously, or placebo for days 1–6. When added to aspirin, dalteparin was associated with a significant relative reduction of 63% in death or nonfatal MI by day 6 (1.8% vs 4.7%, p = 0.001). In addition, significant reductions were observed in the composite secondary endpoints of death, MI, or occurrence of revascularization and death, MI, occurrence of revascularization, or need for infusion of UFH (p < 0.001). However, the advantage at day 6 was lost by day 150 (Fig. 4)

3. In the FRIC study, a phase III trial, patients with unstable angina or non–Q-wave MI were randomized to receive 75 mg/day of aspirin and, in an open-label manner, either dalteparin, 120 IU/kg/12 hr subcutaneously, or UFH, 5000 IU bolus followed by 1000 IU/hr infusion for 48 hr or longer and then 12,500 IU/12 hr subcutaneously for days 1–6. A second randomization assigned patients in a double-blind manner to prolonged treatment through day 40 with either dalteparin, 7500 IU/24 hr subcutaneously, or placebo. Data about the open-label phase (through day 6) suggest that dalteparin is equivalent to UFH (Table 1).

The following conclusions can be drawn from these trials:

1. When added to a regimen of aspirin and standard medical therapy for unstable angina or non–Q-wave MI, LMWH preparations are significantly superior to placebo for preventing death, MI, or recurrent ischemic events during the acute phase of treatment (i.e., first week).

2. The benefit of therapy with LMWHs during the acute phase of treatment of unstable angina or non–Q-wave MI is at least equivalent to that seen with an intravenous infusion of UFH.

Rationale for Use in the Chronic Phase

A sizable proportion of patients with unstable angina or non–Q-wave MI continue to have adverse clinical outcomes despite treatment with aspirin and UFH during the acute

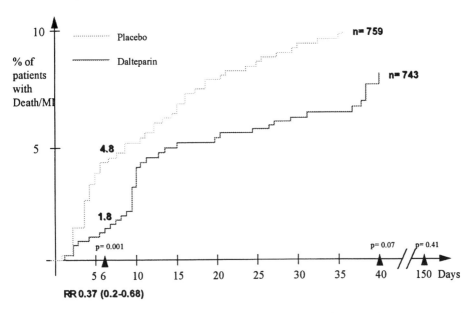

FIGURE 4.   Results of the FRISC Study of dalteparin in patients with unstable angina or non–Q-wave myocardial infarction. (From FRISC Study Group: Low-molecular-weight heparin during instability in coronary artery disease. Lancet 347:561–568, 1996, with permission.)

phase. The incidence of death and nonfatal MI in the early conservative strategy group of TIMI IIIB was 6.1% at hospital discharge; the incidence rose to 7.8% at 42 days and 12.2% at 1 year.[33]

Possible explanations for the loss of initial benefit include rebound activation of the coagulation system after discontinuation of infusions of UFH,[34,35] prolonged activation of the coagulation system for several months beyond the acute event,[36,37] and progression of the severity of coronary stenoses (especially in patients with complex lesions).[38]

Because LMWHs are administered as a subcutaneous injection without anticoagulation monitoring, continued treatment after discharge becomes a possibility. Administration of an LMWH on an outpatient basis during the subacute phase of disease has the potential to reduce the risk of death and MI as well as the need for rehospitalization and revascularization for recurrent angina. This potential is expected to decrease health care costs.

The FRISC investigators administered aspirin and dalteparin, 120 IU/kg/12 hr subcutaneously through day 6 followed by 7500 IU/24 hr subcutaneously through day 40, in patients with unstable angina or non–Q-wave MI. Compared with placebo, statistically significant benefits were observed in terms of composite endpoints through day 6; these benefits, however, were progressively lost by 150 days after randomization. The failure to sustain the early benefits of dalteparin may have been due to an outpatient dose that failed to maintain sufficient anti-Xa activity to prevent thrombosis. Therefore, the benefit of

TABLE 1.   Results of the FRIC Trial

Day 1–6	Dalteparin (n = 751)	UFH (n = 731)	RR	95% CI	p
Composite endpoints: death, myocardial infarction, and revascularization	98 (13.0%)	91 (12.5%)	1.05	0.80–1.37	0.99

UFH = unfractionated heparin, RR = relative response, CI = confidence interval.

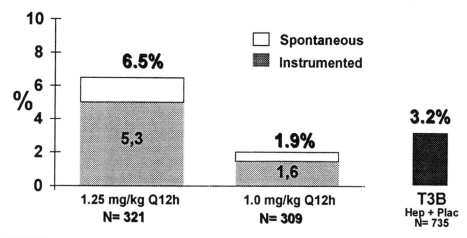

FIGURE 5.   Incidence of major hemorrhage through day 14 in patients with unstable angina or non–Q-wave myocardial infarction treated with two regimens of enoxaparin.

chronic treatment with an LMWH after hospitalization for unstable angina or non–Q-wave myocardial infarction remains to be determined.

The selection of dose for the acute and chronic phases of unstable angina and non–Q-wave MI is critical. The therapeutic index may be narrow, as with heparin in AMI and thrombolytic therapy. Thus, the LMWH enoxaparin was studied in TIMI-11A, a multicenter, open-label dose ranging trial to evaluate the safety and tolerability of 2 doses of enoxaparin in treatment of patients with unstable angina or non–Q-wave MI. All patients received a 2-week treatment consisting of an in-hospital phase with an intravenous bolus of 30 mg of enoxaparin followed by subcutaneous injections every 12 hours of a weight-adjusted dose. After hospital discharge, fixed-dose subcutaneous injections of 60 mg every 12 hours were given to patients ≥ 65 kg and 40 mg every 12 hours to patients < 65 kg. The incidence of major hemorrhage (95% confidence interval) for the 2 regimens is shown in Figure 5.

A significant reduction in the incidence of major hemorrhage was observed with a dose of 1.0 mg/kg/12 hr compared with 1.25 mg/kg/12 hr. Of 170 patients receiving dose 1, in whom anti-Xa levels were available, 14 experienced a major hemorrhage and had significantly higher peak anti-Xa levels (1.74 IU/L) compared with 156 who did not experience major hemorrhage (1.46 IU/ml).

TIMI 11A, in conjunction with other studies (ESSENCE study, with a 1mg/kg/12 hr dose during the acute phase, and TIMI 11B) will identify the benefit of enoxaparin in patients with unstable angina or non–Q-wave MI.

Percutaneous Transluminal Coronary Angioplasty and Stent

The optimal antithrombotic regimen in patients at increased risk for stent thrombosis after deployment of intracoronary stents has not yet been adequately determined. Clinical syndromes associated with intracoronary thrombus and thrombus visualized angiographically increase the risk of acute ischemic complications after intracoronary intervention with PTCA.[39–42]

The theoretical risk of subsequent complete closure in intracoronary stenoses containing thrombus has previously inhibited extensive investigation of stent deployment in patients with AMI. As experience has increased, several recent observational studies have demonstrated the safe and effective use of intracoronary stents in this setting.[43–46]

Since their approval by the Food and Drug Administration (FDA) in 1993 for "bailout" purposes during PTCA, intracoronary stents have been implanted with increasing frequency (from approximately 10,000 in 1994 to 100,000 in 1995), and the indications for their use have expanded significantly beyond the original FDA approval.

Intracoronary stents have been shown to reduce postintervention AMI and urgent revascularization, target vessel revascularization, and restenosis.[47,48] Thrombosis was the Achilles' heel of stenting in the initial trials but has been markedly reduced with the routine use of high-pressure balloon inflations, the combination of aspirin and ticlopidine, and the avoidance of warfarin anticoagulation.[49–52]

Need for Anticoagulant Treatment after Stent Placement

Numerous studies have been published about the need for anticoagulant treatment after stent placement. For instance, in the Intracoronary Stenting and Antithrombotic Regimen (ISAR) trial, 517 patients were randomized to ticlopidine and aspirin or phenprocoumon and aspirin after successful stent implantation.[53] At 30 days, 1.6% of the patients assigned to antiplatelet therapy and 6.2% of the patients assigned to anticoagulant therapy reached the primary endpoint: the composite of cardiac mortality, myocardial infarction, bypass surgery, or repeated angioplasty. Assignment to the antiplatelet group also resulted in a 16% relative risk (95% confidence interval = 0.06–0.36) in the combined clinical endpoint composed of primary cardiac events and noncardiac events (including death, stroke, hemorrhagic events, and peripheral vascular events).

Hall et al. demonstrated the importance of both ticlopidine and aspirin after stent implantation.[54] They randomized 226 patients to either 1 month of ticlopidine combined with only 5 days of aspirin or to more than 1 month of aspirin alone after successful intravascular ultrasound-guided stent implantation. At 1 month, the stent thrombosis rate was 0.8% in the ticlopidine plus aspirin group and 2.9% in the aspirin only group (p = 0.2), and the incidence of cumulative major clinical events (stent thrombosis, death, myocardial infarction, need for reintervention [bypass grafting or PTCA]) was 0.8% and 3.9%, respectively (p = 0.1). Three patients in the ticlopidine plus aspirin group and no patients in the aspirin only group reported medication side effects (p = 0.2). The lack of a significant difference between treatment groups in either stent thrombosis or clinical endpoints may be related to the relatively small study population and/or the low incidence of thrombotic events.

Of note, the ability of heparin to reduce ischemic complications after coronary intervention has not been subjected to a randomized trial. Information is limited largely to retrospective analyses documenting decreased abrupt closure and ischemic complications in patients who receive heparin to maintain a therapeutic activated clotting time (ACT) during intervention.[55–65]

The appropriate duration of heparin therapy after coronary interventions is controversial. Activation of the coagulation system after abrupt cessation of heparin therapy in patients who experience AMI after successful PTCA is particularly problematic.[66] In patients with unstable angina, the benefit of heparin therapy is attenuated by heparin rebound and reactivation of ischemia on discontinuation of heparin. Théroux et al. reported reactivation of unstable angina and myocardial infarction in 14 of 107 patients treated with heparin alone at a median of 9.5 hours after discontinuation of treatment.[67] Logistic regression revealed that cessation of heparin therapy was the most important predictor of reactivation of the disease process.

The **En**oxaparin and **Tic**lopidine after **E**lective **S**tenting (ENTICES) trial demonstrated that subcutaneous LMWH, ticlopidine, and aspirin are easily administered and, compared with standard treatment, reduce stent thrombosis and ischemic clinical events. In this recently completed study, 122 patients scheduled for elective intracoronary stent implantation were randomly assigned in a 2:1 fashion to enoxaparin, ticlopidine, and aspirin or to the conventional treatment regimen of warfarin, heparin, dextran, dipyridamole, and aspirin. Using intention-to-treat analysis, stent thrombosis occurred in 7% of the 43 patients in the conventional treatment group vs. 0% in the 79 patients in the enoxaparin

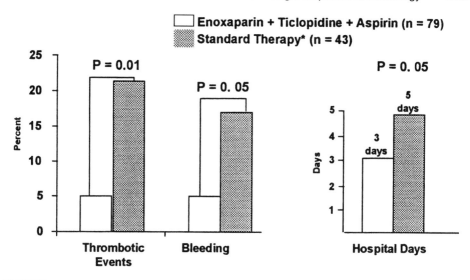

FIGURE 6.   Comparison of standard therapy with a regimen of enoxaparin, ticlopidine, and aspirin in patients scheduled for elective intracoronary stent implantation. (From Zidar J, et al: in press, with permission.)

group. The composite clinical endpoint (death, non-fatal MI, bypass grafting, or repeat PTCA) at 30 days was significantly reduced in patients treated with enoxaparin compared with patients assigned to the standard therapy (5% vs. 21%, respectively; p = 0.01). In addition, there was significant reduction (16% vs. 5%; p = 0.05) in the incidence of hemorrhage or vascular complications (transfusions, pseudoaneurysms, arteriovenous fistulas, or vascular surgery) in favor of the enoxaparin-ticlopidine-aspirin regimen (Fig. 6)

Shortly after the FDA Center for Devices and Radiological Health approved the first intracoronary stent, significant controversy emerged about the five-drug regimen for concomitant use with stent implantation recommended in the stent labeling. Recently, several trials, in addition to ENTICES, have been designed to investigate other regimens for electively implanted stents that may provide greater safety and effectiveness than that currently approved. Until the results of these studies are published, discussions with many interventional cardiologists indicate that the most commonly prescribed concomitant therapy will continue to be an antiplatelet regimen that includes both aspirin and ticlopidine. Although it appears that most interventional cardiologists no longer prescribe the five-drug regimen that included oral antithrombotic therapy with warfarin, some are administering subcutaneous LMWH injections as adjunctive antithrombotic therapy in selected cases. Therefore, further studies are necessary to determine whether the addition of LMWH to the currently prescribed antiplatelet regimen of aspirin and ticlopidine provides a significant advantage for most patients who are at an increased risk for stent thrombosis. To achieve this goal without diluting the results with multiple study-group combinations, only patients who have already started a standard antiplatelet regimen that includes both aspirin and ticlopidine need to be randomly assigned to one of the two treatment groups, LMWH or placebo.

Although it is recognized that abciximab (7E3) and other agents may prove to be appropriate for use in this patient population, their safety and efficacy have not yet been adequately investigated. However, after the publication of EPIC, EPILOG, and CAPTURE studies in patients with unstable angina and PTCA patients, as with thrombolytic therapy in patients with MI, the therapeutic index of UFH is very limited (high rate of bleeding in

EPIC trial with high dose of UFH and lower rate with lower and weight-adjusted doses). The potential advantages of LMWH in terms of pharmacokinetics and pharmacodynamics have to be explored in combination with abciximab.

CONCLUSION

LMWHs offer advantages in comparison with UFH in prevention and treatment of DVT. Therefore, they are likely to offer some advantages in arterial diseases, particularly coronary artery disease.

Each LMWH has to demonstrate its efficacy/safety ratio in patients with arterial disease. However, it is likely that the patient will be the winner because of:

1. Shorter hospital stays
2. Fewer days in intensive care
3. No need for routine laboratory monitoring of anticoagulation
4. Subcutaneous as opposed to intravenous injection

A tendency to "pacify" the arterial disease may be achievable with LMWHs. With UFH it is impossible to prolong the treatment. However, the interactions of LMWHs with the endothelium, platelets, and fibrinolytic system need to be studied in cardiovascular interventions; the results may indicate that LMWHs provide an interesting alternative to UFH.

REFERENCES

1. Elliot A, for the TIMI 9B Investigators: Hirudin in acute myocardial infarction. Thrombolysis and Thrombin Inhibition in Myocardial Infarction (TIMI) 9B Trial. Circulation 94:911–921, 1996.
2. Bittle JA, et al: Treatment with Bivalorudin (hirulog) as compared with heparin during coronary angioplasty for unstable angina. N Engl J Med 333:764–769, 1995.
3. Bergqvist D, et al: Low-molecular-weight heparin (enoxaparin) as prophylaxis against venous thromboembolism after total hip replacement. N Engl J Med 334, 1996.
4. Simonneau G, Charbonnier B, Decousus H, et al: Subcutaneous low molecular weight heparin compared with continuous intravenous unfractionated heparin in the treatment of proximal deep vein thrombosis. Arch Intern Med July 12, 1993.
5. Ofosu FA: Pharmacology of unfractionated and low-molecular-weight heparins. In Bounameaux H (ed): Low-Molecular-Weight Heparins in Prophylaxis and Therapy of Thromboembolic Diseases. New York, Marcel Dekker, 1994.
6. Warkentin TE, et al: Heparin-induced thrombocytopenia in patients treated with low-molecular-weight heparin or unfractioned heparin. N Engl J Med 333, 1995.
7. Warkentin TE, Kelton JG: In Bounameaux H (ed): Low-Molecular-Weight Heparins in Prophylaxis and Therapy of Thromboembolic Diseases. New York, Marcel Dekker, 1994.
8. Planes A, Vochelle N, Darmon J-Y, et al: Risk of deep-venous thrombosis after hospital discharge in patients having undergone total hip replacement: Double-blind randomised comparison of enoxaparin versus placebo. Lancet ii:348, 1996.
9. Levine M, et al: A comparison of low-molecular-weight heparin administered primarily at home with unfractioned heparin administered in the hospital for proximal deep-vein thrombosis. N Engl J Med 334, 1996.
10. Latour JG, et. al, in press, 1996.
11. Cairns J, Lewis HD Jr, Meade TW, et al: Antithrombotic agents in coronary artery disease. Circulation 95:380–400, 1995.
12. Loscalzo J: Thrombin inhibitors in fibrinolysis. Circulation 94:863–865, 1996.
13. GUSTO Angiographic Investigators: The comparative effects of tissue plasminogen activator, streptokinase, or both on coronary artery patency, ventricular function and survival in acute myocardial infarction. N Engl J Med 329:1615–1622, 1993.
14. Bode CH, Smalling RW, Berg G, et al, for the RAPID II Investigators: Randomized comparison of coronary thrombolysis achieved with double-bolus reteplase (recombinant plasminogen activator) and front-loaded, accelerated alteplase (recombinant tissue plasminogen activator) in patients with acute myocardial infarction. Circulation 94:5, 1996.
15. Antman EM, for the TIMI 9B Investigators: Hirudin in acute myocardial infarction: Thrombolysis and Thrombin Inhibition in Myocardial Infarction (TIMI) 9B Trial. Circulation 94:5, 1996.
16. Hsia J, Hamilton P, Kleiman N, et al, for the Heparin-Aspirin Reperfusion Trial (HART) Investigators: N Engl J Med 323:1433–1437, 1990.
17. Randomized comparison of coronary thrombolysis achieved with double-bolus reteplase and front load, accelerated alteplase in patients with acute myocardial infarction. Circulation 94:891–898, 1996.

18. Leadley R, et al: Superiority of enoxaparin over heparin in "in vivo" model of arterial thrombosis/thrombolysis in terms of efficacy and safety. Thromb Haemost 69:454–459, 1993.
19. Brieger DB, Dawes J: Persistence and endothelial sequestration of low molecular weight heparin [abstract]. Circulation 90 (Pt 2):969, 1994.
20. Lewis HD Jr, Davis JW, Archibald DG, et al: Protective effects of aspirin against acute myocardial infarction and death in men with unstable angina. N Engl J Med 309:396–403, 1983.
21. Cairns JA, Gent M, Singer J, et al: Aspirin, sulfinpyrazone or both in unstable angina: Results of a Canadian multicenter trial. N Engl J Med 313:1369–1375, 1985.
22. Wallentin L, for the RISC Group: Risk of myocardial infarction and death during treatment with low dose aspirin and intravenous heparin in men with unstable coronary artery disease. Lancet 336:827–830, 1990.
23. Balsano F, Rizzon P, Violi F, et al, for the STAI Group: Antiplatelet treatment with ticlopidine in unstable angina: A controlled multicenter clinical trial. Circulation 82:17–26, 1990.
24. Williams DO, Kirby MG, McPherson K: Anticoagulant treatment in unstable angina. Br J Clin Pract 40:114–116, 1986.
25. Theroux P, Ouimet H, McCans J, et al: Aspirin, heparin, or both to treat acute unstable angina. N Engl J Med 319:1105–1111, 1988.
26. Neri-Serneri GG, Gensini GF, Poggesi L, et al: Effect of heparin, aspirin, or alteplase in reduction of myocardial ischemia in refractory unstable angina. Lancet 335:615–618, 1990.
27. Braunwald E, Mark DB, Jones RH, et al: Unstable Angina: Diagnosis and Management. Clinical Practice Guideline No. 10. AHCPR Publication No. 94-0602. Rockville, MD, Agency for Health Care Policy and Research and the National Heart, Lung, and Blood Institute, Public Health Service, U.S. Department of Health and Human Services, 1994.
28. Cohen M, Adams P, Parry G, et al: Combination antithrombotic therapy in unstable rest angina and non–Q-wave infarction in non prior aspirin users. Circulation 89:81–88, 1994.
29. Hirsh J, Levine M: Low molecular weight heparin. Blood 79:1–17, 1993.
30. Dawes J, Pavuk N: Sequestration of therapeutic glycosaminoglycans by plasma fibrinonectin [abstract]. Thromb Haemost 65(Suppl 1):929, 1991.
31. Gurfinkel EP, Manos EJ, Mejail RI, et al: Low molecular weight heparin versus regular heparin or aspirin in the treatment of unstable angina and silent ischemia. J Am Coll Cadiol 26:313–318, 1995.
32. FRISC Study Group: Low-molecular-weight heparin during instability in coronary artery disease. Lancet 347:561–568, 1996.
33. TIMI IIIB Investigators: Effects of tissue plasminogen activator and a comparison of early invasive and conservative strategies in unstable angina and non–Q-wave myocardial infarction: Results of the TIMI IIIB trial. Circulation 89:1545–1556, 1994.
34. Theroux P, Waters D, Lam J, et al: Reactivation of unstable angina after the discontinuation of heparin. N Engl J Med 327:141–145, 1992.
35. Granger CB, Miller JM, Bovill, EG, et al: Rebound increase in thrombin generation and activity after cessation of intravenous heparin in patients with acute coronary syndromes. Circulation 91:1929, 1995
36. Merlini PA, Bauer KA, Oltrona L, et al: Persistent activation of coagulation mechanism in unstable angina and myocardial infarction. Circulation 90:61, 1994.
37. Hoffmeister H, Jur M, Wendel H, et al: Alterations of coagulation and fibrinolytic and kallikrein-kinin systems in the acute and postacute phases in patients with unstable angina. Circulation 91:2520, 1995.
38. Kaski J, Chester M, Chen L, et al: Rapid angiographic progression of coronary artery disease in patients with angina pectoris. The role of complex stenosis morphology. Circulation 92:2058, 1995.
39. Lincoff AM, Popma JJ, Ellis SG, et al: Abrupt vessel closure complicating coronary angioplasty: Clinical, angiographic and therapeutic profile. J Am Coll Cardiol 19:926–935, 1992.
40. Ellis SG, Roubin GS, King SB, et al: Angiographic and clinical predictors of acute closure after native vessel coronary angioplasty. Circulation 77:372–379, 1988.
41. Reeder GS, Bryant SC, Suman VJ, Holmes DR Jr: Intracoronary thrombus: Still a risk factor for PTCA failure? Cathet Cardiovasc Diagn 34:191–195, 1995.
42. Tenaglia AN, Fortin DF, Califf RM, et al: Predicting the risk of abrupt vessel closure after angioplasty in an individual patient. J Am Coll Cardiol 24:1004–1011, 1994.
43. Rodriguez AE, Fernandez M, Santaera O, et al: Coronary stenting in patients undergoing percutaneous transluminal coronary angioplasty during acute myocardial infarction. Am J Cardiol 77:684–689, 1996.
44. Steinhubl SR, Moliterno DJ, Teirstein PS, et al: Stenting for acute myocardial infarction: The early United States multicenter experience. J Am Coll Cardiol 27:279A, 1996.
45. Wong PH, Wong CM: Intracoronary stenting in acute myocardial infarction. Cathet Cardiovasc Diagn 33:39–45, 1994.
46. Walton AS, Oesterle SN, Yeung AC: Coronary artery stenting for acute closure complicating primary angioplasty for acute myocardial infarction. Cathet Cardiovasc Diagn 34:142–146, 1995.
47. Fischman DL, Leon MB, Baim DS, et al: A randomized comparison of coronary-stent placement and balloon angioplasty in the treatment of coronary artery disease. Stent Restenosis Study Investigators. N Engl J Med 331:496–501, 1994.

48. Serruys PW, de Jaegere P, Kiemeneij F, et al: A comparison of balloon-expandable-stent implantation with balloon angioplasty in patients with coronary artery disease. Benestent Study Group. N Engl J Med 331: 489–495, 1994.

49. Colombo A, Hall P, Nakamura S, et al: Intracoronary stenting without anticoagulation accomplished with intravascular ultrasound guidance. Circulation 91:1676–1688, 1995.

50. Barragan P, Sainsous J, Silvestri M, et al: Ticlopidine and subcutaneous heparin as an alternative regimen following coronary stenting. Cathet Cardiovasc Diagn 32:133–138, 1994.

51. Morice MC, Bourdonnec C, Lefevre T, et al: Coronary stenting without coumadin. Circulation 90:1–125, 1994.

52. Jordan C, Carvalho H, Fajadet J, et al: Reduction of subacute thrombosis rate after coronary stenting using a new anticoagulation protocol. Circulation 90:1–125, 1994.

53. Schomig A, Neumann F, Kastrati A, et al: A randomized comparison of antiplatelet and anticoagulant therapy after the placement of coronary-artery stents. N Engl J Med 334:1084–1089, 1996.

54. Hall P, Nakamura S, Maiello L, et al: A randomized comparison of combined ticlopidine and aspirin therapy versus aspirin therapy alone after successful intravascular ultrasound-guided stent implantation. Circulation 93:215–222, 1996.

55. McGarry TF J., Gottlieb RS, Morganroth J, et al: The relationship of anticoagulation level and complications after successful percutaneous transluminal coronary angioplasty. Am Heart J 123:1445–1451, 1992.

56. Dougherty KG, Marsh KC, Edelman SK, et al: Relationship between procedural activated clotting time and in-hospital post-PTCA outcome. Circulation 82:189-III, 1990.

57. Rath B, Bennett DH: Monitoring the effect of heparin by measurement of activated clotting time during and after percutaneous transluminal coronary angioplasty. Br Heart J 63:18–21, 1990.

58. Vaitkus PT, Herrmann HC, Laskey WK: Management and immediate outcome of patients with intracoronary thrombus during percutaneous transluminal coronary angioplasty. Am Heart J 124:1–8, 1992.

59. Gabliani G, Deligonul U, Kern MJ, Vandormael M: Acute coronary occlusion occurring after successful percutaneous transluminal coronary angioplasty: Temporal relationship to discontinuation of anticoagulation. Am Heart J 116:696–700, 1988.

60. Ogilby JD, Kopelman HA, Klein LW, Agarwal JB: Adequate heparinization during PTCA: assessment using activated clotting times. Cathet Cardiovasc Diagn 18:206–209, 1989.

61. Satler LF, Leon MB, Kent KM, Pichard AD: Strategies for acute occlusion after coronary angioplasty. J Am Coll Cardiol 19:936–938, 1992.

62. Ferguson JJ, Dougherty KG, Gaos CM, et al: Relation between procedural activated coagulation time and outcome after percutaneous transluminal coronary angioplasty. J Am Coll Cardiol 23:1061–1065, 1994.

63. Narins CR, Hillegass WB, Nelson CL, et al: Relation between activated clotting time during angioplasty and abrupt closure. Circulation 93:667–671, 1996.

64. Mooney MR, Mooney JF, Goldenberg IF, et al: Percutaneous transluminal coronary angioplasty in the setting of large intracoronary thrombi. Am J Cardiol 65:427–431, 1990.

65. Popma JJ, Coller BS, Ohman EM, et al: Antithrombotic therapy in patients undergoing coronary angioplasty. Chest 108:486S–501S, 1995.

66. Granger CB, Miller JM, Bovill EG, et al: Rebound increase in thrombin generation and activity after cessation of intravenous heparin in patients with acute coronary syndromes. Circulation 91:1929–1935, 1995.

67. Theroux P, Waters D, Lam J, et al: Reactivation of unstable angina after the discontinuation of heparin. N Engl J Med 327:141–145, 1992.

CHAPTER 38

Low-Molecular-Weight Heparin in the Treatment of Deep Vein Thrombosis

EVI KALODIKI, M.D., B.A.
ANDREW N. NICOLAIDES, M.S., FRCS, FRCSE

TREATMENT OF THROMBOEMBOLISM

Epidemiologic data indicate that the annual incidence of thromboembolism per 100,000 of the population is approximately 160 for deep venous thrombosis (DVT), 20 for symptomatic nonfatal pulmonary embolism (PE), and 50 for fatal autopsy-detected PE.[3,50,51,62] If DVT is suspected, it should be diagnosed with objective methods before treatment begins because anticoagulants must be given over the long term, monitoring is expensive, and treatment is not without risk.[44] At therapeutic dosages, unfractionated heparin (UFH) and low-molecular-weight heparins (LMWHs) are associated with a 5% risk of major hemorrhage, whereas the risk of major hemorrhage with coumarins is 1% per month.[7]

It is believed that thrombi in proximal veins are particularly likely to embolize.[58] Inadequate anticoagulant therapy carries an overall 26% risk of recurrent thromboembolism in all patients with DVT, whereas the risk for patients with proximal DVT is 47%.[35] In ambulatory patients, thrombi confined to the calf can be safely kept under observation and treated only if they propagate to the popliteal or more proximal veins.[34,36] In immobile patients, however, treatment is essential to prevent propagation.

The aim of treatment in patients with acute proximal DVT is to prevent propagation of the thrombus, to limit leg edema, to reduce the symptomatic recurrence of DVT and PE, and to limit the severity of the postthrombotic syndrome.[27] Until recently the following options were available for treating thromboembolism: (1) anticoagulants (UFH, initially either subcutaneously or intravenously, overlapped and followed by 3–6 months of oral anticoagulants), and (2) surgical intervention (thrombectomy, pulmonary embolectomy, or insertion of inferior vena cava filters). However, increasing experience with LMWHs seems promising. The duration of therapy depends on the magnitude of thrombosis and the patient's risk factors. Thus warfarin is recommended for 3 months in patients with DVT of the calf and for 3–6 months in patients with proximal DVT or PE.[38]

LOW-MOLECULAR-WEIGHT HEPARINS: CHARACTERISTICS

The recently prepared low-molecular-weight derivatives of commercial heparin[27] opened a new and exciting chapter in the management of thromboembolism. LMWHs have a mean molecular weight of 4,000–5,000 Da compared with 12,000–16,000 Da for UFH.[69,76]

In the mid 1970s it was observed that with reduction in molecular weight LMWHs prepared from standard heparin progressively lose their ability to prolong the activated partial thromboplastin time (APTT) but retain their ability to inhibit activated factor X (factor Xa).[4,40] In the early 1980s experimental models demonstrated that for an equivalent antithrombotic effect, LMWHs produce less bleeding than subcutaneous heparins.[6,11,12,18,30]

All LMWHs are readily absorbed from subcutaneous tissue and are less bound to the endothelium than UFH.[76] They have a much longer plasma half-life and better bioavailability at low doses than heparin[5a,9,23,56,76] as well as a more predictable dose-response relationship.[25] These properties allow LMWHs to be administered once or twice daily without laboratory monitoring.

In summary, low-molecular-weight heparins have the following advantages[20]:
1. High antithrombotic–low anticoagulant index
2. Sustained antithrombotic action (1 dose daily compared with other heparins)
3. Subcutaneous administration (thereby dispensing with the need for highly trained personnel)
4. Less platelet interaction than heparin and hence reduced risk of thrombocytopenia
5. Lesser degree of neutralization by endogenous antiheparin agents
6. Possibly no need for monitoring in prophylaxis
7. Non–antithrombin III-mediated anticoagulant and antithrombotic actions

The risk of thrombocytopenia, always a concern with UFHs, appears to be sporadic,[16] but the platelet count must be regularly monitored during LMWH therapy.[46,73] LMWHs have been administered successfully in patients with heparin-induced thrombocytopenia.[14,48] A rare case of urticaria and angioedema induced by LMWH has been reported.[64]

Although sharing a number of common properties, LMWHs of various manufacturers are produced to different specifications; thus they are not comparable and are considered to be individual products with different pharmacologic and clinical properties.[75,78] Differences include (1) molecular weight distribution profiles, (2) specific activities (anti-Xa to anti-IIa), (3) rates of plasma clearance, and (4) recommended dosage regimens. Therefore, until more information about their relative safety and efficacy is available, LMWHs should be considered to be distinct and individual compounds.[28,78]

So far LMWHs have been found to be at least as effective as UFH for prophylaxis in general surgery, and for total hip replacement they may even be superior, as indicated by a large number of studies.[41,47,63] Furthermore, a multicenter study involving 4,498 patients undergoing general surgery found that LMWH reduced not only the incidence of fatal PE but also the overall surgical mortality rate compared with controls without prophylaxis.[65]

For the treatment of established DVT, various studies involving small numbers of patients evaluated the efficacy of LMWHs compared with standard UFH.[25,26,33,53,67,70] These studies provided data (largely based on venographic observations) suggesting that subcutaneous LMWHs are at least as effective and safe as continuous intravenous UFH. More recently, the results of 14 major randomized trials[1,8,10,15,19,22,29,37,45,49,52,54,68,71] have shown that LMWHs are highly effective in the initial treatment of established DVT and are superior to standard UFH in the following areas:
• Superior[10,15,54,71] or equal[8,19,22,29,52] thrombolysis on repeat venography
• Fewer bleeding complications[1,10,19,29,37,45,54,68]
• Reduced mortality at 90 days, particularly in patients with cancer[37,68]
• Reduced recurrence of DVT[1,8,10,19,29,37,45,49,68]
• No need for monitoring; hence the potential for treatment in an outpatient setting[1,8,10,15,19,29,37,45,49,52,54,68,71]

More specifically, in the study by Bratt et al.,[8] in which 54 patients were originally treated with high doses (240 anti-Xa U/12 hr) of LMWH (Fragmin), an adjustment was needed as bleeding complications occurred.[53] After adjusting the dose to 120 anti-Xa U/kg/12 hr, the mean heparin activity was still higher in group A patients treated with LMWH (0.9–1.2 anti-Xa U/ml) than in group B patients treated with UFH (0.5–0.7 anti-Xa U/ml). Phlebography showed progression of thrombus size in 3 patients in group B (11%) compared with no patients in group A and improvement in 14 patients in group B (48%) compared with 10 patients (77%) in group A. The mean decrease in thrombus size (Marder score)[55] was the same. Antithrombin III decreased significantly in group B, and there was no difference in mean capillary bleeding time. The results of this study showed that Fragmin (in a dose of 120 anti-Xa U/kg/12 hr) and UFH were equally effective in patients with DVT and also that bleeding complications may occur with doses of LMWH as high as 240 anti-Xa U/kg/12 hr. In subsequent studies, the investigators randomly allocated patients with DVT (as established by venography) into two groups: group A was treated with the LMWH under investigation and group B was treated with UFH.

In the study by Holm et al.,[29] 56 patients were randomized into two groups: group A received subcutaneous LMWH (Fragmin), and group B received subcutaneous UFH. Both groups were injected twice daily, and initial doses were determined according to age and sex (disregarding body weight). The dose was adjusted when the peak plasma concentration of heparin fell outside the desired range of 0.5–0.8 anti-Xa U/ml. The correlation between the injected dose (U/kg body weight) and heparin concentration was higher in group A (r = 0.59) than in group B (r = 0.38). The study demonstrated that the initial dose of LMWH needed to obtain therapeutic concentration should be around 100 anti-Xa U/kg/12 hr. When this therapeutic strategy was followed in a group of 15 patients, the peak heparin concentration on day 2 ranged from 0.4–0.75 anti-Xa U/ml; adjustment was required in only 3 patients. Day-to-day variation in peak heparin activity in individual patients had a coefficient of variation of 12% without accumulation. This study confirmed that the therapeutic dose of Fragmin should be 100–120 anti-Xa U/kg/12 hr and indicated that plasma heparin concentration may be more predictable with LMWH than with UFH.

In the study of Faivre et al.,[19] 68 patients with venographically proven DVT were randomized into 2 groups: 33 patients in group A received a fixed subcutaneous dose of 750 anti-Xa U of ultra LMWH (CY 222), and 35 patients in group B received standard UFH in doses of 500 IU/kg/24 hr. Both treatments were given for 10 days in two daily subcutaneous injections. A second phlebography was performed on the last day of treatment. No hemorrhagic complications were observed in group A, whereas 3 cases were observed in group B. The initial phlebographic score and the location of the DVT lesions were the same in both groups. Angiographic improvement, with more than 30% thrombolysis, was obtained at the end of treatment in 64% of patients in group A and 65% in group B. Thrombus extension was demonstrated in only 2 patients in group B. The initial score remained unchanged in one-third of patients in both groups. The APTT was prolonged (2 or 3 times that of the control) in group B and unchanged in group A, whereas anti-Xa activity was significantly higher in group A than in group B. The results of this study showed that two daily subcutaneous injections of LMWH and UFH were equally effective in patients with acute DVT and that LMWH appeared to be safer than UFH.

In the study of Albada et al.,[1] 194 patients with acute DVT were randomized into 2 groups: 96 patients in group A received LMWH (Fragmin), and 98 patients in group B received UFH. Both groups received treatment for 5–10 days. Doses were adjusted to maintain anti-Xa levels of 0.3–0.6 U/ml for patients with high risk of bleeding and 0.4–0.9 U/ml for low-risk patients. Administration of UFH was stopped when a therapeutic level of anticoagulation (International Normalized Ratio [INR] > 3.5) was reached with coumarins. Ten patients in group A and 13 patients in group B had major bleeding complications. The combined incidence of major and minor bleeding complications decreased from 48.9% to 38.5%, corresponding to a reduction of 21.2% in relative bleeding risk. No difference was seen in recurrent PE. The results of this study showed that Fragmin given in adjusted, continuous intravenous doses of 15.000 anti-Xa U/24 hr is as safe and effective as intravenous UFH. The results also showed a trend in risk reduction for bleeding in favor of LMWHs, although the reduction was smaller than expected.

In the French Multicenter Study,[22] 66 patients with phlebographically verified DVT were randomized into 2 groups: patients in group A initially received subcutaneous Fragmin at a dose of 100 anti-Xa U/kg/12 hr; further doses were adjusted in accordance with anti-Xa activity to 0.5–0.8 U/ml. Patients in group B initially received continuous intravenous UFH at a dose of 240 IU/kg/12 hr; the dose was then adjusted to achieve a daily APTT of 1.5–3 times that of the control. Repeat phlebography after 10 days showed improvement in 71% in group A and 79.3% in group B (no statistical significance), whereas propagation was seen in 6.4% and 3.4% of patients, respectively (no statistical significance). The need for dosage adjustments was less and the stability of biologic tests was better in the LMWH-treated group.

In a more recent study by Bratt et al.,[10] 110 consecutive patients with phlebographically verified DVT (36% distal and 64% proximal) were randomized into 2 groups: 55 patients in group A were treated with subcutaneous Fragmin at a dose of 120 anti-Xa U/kg/12 hr and 55 in group B with continuous intravenous UFH at a dose of 480 IU/kg/24 hr. The LMWH doses were adjusted to achieve an anti-Xa activity of 0.2–0.4 U/ml before injection and no greater than 1.5 U/ml 4 hours after the morning injection. The UFH dose was modified to prolong the APTT to 2–3 times that of the controls. Repeat phlebography after 5–7 days showed improvement in 34 of the 45 patients in group A (76%) and in 30 of the 49 patients in group B (61%), whereas propagation was seen in 2 (4%) and 3 patients (6%), respectively. The mean Marder scores[55] decreased in both groups but not to a statistically significant extent. Two patients in group B had major bleeding complications compared with none in group A. During 2-year follow-up, thrombosis recurred in 4 patients in group A and 6 in group B, whereas postthrombotic symptoms and signs were similar in both groups.

In the study of Simonneau et al.,[71] 134 patients with venographically proven proximal DVT were randomized into two groups: 67 in group A received the LMWH Enoxaparin at a fixed dose of 1 mg/kg/12 hr, and 67 patients in group B received a continuous intravenous infusion of UFH adjusted to maintain the APTT at 2–3 times that of controls. Venographic assessment of thrombus size evolution between days 0 and 10, using the Arnesen score,[5] showed that Enoxaparin was superior to UFH (p < 0.002). There were no serious bleeding complications in either group. The results of this study showed that Enoxaparin in a fixed dose of 1mg/kg/12 hr is as effective and safe as UFH.

In the Collaborative European Multicenter Study,[15] 166 patients with venographically proven DVT were randomized into 2 groups: 85 patients in group A received the LMWH Fraxiparine (CY 216) at a daily subcutaneous dose of 30,000 IU (255 Institute Choay anti-Xa U/kg/12 hr), and 81 patients in group B received continuous UFH at a dose of 34,000 anti-Xa IU/24 hr. Patients were from both medical and surgical wards and had leg venography and lung scans on days 0 and 10. Outcome was assessed at the twelfth week according to the incidence of clinical symptoms of recurrent thromboembolism. On day 10 there was venographically proven improvement in both groups, but improvement was more significant in group A (for the Marder score,[55] p = 0.02; for the Arnesen score,[5] p=0.03). Recanalization of proximal DVT and reduction of thrombus size in the medical subgroup were also significantly higher in group A, whereas the incidence of propagation was similar. The decrease in pulmonary vascular obstruction seen on pulmonary scans at day 10 was similar in both groups. Recurrent thromboembolism and hemorrhagic complications were also similar at 10 days. Long-term follow-up revealed similar rates of death and recurrence. The results of this study showed that Fraxiparine is as safe and effective as UFH and improves the venographic picture of DVT without significantly prolonging the coagulation parameters.

In the Polish Multicenter Study,[54] 134 consecutive patients with phlebographically proven DVT were randomized into 2 groups: 68 patients in group A received a fixed subcutaneous dose of the LMWH Fraxiparine twice daily, and 66 patients in group B received UFH in a subcutaneous dose adjusted to achieve an APTT of 1.5–2.5 times the pretreatment value. Treatment continued for 10 days and was followed by oral anticoagulants. Phlebograms were performed on day 10. The mean phlebographic score was significantly decreased in both groups (p < 0.001) compared with baseline, but no significant differences in the score were observed between the two groups. Improvement was noted in 45 of the 68 patients (66%) in group A compared with 32 of the 66 patients (48%) in group B, but the difference did not reach statistical significance. Thrombus size was increased in 10 patients (15%) in group A and 12 (18%) in group B (no statistical significance). No thromboembolic complications occurred in group A, whereas 1 nonfatal PE and 1 major bleeding episode were observed in group B. During 3-month follow-up, 2 rethromboses occurred in group B compared with none in group A. The results of this study showed that subcutaneous Fraxiparine at a fixed dose is as safe and at least as effective as adjusted subcutaneous UFH in the treatment of DVT.

In the study of Prandoni et al.,[68] 170 consecutive symptomatic patients with venographically proven proximal deep vein thrombosis were randomized into 2 groups: 85 patients in group A received the LMWH Fraxiparine in a subcutaneous, twice-daily dose adjusted to body weight (0.5 ml/kg for patients < 55 kg; 0.6 ml/kg for patients 55–80 kg; and 0.7 ml/kg for patients > 80 kg), and 85 patients in group B received UFH in a dose adjusted to achieve an APTT of 1.5–2.0 times the pretreatment value. Treatment lasted 10 days; oral coumarin was started on day 7 and continued for at least 3 months. There was a tendency (although not statistically significant) for better results in group A in terms of recurrent thromboembolism (7% vs. 14%), bleeding complications (1.1% vs. 3.5%), and thrombocytopenia (0% vs. 2.3%), whereas the venographic score and death rate at 6-month follow-up were similar in both groups. An interesting observation was the incidence of death among patients with cancer: there was 1 death among the 15 patients with cancer treated with LMWH compared with 8 deaths among the 18 patients with cancer treated with UFH. The results of this study confirmed that a fixed subcutaneous dose of Fraxiparine is at least as effective and safe as an adjusted intravenous dose of UFH for the initial treatment of symptomatic proximal DVT, whereas cancer patients treated with LMWHs appear to have a survival advantage over those treated with UFH.

In the multicenter study of Hull et al.,[37] 432 patients with venographically proven proximal DVT were randomized into 2 groups: 213 patients in group A received the LMWH Logiparin in a fixed subcutaneous dose of 175 International Factor Xa Inhibitory Units IU/kg/24 hr, and 219 patients in group B received an adjusted dose of continuous intravenous UFH. Both groups received warfarin sodium in a dose of at least 10 mg/24 hr, beginning on the second day of therapy and then adjusted daily to maintain the INR between 2 and 3. The differences between group A and group B were significant in terms of major bleeding associated with initial therapy (0.5% vs. 5.0%, respectively; p = 0.006; risk reduction of 91%) and number of deaths (4.7% vs. 9.6%, respectively; p = 0.049; risk reduction of 51%), but the advantage of group A in terms of major bleeding was lost during long-term therapy. In addition, group A showed a tendency for better results in terms of recurrent thromboembolic complications (2.8% vs. 6.9%, p = 0.07). Among patients with cancer, death occurred in 6 of the 47 treated with LMWHs compared with 13 of the 49 treated with UFH, suggesting that LMWHs may have some antineoplastic action. The results of this study confirmed that Logiparin in a once-daily, fixed subcutaneous dose (175 International Factor Xa Inhibitory Units/kg) is at least as effective and safe as classic intravenous UFH for the treatment of uncomplicated acute proximal DVT.

In the Swedish Multicenter Study of Lindmarker et al.,[52] 204 patients with venographically confirmed DVT (58%, proximal; 42%, distal) after a 24-hour initial treatment with intravenous UFH were randomized into 2 groups: 101 patients in group A received the LMWH Fragmin in a fixed subcutaneous dose of 200 IU/kg/24 hr and 103 patients in group B received an adjusted dose of continuous intravenous UFH to achieve an APTT of 1.5–3.0 times that of the control. Warfarin sodium was initiated in a dose of 10–15 mg on the day that venography was performed and continued for at least 3 months. Patients were followed for 6 months. Both groups had repeat venography at the end of the treatment (days 5–9). There were no significant differences in the change in mean Marder score between the two groups.[55] No major bleeding events, symptomatic PE, symptomatic thrombosis progression, or death occurred during hospitalization. The results of this study showed that Fragmin in a fixed subcutaneous dose adjusted for body weight is as effective and safe as continuous intravenous UFH for treatment of DVT.

Two studies addressed the question of the safety and efficacy of LMWH administered at home for the treatment of venographically proven proximal DVT. Levine et al.,[49] randomized their patients into 2 groups: 247 patients in group A received the LMWH Enoxaparin, 1mg/kg/12 hr subcutaneously, and 253 patients in group B received intravenous UFH. All patients received warfarin on the second day. Thromboembolism recurred in 5.3% of patients in group A and 6.7% of patients in group B (p = 0.57). There was no statistically significant difference in bleeding between the two groups. After randomization patients in group A spent a mean of 1.1 days in hospital compared with 6.5 days for group B; 120 patients in group A required no hospitalization. The results of this study show that LMWH can be used safely and effectively to treat patients with proximal DVT at home.

In the study of Koopman et al.,[45] patients were randomized into two groups: 202 patients in group A received the LMWH nadroparin-Ca (Fraxiparine) in a twice-daily dose adjusted to body weight, and 198 in group B received UFH in an intravenous dose adjusted to achieve an APTT of 1.5–2.0 times the pretreatment value. Oral anticoagulant treatment was initiated on the first day and continued for 3 months. All patients were contacted daily during the initial treatment and at 4, 12, and 24 weeks. Thromboembolism recurred in 6.9% of patients in group A and 8.6% of patients in group B. Major bleeding occurred in 0.5% in group A and 2% in group B. Among patients in group A, 36% required no hospitalization, and 40% were discharged early. Quality of life over time improved in both groups, but patients in group A had better scores for physical activity (p = 0.002) and social functioning (p < 0.001) at the end of the initial treatment, which lasted a mean of 6 days in each group. The results of this study confirm that LMWH for the initial treatment of proximal DVT in the home is feasible, safe, and effective. This and the results of the previous study have obvious implications for cost effectiveness in the avoidance of unnecessary hospitalization.

In addition to the above studies, several other studies, either dose-finding[2,31,42] or open (using one of the established preparations),[21,24,39,77] have been reported. Three studies[17,57,66] used different LMWHs in healthy volunteers to compare certain properties by measuring anticoagulant activities. In the study by Pindur et al.,[66] three different LMWHs were administered and UFH was used as a control. The authors concluded that in LMWH-treated individuals, the anti-Xa activity, as measured by the chromogenic substrate assay and Heptest, revealed maximal correlation (r = 0.51), whereas in UFH-treated individuals, peak correlation (r = 0.75) was observed between APTT and thrombin time (TT). In addition, anticoagulant activity as measured by Heptest was significantly influenced by body weight. In the study by Eriksson et al.,[17] the bioavailability of three LMWHs was compared with that of UFH. Using chromogenic substrate methods, the anti-Xa peak activity (C_{max}) and the area under the curve (AUC) were found to be highest for Clexane and Fragmin and lower for Logiparin and UFH; no bioequivalence was found in terms of anti-IIa activity. Fragmin had values for C_{max} and AUC almost double those of the other drugs. However, the clinical significance of these results remains unclear and can be established only by comparative clinical studies. Mismetti et al.,[57] who analyzed the parameters of heparin activity (i.e., APTT,

TT, prothrombin time [PT], and levels of tissue factor pathway inhibitor [TFPI]) found that the biologic anticoagulant effect of 200 IU anti-Xa/kg of Dalteparin appeared to be higher after an 8 PM injection than after an 8 AM injection ($p < 0.05$), whereas no chronopharmacologic variation of anti-factor Xa activity was observed.

The original rationale that fragments with high anti-factor Xa activity and anti-factor Xa/anti-factor IIa ratio would retain optimal antithrombotic activity with greatly reduced prohemorrhagic action appears to have been an oversimplification. In practice, anti-factor Xa activity is not the only determinant of the antithrombotic effect, nor is anti-factor IIa activity a good predictor of hemorrhage.[13]

UNANSWERED QUESTIONS

Taken together, the results of all major trials provide strong evidence that LMWHs in adjusted doses are as effective and safe as UFH for initial treatment of proximal DVT. These trials have provided data about dose adjustment (Table 1) and have established eligibility criteria (Table 2). They also have improved characterization of complications and outcome assessment. However, they did not objectively document the incidence of symptomatic recurrent venous thromboembolism during both initial treatment and follow-up. Using venography as the definitive follow-up investigation, no assessment of thrombus propagation or reduction can be accurately and repeatedly obtained because venography is invasive and carries an inherent risk of causing thrombosis.[74] Furthermore, venous hemodynamic studies were not performed; therefore, the efficacy of LMWHs in preventing the postthrombotic sequelae of swelling, skin changes, and ulceration is unknown. Finally, no study of the efficacy of blood monitoring tests was performed; in some studies, only the factor Xa inhibition activity was evaluated.

THE FUTURE

One major trial currently in progress, the Canadian Multicentre Study, is trying to elucidate the unanswered questions regarding LMWHs vs. UFH as the initial treatment of established proximal DVT (R.D. Hull, personal communication). The primary aim is to determine whether LMWHs are more effective in reducing the incidence of death, recurrent venous thromboembolism, and hemorrhagic complications during both initial treatment and 3-month follow-up. Another aim is to determine whether such LMWH therapy is more cost-effective than present methods of standard care. The hypothesis is that LMWHs can reduce the incidence of both death and thromboembolic events. The criteria for ineligibility are similar to those in Table 2, whereas the effectiveness of treatment will be assessed by the following parameters: death at 12 weeks, recurrent thromboembolism, bleeding complications, and thrombocytopenia. A cost-effectiveness study also will be performed. As in all previous studies, however, the investigators do not assess the effect of treatment on venous hemodynamics and its potential to prevent postthrombotic syndrome; there is also a need to determine whether the use of subcutaneous LMWHs for a prolonged period (i.e., 90 days) is more effective in preventing the hemodynamic disturbances (which are associated with or produce the postthrombotic sequelae of swelling, skin changes, and ulceration) than the currently used standard treatment.

Finally, other issues also need to be clarified: determination of the hematologic changes associated with the two treatments; identification of any relation between hematological changes and recurrence rate or incidence of hemorrhagic complications; identification of efficient blood monitoring tests; and determination of the feasibility of early discharge from hospital with its implications for cost-effectiveness.

The attractive hypothesis is that prolonged (90-day) treatment of proximal DVT by therapeutic doses of LMWHs may be more effective in preventing the hemodynamic changes associated with or producing postthrombotic syndrome than the currently prescribed regimen of 5 days of intravenous UFH followed by 3 months of oral anticoagulants.

TABLE 1.   Low-Molecular-Weight Heparins in Patients with Established Deep Vein Thrombosis

Authors	LMWH	Dose	Administration
Bratt et al., 1985	Fragmin	240 Anti-Xa U/kg/12 hr 120 Anti-Xa U/kg/12 hr	Intravenous, twice daily Intravenous, twice daily
Holm et al., 1986	Fragmin	*Anti-Xa U/kg/ 12 hr	Subcutaneous, twice daily
Bratt et al., 1990	Fragmin	120 Anti-Xa U/kg/12 hr	Subcutaneous, twice daily
Albada et al., 1989	Fragmin	15,000 Anti-Xa U/kg/24 hr	Intravenous, continuous
Lindmarker et al., 1994	Fragmin	200 IU/kg/24 hr	Subcutaneous, once daily
Huet et al., 1990	Enoxaparin	1 mg/kg/ 12 hr	Subcutaneous, twice daily
Simmoneau et al., 1991	Enoxaparin	1 mg/kg/ 12 hr	Subcutaneous, twice daily
Levine et al., 1996	Enoxaparin	1 mg/kg/ 12 hr	Subcutaneous, twice daily
Duroux et al., 1991	Fraxiparin	255 Anti-Xa U/kg/12 hr	Subcutaneous, twice daily
Lopaciuk et al., 1992	Fraxiparin	255 Anti-Xa U/kg/12 hr	Subcutaneous, twice daily
Prandoni et al., 1992	Fraxiparin	255 Anti-Xa U/kg/12 hr	Subcutaneous, twice daily
Hull et al., 1992	Logiparin	175 Int Factor Xa U/kg/24 hr	Subcutaneous, once daily, fixed dose
Faivre et al., 1987	CY 222	750 Anti-Xa U/kg/24 hr	Subcutaneous, twice daily, fixed dose

LMWH = low-molecular-weight heparin.
* Dose adjusted for age and gender.

The different structure of thrombus in the presence of LMWHs may be a factor. Because treatment with LMWH has a low complication rate and requires no monitoring, its use may reduce hospital stay by 3–4 days.

In recent years colorflow duplex imaging (CFDI) has proved to be a unique tool for the imaging and accurate and repeatable evaluation of the functional anatomy of the venous system of the legs.[43,72] Future studies should use this method to identify the presence, anatomic extent, and propagation of thrombus and the presence or absence of recanalization and reflux. Currently venous hemodynamics are uniquely evaluated with air plethysmography (APG),[60,61] which provides a quantitative analysis that cannot be obtained by venography. APG can assess the severity of obstruction, as indicated by the outflow fraction with and without occlusion of the superficial veins at the level of the knee; it can also assess the severity of reflux, as indicated by the venous filling index. Furthermore, APG can identify the efficacy of calf muscle pump function, as shown by the ejection fraction, and the degree of venous hypertension, as indicated by the residual volume fraction, which is linearly related to ambulatory venous pressure.

TABLE 2.   Contraindications to Treatment with Low-Molecular-Weight Heparins

1. Age less than 18 years
2. Suspected pulmonary embolism at referral
3. Venous thrombosis at the same leg in the past two years
4. Familial bleeding diathesis or active bleeding contraindicating anticoagulant therapy
5. Ongoing anticoagulant therapy at time of referral
6. Known allergy to heparin, warfarin sodium, or bisulfate (stabilizer contained in LMWHs)
7. History of heparin-associated thrombocytopenia
8. Pregnancy
9. Hepatic encephalopathy
10. Severe malignant hypertension (systolic blood pressure >250 mmHg, diastolic >130 mmHg)
11. Residence far from the hospital
12. Inability or refusal to give signed informed consent

Finally, in recent years important steps have been made toward understanding of the coagulation system.[59] Hypercoagulable states (i.e., disorders characterized by an increased risk of thromboembolism) may be inherited or secondary. Inherited disorders include deficiencies of antithrombin III, protein C, and protein S, whereas secondary disorders are associated with antiphospholipid syndrome, heparin-induced thrombopathy, myeloproliferative syndromes, and cancer.[59]

CONCLUSION

All major trials provide strong evidence that, for the initial treatment of DVT, LMWHs in adjusted doses are as effective and safe as UFH and show overall superiority in terms of more effective thrombolysis, fewer bleeding complications (21–91% risk reduction), reduced mortality (51%), and reduced recurrence of DVT (61%) and PE at 90-day follow-up. In addition, LMWHS do not require monitoring. However, long-term evaluations of mortality rates, recurrent venous thromboembolism, blood monitoring tests, thrombus propagation or reduction, and venous hemodynamics are open issues.

REFERENCES

1. Albada J, Nieuwenhuis HK, Sixma JJ: Treatment of acute venous thromboembolism with low molecular weight heparin (Fragmin): Results of a double-blind randomised study. Circulation 80:935–940, 1989.
2. Alhenc-Gelas M, Jestin Le Guernic C, Vitoux JF, et al: Adjusted versus fixed doses of the low-molecular-weight heparin Fragmin in the treatment of deep vein thrombosis. Fragmin Study Group. Thromb Haemost 71:698–702, 1994.
3. Anderson FA, Wheeler HB, Goldberg RJ, et al: The prevalence of risk factors for venous thromboembolism among hospital patients. Arch Intern Med 152:1660–1664, 1992.
4. Andersson L-O, Barrowcliffe TW, Holmer E, et al: Anticoagulant properties of heparin fractionated by affinity chromatography on matrix-bound antithrombin III and by gel filtration. Thromb Res 9:575–583, 1976.
5. Arnesen H, Heilo A, Jacobsen E, et al: A prospective study of streptokinase and heparin in the treatment of deep vein thrombosis. Acta Med Scand 203:457–463, 1978.
5a. Bara L, Billaud E, Gramond G, et al: Comparative pharmacokinetics of low molecular weight heparin (PK 10169) and unfractionated heparin after intravenous and subcutaneous administration. Thromb Res 39:631–636, 1985.
6. Bergqvist D, Nilsson B, Hedner U, et al: The effect of heparin fragments of different molecular weights on experimental thrombosis and hemostasis. Thromb Res 38:589–601, 1985.
7. Bounameaux H: Hemorrhagic complications of anticoagulants in angiology. J Mal Vasc 19(2):98–102, 1994.
8. Bratt G, Tornebohm E, Granqvist S, et al: A comparison between low molecular weight heparin (Kabi 2165) and standard heparin in the intravenous treatment of deep vein thrombosis. Thromb Haemost 54:813–817, 1985.
9. Bratt G, Tornebohm E, Widlund L, Lockner D: Low molecular weight heparin (Kabi 2165; Fragmin): Pharmacokinetics after intravenous and subcutaneous administration in human volunteers. Thromb Res 42:613–620, 1986.
10. Bratt G, Aberg W, Johansson M, et al: Two daily subcutaneous injections of fragmin as compared with intravenous standard heparin in the treatment of deep venous thrombosis (DVT). Thromb Haemost 64:506–510, 1990.
11. Cade JF, Buchanan MR, Boneu B, et al: A comparison of the antithrombotic and haemorrhagic effects of low molecular weight heparin fractions: The influence of the method of preparation. Thromb Res 35:613–625, 1984.
12. Carter CJ, Kelton JG, Hirsh J, et al: The relationship between the hemorrhagic and antithrombotic properties of low molecular weight heparin in rabbits. Blood 59:1239–1245, 1982.
13. Coccheri S: Low molecular weight heparins: an introduction. Haemostasis 20(Suppl 1):74–80, 1990.
14. Drakos P, Uziely B, Nagler A, et al: Successful administration of low molecular weight heparin in a patient with heparin-induced thrombocytopenia and coumarin-induced skin necrosis. Haemostasis 23(5):259–262, 1993.
15. Duroux P, Becle A: A Collaborative European Multicentre Study. A randomised trial of subcutaneous low molecular weight heparin (CY 216) compared with intravenous unfractionated heparin in the treatment of deep vein thrombosis. Thromb Haemost 65:251–256, 1991.
16. Eichinger S, Kyrle PA, Brenner B, et al: Thrombocytopenia associated with low molecular weight heparin. Lancet 337:1425–1426, 1991.
17. Eriksson BI, Soderberg K, Widlund L, et al: A comparative study of three low-molecular weight heparins (LMWH) and unfractionated heparin (UH) in healthy volunteers. Thromb Haemost 73:398–401, 1995.
18. Esquivel CO, Bergqvist D, Bjorck C-G, Nilsson B: Comparison between commercial heparin, low molecular weight heparin and pentosan polysulfate on hemostasis and platelets in vivo. Thromb Res 28:389–399, 1982.

19. Faivre R, Neuhart E, Kieffer Y, et al: Subcutaneous administration of a low molecular weight heparin CY222 compared with subcutaneous administration of standard heparin in patients with acute deep vein thrombosis [abstract]. Thromb Haemost 58(Suppl):120S, 1987.

20. Fareed J, Hoppensteadt D, Wallenga JM, Pifarré R: An overview of current anticoagulant and antithrombotic drugs. In Pifarré R (ed): Anticoagulation, Hemostasis and Blood Preservation in Cardiovascular Surgery. Philadelphia, Hanley & Belfus, 1993.

21. Fiessinger JN, Paul JF, Alhenc-Gelas M, et al: Treatment of venous thrombosis with low molecular weight heparin and fluindione. Presse Med 21(2):65–68, 1992.

22. French Multicenter Study: Treatment of deep venous thrombosis. Comparative study of a low molecular weight heparin fragment (Fragmin) by the subcutaneous route and standard heparin by the continuous intravenous route. Rev Med Interne 10:375–381, 1989.

23. Frydman AM, Bara L, Le-Roux Y, et al: The antithrombotic activity and pharmacokinetics of Enoxaparin, a low molecular heparin, in humans given single subcutaneous dose of 20 to 80 mg. J Clin Pharmacol 28:609–618, 1988.

24. Hallert C, Blomqvist K: Simplified ambulatory treatment of thrombosis. A daily dosage of subcutaneous low-molecular-weight heparin. Lakartidningen 92:3011–3013, 1995.

25. Handeland GF, Abildgaard U, Holm HA, Arnesen KE: Dose adjusted heparin treatment of deep vein thrombosis: A comparison of unfractioned and low molecular weight heparin. Eur J Clin Pharmacol 39:107–112, 1990.

26. Harenberg J, Huck K, Bratsch H, et al: Therapeutic application of subcutaneous low molecular weight heparin in acute venous thrombosis. Haemostasis 20(Suppl 1):205–219, 1990.

27. Hirsh J: Heparin. N Engl J Med 324:1565–1574, 1991.

28. Hirsh J, Levine MN: Low molecular weight heparin. Blood 79:1–17, 1992.

29. Holm HA, Ly B, Handeland GF, et al: Subcutaneous heparin treatment of deep venous thrombosis: A comparison of unfractioned and low molecular weight heparin. Haemostasis 16(Suppl 20):30–37, 1986.

30. Holmer E, Mattsson C, Nilsson S: Anticoagulant and antithrombotic effects of heparin and low molecular weight heparin fragments in rabbits. Thromb Res 25:475–485, 1982.

31. Holmström M, Berglund MC, Granquist S, et al: Fragmin once or twice daily subcutaneously in the treatment of deep venous thrombosis of the leg. Thromb Res 67:49–55, 1992.

32. Hoppensteadt D, Walenga JM, Fareed J: Low molecular weight heparins: An objective overview. Clin Pharmacol Drugs Aging 2:406–422, 1992.

33. Huet Y, Janvier G, Bendriss PH, et al: Treatment of established venous thromboembolism with enoxaparin: Preliminary report. Acta Chir Scand Suppl 556:116–120, 1990.

34. Huisman M, Buller HR, ten Cate JW, Vreeken J: Serial impedance plethysmography for suspected deep venous thrombosis in outpatients. The Amsterdam general practitioner study. N Engl J Med 314:823–828, 1986.

35. Hull RD, Delmore T, Genton E, et al: Warfarin sodium versus low-dose heparin in the long-term treatment of venous thrombosis. N Engl J Med 301:855–858, 1979.

36. Hull RD, Hirsh J, Carter CJ, et al: Diagnostic efficacy of impedance plethysmography for clinically suspected deep-vein thrombosis. Ann Intern Med 102:21–28, 1985.

37. Hull RD, Raskob GE, Pineo GF, et al: Subcutaneous low molecular weight heparin compared with continous intravenous heparin in the treatment of proximal vein thrombosis. N Engl J Med 326:975–982, 1992.

38. Hull RD: Anticoagulant therapy. In Bergqvist D, Comerota AJ, Nicolaides AN, Scurr JH (eds): Prevention of Venous Thromboembolism. London, Med-Orion, 1994, pp 429–442.

39. Janvier G, Freyburger G, Winnock S, et al: An open trial of enoxaparin in the treatment of deep vein thrombosis of the leg. Haemostasis 21(3):161–168, 1991.

40. Johnson EA, Kirkwood TBL, Stirling Y, Perez-Requejo JL: Four heparin preparations: Anti-Xa potentiating effect of heparin after subcutaneous injection. Thromb Haemost 35:586–591, 1976.

41. Jorgensen LN, Wille-Jorgensen P, Hauch O: Prophylaxis of postoperative thromboembolism with low molecular weight heparins. A review. Br J Surg 80:689–704, 1993.

42. Kakkar VV, Kakkar S, Sanderson RM, Peers CE: Efficacy and safety of two regiments of low molecular weight heparin fragment (Fragmin) in preventing venous thromboembolism. Haemostasis 16:19–24, 1986.

43. Kalodiki E, Marston R, Volteas N, et al: The combination of liquid crystal thermography and duplex scanning in the diagnosis of deep vein thrombosis. Eur J Vasc Surg 6:311–316, 1992.

44. Kalodiki E: The diagnosis of deep venous thrombosis. Postgrad Surg Middle East 6:4–8, 1996.

45. Koopman MMW, Prandoni P, Piovella F, et al, for the TASMAN study group: Treatment of venous thrombosis with intravenous unfractionated heparin administered in the hospital as compared with subcutaneous low-molecular-weight heparin administered at home. N Engl J Med 334:677–681, 1996.

46. Lecompte T, Kai Luo S, Stieltjes N, et al: Thrombocytopenia associated with low molecular weight heparin. Lancet 338:1217, 1991.

47. Leizorovicz A, Haugh MC, Chapuis F-R, et al: Low molecular weight heparin in prevention of perioperative thrombosis. BMJ 305:913–920, 1992.

48. Leroy J, Leclerc MH, Delahousse B, et al: Treatment of heparin-associated thrombocytopenia and thrombosis with low molecular weight heparin (CY 216). Semin Thromb Hemost 11:326–329, 1985.

49. Levine M, Gent M, Hirsh J, et al: A comparison of low-molecular-weight heparin administered primarily at home with unfractionated heparin administered in the hospital for proximal deep-vein thrombosis. N Engl J Med 334:677–681, 1996.

50. Lindblad B, Eriksson A, Bergqvist D: Autopsy-verified pulmonary embolism in a surgical department: Analysis of the period from 1951 to 1988. Br J Surg 78:849–852, 1991.

51. Lindblad B, Sternby NH, Bergqvist D: Incidence of venous thromboembolism verified by necropsy over 30 years. BMJ 302:709–711, 1991.

52. Lindmarker P, Holmstrom M, Granqvist S, et al: Comparison of once-daily subcutaneous Fragmin with continuous intravenous unfractionated heparin in the treatment of deep vein thrombosis. Thromb Haemost 72:186–190, 1994.

53. Lockner D, Bratt G, Tornebohm E, et al: Intravenous and subcutaneous administration of Fragmin in deep vein thrombosis. Haemostasis 16(Suppl 2):25–29, 1986.

54. Lopaciuk S, Meissner AJ, Filipecki S, et al: Subcutaneous low molecular heparin versus subcutaneous unfractioned heparin in the treatment of deep vein thrombosis: A Polish multicenter study. Thromb Haemost 68:14–18, 1992.

55. Marder VJ, Soulen RL, Atichartakarn V, et al: Quantitative venographic assessment of deep vein thrombosis in the evaluation of streptokinase and heparin therapy. J Lab Clin Med 89:1018–1029, 1977.

56. Matzsch T, Bergqvist D, Hedner U, Ostergaard P: Effects of an enzymatically depolymerized heparin as compared with conventional heparin in healthy volunteers. Thromb Haemost 57:97–101, 1987.

57. Mismetti P, Reynaud J, Tardy-Ponce B, et al: Chrono-pharmacological study of once daily curative dose of a low molecular weight heparin (200 IU antiXa/kg of Dalteparin) in ten healthy volunteers. Thromb Haemost 74:660–666, 1995.

58. Moser KM, LeMoine JR. Is embolic risk conditioned by location of deep venous thrombosis? Ann Intern Med 94:439–444, 1981.

59. Nachman RL, Silverstein R: Hypercoagulable states. Ann Intern Med 119:819–827, 1993.

60. Nicolaides AN, Christopoulos D: Quantification of venous reflux and outflow obstruction with air-plethysmography. In Bernstein EF (ed): Vascular Diagnosis. St. Louis, Mosby,1993, pp 915–921.

61. Nicolaides AN, Kalodiki E, Christopoulos D, et al: Diagnosis of deep vein thrombosis by air-plethysmography. In Bernstein EF (ed): Vascular Diagnosis. St. Louis, Mosby,1993, pp 830–831.

62. Nordstrom M, Lindblad B, Bergqvist D, Kjellstrom T: A prospective study of the incidence of deep-vein thrombosis within a defined urban population. J Intern Med 232:155–160, 1992.

63. Nurmohamed MT, Rosendaal FR, Büller HR, et al: Low molecular weight heparin versus standard heparin in general and orthopaedic surgery: A meta-analysis. Lancet 340:152–156, 1992.

64. Odeh M, Oliven A: Urticaria and angioedema induced by low molecular weight heparin. Lancet 340:972–973, 1992.

65. Pezzuoli G, Neri Serneri GG, Settembrini P, et al, and the STEP Study Group: Prophylaxis of fatal pulmonary embolism in general surgery using LMWH Cy 216: A multicentre, double blind, randomised, controlled clinical trial versus placebo (STEP). Int Surg 74:205–210, 1989.

66. Pindur G, Heiden M, Kohler M: Comparison of low molecular weight heparins and unfractionated heparin after successive subcutaneous administration. A randomized controlled study in healthy volunteers. Arznei-mittelforschung 43:542–547, 1993.

67. Prandoni P, Vigo M, Cattelan AM, Ruol A: Treatment of deep venous thrombosis by fixed doses of low molecular heparin (CY 216). Haemostasis 20(Suppl 1):220–223, 1990.

68. Prandoni P, Lensing AWA, Büller HR, et al: Comparison of subcutaneous low molecular weight heparin with intravenous standard heparin in proximal deep vein thrombosis. Lancet 339:441–445, 1992.

69. Saltzman EW: Low molecular weight heparin. Is small beautiful? N Engl J Med 315:957–959, 1986.

70. Siegbahn A, Y-Hassan S, Boberg J, et al: Subcutaneous treatment of deep venous thrombosis with low molecular weight heparin. A dose finding study with LMWH-Novo. Thromb Res 55:767–778, 1989.

71. Simonneau G, for the TVPENOX group study: Subcutaneous fixed dose of enoxaparin versus intravenous adjusted dose of unfractionated heparin in the treatment of deep venous thrombosis. Thromb Haemost 65(Suppl):754, 1991.

72. Sumner DS, Mattos MA: Diagnosis of deep vein thrombosis with real-time color and duplex scanning. In Bernstein EF (ed): Vascular Diagnosis. St. Louis, Mosby, 1993.

73. Tardy B, Tardy-Poncet B, Zeni F, et al: Thrombocytopenia associated with low molecular weight heparin. Lancet 338:1217, 1991.

74. ten Cate JW, Prins MH: Major orthopaedic surgery and post-discharge DVT. Lancet 348:209–210, 1996.

75. Thomas DP, Barrowcliffe TW, Curtis AD: Low molecular weight heparin: A better drug? Haemostasis 16(2):87–92, 1986.

76. Verstraete M: Pharmacotherapeutic aspects of unfractionated and low molecular weight heparin. Drugs 40:498–530, 1990.

77. Wattrisse G, Lecoutre D, Groux-Pante C, Dufossez F: An open study on the efficacy and tolerance of a low molecular weight heparin (CY 216) in the therapeutic treatment of deep venous thrombi in orthopedics. Can Anesthesiol 40:37–42, 1992.

78. Wolf H: Low-molecular-weight heparin. Med Clin North Am 78:733–743, 1994.

Epilogue
Management of Thrombotic and Cardiovascular Disorders in the Year 2000

Over the past few years, interest in anticoagulant drugs has grown significantly, as evidenced by a constant increase in the number of drugs introduced for both preclinical and clinical development. The excellent scientific research and development activities in the laboratories of the pharmaceutical industry have resulted in a steady flow of new products from various groups. Several new antithrombotics and anticoagulants have been introduced during the past five years for clinical evaluation. Third-party validation of developed products and well-designed clinical trials have been carried out in various academic medical centers. The results of these studies also constitute a significant portion of the progress reported at scientific meetings, and many important results have become available since the inception of this publication. Through its fast-track drug approval and revised policies, the Food and Drug Administration (FDA) has provided expeditious mechanisms to the pharmaceutical industry, along with open-platform meetings to discuss regulatory issues in the optimal development of newer anticoagulant, antithrombotic, and thrombolytic drugs. The FDA and its representatives have continually contributed to the timely availability of new drugs by providing input at various stages of drug development. This input also has helped to clarify various issues related to new drug development and, in fact, has accelerated the approval process for many newer drugs, such as the low-molecular-weight heparins (LMWHs), ReoPro, and recombinant hirudin.

Although heparin remains the sole anticoagulant used for cardiovascular surgical procedures, the introduction of LMWH has added a new dimension to the overall management of thrombotic and cardiovascular disorders. Evidently, the LMWHs have achieved gold standard status in the management of thromboembolic disorders and now challenge other treatments, such as oral anticoagulants, for various indications. At the most recent meeting of the American Heart Association (New Orleans, November 1996), cardiologists revealed supportive data for the polytherapeutic use of LMWHs in the management of coronary syndromes, thrombotic stroke, and malignancy associated with thrombotic events. Antithrombin agents such as hirudin also have been compared with LMWHs for postsurgical prophylaxis of thromboembolism. Initial reports indicate favorable results with the use of polyethylene glycol-coupled (PEG) hirudin for treatment of coronary syndromes. In addition to the development of LMWHs, understanding of the mechanisms of their antithrombotic actions and the relevance of their structural components has led to the development of synthetic analogs of heparin fragments. One remarkable approach based on elucidation of the structure of heparin has led to the synthesis of oligosaccharides with high affinity for antithrombin III (AT III). Synthetic pentasaccharide is under evaluation in clinical trials for both thromboembolic and coronary indications. A recent report describes its use in percutaneous transluminal coronary angioplasty (PTCA). This report represents the first clinical trial of the pentasaccharide in coronary syndromes.

There is much discussion of how LMWHs mediate their effects. In addition to potentiation of AT III, several other mechanisms have been identified, including release of tissue factor pathway inhibitor (TFPI), vascular effects, profibrinolytic effects, platelet selectin modulation, and growth factor modulation. Clinical trials in Europe have shown that subcutaneous LMWH, given once or twice daily, is at least as safe and effective as continuous intravenous heparin in the prevention of recurrent venous thromboembolism and is associated with reduced bleeding and lower mortality rates. Several recent studies have shown that home administration of LMWH is as safe and effective as hospital administration of intravenous heparin in patients with proximal venous thrombosis. Initial evidence clearly suggests that LMWH may be a useful alternative to heparin in patients with pulmonary embolism. LMWHs also may be useful alternatives to heparin for arterial indications, such as treatment of unstable angina and stroke and maintenance of peripheral arterial grafts. Recognizing the usefulness of LMWHs, the pharmaceutical industry has focused its attention on their use in the management of ischemic and thrombotic stroke. The initial results of clinical trials are promising. Thus, in the near future, the use of LMWH for prevention of thrombotic or ischemic stroke will be an important goal. The success of early clinical trials also suggests that LMWH may be useful in the management of primary and secondary ischemic or thrombotic stroke.

Although LMWHs are proving to be as effective as and safer than heparin for various indications, it is important to realize that differences in the manufacture of various LMWHs lead to differences in their pharmacologic profile. Although these differences have not been clinically validated, each of the LMWHs is expected to exhibit its own therapeutic index in a given clinical setting. Thus, the interchange of LMWHs based on equivalent gravimetric or biologic potency of standardized dosages may not be feasible. Because of the newer indications and the length of therapy, some additional issues related to the optimal use of LMWHs remain to be addressed. Examples include monitoring, control of bleeding, and drug interactions. Clinical trials have been designed to obtain information related to these issues. The differential clinical efficacy of various LMWHs was evident in the trials carried out with Fragmin (FRISC and FRIC) and enoxaparin (ESSENCE).

Economic analyses of the treatment cost of heparin vs. LMWH in various clinical settings show that although the cost of LMWH is marginally higher than the cost of heparin ($40–150), the expected reduction in costs for all treatment-related clinical events is much higher for LMWHs ($350–2700) than for heparin. Thus, LMWHs are an attractive alternative in an era of managed care health reform. Individual economic analysis for specific indications may provide additional information about reduced costs with the use of LMWHs for long-term outpatient treatment of such syndromes as unstable angina and ischemic cerebral events.

In the search for antiplatelet agents to be used as antithrombotic drugs, it was recognized that the platelet glycoprotein IIb/IIIa (GPIIb/IIIa) plays a key role in the final common pathway for platelet aggregation. Several reports have become available recently. Many synthetic GPIIb/IIIa inhibitors are currently under clinical development for various indications. In the EPIC trial, ReoPro (an anti-GPIIb/IIIa Fab) has been shown to reduce thrombotic events after PTCA. In the EPILOG study, the combined effects of ReoPro and heparin resulted in inhibition of restenosis. Many of the GPIIa/IIIb inhibitors, including ReoPro, also have been found to inhibit the vitronectin receptor ($\alpha_v\beta_3$ integrin), which is implicated in endothelial and smooth muscle cell migration. Thus, these agents exhibit multiple effects in addition to their antiplatelet functions. Another application of GPIIb/IIIa inhibitors is as alternative agents to aspirin in the management of unstable angina, non-Q wave myocardial infarction, and ischemic or thrombotic stroke. The mechanism of the antiplatelet action of the synthetic GPIIb/IIIa inhibitors and antibodies may be the same; however, major differences have been noted in their safety and efficacy. An emerging problem is therapeutic monitoring, which is being addressed with point-of-care systems. Thus, major clinical breakthroughs are expected with the use of these inhibitors in the management of cerebrovascular and cardiovascular disorders. The introduction of novel antiplatelet drugs has added a new dimension to the management of arterial thrombosis—in particular, thrombotic stroke. The availability of specific antagonists of the adenosine diphosphate (ADP) receptor (e.g., ticlopidine) has provided a new approach for several cardiovascular and cerebrovascular indications. The second-generation ADP receptor-blocking agents (e.g., clopidogrel) underwent extensive clinical trials to test their therapeutic efficacy in combined cardiovascular and cerebrovascular endpoints. The comparative results, reported at a recent meeting of the American Heart Association, favored clopidogrel.

Understanding of the coagulation process has led to the identification of thrombin as a key enzyme in thrombogenic processes. Several direct thrombin inhibitors have been developed over the past few years by different methods. Hirudin, the leech-derived protein, has been compared with heparin for various procedures in numerous clinical settings, including treatment and prophylaxis of venous and arterial thrombotic disorders. The use of hirudin has been reported to be associated with increased risk of bleeding, indicating that better monitoring and dose-adjustment protocols are needed as well as antidotes. So far, clinical trials comparing hirudin and heparin as adjuncts in thrombolytic therapy in myocardial infarction (TIMI 9B) and acute coronary syndromes (GUSTO IIb) have shown hirudin to be marginally (if at all) superior to heparin.

Recently several reports comparing the effects of heparin and hirudin on various parameters have become available. A study comparing heparin and recombinant hirudin for the prophylaxis of deep venous thrombosis (DVT) provided impressive data in favor of hirudin. In a second study, LMWH also was compared with hirudin for postsurgical prophylaxis of DVT. The results favored hirudin. Both studies emphasize an important point about the validity of well-designed clinical trials. It is important to understand that the efficacy and safety of a new drug may not be determined by trials for a single indication. Therefore, clinical trials are needed for various specific indications.

Argatroban, another smaller thrombin inhibitor, is currently under clinical development for various indications. It has been used successfully in Japan for over a decade in the treatment of thrombotic disorders. Several clinical trials in both Europe and the United States have been designed to investigate its use as an alternative to heparin in heparin-compromised patients and as a prophylactic agent to reduce late restenosis after PTCA and coronary directional atherectomy (CDA). Argatroban was successfully used for the management of anticoagulation in patients with heparin-induced thrombocytopenia and as a substitute for heparin in PTCA. Since the half-life of argatroban is rather short, it has been administered via infusion protocols. For therapeutic anticoagulation, a level of 1–2 μg/ml is indicated, whereas for interventional cardiologic procedures a level of 3–7 μg/ml is maintained.

Because of their weaker anticoagulant effects in global clotting tests, direct factor Xa inhibitors were not considered desirable anticoagulant and antithrombotic agents for developmental purposes. However, because of the favorable clinical results with pentasaccharide, strong interest in synthetic anti-factor Xa drugs has reemerged. These agents may be useful in the prophylaxis of both arterial and venous thrombotic disorders and may offer a greater margin of safety than existing drugs. Additional advantages of direct thrombin and factor Xa inhibitors over heparin include subcutaneous and oral bioavailability. Although their biologic half-life is usually under 30 minutes, coupling to larger agents such as dextran or albumin can prolong their half-life without affecting their pharmacologic actions. Questions about monitoring and antagonism will have to be answered before thrombin and factor Xa inhibitors can be widely explored in clinical settings. Depending on their specificity for thrombin or factor Xa, they may be used as adjuncts with other classes of drugs, such as thrombolytic agents for treatment of acute myocardial infarction. Low-molecular-weight thrombin and factor Xa inhibitors also may be used for localized delivery, stenting, and transdermal delivery.

Because of their better bioavailability, cothrombin and factor Xa inhibitors in combination may be more useful than the single agents. Optimal combinations for specific indications may be considered. As in the clinical development of LMWHs, thrombin and factor Xa inhibitors should be compared with heparin in terms of safety, efficacy, and cost.

Newer developments in thrombolytic therapy include recombinant tissue plasminogen activators (tPAs). Bolus-injectable Reptilase is an unglycosylated plasminogen activator consisting of the Kringle 2 and protease domain of tPA with a 3–4-fold longer half-life than tPA. The INJECT trial demonstrated that Reptilase is superior to streptokinase for management of heart failure. Difference variants of wild-type (wt) tPA, recombinant staphylokinase, and RTSPAα1 and 2 (vampire bat tPA) also have undergone clinical trials. Recombinant urokinase and prourokinase are now expressed in mammalian cell lines and are undergoing active clinical development. Molecular engineering of the wt recombinant tPA extended the biologic half-life for bolus dosing, whereas staphylokinase and vampire bat plasminogen activator exhibited fibrin specificity. The thrombolytic agents also have found a place in the management of acute thrombotic stroke. Optimal approaches to improve the safety/efficacy index are currently under investigation. The next few years will witness the emergence of longer-acting thrombolytics to facilitate bolus dosing and improved specificity for fibrin and other receptors to target thrombotic sites. Newer indications for thrombolytic therapy, such as stroke and microangiographic syndromes, will be pursued.

Restenosis after cardiac interventions remains a major challenge. An optimal therapeutic approach is still unavailable despite major scientific and financial undertakings. Even with the introduction of newer interventional cardiovascular and peripheral vascular procedures, late restenosis is commonly seen at a rate of 10–60%. Although the claimed efficacy of cardiovascular interventions exceeds that of medical and surgical approaches, restenosis is a major problem, resulting in angina and myocardial infarction. Several newer anticoagulant and antithrombotic drugs have been used to reduce restenosis. However, these approaches have met with limited success. Recent results with GPIIb/IIIa-targeting antibodies have been encouraging. With a better understanding of the pathophysiology of restenosis, improved drugs can be developed. Anticoagulant drugs such as LMWHs and PEG hirudin may prove useful. Mechanical devices such as stents and localized and programmed delivery of drugs may be expected to improve outcomes. Although monotherapy may be useful in the control of abrupt closure and subchronic occlusion, its role in late restenosis may be limited. Combined pharmacologic and mechanical approaches, coupled with specialized delivery, already have provided favorable results.

The remainder of the 1990s will witness dramatic developments in the management of thrombotic and cardiovascular disorders. Synthetic and recombinant approaches will provide cost-effective and clinically useful drugs. LMWHs and synthetic heparin analogs are expected to have significant effects on the overall management of thrombotic and cardiovascular disorders. Factors such as managed care, regulatory issues, polytherapy, and combined pharmacologic and mechanical approaches will redirect the focus in management of DVt, thromboembolism, myocardial infarction, and thrombotic stroke. The direct thrombin agents such as hirudin and PEG hirudin will be of great value for surgical anticoagulation and various acute indications. Postsurgical control of thrombotic processes may require combination therapy and LMWHs.

Conventional drugs such as heparin, oral anticoagulants, and aspirin will remain the gold standards despite their known drawbacks. They require further optimization and can be used for various indications in a cost-effective manner. The newer drugs, however, provide alternatives that in the next few years may lead to improved, cost-compliant treatments.

R. Pifarré
J. Fareed
January 1997

Index

Entries in **boldface type** indicate complete chapters.

Divorce, effect on ownership, as community property, 71; as tenants by the entirety, 71

Doctrine of prior appropriation: a legal philosophy that allows a first user to continue diverting water, 17

Documentary tax: a fee or tax on deeds and other documents payable at the time of recordation, 271, 292-93

Documents other than maps (in land description), 31-32

Dollar value, *table,* 558

Dominant estate: the parcel of land which benefits from an easement, 47

Door details, *illustrated,* 539, 545

Double declining balance: depreciation at twice normal rates for income tax purposes, 515

Dower: the legal right of a widow to a portion of her deceased husband's real property, 41, 53-54, 59; by states, *table,* 55; waiver of, 65

Down payment, FHA, 218; GI Bill and, 221-22

Downside risk: the possibility that an investor will lose his money in an investment, 511; *see also* **Risk**

Drilling rights. *See* **Subsurface right**

Dry rot: a decay of wood that usually results from alternate soaking and drying over a long period, 157

Dual agency (divided agency): representation of two or more parties in a transaction by the same agent, 373, 387-88; *see also* **Agency**

Due-on-sale clause. *See* **Alienation clause**

Duration of estates, 57-58

Duress: the application of force to obtain an agreement, 131, 139

Earnest money deposit: money that accompanies an offer to purchase as evidence of good faith, 149, 151, 158, 297, 389; disposition of, 144, 397-98; return of, 168, 452

Earth's center, 14, 446

Easement: the right or privilege one party has to use land belonging to another for a special purpose not inconsistent with the owner's use of the land, 41, 46-48, 59, 61; dominant estate, 47; granting, by quit-claim deed, 92; party wall, 48; servient estate, 47; termination, 48

Easement appurtenant: an easement that runs with the land, 47

Easement by necessity: an easement created by law usually for the right to travel to a landlocked parcel of land, 46

Easement by prescription: acquisition of an easement by prolonged use, 46, 99-100

Easement in gross: an easement given to a person or business, 47

Economic base: the ability of a region to export goods and services to other regions and receive money in return, 485-87

Economic characteristics of land, 35-37

Economic obsolescence, 355, 357

Economic rent: the amount of rent a property could command in the open market, 327; *see also* **Rent**

Economy, effect on real estate prices, 485-507

Education, real estate, career in, 10

Education requirements, 413-14, 430; for GRI designation, 440; by states, *table,* 414-15

Educational Testing Service (ETS): a private firm that writes, administers and grades real estate license examinations in 30 states, 417

Effective yield: a return on investment calculation that considers the price paid, the time held and the interest rate, 226-27

Ellwood Tables, 361

Emblements: annual plantings that require cultivation, 16

Eminent domain: the right of government to take privately held land for public use, provided fair compensation is paid, 41, 42, 43, 59, 327

Sale and leaseback: owner-occupant sells his property and then remains as a tenant, 267

Sale of property, held by tenants in common, 66-67

Sales contracts, 149-71; *illustrated* purchase contract, 150-56, 160-63; purpose of, 149-50

Salesman or Salesperson: a person employed by a broker to list, negotiate, sell, or lease real property for others, 409; affiliating with a broker, 429-33; as sub-agent of a broker, 393; Canon of Ethics for, 421-25; career opportunities, 5-7, 10-11; compensation, 374, 430-31, 432; defined, 411; education requirements, 410, 413-14, 430; independent contractor issue, 433-34; licensing requirements, 412-14; limited, 411-12

Salvage value: the price that can be expected for an improvement that is to be removed and used elsewhere, 368

Sandwich lease: a leasehold interest lying between the owner of a property and its actual user, 57, 319, 326; *see also* **Lease**

Satisfaction of mortgage: a certificate from the lender stating that the loan has been repaid, 186-87

Savings and loan associations, 235-40, 242; growth, 236-38; history, 235-36; money market certificates, 240; regulation, 225, 238-39; variable-rate mortgage, 253

Savings certificates (time deposits), 239; banks, 242; money market certificates, 240, 498-99; savings and loans, 239-40

Scarcity, 366; of land, 35

Scheduled gross (projected gross): the estimated rent that a fully-occupied property can be expected to produce on an annual basis, 358; *illustrated* example, 341, 358; sample statement of, 359

Seal: a hot wax, paper, or embossed seal, or the word "seal," or "L.S." placed on a document, 88

Second mortgage: one which ranks immediately behind the first mortgage in priority, 188-89

Secondary mortgage market, 246-49; FHLMC, 248, 249; FNMA, 246-47, 249;

GNMA, 247-48, 249; MGIC, 248-49; real estate market impact, 499-500

Section: a unit of land in the rectangular survey system that is one mile long on each of its four sides and contains 640 acres, 26, 27-28; subdivision of, 27, 28

Section 203(b): FHA home insurance program, 219-20; *see also* **Federal Housing Authority**

Secular events, 497

Seizin. *See* **Covenant of seizin**

Seller's affidavit of title: a document provided by the seller at the settlement meeting stating that he has done nothing to encumber title since the title search was made, 293, 295-96

Seller's closing statement: an accounting of the seller's money at settlement, 309-11

Seller's market: one with few sellers and many buyers, 368-69

Seller's points: loan discount points paid by a seller so that a buyer can obtain a loan, 228

Seller's responsibilities, at closing, 294-95

Senior mortgage: the mortgage against a property that holds first priority in the event of foreclosure, 188-89

Sensitivity to credit. *See* **Credit availability**

Separate property: the cubicle of air space that the condominium owner's unit occupies, 446; spouse-owned property that is exempt from community property status, 71-72

Service fees (management), 531-32

Service industry: an industry that produces goods and services to sell to local residents, 485, 486

Service the loan. *See* **Loan servicing**

Servient estate: the land on which an easement exists in favor of a dominant estate, 47

Settlement: the day on which title is conveyed, 293; *see also* **Title closing**

Settlement funds, 257, 295

Settlement meeting: a meeting at which the seller delivers his deed to the buyer, the buyer pays for the property, and all other matters pertaining to the sale are concluded, 293, 295-97